14TH EDITION

Harrison's

PRINCIPLES of INTERNAL MEDICINE

COMPANION HANDBOOK

EDITORS

14TH EDITION

Harrison's

PRINCIPLES of INTERNAL MEDICINE

COMPANION HANDBOOK

EDITORS

Anthony S. Fauci, MD

Eugene Braunwald, AB, MD, MA(Hon), MD(Hon), ScD(Hon)

Kurt J. Isselbacher, AB, MD

Jean D. Wilson, MD

Joseph B. Martin, MD, PhD, FRCP(C), MA(Hon)

Dennis L. Kasper, MD, MA(Hon)

Stephen L. Hauser, MD

Dan L. Longo, AB, MD, FACP

McGraw-Hill
HEALTH PROFESSIONS DIVISION

New York St. Louis San Francisco Auckland Bogotá
Caracas Lisbon London Madrid Mexico City Milan Montreal
New Delhi San Juan Singapore Sydney Tokyo Toronto

McGraw-Hill

*A Division of The **McGraw·Hill** Companies*

Harrison's
PRINCIPLES OF INTERNAL MEDICINE
Fourteenth Edition
COMPANION HANDBOOK
Copyright © 1998, 1995, 1991, 1988 by *The McGraw-Hill Companies*. All rights reserved. Printed in the United States of America. Except as permitted under the United States Copyright Act of 1976, no part of this publication may be reproduced or distributed in any form or by any means, or stored in a data base or retrieval system, without the prior written consent of the author.

2 3 4 5 6 7 8 9 0   DOCDOC   9 9 8

ISBN 0-07-021530-8

This book was set in Times New Roman by Monotype Composition Company. The editors were J. Dereck Jeffers, Martin J. Wonsiewicz, and Mariapaz Ramos Englis; the production supervisor was Helene Landers; the designer was Marsha Cohen. The index was prepared by Irving Conde Tullar.
R. R. Donnelley & Sons, Inc., was printer and binder.

Library of Congress Cataloging-in-Publication Data
Harrison's principles of internal medicine, fourteenth edition.
    Companion handbook / editors, Anthony S. Fauci . . . [et al.].
        p.   cm.
    An extension of: Harrison's principles of internal medicine, 14th ed. © 1998.
    Includes bibliographical references and index.
    ISBN 0-07-021530-8
    1. Internal medicine—Handbooks, manuals, etc.   I. Fauci, Anthony S.   II. Principles of internal medicine, 14th ed.
    [DNLM: 1. Internal Medicine—handbooks.   WB 115 H322 1998 Suppl.]
RC46.H333   1998 Suppl. 2
616—DC21
DNLM/DLC
for Library of Congress   97-42634
                                                                          CIP

ABBREVIATED CONTENTS

NOTICE

Medicine is an ever-changing science. As new research and clinical experience broaden our knowledge, changes in treatment and drug therapy are required. The editors and the publisher of this work have checked with sources believed to be reliable in their efforts to provide information that is complete and generally in accord with the standards accepted at the time of publication. However, in view of the possibility of human error or changes in medical sciences, neither the editors nor the publisher nor any other party who has been involved in the preparation or publication of this work warrants that the information contained herein is in every respect accurate or complete, and they are not responsible for any errors or omissions or the results obtained from the use of such information. Readers are encouraged to confirm the information contained herein with other sources. For example and in particular, readers are advised to check the product information sheet included in the package of each drug they plan to administer to be certain that the information contained in this book is accurate and that changes have not been made in the recommended dose or in the contraindications for administration. This recommendation is particularly important in connection with new or infrequently used drugs.

CONTENTS

SECTION 1

IMPORTANT SIGNS AND SYMPTOMS

SECTION 5

HEMATOLOGY AND ONCOLOGY

SECTION 6

INFECTIOUS DISEASES

SECTION 7

CARDIOVASCULAR DISEASES

SECTION 8

RESPIRATORY DISEASES

SECTION 9

RENAL DISEASES

SECTION 13

NEUROLOGY

CONTRIBUTORS

Numbers in brackets refer to the chapters written or co-written by the contributor.

BRUCE T. ADORNATO, MD
Director, Stanford Health Services Sleep Disorders Center, San Francisco; Clinical Associate Professor of Neurology, Stanford University, Stanford [187]

EUGENE BRAUNWALD, MD, MD(Hon), ScD(Hon)
Distinguished Hersey Professor of Medicine, Faculty Dean for Academic Programs at Brigham and Women's Hospital and Massachusetts General Hospital, Harvard Medical School; Vice-President for Academic Programs, Partners HealthCare System, Boston [2, 14–17, 27–29, 104–117, 196]

GLENN CHERTOW, MD, MPH
Assistant Professor of Medicine, Instructor in Surgery, Harvard Medical School; Assistant Director of Dialysis, Renal Division, Metabolic Support Services, Brigham and Women's Hospital, Boston [24, 25, 128–133, 135–137]

ROBERT L. DERESIEWICZ, MD
Assistant Professor of Medicine, Harvard Medical School; Associate Physician, Channing Laboratory and the Division of Infectious Diseases, Brigham and Women's Hospital, Boston [40, 68, 72, 75, 81, 85, 88, 89, 91, 100, 102, 103, 134]

ROBERT L. DOBBINS, MD, PhD
Research Fellow, Department of Internal Medicine, The University of Texas Southwestern Medical Center, Dallas [19, 34, 35, 44–47, 160–170]

JOHN W. ENGSTROM, MD
Associate Professor and Vice-Chairman, Department of Neurology, University of California-San Francisco, San Francisco [4, 5, 67, 175, 179, 180, 186, 189, 191]

ANTHONY S. FAUCI, MD
Chief, Laboratory of Immunoregulation; Director, National Institute of Allergy and Infectious Diseases, National Institutes of Health, Bethesda [7, 8, 38, 39, 42, 43, 78, 148–159]

HOWARD L. FIELDS, MD, PhD
Professor of Neurology and Physiology, University of California-San Francisco, San Francisco [1]

LAWRENCE FRIEDMAN, MD
Associate Professor of Medicine, Harvard Medical School; Associate Physician, Massachusetts General Hospital, Boston [21, 23, 138, 141, 144–147]

DARYL R. GRESS, MD
Assistant Professor of Neurology, University of California-San Francisco, San Francisco [30, 174]

STEPHEN L. HAUSER, MD
Chairman and Betty Anker Fife Professor, Department of Neurology, University of California-San Francisco, San Francisco [178, 181, 188, 191]

JONATHAN C. HORTON, MD, PhD
Associate Professor of Ophthalmology, Neurology, and Physiology, University of California-San Francisco, San Francisco [11]

KURT J. ISSELBACHER, AB, MD
Mallinckrodt Professor of Medicine, Harvard Medical School; Physician and Director, Massachusetts General Hospital Cancer Center, Boston [3, 18, 20–23, 138–147]

LEE KAPLAN, MD
Assistant Professor of Medicine, Harvard Medical School; Associate Chief for Research, Gastrointestinal Unit, Massachusetts General Hospital, Boston [3, 20, 22]

DENNIS L. KASPER, MD, MA(Hon)
William Ellery Channing Professor of Medicine, Professor of Microbiology and Molecular Genetics, and Executive Dean for Academic Programs, Harvard Medical School; Director, Channing Laboratory, and Co-Director, Division of Infectious Diseases, Brigham and Women's Hospital, Boston [73, 84, 87, 90, 92, 93, 97, 99]

WALTER J. KOROSHETZ, MD
Associate Professor of Neurology, Massachusetts General Hospital, Harvard Medical School, Boston [10, 13, 31, 185]

CAROL LANGFORD, MD
National Institute of Allergy and Infectious Diseases, National Institutes of Health, Bethesda [7. 8, 42, 43, 150–159]

LEONARD LILLY, MD
Associate Professor of Medicine, Harvard Medical School; Physician, Cardiovascular Division, Brigham and Women's Hospital, Boston [2, 17, 27–29, 104–116]

DAN L. LONGO, AB, MD, FACP
Scientific Director, National Institute on Aging, National Institutes of Health, Gerontology Research Center, Bethesda and Baltimore [26, 36, 48–66]

DANIEL H. LOWENSTEIN, MD
Associate Professor of Neurology, Anatomy, and Neurosurgery; Robert B. and Ellinor Aird Chair in Neurology; University of California-San Francisco, San Francisco [9, 32, 173]

LAWRENCE C. MADOFF, MD
Assistant Professor of Medicine, Harvard Medical School; Channing Laboratory, Brigham and Women's Hospital; Division of Infectious Diseases, Beth Israel Deaconess Medical Center, Boston [6, 41, 69–71, 74, 76, 77, 79, 80, 82, 83, 86, 94–96, 98, 101, 122]

JOSEPH B. MARTIN, MD, PhD, FRCP (C), MA(Hon)
Dean of the Faculty of Medicine, Caroline Shields Walker Professor of Clinical Neuroscience and Neurobiology, Harvard Medical School, Boston [172, 176, 177, 181–187, 190]

NORMAN NISHIOKA, MD
Assistant Professor of Medicine, Harvard Medical School; Associate Physician in Medicine, Massachusetts General Hospital, Boston [18, 142, 143]

ANN N. PONCELET, MD
Assistant Clinical Professor of Neurology, University of California-San Francisco, San Francisco [172]

THOMAS A. RANDO, MD, PhD
Assistant Professor of Neurology, Stanford University Medical Center, Stanford [12, 37, 190]

MICHAEL SNELLER, MD
National Institute of Allergy and Infectious Diseases, National Institutes of Health, Bethesda [38, 39, 78, 148, 149]

KENNETH L. TYLER, MD
Professor of Neurology, Medicine, and Microbiology & Immunology, University of Colorado Health Sciences Center; Chief, Neurology Service, Veterans Affairs Medical Center, Denver [171, 176, 177, 182, 183]

SOPHIA VINOGRADOV, MD
Assistant Professor of Psychiatry, Department of Psychiatry, University of California-San Francisco, San Francisco [192–195]

J. WOODROW WEISS, MD
Associate Professor of Medicine, Harvard Medical School; Medical Director of the Pulmonary MICU, Beth Israel–Deaconess Medical Center, Boston [14–16, 118–121, 123–127]

JEAN D. WILSON, MD
Charles Cameron Sprague Distinguished Chair and Clinical Professor of Internal Medicine, The University of Texas Southwestern Medical Center, Dallas [19, 33, 34, 35, 44–47, 160–170, 197]

PREFACE

It would certainly be ideal to have a copy of the 14th edition of *Harrison's Principles of Internal Medicine (HPIM)* available at all times. This is particularly true for students and residents who are constantly on the move from outpatient clinics to inpatient wards to emergency rooms and other specialized facilities. However, the sheer weight and size of the book make this quite impractical. It is for this reason that the Editors have condensed the clinical portions of *HPIM* into this pocket-sized *Companion Handbook* that contains key features of the diagnosis and treatment of the major diseases that are likely to be encountered on a medical service. We have developed this handbook with the able assistance of selected contributors.

HPIM is updated every 3 to 4 years and the total amount of information continues to grow. It has been a challenge to distill the broad field of internal medicine with each new edition in which we provide a solid base of classic and established principles while providing important updates in pathogenesis, treatment, and prevention of a broad range of diseases. In the *Companion Handbook,* we try to distill this body of knowledge even further so that summaries of this important information can be available to the student and resident within the easy reach of a coat pocket.

The purpose of the *Companion Handbook* is to provide on-the-spot summaries in preparation for a more in-depth analysis of the clinical problem. Therefore, it is important to point out that this book is not considered to be a replacement for a full textbook of medicine. Rather, it is an extension of the fourteenth edition of *HPIM*. The amount and depth of material are not adequate to stand on their own; however, it is an excellent introduction to or reminder of some aspects of clinical medicine. It has been written with easy reference to the full text of *HPIM* and it is recommended that the full textbook be consulted as soon as time permits. Thus, we consider *HPIM* and the *Companion Handbook* as a combination that is complementary, but not interchangeable.

THE EDITORS

14TH EDITION

Harrison's

PRINCIPLES of INTERNAL MEDICINE

COMPANION HANDBOOK

1

PAIN AND ITS MANAGEMENT

Pain is the most common symptom of disease. Management depends on determining its cause and alleviating triggering and potentiating factors.

Organization of Pain Pathways

(See HPIM-14, Fig. 12-1.) Pain-producing (nociceptive) sensory stimuli in skin and viscera activate peripheral nerve endings of primary afferent neurons, which synapse on second-order neurons in cord or medulla. These second-order neurons form crossed ascending pathways that reach the thalamus and are projected to somatosensory cortex. Parallel ascending neurons connect with brainstem nuclei and ventrocaudal and medial thalamic nuclei. These parallel pathways project to the limbic system and underlie the emotional aspect of pain. Pain transmission is regulated at the dorsal horn level by descending bulbospinal pathways that contain serotonin, norepinephrine, and several neuropeptides.

Agents that modify pain perception may act to reduce tissue inflammation (glucocorticoids, NSAIDs, prostaglandin synthesis inhibitors), to interfere with pain transmission (narcotics), or to enhance descending modulation (narcotics and antidepressants). Anticonvulsants (gabapentin, carbamazepine) may be effective for aberrant pain sensations arising from peripheral nerve injury.

Evaluation

Pain may be of *somatic* (skin, joints, muscles), *visceral*, or *neuropathic* (injury to nerves, spinal cord pathways, or thalamus) origin. Characteristics of each are summarized in Table 1-1.

Sensory symptoms and signs in neuropathic pain are described by the following definitions: *neuralgia:* pain in distribution of a single nerve, as in trigeminal neuralgia; *dysesthesia:* spontaneous, unpleasant, abnormal sensations; *hyperalgesia* and *hyperesthesia:* exaggerated responses to nociceptive or touch stimulus, respectively; *allodynia:* perception of light mechanical stimuli as painful, as when vibration evokes painful sensation. Reduced pain perception is called *hypalgesia* or, when absent,

1

Table 1-1

Characteristics of Nociceptive and Neuropathic Pain

Nociceptive pain
    Nociceptive stimulus usually evident
    Usually well localized
    Similar to other somatic pains in pt's experience
    Relieved by anti-inflammatory or narcotic analgesics
Visceral pain
    Most commonly activated by inflammation
    Pain poorly localized and usually referred
    Associated with diffuse discomfort, e.g., nausea, bloating
    Relieved by narcotic analgesics
Neuropathic pain
    No obvious nociceptive stimulus
    Associated evidence of nerve damage, e.g., sensory impairment
    Unusual, dissimilar from somatic pain, often shooting or electrical quality
    Only partially relieved by narcotic analgesics, may respond to antiarrhythmics or anticonvulsants

analgesia. Causalgia is continuous severe burning pain with indistinct boundaries and accompanying sympathetic nervous system dysfunction (sweating vascular, skin, and hair changes—sympathetic dystrophy) that occurs after injury to a peripheral nerve.

℞ TREATMENT

    Acute Somatic Pain   If moderate, it can usually be effectively treated with nonnarcotic analgesic agents (Table 1-2). Narcotic analgesics are usually required for relief of severe pain.

    Neuropathic Pain   Often chronic; management is particularly difficult. The following drugs, in combination with careful assessment of underlying factors that contribute to pain (depression, "compensation neurosis"), may be beneficial:

    1.   *Anticonvulsants:* In pts with neuropathic pain and little or no evidence of sympathetic dysfunction; diabetic neuropathy, trigeminal neuralgia (tic douloureux, postherpetic neuralgia).

    2.   *Antidepressants:* Pharmacologic effects include facili-

Table 1-2

Drugs for Relief of Pain

NONNARCOTIC ANALGESICS: USUAL DOSES AND INTERVALS

Generic Name	Dose, mg	Interval	Comments
Acetylsalicylic acid	650 PO	q4h	Enteric-coated preparation available
Acetaminophen	650 PO	q4h	Side effects uncommon
Ibuprofen	400 PO	q4–6h	Available without prescription
Naproxen	250–500 PO	q12h	Delayed effects may be due to long half-life
Fenoprofen	200 PO	q4–6h	—
Indomethacin	25–50 PO	q8h	Gastrointestinal side effects common
Ketorolac	15–60 IM	q4–6h	Available for parenteral use (IM)

NARCOTIC ANALGESICS: USUAL DOSES AND INTERVALS

Generic Name	Parenteral Dose, mg	PO Dose, mg	Comments
Codeine	30–60	30–60 q4h	Nausea common
Oxycodone	—	5–10 q4–6h	Usually available with acetaminophen or aspirin
Morphine	5–10 q4h	30–60 q4h	—
Morphine, sustained release	—	60–180 bid to tid	Oral slow-release preparation
Hydromorphone	1–2 q4h	2–4 q4h	Shorter acting than morphine sulfate
Levorphanol	2 q6–8h	4 q6–8h	Longer acting than morphine sulfate; absorbed well PO
Methadone	10 q6–8h	5–20 q6–8h	Delayed sedation due to long half-life
Meperidine	75–100 q3–4h	300 q4h	Poorly absorbed PO; normeperidine a toxic metabolite
Butorphanol	—	1–2 q4h	Intranasal spray
Fentanyl	—	—	Transdermal patch
Tramadol	—	50–100 q4h	Some biogenic amine uptake blockade

3

Table 1-2 (Continued)

Drugs for Relief of Pain

ANTICONVULSANTS AND ANTIARRHYTHMICS

Generic Name	PO Dose, mg	Interval
Phenytoin	300	daily/qhs
Carbamazepine	200–300	q6h
Clonazepam	1	q6h
Mexiletine	150–300	q6–12h
Gabapentin	100–600	q6h

TRICYCLIC ANTIDEPRESSANTS

Generic Name	Uptake Blockade		Sedative Potency	Anticholinergic Potency	Orthostatic Hypotension	Cardiac Arrhythmia	Average Dose, mg/d	Range, mg/d
	5HT	NE						
Doxepin	++	+	High	Moderate	Moderate	Less	200	75–400
Amitriptyline	++++	++	High	Highest	Moderate	Yes	150	25–300
Imipramine	++++	++	Moderate	Moderate	High	Yes	200	75–400
Nortriptyline	+++	++	Moderate	Moderate	Low	Yes	100	40–150
Desipramine	+++	++++	Low	Low	Low	Yes	150	50–300
Venlafaxine	++	+	None	None	None	No	150	37.5–300

tation of monoamine neurotransmitters by inhibition of transmitter reuptake. Are useful in management of pts with chronic pain, including headache, diabetic neuropathy, postherpetic neuralgia, atypical facial pain (see Chap. 4), chronic low back pain (see Chap. 5).

CHRONIC PAIN   The problem is often difficult to diagnose, and pts may appear emotionally distraught. Psychological evaluation and behaviorally based treatment paradigms are frequently helpful, particularly in a multidisciplinary pain management center.

Several factors can cause perpetuate, or exacerbate chronic pain: (1) painful disease for which there is no cure (e.g., arthritis, cancer, migraine headaches, diabetic neuropathy); (2) neural factors initiated by a bodily disease that persist after the disease has resolved (e.g., damaged sensory or sympathetic nerves); (3) psychological conditions.

Pay special attention to the medical history and to depression. Major depression is common, treatable, and potentially fatal (suicide).

[R_x] **TREATMENT**

After evaluation, an explicit treatment plan should be developed for pt, including specific and realistic goals for therapy, e.g., getting a good night's sleep, being able to go shopping, or returning to work. A multidisciplinary approach that utilizes medications, counseling, physical therapy, nerve blocks, and even surgery may be required to improve pt's quality of life. Some pts may require referral to a pain clinic; for others, pharmacologic management alone can provide significant help.

For a more detailed discussion, see Fields HL, Martin JB: Pain: Pathophysiology and Management, Chap. 12, p. 53, in HPIM-14.

2

CHEST PAIN

There is little correlation between the severity of chest pain and the seriousness of its cause.

POTENTIALLY SERIOUS CAUSES

The differential diagnosis of chest pain is shown in Fig. 2-1. It is useful to characterize the chest pain as (1) new, acute, and ongoing; (2) recurrent, episodic; and (3) persistent, sometimes for days (Table 2-1).

MYOCARDIAL ISCHEMIA *Angina Pectoris* (Chap. 114) Substernal pressure, squeezing, constriction, with radiation typically to left arm; usually on exertion, especially after meals or with emotional arousal. Characteristically relieved by rest and nitroglycerin.

Acute Myocardial Infarction (Chap. 113) Similar to angina but usually more severe, of longer duration ($\geq$30 min), and not immediately relieved by rest or nitroglycerin. S_3 and S_4 common.

PULMONARY EMBOLISM (Chap. 123) May be substernal or lateral, pleuritic in nature, and associated with hemoptysis, tachycardia, and hypoxemia.

AORTIC DISSECTION (Chap. 116) Very severe, in center of chest, a "ripping" quality, radiates to back, not affected by changes in position. May be associated with weak or absent peripheral pulses.

MEDIASTINAL EMPHYSEMA Sharp, intense, localized to substernal region; often associated with audible crepitus.

ACUTE PERICARDITIS (Chap. 112) Usually steady, crushing, substernal; often has pleuritic component aggravated by cough, deep inspiration, supine position, and relieved by sitting upright; one-, two-, or three-component pericardial friction rub often audible.

PLEURISY Due to inflammation; less commonly tumor and pneumothorax. Usually unilateral, knifelike, superficial, aggravated by cough and respiration.

LESS SERIOUS CAUSES

COSTOCHONDRAL PAIN In anterior chest, usually sharply localized, may be brief and darting or a persistent dull ache. Can be reproduced by pressure on costochondral and/or

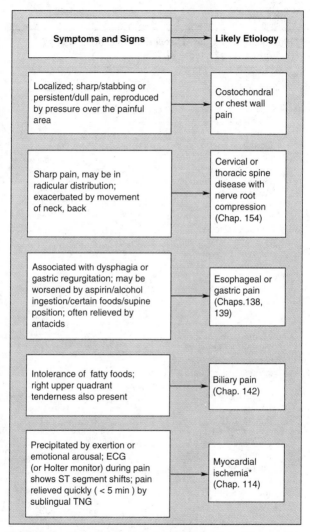

FIGURE 2-1 Differential diagnosis of recurrent chest pain. *If myocardial ischemia suspected, also consider aortic valve disease (Chap. 110) and hypertrophic obstructive cardiomyopathy (Chap. 111) if systolic murmur present.

Table 2-1

Some Causes of Chest Discomfort and the Types of Discomfort Associated with Them

Cause	New, Acute, Often Ongoing	Recurrent Episodic	Persistent, Even for Days
Cardiac			
Coronary artery disease	+	+	—
Aortic stenosis	—	+	—
Hypertrophic cardiomyopathy	—	+	—
Pericarditis	+	+	+
Vascular			
Aortic dissection	+	—	—
Pulmonary embolism	+	+	—
Pulmonary hypertension	+	+	—
Pulmonary			
Pleuritis or pneumonia	+	+	+
Tracheobronchitis	+	+	+
Pneumothorax	+	—	+
Mediastinitis or mediastinal emphysema	+	—	+
Gastrointestinal			
Esophageal reflux or spasm	+	+	+
Peptic ulcer disease	+	+	—
Biliary disease	+	+	—
Pancreatitis		+	+
Musculoskeletal			
Cervical disk disease	—	+	+
Arthritis of the shoulder spine	—	+	+
Costochondritis	+	+	+
Intercostal muscle cramps	+	+	+
Subacromial bursitis	+	+	+
Other			
Disorders of the breast	—	+	+
Herpes zoster	+	—	+
Emotional	+	+	+

	Acute myocardial infarction (Chap. 113)	Aortic dissection (Chap. 116)	Acute pericarditis (Chap. 112)	Pulmonary embolism (Chap. 123)	Acute pneumothorax (Chap. 125)	Rupture of esophagus
Description of pain	Oppressive, constrictive, or squeezing; may radiate to arm(s), neck, back	"Tearing" or "ripping"; may travel from anterior chest to mid-back	Crushing, sharp, pleuritic; relieved by sitting forward	Pleuritic, sharp; possibly accompanied by cough/hemoptysis	Very sharp, pleuritic	Intense substernal and epigastric; accompanied by vomiting ± hematemesis
Background history	Less severe, similar pain on exertion; + coronary risk factors (Chap. 114)	Hypertension or Marfan syndrome (Chap. 150)	Recent upper respiratory tract infection, or other conditions which predispose to pericarditis (Chap. 112)	Recent surgery or other immobilization	Recent chest trauma, or history of chronic obstructive lung disease	Recent recurrent vomiting/retching
Key Physical findings	Diaphoresis, pallor; S4 common; S3 less common	Weak, asymmetric peripheral pulses; possible diastolic murmur of aortic insufficiency (Chap. 110)	Pericardial friction rub (usually 3 components, best heard by sitting patient forward)	Tachypnea; possible pleural friction rub	Tachypnea; breath sounds & hyperresonance over affected lung field	Subcutaneous emphysema; audible crepitus adjacent to the sternum
Consider						
Confirmatory Tests	• Serial ECGs • Serial cardiac enzymes (esp. CK, LDH)	• CXR – widened mediastinal silhouette • MRI, CT, or transesophageal echogram: intimal flap visualized • Aortic angiogram: definitive diagnosis	• ECG: diffuse ST elevation and PR Segment depression • Echogram: pericardial effusion often visualized	• Arterial blood gas: hypoxemia & respiratory alkalosis • Lung scan: V/Q mismatch • Pulmonary angiogram: arterial luminal filling defects	• CXR: radiolucency within pleural space; poss. collapse of adjacent lung segment; if tension pneumothorax, mediastinum is shifted to opp. side	• CXR: pneumomediastinum • Esophageal endoscopy is diagnostic

FIGURE 2-2 Differential diagnosis of acute chest pain.

9

chondrosternal junctions. In Tietze's syndrome (costochondritis), joints are swollen, red, and tender.

CHEST WALL PAIN   Due to strain of muscles or ligaments from excessive exercise or rib fracture from trauma; accompanied by local tenderness.

ESOPHAGEAL PAIN   Deep thoracic discomfort; may be accompanied by dysphagia and regurgitation.

EMOTIONAL DISORDERS   Prolonged ache or dartlike, brief, flashing pain; associated with fatigue, emotional strain.

OTHER CAUSES

(1) Cervical disk; (2) osteoarthritis of cervical or thoracic spine; (3) abdominal disorders: peptic ulcer, hiatus hernia, pancreatitis, biliary colic; (4) tracheobronchitis, pneumonia; (5) diseases of the breast (inflammation, tumor); (6) intercostal neuritis (herpes zoster).

―――――――― *Approach to the Patient* ――――――――

A meticulous history of the behavior of pain, what precipitates it and what relieves it, aids diagnosis of recurrent chest pain. Fig. 2-2 presents clues to diagnosis and workup of acute, life-threatening chest pain.

For a more detailed discussion, see Goldman L: Chest Discomfort and Palpitation, Chap. 13, p. 58, in HPIM-14.

3

ABDOMINAL PAIN

Numerous causes, ranging from acute, life-threatening emergencies to chronic functional disease and disorders of several organ systems, can generate abdominal pain. Evaluation of acute pain requires rapid assessment of likely causes and early initiation of appropriate therapy. A more detailed and leisurely approach to diagnosis may be followed in less acute situations. Table 3-1 lists the common causes of abdominal pain.

_____ *Approach to the Patient* _____

History

Extremely important. Physical examination may be unrevealing or misleading and laboratory and radiologic exams delayed or unhelpful.

Characteristic Features of Abdominal Pain

Duration and Pattern Provide clues to nature and severity, although acute abdominal crisis may occasionally present insidiously or on background of chronic pain.

Type and location provide rough guide to nature of disease. *Visceral pain* (due to distention of a hollow viscus) localizes poorly and is often perceived in the midline. Intestinal pain tends to be crampy; when originating proximal to the ileocecal valve, it usually localizes above and around the umbilicus. Pain of colonic origin is perceived in the hypogastrium and lower quadrants. Pain from biliary or ureteral obstruction often causes pts to writhe in discomfort. *Somatic pain* (due to peritoneal inflammation) is usually sharper and more precisely localized to the diseased region (e.g., acute appendicitis, capsular distention of liver, kidney, or spleen), exacerbated by movement, causing pts to remain still. Pattern of radiation may be helpful: right shoulder (hepatobiliary origin), left shoulder (splenic), midback (pancreatic), flank (proximal urinary tract), groin (genital or distal urinary tract).

Factors That Precipitate or Relieve Pain Relationship to eating (e.g., upper GI, biliary, pancreatic, ischemic bowel disease), defecation (colorectal), urination (genitourinary or colorectal), respiratory (pleuropulmonary, hepatobiliary), position (pancreatic, gastroesophageal reflux, musculoskeletal), menstrual cycle/menarche (tuboovarian, endometrial, including endometriosis), exertion (coronary/intestinal ischemia, musculoskeletal), medication/specific foods (motility disorders, food intolerance, gastroesophageal reflux, porphyria, adrenal insuf-

Table 3-1

Common Etiologies of Abdominal Pain

Mucosal or muscle inflammation in hollow viscera: Peptic disease (ulcers, erosions, inflammation), hemorrhagic gastritis, gastroesophageal reflux, appendicitis, diverticulitis, cholecystitis, cholangitis, inflammatory bowel diseases (Crohn's, ulcerative colitis), infectious gastroenteritis, mesenteric lymphadenitis, colitis, cystitis, or pyelonephritis

Visceral spasm or distention: Intestinal obstruction (adhesions, tumor, intussusception), appendiceal obstruction with appendicitis, strangulation of hernia, irritable bowel syndrome (muscle hypertrophy and spasm), acute biliary obstruction, pancreatic ductal obstruction (chronic pancreatitis, stone), ureteral obstruction (kidney stone, blood clot), fallopian tubes (tubal pregnancy)

Vascular disorder: Mesenteric thromboembolic disease (arterial or venous), arterial dissection or rupture (e.g., aortic aneurysm), occlusion from external pressure or torsion (e.g., volvulus, hernia, tumor, adhesions, intussusception), hemoglobinopathy (esp. sickle cell disease)

Distention or inflammation of visceral surfaces: Hepatic capsule (hepatitis, hemorrhage, tumor, Budd-Chiari syndrome, Fitz-Hugh–Curtis syndrome), renal capsule (tumor, infection, infarction, venous occlusion), splenic capsule (hemorrhage, abscess, infarction), pancreas (pancreatitis, pseudocyst, abscess, tumor), ovary (hemorrhage into cyst, ectopic pregnancy, abscess)

Peritoneal inflammation: Bacterial infection (perforated viscus, pelvic inflammatory disease, infected ascites), intestinal infarction, chemical irritation, pancreatitis, perforated viscus (esp. stomach and duodenum, mittelschmerz), reactive inflammation (neighboring abscess, incl. diverticulitis, pleuropulmonary infection or inflammation), serositis (collagen-vascular diseases, familial Mediterranean fever)

Abdominal wall disorders: Trauma, hernias, muscle inflammation or infection, hematoma (trauma, anticoagulant therapy), traction from mesentery (e.g., adhesions)

Toxins: Lead poisoning, black widow spider bite

Metabolic disorders: Uremia, ketoacidosis (diabetic, alcoholic), Addisonian crisis, porphyria, angioedema (C1 esterase deficiency), narcotic withdrawal

Neurologic: Herpes zoster, tabes dorsalis, causalgia, compression or inflammation of spinal roots, (e.g., arthritis, herniated disk, tumor, abscess), psychogenic

Referred pain: From heart, lungs, esophagus, genitalia (e.g., cardiac ischemia, pneumonia, pneumothorax, pulmonary embolism, esophagitis, esophageal spasm, esophageal rupture)

ficiency, ketoacidosis, toxins), and stress (motility disorders, nonulcer dyspepsia, irritable bowel syndrome).

Associated Symptoms Fevers/chills (infection, inflammatory disease, infarction), weight loss (tumor, inflammatory diseases, malabsorption, ischemia), nausea/vomiting (obstruction, infection, inflammatory disease, metabolic disease), dysphagia/odynophagia (esophageal), early satiety (gastric), hematemesis (esophageal, gastric, duodenal), constipation (colorectal, perianal, genitourinary), jaundice (hepatobiliary, hemolytic), diarrhea (inflammatory disease, infection, malabsorption, secretory tumors, ischemia, genitourinary), dysuria/hematuria/vaginal or penile discharge (genitourinary), hematochezia (colorectal, or, rarely, urinary), skin/joint/eye disorders (inflammatory disease, bacterial or viral infection).

Predisposing Factors Family history (inflammatory disease, tumors, pancreatitis), hypertension and atherosclerotic disease (ischemia), diabetes mellitus (motility disorders, ketoacidosis), connective tissue disease (motility disorders, serositis), depression (motility disorders, tumors), smoking (ischemia), recent smoking cessation (inflammatory disease), ethanol (motility disorders, hepatobiliary, pancreatic, gastritis, peptic ulcer disease).

Physical Examination

Evaluate abdomen for prior trauma or surgery, current trauma; abdominal distention, fluid, or air; direct, rebound, and referred tenderness; liver and spleen size; masses, bruits, altered bowel sounds, hernias, arterial masses. Rectal examination for presence and location of tenderness, masses, blood (gross or occult). Pelvic examination in women is essential. *General examination*: evaluate for evidence of hemodynamic instability, acid-base disturbances, nutritional deficiency, coagulopathy, arterial occlusive disease, stigmata of liver disease, cardiac dysfunction, lymphadenopathy, and skin lesions.

Routine Laboratory and Radiologic Studies

Choices depend on clinical setting (esp. severity of pain, rapidity of onset). May include CBC, serum electrolytes, coagulation parameters, serum glucose, and biochemical tests of liver, kidney, and pancreatic function; CXR to determine the presence of diseases involving heart, lung, mediastinum, and pleura; ECG is helpful to exclude referred pain from cardiac disease; plain abdominal radiographs to evaluate bowel displacement, intestinal distention, fluid and gas pattern, free peritoneal air, liver size, and abdominal calcifications (e.g., gallstones, renal stones, chronic pancreatitis).

Special Studies

May include abdominal ultrasonography (to visualize biliary ducts, gallbladder, liver, pancreas, and kidneys); CT to identify masses, abscesses, evidence of inflammation (bowel wall thickening, mesenteric "stranding," lymphadenopathy), aortic aneurysm; barium contrast radiographs (barium swallow, upper GI series, small bowel follow-through, barium enema; upper GI endoscopy, sigmoidoscopy, or colonoscopy; cholangiography (endoscopic, percutaneous, or via MRI), angiography (direct or via CT or MRI), and radionuclide scanning. In selected cases, percutaneous biopsy, laparoscopy, and exploratory laparotomy may be required.

ACUTE, CATASTROPHIC ABDOMINAL PAIN

Intense abdominal pain of acute onset or pain associated with syncope, hypotension, or toxic appearance necessitates rapid yet orderly evaluation. Consider obstruction, perforation, or rupture of hollow viscus, dissection or rupture of major blood vessels (esp. aortic aneurysm), ulceration, abdominal sepsis, ketoacidosis, and adrenal crisis.

BRIEF HISTORY AND PHYSICAL EXAMINATION
Should focus on presence of fever or hypothermia, hyperventilation, cyanosis, direct or rebound abdominal tenderness, pulsating abdominal mass, abdominal bruits, ascites, rectal blood, rectal or pelvic tenderness, and evidence of coagulopathy. Useful laboratory studies include hematocrit (may be normal with acute hemorrhage or misleadingly high with dehydration), WBC, arterial blood gases, serum electrolytes, BUN, creatinine, glucose, lipase or amylase, and UA. Radiologic studies should include supine and upright abdominal films (left lateral decubitus view if upright unobtainable) to evaluate bowel caliber and presence of free peritoneal air, cross-table lateral film to assess aortic diameter. CT (when available) to detect evidence of bowel perforation, inflammation, solid organ infarction, retroperitoneal bleeding, abscess, or tumor. Abdominal paracentesis (or peritoneal lavage in cases of trauma) to detect evidence of bleeding or spontaneous peritonitis. Abdominal ultrasound (when available) to disclose evidence of abscess, cholecystitis, biliary obstruction, or hematoma and to determine aortic diameter.

℞ TREATMENT

Should include intravenous fluids, correction of life-threatening acid-base disturbances, and assessment of need for emergent surgery; careful follow-up with frequent reexamination (when possible, by the same examiner) is essential. Narcotic analgesics may best be withheld pending establishment of diagnosis and therapeutic plan, since masking of diagnostic signs may delay needed intervention.

For a more detailed discussion, see Silen W: Abdominal Pain, Chap. 14, p. 65, in HPIM-14.

HEADACHE AND FACIAL PAIN

Clinical Considerations

The causes of headache are summarized in Table 4-1. First step in clinical evaluation—distinguishing benign from serious etiologies. New-onset headache raises suspicion for a serious cause. Associated amenorrhea or galactorrhea—consider polycystic ovary syndrome or prolactin-secreting pituitary adenoma. New headache in patient with malignancy—consider cerebral metastasis or carcinomatous meningitis. Accentuation of pain with eye movements—consider meningitis. Head pain following bending, lifting, or coughing—consider posterior fossa mass.

Quality and intensity of pain rarely have *diagnostic* value. Headache location can suggest involvement of local structures (temporal pain in giant cell arteritis, facial pain in sinusitis). Ruptured aneurysm (instant onset), cluster headache (peak over 3–5 min), and migraine (onset over minutes to hours) differ in time-intensity course. Therapeutic trials of medication do *not* provide diagnostic information due to high frequency of placebo responders (~30%). Provocation by environmental factors suggests a benign cause.

Most common cause of facial pain is dental; triggered by hot, cold, or sweet foods. Facial neuralgias (trigeminal and glossopharyngeal) consist of paroxysmal, fleeting, electric shock–like episodes of pain.

Table 4-1

The Classification of Headache

1. Migraine
   Migraine without aura
   Migraine with aura
   Ophthalmoplegic migraine
   Retinal migraine
   Childhood periodic syndromes that may be precursors to or associated with migraine
   Migrainous disorder not fulfilling above criteria
2. Tension-type headache
   Episodic tension-type headache
   Chronic tension-type headache
3. Cluster headache and chronic paroxysmal hemicrania
   Cluster headache
   Chronic paroxysmal hemicrania
4. Miscellaneous headaches not associated with structural lesion
   Idiopathic stabbing headache
   External compression headache
   Cold stimulus headache
   Benign cough headache
   Benign exertional headache
   Headache associated with sexual activity
5. Headache associated with head trauma
   Acute posttraumatic headache
   Chronic posttraumatic headache
6. Headache associated with vascular disorders
   Acute ischemic cerebrovascular disorder
   Intracranial hematoma
   Subarachnoid hemorrhage
   Unruptured vascular malformation
   Arteritis
   Carotid or vertebral artery pain
   Venous thrombosis
   Arterial hypertension
   Other vascular disorder
7. Headache associated with nonvascular intracranial disorder
   High CSF pressure
   Low CSF pressure
   Intracranial infection
   Sarcoidosis and other noninfectious inflammatory diseases
   Related to intrathecal injections

(continued)

Table 4-1 (*Continued*)

The Classification of Headache

Headache associated with nonvascular intracranial disorder (cont.)
  Intracranial neoplasm
  Associated with other intracranial disorder
8. Headache associated with substances or their withdrawal
  Headache induced by acute substance use or exposure
  Headache induced by chronic substance use or exposure
  Headache from substance withdrawal (acute use)
  Headache from substance withdrawal (chronic use)
9. Headache associated with noncephalic infection
  Viral infection
  Bacterial infection
  Other infection
10. Headache associated with metabolic disorder
  Hypoxia
  Hypercapnia
  Mixed hypoxia and hypercapnia
  Hypoglycemia
  Dialysis
  Other metabolic abnormality
11. Headache or facial pain associated with disorder of facial or cranial structures
  Cranial bone
  Eyes
  Ears
  Nose and sinuses
  Teeth, jaws, and related structures
  Temporomandibular joint disease
12. Cranial neuralgias, nerve trunk pain, and deafferentation pain
  Persistent (in contrast to ticlike) pain of cranial nerve origin
  Trigeminal neuralgia
  Glossopharyngeal neuralgia
  Nervus intermedius neuralgia
  Superior laryngeal neuralgia
  Occipital neuralgia
  Central causes of head and facial pain other than tic douloureux
13. Headache not classifiable

SOURCE: Raskin: HPIM, 14/e, p. 69.

MIGRAINE

CLASSIC MIGRAINE   Onset usually in childhood, adolescence, or early adulthood. First attacks occurring in adults after age 50 are described. Family history is often positive, and migraine is more common in women. Classic triad: visual scotomata or scintillations, unilateral throbbing headache, accompanied by nausea and vomiting. An attack lasting 2–6 h is common, with relief after sleep. Attacks may be triggered by wine, cheese, chocolate, contraceptives, stress, exercise, or travel.

COMMON MIGRAINE   Unilateral or bilateral headache with nausea, but rarely with vomiting or visual complaints. More common in women. Onset is usually more gradual than in classic migraine, and pain becomes more generalized and may persist for hours or days.

℞ **TREATMENT**

Three approaches to migraine treatment: removal of environmental precipitants (i.e., sleep deprivation, skipping meals, specific medications, foods, or wine), pharmacologic treatment of acute attacks, and prophylaxis (Table 4-2). Drug treatment necessary for most migraine pts: (1) response rates vary from 60–90%, (2) initial choice of drug is largely empiric, (3) effect of prophylactic treatment may take several months to assess with each drug, (4) patience is required by both physician and pt. Choice of individual drugs is influenced by pt's age, coexisting illnesses, and side effect profile; for prophylaxis, amitriptyline is a good first choice in young people with difficulty falling asleep, ergonovine is also well-tolerated in young pts, whereas verapamil often is the first choice in the elderly.

CLUSTER HEADACHE   Characterized by recurrent, nocturnal, unilateral, retroorbital searing pain. Typically a young male (90%) awakens 2–4 h after sleep onset with severe pain, accompanied by unilateral lacrimation, and nasal and conjunctival congestion. Visual complaints or nausea and vomiting are rare. Pain lasts 20–60 min and subsides quickly but tends to recur at the same time of night or several times each 24 h over several weeks (a cluster). A pain-free period of months or years may be followed by another cluster of headaches. Alcohol provokes attacks in 70%. Prophylaxis with lithium, 600–900 mg qd, or prednisone, 60 mg for 7 d followed by a rapid taper. Ergotamine, 1 mg suppository 1–2 h before expected attack, may prevent daily episode.

Table 4-2

Migraine Treatment

ACUTE

Drug	Initial Dose, mg	Frequency	Common Side-Effects
Ibuprofen	400–800 PO	qid	GI, dizziness, rash
Naproxen	375–750 PO	bid	GI, dizziness, rash
Aspirin	325–650 PO	qid	GI
Acetaminophen	325–650 PO	qid	—
Midrin	1–2 tablets PO	q1h*	Vasoconstriction, dizziness
Ergotamine	1–2	q 30 min†	Vasoconstriction, GI, cramps, paresthesia
Sumatriptan	6–12 SC; 25–100 PO	2 doses/day	Vasoconstriction
Dihydroergotamine	0.2–1.0 IV or IM	q 1 h × 3	GI, leg pain, paresthesia

PROPHYLAXIS

Drug	Total Oral Daily Dose, mg	Frequency	Common Side-Effects
Amitriptyline	10–175‡	qhs	Sedation, dry mouth
Propranolol	40–320	bid	Lethargy, insomnia
Verapamil SR	180–480	qd	Constipation, light-headedness, nausea, hypotension
Valproate	500–1500	bid-qid	Nausea, tremor, hair loss
Ergonovine	0.4–2.0	tid†	Nausea, abdominal pain

* Total = 5 tablets/12 h; † Total = 6 mg/d
‡ Begin 10–25 mg qhs; increase by 10–25 mg qhs each week to 100–150 m maximum

TENSION HEADACHE   Onset in adolescence/young adulthood. Pain is holocephalic, as pressure or a tight band, but may be throbbing. Tends to occur late in day; related often to stress. May persist for hours or days. Distinction from common migraine may be impossible; treatment as for migraine (Table 4-2).

OTHER HEADACHE TYPES

TEMPORAL ARTERITIS   Elderly patients; two-thirds are women. Untreated—blindness due to ophthalmic artery involvement. Symptoms—headache, jaw claudication, proximal limb aching, visual obscuration, fever, or weight loss. Pain dull; superimposed episodic, lancinating pains. Scalp tenderness common; brushing hair may be painful. ESR usually elevated; temporal artery biopsy for diagnosis. *Treatment:* glucocorticoids.

COUGH HEADACHE   Transient severe head pain with coughing, bending, lifting, sneezing, or stooping; lasts from seconds to several minutes; men > women. Usually benign; consider posterior fossa mass lesion (~25%).

BRAIN TUMOR   Vomiting preceding headache suggests posterior fossa tumor. Sleep disturbance in 10%; worse at night if associated with elevated intracranial pressure. Nonspecific headache initial complaint in 30%.

PSEUDOTUMOR CEREBRI (BENIGN INTRACRANIAL HYPERTENSION)   Elevated intracranial pressure from impaired CSF reabsorption by arachnoid villi. Headache, papilledema, without focal neurologic signs. Most pts are young, female, obese. *Treatment:* acetazolamide (125–250 mg PO tid); repeat LP; in severe cases, optic nerve fenestration.

POST-CONCUSSION HEADACHE   Common following motor vehicle collisions, other head trauma; severe injury or loss of consciousness often not present. Symptoms of headache, dizziness, vertigo, or impaired memory; typically remits after several weeks to months. Neurologic examination and neuroimaging studies normal. Not a functional disorder; cause unknown.

LUMBAR PUNCTURE HEADACHE   Caused by reduced intracranial pressure; typical onset 24–48 h after puncture. Posi set when pt sits or stands, relief by lying flat. Most pontaneously in 1 week or less; epidural blood in refractory cases.

FACIAL PAIN

TRIGEMINAL NEURALGIA Lancinating pains lasting seconds; maxillary > mandibular distribution of trigeminal nerve. Most cases are idiopathic; pts under age 50 at risk for structural cause (multiple sclerosis, vascular anomaly, tumor). *Treatment:* carbamazepine (400–1600 mg/d) usually effective; phenytoin, baclofen, and valproic acid are other options.

POSTHERPETIC NEURALGIA Pain following skin rash of herpes zoster; may be associated with sensory loss. Pain usually resolves over weeks.

OCCIPITAL NEURALGIA Entrapment of greater occipital nerve at exit from skull; unilateral, lancinating occipital pain. Percussion over exit point of greater occipital nerve may elicit symptoms. *Treatment:* block-injection of steroid and local anesthetic.

For a more detailed discussion, see Raskin NH: Headache, Chap. 15, p. 68, and Migraine and the Cluster Headache Syndrome, Chap. 364, p. 2307, in HPIM-14.

5

LOW BACK PAIN

Anatomy

Vertebral bodies and disks function to absorb the shock of body movements. Posteriorly, vertebral processes and arches protect the nerve roots within the lumbar spinal canal, provide sites for attachment of muscles and ligaments, and produce a system of levers and pulleys that results in spine movements. Lumbar roots exit a level below their respective vertebral bodies; spinal cord ends at L1 or L2 level of the bony spine. Lumbar roots follow a long course within spinal canal and can be injured from the upper lumbar spine to their exit. Many spine structures are pain-sensitive; sources of low back pain (LBP) include vertebral body periosteum, dura, facet joints, annulus fibrosus of the intervertebral disk, epidural veins, and the posterior longitudinal ligament.

Clinical Features

CLASSIFICATION   Five types of low back pain:

- *Local pain*—caused by activation of local, pain-sensitive nerve endings near affected part of the spine (i.e., tears, stretching).
- *Pain referred to the spine*—typically abdominal or pelvic and back pain unaffected by spine movement.
- *Pain of spine origin*—restricted to the back or referred to lower limbs. Diseases of upper lumbar spine refer pain to upper lumbar region, groin, or anterior thighs. Diseases of lower lumbar spine refer pain to buttocks or posterior thighs.
- *Radicular pain*—radiates from spine to leg in territory of a specific nerve root. Coughing, sneezing, lifting heavy objects, or straining at stool often elicits pain; description of pain fails to distinguish between pain of spine and nerve root origins.
- *Pain associated with muscle spasm*—diverse origin; accompanied by taut paraspinal muscles.

EXAMINATION   General examination includes abdomen, pelvis, and rectum to search for visceral sources of pain. Inspection may reveal scoliosis or muscle spasm. Palpation may elicit pain over a diseased spine segment. Pain from hip may be confused with spine pain. Manual internal/external rotation at hip (knee and hip in flexion) may reproduce the pain. *Straight-leg raising (SLR) sign*—elicited by passive flexion of leg on abdomen with knee extended; pt in sitting or supine position; maneuver stretches L5/S1 nerve roots and sciatic nerve passing posterior to the hip; SLR is positive if maneuver reproduces the pain. *Crossed SLR sign*—positive when SLR on one leg reproduces symptoms in opposite leg or buttocks; nerve/nerve root lesion is on the painful side. *Reverse SLR sign*—elicited by passive extension of leg on trunk with the knee extended and pt prone or standing beside exam table; maneuver stretches L2-L4 nerve roots and femoral nerve passing anterior to the hip. Neurologic exam—search for focal atrophy, weakness, reflex loss, diminished sensation in a dermatomal distribution; with trauma, important to avoid nerve root injury from manipulating legs. Findings on radiculopathy are summarized in Table 5-1.

LABORATORY STUDIES   "Routine" laboratory studies and lumbar spine x-rays—rarely needed for acute LBP but are indicated when risk factors for serious underlying disease are present (Table 5-2). MRI and CT-myelography are tests of choice for anatomic definition of spine disease.

Causes of Low Back Pain

1.   *Lumbar disk disease*—common cause of low back and leg pain; usually at L4-L5 or L5-S1 levels. Dermatomal sensory loss, asymmetric reduction or loss of deep tendon reflexes, or myotomal pattern of weakness more informative than pain pattern for localization. Usually unilateral; bilateral nerve root involvement—seen with large central disk herniations compressing multiple nerve roots—may cause cauda equina syndrome. Five potential indications for lumbar disk surgery: (a) progressive motor weakness from nerve root injury; (b) progressive motor impairment demonstrable by electromyography; (c) abnormal bowel or bladder function; (d) incapacitating nerve root pain despite conservative treatment over 4 weeks; and (e) recurrent incapacitating pain despite conservative treatment. The latter two criteria are controversial.

2.   *Spinal stenosis*—a narrowed spinal canal producing back and bilateral leg pain induced by walking or standing and relieved by sitting or supine position. Unlike vascular claudication, symptoms are provoked by standing without walking. Unlike lumbar disk disease, symptoms are relieved by sitting. Focal neurologic deficits common; severe neurologic deficits (paralysis, incontinence) rare. Results from acquired (75%), congenital, or mixed acquired/congenital factors. Symptomatic treatment adequate for mild disease; surgery often indicated when pain interferes with activities of daily living or when focal neurologic signs present. Surgery successful in 65–80%, but 25% develop recurrent stenosis within 5 years.

Table 5-1

Lumbosacral Radiculopathy—Neurologic Findings

Lumbosacral Nerve Roots	Reflex	Sensory	Motor	Pain Distribution
L2†	—	Upper anterior thigh	Psoas* (hip flexion)	Anterior thigh
L3†	—	Lower anterior thigh Anterior knee	Psoas* (hip flexion) Quadriceps (knee extension) Thigh adduction	Anterior thigh, knee
L4†	Quadriceps (knee)	Medial calf	Quadriceps* (knee extension) Thigh adduction Tibialis anterior (foot dorsiflexion)	Knee, medial calf
L5‡	—	Dorsal surface—foot Lateral calf	Peroneii* (foot eversion) Tibialis anterior (foot dorsiflexion) Gluteus medius (hip abduction) Toe dorsiflexors	Lateral calf, dorsal foot, posterolateral thigh, buttocks

| S1† | Gastrocnemius/soleus (ankle) | Plantar surface—foot
Lateral aspect—foot
Abductor hallucis
(Toe flexors)
Gluteus maximus
(Hip extension) | Gastrocnemius/soleus* (foot plantar flexion) | Bottom foot, posterior calf, posterior thigh, buttocks |

† Reverse straight-leg raising sign present—see "Examination."
‡ Straight-leg raising sign present—see "Examination."
* These muscles receive the majority of innervation from the root in the same horizontal row.

25

Table 5-2

Risk Factors for Possible Serious Causes of Acute LBP

HISTORY

Pain worse at rest or at night
Prior history of cancer
History of chronic infection (esp. pulmonary, urinary tract, or skin)
History of trauma
Age >50 years
Intravenous drug use
Glucocorticoid use
Rapidly progressive neurologic deficit

EXAMINATION

Unexplained fever
Unexplained weight loss
Straight-leg raising sign
Percussion tenderness—low spine or costovertebral angle
Abdominal, rectal, or pelvic mass
Rapidly progresive focal neurologic deficit (e.g., sensory loss, leg weakness, asymmetric or absent leg reflexes, abnormal bladder function)

3. *Trauma—low back strain* or *sprain* used to describe minor, self-limited injuries associated with LBP. Vertebral fractures from trauma result in wedging or compression of vertebral bodies; *burst fractures* involving anterior and posterior spine elements can occur. Neurologic impairment common with vertebral fractures; early treatment produces better outcome. Most common cause of nontraumatic fracture is osteoporosis. Osteomalacia, hyperparathyroidism, hyperthyroidsm, multiple myeloma, metastatic carcinoma, or glucocorticoid use may predispose vertebral body to fracture. Clinical content, exam findings, and spine x-rays extablish the diagnosis.

4. *Spondylolisthesis*—slippage of anterior spine (vertebral bodies, pedicles, superior facets) forward, leaving posterior elements behind; L5-S1 > L4-L5 levels; can produce LBP or radiculopathy/cauda equina syndrome.

5. *Osteoarthritis* of lumbosacral spine increases with age. Back pain induced by spine movement; severity of radiologic findings do not correlate to severity of pain. *Facet syndrome*—radicular symptoms and signs, nerve root compression by unilateral facet hypertrophy. Foraminotomy and facetectomy—long-

term pain relief in 80-90%. Loss of intervertebral disk height reduces vertical dimensions of intervertebral foramen; descending pedicle can compress the exiting nerve root.

6.   *Vertebral metastases*—back pain is most common neurologic symptom in pts with *systemic cancer*. Metastatic carcinoma, multiple myeloma, and lymphomas frequently involve spine. LBP may be presenting symptom of cancer; pain typically unrelieved by rest. MRI or CT-myelography demonstrate spinal metastasis; the disk space is spared.

7.   *Infection: vertebral osteomyelitis*—LBP unrelieved by rest; focal spine tenderness and elevated ESR. Primary source of infection (lung, urinary tract, or skin) found in 40%; *Staphylococcus* species most common. Destruction of the vertebral bodies *and* disk space common. *Lumbar spinal epidural abscess* presents as back pain and fever; exam may be normal or show radicular findings or cauda equina syndrome; abscess extent best defined by MRI.

8.   *Lumbar arachnoiditis* may follow inflammatory response to local tissue injury within subarachnoid space; fibrosis results in clumping of nerve roots, best seen by MRI; treatment is unsatisfactory.

9.   *Immune disorders*—ankylosing spondylitis, rheumatoid arthritis, Reiter's syndrome, psoriatic arthritis, and chronic inflammatory bowel disease. *Ankylosing spondylitis*—typically a male <40 years with nocturnal back pain; pain unrelieved by rest but improves with exercise.

10.   *Osteoporosis*—loss of bone substance resulting from hyperparathyroidism, chronic steroid use, immobilization, or other medical disorders. Sole manifestation may be LBP exacerbated by movement.

11.   *Visceral diseases* (Table 5-3)—pelvic diseases refer pain to sacral region, lower abdominal diseases to lumbar region, upper abdominal diseases to lower thoracic or upper lumbar spine. Local signs are absent; normal movements of the spine are painless. Isolated LBP—20% of pts with contained rupture of abdominal aortic aneurysm.

12.   *Others*—chronic LBP with no clear cause; poor posture, compensation hysteria, malingering, substance abuse, chronic anxiety, and states of depression may be associated. A history of psychiatric illness may antedate LBP.

R̶x̶ TREATMENT

   Acute Low Back Pain (ABP)   Defined as pain of less than 3 months' duration; full recovery occurs in 85%. Management controversial; few well-controlled clinical trials exist. Proposed algorithms presented in Figs. 5-1 and 5-2. Entry begins

Table 5-3

Visceral Causes of Low Back Pain

Stomach (posterior wall)—ulcer/tumor
Gallbladder—gallstones
Pancreas—tumor, cyst, pancreatitis
Retroperitoneal—hemorrhage, tumor, pyelonephritis
Vascular—abdominal aortic aneurysm, renal artery and vein thrombosis
Colon—colitis, diverticulitis, neoplasm
Uterosacral ligaments—endometriosis, carcinoma
Uterine malposition
Menstrual pain
Neoplastic infiltration of nerves
Radiation neurosis of tumors/nerves
Prostate—carcinoma, prostatitis
Kidney—renal stones, inflammatory disease, neoplasm, infection

with adults having <3 months activity intolerance due to ABP or back-related leg symptoms. Medical history and physical exam used to search for "risk factors" (Table 5-2); if absent, initial treatment is symptomatic and no diagnostic tests necessary (Fig. 5-1). Spine infections, fractures, tumors, or rapidly progressive neurologic deficits require urgent diagnostic evaluation. Pts with no risk factors and no improvement over 4 weks are subdivided by the presence/absence of leg symptoms (Fig. 5-2) and managed accordingly. Extensive clinical data are obtained prior to spine surgery consultation for ABP

Clinical trials do not show benefit from bed rest >2 days. Possible benefits of early activity—cardiovascular conditioning, disk and cartilage nutrition, bone and muscle strength, increased endorphin levels. Well-designed studies of traction fail to show a benefit. Proof is lacking to support treatment of ABP with acupuncture, ultrasound, diathermy, transcutaneous electrical nerve stimulation, massage, biofeedback, or electrical stimulation. Self-application of ice or heat or use of shoe insoles is optional given low cost and risk; benefit of exercises or posture modification uncertain. Spinal manipulation may lessen pain and improve function; treatment >1 month or in radiculopathy is of unknown value and carries risk. Temporary

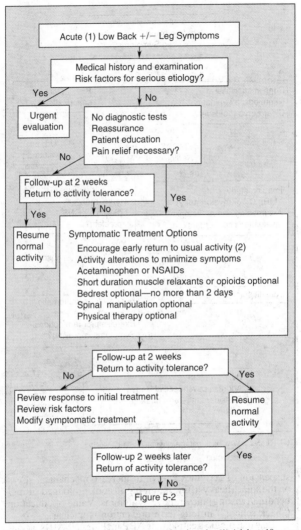

FIGURE 5-1 Low back pain management: first 4 weeks. (1) Adults ≥18 years old, symptoms <3 mos. (2) Excluding heavy manual labor.

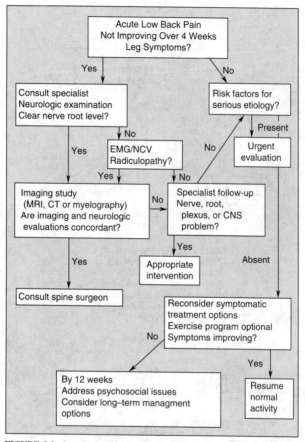

FIGURE 5-2 Low back pain management: 4–12 weeks.

suspension of activities known to increase mechanical stress on the spine (heavy lifting, straining at stool, prolonged sitting/bending/twisting) may relieve symptoms. Value of education ("back school") in long-term prevention is unclear.

Pharmacologic treatment of ABP includes NSAIDs, acetaminophen, muscle relaxants, and opioids. NSAIDs and acetaminophen are superior to placebo for ABP relief. Muscle relaxants provide short-term benefit (4–7 days), but drowsiness limits use during the day for active pts. Opioids are not superior to NSAIDs or acetaminophen in the treatment of ABP. Epidural anesthetics, steroids, opioids, or tricyclic antidepressants are not indicated as initial treatment.

Chronic low back pain (CLBP)   Defined as pain lasting longer than 3 months; differential diagnosis includes most conditions described above. Management is complex and not amenable to a simple algorithmic approach. Treatment based upon identification of underlying cause; when specific cause not found, conservative management necessary. Pharmacologic and comfort measures similar to those described for ABP. Exercise ("work hardening") regimens effective in returning some pts to work, diminishing pain, and improving walking distances.

CLBP causes can be clarified by neuroimaging and neurophysiologic (nerve conduction velocity/EMG) studies; diagnosis of radiculopathy secure when results concordant with findings on neurologic examination. Surgical intervention based upon neuroimaging alone not recommended: 25% of asymptomatic young adults have a herniated lumbar disk by CT or MRI.

For more detailed discussion, see Engstrom JW, Bradford DS: Back and Neck Pain, Chap. 16, p. 73, in HPIM-14.

6

FEVER AND HYPERTHERMIA

Fever is an abnormal elevation of body temperature due to a change in the hypothalamic thermoregulatory center. Although "normal" temperature is said to be 37°C, the maximal normal temperature ranges from 37.2°C (98.9°F) at 6 A.M. to 37.7°C (99.9°F) at 4 P.M. Fever is caused by a resetting of the hypothalamic "setpoint" by prostaglandins (especially PGE_2), a process mediated by cytokines. Few signs and symptoms in medicine suggest as many diagnostic possibilities as fever. Hyperthermia without fever may result from failure to dissipate body heat adequately (e.g., in a hot environment) or from drugs (e.g., neuroleptic malignant syndrome caused by phenothiazines and other neuroleptics, malignant hyperthermia caused by inhalation anesthetics or succinylcholine in genetically susceptible individuals). True fever may result from infection, immune phenomena, vascular inflammation or thrombosis, infarction or trauma, granulomatous diseases (e.g., sarcoid), inflammatory bowel disease, neoplasms (especially Hodgkin's disease, lymphoma, leukemia, renal cell carcinoma, and hepatoma), or acute metabolic disorders (e.g., thyroid crisis, addisonian crisis).

Clinical Manifestations

In addition to an elevated body temperature, patients with fever may develop generalized symptoms such as myalgias, arthralgias, anorexia, and somnolence. Chills—a sensation of cold—occur with most fevers. Rigors—profound chills—are associated with piloerection, chattering of the teeth, and severe shivering. Sweats accompany the activation of heat-loss mechanisms. Alterations in mental status, including delirium and convulsions, are most common among the very young, the very old, and the debilitated.

Diagnosis

With such a vast differential diagnosis, fever requires careful clinical evaluation. A detailed history must be obtained, including present illness and medical, social and travel, and family history. A meticulous physical exam must be performed and repeated on a regular basis. The lab workup must be individualized in light of the clinical circumstances. It should always include a CBC with differential and examination of any abnormal fluid collection (joint, pleural fluid). Other tests to consider include ESR determination, UA, LFTs, and cultures of blood, urine, sputum, or stool. Radiologic tests may include plain radiography, MRI and CT scanning (for detection of abscesses), and radionuclide scanning (esp. tagged WBC scanning). If no diagnosis can be made on the basis of less invasive tests, tissue must be obtained for biopsy, particularly from any abnormal organ; bone marrow biopsy may be useful, esp. for pts with anemia.

Fever of Unknown Origin (FUO)

Classic FUO is diagnosed when fever of >38.3°C (101°F) develops on several occasions over the course of >2 weeks and when 1 week of study in the hospital or three outpatient visits fail to result in a diagnosis. Most cases of FUO are due to infection, neoplasm, or collagen-vascular disease. Other causes include drugs, granulomatous diseases, inflammatory bowel disease, pulmonary embolism, factitious fever, erythema multiforme, familial Mediterranean fever, Behçet's syndrome, Fabry's disease, and Whipple's disease. FUO prolonged beyond 6 months is much less commonly due to infection and more often due to unusual or undetermined causes. When no cause can be identified, the prognosis is usually favorable. Other specialized categories of FUO have been established for certain populations of pts (Table 6-1).

Rx **TREATMENT**

The first decision to make is whether an elevation in body temperature reflects fever or hyperthermia. The latter condition is an elevation of the core temperature without an elevation of the hypothalamic setpoint, most commonly due to inadequate heat dissipation. By definition, hyperthermia does not respond to attempts to reset the already-normal hypothalamic setpoint (e.g., with acetaminophen) but does respond to physical cooling with measures such as sponging, fans, cooling blankets, and even ice baths. These measures should be instituted immediately in hyperthermia, and IV fluids should be administered. If insufficient cooling is achieved with these methods, gastric or peritoneal lavage with iced saline can be initiated; in extreme circumstances, hemodialysis or cardiopulmonary bypass with cooling of the blood can be undertaken. Malignant hyperthermia, neuroleptic malignant syndrome, drug-induced hyperthermia, and perhaps hyperthermia due to thyrotoxicosis respond to dantrolene (1–2.5 mg/kg IV q6h). Procainamide should be administered to pts with malignant hyperthermia because of the high risk of ventricular fibrillation in this syndrome.

High fever (>41°C) should be managed with antipyretics and with physical cooling with a cooling blanket or sponge bath. Low-grade or mild fevers do not necessarily require treatment except in pregnant women, children with febrile

Table 6-1

Categories of FUO*

Feature	Category of FUO			
	Nosocomial	Neutropenic	HIV-Associated	Classic
Patient's situation	Hospitalized, acute care, no infection when admitted	Neutrophil count either less than 500/μL or expected to reach that level in 1–2 days	Confirmed HIV-positive	All others with fevers for ≥3 weeks
Duration of illness while under investigation	3 days†	3 days†	3 days† (or 4 weeks as outpatient)	3 days† or three outpatient visits
Examples of cause	Septic thrombophlebitis, sinusitis, *Clostridium difficile* colitis, drug fever	Perianal infection, aspergillosis, candidemia	MAI‡ infection, tuberculosis, non-Hodgkin's lymphoma, drug fever	Infections, malignancy, inflammatory diseases, drug fever

* All require temperatures of ≥38.3°C (101°F) on several occasions.
† Includes at least 2 days' incubation of microbiology cultures.
‡ *M. avium/M. intracellulare.*

SOURCE: Gelfand J, Dinarello C: HPIM-14, p. 781 (modified from Durack and Street).

seizures, or pts with impaired cardiac, pulmonary, or cerebral function. Indeed, fever may have beneficial effects, inhibiting the growth of certain pathogens and enhancing the immune response. Acetaminophen (0.65 g) given every 3 h around the clock (rather than intermittently, which aggravates symptoms of sweats and chills) is effective for the management of most fever and is preferred because it does not (1) mask signs of inflammation that might indicate a cause of the fever, (2) impair platelet function, and (3) cause Reye's syndrome in children. NSAIDs and aspirin have anti-inflammatory as well as antipyretic effects. NSAIDs may be particularly useful in the management of fever due to malignancy. Choices about specific therapy must consider the probability of a diagnosis, the risk of not treating, and the risk of treatment. If bacterial sepsis is suspected, prompt treatment with antimicrobials should be initiated. In immunocompetent adults, gram-positive infection, gram-negative rod infection, and meningococcal infection can be covered by a variety of antibiotics including imipenem, ticarcillin/clavulanate, or a third-generation cephalosporin. Patients with neutropenia and fever should be treated empirically, usually with a combination of an aminoglycoside and an antipseudomonal antibiotic or with imipenem or ceftazidime alone. Other syndromes that, if suspected, require prompt empiric treatment (i.e., treatment before a specific diagnosis can be made) include rickettsial diseases, bacterial meningitis, bacterial infection in splenectomized pts, malaria, and typhoidal syndromes.

For a more detailed discussion see Gelfand JA, Dinarello CA: Fever and Hyperthermia, Chap. 17, p. 84, in HPIM-14.

SKIN RASH

Alterations in the appearance of the skin are most commonly manifestations of disorders that primarily affect or are limited to the skin; however, they may also indicate the presence of systemic disease. For this reason, it is extremely important that the physician have an organized approach to the differential diagnosis, evaluation, and treatment of skin conditions.

Approach to the Patient

In the pt who presents with a skin rash, it is beneficial to begin the evaluation with a thorough cutaneous exam. From these objective findings a differential diagnosis can be generated and then combined with information from a careful history to narrow the diagnostic approach. Laboratory or diagnostic procedures are used when appropriate to clarify the diagnosis.

Physical Examination (See Chap. 42)

Besides the usual goals of the physical exam, the characteristics of the skin lesion(s) should be assessed and described:

- Distribution—location can provide important clues to the diagnosis
- Arrangement and shape
- Nature of the primary lesion—the primary lesion should be carefully described (e.g., macule, papule, vesicle) and characterized with regard to color, size, topography (raised or flat), etc.
- Secondary changes—changes in area of primary pathology often due to secondary events (e.g., scaling, crusting, excoriation)

History (See Chap. 42)

- Evolution of lesions (site of onset, manner of progression, duration)
- Cutaneous and systemic symptoms
- Current or recent medications
- Ongoing or previous illnesses
- Allergies
- Photosensitivity
- Review of systems

Additional Diagnostic Techniques (See Chap. 42)

Occasionally helpful in the diagnosis of the rash are the following:

- Skin biopsy
- KOH preparation to elucidate possible fungal etiology
- Tzanck smear to detect evidence of herpesvirus infection
- Diascopy to evaluate blanching of vascular lesions
- Examination under Wood's (UV) light
- Patch tests to evaluate cutaneous sensitivity to specific antigens

---

For a more detailed discussion, see Lawley TJ, Yancey KB: Approach to the Patient with Skin Disorders, Chap. 54, p. 294, in HPIM-14.

8

PAIN OR SWELLING OF JOINTS

Musculoskeletal complaints are extremely common in outpatient medical practice and are among the leading causes of disability and absenteeism from work. Pain in the joints must be evaluated in a uniform, thorough, and logical fashion to ensure the best chance of accurate diagnosis and to plan appropriate follow-up testing and therapy. Joint pain and swelling may be manifestations of disorders affecting primarily the musculoskeletal system or may reflect systemic disease.

Goals for the Initial Assessment of a Musculoskeletal Complaint (See Fig. 8-1)

1. *Articular versus nonarticular.* Is the pain located in a joint or in a periarticular structure such as soft tissue or muscle?
2. *Inflammatory versus noninflammatory.* Inflammatory disease is suggested by local signs of inflammation (erythema, warmth, swelling), systemic features (morning stiffness, fatigue, fever, weight loss), or laboratory evidence of inflammation (thrombocytosis, elevated ESR or C-reactive protein).

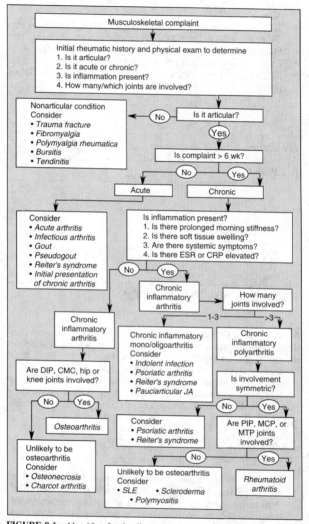

FIGURE 8-1 Algorithm for the diagnosis of musculoskeletal complaints. An approach to formulating a differential diagnosis (shown in italics). (ESR, erythrocyte sedimentation rate; CRP, C-reactive protein; DIP, distal interphalangeal; CMC, carpometacarpal; PIP, proximal interphalangeal; MCP, metacarpophalangeal; MTP, metatarsophalangeal; PMR, polymyalgia rheumatica; SLE, systemic lupus erythematosus; JA, juvenile arthritis.)

3.   *Acute (6 weeks or less) versus chronic.*
4.   *Localized versus systemic.*

Historic Features

*   Age, sex, race, and family history.
*   Duration of symptoms: acute versus chronic.
*   Number and distribution of involved structures: monarticular (one joint), oligoarticular (2–3 joints), polyarticular (>3 joints); symmetry.
*   Other articular features: morning stiffness, effect of movement, features that improve/worsen Sx, migratory pain, Sx intermittent/continuous.
*   Extraarticular Sx: e.g., fever, rash, weight loss, visual change, dyspnea, diarrhea, dysuria, numbness, weakness.
*   Recent events: e.g., trauma, drug administration, travel, other illnesses.

Physical Examination

Complete examination is essential: particular attention to skin, mucous membranes, nails (may reveal characteristic pitting in psoriasis), eyes. Careful and thorough examination of involved and uninvolved joints and periarticular structures; this should proceed in an organized fashion from head to foot or from extremities inward toward axial skeleton; special attention should be paid to identifying the presence or absence of

*   Warmth and/or erythema
*   Swelling
*   Synovial thickening
*   Subluxation, dislocation, joint deformity
*   Joint instability
*   Limitations to active and passive range of motion
*   Crepitus
*   Periarticular changes
*   Muscular changes including weakness, atrophy

Laboratory Investigations

Additional evaluation usually indicated for monarticular, traumatic, inflammatory, or chronic conditions or for conditions accompanied by neurologic changes or systemic manifestations.

*   For all evaluations: include CBC, ESR, or C-reactive protein.
*   Should be performed where there are suggestive clinical features: rheumatoid factor, ANA, ANCA, antistreptolysin O titer, Lyme antibodies.
*   Where systemic disease present or suspected: renal/hepatic function tests, UA.

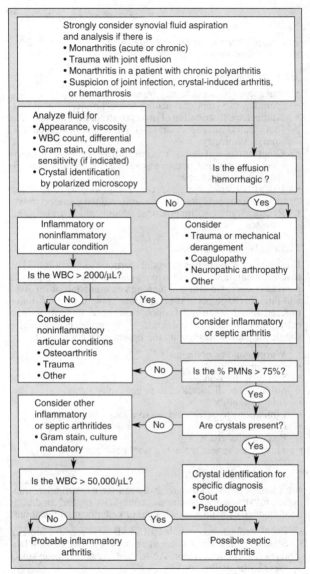

FIGURE 8-2 Algorithmic approach to the use and interpretation of synovial fluid aspiration and analysis.

- Uric acid—useful only when gout diagnosed and therapy contemplated.
- CPK, aldolase—consider with muscle pain, weakness.
- Synovial fluid aspiration and analysis: always indicated for acute monarthritis or when infectious or crystal-induced arthropathy is suspected. Should be examined for (1) appearance, viscosity; (2) cell count and differential (suspect septic joint if WBC count >50,000/μL); (3) crystals using polarizing microscope; (4) Gram's stain, cultures (Fig. 8-2).

Diagnostic Imaging

Plain radiographs should be considered for

- Trauma
- Suspected chronic infection
- Progressive disability
- Monarticular involvement
- Baseline assessment of a chronic process
- When therapeutic alterations are considered

Additional imaging procedures, including ultrasound, radionuclide scintigraphy, CT, and MRI may be helpful in selected clinical settings.

Special Considerations in the Elderly Patient

The evaluation of joint and musculoskeletal disorders in the elderly pt presents a special challenge given the frequently insidious onset and chronicity of disease in this age group, the confounding effect of other medical conditions, and the increased variability of many diagnostic tests in the geriatric population. Although virtually all musculoskeletal conditions may afflict the elderly, certain disorders are especially frequent. Special attention should be paid to identifying the potential rheumatic consequences of intercurrent medical conditions and therapies when evaluating the geriatric pt with musculoskeletal complaints.

For a more detailed discussion, see Cush JJ, Lipsky PE: Approach to Articular and Musculoskeletal Disorders, Chap. 321, p. 1928, in HPIM-14.

9

SYNCOPE AND SEIZURES

Syncope

Loss of consciousness due to hypoperfusion of the entire brain or the brainstem reticular activating system. Prodromal symptoms include light-headedness, weakness, nausea, dimming vision, ringing in ears, or sweating. Occasionally occurs so rapidly that there is no warning. Pt appears pallid and has a faint, rapid, or irregular pulse; spontaneous myoclonic or clonic movements may occur for 5–10 s. Recovery of consciousness is prompt if the pt is horizontal and cerebral perfusion is restored. Usually no persistent symptoms beyond 5 min.

Faintness

The prodromal symptoms that precede the loss of consciousness in syncope (i.e., presyncope).

Seizure

A paroxysmal event due to abnormal, excessive, hypersynchronous discharges from an aggregate of CNS neurons. Clinical manifestations depend on the distribution of discharges and range from loss of consciousness with convulsive activity to experiential phenomena not readily discernible by an observer.

Features Distinguishing Syncope from Seizure

The differential diagnosis is often between syncope and a generalized, convulsive seizure. Syncope is more likely if the event was provoked by acute pain or anxiety or occurred immediately after arising from a lying or sitting position. Seizures are typically not related to posture. Pts with syncope often describe a stereotyped transition from consciousness to unconsciousness that develops over a few seconds. Seizures occur either very abruptly without a transition or are preceded by premonitory symptoms such as an epigastric rising sensation, preception of odd odors, or racing thoughts. Pallor is seen during syncope; cyanosis is usually seen during a seizure. The duration of unconsciousness is usually very brief (i.e., seconds) in syncope and more prolonged (i.e., >5 min) in a seizure. Injury from falling is common in seizure, rare in syncope. Full return to alertness is typically within minutes after syncope and spans many minutes to hours after a seizure. Headache or incontinence may be observed following either a seizure or syncope and are not useful distinguishing features.

Table 9-1

Causes of Syncope and Presyncope

I. Reduced blood flow to the entire central nervous system
  A. Inadequate vasoconstrictor mechanisms
    1. Vasovagal (vasodepressor)
    2. Autonomic insufficiency (e.g., primary, neuropathic, pharmacologic, surgical, Shy-Drager syndrome)
  B. Hypovolemia
    1. Dehydration
    2. Blood loss (e.g., gastrointestinal hemorrhage)
    3. Diuretic overuse
  C. Mechanical reduction of venous return
    1. Valsalva maneuver
    2. Cough
    3. Micturition
  D. Reduced cardiac output
    1. Obstruction of left ventricular outflow (e.g., aortic stenosis, hypertrophic subaortic stenosis, atrial myxoma, ball valve thrombus)
    2. Obstruction of pulmonary flow (e.g., pulmonic stenosis, primary pulmonary hypertension, pulmonary embolism, tetralogy of Fallot)
    3. Myocardial (e.g., pump failure due to myocardial ischemia or infarction)
    4. Pericardial (e.g., cardiac tamponade)
  E. Arrhythmias
    1. Bradyarrhythmias
      a. Sinus bradycardia, sinoatrial block, sinus arrest
      b. Atrioventricular (AV) block (second- and third-degree)
      c. Ventricular asystole
    2. Tachyarrhythmias
      a. Supraventricular tachycardia without AV block
      b. Ventricular tachycardia
    3. Sick-sinus syndrome

(continued)

Table 9-1 (*Continued*)

Causes of Syncope and Presyncope

II. Reduced blood flow or related effects on the brain-
   stem reticular activating system
   A. Transient ischemic attacks (TIA)
      1. Basilar artery embolus
      2. Vertebrobasilar insufficiency
   B. Other
      1. Basilar migraine
      2. Third ventricular cyst
III. Altered state of blood supplied to the brain
   A. Hypoxia
   B. Anemia
   C. Hyperventilation
   D. Hypoglycemia

Etiology of Syncope

Most often due to processes resulting in reduced cerebral blood
flow (see Table 9-1).

For a more detailed discussion, see Daroff RB, Martin JB:
Faintness, Syncope, Dizziness, and Vertigo, Chap. 20, p. 100;
and Lowenstein DH: Seizures and Epilepsy, Chap. 365, p. 2311,
in HPIM-14.

10

DIZZINESS AND VERTIGO

Patients use the term *dizziness* to describe several unusual head sensations or gait unsteadiness. With a careful history, pt's symptoms can be placed into more specific neurologic categories, of which faintness and vertigo are most important.

Definitions

FAINTNESS A symptom of insufficient blood, oxygen or, rarely, glucose supply to the brain. Usually described as light-headedness followed by visual blurring and postural swaying. Occurs with hyperventilation, hypoglycemia, and prior to a syncopal event (Chap. 9). Light-headedness can also occur as an aura before a seizure. Chronic light-headedness is a common somatic complaint in patients with depression.

VERTIGO The illusion of self or environmental movement, most commonly a sensation of spinning. Physiologic vertigo is due to unfamiliar head movement or visual-proprioceptive-vestibular mismatch, i.e., seasickness, height vertigo, visual vertigo. True vertigo almost never occurs in the presyncopal state.

PATHOLOGIC VERTIGO Caused by abnormalities of visual, somatosensory, or vestibular inputs, most commonly the latter. Frequently accompanied by nausea, postural unsteadiness, and gait ataxia, vertigo is provoked or worsened by head movement. May be caused by peripheral (labyrinth or eighth nerve) or CNS lesion. The distinction is prognostically important.

Peripheral Vertigo

Usually severe, accompanied by nausea and emesis. Tinnitus, a feeling of ear fullness, or hearing loss may occur. Pt may be pale and diaphoretic. A characteristic jerk nystagmus is almost always present. The nystagmus does not change direction with a change in direction of gaze, it is horizontal with a torsional component, and has its fast phase to side of normal ear. It is inhibited by visual fixation. Pt senses spinning motion in direction of slow phase and falls or mispoints to that side. Usually no other neurologic abnormalities.

ETIOLOGY Peripheral vertigo is common and usually episodic because central compensatory mechanisms ultimately diminish it. An attack of acute peripheral vestibulopathy may be followed by multiple recurrent episodes. Common causes of peripheral vertigo include recent head trauma, labyrinthine infection, toxins, Ménière's disease (recurrent vertigo accompanied by tinnitus and deafness), and acoustic neuroma. The latter may also cause hearing loss, facial weakness, and facial sensory loss due to involvement of cranial nerves V and VII. Drug toxicity (streptomycin, gentamicin, neomycin) can cause peripheral vestibulopathy. Psychogenic vertigo should be suspected in pts with chronic incapacitating vertigo who also have agoraphobia, a normal neurologic exam, and no nystagmus.

Central Vertigo

Identified by associated abnormal brainstem or cerebellar signs such as dysarthria, diplopia, paresthesia, headache, weakness, limb ataxia. The nystagmus can take almost any form, i.e., vertical or multidirectional, but is often purely horizontal without a torsional component. Central nystagmus is not inhibited by fixation. Central vertigo may be chronic or mild and is less likely to be accompanied by tinnitus or hearing loss. It is usually a sign of brainstem dysfunction and may be due to demyelinating, vascular, or neoplastic disease. Rarely, it occurs as a manifestation of temporal lobe epilepsy.

Evaluation

The "dizzy" pt usually requires provocative tests to reproduce the symptoms. Valsalva maneuver, hyperventilation, or postural changes may reproduce faintness. Rapid rotation of pt in a swivel chair may reproduce vertigo. Benign positional vertigo is identified by positioning the turned head of a recumbent pt in extension over the edge of the bed to elicit vertigo and a characteristic type of nystagmus. If pt does not exhibit signs of peripheral vertigo or has other neurologic abnormalities, then prompt evaluation for central pathology is indicated, i.e., CT or MRI scan of the posterior fossa, electronystagmography, evoked potential tests, or vertebrobasilar angiography.

℞ TREATMENT

For acute vertigo, bed rest and vestibular suppressant drugs such as antihistamines (meclizine, dimenhydrinate, promethazine), anticholinergics (scopolamine), or hypnotics. Ménière's may respond to a low-salt diet with a diuretic. A mild vestibular exercise program is prescribed for pts with a prolonged episode of peripheral vertigo to induce central compensatory mechanisms. Pts with central vertigo should be carefully evaluated for potentially life-threatening brainstem lesions.

For a more detailed discussion, see Daroff RB, Martin JB: Faintness, Syncope, Dizziness, and Vertigo, Chap. 20, p. 100, in HPIM-14.

11

VISUAL LOSS AND DISORDERS OF OCULAR MOTILITY

Clinical Assessment

Accurate measurement of visual acuity in each eye (with glasses) is of primary importance. Additional assessments include testing of pupils, eye movements, ocular alignment, and visual fields. Slit-lamp examination can exclude corneal infection, trauma, glaucoma, uveitis, and cataract. Ophthalmoscopic exam to inspect the optic disc and retina often requires pupillary dilation using 1% topicamide and 2.5% phenylephrine; the risk of provoking an attack of narrow-angle glaucoma is remote.

Visual field mapping by finger confrontation permits localization of lesions in the visual pathway (Fig. 11-1); formal testing using a perimeter may be necessary. The goal is to determine whether the lesion is anterior, at, or posterior to the optic chiasm. A scotoma confined to one eye is caused by an anterior lesion affecting the optic nerve or globe; the *swinging flashlight test may reveal an afferent pupil defect*. History and ocular exam are usually sufficient for diagnosis. If a bitemporal hemianopia is present, the lesion is located at the optic chiasm (e.g., pituitary adenoma, meningioma). Homonymous visual field loss signals a retrochiasmal lesion, affecting either the optic tract, lateral geniculate body, optic radiations, or visual cortex (e.g., stroke, tumor, abscess). Neuroimaging is recommended for any pt with a bitemporal or homonymous hemianopia.

Transient or Sudden Visual Loss

Amaurosis fugax or *transient monocular blindness* usually occurs from a retinal embolus or severe ipsilateral carotid stenosis.

OPTIC NERVE OR RETINA

Central scotoma (Optic neuritis; macular degeneration)

Arcuate scotoma (AION, glaucoma, branch retinal artery or vein occlusion)

Altitudinal field defect (AION; retinal artery branch occlusion)

Centrocecal scotoma (Optic neuritis; toxic, nutritional, or hereditary optic neuropathy)

Generalized constriction (Papilledema, retinitis pigmentosa)

OPTIC CHIASM

Bitemporal hemianopia (Optic chiasm compression by pituitary tumor, meningioma)

RETRO-CHIASMAL PATHWAY

Homonymous hemianopia (Lesion of optic tract, lateral geniculate body, optic radiations, or visual cortex)

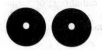

Homonymous quadrantopia ("Pie in the Sky") (Lesion of optic radiations in temporal lobe)

Macular sparing (Bilateral visual cortex lesions)

FIGURE 11-1 Deficits in visual fields caused by lesions affecting visual pathways.

Prolonged occlusion of the central retinal artery results in the classic fundus appearance of a milky, infarcted retina with a cherry-red fovea. Any pt with compromise of the retinal circulation should be evaluated promptly for stroke factors (e.g., carotid atheromata, heart disease, atrial fibrillation). *Vertebrobasilar insufficiency* or emboli can be confused with amaurosis fugax, because many pts mistakenly ascribe symptoms to their left or right eye, when in fact they are occurring in the left or right hemifield of both eyes. Interruption of blood flow to the visual cortex causes sudden graying of vision, occasionally with flashing lights or other symptoms that mimic *migraine.* The history may be the only guide to the correct diagnosis. Pts should be questioned about the precise pattern and duration of visual loss and about other neurologic symptoms such as diplopia, vertigo, numbness, or weakness, which may help decide between compromise of the anterior or posterior cerebral circulation.

Malignant hypertension can cause visual loss from exudates, hemorrhages, cotton wool spots (focal nerve fiber layer infarcts), and optic disc edema. In *central* or *branch retinal vein occlusion,* the fundus exam reveals engorged, dusky veins with extensive retinal bleeding. In *age-related macular degeneration,* characterized by extensive drusen and scarring of the pigment epithelium, leakage of blood or fluid from subretinal neovascular membranes can produce sudden central visual loss. Flashing lights and floaters may indicate a fresh *vitreous detachment.* Separation of the vitreous from the retina is a frequent involutional event in the elderly. It is not harmful unless it creates sufficient traction to produce a *retinal detachment. Vitreous hemorrhage* may occur in diabetic patients from retinal neovascularization.

Papilledema refers to bilateral optic disc edema from raised intracranial pressure. Transient visual obscurations are common, but visual acuity is not affected unless the papilledema is severe, long-standing, or accompanied by macular exudates or hemorrhage. Neuroimaging should be obtained to exclude an intracranial mass. If negative, a lumbar puncture is required to confirm elevation of the intracranial pressure. *Optic neuritis* is a common cause of monocular optic disc swelling and visual loss, although it rarely affects both eyes. If the site of inflammation is retrobulbar, the fundus will appear normal on initial exam. The typical pt is female, aged 15–45, with pain provoked by eye movements. Glucocorticoids, consisting of intravenous methylprednisolone followed by oral prednisone (see Table 178-3), may hasten recovery in severely affected pts. *Anterior ischemic optic neuropathy* (AION) is an infarction of the optic nervehead due to inadequate perfusion via the posterior ciliary arteries. Pts have sudden visual loss, often upon awakening, and painless swelling of the optic disc. It is important to differentiate between nonarteritic (idiopathic) AION and arteritic AION. The latter is caused by temporal arteritis and requires immediate steroid therapy. A sedimentation rate should be checked in any elderly pt with acute optic disc swelling or symptoms suggestive of polymyalgia rheumatica.

Diplopia

If the pt has diplopia while being examined, motility testing will usually reveal a deficiency in ocular excursions. However, if the degree of angular separation between the double images is small, the limitation of eye movements may be subtle and difficult to detect. In this situation, the cover test is useful. While the pt is fixating upon a distant target, one eye is covered while observing the other eye for a movement of redress as it takes up fixation. If none is seen, the procedure is repeated upon the fellow eye. In pts with genuine diplopia, this test should reveal ocular malalignment, especially if the pt's head is turned or tilted in the position that gives rise to the worst symptoms.

The most frequent causes of diplopia are summarized in Table 11-1. The physical findings in isolated ocular motor nerve palsies are:

- CN III: Ptosis and deviation of the eye down and outwards, causing vertical and horizontal diplopia. Pupil dilation suggests direct compression of the third nerve; if present, the possibility of an aneurysm of the posterior communicating artery must be considered urgently.
- CN IV: Vertical diplopia with cyclotorsion; the affected eye is slightly elevated, and limitation of depression is seen when the eye is held in adduction. The pt may assume a head tilt to the opposite side (e.g., left head tilt in right fourth nerve paresis).
- CN VI: Horizontal diplopia with crossed eyes; the affected eye cannot abduct.

Isolated ocular motor nerve palsies often occur in pts with hypertension or diabetes. They usually resolve spontaneously over several months. The apparent occurrence of multiple ocular motor nerve palsies, or diffuse ophthalmoplegia, raises the possibility of myasthenia gravis. In this disease, the pupils are always normal. Systemic weakness may be absent. Diplopia that cannot be explained by a single ocular motor nerve palsy may also be caused by carcinomatous or fungal meningitis, Graves' disease, Guillain-Barré syndrome, Fisher's syndrome, or Tolosa-Hunt syndrome.

Table 11-1

Common Causes of Diplopia

Brainstem stroke (skew deviation, nuclear or fascicular palsy)

Microvascular infarction (III, IV, VI nerve palsy)

Tumor (brainstem, cavernous sinus, superior orbital fissure, orbit)

Multiple sclerosis (internuclear ophthalmoplegia, ocular motor nerve palsy)

Aneurysm (III nerve)

Raised intracranial pressure (VI nerve)

Postviral inflammation

Meningitis (bacterial, fungal, granulomatosis, neoplastic)

Carotid-cavernous fistula or thrombosis

Herpes zoster

Tolosa-Hunt syndrome

Wernicke-Korsakoff syndrome

Botulism

Myasthenia gravis

Guillain-Barré or Fisher syndrome

Graves' disease

Orbital pseudotumor

Orbital myositis

Trauma

Orbital cellulitis

For a more detailed discussion, see Horton JC: Disorders of the Eye, Chap. 28, p. 159, in HPIM-14.

12

PARALYSIS AND MOVEMENT DISORDERS

PARALYSIS OR WEAKNESS

GENERAL CONSIDERATIONS   The loss of power or control of voluntary muscle is usually described by pts as "weakness" or as some difficulty that can be interpreted as "loss of dexterity." The diagnostic approach to such a problem begins first and most importantly in determining which part of the nervous system is involved. It is important to distinguish weakness arising from disorders of upper motor neurons (i.e., motor neurons in the cerebral cortex and their axons that descend through the subcortical white matter, the internal capsule, the brainstem, and down the spinal cord) from that arising from disorders of the motor unit. (i.e., the lower motor neurons in the ventral horn of the spinal cord and their axons in the spinal roots and peripheral nerves, the neuromuscular junction, and the skeletal muscle). In general:

- *Upper motor neuron dysfunction:* increased muscle tone (spasticity), brisk deep tendon reflexes, and Babinski's sign.
- *Lower motor neuron dysfunction:* reduced muscle tone, diminished reflexes, and muscle atrophy.

Table 12-1 presents patterns of weakness and signs associated with weakness arising from lesions of different parts of the nervous system. Table 12-2 lists common causes of weakness by the primary site of pathology.

EVALUATION   The history should focus on the tempo of development of weakness, the presence of sensory and other neurologic symptoms, medication history, predisposing medical conditions, and family history. The physical exam should primarily focus on the localization of the abnormality by criteria such as described above and in Table 12-1.

For disorders of the brain or spinal cord, radiologic investigation with MRI, CT, or myelography is essential to distinguish various causes, especially structural and demyelinative lesions; LP may be diagnostic for demyelinating and infectious processes, serum and urine studies for nutritional and toxic causes; biopsy of mass lesions is often necessary for diagnosis and to differentiate neoplastic from infectious causes.

For disorders of the motor unit, an EMG and nerve conduction studies are critical to discrimination between abnormalities of different components of the motor unit. MRI or myelography are important for structural causes of nerve root disorders; serum

Table 12-1

Clinical Differentiation of Weakness Arising from Different Areas of the Nervous System

Location of Lesion	Pattern of Weakness	Associated Signs
UPPER MOTOR NEURON		
Cerebral cortex	Hemiparesis (face and arm predominantly, or leg predominantly)	Hemisensory loss, seizures, homonymous hemianopia or quadrantopia, aphasia, apraxias, gaze preference
Internal capsule	Hemiparesis (face, arm, leg may be equally affected)	Hemisensory deficit; homonymous hemianopia or quadrantopia
Brainstem	Hemiparesis (arm and leg; face may not be involved at all)	Vertigo, nausea and vomiting, ataxia and dysarthria, eye movement abnormalities, cranial nerve dysfunction, altered level of consciousness, Horner's syndrome
Spinal cord	Quadriparesis if midcervical or above; Paraparesis if low cervical or thoracic	Sensory level; bowel and bladder dysfunction
	Hemiparesis below level of lesion (Brown-Séquard)	Contralateral sensory loss below level of lesion
MOTOR UNIT		
Spinal motor neuron	Diffuse weakness, may involve control of speech and swallowing	Muscle fasciculations and atrophy; no sensory loss
Spinal root	Radicular pattern of weakness	Dermatomal sensory loss; radicular pain common with compressive lesions

(continued)

Table 12-1 (*Continued*)

Clinical Differentiation of Weakness Arising from Different Areas of the Nervous System

Location of Lesion	Pattern of Weakness	Associated Signs
Peripheral nerve		
Polyneuropathy	Distal weakness, usually feet more than hands; usually symmetric	Distal sensory loss, usually feet more than hands
Mononeuropathy	Weakness in distribution of single nerve	Sensory loss in distribution of single nerve
Neuromuscular junction	Fatigable weakness, usually with ocular involvement producing diplopia and ptosis	No sensory loss; no reflex changes
Muscle	Proximal weakness	No sensory loss; diminished reflexes only when severe; may have muscle tenderness

and urine studies for systemic diseases may be complemented by CSF examination; serum CPK is a very useful indicator of muscle diseases; nerve biopsy is rarely useful, but muscle biopsy is diagnostic for many muscle diseases.

MOVEMENT DISORDERS

Movement disorders are often divided into akinetic rigid forms, in which there is muscle rigidity and slowness of movement, and hyperkinetic forms, in which there are involuntary movements. In either case, *preservation of strength* is the rule.

Most movement disorders arise from dysfunction of the circuitry in the basal ganglia and can occur by virtually any pathogenetic mechanism. Most commonly, the causes are degenerative diseases (hereditary and "idiopathic"), drug-induced, organ system failure, CNS infection, and ischemia of the basal ganglia. Below are brief synopses of the clinical aspects of major categories of movement disorders.

Table 12-2

Common Causes of Weakness

UPPER MOTOR NEURON

Cortex: ischemia; hemorrhage; intrinsic mass lesion (primary or metastatic cancer, abscess); extrinsic mass lesion (subdural hematoma); degenerative (amyotrophic lateral sclerosis)

Subcortical white matter/internal capsule: ischemia; hemorrhage; intrinsic mass lesion (primary or metastatic cancer, abscess); immunologic (multiple sclerosis); infectious (progressive multifocal leukoencephalopathy)

Brainstem: ischemia; immunologic (multiple sclerosis)

Spinal cord: extrinsic compression (cervical spondylosis, metastatic cancer, epidural abscess); immunologic (multiple sclerosis, transverse myelitis); infectious (AIDS-associated myelopathy, HTLV-1–associated myelopathy, tabes dorsalis); nutritional deficiency (subacute combined degeneration)

MOTOR UNIT

Spinal motor neuron: degenerative (amyotrophic lateral sclerosis); infectious (poliomyelitis)

Spinal root: compressive (degenerative disc disease); immunologic (Guillain-Barré syndrome); infectious (AIDS-associated polyradiculopathy, Lyme disease)

Peripheral nerve: metabolic (diabetes mellitus, uremia, porphyria); toxic (ethanol, heavy metals,*many* drugs, diphtheria); nutritional (B_{12} deficiency); inflammatory (polyarteritis nodosa); hereditary (Charcot-Marie-Tooth); immunologic (paraneoplastic, paraproteinemia); infectious (AIDS-associated polyneuropathies and mononeuritis multiplex); compressive (entrapment)

Neuromuscular junction: immunologic (myasthenia gravis); toxic (botulism, aminoglycosides)

Muscle: inflammatory (polymyositis, inclusion body myositis); degenerative (muscular dystrophy); toxic (glucocorticoids, ethanol, AZT); infectious (trichinosis); metabolic (hypothyroid, periodic paralyses); congenital (central core disease)

BRADYKINESIA Inability to initiate changes in activity or perform ordinary volitional movements rapidly and easily. There are slowness of movement and paucity of automatic motions such as arm swinging while walking and eye blinking. Usually indicative of Parkinson's disease.

TREMOR Rhythmic oscillation of a part of the body about a fixed point, usually involving the distal limbs and less commonly the head, tongue, and jaw. May be divided according to relationship to posture and amplitude. Most common—a coarse tremor at rest, 4–5 beats/s, usually indicative of Parkinson's disease; a fine postural tremor of 8–10 beats/s, which may be an exaggeration of normal physiologic tremor or indicative of familial essential tremor. The latter often responds to propranolol or primidone.

ASTERIXIS Brief, arrhythmic interruptions of sustained voluntary muscle contraction, usually observed as a brief lapse of posture of wrists in dorsiflexion with arms outstretched. This "liver flap" may be seen in any diffuse encephalopathy related to drug intoxication, organ system failure, or CNS infection. Only therapy is correction of underlying disorder.

MYOCLONUS Brief, arrhythmic muscle contractions, or twitches. Like asterixis, usually indicative of a diffuse encephalopathy; sometimes seen after cardiac arrest when diffuse cerebral hypoxia may lead to multifocal myoclonus. Clonazepam, valproate, or baclofen have been effective therapies.

DYSTONIA Involuntary, sustained posture or slowly changing involuntary postures. Postures attained are often bizarre with forceful extensions and twisting about individual joints. Dystonias may be generalized or focal (e.g., spasmodic torticollis, blepharospasm). Symptomatic benefit has been achieved with high doses of anticholinergics, benzodiazepines, baclofen, and anticonvulsants. Local injection of botulinum toxin is effective in certain focal dystonias.

CHOREOATHETOSIS A combination of *chorea* (rapid, jerky movements) and *athetosis* (slow writhing movements). The two usually exist together though one may be more prominent. Choreic movements are the predominant involuntary movements in rheumatic (Sydenham's) chorea and Huntington's disease. Athetosis is prominent in some forms of cerebral palsy. Chronic neuroleptic use may lead to tardive dyskinesia, in which choreoathetotic movements are usually restricted to the buccal, lingual, and mandibular areas. While often ineffective, treatments to suppress choreoathetotic movements include benzodiazepines, reserpine, and low-dose neuroleptics.

TICS Stereotypical, purposeless movements such as eye blinks, sniffling, and clearing of the throat. Gilles de la Tourette syndrome is a rare but severe multiple tic disorder that may involve motor tics (especially twitches of the face, neck, and shoulders), vocal tics (grunts, words), and "behavioral tics" (coprolalia, echolalia). The cause is unknown. Treatment with haloperidol usually reduces the frequency and severity of the tics.

For a more detailed discussion, see Olney RK, Aminoff MJ: Weakness, Abnormal Movements, and Imbalance, Chap. 21, p. 107, in HPIM-14.

13

ALTERATIONS IN CONSCIOUSNESS (CONFUSION, STUPOR, AND COMA)

Disorders of consciousness are common in medical practice. Assessment of consciousness abnormalities should determine whether there is a change in *level* of consciousness (drowsy, stuporous, comatose) and/or *content* of consciousness (confusion, perseveration, hallucinations). *Confusion* is a lack of clarity in thinking with inattentiveness; *stupor*, a state in which vigorous stimuli are needed to elicit a response; *coma*, a condition of unresponsiveness. Pts in such states are usually seriously ill, and etiologic factors must be assessed.

_____ *Approach to the Patient* _____

1. Support the pt's vital functions.
2. Administer glucose, thiamine, and naloxone if etiology is not clear.
3. Utilize history, examination, and laboratory and radiologic information to establish the cause of the disorder rapidly.
4. Provide the appropriate medical and surgical treatment.

History

Pt should be aroused, if possible, and questioned regarding use of insulin, narcotics, anticoagulants, other prescription drugs, suicidal intent, recent trauma, headache, epilepsy, significant medical problems, and preceding symptoms. Witnesses and family members should be interrogated, often by phone. History of sudden headache followed by loss of consciousness suggests intracranial hemorrhage; preceding vertigo, nausea, diplopia, ataxia, hemisensory disorder suggest basilar insufficiency; chest pain, palpitations, and faintness suggest cardiovascular cause.

Immediate Assessment

Vital signs should be evaluated, and appropriate support initiated. Blood should be drawn for glucose, Na, K, Ca, BUN, ammonia, alcohol, liver transaminase levels; also screen for presence of toxins. Fever, especially with petechial rash, should suggest meningitis. Fever with dry skin suggests heat shock or intoxication with anticholinergics. Hypothermia suggests myxedema, intoxication, sepsis, exposure, or hypoglycemia. Marked hypertension occurs with increased intracranial pressure and hypertensive encephalopathy.

Neurologic Evaluation

Focus on establishing pt's best level of function and uncovering signs that enable a specific diagnosis. Although confused states may occur with unilateral cerebral lesions, stupor and coma are signs of bihemispheral dysfunction or damage to midbrain-tegmentum (reticular activating system).

RESPONSIVENESS Stimuli of increasing intensity are applied to body parts to gauge the degree of unresponsiveness and any asymmetry in sensory or motor function. Motor responses may be purposeful or reflexive. Spontaneous flexion of elbows with leg extension, termed *decortication*, accompanies severe damage to contralateral hemisphere above midbrain. Interval rotation of the arms with extension of elbows, wrists, and legs, termed *decerebration*, suggests damage to diencephalon or midbrain. Postural reflexes can occur in profound encephalopathic states.

PUPILS In pts with coma, equal, round, reactive pupils exclude midbrain damage as cause and suggest a metabolic abnormality. Pinpoint pupils occur in narcotic overdose (except meperidine, which causes midsize pupils). Small pupils also occur with hydrocephalus and thalamic or pontine damage. A unilateral, enlarged, often oval, poorly reactive pupil is caused by midbrain lesions or compression of third cranial nerve, as occurs in transtentorial herniation. Bilaterally dilated, unreactive pupils indicate severe bilateral midbrain damage, anticholinergic overdose, or ocular trauma.

EYE MOVEMENT Spontaneous and reflex eye movements should be examined for limitations of ocular movement, involuntary movements, and misalignment of ocular axes. Intermittent horizontal divergence is common in drowsiness. Slow, to-and-fro horizontal movements suggest bihemispheric dysfunction. An *adducted* eye at rest with impaired ability to turn eye laterally indicates an abducens (VI) nerve palsy, common in raised intracranial pressure or pontine damage. The eye with a dilated, unreactive pupil often is *abducted* at rest and cannot adduct fully due to third nerve dysfunction, as occurs with transtentorial herniation. Vertical separation of ocular axes, *skew deviation*, occurs in pontine or cerebellar lesions. *Doll's head maneuver* and *cold caloric*–induced eye movements allow accurate diagnosis of gaze or cranial nerve palsies in pts who do not move their eyes purposefully. Oculocephalic reflex is tested by observing eye movements in response to lateral rotation of head (significant neck injury is a contraindication). Loose movement of eyes with the doll's head maneuver occurs in bihemispheric dysfunction. In comatose pts with an intact brainstem, raising head to 60° above the horizontal and irrigating external auditory canal with ice water causes tonic deviation of gaze to irrigated ear. In conscious pts, it causes nystagmus, vertigo, and emesis.

RESPIRATION Respiratory pattern may suggest site of neurologic damage. Cheyne-Stokes (periodic) breathing occurs in bihemispheric dysfunction and is common in metabolic encephaopathies. Respiratory patterns composed of gasps or apneustic breathing are indicative of lower brainstem damage; such pts usually require intubation and ventilatory assistance.

OTHER Comatose pt's best motor and sensory function should be assessed by testing reflex responses to noxious stimuli; carefully note any asymmetric responses, which suggest a focal lesion. If possible, pt with disordered consciousness should have gait examined. Ataxia may be the prominent neurologic finding in a stuporous pt with a cerebellar mass.

Radiologic Examination

Lesions causing raised intracranial pressure commonly cause impaired consciousness. CT or MRI scans of the brain are often abnormal in coma but are not usually diagnostic in pts with metabolic encephalopathy, meningitis, early infarction, early encephalitis, diffuse anoxic injury, or drug overdose. Postponing appropriate therapy in these pts while awaiting a CT or MRI scan may be deleterious. Pts with disordered consciousness due to high intracranial pressure can deteriorate rapidly; emergent CT study is necessary to confirm presence of mass effect and to guide surgical decompression. CT scan is normal in some pts with subarachnoid hemorrhage; the diagnosis then rests on clinical history combined with RBC in spinal fluid. Cerebral angiography or magnetic resonance angiography is frequently necessary to establish basilar artery insufficiency as cause of coma in pts with brainstem signs.

Brain Death

This results from total cessation of cerebral function and blood flow at a time when cardiopulmonary function continues but is dependent on ventilatory assistance. EEG is isoelectric at high gain, pt is unresponsive, brainstem reflexes are absent, drug toxicity and hypothermia are excluded. Diagnosis should be made only if the state persists for some agreed upon period, 6–24 h. Demonstration of apnea requires that the P_{CO_2} be high enough to stimulate respiration, while P_{O_2} and bp are maintained.

For a more detailed discussion, see Ropper AH, Martin JB: Acute Confusional States and Coma, Chap. 24, p. 125, HPIM-14.

14

DYSPNEA

Definition

An abnormally uncomfortable awareness of breathing; intensity can be quantified by establishing the amount of physical exertion necessary to produce the sensation.

Causes

HEART DISEASE   Dyspnea is due to ↑ pulmonary capillary pressure, left atrial hypertension, and sometimes fatigue of respiratory muscles. Vital capacity and lung compliance are ↓ and airway resistance ↑. Begins as exertional breathlessness → orthopnea → paroxysmal nocturnal dyspnea and dyspnea at rest. Diagnosis depends on recognition of heart disease, e.g., Hx of MI, presence of S_3, S_4, murmurs, cardiomegaly, jugular vein distention, hepatomegaly, and peripheral edema (see Chap. 108).

OBSTRUCTIVE DISEASE OF THE AIRWAYS   May occur with obstruction anywhere from extrathoracic airways to lung periphery. Acute dyspnea with difficulty *inhaling* suggests *upper* airway obstruction. Physical exam may reveal inspiratory stridor and retraction of supraclavicular fossae. Acute intermittent dyspnea with expiratory wheezing suggests reversible intrathoracic obstruction due to asthma. Chronic, slowly progressive exertional dyspnea characterizes emphysema and CHF. Chronic cough with expectoration is typical of chronic bronchitis and bronchiectasis.

DIFFUSE PARENCHYMAL LUNG DISEASES   Many parenchymal lung diseases, ranging from sarcoidosis to the pneumoconioses, may cause dyspnea. Dyspnea is usually related to exertion early in the course of the illness. Physical exam typically reveals late tachypnea and inspiratory rales.

PULMONARY EMBOLISM   (See Chap. 123) Repeated discrete episodes of dyspnea may occur with recurrent pulmonary emboli, but others describe slowly progressive dyspnea without abrupt worsening; tachypnea is frequent. Finding of deep venous thrombosis often absent in chronic pulmonary embolism

DISEASE OF THE CHEST WALL OR RESPIRATORY MUSCLES   Severe kyphoscoliosis may produce chronic dyspnea, often with chronic cor pulmonale. The spinal deformity must be severe before respiratory function is compromised. Pts with bilateral diaphragmatic paralysis appear normal while standing, but complain of severe orthopnea and display paradoxical abnormal respiratory movement when supine.

_____ *Approach to the Patient* _____

Elicit a description of the amount of physical exertion necessary to produce the sensation and whether it varies under different conditions.

- If acute upper airway obstruction is suspected, lateral neck films or a fiberoptic exam of upper airway may be helpful. Pt should be accompanied by a physician adept in all aspects of airway management during the evaluation. With chronic upper airway obstruction the respiratory flow-volume curve may show inspiratory cutoff of flow, suggesting variable extrathoracic obstruction.
- Dyspnea due to emphysema is reflected in a reduction in expiratory flow rates (FEV_1).
- Pts with intermittent dyspnea due to asthma may have normal pulmonary function if tested when asymptomatic.
- Cardiac dyspnea usually begins as breathlessness on strenuous exertion with gradual (months-to-years) progression to dyspnea at rest.
- Pts with dyspnea due to both cardiac and pulmonary diseases may report orthopnea. Paroxysmal nocturnal dyspnea occurring after awakening from sleep is characteristic of CHF.
- Dyspnea of chronic obstructive lung disease tends to develop more gradually than that of heart disease.
- PFTs should be performed when etiology is not clear. When the diagnosis remains obscure a pulmonary stress test is often useful.
- Management depends on elucidating etiology.

_____

Differentiation between cardiac and pulmonary dyspnea is summarized in Table 14-1.

Table 14-1

Differentiation between Cardiac and Pulmonary Dyspnea

1. *Careful history:* Dyspnea of lung disease usually more gradual in onset than that of heart disease; nocturnal exacerbations common with each.
2. *Examination:* Usually obvious evidence of cardiac or pulmonary disease. Findings may be absent at rest when symptoms are present only with exertion.
3. *Pulmonary function tests:* Pulmonary disease rarely causes dyspnea unless tests of obstructive disease (FEV_1, FEV_1/FVC) or restrictive disease (total lung capacity) are reduced (<80% predicted).
4. *Ventricular performance:* LV ejection fraction at rest and/or during exercise usually depressed in cardiac dyspnea.

For a more detailed discussion, see Ingram RH Jr, Braunwald E: Dyspnea and Pulmonary Edema, Chap. 32, p. 190, in HPIM-14.

15

COUGH AND HEMOPTYSIS

COUGH

Produced by inflammatory, mechanical, chemical, and thermal stimulation of cough receptors.

ETIOLOGY

Inflammatory   Edema and hyperemia of airways and alveoli due to laryngitis, tracheitis, bronchitis, bronchiolitis, pneumonitis, lung abscess.

Mechanical   Inhalation of particulates (dust) or compression of airways (pulmonary neoplasms, foreign bodies, granulomas, bronchospasm).

Chemical Inhalation of irritant fumes, including cigarette smoke.

Thermal Inhalation of cold or very hot air.

———————— *Approach to the Patient* ————————

Diagnosis (Fig. 15-1) *History* should consider: (1) duration—acute or chronic; (2) presence of fever or wheezing; (3) sputum quantity and character; (4) temporal or seasonal pattern; (5) risk factors for underlying disease; and (6) past medical history. Short duration with associated fever suggests acute viral or bacterial infection. Persistent cough after viral illness suggests postinflammatory cough. Postnasal drip is a common cause of chronic cough. Nocturnal cough may indicate chronic sinus drainage or esophageal reflux. Change in sputum character, color, or volume in a smoker with "smoker's cough" necessitates investigation. Seasonal cough may indicate "cough asthma." Environmental exposures may suggest occupational asthma or interstitial lung disease. Past history of recurrent pneumonias may indicate bronchiectasis, particularly if associated with purulent or copious sputum production. A change in the character of chronic cigarette cough raises suspicion of bronchogenic carcinoma.

Physical exam should assess upper and lower airways and lung parenchyma. Stridor suggests upper airway obstruction; wheezing suggests bronchospasm as the cause of cough. Midinspiratory crackles indicate airways disease (e.g., chronic bronchitis); fine end-inspiratory crackles occur in interstitial fibrosis and heart failure. *CXR* may show neoplasm, infection, interstitial disease or the hilar adenopathy of sarcoidosis. PFTs may reveal obstruction or restriction. *Sputum exam* can indicate malignancy or infection.

—————————————————————————————

COMPLICATIONS   (1) Syncope, due to transient decrease in venous return; (2) rupture of an emphysematous bleb with pneumothorax; (3) rib fractures—may occur in otherwise normal individuals.

℞ **TREATMENT**
When possible, therapy of cough is that of underlying disease. If no cause can be found, an irritative nonproductive cough may be suppressed with a narcotic antitussive agent such as codeine, 15–30 mg up to qid, or a nonnarcotic such as dextromethorphan (15 mg qid). Cough productive of significant volumes of sputum should generally not be suppressed. Sputum clearance can be facilitated with adequate hydration,

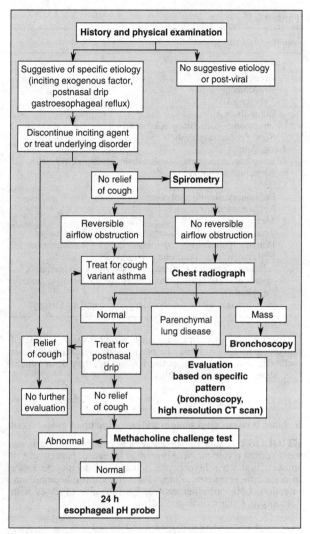

FIGURE 15-1 An algorithm for the evaluation of chronic cough.

Table 15-1

Causes of Hemoptysis

> Inflammatory
>   Bronchitis
>   Bronchiectasis
>   Tuberculosis
>   Lung abscess
>   Pneumonia, particularly *Klebsiella*
>   Septic pulmonary embolism
> Neoplastic
>   Lung cancer: squamous cell, adenocarcinoma, oat cell
>   Bronchial adenoma
> Other
>   Pulmonary thromboembolism
>   Left ventricular failure
>   Mitral stenosis
>   Traumatic, including foreign body and lung contusion
>   Primary pulmonary hypertension; AV malformation;
>   Eisenmenger's syndrome; pulmonary vasculitis, in-
>   cluding Wegener's granulomatosis and Goodpasture's
>   syndrome; idiopathic pulmonary hemosiderosis; and
>   amyloid
>   Hemorrhagic diathesis, including anticoagulant therapy

expectorants, and ultrasonic mist humidification. Iodinated glycerol (30 mg qid) may be particularly useful in asthma or chronic bronchitis. Guaifensin, 100 mg tid, may be of benefit in acute or chronic bronchitis.

HEMOPTYSIS

Includes both streaked sputum and coughing up of gross blood.

ETIOLOGY (Table 15-1) Bronchitis and bronchiectasis are most common causes. Neoplasm may be cause, particularly in smokers and when hemoptysis is persistent. Hemoptysis rare in metastatic neoplasm to lung. Pulmonary thromboembolism, infection, CHF are other causes. Five to 15% of cases with hemoptysis remain undiagnosed.

_____ *Approach to the Patient* _____

Diagnosis (Fig. 15-2) Essential to determine that blood is coming from respiratory tract. Often frothy, may be preceded

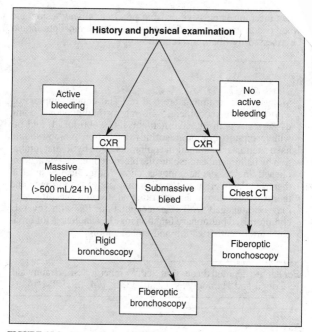

FIGURE 15-2 Diagnostic approach to hemoptysis.

by a desire to cough. History may suggest diagnosis: chronic hemoptysis in otherwise asymptomatic young woman suggests bronchial adenoma; recurrent hemoptysis in pts with chronic copious sputum production suggests bronchiectasis; hemoptysis, weight loss, and anorexia in a smoker suggest carcinoma; hemoptysis with acute pleuritic pain suggests infarction.

Physical exam may also suggest diagnosis: pleural friction rub raises possibility of pulmonary embolism or some other pleural-based lesion (lung abscess, coccidioidomycosis cavity, vasculitis); diastolic rumble suggests mitral stenosis; localized wheeze suggests bronchogenic carcinoma. Initial evaluation includes CXR. A normal CXR does not exclude tumor or bronchiectasis as a source of bleeding. The CXR may show an air-fluid level suggesting an abscess or atelectasis distal to an obstructing carcinoma.

Most pts should then have chest CT scan followed by bronchoscopy. While rigid bronchoscopy is particularly helpful when bleeding is massive or from proximal airway lesion and when endotracheal intubation is contemplated, most pts should be assessed by fiberoptic bronchoscopy.

℞ TREATMENT

Mainstays of treatment are bed rest and cough suppression with an opiate (codeine, 15–30 mg, or hydrocodone, 5 mg q4–6h). Pts with massive hemoptysis (>600 mL/d) and pts with respiratory compromise due to aspiration of blood should have suction and intubation equipment close by so that intubation by balloon tube to isolate the bleeding lung can be accomplished. In massive hemoptysis, choice of medical or surgical therapy relates often to the anatomic site of hemorrhage and the pt's baseline pulmonary function. Central bleeding sites may be managed with laser coagulation. Pts with severely compromised pulmonary function may be candidates for bronchial artery catherization and embolization.

For a more detailed discussion, see Weinberger, SE, Braunwald, E: Cough and Hemoptysis, Chap. 33, p. 194, in HPIM-14.

16

CYANOSIS

The circulating quantity of reduced hemoglobin is elevated [>50 g/L (>5 g/dL)] resulting in bluish discoloration of the skin and/or mucous membranes.

CENTRAL CYANOSIS

Results from arterial desaturation. Usually evident when arterial saturation is 85% or less. Particularly in dark skinned individuals, cyanosis may not be detected until saturation is 75%.

1. *Impaired pulmonary function:* Poorly ventilated alveoli or impaired oxygen diffusion; most frequent in pneumonia,

pulmonary edema, and chronic obstructive pulmonary disease (COPD); in COPD with cyanosis, polycythemia is often present.

2. *Anatomic vascular shunting:* Shunting of desaturated venous blood into the arterial circulation may result from congenital heart disease or pulmonary AV fistula.

3. *Decreased inspired O_2:* Cyanosis may develop in ascents to altitudes >2400 m (>8000 ft).

4. *Abnormal hemoglobins:* Methemoglobinemia, sulfhemoglobinemia, and mutant hemoglobins with low oxygen affinity (see HPIM-14, Chap. 107).

PERIPHERAL CYANOSIS

Occurs with normal arterial O_2 saturation with increased extraction of O_2 from capillary blood caused by decreased localized blood flow. Vasoconstriction due to cold exposure, decreased cardiac output (in shock, Chap. 28), and peripheral vascular disease (Chap. 117) with arterial obstruction or vasospasm (Table 16-1). Local (e.g., thrombophlebitis) or central (e.g., constrictive pericarditis) venous hypertension intensifies cyanosis.

———— *Approach to the Patient* ————

- Inquire about duration (cyanosis since birth suggests congenital heart disease) and exposures (drugs or chemicals that result in abnormal hemoglobins).
- Differentiate central from peripheral cyanosis by examining nailbeds, lips, and mucous membranes. Peripheral cyanosis may resolve with gentle warming of extremities.
- Check for clubbing of fingers and toes; clubbing is the selective enlargement of the distal segments of fingers and toes. Clubbing may be hereditary, idiopathic, or acquired and is associated with a variety of disorders. Combination of clubbing and cyanosis is frequent in congenital heart disease and occasionally with pulmonary disease (lung abscess, pulmonary AV shunts but *not* with uncomplicated obstructive lung disease).
- Examine chest for evidence of pulmonary disease, pulmonary edema, or murmurs associated with congenital heart disease.
- If cyanosis is localized to an extremity, evaluate for peripheral vascular obstruction.
- Obtain arterial blood gas to measure systemic O_2 saturation. Repeat while patient inhales 100% O_2; if saturation fails to increase to >95%, intravascular shunting of blood bypassing the lungs is likely (e.g., right-to-left intracardiac shunts).

Table 16-1

Causes of cyanosis

I. Central Cyanosis
    A. Decreased arterial oxygen saturation
        1. Decreased atmospheric pressure—high
            altitude
        2. Impaired pulmonary function
           a. Alveolar hypoventilation
           b. Uneven relationships between pulmonary
              ventilation and perfusion (perfusion of
              hypoventilated alveoli)
           c. Impaired oxygen diffusion
        3. Anatomic shunts
           a. Certain types of congenital heart disease
           b. Pulmonary arteriovenous fistulas
           c. Multiple small intrapulmonary shunts
        4. Hemoglobin with low affinity for oxygen
    B. Hemoglobin abnormalities
        1. Methemoglobinemia—hereditary, acquired
        2. Sulfhemoglobinemia—acquired
        3. Carboxyhemoglobinemia (not true cyanosis)
II. Peripheral cyanosis
    A. Reduced cardiac output
    B. Cold exposure
    C. Redistribution of blood flow from extremities
    D. Arterial obstruction
    E. Venous obstruction

- Evaluate abnormal hemoglobins by hemoglobin electrophoresis and measurement of methemoglobin level.

For a more detailed discussion, see Braunwald E: Hypoxia, Polycythemia, and Cyanosis, Chap. 36, p. 205, in HPIM-14.

17

EDEMA

Definition

Soft tissue swelling due to abnormal expansion of interstitial fluid volume. Edema fluid is a plasma transudate that accumulates when movement of fluid from vascular to interstitial space is favored. Since detectable generalized edema in the adult reflects a gain of ≥ 3 L, renal retention of salt and water is necessary for edema to occur. Distribution of edema can be an important guide to cause.

LOCALIZED EDEMA   Limited to a particular organ or vascular bed; easily distinguished from generalized edema. Unilateral extremity edema is usually due to venous or lymphatic obstruction (e.g., deep venous thrombosis, tumor obstruction, primary lymphedema). Stasis edema of a paralyzed lower extremity also may occur. Allergic reactions ("angioedema") and superior vena caval obstruction are causes of localized facial edema. Bilateral lower extremity edema may have localized causes: e.g., inferior vena caval obstruction, compression due to ascites, abdominal mass. Ascites (fluid in peritoneal cavity) and hydrothorax (in pleural space) may also present as isolated localized edema, due to inflammation or neoplasm.

GENERALIZED EDEMA (See Fig. 17-1)   Soft tissue swelling of most or all regions of the body. Bilateral lower extremity swelling, more pronounced after standing for several hours, and pulmonary edema are usually cardiac in origin. Periorbital edema noted on awakening often results from renal disease and impaired Na excretion. Ascites and edema of lower extremities and scrotum are frequent in cirrhosis or CHF. In *CHF*, diminished cardiac output and effective arterial blood volume result in both decreased renal perfusion and increased venous pressure with resultant renal Na retention due to renal vasoconstriction, intrarenal blood flow redistribution, and secondary hyperaldosteronism.

In *cirrhosis*, arteriovenous shunts lower effective renal perfusion, resulting in Na retention. Ascites accumulates when increased intrahepatic vascular resistance produces portal hypertension. Reduced serum albumin and increased abdominal pressure promote lower extremity edema.

In *nephrotic syndrome*, massive renal loss of albumin lowers plasma oncotic pressure, promoting fluid transudation into interstitium; lowering of effective blood volume stimulates renal Na retention.

In acute or chronic *renal failure*, edema occurs if Na intake

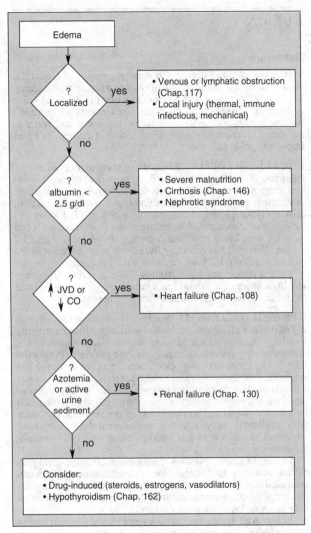

FIGURE 17-1 Diagnostic approach to edema. JVD, jugular venous distention; CO, cardiac output.

exceeds kidney's ability to excrete Na secondary to marked reductions in glomerular filtration. Severe *hypoalbuminemia* [<25 g/L (2.5 g/dL)] of any cause (e.g., nephrosis, nutritional deficiency states, chronic liver disease) may lower plasma oncotic pressure sufficiently to cause edema.

Less common causes of generalized edema: *idiopathic edema*, a syndrome of recurrent rapid weight gain and edema in women of reproductive age; *hypothyroidism*, in which myxedema is typically located in pretibial region; *drugs* such as steroids, estrogens, and vasodilators; *pregnancy*; *refeeding* after starvation.

℞ TREATMENT

Primary management is to identify and treat the underlying cause of edema (Fig. 17-1).

Dietary Na restriction (<500 mg/d) may prevent further edema formation. Bed rest enhances response to salt restriction in CHF and cirrhosis. Supportive stockings and elevation of edematous lower extremities will help mobilize interstitial fluid. If severe hyponatremia (<132 mmol/L) is present, water intake also should be reduced (<1500 mL/d). Diuretics (Table 17-1) are indicated for marked peripheral edema, pulmonary edema, CHF, inadequate dietary salt restriction. Complications are listed in Table 17-2. Weight loss by diuretics should be limited to 1–1.5 kg/d. Metolazone may be added to loop diuretics for enhanced effect. Note that intestinal edema may impair absorption of oral diuretics and reduce effectiveness. When desired weight is achieved, diuretic doses should be reduced.

In *CHF* (Chap. 108), avoid overdiuresis because it may bring a fall in cardiac output and prerenal azotemia. Avoid diuretic-induced hypokalemia, which predisposes to digitalis toxicity.

In *cirrhosis*, spironolactone is the diuretic of choice but may produce acidosis and hyperkalemia. Thiazides or small doses of loop diuretics also may be added. However, renal failure may result from volume depletion. Overdiuresis may result in hyponatremia and alkalosis, which may worsen hepatic encephalopathy (Chap. 146).

In *nephrotic syndrome*, albumin infusion should be limited to very severe cases (pts with associated hypotension), since rapid renal excretion prevents any sustained rise in serum albumin.

Table 17-1

Diuretics for Edema (See also Table 17-2)

Drug	Usual Dose	Comments
LOOP (MAY BE ADMINISTERED PO OR IV)		
Furosemide	40–120 mg qd or bid	Short-acting; potent; effective with low GFR
Bumetanide	0.5–2 mg qd or bid	May be used if allergic to furosemide
Ethacrynic acid	50–200 mg qd	Longer-acting
DISTAL, K-LOSING		
Hydrochlorothiazide	25–200 mg	First choice; causes hypokalemia; need GFR > 25 mL/min
Chlorthalidone	100 mg qd or qod	Long-acting (up to 72 h); hypokalemia; need GFR > 25 mL/min
Metolazone	1–10 mg qd	Long-acting; hypokalemia; effective with low GFR, especially when combined with a loop diuretic
DISTAL, K-SPARING		
Spironolactone	25–100 mg qid	Hyperkalemia; acidosis; blocks aldosterone; gynecomastia, impotence, amenorrhea; onset takes 2–3 days; avoid use in renal failure or in combination with ACE inhibitors or potassium supplements
Amiloride	5–10 mg qd or bid	Hyperkalemia; once daily; less potent than spironolactone
Triamterene	100 mg bid	Hyperkalemia; less potent than spironolactone; renal stones

Table 17-2

Complications of Diuretics

Common	Uncommon
Volume depletion	Interstitial nephritis
Prerenal azotemia	(thiazides, furosemide)
Potassium depletion	Pancreatitis (thiazides)
Hyponatremia (thiazides)	Loss of hearing (loop
Metabolic alkalosis	diuretics)
Hypercholesterolemia	Anemia, leukopenia,
Hyperglycemia (thiazides)	thrombocytopenia
Hyperkalemia (K-sparing)	(thiazides)
Hypomagnesemia	
Hyperuricemia	
Hypercalcemia (thiazides)	
GI complaints	
Rash (thiazides)	

For a more detailed discussion, see Braunwald E: Edema, Chap. 37, p. 210, in HPIM-14.

18

NAUSEA AND VOMITING

Definition

Nausea refers to the imminent desire to vomit and often precedes or accompanies vomiting. *Vomiting* refers to the forceful expulsion of gastric contents through the mouth. Retching refers to labored rhythmic respiratory activity that precedes emesis. *Regurgitation* refers to the gentle expulsion of gastric contents in the absence of nausea and abdominal diaphragmatic muscular contraction. *Rumination* refers to the regurgitation, rechewing, and reswallowing of food from the stomach.

Pathophysiology

Gastric contents are propelled into the esophagus when there is relaxation of the gastric fundus and gastroesophageal sphincter followed by a rapid increase in intraabdominal pressure produced by contraction of the abdominal and diaphragmatic musculature. Increased intrathoracic pressure results in further movement of the material to the mouth. Reflex elevation of the soft palate and closure of the glottis protects the nasopharynx and trachea and completes the act of vomiting. Vomiting is controlled by two brainstem areas, the vomiting center and chemoreceptor trigger zone. Activation of the chemoreceptor trigger zone results in impulses to the vomiting center, which controls the physical act of vomiting.

Etiology

Nausea and vomiting are manifestations of a large number of disorders. Clinical classification:

- Acute abdominal emergency: appendicitis, acute cholecystitis, acute intestinal obstruction (adhesions, malignancy, hernia, volvulus), acute peritonitis.
- Chronic indigestion: peptic ulcer disease, aerophagia.
- Disordered GI motility: gastroparesis (postvagotomy, diabetic, ischemic, idiopathic), abnormal gastric myoelectric activity ("dysrhythmia"), achalasia, intestinal pseudoobstruction.
- Infections: bacterial, viral, and parasitic infections of the GI tract. Systemic infection with fever not involving the GI tract directly, especially in children.
- CNS disorders: increased intracranial pressure (neoplasms, encephalitis, hydrocephalus) may result in vomiting, often of a projectile nature. Migraine headaches, tabetic crises, and acute meningitis can be accompanied by nausea and vomiting. Labyrinthine disorders (acute labyrinthitis, Mé-

nière's disease) that underlie vertigo are often associated with nausea and vomiting.
- Cardiac: acute myocardial infarction (esp. posterior or transmural MI) and congestive heart failure.
- Metabolic and endocrine disorders: diabetic ketoacidosis, adrenal insufficiency, hyperthyroid crisis, pregnancy, uremia, hypo- and hyperparathyroidism.
- Cancer, especially widespread disease, often produces nausea and vomiting.
- Medicines/toxins: nausea is a common side effect of many medications and toxins. Enterotoxins produced by bacteria cause food poisoning.
- Psychogenic: emotional upset, anorexia, bulimia.
- GI hemorrhage: blood in the stomach from any cause can result in nausea and vomiting.

Evaluation

The history, including a careful drug history, and the timing and character of the vomitus can be helpful. For example, vomiting that occurs predominantly in the morning is often seen in pregnancy, uremia, and alcoholic gastritis; feculent emesis implies distal intestinal obstruction or gastrocolic fistula; projectile vomiting suggests increased intracranial pressure; vomiting during or shortly after a meal may be due to psychogenic causes or peptic ulcer disease. Associated symptoms also may be helpful: vertigo and tinnitus in Ménière's disease, relief of abdominal pain with vomiting in peptic ulcer, and early satiety in gastroparesis. Plain radiographs can suggest diagnoses such as intestinal obstruction. The upper GI series assesses motility of the proximal GI tract as well as the mucosa. Other studies may be indicated such as gastric emptying scans (diabetic gastroparesis) and CT scan of the brain.

Complications

Rupture of the esophagus (Boerhaave's syndrome), hematemesis from a mucosal tear (Mallory-Weiss syndrome), dehydration, malnutrition, dental caries, metabolic alkalosis, hypokalemia, and aspiration pneumonitis.

Rx TREATMENT

This should be directed toward correcting the specific cause. The effectiveness of antiemetic medications depends on etiology of symptoms, pt responsiveness, and side effects. Antihistamines such as dimenhydrinate and promethazine hydrochloride are effective for nausea due to inner ear dysfunction.

Anticholinergics such as scopolamine are effective for nausea associated with motion sickness. Haloperidol and phenothiazine derivatives such as prochlorperazine are often effective in controlling mild nausea and vomiting, but sedation, hypotension, and parkinsonian symptoms are common side effects. Selective dopamine antagonists such as metoclopramide may be superior to the phenothiazines in treating severe nausea and vomiting and are particularly useful in treatment of gastroparesis. Intravenous metoclopramide may be effective as prophylaxis against nausea when given prior to chemotherapy. Cisapride exerts peripheral antiemetic effects but is devoid of the CNS effects of metoclopramide. Ondansetron and dronabinal are used for treating nausea and vomiting associated with cancer chemotherapy. Erythromycin is effective in some pts with gastroparesis.

For a more detailed discussion, see Friedman LS, Isselbacher KJ: Nausea, Vomiting, and Indigestion, Chap. 41, p. 230, in HPIM-14.

19

WEIGHT GAIN AND WEIGHT LOSS

In normal persons weight is stable over long periods because hypothalamic signals match intake to energy expenditure. The system is so effective that an unintentional change in body weight of 5% or more may be significant. Changes in weight can involve body fluid or tissue mass. Rapid fluctuations of weight over days suggest loss or gain of fluid, whereas long-term changes usually involve tissue mass.

WEIGHT GAIN

Weight gain due to fluid accumulation can occur with CHF, nephrosis, or renal failure. However, weight gain is most commonly due to increased tissue mass. The usual diagnosis is simple obesity due to overeating coupled with inadequate physical activity. The history may be misleading, and energy intake should be documented by calorie counts. However, the disorder is multifactorial in origin, and identification of leptin, the hormone produced by the adipocyte, has provided new insight into the neurohormonal regulation of satiety. Secondary causes of obesity include Cushing's syndrome, hypothyroidism, and hypogonadism. Insulin-secreting tumors also can cause overeating, and rarely, neoplasms of the CNS such as craniopharyngiomas cause a central drive to overeat. Congenital disorders such as Prader-Willi and Laurence-Moon-Biedl syndromes cause obesity early in life. Obesity predisposes to diseases such as diabetes mellitus, cholelithiasis, degenerative joint disease, hyperlipidemia, hypertension, and sleep apnea. A primary cause of secondary weight gain may be apparent in the initial diagnostic evaluation; if not, dietary intervention should be started.

WEIGHT LOSS

Weight can be lost as a result of increased energy expenditure, loss of energy in the stool or urine, or decreased food intake. Unintentional weight loss is usually an indication of serious disease and requires careful evaluation and follow-up. In young persons the most likely causes are diabetes mellitus, hyperthyroidism, anorexia nervosa, or infection such as HIV. In older persons cancer is the most common cause followed by depression and dementia.

The evaluation of weight loss begins with a careful history, physical examination, and first-phase laboratory assessment that should include HIV testing for those at risk (Table 19-1). When such an assessment is followed by judicious use of second-phase tests to confirm initial suspicions, the cause of weight loss can usually be identified. In individuals with normal or increased food intake, the most common diagnoses include hyperthyroidism, pheochromocytoma, excessive exercise (ballet dancers, long distance runners), diabetes mellitus, or intestinal malabsorption. Weight loss associated with diminished food intake can be due to malignancy, HIV, tuberculosis, endocarditis, hypercalcemic states such as hyperparathyroidism, uremia, anorexia nervosa, gastrointestinal obstruction, adrenal insufficiency, pernicious anemia, dementia, or depression.

Table 19-1

Screening Tests for Involuntary Weight Loss

1. First-phase screen*
   a. CBC, ESR
   b. Urinalysis
   c. Multiphase chemical screen (SMA 20)
   d. TSH
   e. HIV test for persons at risk
   f. Chest x-ray
   g. Stool for occult blood
2. Second-phase screen
   a. Abdominal CT scan
   b. Mammography, serum protein electrophoresis, parathyroid hormone, human PTH-related peptide, ACE, and 1,25-dihydroxycholecalciferol if hypercalcemia is present
   c. Colonoscopy if iron-deficiency anemia or melena is found or inflammatory bowel disease is suspected
   d. Upper endoscopy for upper GI bleeding or dysphagia
   e. Short ACTH test for weakness, pigmentation, or hyponatremia/hyperkalemia
   f. Blood cultures for fever of unknown origin with weight loss
   g. Bone marrow biopsy with culture for febrile weight loss with negative blood cultures
   h. 72-h stool fat for weight loss with chronic diarrhea
   i. Head CT or MRI for weight loss with headache, neurologic symptoms, or endocrine deficiency
   j. Spinal MRI if examination suggests paraspinal disease.
   k. Vitamin B_{12}

* First-phase and second-phase screens are arbitrary definitions. The history and physical examination together with initial laboratory tests may move a second-phase test to an early time point. The suggested order is for true occult disease.

SOURCE: Foster, DW: HPIM-14, p. 246.

For a more detailed discussion, see Foster DW: Gain and Loss in Weight, Chap. 43, p. 244, in HPIM-14.

20

DIARRHEA, CONSTIPATION, AND MALABSORPTION

NORMAL GASTROINTESTINAL FUNCTION

ABSORPTION OF FLUID AND ELECTROLYTES   Fluid delivery to the GI tract is 8–10 L/d, including 2 L/d ingested; most is absorbed in small bowel. Colonic absorption is normally 0.05–2 L/d, with capacity for 6 L/d if required. Intestinal water absorption passively follows active transport of Na^+, Cl^-, glucose, and bile salts. Additional transport mechanisms include Cl^-/HCO_3^- exchange, Na^+/H^+ exchange, H^+, K^+, Cl^-, and HCO_3^- secretion, Na^+-glucose cotransport, and active Na^+ transport across the basolateral membrane by Na^+, K^+-ATPase.

NUTRIENT ABSORPTION   (1) Proximal small intestine: iron, calcium, folate, fats (after hydrolysis of triglycerides to fatty acids by pancreatic lipase and colipase), proteins (after hydrolysis by pancreatic and intestinal peptidases), carbohydrates (after hydrolysis by amylases and disaccharidases); triglycerides absorbed as micelles after solubilization by bile salts; amino acids and dipeptides absorbed via specific carriers; sugars absorbed by active transport. (2) Distal small intestine: vitamin B_{12}, bile salts, water. (3) Colon: water, electrolytes.

INTESTINAL MOTILITY   Allows propulsion of intestinal contents from stomach to anus and separation of components to facilitate nutrient absorption. Propulsion is controlled by neural, myogenic, and hormonal mechanisms; mediated by migrating motor complex, an organized wave of neuromuscular activity that originates in the distal stomach during fasting and migrates slowly down the small intestine. Colonic motility is mediated by local peristalsis to propel feces. Defecation is effected by relaxation of internal anal sphincter in response to rectal distention, with voluntary control by contraction of external anal sphincter.

DIARRHEA

PHYSIOLOGY   Formally defined as fecal output greater than 200 g/d on low-fiber (western) diet; also frequently used to connote loose or watery stools. Mediated by one or more of the following mechanisms:

Osmotic Diarrhea   Nonabsorbed solutes increase intraluminal oncotic pressure, causing outpouring of water; usually ceases with fasting; stool osmolal gap greater than 40 (see below). Causes include disaccharidase (e.g., lactase) deficiencies, pancreatic insufficiency, bacterial overgrowth, lactulose or sorbitol ingestion, polyvalent laxative abuse, celiac or tropical sprue, and short bowel syndrome. Lactase deficiency can be either primary (more prevalent in blacks and Asians, usually presenting in early adulthood) or secondary (from viral, bacterial, or protozoal gastroenteritis, celiac or tropical sprue, or kwashiorkor).

Secretory Diarrhea Active ion secretion causes obligatory water loss; diarrhea is usually watery, often profuse, unaffected by fasting; stool Na^+ and K^+ are elevated with osmolal gap less than 40. Causes include viral infections (e.g., rotavirus, Norwalk virus), bacterial infections (e.g., cholera, enterotoxigenic *E. coli, Staphylococcus aureus*), protozoa (e.g., *Giardia, Isospora, Cryptosporidium*), AIDS-associated disorders (including mycobacterial and HIV-induced), medications (e.g., theophylline, colchicine, prostaglandins, diuretics), Zollinger-Ellison syndrome (excess gastrin production), vasoactive intestinal peptide (VIP)-producing tumors, carcinoid tumors (histamine and serotonin), medullary thyroid carcinoma (prostaglandins and calcitonin), systemic mastocytosis, basophilic leukemia, distal colonic villous adenomas (direct secretion of potassium-rich fluid), collagenous and microscopic colitis, and cholerrheic diarrhea (from ileal malabsorption of bile salts).

Exudative Inflammation, necrosis, and sloughing of colonic mucosa; may include component of secretory diarrhea due to prostaglandin release by inflammatory cells; stools usually contain PMNs as well as occult or gross blood. Causes include bacterial infections [e.g., *Campylobacter, Salmonella, Shigella, Yersinia*, invasive or enterotoxigenic *E. coli, Vibrio parahemolyticus, Clostridium difficile* colitis (frequently antibiotic-induced)], colonic parasites (e.g., *Entamoeba histolytica*), Crohn's disease, ulcerative proctocolitis, idiopathic inflammatory bowel disease, radiation enterocolitis, cancer chemotherapeutic agents, and intestinal ischemia.

Altered Intestinal Motility Alteration of coordinated control of intestinal propulsion; diarrhea often intermittent or alternating with constipation. Causes include diabetes mellitus, adrenal insufficiency, hyperthyroidism, collagen-vascular diseases, parasitic infestations, gastrin and VIP hypersecretory states, amyloidosis, laxatives (esp. magnesium-containing agents), antibiotics (esp. erythromycin), cholinergic agents, primary neurologic dysfunction (e.g., Parkinson's disease, traumatic neuropathy), fecal impaction, diverticular disease, and irritable bowel syndrome. Blood in intestinal lumen is cathartic, and major upper GI bleeding leads to diarrhea from increased motility.

Decreased Absorptive Surface   Usually arises from surgical manipulation (e.g., extensive bowel resection or rearrangement) that leaves inadequate absorptive surface for fat and carbohydrate digestion and fluid and electrolyte absorption; occurs spontaneously from enteroenteric fistulas (esp. gastrocolic).

EVALUATION   *History*   Diarrhea must be distinguished from fecal incontinence, change in stool caliber, rectal bleeding, and small, frequent, but otherwise normal stools. Careful medication history is essential. Alternating diarrhea and constipation suggests fixed colonic obstruction (e.g., from carcinoma) or irritable bowel syndrome. A sudden, acute course, often with nausea, vomiting, and fever, is typical of viral and bacterial infections, diverticulitis, ischemia, radiation enterocolitis, or drug-induced diarrhea and may be the initial presentation of inflammatory bowel disease. A longer, more insidious course suggests malabsorption, inflammatory bowel disease, metabolic or endocrine disturbance, pancreatic insufficiency, laxative abuse, ischemia, neoplasm (hypersecretory state or partial obstruction), or irritable bowel syndrome. Parasitic and certain forms of bacterial enteritis also can produce chronic symptoms. Particularly foul-smelling or oily stool suggests fat malabsorption. Fecal impaction may cause apparent diarrhea because only liquids pass partial obstruction. Several infectious causes of diarrhea are associated with an immunocompromised state (see Table 20-1).

Physical Examination   Signs of dehydration are often prominent in severe, acute diarrhea. Fever and abdominal tenderness suggest infection or inflammatory disease but are often absent in viral enteritis. Evidence of malnutrition suggests chronic course. Certain signs are frequently associated with specific deficiency states secondary to malabsorption (e.g., cheilosis with riboflavin deficiency, glossitis with B_{12}, folate deficiency).

Stool Examination   Culture for bacterial pathogens, examination for leukocytes, measurement of *Clostridium difficile* toxin, and examination for ova and parasites are important components of evaluation of pts with severe, protracted, or bloody diarrhea. Presence of blood (fecal occult blood test) or leukocytes (Wright's stain) suggests inflammation (e.g., ulcerative colitis, Crohn's disease, infection, or ischemia). Gram's stain of stool can be diagnostic of *Staphylococcus*, *Campylobacter*, or *Candida* infection. Steatorrhea (determined with Su-

Table 20-1

Infectious Causes of Diarrhea in Patients with AIDS

NONOPPORTUNISTIC PATHOGENS

> *Shigella*
> *Salmonella*
> *Campylobacter*
> *Entamoeba histolytica*
> *Chlamydia*
> *Neisseria gonorrhoeae*
> *Treponema pallidum* and other spirochetes
> *Giardia lamblia*

OPPORTUNISTIC PATHOGENS

Protozoa
  Cryptosporidium
  Isospora belli
  Microsporidia
  Blastocystis hominis
Viruses
  Cytomegalovirus
  Herpes simplex
  Adenovirus
  Human immunodeficiency virus
Bacteria
  Mycobacterium avium complex

---

dan III stain of stool sample or 72-h quantitative fecal fat analysis) suggests malabsorption or pancreatic insufficiency. Measurement of Na^+ and K^+ levels in fecal water helps to distinguish osmotic from other types of diarrhea; osmotic diarrhea is implied by stool osmolal gap >50, where stool osmolal gap = $osmol_{serum} - [2 \times (Na^+ + K^+)_{stool}]$.

Laboratory Studies CBC may indicate anemia (acute or chronic blood loss or malabsorption of iron, folate, or B_{12}), leukocytosis (inflammation), eosinophilia (parasitic, neoplastic, and inflammatory bowel diseases). Serum levels of calcium, albumin, iron, cholesterol, folate, B_{12}, vitamin D, and carotene; serum iron-binding capacity; and prothrombin time can provide evidence of intestinal malabsorption or maldigestion.

Other Studies D-Xylose absorption test is a convenient screen for small-bowel absorptive function. Small-bowel biopsy is especially useful for evaluating intestinal malabsorption. Specialized studies include Schilling test (B_{12} malabsorption), lactose H_2 breath test (carbohydrate malabsorption), [^{14}C]xylose and lactulose H_2 breath tests (bacterial overgrowth), glycocholic breath test (ileal malabsorption), triolein breath test (fat malabsorption), and bentiromide and secretin tests (pancreatic insufficiency). Sigmoidoscopy or colonoscopy with biopsy is useful in the diagnosis of colitis (esp. pseudomembranous, ischemic, microscopic); it may not allow distinction between infectious and noninfectious (esp. idiopathic ulcerative) colitis. Barium contrast x-ray studies may suggest malabsorption (thickened bowel folds), inflammatory bowel disease (ileitis or colitis), tuberculosis (ileocecal inflammation), neoplasm, intestinal fistula, or motility disorders.

℞ TREATMENT

Varies widely depending on etiology. Table 20-2 lists treatment options for common causes of diarrhea. In addition, symptomatic therapy includes vigorous rehydration (IV or with oral glucose-electrolyte solutions), electrolyte replacement, binders of osmotically active substances (e.g., kaolin-pectin), and opiates to decrease bowel motility (e.g., loperamide, diphenoxylate); opiates may be contraindicated in infectious or inflammatory causes of diarrhea.

MALABSORPTION SYNDROMES

Intestinal malabsorption of ingested nutrients may produce osmotic diarrhea, steatorrhea, or specific deficiencies (e.g., iron, folate, B_{12}, vitamins A, D, E, and K). Table 20-3 lists common causes of intestinal malabsorption. Protein-losing enteropathy may result from several causes of malabsorption; it is associated with hypoalbuminemia and can be detected by measuring stool α_1-antitrypsin or radiolabeled albumin levels. Therapy is directed at the underlying disease.

CONSTIPATION

Defined as decrease in frequency of stools to <1 per week or difficulty in defecation; may result in abdominal pain, distention, and fecal impaction, with consequent obstruction or, rarely, perforation. A frequent and often subjective complaint. Contributory factors may include inactivity, low-roughage diet, and inadequate allotment of time for defecation.

SPECIFIC CAUSES Altered colonic motility due to neurologic dysfunction (diabetes mellitus, spinal cord injury, multiple sclerosis, Chagas disease, Hirschsprung's disease, chronic idio-

Table 20-2

Treatment of Common Causes of Diarrhea

Infectious (uncomplicated enteritis or colitis)
    Viral
        Rotavirus, Norwalk virus, unclassified enteritis—
          symptomatic therapy only
        AIDS-associated—symptomatic therapy; octreotide
          possibly helpful
    Bacterial
        Staphylococcus, *Yersinia enterocolitica*, salmonellae,
          Vibrio—supportive therapy; avoid opiates
        Enterotoxigenic *E. coli*, traveler's diarrhea—bismuth
          subsalicylate; trimethoprim/sulfamethoxazole; doxy-
          cycline, ciprofloxacin
        Shigella—bismuth subsalicylate; ampicillin
        Campylobacter—symptomatic therapy; erythromycin
        Clostridium difficile—metronidazole; oral vanco-
          mycin
    Protozoan
        Giardia—metronidazole; quinacrine
        Cryptosporidium—symptomatic therapy; spiramycin
        Entamoeba histolytica—metronidazole; iodoquinone
Inflammatory
    Crohn's disease—glucocorticoids, aminosalicylates
        (esp. for colitis), metronidazole, azathioprine (or 6-
        mercaptopurine), methotrexate
    Ulcerative proctocolitis—glucocorticoids (oral or rec-
        tal), aminosalicylates (oral or rectal)
    Diverticulitis—tetracycline
Malabsorptive
    Pancreatic insufficiency—low-fat diet, pancreatic en-
        zyme replacement
    Lactase deficiency—lactose-free diet; lactase prepara-
        tions (e.g., Lactaid)
    Nontropical (celiac) sprue (gluten-sensitive enteropa-
        thy)—gluten-free diet; glucocorticoids for refractory
        disease
    Bacterial overgrowth, tropical sprue—tetracycline (with
        folic acid for sprue)
    Short-bowel syndrome—symptomatic therapy; opiates,
        elemental diet, medium-chain triglycerides; octreotide
        possibly helpful
    Postgastrectomy—symptomatic therapy; frequent small
        meals; low-carbohydrate diet; octreotide for dumping
        syndrome

(continued)

Table 20-2 (*Continued*)

Treatment of Common Causes of Diarrhea

    Postileal resection—symptomatic therapy; cholestyramine

    Lymphangiectasia—medium-chain triglycerides; treat underlying disease if possible

Endocrine

    Adrenal insufficiency, hyperkalemia, hypocalcemia, thyrotoxicosis, diabetes mellitus—treat underlying disorder

Neoplastic

    Gastrinoma (Zollinger-Ellison)—H_2-receptor blockers, proton pump inhibitors, gastrectomy, tumor resection

    Carcinoid syndrome—symptomatic therapy; resection/tumor ablation, octreotide

    Secretory villous adenoma—resection

Ischemic

    Supportive therapy; avoid opiates; resection of nonviable bowel

Radiation-induced

    Symptomatic therapy; opiates

Irritable bowel disease

    High-fiber diet, bulk producing agents, anticholinergic agents

---

pathic intestinal pseudoobstruction, idiopathic megacolon), scleroderma, drugs (esp. anticholinergic agents, opiates, aluminum- or calcium-based antacids, calcium channel blockers, iron supplements, sucralfate), hypothyroidism, Cushing's syndrome, hypokalemia, hypercalcemia, dehydration, mechanical causes (colorectal tumors, diverticulitis, volvulus, hernias, intussusception), and anorectal pain (from fissures, hemorrhoids, abscesses, or proctitis) leading to retention, constipation, and fecal impaction.

℞ **TREATMENT**

In absence of identifiable cause, constipation may improve with reassurance, exercise, increased dietary fiber, bulking agents (e.g., psyllium), and increased fluid intake. Specific therapies include removal of bowel obstruction (fecolith, tumor), discontinuance of nonessential hypomotility agents (esp. aluminum- or calcium-containing antacids, opiates). For symptomatic relief, magnesium-containing agents or other cathartics are occasionally needed. With severe hypo- or dys-motility or in presence of opiates, osmotically active agents (e.g., oral lactulose, intestinal polyethylene glycol–containing lavage solutions) and oral or rectal emollient laxatives (e.g., docusate salts) and mineral oil are most effective.

Table 20-3

Common Causes of Malabsorption

Maldigestion: Chronic pancreatitis, cystic fibrosis, pancreatic carcinoma

Bile salt deficiency: Cirrhosis, cholestasis, bacterial overgrowth (blind loop syndromes, intestinal diverticula, hypomotility disorders), impaired ileal reabsorption (resection, Crohn's disease), bile salt binders (cholestyramine, calcium carbonate, neomycin)

Inadequate absorptive surface: Massive intestinal resection, gastrocolic fistula, jejunoileal bypass

Lymphatic obstruction: Lymphoma, Whipple's disease, intestinal lymphangiectasia

Vascular disease: Constrictive pericarditis, right-sided heart failure, mesenteric arterial or venous insufficiency

Mucosal disease: Infection (esp. *Giardia*, Whipple's disease, tropical sprue), inflammatory diseases (esp. Crohn's disease), radiation enteritis, eosinophilic enteritis, ulcerative jejunitis, mastocytosis, tropical sprue, infiltrative disorders (amyloidosis, scleroderma, lymphoma, collagenous sprue, microscopic colitis), biochemical abnormalities (gluten-sensitive enteropathy, disaccharidase deficiency, hypogamma-globulinemia, abetalipoproteinemia, amino acid transport deficiencies), endocrine disorders (diabetes mellitus, hypoparathyroidism, adrenal insufficiency, hyperthyroidism, Zollinger-Ellison syndrome, carcinoid syndrome)

For a more detailed discussion, see Friedman LS, Isselbacher KJ: Diarrhea and Constipation, Chap. 42, p. 236; and Greenberger NJ, Isselbacher KJ: Disorders of Absorption, Chap. 285, p. 1616, in HPIM-14.

21

GASTROINTESTINAL BLEEDING

PRESENTATION

1. *Hematemesis:* Vomiting of blood or altered blood ("coffee grounds") indicates bleeding proximal to ligament of Treitz.
2. *Melena:* Altered (black) blood per rectum (≥ 100 mL blood required for one melenic stool) usually indicates bleeding proximal to ligament of Treitz but may be as distal as ascending colon; pseudomelena may be caused by ingestion of iron, bismuth, licorice, beets, blueberries, charcoal.
3. *Hematochezia:* Bright red or maroon rectal bleeding usually implies bleeding beyond ligament of Treitz but may be due to rapid upper GI bleeding (≥ 1000 mL).
4. *Positive fecal occult blood test* (see Chap. 50).
5. *Iron deficiency anemia* (see Chap. 48).

HEMODYNAMIC CHANGES　Orthostatic drop in bp >10 mmHg usually indicates $>20\%$ reduction in blood volume ($\pm$ syncope, light-headedness, nausea, sweating, thirst).

SHOCK　bp < 100 mmHg systolic usually indicates $>30\%$ reduction in blood volume ($\pm$ pallor, cool skin).

LABORATORY CHANGES　Hematocrit may not reflect extent of blood loss because of delayed equilibration with extravascular fluid. Mild leukocytosis and thrombocytosis. Elevated BUN is common in upper GI bleeding.

ADVERSE PROGNOSTIC SIGNS　Age >60, associated illnesses, coagulopathy, immunosuppression, presentation with shock, rebleeding, onset of bleeding in hospital, variceal bleeding, endoscopic stigmata of recent bleeding, [e.g., "visible vessel" in ulcer base (see below)].

UPPER GI BLEEDING

CAUSES *Common*　Peptic ulcer, gastropathy (alcohol, aspirin, NSAIDs, stress), esophagitis, Mallory-Weiss tear (mucosal tear at gastroesophageal junction due to retching), gastroesophageal varices.

Less Common　Swallowed blood (nosebleed); esophageal, gastric, or intestinal neoplasm; anticoagulant and fibrinolytic therapy; hypertrophic gastropathy (Ménétrier's disease); aortic aneurysm; aortoenteric fistula (from aortic graft); AV malformation; telangiectases (Osler-Rendu-Weber syndrome); Dieulafoy lesion (ectatic submucosal vessel); vasculitis; connective tissue disease (pseudoxanthoma elasticum, Ehlers-Danlos syndrome);

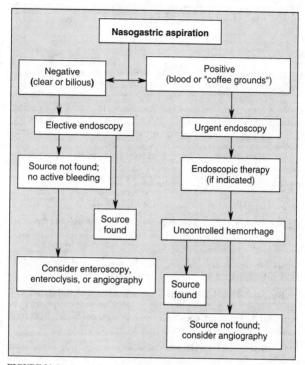

FIGURE 21-1   Approach to the patient with acute upper GI bleeding. (*Request surgical consultation early, in event operative intervention is required.) (Reproduced from Epstein A, Isselbacher KJ, HPIM-14, p. 248.)

blood dyscrasias; neurofibroma; amyloidosis; hemobilia (biliary origin).

EVALUATION   *After* hemodynamic resuscitation (see below and Fig. 21-1).

- History and physical examination: Drugs (increased risk of upper and lower GI tract bleeding with aspirin and NSAIDs), prior ulcer, bleeding history, family history, features of cirrhosis or vasculitis, etc.
- Nasogastric aspirate for blood, if source (upper versus lower) not clear from history; may be falsely negative if bleeding has ceased.

- Upper endoscopy: Accuracy >90%; allows visualization of bleeding site and possibility of therapeutic intervention; mandatory for suspected varices, aortoenteric fistulas; permits identification of "visible vessel" (protruding artery in ulcer crater), which connotes high (~50%) risk of rebleeding.
- Upper GI barium radiography: Accuracy ~80% in identifying a lesion, though does not confirm source of bleeding; acceptable alternative to endoscopy in resolved or chronic low-grade bleeding.
- Selective mesenteric arteriography: When brisk bleeding precludes identification of source at endoscopy.
- Radioisotope scanning (e.g., ^{99m}Tc tagged to red blood cells or albumin); used primarily as screening test to confirm bleeding is rapid enough for arteriography to be of value or when bleeding is intermittent and of unclear origin.

LOWER GI BLEEDING

CAUSES Anal lesions (hemorrhoids, fissures), rectal trauma, proctitis, colitis (ulcerative colitis, Crohn's disease, infectious colitis, ischemic colitis, radiation), colonic polyps, colonic carcinoma, angiodysplasia (vascular ectasia), diverticulosis, intussusception, solitary ulcer, blood dyscrasias, vasculitis, connective-tissue disease, neurofibroma, amyloidosis, anticoagulation.

EVALUATION

- History and physical examination.
- Anoscopy and sigmoidoscopy: Exclude hemorrhoids, fissure, ulcer, proctitis, neoplasm.
- Nasogastric aspirate (if any suspicion of upper GI source, best to do upper endoscopy).
- Colonoscopy: Often test of choice, but may be impossible if bleeding is massive.
- Barium enema: No role in active bleeding.
- Arteriography: When bleeding is severe (requires bleeding rate >0.5 mL/min; may require prestudy radioisotope bleeding scan as above); defines site of bleeding or abnormal vasculature.
- Surgical exploration (last resort).

BLEEDING OF OBSCURE ORIGIN Often small-bowel source. Consider small-bowel enteroclysis x-ray (careful barium radiography via peroral intubation of small bowel), Meckel's scan, enteroscopy (small-bowel endoscopy), or exploratory laparotomy with intraoperative enteroscopy.

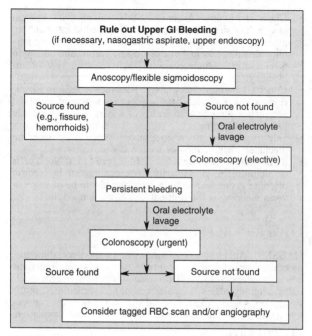

FIGURE 21-2 Approach to the patient with acute lower GI bleeding. (Reproduced from Epstein A, Isselbacher KJ, HPIM-14, p. 249.)

℞ TREATMENT
Of Upper and Lower GI Bleeding (See Fig. 21-2)

- Venous access with large bore IV (14–18 gauge); central venous line for major bleed and pts with cardiac disease; monitor vital signs, urine output, Hct (fall may lag). Gastric lavage of unproven benefit but clears stomach before endoscopy. Iced saline may lyse clots; room-temperature tap water may be preferable. Intubation may be required to protect airway.
- Type and cross match blood (6 units for major bleed).
- Surgical standby when bleeding is massive.
- Support blood pressure with isotonic fluids (normal saline); albumin and fresh frozen plasma in cirrhotics. Packed red blood cells when available (whole blood if massive bleeding); maintain Hct ≥25–30.

- Fresh frozen plasma and vitamin K (10 mg SC or IV) in cirrhotics with coagulopathy.
- IV calcium (e.g., up to 10–20 mL 10% calcium gluconate IV over 10–15 min) if serum calcium falls (due to transfusion of citrated blood). Empirical drug therapy (antacids, H_2 receptor blockers, omeprazole) of unproven benefit.
- Specific measures: *Varices:* IV vasopressin (0.4–0.9 U/min) with nitroglycerin IV, SL, or transdermally to maintain systolic bp >90 mmHg, Blakemore-Sengstaken tube tamponade, endoscopic sclerosis or band ligation; propranolol or nadolol in doses sufficient to cause beta blockade reduces risk of recurrent or initial variceal bleeding (do not use in acute bleed) (see Chap. 147); *ulcer with visible vessel or active bleeding:* endoscopic bipolar, heater-probe, or laser coagulation or injection of epinephrine; *gastritis:* embolization or vasopressin infusion of left gastric artery; *GI telangiectases:* ethinylestradiol/norethisterone (0.05/1.0 mg PO qd) may prevent recurrent bleeding, particularly in pts with chronic renal failure; *diverticulosis:* mesenteric arteriography with intraarterial vasopressin; *angiodysplasia:* colonoscopic bipolar or laser coagulation, may regress with replacement of stenotic aortic valve.
- Indications for emergency surgery: Uncontrolled or prolonged bleeding, severe rebleeding, aortoenteric fistula. For intractable variceal bleeding, consider transjugular intrahepatic portosystemic shunt (TIPS).

For a more detailed discussion, see Epstein A, Isselbacher KJ: Gastrointestinal Bleeding, Chap. 44, p. 246, in HPIM-14.

22

JAUNDICE AND EVALUATION OF LIVER FUNCTION

JAUNDICE

DEFINITION Yellow skin pigmentation caused by elevation in serum bilirubin level (also termed *icterus*); often more easily discernible in sclerae. Jaundice and scleral icterus become clinically evident at a serum bilirubin level of 34–43 μmol/L (2–2.5 mg/dL) (approximately twice normal); yellow skin discoloration also occurs with elevated serum carotene levels but without pigmentation of the sclerae.

BILIRUBIN METABOLISM Bilirubin is the major breakdown product of hemoglobin released from senescent erythrocytes. Initially it is bound to albumin, transported into the liver, conjugated to a water-soluble form (glucuronide) by glucuronosyl transferase, excreted into the bile, and converted to urobilinogen in colon. Urobilinogen is mostly excreted in the stool; a small portion is reabsorbed and excreted by the kidney. Bilirubin can be filtered by the kidney only in its conjugated form (measured as the "direct" fraction); thus increased *direct* serum bilirubin level is associated with bilirubinuria. Increased bilirubin production and excretion (even without hyperbilirubinemia, as in hemolysis) produce elevated urinary urobilinogen levels.

ETIOLOGY Hyperbilirubinemia occurs as a result of (1) overproduction, (2) decreased hepatic uptake, (3) decreased hepatic conjugation (required for excretion), or (4) decreased biliary excretion (see Table 22-1). Jaundice due to decreased hepatic excretory function is often associated with pruritus, probably related to endogenous opioid peptides and abnormal neurotransmission/neuromodulation; these cholestatic disorders include all causes of *conjugated* hyperbilirubinemia except Dubin-Johnson and Rotor syndromes and benign familial cholestasis (in which bilirubin excretion is predominantly disrupted).

EVALUATION Important to determine whether hyperbilirubinemia is primarily conjugated or unconjugated (see Table 22-1). Conjugated hyperbilirubinemia usually results from hepatocellular disease, cholestasis (intrahepatic obstruction), or extrahepatic obstruction. Essential clinical examination includes history (especially duration of jaundice, pruritus, associated pain, fever, weight loss, risk factors for parenterally transmitted diseases, medications, ethanol use, travel history, surgery, pregnancy), physical examination (hepatomegaly, tenderness over

Table 22-1

Causes of Hyperbilirubinemia

PREDOMINANTLY UNCONJUGATED (INDIRECT-
REACTING) BILIRUBIN

Overproduction of bilirubin pigments: Intravascular hemolysis, hematoma resorption, ineffective erythropoiesis
(bone marrow)

Decreased hepatic uptake: Sepsis, prolonged fasting,
right-sided heart failure, drugs (e.g., rifampin, probenecid)

Decreased conjugation: Severe hepatocellular disease
(e.g., hepatitis, cirrhosis), sepsis, drugs (e.g., chloramphenicol, pregnanediol), neonatal jaundice, inherited glucuronosyl transferase deficiency (Gilbert's syndrome,
Crigler-Najjar syndromes type II or I)

PREDOMINANTLY CONJUGATED (DIRECT-
REACTING) BILIRUBIN

Impaired hepatic excretion: Hepatocellular disease (e.g.,
drug-induced, viral, or ischemic hepatitis, cirrhosis),
drug-induced cholestasis (e.g., oral contraceptives, meth-
yltestosterone, chlorpromazine), sepsis, postoperative
state, parenteral nutrition, biliary cirrhosis (primary or
secondary), inherited disorders (Dubin-Johnson syndrome, Rotor syndrome, cholestasis of pregnancy, benign familial recurrent cholestasis)

Biliary obstruction: Biliary cirrhosis (primary or secondary), sclerosing cholangitis, intraluminal mechanical obstruction (e.g., stone, tumor, parasites, stricture, cyst), biliary compression (e.g., pancreatic tumor, portal
lymphadenopathy, pancreatitis)

---

liver, palpable gallbladder, splenomegaly, gynecomastia, testicular atrophy), blood liver tests (see below), and complete blood
count. If liver tests are suggestive of hepatocellular disease,
evaluation should include metabolic and serologic tests and,
possibly, liver biopsy; evidence of cholestasis or extrahepatic
obstruction merits radiologic examination [ultrasound (US), CT,
or MRI] with follow-up biopsy, cholangiography, and drainage
as needed. Conjugated hyperbilirubinemia without other liver
enzyme abnormalities is seen with recent or ongoing sepsis and
Rotor and Dubin-Johnson syndromes.

Table 22-2

Important Causes of Hepatomegaly

Vascular congestion: Right-sided heart failure (including tricuspid valve disease), Budd-Chiari syndrome
Infiltrative disorders: Fatty liver (e.g., ethanol abuse, diabetes, parenteral hyperalimentation, pregnancy), lymphoma or leukemia, extramedullary hematopoiesis, amyloidosis, granulomatous hepatitis (e.g., TB, atypical mycobacteria, sarcoidosis, CMV), hemochromatosis, Gaucher's disease, glycogen storage diseases
Inflammatory disorders: Viral or drug-induced hepatitis, cirrhosis
Tumors: Hepatocellular carcinoma, metastatic cancer, focal nodular hyperplasia, hepatic adenoma
Cysts (e.g., polycystic disease)

HEPATOMEGALY

DEFINITION   Generally a span of greater than 12 cm in the right midclavicular line or a palpable left lobe in the epigastrium. It is important to exclude low-lying liver (e.g., with chronic obstructive pulmonary disease and lung hyperinflation) and other RUQ masses (e.g., enlarged gallbladder or bowel or kidney tumor). Independent assessment of size best obtained from US or CT examination. Contour and texture are important: Focal enlargement or rocklike consistency suggests tumor; tenderness suggests inflammation (e.g., hepatitis) or rapid enlargement (e.g., right-sided heart failure, Budd-Chiari syndrome, fatty infiltration). Cirrhotic livers are usually firm and nodular, often enlarged until late in course. Pulsations frequently connote tricuspid regurgitation. Arterial bruit or hepatic rub suggests tumor. Portal hypertension is occasionally associated with continuous venous hum (see Table 22-2).

BLOOD TESTS OF LIVER FUNCTION

Used to evaluate functional status of liver and to discriminate among different types of liver disease (inflammatory, infiltrative, metabolic, vascular, hepatobiliary; see Table 22-3).

BILIRUBIN   Provides indication of hepatic uptake, metabolic (conjugation) and excretory functions; conjugated fraction (direct-reacting) distinguished from unconjugated by chemical assay (see Table 22-1).

Table 22-3

Patterns of Liver Test Abnormalities

Test	Type of Liver Disease			
	Hepato-cellular	Obstruc-tive	Ischemic	Infiltra-tive
AST, ALT*	↑↑↑	↑	↑ – ↑↑↑	N – ↑
Alkaline phosphatase	↑ – ↑↑	↑↑↑	↑ – ↑↑	↑ – ↑↑↑
5'-Nucleotidase	↑ – ↑↑	↑↑↑	↑	↑ – ↑↑↑
Bilirubin	↑ – ↑↑↑	↑ – ↑↑↑	N – ↑	N
Prothrombin time	↑ – ↑↑↑	N†	N – ↑↑	N
Albumin	N – ↓↓↓	N‡	N – ↓	N

* In *acute complete obstruction*, serum transaminases may rise rapidly and dramatically but return to near normal levels after 1–3 days even in the presence of continued obstruction.

† May increase with prolonged biliary obstruction and secondary biliary cirrhosis.

‡ May decrease with prolonged biliary obstruction and secondary biliary cirrhosis.
NOTE: N, normal; ↑, elevated; ↓, decreased.

AMINOTRANSFERASES (TRANSAMINASES)   Aspartate aminotransferase (AST; SGOT) and alanine aminotransferase (ALT; SGPT); sensitive indicators of liver cell integrity; greatest elevations seen in hepatocellular necrosis (e.g., viral hepatitis, toxic liver injury, circulatory collapse, acute hepatic vein obstruction), occasionally with sudden, complete biliary obstruction (e.g., from gallstone); levels correlate poorly with severity of disease; milder abnormalities in cholestatic, cirrhotic, and infiltrative disease; ALT more specific measure of liver injury, since AST also found in striated muscle; ethanol-induced liver injury usually produces modest increases with more prominent elevation of AST than ALT.

LACTATE DEHYDROGENASE (LDH)   Less specific measure of hepatocellular integrity with little value in evaluation of liver disease.

ALKALINE PHOSPHATASE   Sensitive indicator of cholestasis, biliary obstruction (enzyme increases more quickly than serum bilirubin), and liver infiltration; mild elevations in other forms of liver disease; limited specificity because of wide tissue distribution; elevations also seen in childhood, pregnancy, and bone diseases; tissue-specific isoenzymes can be distinguished by differences in heat stability (liver enzyme activity stable under conditions that destroy bone enzyme activity).

5′-NUCLEOTIDASE (5′-NT)   Pattern of elevation in hepatobiliary disease similar to alkaline phosphatase; has greater specificity for liver disorders; used to determine whether liver is source of elevation in serum alkaline phosphatase, esp. in children, pregnant women, pts with possible concomitant bone disease.

γ-GLUTAMYLTRANSPEPTIDASE   Correlates with serum alkaline phosphatase activity; greater sensitivity for hepatobiliary disease (esp. due to alcoholic liver disease), but also elevated in pancreatic, renal, pulmonary, and cardiac disorders.

PROTHROMBIN TIME (PT) (See also Chap. 52)   Measure of clotting factor activity; prolongation results from clotting-factor deficiency or inactivity; all clotting factors except factor VIII are synthesized in the liver, and deficiency can occur rapidly from widespread liver necrosis, as in hepatitis, toxic injury, or cirrhosis; clotting factors II, VII, IX, X function only in the presence of the fat-soluble vitamin K; PT prolongation from fat malabsorption distinguished from hepatic disease by rapid and complete response to vitamin K replacement.

ALBUMIN   Decreased serum levels result from decreased hepatic synthesis (chronic liver disease or prolonged malnutrition) or excessive losses in urine or stool; insensitive indicator of acute hepatic dysfunction, since serum half-life is 2 to 3 weeks; in pts with chronic liver disease, degree of hypoalbuminemia correlates with severity of liver dysfunction.

GLOBULIN   Mild polyclonal hyperglobulinemia often seen in chronic liver diseases; marked elevation frequently seen in *autoimmune* chronic active hepatitis.

AMMONIA   Elevated blood levels result from deficiency of hepatic detoxification pathways and portal-systemic shunting, as in fulminant hepatitis, hepatotoxin exposure, and severe portal hypertension (e.g., from cirrhosis); for many (but not all) pts, blood ammonia level correlates with degree of portal-systemic encephalopathy; asterixis correlates with encephalopathy more accurately but does not distinguish among several metabolic causes, including hepatic dysfunction, uremia, and hypercarbia.

HEPATOBILIARY IMAGING PROCEDURES

ULTRASONOGRAPHY   Rapid, noninvasive examination of abdominal structures; no radiation exposure; relatively low cost, equipment portable; images and interpretation strongly dependent on expertise of examiner; particularly valuable for detecting biliary duct dilatation and gallbladder stones (>95%); much less sensitive for intraductal stones (~60%); most sensitive means of detecting ascites; moderately sensitive for detecting hepatic masses but excellent for discriminating solid from cystic structures; useful in directing percutaneous needle biopsies of suspicious lesions; Doppler US useful to determine patency and flow in portal, hepatic veins and portal-systemic shunts; imaging improved by presence of ascites but severely hindered by bowel gas; endoscopic US less affected by bowel gas and is sensitive for determination of depth of tumor invasion through bowel wall.

CT   Particularly useful for detecting, differentiating, and directing percutaneous needle biopsy of abdominal masses, cysts, and lymphadenopathy; imaging enhanced by intestinal or intravenous contrast dye and unaffected by intestinal gas; somewhat less sensitive than US for detecting stones in gallbladder but more sensitive for choledocholithiasis; may be useful in distinguishing certain forms of diffuse hepatic disease (e.g., fatty infiltration, iron overload).

MRI   Most sensitive detection of hepatic masses and cysts; allows easy differentiation of hemangiomas from other hepatic tumors; most accurate noninvasive means of assessing hepatic and portal vein patency, vascular invasion by tumor; useful for monitoring iron, copper deposition in liver (e.g., in hemochromatosis, Wilson's disease).

RADIONUCLIDE SCANNING   Using various radiolabeled compounds, different scanning methods allow sensitive assessment of biliary excretion (HIDA, PIPIDA, DISIDA scans), parenchymal changes (technetium sulfur colloid liver/spleen scan), and selected inflammatory and neoplastic processes (gallium scan); HIDA and related scans particularly useful for assessing biliary patency and excluding acute cholecystitis in situations where US is not diagnostic; CT, MRI, and colloid scans have similar sensitivity for detecting liver tumors and metastases; CT and combination of colloidal liver and lung scans sensitive for detecting right subphrenic (suprahepatic) abscesses.

CHOLANGIOGRAPHY   Most sensitive means of detecting biliary ductal calculi, biliary tumors, sclerosing cholangitis, choledochal cysts, fistulas, and bile duct leaks; may be performed via endoscopic (transampullary) or percutaneous (transhepatic) route; allows sampling of bile and ductal epithelium for cytologic analysis and culture; allows placement of biliary drainage catheter, stricture dilatation, and gallstone dissolution; endoscopic route (ERCP) permits manometric evaluation of sphincter of Oddi, sphincterotomy, and stone extraction.

ANGIOGRAPHY Most accurate means of determining portal pressures and assessing patency and direction of flow in portal and hepatic veins; highly sensitive for detecting small vascular lesions and hepatic tumors (esp. primary hepatocellular carcinoma); "gold standard" for differentiating hemangiomas from solid tumors; most accurate means of studying vascular anatomy in preparation for complicated hepatobiliary surgery (e.g., portal-systemic shunting, biliary reconstruction) and determining resectability of hepatobiliary and pancreatic tumors. Similar anatomic information (but not intravascular pressures) can often be obtained noninvasively by CT- and MR-based techniques.

For a more detailed discussion, see Kaplan LM, Isselbacher KJ: Jaundice, Chap. 45, p. 249; and Podolsky DK, Isselbacher KJ: Evaluation of Liver Function, Chap. 292, p. 1663, in HPIM-14.

23

ASCITES

Definition

Accumulation of fluid within the peritoneal cavity. Small amounts may be asymptomatic; increasing amounts cause abdominal distention and discomfort, anorexia, nausea, early satiety, heartburn, flank pain, and respiratory distress.

Detection

PHYSICAL EXAMINATION Detects no less than several 100 mL; bulging flanks, fluid wave, shifting dullness, "puddle sign" (dullness over dependent abdomen with pt on hands and knees). May be associated with penile or scrotal edema, umbilical or inguinal herniation, pleural effusion.

ULTRASONOGRAPHY/CT Very sensitive; able to distinguish fluid from cystic masses.

EVALUATION

Diagnostic paracentesis (50–100 mL) essential; use 22-gauge needle in linea alba 2 cm below umbilicus or with "Z-track" insertion in LLQ or RLQ. Routine evaluation includes inspection, protein, albumin, glucose, cell count and differential, culture, cytology; in selected cases check amylase, LDH, triglycerides, culture for TB. Rarely, laparoscopy or even exploratory laparotomy may be required. Ascites due to CHF (e.g., pericardial constriction) may require evaluation by right-sided heart catheterization.

Differential Diagnosis

More than 90% of cases due to cirrhosis, neoplasm, CHF, tuberculosis.

1. *Diseases of peritoneum*: Infections (bacterial, tuberculous, fungal, parasitic), neoplasms, vasculitis, miscellaneous (Whipple's disease, familial Mediterranean fever, endometriosis, starch peritonitis, etc.).
2. *Diseases not involving peritoneum:* Cirrhosis, CHF, Budd-Chiari syndrome, hepatic venocclusive disease, hypoalbuminemia (nephrotic syndrome, protein-losing enteropathy, malnutrition), miscellaneous (myxedema, ovarian diseases, pancreatic disease, chylous ascites).

Pathophysiologic Classification Using Serum-Ascites Albumin Gradient

Difference in albumin concentrations between serum and ascites as a reflection of imbalances in hydrostatic pressures: *Low gradient* (serum-ascites albumin gradient <1.1): 2° peritonitis, neoplasm, pancreatitis, vasculitis, nephrotic syndrome. *High gradient* (serum-ascites albumin gradient >1.1 suggesting increased hydrostatic pressure): cirrhosis, CHF, Budd-Chiari syndrome.

Representative Fluid Characteristics (See Table 23-1)

CIRRHOTIC ASCITES

PATHOGENESIS Contributing factors: (1) portal hypertension, (2) hypoalbuminemia, (3) increased hepatic lymph formation, (4) renal sodium retention—secondary to hyperaldosteronism, increased sympathetic nervous activity (renin-angiotensin production). Initiating event may be peripheral arterial vasodila-

Table 23-1

Representative Fluid Characteristics

Cause	Appearance	Protein, g/dL	Serum-Ascites Albumin Gradient	Cell Count, per µL		Other
				RBC	WBC	
Cirrhosis	Straw-colored	<2.5	>1.1	Low	<250	—
Neoplasm	Straw-colored, hemorrhagic, mucinous, or chylous	>2.5	Variable	Often high	>1000 (>50% lymphs)	+Cytology
2° Bacterial peritonitis	Turbid or purulent	>2.5	<1.1	Low	>10,000	+Gram's stain, culture (often multiple organisms)
Spontaneous bacterial peritonitis	Turbid or purulent	<2.5	>1.1	Low	>250 polys	+Gram's stain, culture
Tuberculous peritonitis	Clear, hemorrhagic, or chylous	>2.5	<1.1	Occ. high	>1000 (>70% lymphs)	+AFB stain, culture
CHF	Straw-colored, rarely chylous	>2.5	>1.1	Low	>1000 (mesothelial)	—
Pancreatitis	Turbid, hemorrhagic, or chylous	>2.5	<1.1	Variable	Variable	Increased amylase

tion triggered by endotoxin and cytokines and mediated by nitric oxide; results in decreased "effective" plasma volume and activation of compensatory mechanisms to retain renal Na and preserve intravascular volume. In severe ascites, plasma atrial natriuretic factor levels are high but insufficient to cause natriuresis.

R̲x̲ TREATMENT

Maximum mobilization ~700 mL/d (peripheral edema may be mobilized faster).

1. Rigid salt restriction (400 mg Na/d).
2. Fluid restriction of 1–1.5 L only if hyponatremia.
3. Diuretics if no response after 1 week or if urine Na concentration <25 meq/L; spironolactone (mild, potassium-sparing, aldosterone-antagonist) 100 mg/d PO increased by 100 mg q4–5d to maximum of 600 mg/d; furosemide 40–80 mg/d PO or IV may be added if necessary (greater risk of hepatorenal syndrome, encephalopathy), can increase by 40 mg/d to maximum of 240 mg/d until effect achieved or complication occurs. If still no diuresis, add hydrochlorothiazide 50–100 mg PO qd.
4. Monitor weight, urinary Na and K, serum electrolytes, and creatinine.
5. Repeated large-volume paracentesis (5 L) with IV infusions of albumin (10 g/L ascites removed) is preferable for initial management of massive ascites because of fewer side effects than diuretics.
6. In refractory cases, consider transjugular intrahepatic portosystemic shunt (TIPS), though 20–30% risk of encephalopathy and high rate of shunt stenosis and occlusion. Peritoneovenous (LeVeen, Denver) shunt (high complication rate—occlusion, infection, DIC) and side-to-side portacaval shunt (high mortality rate in end-stage cirrhotic pt) have fallen out of favor. Consider liver transplantation in appropriate candidates (Chap. 147).

Complications

SPONTANEOUS BACTERIAL PERITONITIS   Suspect in cirrhotic pt with ascites and fever, abdominal pain, worsening ascites, ileus, hypotension, worsening jaundice, or encephalopathy; low ascitic protein concentration (low opsonic activity) is predisposing factor. Diagnosis suggested by ascitic fluid PMN cell count >250/μL and symptoms or PMN count >500/μL; confirmed by positive culture (usually Enterobacteriaceae, group D streptococci, *Streptococcus pneumoniae*, *S. viridans*).

Initial treatment: Cefotaxime 2 g IV q8h; efficacy demonstrated by marked decrease in ascitic PMN count after 48 h; treat 5–10 days or until ascitic PMN count is normal. Risk of recurrence can be reduced with norfloxacin 400 mg PO qd, trimethoprim-sulfamethexazole 1 double-strength PO bid 5 days a week, or possibly ciprofloxacin 750 mg PO once a week. Consider prophylactic therapy (before first episode of peritonitis) in pts with cirrhotic ascites and an ascitic albumen level <1g/dL.

HEPATORENAL SYNDROME   Progressive renal failure characterized by azotemia, oliguria with urinary sodium concentration <10 mmol/L, hypotension, and lack of response to volume challenge. May be spontaneous or precipitated by bleeding, excessive diuresis, paracentesis, or drugs (aminoglycosides, NSAIDs, ACE inhibitors). Thought to result from altered renal hemodynamics, elevated serum thromboxane and endothelin levels, and decreased urinary prostaglandin levels. Prognosis poor. Treatment: Trial of plasma expansion; TIPS of doubtful benefit; liver transplantation in selected cases.

For a more detailed discussion, see Glickman RM, Isselbacher KJ, Abdominal Swelling and Ascites, Chap. 46, p. 255, in HPIM-14.

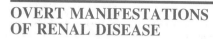

OVERT MANIFESTATIONS OF RENAL DISEASE

ABNORMALITIES OF RENAL FUNCTION

Azotemia is the retention of nitrogenous waste products excreted by the kidney. Increased levels of blood urea nitrogen (BUN) (>30 mg/dL) and creatinine (>1.5 mg/dL) are indicative of impaired renal function. Renal function can be estimated by determining the clearance of creatinine (CL_{cr}) (normal >100 mL/min). CL_{cr} overestimates glomerular filtration rate (GFR), particularly at lower levels. Isotopic markers (e.g., iothalamate) provide more accurate estimates of GFR.

Manifestations of impaired renal function include: volume overload, hypertension, electrolyte abnormalities (e.g., hyperkalemia, hypocalcemia, hyperphosphatemia), metabolic acidosis, and, when severe, "uremia" (one or more of the following: anorexia, lethargy, confusion, asterixis, pleuritis, pericarditis, enteritis, pruritus, sleep and taste disturbance, nitrogenous fetor).

ABNORMALITIES OF URINE VOLUME

OLIGURIA This refers to sparse urine output, usually defined as <400 mL/d. Oligoanuria refers to a more marked reduction in urine output, i.e., <100 mL/d. Anuria indicates the absence of urine output. Oliguria most often occurs in the setting of volume depletion and/or renal hypoperfusion, resulting in "prerenal azotemia" and acute renal failure (Chap. 129). Anuria can be caused by complete bilateral urinary tract obstruction, a vascular catastrophe (dissection or arterial occlusion), renal vein thrombosis, and hypovolemic, cardiogenic, or septic shock. Oliguria is never normal, since at least 400 mL of maximally concentrated urine must be produced to excrete the obligate daily osmolar load.

POLYURIA Polyuria is defined as a urine output >3 L/d. It is often accompanied by nocturia and urinary frequency and must be differentiated from other more common conditions associated with lower urinary tract pathology and urinary urgency or frequency (e.g., cystitis, prostatism). It is often accompanied by hypernatremia (Chap. 25). Polyuria (Table 24-1) can occur as a response to a solute load (e.g., hyperglycemia) or to an abnormality in antidiuretic hormone (ADH) action. Diabetes insipidus is termed *central* if due to the insufficient hypothalamic production of ADH and *nephrogenic* if the result of renal

Table 24-1

Major Causes of Polyuria

Excessive fluid intake	Nephrogenic diabetes insipidus
Primary polydipsia	Lithium exposure
Iatrogenic (intravenous fluids)	Urinary tract obstruction
Therapeutic	Papillary necrosis
Diuretic agents	Reflux nephropathy
Osmotic diuresis	Interstitial nephritis
Hyperglycemia	Hypercalcemia
Azotemia	Central diabetes insipidus
Mannitol	Tumor
Radiocontrast	Postoperative
	Head trauma
	Basilar meningitis
	Neurosarcoidosis

---

insensitivity to the action of ADH. Excess fluid intake can lead to polyuria, but primary polydipsia rarely results in changes in plasma osmolality unless urinary diluting capacity is impaired, as with chronic renal failure.

The approach to the pt with polyuria is shown in Fig. 24-1.

ABNORMALITIES OF URINE COMPOSITION

PROTEINURIA This is the hallmark of glomerular disease. Levels up to 150 mg/d are considered within normal limits. Typical measurements are semi-quantitative, using a moderately sensitive dipstick that estimates protein concentration; therefore, the degree of hydration may influence the dipstick protein determination. Most commercially available urine dipsticks detect albumin and do not detect smaller proteins, such as light chains, that require testing with sulfosalicylic acid. More sensitive assays can be used to detect microalbuminuria in diabetes mellitus.

Urinary protein excretion rates between 500 mg/d and 3 g/d are nonspecific and can be seen in a variety of renal diseases (including hypertensive nephrosclerosis, interstitial nephritis, vascular disease, and other primary renal diseases with little or no glomerular involvement). Lesser degrees of proteinuria (500 mg/d to 1.5 g/d) may be seen after vigorous exercise, changes in body position, fever, or congestive heart failure. Protein excretion rates >3 g/d are termed *nephrotic range* proteinuria

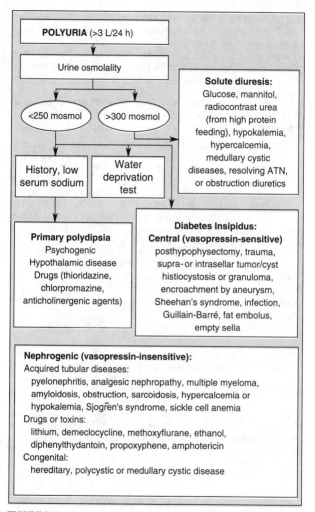

FIGURE 24-1 Approach to the patient with polyuria. (OSM, osmolality; ATN, acute tubular necrosis.)

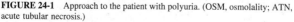

and are accompanied by hypoalbuminemia, hypercholesterolemia, and edema in the nephrotic syndrome. Massive degrees of proteinuria (>10 g/d) can be seen with minimal change disease, primary focal segmental sclerosis, membranous nephropathy, collapsing glomerulopathy, and HIV-associated nephropathy and can be associated with a variety of extrarenal complications (Chap. 132).

Pharmacologic inhibition of ACE or blockade of angiotensin II receptors may reduce proteinuria in some pts. Specific therapy for nephrotic syndrome is discussed in Chap. 132.

HEMATURIA   Gross hematuria refers to the presence of frank blood on voiding and is more characteristic of lower urinary tract disease and/or bleeding diatheses rather than intrinsic renal diseases (Table 24-2). Cyst rupture in polycystic kidney disease and flares of IgA nephropathy are exceptions. Microscopic hematuria ($>1–2$ RBC/high powered field) accompanied by proteinuria, hypertension, and an active urinary sediment (the "nephritic syndrome") is most likely related to an inflammatory glomerulonephritis (Chap. 132).

Free hemoglobin and myoglobin are detected by dipstick; a negative urinary sediment with strongly heme-positive dipstick are characteristic of either hemolysis or rhabdomyolysis, which can be differentiated by clinical history and laboratory testing. Red blood cell casts are not commonly seen but are highly specific for glomerulonephritis.

The approach to the pt with hematuria is shown in Fig. 24-2.

PYURIA   This may accompany hematuria in inflammatory glomerular diseases. Isolated pyuria is most commonly observed in association with an infection of the upper or lower urinary tract. Pyuria may also occur with allergic interstitial nephritis (often with a preponderance of eosinophils), transplant rejection, and noninfectious, nonallergic tubulointerstitial diseases. The finding of "sterile" pyuria (i.e., urinary white blood cells without bacteria) in the appropriate clinical setting should raise suspicion of renal tuberculosis.

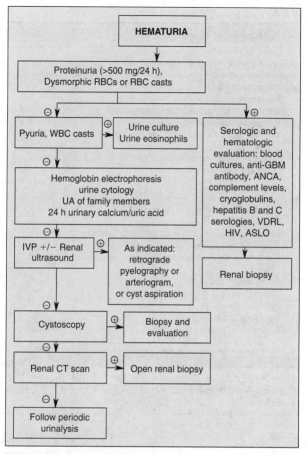

FIGURE 24-2 Approach to the patient with hematuria. (RBC, red blood cell; WBC, white blood cell; GBM, glomerular basement membrane; ANCA, antineutrophil cytoplasmic antibody; VDRL, venereal disease research laboratory; HIV, human immunodeficiency virus; ASLO, antistreptolysin O; UA, urinalysis; IVP, intravenous pyelography; CT, computed tomography.)

Table 24-2

Major Causes of Hematuria

LOWER URINARY TRACT

Bacterial cystitis
Intestitial cystitis
Urethritis (infectious or inflammatory)
Passed or passing kidney stone
Transitional cell carcinoma of bladder or structures
   proximal to it
Squamous cell carcinoma of bladder (e.g., following
   schistosomiasis)

UPPER URINARY TRACT

Renal cell carcinoma
Age-related renal cysts
Other neoplasms (e.g., oncocytoma, hamartoma)
Acquired renal cystic disease
Congenital cystic disease, including autosomal dominant
   form
Glomerular diseases
Intersitial renal diseases
Nephrolithiasis
Pyelonephritis
Renal infarction

For a more detailed discussion, see Denker BM, Brenner BM: Cardinal Manifestations of Renal Disease, Chap. 47, p. 258, in HPIM-14.

ELECTROLYTES/ACID-BASE BALANCE

SODIUM

In most cases, disturbances of sodium concentration [Na$^+$] result from abnormalities of water homeostasis. Disorders of Na$^+$ balance usually lead to hypo- or hypervolemia. Attention to the dysregulation of volume (Na$^+$ balance) and osmolality (water balance) must be considered separately for each pt (see below).

HYPONATREMIA   This is defined as a serum [Na$^+$] <135 mmol/L and is among the most common electrolyte abnormalities encountered in hospitalized pts. Symptoms include confusion, lethargy, and disorientation; if severe (<120 mmol/L) and abrupt, seizures or coma may develop. Hyponatremia is often iatrogenic and almost always the result of an abnormality in the action of antidiuretic hormone (ADH), deemed either "appropriate" or "inappropriate," depending on the associated clinical conditions. The serum [Na$^+$] by itself does not yield diagnostic information regarding the total-body Na$^+$ content. Therefore, a useful way to categorize pts with hyponatremia is to place them into three groups, depending on the volume status (i.e., hypovolemic, euvolemic, and hypervolemic hyponatremia) (Fig. 25-1).

Hypovolemic Hyponatremia   Mild to moderate degree of hyponatremia ([Na$^+$] 125–135 mmol/L) complicate GI fluid or blood loss for two reasons. First, there is activation of the three major "systems" responsive to reduced organ perfusion: the renin-angiotensin-aldosterone axis, the sympathetic nervous system, and ADH. This sets the stage for enhanced renal absorption of solutes and water. Second, replacement fluid before hospitalization or other intervention is usually hypotonic (e.g., water, fruit juices). The optimal treatment of hypovolemic hyponatremia is volume administration, either in the form of colloid or isotonic crystalloid (e.g., 0.9% NaCl or lactated Ringer's solution).

Hypervolemic Hyponatremia   The edematous disorders (CHF, hepatic cirrhosis, and nephrotic syndrome) are often associated with mild to moderate degrees of hyponatremia ([Na$^+$] 125–135 mmol/L); occasionally, pts with severe CHF or cirrhosis may present with serum [Na$^+$] <120 mmol/L. The pathophysiology is similar to that in hypovolemic hyponatremia, except that perfusion is decreased due to (1) reduced cardiac output, (2) arteriovenous shunting, and (3) severe hypoprotein-

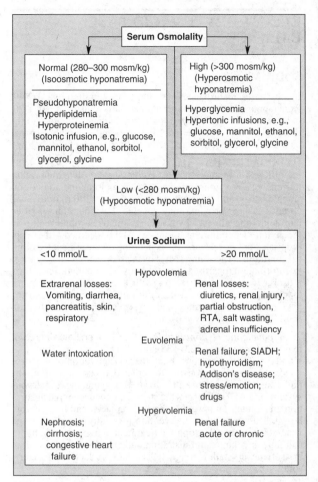

FIGURE 25-1 Evaluation of hyponatremia. RTA, renal tubular acidosis; SIADH, syndrome of inappropriate antidiuretic hormone secretion.

emia, respectively, rather than true volume depletion. The scenario is sometimes referred to as reduced "effective circulating arterial volume." The evolution of hyponatremia is the same: increased water reabsorption due to ADH, complicated by hypotonic fluid replacement. This problem may be compounded by increased thirst in patients with CHF.

Management consists of treatment of the underlying disorder (e.g., afterload reduction in heart failure, large-volume paracentesis in cirrhosis, glucocorticoid therapy in some forms of nephrotic syndrome), Na^+ restriction, diuretic therapy, and, in some pts, H_2O restriction. This approach is quite distinct from that applied to hypovolemic hyponatremia.

Euvolemic Hyponatremia The syndrome of inappropriate ADH secretion (SIADH) characterizes most cases of euvolemic hyponatremia. Common causes of the syndrome are pulmonary (e.g., pneumonia, tuberculosis, pleural effusion) and CNS diseases (e.g., tumor, subarachnoid hemorrhage, meningitis); SIADH also occurs with malignancies (e.g., small cell carcinoma of the lung) and drugs (e.g., chlorpropamide, carbamezapine, narcotic analgesics, cyclophosphamide). Optimal treatment of euvolemic hyponatremia is H_2O restriction to <1 L/d, depending on the severity of the syndrome.

Treatment of Hyponatremia The rate of correction should be relatively slow (0.5 Na^+ mmol/L per h). A useful "rule of thumb" is to limit the change in Na^+ mmol/L to half of the total difference within the first 24 h. More rapid correction has been associated with central pontine myelinolysis, especially if the hyponatremia has been of long standing. More rapid correction (with the potential addition of hypertonic saline to the above-recommended regimens) should be reserved for pts with very severe degrees of hyponatremia and ongoing neurologic compromise (e.g., pt with Na^+ <105 mmol/L in status epilepticus).

HYPERNATREMIA This is rarely associated with hypervolemia, and this association is always iatrogenic, e.g., administration of hypertonic sodium bicarbonate. Rather, hypernatremia is almost always the result of a combined water and volume deficit, with losses of H_2O in excess of Na^+. The most common causes are osmotic diuresis secondary to hyperglycemia, azotemia, or drugs (radiocontrast, mannitol, etc.) or central or nephrogenic diabetes insipidus (DI) (see "Polyuria," Chap. 24). The evaluation of hypernatremia is outlined in Fig. 25-2.

Treatment of Hypernatremia The approach to correction of hypernatremia is outlined in Fig. 25-2 and Table 25-1. As with hyponatremia, it is advisable to correct the water deficit

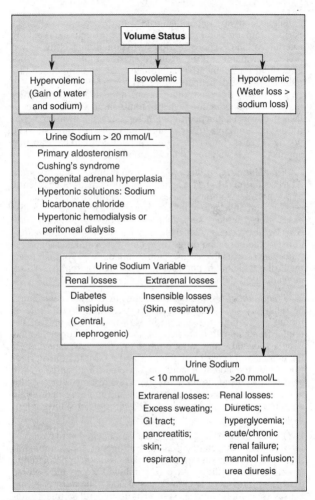

FIGURE 25-2 Evaluation of hypernatremia.

Table 25-1

Correction of Hypernatremia

WATER DEFICIT

---

1. Estimate total-body water (TBW): 50–60% body weight (kg) depending on body composition
2. Calculate free-water deficit: [(NA − 140)/140] × TBW
3. Administer deficit over 48–72 h

ONGOING WATER LOSSES

---

4. Calculate free-water clearance from urinary flow rate (V) and urine (U) Na and K concentrations
$$V − V × (U_{Na} + U_K)/140$$

INSENSIBLE LOSSES

---

5. ~10 mL/kg per day: less if ventilated, more if febrile

TOTAL

---

6. Add components to determine water of D_5W administration rate (typically ~50–250 mL/h)

---

slowly to avoid neurologic compromise. In addition to the water replacement formula provided, other forms of therapy may be helpful in selected cases of hypernatremia. Pts with central DI may respond well to the administration of intranasal desmopressin or to the use of chlorpropamide (if the risk of drug-induced hypoglycemia is not excessive). Pts with nephrogenic DI due to lithium may reduce their polyuria with amiloride (2.5–10 mg/d) or hydrochlorothiazide (12.5–50 mg/d). Paradoxically, the use of diuretics may decrease distal nephron filtrate delivery, thereby reducing free-water losses and polyuria.

POTASSIUM

Since potassium (K^+) is the major intracellular cation, discussion of disorders of K^+ balance must take into consideration changes in the exchange of intra- and extracellular K^+ stores (extracellular K^+ constitutes less than 2% of total-body K^+ content). Insulin, beta$_2$-adrenergic agonists, and alkalosis tend to promote K^+ uptake by cells; acidosis promotes shifting of K^+ out of cells.

HYPOKALEMIA   Major causes of hypokalemia are outlined in Table 25-2. Atrial and ventricular arrhythmias are the major health consequences of hypokalemia. Pts with concurrent mag-

Table 25-2

Causes of Hypokalemia

I. Decreased intake
  A. Starvation
  B. Clay ingestion
II. Redistribution into cells
  A. Acid-base
    1. Metabolic alkalosis
  B. Hormonal
    1. Insulin
    2. Beta$_2$-adrenergic agonists (endogenous or exogenous)
    3. Alpha-adrenergic antagonists
  C. Anabolic state
    1. Vitamin B$_{12}$ or folic acid (red blood cell production)
    2. Granulocyte-macrophage colony stimulating factor
    3. Total parenteral nutrition
  D. Other
    1. Pseudohypokalemia
    2. Hypothermia
    3. Hypokalemic periodic paralysis
III. Increased loss
  A. Nonrenal
    1. Gastrointestinal loss (diarrhea)
    2. Integumentary loss (sweat)
  B. Renal
    1. Increased distal flow; diuretics, osmotic diuresis, salt-wasting nephropathies
    2. Increased secretion of potassium
      a. Mineralocorticoid excess: primary hyperaldosteronism, secondary hyperaldosteronism (malignant hypertension, renin-secreting tumors, renal artery stenosis, hypovolemia), apparent mineralocorticoid excess (licorice, chewing tobacco, carbenoxolone), congenital adrenal hyperplasia, Cushing's syndrome, Bartter's syndrome
      b. Distal delivery of non-reabsorbed anions: vomiting, masogastric suction, proximal (type 2) renal tubular acidosis, diabetic ketoacidosis, glue-sniffing (toluene abuse), penicillin derivatives
      c. Other: amphotericin B, Liddle's syndrome, hypomagnesemia

nesium deficit (e.g., after diuretic therapy) and/or digoxin therapy are at particularly increased risk. Other clinical manifestations include muscle weakness, which may be profound at serum $[K^+]$ <2.5 mmol/L, and, if prolonged, ileus and polyuria. Clinical history and urinary $[K^+]$ are most helpful in distinguishing causes of hypokalemia.

℞ TREATMENT

Hypokalemia is most often managed by correction of the acute underlying disease process (e.g., diarrhea) or withdrawal of an offending medication (e.g., loop or thiazide diuretic), along with oral K^+ supplementation with KCl, or, in rare cases, $KHCO_3$, or K-acetate. Hypokalemia may be refractory to correction in the presence of magnesium deficiency; both cations may need to be supplemented in selected cases (e.g., cisplatin nephrotoxicity). If loop or thiazide diuretic therapy cannot be discontinued, a distal tubular K^+-sparing agent, such as amiloride or spironolactone, can be added to the regimen. ACE inhibition in pts with CHF attenuate diuretic-induced hypokalemia and protect against cardiac arrhythmia. If hypokalemia is severe (<2.5 mmol/L) and/or if oral supplementation is not tolerated, intravenous KCl can be administered through a central vein at rates up to 20 mmol/h), with telemetry and skilled monitoring.

HYPERKALEMIA   Causes are outlined in Table 25-3. In most cases, hyperkalemia is due to decreased K^+ excretion. Drugs can be implicated in many cases. Where the diagnosis is uncertain, calculation of the transtubular K gradient (TTKG) can be helpful. TTKG $= U_K P_{Osm}/P_K U_{Osm}$ (U, urine; P, plasma). TTKG <10 suggests decreased K^+ excretion due to (1) hypoaldosteronism, or (2) renal resistance to the effects of mineralocorticoid. These can be differentiated by the administration of fludrocortisone (florinef) 0.2 mg, with the former increasing K^+ excretion (and decreased TTKG).

℞ TREATMENT

The most important consequence of hyperkalemia is altered cardiac conduction, leading to bradycardic cardiac arrest in severe cases. Hypocalcemia and acidosis accentuate the cardiac effects of hyperkalemia. Figure 25-3 shows serial ECG patterns of hyperkalemia. Stepwise treatment of hyperkalemia is summarized in Table 25-4.

ACID-BASE DISORDERS (See Fig. 25-4)

Regulation of normal pH (7.35–7.45) depends on lungs and kidneys. By the Henderson-Hasselbalch equation, pH is a func-

Table 25-3

Major Causes of Hyperkalemia

I. "Pseudo"-hyperkalemia
  A. Thrombocytosis, leukocytosis, in vitro hemolysis
II. Intra- to extracellular shift
  A. Acidosis
  B. Hyperosmolality; radiocontrast, hypertonic dextrose, mannitol
  C. Beta$_2$-adrenergic antagonists (noncardioselective agents)
  D. Digoxin or ouabain poisoning
  E. Hyperkalemic periodic paralysis
III. Inadequate excretion
  A. Distal K-sparing diuretic agents and analogues
    1. Amiloride, spironolactone, triamterene, trimethoprim
  B. Decreased distal delivery
    1. Congestive heart failure, volume depletion, NSAIDs, cyclosporine
  C. Renal tubular acidosis, type IV
    1. Tubulointerstitial diseases
      a. Reflux nephropathy, pyelonephritis, interstitial nephritis, heavy metal (e.g., Pb) nephropathy
    2. Diabetic glomerulosclerosis
  D. Advanced renal insufficiency with low GFR
  E. Decreased mineralocorticoid effects
    1. Addison's disease, congenital adrenal enzyme deficiency, other forms of adrenal insufficiency (e.g., adrenalitis), heparin, ACE inhibitors, AII antagonists

tion of the ratio of HCO$_3$ (regulated by the kidney) to P$_{CO_2}$ (regulated by the lungs). The HCO$_3$/P$_{CO_2}$ relationship is useful in classifying disorders of acid-base balance. *Acidosis* is due to gain of acid or loss of alkali; causes may be metabolic (fall in serum HCO$_3$) or respiratory (rise in P$_{CO_2}$). *Alkalosis* is due to loss of acid or addition of base and is either metabolic ($\uparrow$ serum HCO$_3$) or respiratory ($\downarrow$ P$_{CO_2}$).

To limit the change in pH, metabolic disorders evoke an immediate compensatory response in ventilation; compensation to respiratory disorders by the kidneys takes days. *Simple* acid-base disorders consist of one primary disturbance and its com-

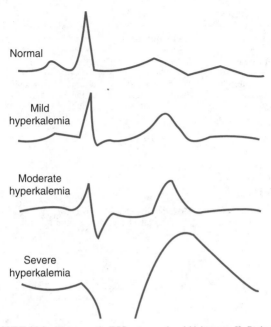

Normal

Mild
hyperkalemia

Moderate
hyperkalemia

Severe
hyperkalemia

FIGURE 25-3 Diagrammatic ECGs at normal and high serum K. Peaked T waves (precordial leads) are followed by diminished R wave, wide QRS, prolonged, P-R, loss of P wave, and ultimately a sine wave.

pensatory response. In *mixed* disorders, a combination of primary disturbances is present.

METABOLIC ACIDOSIS   The low HCO_3 results from the addition of acids (organic or inorganic) or loss of HCO_3. The *causes* of metabolic acidosis are categorized by the anion gap, which equals $Na - (Cl + HCO_3)$ (Table 25-5). *Increased* anion gap acidosis (>12 mmol/L) is due to addition of acid (other than HCl) and unmeasured anions to the body. Causes include ketoacidosis (diabetes mellitus, starvation, alcohol), lactic acidosis, poisoning (salicylates, ethylene glycol, and ethanol), and renal failure. Diagnosis may be made by measuring BUN, creatinine, glucose, lactate, serum ketones, and serum osmolality and obtaining a toxic screen.

Normal anion gap acidoses result from HCO_3 loss from the

Table 25-4

Management of Hyperkalemia

Treatment	Indication	Dose
Calcium gluconate*	K >6.5 mmol/L with advanced ECG changes	10 mL of 10% solution IV over 2–3 min
Insulin + Glucose	Moderate hyperkalemia, peaked T waves only	10 U reg, IV + 50 mL, 50% IV
NaHCO$_3$	Moderate hyperkalemia	90 mmol (2 ampules, IV push over 5 min)
Kayexalate + Sorbitol	Moderate hyperkalemia	Oral: 30 g, with 50 mL 20% sorbitol; rectal: 50 g in 200 mL 20% sorbitol enema, retain 45 min
Furosemide	Moderate hyperkalemia, serum creatinine <265 mmol/L (<3 mg%)	20–40 mg IV push
Dialysis	Hyperkalemia with renal failure	

* Calcium chloride may be preferable in presence of circulatory instability or liver impairment.

Onset	Duration	Mechanism	Note
1–5 min	30 min	Lowers threshold potential. Antagonizes cardiac and neuromuscular toxicity of hyperkalemia.	Fastest action. Monitor ECG. Repeat in 5 min if abnormal ECG persists. Hazardous in presence of digitalis. Correct hyponatremia if present. Follow with other treatment for K.
15–45 min	4–6 h	Moves K into cells.	Glucose unnecessary if blood sugar elevated. Repeat insulin q 15 min with glucose infusion if needed.
Immediate	Short	Moves K into cells.	Most effective when acidosis is present. Of more risk in CHF or hypernatremia. Beware of hypocalcemic tetany.
1 h	4–6 h	Removes K.	Each gram Kayexalate orally removes about 1 mmol K and about 0.5 mmol K when given rectally. Repeat every 4 h. Use with caution in CHF.
15 min	4 h	Kaliuresis.	Most useful if inadequate K excretion contributes to hyperkalemia.
Immediate after start-up	Variable	Removes K.	Hemodialysis most effective. Also improves acidosis.

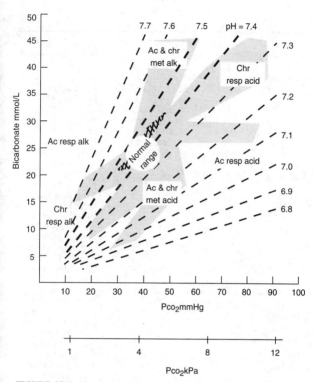

FIGURE 25-4 Nomogram, showing bands for uncomplicated respiratory or metabolic acid-base disturbances in intact subjects. Each "confidence" band represents the mean ±2 SD for the compensatory response of normal subjects or patients to a given primary disorder. Ac, acute; chr, chronic; resp, respiratory; met, metabolic; acid, acidosis; alk, alkalosis. (From Levinsky NG: HPIM-12, p. 290; modified from Arbus GS: Can Med Assoc J 109:291, 1973.)

GI tract or from the kidney, e.g., renal tubular acidosis, urinary obstruction, rapid volume expansion, and administration of NH_4Cl, lysine HCl, or arginine HCl. Calculation of urinary anion gap may be helpful in evaluation of hyperchloremic metabolic acidosis. A negative anion gap suggests GI losses; a positive anion gap suggests altered urinary acidification.

Clinical Features   Include hyperventilation, cardiovascular collapse, and nonspecific symptoms ranging from anorexia to coma.

Table 25-5

Metabolic Acidosis

Non-Anion Gap Acidosis		Anion Gap Acidosis	
Cause	Clue	Cause	Clue
Diarrhea	Hx; ↑ K	DKA	Hyperglyce-mia, ketones
Enterostomy	Drainage		
RTA		RF	Uremia, ↑ BUN, ↑ CR
Proximal	↓ K		
Distal	↓ K; UpH > 5.5	Lactic aci-dosis	Clinical set-ting + ↑ se-rum lactate
Dilutional	Volume expansion	Alcoholic ke-toacidosis	Hx; weak + ketones; + osm gap
Ureterosig-moidostomy	Obstructed il-eal loop		
Hyperalimen-tation	Amino acid infusion	Starvation	Hx; mild aci-dosis; + ke-tones
Acetazolam-ide, NH₄Cl, lysine HCl, arginine HCl	Hx of admin-istration of these agents	Salicylates	Hx; tinnitus; high serum level; + ke-tones
		Methanol	Large AG; retinitis; + toxic screen; + osm gap
		Ethylene glycol	RF, CNS; + toxic screen; crystalluria; + osm gap

RTA, renal tubular acidosis; UpH, urinary pH; DKA, diabetic ketoacidosis; RF, renal failure; AG, anion gap; osm gap, osmolar gap

Table 25-6

Metabolic Alkalosis

Cl Responsive (Low U_α)	Cl Resistant (High U_α)

Gastrointestinal causes:
    Vomiting
    Nasogastric suction
    Chloride-wasting di-
        arrhea
    Villous adenoma of
        colon
Diuretic therapy
Posthypercapnia
Carbenicillin or penicillin
	Adrenal disorders:
	    Hyperaldosteronism
	    Cushing's syndrome (1°,
	        2°, ectopic)
	Exogenous steroids:
	    Gluco- or mineralocor-
	        ticoid
	    Licorice ingestion
	    Carbenoxolone
	Bartter's syndrome
	Refeeding alkalosis
	Alkali ingestion

℞ TREATMENT

Depends on cause and severity. Always correct the underlying disturbance. Administraton of alkali is controversial. It may be reasonable to treat lactic acidosis with intravenous HCO_3 at a rate sufficient to maintain a plasma HCO_3 of 8 to 10 mmol/L and a pH >7.10.

Chronic acidosis is treated when HCO_3 <15 mmol/L or symptoms of anorexia or fatigue are present. Na citrate may be more palatable than oral $NaHCO_3$. Oral therapy with $NaHCO_3$ usually begins with 1 g tid and is titrated *upward* to maintain desired serum HCO_3.

METABOLIC ALKALOSIS   A primary increase in serum HCO_3. Most cases originate with volume concentration and loss of acid from the stomach or kidney. Less commonly, HCO_3 administered or derived from endogenous lactate is the cause and is perpetuated when renal HCO_3 reabsorption continues. In vomiting, Cl loss reduces its availability for renal reabsorption with Na. Enhanced Na avidity due to volume depletion then accelerates HCO_3 reabsorption and sustains the alkalosis. Urine Cl is typically low (<10 mmol/L) (Table 25-6). Alkalosis may also be maintained by hyperaldosteronism, due to enhancement of H secretion and HCO_3 reabsorption. Severe K depletion also causes metabolic alkalosis by increasing HCO_3 reabsorption; urine Cl >20 mmol/L.

Vomiting and nasogastric drainage cause HCl and volume loss, kaliuresis, and alkalosis. Diuretics are a common cause of alkalosis due to volume contraction, Cl depletion, and hypokalemia. Pts with chronic pulmonary disease, high P_{CO_2} and serum HCO_3 levels, whose ventilation is acutely improved, may develop alkalosis.

Excessive mineralocorticoid activity due to Cushing's syndrome (worse in ectopic ACTH or primary hyperaldosteronism) causes metabolic alkalosis not associated with volume or Cl depletion and not responsive to NaCl.

Severe K depletion also causes metabolic alkalosis.

Diagnosis   The Cl on a random urine is useful (Table 25-6) unless diuretics have been administered.

R̲X̲ TREATMENT

Correct the underlying cause. In cases of Cl depletion, administer NaCl; and in hypokalemia, add KCl. Pts with adrenal hyperfunction require treatment of the underlying disorder.

Severe alkalosis may require, in addition, treatment with acidifying agents such as NH_4Cl, HCl, or acetazolamide. The initial amount of H needed (in mmol) should be calculated from $0.5 \times$ (body wt in kg) $\times$ (serum $HCO_3 - 24$).

RESPIRATORY ACIDOSIS   Characterized by CO_2 retention due to ventilatory failure. Causes include sedatives, stroke, chronic pulmonary disease, airway obstruction, severe pulmonary edema, neuromuscular disorders, and cardiopulmonary arrest.

Symptoms   These include confusion, asterixis, and obtundation.

R̲X̲ TREATMENT

The goal is to improve ventilation through pulmonary toilet and reversal of bronchospasm. Intubation may be required in severe acute cases. Acidosis due to hypercapnia is usually mild.

RESPIRATORY ALKALOSIS   Excessive ventilation causes a primary reduction in CO_2 and $\uparrow$ pH in pneumonia, pulmonary edema, interstitial lung disease, asthma. Pain and psychogenic causes are common; other etiologies include fever, hypoxemia, sepsis, delirium tremens, salicylates, hepatic failure, mechanical overventilation, and CNS lesions. Severe respiratory alkalosis may cause seizures, tetany, cardiac arrhythmias, or loss of consciousness.

℞ TREATMENT

Should be directed at the underlying disorders. In psychogenic cases, sedation or a rebreathing bag may be required.

"MIXED" DISORDERS In many circumstances, more than a single acid-base disturbance exists. Examples include combined metabolic and respiratory acidosis with cardiogenic shock; metabolic alkalosis and acidosis in pts with vomiting and diabetic ketoacidosis; metabolic acidosis with respiratory alkalosis in pts with sepsis. The diagnosis may be clinically evident or suggested by relationships between the P_{CO_2} and HCO_3 that are markedly different from those found in simple disorders.

In simple anion-gap acidosis, anion gap increases in proportion to fall in HCO_3. When increase in anion gap occurs despite a normal HCO_3, simultaneous anion-gap acidosis and metabolic alkalosis are suggested. When fall in HCO_3 due to metabolic acidosis is proportionately larger than increase in anion gap, mixed anion gap and non-anion gap metabolic acidosis is suggested.

For a more detailed discussion, see Singer GG, Brenner BM: Fluids and Electrolyte Disturbances, Chap. 49, p. 265; and DuBose TD Jr: Acidosis and Alkalosis, Chap. 50, p. 277, in HPIM-14.

26

LYMPHADENOPATHY AND SPLENOMEGALY

Lymphadenopathy

Exposure to antigen through a break in the skin or mucosa results in antigen being taken up by an antigen-presenting cell and carried via lymphatic channels to the nearest lymph node. Lymph channels course throughout the body except for the brain and the bones. Lymph enters the node through the afferent vessel and leaves through an efferent vessel. As antigen-presenting cells pass through lymph nodes, they present antigen to lymphocytes residing there. Lymphocytes in a node are constantly being replaced by antigen-naive lymphocytes from the blood. They are retained in the node via special homing receptors. B cells populate the lymphoid follicles in the cortex; T cells populate the paracortical regions. When a B cell encounters an antigen to which its surface immunoglobulin can bind, it stays in the follicle for a few days and forms a germinal center where the immunoglobulin gene is mutated in an effort to make an antibody with higher affinity for the antigen. The B cell then migrates to the medullary region, differentiates into a plasma cell, and secretes immunoglobulin into the efferent lymph.

When a T cell in the node encounters an antigen it recognizes, it proliferates and joins the efferent lymph. The efferent lymph laden with antibodies and T cells specific for the inciting antigen passes through several nodes on its way to the thoracic duct, which drains lymph from most of the body. From the thoracic duct, lymph enters the bloodstream at the left subclavian vein. Lymph from the head and neck and the right arm drain into the right subclavian vein. From the bloodstream, the antibody and T cells localize to the cite of infection.

Lymphadenopathy may be caused by infections, immunologic diseases, malignancies, lipid storage diseases, or a number of disorders of uncertain etiology (e.g., sarcoidosis, Castleman's disease) (see Table 61-1, p. 346 in HPIM-14). The two major mechanisms of lymphadenopathy are hyperplasia, in response to immunologic or infectious stimuli, and infiltration, by cancer cells or lipid- or glycoprotein-laden macrophages.

--------------- *Approach to the Patient* ---------------

History Age, occupation, animal exposures, sexual orientation, substance abuse history, medication history, and concomitant symptoms influence diagnostic workup. Adenopathy is more commonly malignant in origin in people over age 40. Farmers have an increased incidence of brucellosis and lymphoma. Male homosexuals may have AIDS-associated adenopathy. Alcohol and tobacco abuse increase risk of malignancy. Phenytoin may induce adenopathy. The concomitant presence of cervical adenopathy with sore throat or with fever, night sweats, and weight loss suggests particular diagnoses (mononucleosis in the former instance, Hodgkin's disease in the latter).

Physical Examination Location of adenopathy, size, node texture, and the presence of tenderness are important in differential diagnosis. Generalized adenopathy (three or more anatomic regions) implies systemic infection or lymphoma. Subclavian or scalene adenopathy is always abnormal and should be biopsied. Nodes larger than 4 cm should be biopsied immediately. Rock hard nodes fixed to surrounding soft tissue are usually a sign of metastatic carcinoma. Tender nodes are most often benign.

Laboratory Tests Usually lab tests are not required in the setting of localized adenopathy. If generalized adenopathy is noted, an excisional node biopsy should be performed for diagnosis, rather than a panoply of laboratory tests.

℞ TREATMENT

Patients over age 40, those with scalene or supraclavicular adenopathy, those with lymph nodes more than 4 cm in diameter, and those with hard nontender nodes should undergo immediate excisional biopsy. In younger patients with smaller nodes that are rubbery in consistency or tender, a period of observation for 7–14 days is reasonable. Empiric antibiotics are not indicated. If the nodes shrink, no further evaluation is necessary. If they enlarge, excisional biopsy is indicated.

Splenomegaly

Just as the lymph nodes are specialized to fight pathogens in the tissues, the spleen is the lymphoid organ specialized to fight bloodborne pathogens. It has no afferent lymphatics. The spleen has specialized areas like the lymph node for making antibodies (follicles) and amplifying antigen-specific T cells (periarteriolar lymphatic sheath, or PALS). In addition, it has a well-developed reticuloendothelial system for removing particles and antibody-coated bacteria. The flow of blood through the spleen permits it to filter pathogens from the blood and to maintain quality control over erythrocytes (RBCs)—those that are old and nondeformable are destroyed, and intracellular inclusions (sometimes including pathogens like babesia and malaria) are culled from the cells in a process called pitting. Under certain conditions, the spleen can generate hematopoietic cells in place of the marrow.

The normal spleen is about 12 cm in length and 7 cm in width and is not normally palpable. Dullness from the spleen can be percussed between the ninth and eleventh ribs with the pt lying on the right side. Palpation is best performed with the pt supine with knees flexed. The spleen may be felt as it descends when the pt inspires. Physical diagnosis is not sensitive. CT or ultrasound are superior tests.

Spleen enlargement occurs by three basic mechanisms: (1) hyperplasia or hypertrophy due to an increase in demand for splenic function (e.g., hereditary spherocytosis where demand for removal of defective RBC is high or immune hyperplasia in response to systemic infection or immune diseases); (2) passive vascular congestion due to portal hypertension, and (3) infiltration with malignant cells, lipid- or glycoprotein-laden macrophages, or amyloid (see Table 61-2 p. 349, in HPIM-14). Massive enlargement, with spleen palpable >8 cm below the left costal margin, usually signifies a lymphoproliferative or myeloproliferative disorder.

Peripheral blood RBC count, WBC count, and platelet count may be normal, decreased, or increased depending on the underlying disorder. Decreases in one or more cell lineages could indicate hypersplenism, increased destruction. In cases with hypersplenism, the spleen is removed and the cytopenia is generally reversed. In the absence of hypersplenism, most causes of splenomegaly are diagnosed on the basis of signs and symptoms and laboratory abnormalities associated with the underlying disorder. Splenectomy is rarely performed for diagnostic purposes.

People who have had splenectomy are at increased risk of sepsis from a variety of organisms including the pneumococcus and *Haemophilus influenzae*. Vaccines for these agents should be given before splenectomy is performed. Splenectomy compromises the immune response to these T-independent antigens.

For a more detailed discussion, see Henry PH, Longo DL: Enlargement of Lymph Nodes and Spleen, Chap. 61, p. 345, in HPIM-14.

27

CARDIOVASCULAR COLLAPSE AND SUDDEN DEATH

Unexpected cardiovascular collapse and death most often result from ventricular fibrillation in pts with underlying coronary artery disease, with or without acute MI. Other common causes are listed in Table 27-1. The arrhythmic causes may be provoked by electrolyte disorders (primarily hypokalemia), hypoxemia, acidosis, or massive sympathetic discharge, as may occur in CNS injury. Immediate institution of cardiopulmonary resuscitation (CPR) followed by advanced life support measures (see below) are mandatory. Ventricular fibrillation, or asystole, without institution of CPR within 4–6 min, usually causes death.

Table 27-1

Differential Diagnosis of Cardiovascular Collapse and Sudden Death

1. Ventricular fibrillation due to:
   Myocardial ischemia (severe coronary artery disease, acute MI)
   Congestive heart failure
   Dilated or hypertrophic cardiomyopathy
   Myocarditis
   Valvular disease [aortic stenosis, mitral valve prolapse (rare)]
   Preexcitation syndromes (Wolff-Parkinson-White)
   Prolonged QT syndromes (congenital, drug-induced)
2. Asystole or severe bradycardia
3. Sudden marked decrease in LV stroke volume from:
   Massive pulmonary embolism
   Cardiac tamponade
   Severe aortic stenosis
4. Sudden marked decrease in intravascular volume, e.g.:
   Ruptured aortic aneurysm
   Aortic dissection

MANAGEMENT OF CARDIAC ARREST

Basic life support (BLS) commences immediately (Fig. 27-1):

1. Open mouth of patient and remove visible debris or dentures. If there is respiratory stridor, consider aspiration of a foreign body and perform Heimlich maneuver.

2. Tilt head backward, lift chin, and begin mouth-to-mouth respiration if rescue equipment is not available (pocket mask is preferable to prevent transmission of infection). The lungs should be inflated once every 5 s when two persons are performing resuscitation or twice in rapid succession every 15 s when one person performs both ventilation and chest compression.

3. If carotid pulse is absent, perform chest compressions (depressing sternum 3–5 cm) at rate of 80–100 per min. For one rescuer, 15 compressions are performed before returning to ventilating twice.

As soon as resuscitation equipment is available, begin advanced life support (Fig. 27-2) with continued chest compressions and ventilation. Although performed as simultaneously as possible, defibrillation takes highest priority, followed by placement of intravenous access and intubation. 100% O_2 should be administered by endotracheal tube or, if rapid intubation cannot be accomplished, by bag-valve-mask device; respirations should not be interrupted for more than 30 s while attempting to intubate. Initial intravenous access should be through the antecubital vein, but if drug administration is ineffective, a central line (internal jugular or subclavian) should be placed. Intravenous $NaHCO_3$ should be administered only if there is persistent severe acidosis (pH < 7.15) despite adequate ventilation. Calcium is *not* routinely administered but should be given to pts with known hypocalcemia, those who have received toxic doses of calcium channel antagonists, or if acute hyperkalemia is thought to be the triggering event for resistant ventricular fibrillation.

FOLLOW-UP

If cardiac arrest was due to ventricular fibrillation in initial hours of an acute MI, follow-up is standard post-MI care (Chap. 113). For other survivors of a ventricular fibrillation arrest, extensive evaluation, including evaluation of coronary anatomy, left ventricular function, and invasive electrophysiologic testing, is recommended. Long-term antiarrhythmic drug therapy, implantation of an automatic defibrillator, and/or cardiac surgery (coronary artery bypass graft, aneurysmectomy, or resection/ablation of arrhythmic foci) may be necessary.

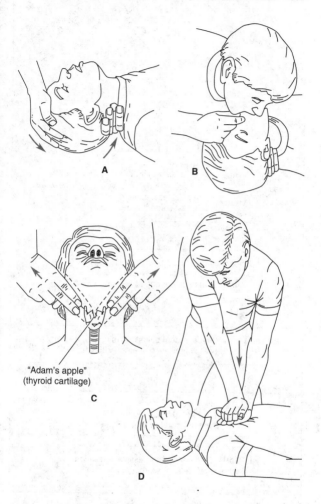

"Adam's apple"
(thyroid cartilage)

FIGURE 27-1   Major steps in cardiopulmonary resuscitation. *A.* Make certain the victim has an open airway. *B.* Start respiratory resuscitation immediately. *C.* Feel for the carotid pulse in the groove alongside the "Adam's apple" or thyroid cartilage. *D.* If pulse is absent, begin cardiac massage. Use 60 compressions/min with one lung inflation after each group of 5 chest compressions. (*From J Henderson, Emergency Medical Guide, 4th ed, New York, McGraw-Hill, 1978.*)

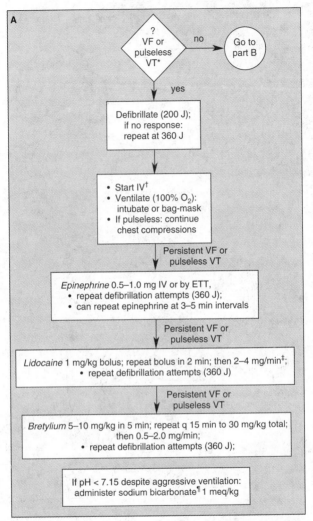

FIGURE 27-2 Advanced life support algorithm. *Rhythm observed by "quick-look" defibrillator paddles; if monitored paddles are not available and patient is pulseless, do blind defibrillation. †Antecubital route preferred; if infusions are not effective, place central (internal jugular, subclavian) line. ‡Procainamide may

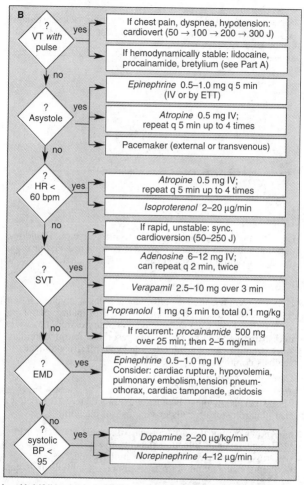

be added if lidocaine is ineffective but loading is prolonged: 500–800 mg, no faster than 20 mg/min, followed by continuous infusion (2–5 mg/min). ¶Do not infuse sodium bicarbonate in same IV line as calcium, epinephrine, or dopamine. ETT, endotracheal tube; VT, ventricular tachycardia; HR, heart rate; SVT, supraventricular tachyarrhythmias; EMD, electromechanical dissociation.

For a more detailed discussion, see Myerburg RJ, Castellanos A: Cardiovascular Collapse, Cardiac Arrest, and Sudden Death, Chap. 39, p. 222, in HPIM-14.

28

SHOCK

Definition

Condition of severe impairment of tissue perfusion. Rapid recognition and treatment are essential to prevent irreversible organ damage. Common causes are listed in Table 28-1.

Clinical Manifestations

Hypotension (systolic bp <90), tachycardia, tachypnea, pallor, restlessness, and altered sensorium; signs of intense peripheral vasoconstriction; weak pulses; cold clammy extremities [*note*: in distributive (e.g., septic) shock, vasodilatation predominates and extremities are warm]. Oliguria (<20 mL/h) and metabolic acidosis common.

Approach to the Patient

Tissue perfusion must be restored immediately (see below); also obtain history for underlying cause, including

- Known cardiac disease (coronary disease, CHF, pericarditis)
- Recent fever or infection (leading to sepsis)
- Drugs, i.e., excess diuretics or antihypertensives
- Predisposing conditions for pulmonary embolism (Chap. 123)
- Possible bleeding from any site, particularly GI tract.

Physical Examination

- Jugular veins are flat in oligemic or distributive shock; jugular venous distention (JVD) suggests cardiogenic shock; JVD

Table 28-1

Common Forms of Shock

Oligemic shock
  Hemorrhage
  Volume depletion (e.g., vomiting, diarrhea, diuretic over-usage, ketoacidosis)
  Internal sequestration (ascites, pancreatitis, intestinal obstruction)
Cardiogenic shock
  Myopathic (acute MI, dilated cardiomyopathy)
  Mechanical (acute mitral regurgitation, ventricular septal defect, severe aortic stenosis)
  Arrhythmic
Extracardiac obstructive shock
  Pericardial tamponade
  Massive pulmonary embolism
  Tension pneumothorax
Distributive shock (profound decrease in systemic vascular tone)
  Sepsis
  Toxic overdoses
  Anaphylaxis
  Neurogenic (e.g., spinal cord injury)
  Endocrinologic (Addison's disease, myxedema)

in presence of paradoxical pulse (Chap. 104) may reflect cardiac tamponade (Chap. 112).
- Look for evidence of CHF (Chap. 108), murmurs of aortic stenosis, acute regurgitation (mitral or aortic), ventricular septal defect.
- Check for asymmetry of pulses (aortic dissection).
- Tenderness or rebound in abdomen may indicate peritonitis or pancreatitis; high-pitched bowel sounds suggest intestinal obstruction. Perform stool guaiac to rule out GI bleeding.
- Fever and chills usually accompany septic shock. Sepsis may not cause fever in elderly, uremic, or alcoholic patients.
- Skin lesion may suggest specific pathogens in septic shock: petechiae or purpura (*Neisseria meningitidis*), ecythyma gangrenosum (*Pseudomonas aeruginosa*), generalized erythroderma (toxic shock due to *Staphylococcus aureus* or *Streptococcus pyogenes*).

Laboratory

Obtain hematocrit, WBC, electrolytes. If actively bleeding, check platelet count, PT, PTT, DIC screen. Arterial blood gas usually shows metabolic acidosis (in septic shock, respiratory alkalosis precedes metabolic acidosis). If sepsis suspected, draw blood cultures, perform urinalysis, and obtain Gram stain and cultures of sputum, urine, and other suspected sites.

Obtain ECG (myocardial ischemia or acute arrhythmia), chest x-ray (CHF, tension pneumothorax, aortic dissection, pneumonia). Echocardiogram may be helpful (cardiac tamponade, CHF). Central venous pressure or pulmonary capillary wedge (PCW) pressure measurements may be necessary to distinguish between the different categories of shock (Table 28-2): Mean PCW <6 mmHg suggests oligemic or distributive shock; PCW >20 mmHg suggests left ventricular failure. Cardiac output is decreased in patients with cardiogenic and oligemic shock, and usually increased initially in septic shock.

Table 28-2

Hemodynamic Profiles in Shock States

Diagnosis	PCW Pressure	Cardiac Output (CO)	Systemic Vascular Resistance	Comments
Cardiogenic shock	↑	↓	↑	PCW is normal or ↓ in RV infarction
Extracardiac obstructive shock				
Cardiac tamponade	↑	↓	↑	Equalization of intracardiac diastolic pressures
Massive pulmonary embolus	Normal or ↓	↓	↓	Right-sided cardiac pressures may be elevated
Oligemic shock	↓	↓	↑	
Distributive shock	↓	↑	↓	CO may ↓ later if sepsis results in LV dysfunction

℞ TREATMENT

Aimed at rapid improvement of tissue hypoperfusion and respiratory impairment:

1. Serial measurements of bp (intraarterial line preferred), heart rate, continuous ECG monitor, urine output, pulse oximetry, blood studies: Hct, electrolytes, creatinine, BUN, ABGs, calcium, phosphate, lactate, urine Na concentration (<20 mmol/L suggests volume depletion). Continuous monitoring of CVP and/or pulmonary artery pressure, with serial PCW pressures.

2. Augment systolic bp to >100 mmHg: (a) place in reverse Trendelenburg position; (b) IV volume infusion (500 mL bolus), unless PCW >20 mmHg (begin with normal saline, then whole blood, dextran, or packed RBCs, if anemic); (c) vasoactive drugs are added after intravascular volume is optimized; administer vasopressors (Table 28-3) if systemic vascular resistance (SVR) is decreased (begin with dopamine; for persistent hypotension add norepinephrine or phenylephrine); vasodilators (see Table 108-1) if SVR is elevated, as long as systolic bp >90 mmHg; (d) if CHF present, add inotropic agents (usually dobutamine) (Chap. 108); aim to maintain cardiac index >2.2 (L/m^2)/min [>4.0 (L/m^2)/min in septic shock].

3. Administer 100% O_2; intubate with mechanical ventilation if P_{O_2} <70 mmHg.

4. If severe metabolic acidosis present (pH < 7.15), administer $NaHCO_3$ (44.6–89.2 mmol).

5. Identify and treat underlying cause of shock. Cardiogenic shock in acute MI is discussed in Chap. 113.

Septic shock can rapidly result in the acute respiratory distress syndrome, acute tubular necrosis, DIC, multiple organ failure, or death. Successful management relies on immediate hemodynamic and respiratory support and eliminating the infecting organism. A Gram stain of the primary site of infection, if known, helps to direct antimicrobial therapy. In overwhelming sepsis (e.g., pneumococcal bacteremia in a splenectomized patient), the organism may sometimes be identified on buffy coat smear of peripheral blood. If no source of infection identified, initiate empirical antibiotic therapy after cultures of potentially infected tissues are obtained (e.g., blood, urine, sputum, pleural effusion, CSF).

It is essential to drain foci of septic material. Potentially infected intravenous or urinary catheters should be removed and cultured. Look for occult sites of infection, e.g., sinusitis, perianal abscess, dental abscess, infected decubitus ulcer. In

Table 28-3

Vasopressors Used in Shock States*

Drug	Dose, (μg/kg)/min	Notes
Dopamine	1–5	Facilitates diuresis
	5–10	Positive inotropic and chronotropic effects; most useful agent in shock states in this and higher dose range
	10–20	Generalized vasoconstriction (decreases renal perfusion)
Norepinephrine	2–8	Potent vasoconstrictor; moderate inotropic effect; may result in myocardial ischemia/arrhythmias; may be useful in cardiogenic shock with reduced SVR but should generally be reserved for refractory hypotension
Dobutamine	1–10	Primarily for cardiogenic shock (Chap. 113): positive inotrope; lacks vasoconstrictor activity; most useful when only mild hypotension present and avoidance of tachycardia desired
Phenylephrine	20–200	Potent vasoconstrictor without inotropic effect; may be useful in distributive (septic) shock

*Isoproterenol not recommended in shock states because of potential hypotension and arrhythmogenic effects.

suspected urosepsis, a renal or perinephric abscess can be evaluated by ultrasound, CT, or MRI.

Hemodynamic support must be provided as in other causes of shock to maintain tissue perfusion. Large volumes of intravascular fluid are often necessary and should be gauged by the PCW pressure (desired range 12–15 mmHg) or CVP (desired range 10–12 cmH$_2$O) and urinary output (aim for ≥30 mL/h). Maintain systolic bp ≤90 mmHg by repleting intravascular volume and, if necessary, by vasopressors (see Table 28-3): dopamine 5–10 (μg/kg)/min, followed, if needed, by norepinephrine or phenylephrine.

Consider the possible complication of adrenal insufficiency if patient has septic shock with fulminant *N. meningitidis* infection, refractory hypotension, recent glucocorticoid use, disseminated tuberculosis, or AIDS. Administer hydrocortisone 50 mg IV q6h while evaluating this possibility (Chap. 163).

For a more detailed discussion, see Hollenberg S, Parrillo JE: Shock, Chap. 38, p. 214; and Munford RS: Sepsis and Septic Shock, Chap. 124, p. 776, in HPIM-14.

29

ACUTE PULMONARY EDEMA

Life-threatening, acute development of alveolar lung edema is most often due to (1) elevation of hydrostatic pressure in the pulmonary capillaries (left heart failure, mitral stenosis) or (2) increased permeability of the pulmonary alveolar-capillary membrane. Specific precipitants (Table 29-1) result in cardiogenic pulmonary edema in pts with previously compensated CHF or without previous cardiac history.

Physical Findings

Patient appears severely ill, sitting bolt upright, tachypneic, dyspneic, with marked perspiration; cyanosis may be present. Bilateral pulmonary rales; third heart sound may be present. The sputum is frothy and blood-tinged.

Laboratory Data

In early stages, arterial blood gas measurements demonstrate reductions of both Pa_{O_2} and Pa_{CO_2}; later, with progressive respiratory failure, hypercapnia develops with progressive acidemia. CXR shows pulmonary vascular redistribution, diffuse haziness in the lung fields with perihilar "butterfly" appearance.

 TREATMENT

Immediate, aggressive therapy is mandatory for survival. The following measures should be instituted nearly simultaneously:

1. Seat patient upright to reduce venous return.
2. Administer 100% O_2 by mask to achieve $Pa_{O_2} > 60$ mmHg.
3. Intravenous loop diuretic (furosemide 40–100 mg or bumetanide 1 mg); use lower dose if patient does not take diuretics chronically.
4. Morphine 2–5 mg IV (repetitively); assess frequently for hypotension or respiratory depression; naloxone should be available to reverse effects of morphine, if necessary.
5. Afterload reduction [IV sodium nitroprusside (20–300 μg/min) if systolic bp > 100 mmHg]; arterial line should be placed for continuous bp monitoring.

Additional therapy may be required if rapid improvement does not ensue:

1. Inotropic agents, such as dobutamine (Chap. 28), may be helpful in cardiogenic pulmonary edema with shock.

Table 29-1

Precipitants of Acute Pulmonary Edema

Acute tachy- or bradyarrhythmia
Infection, fever
Acute MI
Severe hypertension
Acute mitral or aortic regurgitation
Increased circulating volume (Na ingestion, blood transfusion, pregnancy)
Increased metabolic demands (exercise, hyperthyroidism)
Pulmonary embolism
Noncompliance (sudden discontinuation) of chronic CHF medications

---

2. Aminophylline [6 mg/kg IV over 20 min, then 0.2–0.5 (mg/kg)/h] reduces bronchospasm and augments myocardial contractility and diuresis; can be used as initial therapy, in place of morphine, if not clear whether dyspnea is due to pulmonary edema or severe obstructive lung disease, before CXR is obtained.
3. If rapid diuresis does not follow diuretic administration, intravascular volume can be reduced by phlebotomy (removal of ~250 mL through antecubital vein) or by placement of rotating tourniquets on the extremities.
4. For persistent hypoxemia or hypercapnia, intubation may be required.

The precipitating cause of pulmonary edema (Table 29-1) should be sought and treated, particularly acute arrhythmias or infection.

Several noncardiogenic conditions may result in pulmonary edema (Table 29-2) in the absence of left heart dysfunction; therapy is directed toward the primary condition.

Table 29-2

Examples of Noncardiogenic Pulmonary Edema

Decreased plasma oncotic pressure
  Hypoalbuminemia

Excessive alveolar-capillary permeability
  Diffuse pulmonary infection
  Inhaled toxins (e.g., phosgene, smoke)
  Gram-negative sepsis or endotoxemia
  Aspiration pneumonia
  Thermal or radiation lung injury
  Disseminated intravascular coagulation
  Acute hemorrhagic pancreatitis

Lymphatic insufficiency
  After lung transplantation
  Lymphangitic carcinomatosis

Unknown mechanism
  High-altitude exposure
  Acute CNS disorders
  Narcotic overdose
  Following cardiopulmonary bypass

For a more detailed discussion, see Ingram RH Jr, Braunwald E: Dyspnea and Pulmonary Edema, Chap. 32, p. 190, in HPIM-14.

30

EMERGENCY ROOM EVALUATION OF STROKE

Stroke is a clinical term applied to a neurologic deficit due to cerebrovascular disease. For a detailed discussion of stroke see Chap. 174. This chapter deals with the ER evaluation of pts suspected of having a stroke. Two goals of management for acute neurologic deficits: (1) to distinguish stroke from conditions that mimic stroke, and (2) to intervene rapidly to improve outcome. Ischemia accounts for the vast majority of acute strokes; approximately 20% are due to primary hemorrhage. An ischemic deficit that rapidly resolves is termed a *transient ischemic attack* (TIA); 24 h has historically been held as the boundary between TIA and stroke. These clinical terms do not coincide perfectly with reversible tissue ischemia and infarction; at presentation, it is usually not possible to identify pts with reversible tissue ischemia.

DIFFERENTIAL DIAGNOSIS OF ACUTE STROKE

When a pt presents with an acute neurologic deficit, stroke should be a prime consideration. However, other conditions can mimic this syndrome, including the following:

1. *Metabolic disturbances:* Metabolic disturbances, especially hyponatremia, hypoglycemia, and nonketotic hyperosmolar hyperglycemia, may produce asymmetric neurologic signs; all pts should have tests of serum electrolytes and glucose.

2. *Intracerebral mass lesions:* Mass lesions such as brain tumors and abscesses may present suddenly, presumably from compression of local vascular structures or sudden expansion from hemorrhage. A head CT scan will usually identify the mass lesion.

3. *Expanding extracerebral masses:* Extracerebral masses (e.g., subdural hematoma or epidural hematoma) may present with sudden onset of neurologic deficit. Usually there is a history of trauma; diagnosis is made by CT scan.

4. *Postseizure paralysis:* If a pt presents with an altered level of consciousness and an asymmetric motor exam, the possibility of a postictal (Todd) paralysis should be considered. This diagnosis is supported by a history of a seizure disorder, a witnessed seizure, or clearance of the mental status and the motor disorder in a matter of hours. Altered consciousness is rare with a TIA.

5. *Acute mononeuropathies:* Certain mononeuropathies, especially Bell's palsy, radial nerve palsy, and peroneal nerve

palsy, may be mistaken for a minor stroke. A detailed neurologic exam will reveal that the pattern of weakness and numbness is in the distribution of a cranial or peripheral nerve.

6.   *Migraine:* Complicated migraine can be associated with visual loss, hemiparesis, sensory loss, vertigo, dysarthria or confusion. Useful is a prior history of similar spells and an associated typical headache. In the ER, complicated migraine is generally a diagnosis of exclusion.

7.   *Psychogenic causes:* Numerous psychiatric disorders, including hysteria, malingering, and catatonia, may appear abruptly. The absence of nonvolitional physical signs (especially reflex changes), normal radiologic and laboratory studies, and a known history of a specific psychiatric disorder may all point to a psychogenic cause, which still should be a diagnosis of exclusion.

STROKE SYNDROMES: EARLY INTERVENTION

All efforts must first be directed to minimize the extent of tissue injury, then to reduce the risk of recurrent events.

ACUTE STROKE INTERVENTION   Assure adequate oxygenation and hemodynamic stability. The bp should not be acutely lowered unless extremely elevated (systolic >220 mmHg), and then only with agents that allow gradual, predictable control. A head CT without contrast is required on an urgent basis, not to visualize infarction but to exclude hemorrhage or other lesions.

ISCHEMIC STROKE   Acute intervention is indicated for pts with ischemic deficits who present to the ER within 3 h of their onset. Thrombolytic therapy is approved for use in this interval, provided hemorrhage has been excluded; IV recombinant tissue plasminogen activator improves neurologic outcome, and other thrombolytic treatments are currently in trial.

The role of anticoagulation in acute stroke is uncertain; many clinicians consider heparin for prevention of recurrent events in pts with transient, or mild to moderate, deficits related to emboli from a cardiac or carotid source.

Pts frequently present to the ER with a history suggestive of TIA. When there is suspicion of underlying carotid stenosis, atrial fibrillation, or other stroke mechanism with high risk of recurrent events, acute heparinization and admission to hospital are advisable.

HEMORRHAGE   Subarachnoid hemorrhage (SAH) is associated with sudden and severe headache. The head CT is usually diagnostic, although occasional cases require lumbar puncture for diagnosis. The aim of acute management is bp control to limit risk of rebleeding. The bp can be lowered to systolic <150 mmHg if pt is awake or intracranial pressure is monitored to assure preservation of adequate cerebral perfusion pressure >60 mmHg (cerebral perfusion pressure = mean arterial pressure − intracranial pressure). Vasospasm may occur between days 4 and 14 after hemorrhage and lead to ischemia and stroke. Pts seen in this interval should not have aggressive lowering of bp until evaluation is completed. Seizures are infrequent following SAH but may precipitate rebleeding; thus anticonvulsants are employed through the acute period. Nimodipine is usually begun as soon as diagnosis of SAH is made to help prevent neurologic deficit related to vasospasm. Emergent neurosurgical consultation or referral is necessary, as early aneurysm treatment is optimal.

Intraparenchymal cerebellar hemorrhage usually presents with headache and difficulty walking; ER evaluation should include gait testing. Head CT confirms the diagnosis. These lesions can lead to acute hydrocephalus and brainstem compression with rapid progression to death. Neurosurgical consultation should be sought, as clot evacuation is often necessary and associated with good recovery.

Hemorrhage deep in the cerebral nuclei such as the thalamus or basal ganglia is typically related to long-standing hypertension. Neurosurgical management of hydrocephalus may be necessary, although evacuation of the clot is usually not done.

PREVENTION OF RECURRENT STROKE

For most pts with stroke, the cause is a generalized vascular disorder associated with a chronic condition such as smoking, chronic hypertension, elevated cholesterol and lipids, or diabetes mellitus. Treatment of these conditions clearly reduces the risk for subsequent stroke in the years ahead; all pts require a comprehensive review of stroke risk factors and incorporation of risk-reduction measures into their primary health care program. However, some causes carry a substantial risk of recurrence in the days or weeks ahead and should be considered for every pt. In the ER, the laboratory evaluation of all pts with an acute stroke should include, as a minimum, a CBC, platelet count, serum electrolytes and glucose, PT/PTT, ESR, VDRL, and ECG. Additional tests depend on suspicion of the following etiologies:

ISCHEMIC STROKE Emboli, particularly from a cardiac source, carry a high risk of recurrence. Predisposing conditions such as rheumatic heart disease, atrial fibrillation, endocarditis (infective and noninfective), prior myocardial infarction, prosthetic heart valve, patent foramen ovale, and mitral valve prolapse are all associated with embolic strokes. If cardioembolic stroke is suspected by history and physical exam, an echocardiogram, blood cultures, and possibly a Holter monitor should be performed. Treatment should be directed at the cause, with anticoagulation, antiarrhythmic therapy, or antibiotics, either alone or in combination. Certain hematologic conditions, such as hypercoagulable states (e.g., associated with pregnancy, cancer, paraproteinemia), hyperviscosity syndromes (e.g., polycythemia, leukocytosis, thrombocytosis), and sickle cell disease, predispose to intravascular thrombosis and embolization. Although many of these conditions will be detected in routine blood tests, some of the hypercoagulable states are clinical associations without confirmatory laboratory tests. Heparin therapy may be useful for some hypercoagulable states. For hyperviscosity syndromes, cerebral ischemia from polycythemia may respond to venesection; other proliferative disorders require chemotherapy. Disorders of blood vessels such as cerebral vasculitis and fibromuscular dysplasia may also predispose to recurrent strokes; blood tests such as ESR, VDRL, and ANA and urine tests for cocaine and amphetamines may indicate specific etiologies, but cerebral angiography is necessary to confirm the diagnosis of a vasculopathy. Immune suppressive treatment is indicated for vasculitis, and antibiotic therapy for infectious etiologies. For noninflammatory vascular conditions, surgical treatment or angioplasty of the abnormal vascular structure may be indicated.

HEMORRHAGE The risk of recurrence is high if a hemorrhage occurs because of a primary defect in blood clotting arising from either a platelet disorder [e.g., thrombocytopenia, as with thrombotic and idiopathic thrombocytopenic purpura (ITP), or antiplatelet therapy] or a disorder of coagulation (e.g., hemophilia, DIC, anticoagulation therapy). These diagnoses should be considered when there is a history of a bleeding tendency, a history of antiplatelet or anticoagulation treatment, or abnormalities of the platelet count or blood coagulation studies. Therapy is aimed at restoring normal clotting function (e.g., platelet transfusion for thrombocytopenia, fresh frozen plasma and vitamin K for oral anticoagulation therapy) as well as treatment of the underlying cause (e.g., DIC, ITP) of the clotting disorder.

For a more detailed discussion, see Easton JD, Hauser SL, Martin JB: Cerebrovascular Diseases, Chap. 366, p. 2325, in HPIM-14.

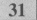
INCREASED INTRACRANIAL PRESSURE AND HEAD TRAUMA

Increased Intracranial Pressure

A limited volume of extra tissue, blood, CSF, or edema fluid can be added to the intracranial contents without raising the intracranial pressure (ICP). Pts will deteriorate and may die when ICP reaches levels that compromise cerebral perfusion or causes a shift in intracranial contents that distorts vital brainstem centers.

CLINICAL MANIFESTATIONS Symptoms of high ICP include headache (especially a constant ache that is worse upon awakening), nausea, emesis, drowsiness, diplopia, and blurred vision. Papilledema and sixth nerve palsies are common. If not controlled, then cerebral hypoperfusion, pupillary dilatation, coma, decerebrate posturing, abnormal respirations, systemic hypertension, and bradycardia may result.

A posterior fossa mass, which may initially cause ataxia, stiff neck, and nausea, is especially dangerous because it can compress vital brainstem structures and cause obstructive hydrocephalus. Masses that cause raised ICP also distort midbrain and diencephalic anatomy, leading to stupor and coma. Brain tissue is pushed away from the mass against fixed intracranial structures and into spaces not normally occupied. Herniation syndromes include (1) medial cortex displaced under the midline falx → anterior or posterior cerebral artery occlusion and stroke; (2) uncus displaced through the tentorium, compressing the third cranial nerve and pushing the cerebral peduncle against the tentorium → ipsilateral pupillary dilatation, contralateral hemiparesis, and posterior cerebral artery occlusion; (3) cerebellar tonsils displaced into the foramen magnum, causing medullary compression, → cardiorespiratory collapse; and (4) downward displacement of the diencephalon through the tentorium.

Rx **TREATMENT**
Cerebral perfusion pressure (CPP) = BP − ICP. Global cerebral ischemia occurs when CPP <45 mmHg. Hypertension should be treated carefully, if at all. Hypertensive therapy is used to maintain CPP >60 mmHg in pts with head trauma. Careful intubation (without causing gagging or coughing) allows controlled hyperventilation to lower ICP quickly. The arterial P_{CO_2} should be maintained around 30 mmHg. Mannitol (1 g/kg) lowers ICP by decreasing interstitial brain fluid. Lasix is somewhat less effective. Free H_2O should be restricted.

Pt's head should be elevated to 45 degrees. Treat fever aggressively.

EVALUATION OF PATIENT After stabilization and initiation of the above therapies, a CT scan (or MRI, if feasible) is performed to delineate the cause of the elevated ICP. Emergency surgical intervention is sometimes necessary to decompress the intracranial contents. Hydrocephalus, cerebellar stroke with edema, surgically accessible cerebral hemorrhage or tumor, and subdural or epidural hemorrhage often require lifesaving neurosurgery. ICP monitoring can guide medical and surgical decisions in pts with cerebral edema due to stroke, head trauma, Reye's syndrome, and intracerebral hemorrhage. High doses of barbiturates may decrease ICP in otherwise refractory pts, and in these pts ICP monitoring is obligatory.

Trauma to the CNS

Head trauma can cause immediate loss of consciousness. If transient and unaccompanied by other serious brain pathology, it is called *concussion*. Prolonged alterations in consciousness may be due to parenchymal, subdural, or epidural hematoma or to diffuse shearing of axons in the white matter. Skull fracture should be suspected in pts with CSF rhinorrhea, hemotympanum, and periorbital or mastoid ecchymoses. Spinal cord trauma can cause transient loss of function or a permanent loss of motor, sensory, and autonomic function below the damaged spinal level. (See also Chap. 4.)

℞ TREATMENT

The neck should be immobilized and spine kept straight; vital functions should be stabilized. An initial neurologic exam should determine the level of consciousness, visual acuity, cranial nerve palsies, gross motor and sensory deficits, presence of blood in the middle ear, visible evidence of head trauma, and presence of pain over spine. Cervical spine films should be evaluated before neck is freed. Dysfunction below a spinal level suggests cord injury; lesions at the C5 level or above can threaten respiratory function. If x-rays show aberration of vertebral alignment, then reduction should be quickly undertaken. Spinal CT scan, MRI, or myelography may show evidence of reversible cord compression. The pt with minor head injury who is alert and attentive after short period of unconsciousness (<1 min) sometimes has headache with a single episode of emesis or mild vertigo. Head injury of intermediate severity causes more prolonged loss of consciousness followed by persistent emesis and change in mental state. CT scan or MRI is required to exclude subdural or epidural hematoma and to define extent of contusions and posttraumatic edema. CT scan may be normal in comatose pts with axonal shearing lesions in cerebral white matter. Pts with intermediate head injury require medical observation to detect increasing drowsiness, respiratory dysfunction, and pupillary enlargement, as well as to ensure fluid restriction. Management of pts with raised ICP due to head injury is outlined above.

For a more detailed discussion, see Ropper AH: Traumatic Injuries of the Head and Spine, Chap. 374, p. 2390, in HPIM-14.

STATUS EPILEPTICUS

Definition

Continuous seizures or repetitive, discrete seizures with impaired consciousness in the interictal period. Condition may occur with all kinds of seizures: grand mal (tonic-clonic) status, myoclonic status, petit mal status, and temporal lobe (complex partial) status. Generalized, tonic-clonic seizures are most common and are usually clinically obvious early in the course. After 30–45 min, the signs may become increasingly subtle and include mild clonic movements of the fingers or fine, rapid movements of the eyes. In some situations, EEG may be the only method of diagnosis. Generalized status may be life-threatening when accompanied by hyperpyrexia, acidosis (from prolonged muscle activity), or respiratory or cardiovascular compromise. Irreversible neuronal injury may occur when tonic-clonic seizures persist for more than 2 h.

Etiology

Principal causes of tonic-clonic status are antiepileptic drug withdrawal or noncompliance, alcohol-related, refractory epilepsy, CNS infection, drug toxicity, metabolic disturbances, CNS tumors, cerebrovascular disease, and head trauma.

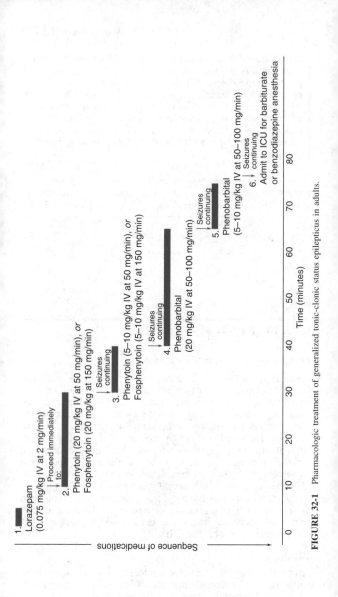

FIGURE 32-1 Pharmacologic treatment of generalized tonic-clonic status epilepticus in adults.

Sequence of medications →

1. Lorazepam (0.075 mg/kg IV at 2 mg/min)
   Proceed immediately to:
2. Phenytoin (20 mg/kg IV at 50 mg/min), or Fosphenytoin (20 mg/kg at 150 mg/min)
   → Seizures continuing
3. Phenytoin (5–10 mg/kg IV at 50 mg/min), or Fosphenytoin (5–10 mg/kg IV at 150 mg/min)
   → Seizures continuing
4. Phenobarbital (20 mg/kg IV at 50–100 mg/min)
   → Seizures continuing
5. Phenobarbital (5–10 mg/kg IV at 50–100 mg/min)
   → Seizures continuing
6. Admit to ICU for barbiturate or benzodiazepine anesthesia

Time (minutes)
0   10   20   30   40   50   60   70   80

℞ TREATMENT

Generalized tonic-clonic status epilepticus is a medical emergency. Pts must be evaluated promptly and appropriate therapy instituted without delay. In parallel, it is essential to determine the cause of the seizures to prevent recurrence and treat any underlying abnormalities.

1. Assess carefully for evidence of respiratory or cardiovascular insufficiency. With careful monitoring and standard airway protection, pts usually do not require intubation (if intubation is necessary, use short-acting paralytics). Treat hyperthermia. Establish IV and administer 50 mL 50% dextrose in water, 100 mg thiamine, and 0.4 mg naloxone (Narcan).

2. Do a brief medical and neurologic examination; send samples for laboratory studies aimed at identifying metabolic abnormalities (CBC with differential, serum electrolytes including calcium, liver and renal function tests, toxicology if indicated).

3. Administer lorazepam, 0.075 mg/kg (3–6 mg) at 2 mg/min (see Fig. 32-1). Repeat after 5 min if seizures persist.

4. Immediately after first lorazepam dose, administer phenytoin, 20 mg/kg (1000–1500 mg) IV slowly over 20 min (50 mg/min) *or* fosphenytoin, 20 mg/kg (150 mg/min). Monitor bp, ECG, and, if possible, EEG during infusion. Phenytoin can cause precipitous fall in bp if given too quickly, especially in elderly pts. (Do not administer phenytoin with 5% dextrose in water—phenytoin precipitates at low pH. This is not a problem with fosphenytoin.) If seizures are not controlled, a repeat bolus of phenytoin (7 mg/kg) *or* fosphenytoin (7 mg/kg) may be given.

5. If seizures persist, administer phenobarbital 20 mg/kg (1000–1500 mg) slowly over 30 min. Endotracheal intubation will often be required by this stage. If seizures continue, give additional dose of phenobarbital (7 mg/kg).

6. If seizures remain refractory after 60–90 min, consider placing pt in midazolam, propofol, or pentobarbital coma. Consultation with a neurologist and anesthesiologist is advised.

Prognosis

The mortality rate is 20% in tonic-clonic status, and the incidence of permanent neurologic sequelae is another 10–30%.

For a more detailed discussion, see Lowenstein DH: Seizures and Epilepsy, Chap. 365, p. 2311, in HPIM-14.

33

POISONING AND ITS MANAGEMENT

Chemical exposures result in an estimated 5 million requests in the U.S. for medical advice or treatment each year, and about 5% of victims of chemical exposure require hospitalization. Suicide attempts account for most serious or fatal poisonings. About 5% of ICU admissions and 30% of psychiatric admissions are poison victims. The diagnosis must be considered in any pt who presents with coma, seizure, or acute renal, hepatic, or bone marrow failure.

DIAGNOSIS

The correct diagnosis can usually be reached by history, physical exam, and laboratory evaluation. Initial assessment of vital signs, cardiopulmonary status, and neurologic function determines the need for immediate supportive treatment. All available sources should be used to determine the exact nature of the ingestion or exposure. The Physicians Desk Reference, regional poison control centers, and local/hospital pharmacies may be useful for identification of ingredients and potential effects of toxins.

 TREATMENT

Goals of therapy include support of vital signs, prevention of further absorption, enhancement of elimination, administration of specific antidotes, and prevention of reexposure. Fundamentals of poisoning management are listed in Table 33-1. Treatment is usually initiated before routine and toxicologic data are known. All symptomatic patients need large-bore IV access, supplemental O_2, cardiac monitoring, continuous observation, and, if mental status is altered, 100 mg thiamine (IM or IV), 1 ampule of 50% dextrose in water, and 4 mg of naloxone along with specific antidotes as indicated. Unconscious pts should be intubated. Activated charcoal may be given PO or via a large-bore gastric tube; gastric lavage requires an orogastric tube. Severity of poisoning determines the management. Suicidal pts require constant observation by qualified personnel.

Supportive Care Airway protection is mandatory. Gag reflex alone is not a reliable indicator of the need for intubation. Need for O_2 supplementation and ventilatory support can be assessed by measurement of arterial blood gases. Drug-induced pulmonary edema is usually secondary to hypoxia, but myocardial depression may contribute. Measurement of

Table 33-1

Fundamentals of Poisoning Management

SUPPORTIVE CARE

Airway protection	Treatment of seizures
Oxygenation/ventilation	Correction of temperature
Treatment of arrhythmias	abnormalities
Hemodynamic support	Correction of metabolic
	derangements
	Prevention of secondary
	complications

PREVENTION OF FURTHER POISON ABSORPTION

Gastrointestinal	Decontamination of other
decontamination	sites
Syrup of ipecac–induced	Eye decontamination
emesis	Skin decontamination
Gastric lavage	Body cavity evacuation
Activated charcoal	
Whole bowel irrigation	
Catharsis	
Dilution	
Endoscopic/surgical	
removal	

ENHANCEMENT OF POISON ELIMINATION

Multiple-dose activated	Extracorporeal removal
charcoal	Peritoneal dialysis
Forced diuresis	Hemodialysis
Alteration of urinary pH	Hemoperfusion
Chelation	Hemofiltration
	Plasmapheresis
	Exchange transfusion
	Hyperbaric oxgenation

ADMINISTRATION OF ANTIDOTES

Neutralization by	Metabolic antagonism
antibodies	Physiologic antagonism
Neutralization by chemical	
binding	

PREVENTION OF REEXPOSURE

Adult education	Notification of regulatory
Child-proofing	agencies
	Psychiatric referral

SOURCE: Modified from Linden CH, Lovejoy FH: HPIM-14, p. 2526.

pulmonary artery pressure may be necessary to establish etiology. Electrolyte imbalances should be corrected as soon as possible.

Supraventricular tachycardia (SVT) with hypertension and CNS excitation is almost always due to sympathetic, anticholinergic, or hallucinogenic stimulation or to drug withdrawal. Treatment is indicated if associated with hemodynamic instability, chest pain, or ischemia on ECG. Treatment with combined alpha and beta blockers or combinations of beta blocker and vasodilator is indicated in severe sympathetic hyperactivity. Physostigmine is useful for anticholinergic hyperactivity. SVT without hypertension usually responds to fluid administration.

Ventricular tachycardia (VT) can be caused by sympathetic stimulation, myocardial membrane destabilization, or metabolic derangements. Lidocaine and phenytoin are generally safe. Drugs that prolong the QT interval (quinidine, procainamide) should not be used in VT due to tricyclic antidepressant overdose. Magnesium sulfate and overdrive pacing (by isoproterenol or a pacemaker) may be useful for torsades de pointes. Arrhythmias may be resistant to therapy until underlying acid-base and electrolyte derangements, hypoxia, and hypothermia are corrected. It is acceptable to observe hemodynamically stable pts without pharmacologic intervention.

Seizures are best treated with γ-aminobutyric acid agonists such as benzodiazepines or barbiturates. Barbiturates should only be given after intubation. Seizures caused by isoniazid overdose may respond only to large doses of pyridoxine IV. Seizures from beta blockers or tricyclic antidepressants may require phenytoin and benzodiazepines.

Prevention of Poison Absorption   Syrup of ipecac is administered orally in doses of 30 mL for adults, 15 mL for children, and 10 mL for infants. Vomiting should occur within 20 min. Ipecac is contraindicated with marginal airway patency, CNS depression, recent GI surgery, seizures, corrosive (lye) ingestion, petroleum hydrocarbon ingestion, and rapidly acting CNS poisons (camphor, cyanide, tricyclic antidepressants, propoxyphene, strychnine). Ipecac is particularly useful in the field.

Gastric lavage is performed using a 28F orogastric tube in children and a 40F orogastric tube in adults. Saline or tap water may be used in adults or children (use saline in infants). Place pt in Trendelenburg and left lateral decubitus position to minimize aspiration (occurs in 10% of pts). Lavage is contraindicated with corrosives and petroleum distillate hydrocarbons because of risk of aspiration-induced pneumonia and gastroesophageal perforation.

Activated charcoal is given orally or by nasogastric or orogastric tube in doses of 1–2 g/kg of body weight, using 8 mL of diluent per gram of charcoal. Premixed formulations are usually available in emergency rooms. The agent may be given with a cathartic (sorbitol) to speed elimination. In pts treated within 1 h, lavage followed by charcoal is more effective than charcoal alone. Charcoal may inhibit absorption of other orally administered agents and is contraindicated in pts with corrosive ingestion.

Whole-bowel irrigation may be useful with ingestions of foreign-bodies, drug packets, and slow-release medications. Golytely is given orally or by gastric tube up to a rate of 0.5 L/h. Cathartic salts (magnesium citrate) and saccharides (sorbitol, mannitol) promote evacuation of the rectum. Dilution of corrosive acids and alkali is accomplished by having pt drink 5 mL water/kg. Endoscopy or surgical intervention may be required in large foreign-body ingestion, heavy metal ingestion, and when ingested drug packets leak or rupture.

Skin and eyes are decontaminated by washing with copious amounts of water or saline.

Enhancement of Elimination   Activated charcoal in repeated doses of 1 g/kg q2–4h is useful for ingestions of drugs with enteral circulation such as carbamazepine, dapsone, diazepam, digoxin, glutethimide, meprobamate, methotrexate, phenobarbital, phenytoin, salicylate, theophylline, and valproic acid.

Forced alkaline diuresis enhances the elimination of chlorphenoxyacetic acid herbicides, chlorpropamide, diflunisal, fluoride, methotrexate, phenobarbital, sulfonamides, and salicylates. Sodium bicarbonate, 1–2 ampules per liter of 0.45% NaCl, is given at a rate sufficient to maintain urine pH ≥7.5 and urine output at 3–6 mL/kg per h. Acid diuresis is no longer recommended. Saline diuresis may enhance elimination of bromide, calcium, fluoride, lithium, meprobamate, potassium, and isoniazid; contraindications include CHF, renal failure, and cerebral edema.

Peritoneal dialysis or hemodialysis may be useful in severe poisoning due to barbiturates, bromide, chloral hydrate, ethanol, ethylene glycol, isopropyl alcohol, lithium, heavy metals, methanol, procainamide, and salicylate. Hemoperfusion may be indicated for chloramphenicol, disopyramide, and hypnotic sedative overdose. Exchange transfusion removes poisons affecting red blood cells.

SPECIFIC POISONS

ACETAMINOPHEN   A dose of ≥140 mg/kg of acetaminophen saturates metabolism to sulfate and glucuronide metabolites, resulting in increased metabolism of acetaminophen to mercapturic acid. Nonspecific toxic manifestations (and not predictive of hepatic toxicity) include nausea, vomiting, diaphoresis, and pallor 2–4 h after ingestion. Laboratory evidence of hepatotoxicity includes elevation of AST, ALT, and, in severe cases, PT and bilirubin, with ultimate hyperammonemia. A serum acetaminophen level drawn 4–24 h after ingestion is compared with the Rumack-Matthew nomogram for purposes of predicting risk (Fig. 33-1).

Initial therapy consists of lavage and activated charcoal, then *N*-acetylcysteine therapy, which is indicated up to 24 h after ingestion. Loading dose is 140 mg/kg PO, followed by 70 mg/kg PO q4h for 17 doses. Therapy should be started immediately and may be discontinued when serum level is below toxic range.

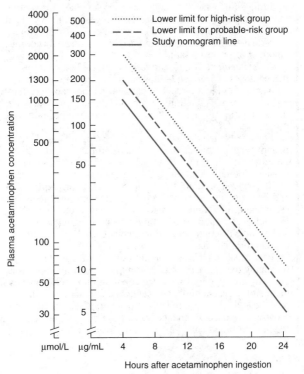

FIGURE 33-1 Nomogram to define risk according to initial plasma acetaminophen concentration. (After Rumack BH, Matthew H: Pediatrics 55:871, 1975.)

ALKALI AND ACID Alkalis include industrial-strength bleach, drain cleaners (sodium hydroxide), surface cleaners (ammonia, phosphates), laundry and dishwashing detergents (phosphates, carbonates), disk batteries, denture cleaners (borates, phosphates, carbonates) and Clinitest tablets (sodium hydroxide). Common acids include toilet bowl cleaners (hydrofluoric, phosphoric, and sulfuric acids), soldering fluxes (hydrochloric acid), antirust compounds (hydrofluoric and oxalic acids), automobile battery fluid (sulfuric acid), and stone cleaners (hydrofluoric and nitric acids). Clinical signs include burns, pain, drooling, vomiting of blood or mucus, and ulceration. Lack of oral manifestations does not rule out esophageal involvement. The esophagus and stomach can perforate, and aspiration can cause fulminant tracheitis.

Endoscopy is safe within 48 h of ingestion to document site and severity of injury.

Immediate treatment consists of dilution with milk or water. Glucocorticoids should be given within 48 h to pts with alkali (not acid) burns of the esophagus and continued for at least 2 weeks. Antacids may be useful for stomach burns.

ANTIARRYTHMIC DRUGS Acute ingestion of $>2 \times$ usual daily dose is potentially toxic and causes symptoms within 1 h. Manifestations include nausea, vomiting, diarrhea, lethargy, confusion, ataxia, bradycardia, hypotension, and cardiovascular collapse. Anticholinergic effects are seen with disopyramide ingestion. Quinidine and class IB agents (lidocaine, mexiletine, phenytoin, tocainide) can cause agitation, dysphoria, and seizures. Ventricular fibrillation (including torsades de pointes) and QT prolongation are characteristic of class IA (disopyramide, procainamide, quinidine) and IC (encainide, moricizine, propafenone, flecainide) poisonings. Myocardial depression may precipitate pulmonary edema.

Treatment consists of GI decontamination and supportive therapy. Persistent hypotension and bradycardia may require monitoring of pulmonary artery pressure, cardiac pacing, intraaortic balloon pump counterpulsation, and cardiopulmonary bypass. Ventricular tachyarrhythmias are treated with lidocaine and bretylium. Sodium bicarbonate or lactate may be useful in class IA or IC overdoses. Torsades de pointes is treated with magnesium sulfate (4 g or 40 mL of 10% solution IV over 10–20 min) or overdrive pacing (with isoproterenol or pacemaker).

ANTICHOLINERGIC AGENTS Antimuscarinic agents inhibit acetylcholine in the CNS and parasympathetic postganglionic muscarinic neuroreceptors and include antihistamines (H_1-receptor blockers and over-the-counter hypnotics), belladonna alkaloids (atropine, glycopyrrolate, homatropine, yoscine, ipatropium, scopolamine), Parkinsonian drugs (benztropine, biperiden, trihexyphenidyl), mydriatics (cyclopentolate, tropicamide), phenothizaines, skeletal muscle relaxants (cyclobenzaprine, orphenadrine), smooth-muscle relaxants (clinidinium, dicyclomine, isometheptene, oxybutynin), tricyclic antidepressants, and a variety of plants (stramonium, jimsonweed) and mushrooms. Manifestations begin 1 h to 3 d after ingestion; agitation, ataxia, confusion, delirium, hallucinations, and choreoathetosis can lead to lethargy, respiratory depression, and coma.

Treatment involves GI decontamination, supportive measures, and in severe cases the acetylcholinesterase inhibitor physostigmine; 1 to 2 mg is given IV over 2 min, and the dose may be repeated for incomplete response or recurrent toxicity. Physostigmine is contraindicated in the presence of cardiac conduction defects or ventricular arrhythmias.

ARSENIC Poisoning can occur from natural sources (contamination of deep-water wells); from occupational exposure (a byproduct of the smelting of ores and use in the microelectronic industry); commercial use of arsenic in wood preservatives, pesticides, herbicides, fungicides, and paints; and through foods and tobacco treated with arsenic-containing pesticides. Acute poisoning causes hemorrhagic gastroenteritis, fluid loss, and hypotension followed by delayed cardiomyopathy, delirium, coma, and seizures. Acute tubular necrosis and hemolysis may develop. Arsine gas causes severe hemolysis. Chronic exposure causes skin and nail changes (hyperkeratosis, hyperpigmentation, exfoliative dermatitis, and transverse white striae of the fingernails), sensory and motor polyneuritis that may lead to paralysis, and inflammation of the respiratory mucosa. Chronic exposure is associated with increased risk of skin cancer and possibly of systemic cancers and with vasospasm and peripheral vascular insufficiency.

Treatment of acute ingestion includes ipecac-induced vomiting, gastric lavage, activated charcoal with a cathartic, aggressive administration of intravenous fluids and electrolyte correction, and dimercaprol IM at an initial dose of 3–5 mg/kg every 4h for 2 d, every 6 h on d 3, and every 12 h for 7 d. Succimer is an alternative agent if adverse reactions develop to dimercaprol. With renal failure doses should be adjusted carefully. Other than avoidance of additional exposure, specific therapy is not of proven benefit for chronic arsenic toxicity.

BARBITURATES Overdose may result in confusion, lethargy, coma, hypotension, hypothermia, pulmonary edema, and death.

Treatment consists of GI decontamination and repetitive charcoal administration for long-acting barbiturates. Renal excretion of phenobarbital is enhanced by alkalinization of urine to a pH of 8 and by saline diuresis. Hemoperfusion and hemodialysis can be used in severe poisoning with short- or long-acting barbiturates.

BENZODIAZEPINES Long-acting agents include chlordiazepoxide, clonazepan, clorazepate, diazepam, flurazepam, prazepam, and quazepam; short-acting drugs include alprazolam, lorazepam, and oxazepam; and ultrashort acting agents include estazolam, midazolam, temazepam, and triazolam. Effects may begin within 30 min of overdosage and include weakness, ataxia, drowsiness, coma, and respiratory depression. Pupils are constricted and do not respond to naloxone.

Treatment includes GI decontamination and support of vital signs. Flumazenil, a competitive benzodiazepine-receptor antagonist, can reverse CNS and respiratory depression and is given IV in incremental doses of 0.2, 0.3, and 0.5 mg at 1-min intervals until the desired effect is achieved or a total dose of 3 to 5 mg is given; flumazenil must be used with caution in pts who have benzodiazepine dependency or have coingested stimulants and benzodiazepines.

BETA-ADRENERGIC BLOCKING AGENTS Some beta blockers are cardioselective (acebutolol, betaxolol, metroprolol), some have sympathomimetic activity (acebutolol, cartelol, pindolol, timolol, possibly penbutolol), and some have quinidine-like effects (acebutolol, metoprolol, pindolol, propranolol, sotalol, possibly betaxolol). Toxicity is usually manifest within 30 min of ingestion. Symptoms include nausea, vomiting, diarrhea, bradycardia, hypotension, and CNS depression. Agents with intrinsic sympathomimetic activity can cause hypertension and tachycardia. Bronchospasm and pulmonary edema may occur. Hyperkalemia, hypoglycemia, metabolic acidosis, all degrees of AV block, bundle branch block, QRS prolongation, ventricular tachyarrhythmias, torsades de pointes, and asystole may occur.

Treatment includes GI decontamination, supportive measures, and administration of calcium (10% chloride or gluconate salt solution, IV 0.2 mL/kg, up to 10 mL) and glucagon (5–10 mg IV, then infusion of 1–5 mg/L). Cardiac pacing or an intraaortic balloon pump may be required. Bronchospasm is treated with inhaled beta agonists.

CADMIUM Foods can be contaminated with cadmium from sewage, polluted ground water, or mining effluents. Airborne cadmium can be released from smelting or incineration of wastes containing plastics and batteries, and occupational exposure occurs in the metal-plating, pigment, battery, and plastics industries. Acute inhalation can cause pleuritic chest pain, dyspnea, cyanosis, fever, tachycardia, nausea, and pulmonary edema. Ingestion can cause severe nausea, vomiting, salivation, abdominal cramps, and diarrhea. Chronic exposure causes anosmia, microcytic hypochromic anemia, renal tubular dysfunction with proteinuria, and osteomalacia with pseudofractures.

Treatment involves avoidance of further exposure and supportive therapy. Chelation therapy is not useful, and dimercaprol may worsen nephrotoxicity and is contraindicated. Succimer is useful in cadmium toxicity in animals and may be useful for the disorder in humans.

CALCIUM CHANNEL BLOCKERS   These agents include amlodipine, bepridil, diltiazem, felodipine, flunarizine, isradipine, lacidipine, nicardipine, nifedipine, nimodipine, nisoldipine, nitrendipine, and verapamil. Toxicity usually develops within 30–60 min following ingestion of 5–10 × usual dose. Manifestations include confusion, drowsiness, coma, seizure, hypotension, bradycardia, cyanosis, and pulmonary edema. ECG findings include all degrees of AV block, prolonged QRS and QT intervals, ischemia or infarction, and asystole. Metabolic acidosis and hyperglycemia may result.

Treatment consists of GI decontamination, supportive care, calcium and glucagon (as above). Electrical pacing or intraaortic balloon pump may be required, and persistent hypotension may require vasopressors.

CARBON MONOXIDE (CO)   CO binds to hemoglobin (forming carboxyhemoglobin) with an affinity 200 times that of O_2 and hence causes cellular anoxia. Once exposure is discontinued, CO is excreted via the lungs with a half-life of 4–6 h. The half-life decreases to 40–80 min with 100% O_2 therapy and to 15–30 min with hyperbaric O_2. Manifestations include shortness of breath, dyspnea, tachypnea, headache, nausea, vomiting, emotional lability, confusion, impaired judgment, and clumsiness. Pulmonary edema, aspiration pneumonia, arrhythmias, and hypotension may occur. The "cherry red" color of skin and mucous membranes is rare; cyanosis is usual.

Treatment consists of giving 100% O_2 via a tightly fitting mask until CO levels are less than 10% and all symptoms have resolved. Hyperbaric O_2 is recommended for comatose pts with CO levels ≥40%, for pts with CO levels ≥25% who also have seizures or intractable arrhythmias, and for pts with delayed onset of sequelae. Pts with loss of consciousness are at risk for neuropsychiatric sequelae 1 to 3 weeks later.

CYANIDE   Cyanide blocks electron transport, resulting in decreased oxidative metabolism and oxidative utilization, decreased ATP production, and lactic acidosis. Lethal dose is

200–300 mg of sodium cyanide and 500 mg of hydrocyanic acid. Early effects include headache, vertigo, excitement, anxiety, burning of mouth and throat, dyspnea, tachycardia, hypertension, nausea, vomiting, and diaphoresis. Breath may have a bitter almond odor. Later effects include coma, seizures, opisthotonos, trismus, paralysis, respiratory depression, arrhythmias, hypotension, and death.

Treatment should begin immediately based on history. Supportive measures, 100% O_2, and GI decontamination are begun concurrently with specific therapy. Amyl nitrite is inhaled for 30 s each min, and a new ampule is broken q3 min. (Nitrite produces methemoglobinemia, which has a higher affinity for cyanide and promotes release from peripheral sites.) Sodium nitrite is then given as a 3% solution IV at a rate of 2.5–5.0 mL/min up to a total dose of 10–15 mL. Then, 50 ml of 25% sodium thiosulfate is given IV over 1–2 min, producing sodium thiocyanate, which is excreted in urine. (Children should be given 0.33 mL/kg sodium nitrite and 1.65 mL/kg sodium thiosulfate.) If symptoms persist, repeat half the dose of sodium nitrite and sodium thiosulfate.

DIGOXIN   Poisoning with digitalis occurs with therapeutic or suicidal use of digoxin and with plant (oleander) ingestion. Symptoms include vomiting, confusion, delirium, hallucinations, blurred vision, disturbed color perception (yellow vision), photophobia, all types of arrhythmias, and all degrees of AV block. The combination of SVT and AV block suggests digitalis toxicity. Hypokalemia is common with chronic intoxication, while hyperkalemia occurs with acute overdosage.

GI decontamination is done carefully to avoid vagal stimulation, repeated doses of activated charcoal are given, and hyperkalemia is treated with Kayexalate, insulin, and glucose. Atropine and electrical pacing may be required. In severe poisoning digoxin antibodies are given; dosage (in 40-mg vials) is calculated by dividing ingested dose of digoxin (mg) by 0.6 mg/vial. If dose and serum levels are unknown, give 5–10 vials to an adult.

ETHYLENE GLYCOL   Ethylene glycol is used as a solvent for paints, plastics, and pharmaceuticals and in the manufacture of explosives, fire extinguishers, foams, hydraulic fluids, windshield cleaners, radiator antifreeze, and de-icer preparations. As little as 120 mg or 0.1 mL/kg can be hazardous. Manifestations include nausea, vomiting, slurred speech, ataxia, nystagmus, lethargy, sweet breath odor, coma, seizures, cardiovascular collapse, and death. Hypocalcemia occurs in half of pts. Anion-gap metabolic acidosis, elevated serum osmolality, and oxalate crystalluria suggest the diagnosis. Renal failure may result from glycolic acid production.

GI lavage should be followed by activated charcoal, and airway protection should be initiated immediately. Calcium salts should be given IV at a rate of 1 mL/min for a total dose of 7–14 mL (10% solution diluted 10:1). Metabolic acidosis should be treated with sodium bicarbonate. Phenytoin and benzodiazepines are given for seizures. Ethanol is administered when ethylene glycol level is >3 mmol/L (>20 mg/dL) and acidosis is present; ethanol is given as follows: the loading dose is 10 mL/kg of 10% ethanol IV or 1 mL/kg of 95% ethanol PO; the maintenance dose is 1.5 (mL/kg)/h of 10% ethanol IV and 3 (mL/kg)/h of 10% ethanol during dialysis. A serum ethanol level of ≥20 mmol/L (≥100 mg/dL) is required to inhibit alcohol dehydrogenase. Hemodialysis is indicated in cases not responding to above therapy, when serum levels are ≥8 mmol/L (≥50 mg/dL), and for renal failure. Give thiamine and pyridoxine supplements.

HALLUCINOGENS   Mescaline, lysergic acid (LSD), and psilocybin cause disorders of mood, thought, and perception lasting 4–6 h. Psilocybin can cause fever, hypotension, and seizures. Symptoms include mydriasis, conjunctival injection, piloerection, hypertension, tachycardia, tachypnea, anorexia, tremors, and hyperreflexia.

Treatment is nonspecific: a calm environment, benzodiazepines for acute panic reactions, and haloperidol for psychotic reactions.

HYDROCARBONS   Forms include aromatic hydrocarbons (xylene, toluene), halogenated hydrocarbons (carbon tetrachloride, trichlorethane), and petroleum distillate hydrocarbons (gasoline, lacquer thinner, mineral seal oil, kerosene, lighter fluid). All cause CNS excitation at low dose and depression at high doses. Other manifestations include nausea, vomiting, diarrhea, abdominal pain, renal tubular acidosis, bone marrow suppression, respiratory distress, rhabdomyolysis, psychosis and cerebral atrophy, and mucosal burns.

Prompt gastric lavage is required for aromatic hydrocarbons, but gastric lavage, ipecac, and activated charcoal are contraindicated for petroleum distillate hydrocarbons. Supportive care involves oxygen, respiratory support; monitoring of liver, renal, and myocardial function; and correction of metabolic abnormalities.

HYDROGEN SULFIDE   Hydrogens sulfide is encountered in the petroleum and mining industries, tanning of leather, vulcanization of rubber, production of synthetic fabrics, refining of metal, production of heavy water for atomic reactors, and manufacture of glue and felt. The chemical is malodorous (rotten eggs) and irritative, producing rhinitis, conjunctivitis, and pharyngitis. Headache, vertigo, nausea, confusion, seizures, and coma may ensue. Respiratory depression causes hypoxia, cyanosis, and metabolic acidosis.

Treatment includes maintenance of airway, 100% O_2, amyl and sodium nitrite (as for cyanide poisoning) when pts do not respond to oxygen, and hyperbaric O_2 in refractory cases.

IRON Ferrous iron injures mitochondria, causes lipid peroxidation, and results in renal, tubular, and hepatic necrosis and occasionally in myocardial and pulmonary injury. Ingestion of 20 mg/kg causes GI symptoms, and 60 mg/kg causes fever, hyperglycemia, leukocytosis, lethargy, hypotension, metabolic acidosis, seizures, coma, vascular collapse, jaundice, elevated liver enzymes, prolongation of PT, and hyperammonemia. X-ray may identify iron tablets in stomach. Serum iron levels greater than iron-binding capacity indicate serious toxicity. A positive urine deferoxamine provocative test (50 mg/kg IV or IM up to 1 g) is a vin rosé color that indicates presence of ferrioxamine.

Ipecac or lavage is administered, followed by x-ray to check adequacy of decontamination. Charcoal is ineffective. Deferoxamine is infused at 10–15 (mg/kg)/h (up to 1–2 g) if iron exceeds binding capacity. If iron level is >180 μmol/L (>1000 μg/dL), larger doses of deferoxamine can be given, followed by exchange transfusion or plasmapheresis to remove deferoxamine complex.

ISONIAZID Acute overdose decreases synthesis of γ-aminobutyric acid and causes CNS stimulation. Symptoms begin within 30 min of ingestion and include nausea, vomiting, dizziness, slurred speech, coma, seizures, and metabolic acidosis.

Prompt GI decontamination is followed by activated charcoal. Pyridoxine (vitamin B_6) should be given slowly IV in weight equivalency to ingested dose of isoniazid. If dose is not known, give 5 g pyridoxine IV over 30 min as a 5–10% solution.

ISOPROPYL ALCOHOL Isopropyl alcohol is present in rubbing alcohol, solvents, aftershave lotions, antifreeze, and window cleaners. Its metabolite acetone is found in cleaners, solvents, and nail polish removers. Manifestations begin promptly and include vomiting, abdominal pain, hematemesis, myopathy, headache, dizziness, confusion, coma, respiratory depression, hypothermia, and hypotension. Hypoglycemia, anion gap (small) metabolic acidosis, elevated serum osmolality, false elevations of serum creatinine, and hemolytic anemia may be present.

Treatment consists of GI decontamination and supportive measures. Activated charcoal is not effective. Dialysis may be needed in severe cases.

LEAD Exposure to lead occurs through paints, cans, plumbing fixtures, leaded gasolines, vegetables grown in lead-contaminated soils, improperly glazed ceramics, lead-containing glass, and industrial sources such as battery manufacturing, demolition of lead-contaminated buildings, and the ceramics industry. Manifestations in childhood include abdominal pain followed by lethargy, anorexia, anemia, ataxia, and slurred speech. Severe manifestations include convulsions, coma, generalized cerebral edema, and renal failure. Impairment of cognition is dose-dependent. In adults symptoms of chronic exposure include abdominal pain, headache, irritability, joint pain, fatigue, anemia, motor neuropathy, and deficits in memory. Encephalopathy is rare. A "lead line" may appear at the gingiva-tooth border. Chronic, low-level exposure can cause interstitial nephritis, tubular damage, hyperuricemia, and decreased glomerular filtration. Elevation of bone lead level is a risk for anemia and hypertension.

Treatment first involves prevention of further exposure and the use of chelating agents such as edetate calcium disodium, dimercaptol, penicillamine, and succimer. Chelation may or may not improve subclinical manifestations such as impaired cognition.

LITHIUM Manifestations begin within 2–4 h of ingestion and include nausea, vomiting, diarrhea, weakness, fasciculations, twitching, ataxia, tremor, myoclonus, choreoathetosis, seizures, confusion, coma, and cardiovascular collapse. Laboratory abnormalities include leukocytosis, hyperglycemia, albuminuria, glycosuria, nephrogenic diabetes insipidus, ECG changes (AV block, prolonged QT), and ventricular arrhythmias.

Within 2–4 h of ingestion lavage and bowel irrigation should be performed. Charcoal is not effective. Serial serum lithium levels should be measured until trend is downward. Supportive care includes saline diuresis and alkalinization of the urine for levels >2–3 mmol/L. Hemodialysis is indicated for acute or chronic intoxication with symptoms and/or a serum level >3 mmol/L.

MERCURY Mercury is used in thermometers, dental amalgams, and some batteries and is combined with other chemicals to form inorganic or organic mercury compounds. Fish can concentrate mercury at high levels, and occupational exposure continues in some chemical, metal-processing; electrical and automotive manufacturing; building industries; and medical and dental services (e.g., ordinary dental amalgam). Inhalation of mercury vapor causes diffuse infiltrates or a pneumonitis, respiratory distress, pulmonary edema, fibrosis, and desquamation of the bronchiolar epithelium. Neurologic manifestations include tremors, emotional lability, and polyneuropathy. Chronic exposure to metallic mercury produces intention tremor and erethism (excitability, memory loss, insomnia, timidity, and sometimes delirium); acute high-dose ingestion of metallic mercury may lead to hematemesis and abdominal pain, acute renal failure, and cardiovascular collapse. Organic mercury compounds can cause a neurotoxicity characterized by paresthesia; impaired vision, hearing, taste, and smell; unsteadiness of gait; weakness; memory loss; and depression. Exposed mothers give birth to infants with mental retardation and multiple neurologic derangements.

Treatment acutely involves emesis or gastric lavage followed by the oral administration of polythiol resins to bind mercury in the GI tract. Chelating agents include dimercaprol, succimer, and penicillamine. Acute poisoning is treated with dimercaprol in divided doses IM not exceeding 24 mg/kg per d; 5-day courses are usually separated by rest periods. *N*-acetyl penicillamine is also useful at a dose of 30 mg/kg per day in divided doses. Peritoneal dialysis, hemodialysis, and extracorporeal hemodialysis with succimer have been used for renal failure. Chronic inorganic mercury poisoning is best treated with acetyl penicillamine.

METHANOL Methanol is a component of shellacs, varnishes, paint removers, Sterno, windshield-washer solutions, copy machine fluid, and denaturants for ethanol. It is metabolized to formic acid, which causes metabolic acidosis. Manifestations begin within 1–2 h of ingestion and include nausea, vomiting, abdominal pain, headache, vertigo, confusion, obtundation, and ethanol-like intoxication. Late manifestations are due to formic acid and include an anion-gap metabolic acidosis, coma, seizures, and death. Ophthalmic manifestations 15–19 h after ingestion include clouding, diminished acuity, dancing and flashing spots, dilated or fixed pupils, hyperemia of the disc, retinal edema, and blindness.

Gastric aspiration should be undertaken. Activated charcoal is not effective. Acidosis is corrected with sodium bicarbonate. Seizures respond to diazepam and phenytoin. Ethanol therapy (as described for ethylene glycol) is indicated in pts with visual symptoms or a methanol level >6 mmol/L (>20 mg/dL). Therapy with ethanol is continued until the methanol level falls below 6 mmol/L. Hemodialysis is indicated when visual signs are present or when metabolic acidosis is unresponsive to sodium bicarbonate.

METHEMOGLOBINEMIA Chemicals that oxidize ferrous hemoglobin (Fe^{2+}) to its ferric (Fe^{3+}) state include aniline, aminophenols, aminophenones, chlorates, dapsone, local anesthetics, nitrates, nitrites, nitroglycerine, naphthalene, nitrobenzene, nitrogen oxides, phenazopyridine, primaquine, and sulfonamides. Cyanosis occurs with methemoglobin levels >15%. When levels exceed 20–30%, symptoms include fatigue, headache, dizziness, tachycardia, and weakness. At levels >45%, dyspnea, bradycardia, hypoxia, acidosis, seizures, coma, and arrhythmias occur. Death usually occurs with levels >70%. Hemolytic anemia may lead to hyperkalemia and renal failure 1–3 d after exposure. Cyanosis in conjunction with a normal Pa_{O_2} and decreased O_2 saturation (measured by oximeter) and "chocolate brown" blood suggest the diagnosis. The chocolate color does not redden with exposure to O_2 but fades when exposed to 10% potassium cyanide.

Ingested toxins should be removed by lavage followed by charcoal and cathartics. Methylene blue is indicated for methemoglobin level >30 g/L or methemoglobinemia with hypoxia. Dosage is 1–2 mg/kg as a 1% solution over 5 min. Additional doses may be needed. Methylene blue is contraindicated in G6PD deficiency. Administration of 100% O_2 and packed red blood cell transfusion to a hemoglobin level of 150 g/L can enhance O_2 carrying capacity of the blood. Exchange transfusions may be indicated in G6PD-deficient pts.

MONOAMINE OXIDASE (MAO) INHIBITORS MAO inhibitors include furzolidone, isocarboxazid, nialamide, pargyline, phenelizine, procarbazine, and tranylcypromine. Manifestations are apparent within 6–12 h of ingestion and include CNS stimulation, fever, tachycardia, tachypnea, hypertension, nausea, vomiting, dilated pupils with nystagmus, and papilledema. Fasciculations, twitching, tremor, and rigidity may be present.

GI decontamination should be followed by activated charcoal and cathartics. Dantrolene (2.5 mg/kg PO or IV q6h) may be effective for hyperthermia. Control of hypertension may require nitroprusside, and tachycardia may require propranolol. Hypotension should be treated with fluids and cautious use of pressors. Seizures are treated with benzodiazepines and phenytoin. In severe cases hyperthermia may require external cooling, and neuromuscular paralysis may be necessary for agitation.

MUSCLE RELAXANTS Manifestations of poisoning by carisoprodol, chlorphenesin, chlorzoxazone, and methocarbamol include nausea, vomiting, dizziness, headache, nystagmus, hypotonia, and CNS depression. Cyclobenzaprine and orphenadrine cause agitation, hallucinations, seizures, stupor, coma, and hypotension. Orphenadrine can also cause ventricular tachyarrhythmias. Baclofen causes CNS depression, hypothermia, excitability, delirium, myoclonus, seizures, conduction abnormalities, arrhythmias, and hypotension.

Prompt GI decontamination, single-dose activated charcoal (repeated for baclofen overdose), and cathartics are indicated. Physostigmine (1–2 mg IV over 2–5 min) is useful for anticholinergic effects.

NONSTEROIDAL ANTI-INFLAMMATORY DRUGS (NSAIDs) All NSAIDs may cause gastroenteritis, drowsiness, headache, glycosuria, hematuria, and proteinuria. Ibuprofen toxicity is usually mild but can cause metabolic acidosis, coma, and seizures. Diflunisal produces, in addition, hyperventilation, tachycardia, and diaphoresis; fenoprofen is nephrotoxic. Seizures occur with mefenamic acid and phenylbutazone and rarely with ketoprofen and naproxen. Coma, respiratory depression, and cardiovascular collapse can occur with mefenamic acid and phenylbutazone.

Gastric lavage, activated charcoal, and cathartics are indicated, and charcoal should be repeated with indomethacin, phenylbutazone, and piroxicam ingestions. Hemodialysis is not efficient because of protein binding but may be useful with severe toxicity.

ORGANOPHOSPHATE AND CARBAMATE INSECTICIDES Organophosphates (chlorpyrifos, phosphorothioic acid, dichlorvos, fenthion, malathion, parathion, sarin, and numerous others) irreversibly inhibit acetylcholinesterase and cause accumulation of acetylcholine at muscarinic and nicotinic synapses. Carbamates (carbaryl, aldicarb, propoxur, and bendicarb) reversibly inhibit acetylcholinesterase; therapeutic carbonates include ambenonium, neostigmine, physostigmine, and pyridostigmine. Both types are absorbed through the skin, lungs, and GI tract and produce nausea, vomiting, abdominal cramps, urinary and fecal incontinence, increased bronchial secretions, coughing, sweating, salivation, lacrimation, and miosis; carbamates are shorter acting. Bradycardia, conduction blocks, hypotension, twitching, fasciculations, weakness, respiratory depression, seizures, confusion, and coma may result. A decrease in cholinesterase activity ≥50% in plasma or red cells is diagnostic.

Treatment begins with washing exposed surfaces with soap and water and, in cases of ingestion, GI decontamination, then activated charcoal. Atropine 0.5–2 mg is given IV q15 min until complete atropinization is achieved (dry mouth). Pralidoxime (2-PAM), 1–2 g IV over several minutes, can be repeated q8h until nicotinic symptoms resolve. Use of 2-PAM in carbamate poisoning is controversial.

PHENOTHIAZINES   The phenothiazines chlorpromazine, fluphenazine, mesoridazine, perphenazine, prochlorperazine, promazine, promethazine, and thioridazine and pharmacologically similar agents such as haloperidol, loxapine, pimozide, and thiothixene are CNS depressants and can cause lethargy, obtundation, respiratory depression, and coma. Pupils are often constricted. Hypothermia, hypotension, SVT, AV block, arrhythmias (including torsades de pointes), prolongation of PR, QRS, and QT intervals, and T-wave abnormalities are seen. Malignant neuroleptic syndrome occurs rarely. With dystonic reactions symptoms include rigidity, opisthotonos, stiff neck, hyperreflexia, irritability, dystonia, fixed speech, torticollis, tremors, trismus, and oculogyric crisis.

Treatment of overdose includes GI decontamination, then a single dose of activated charcoal. Seizures should be treated with phenytoin; hypotension responds to volume expansion and alpha agonists. Sodium bicarbonate is given for metabolic acidosis. Avoid the use of procainamide, quinidine, or any agent that prolongs cardiac repolarization. Neuroleptic malignant syndrome is treated with dantrolene and bromocriptine. Acute dystonic reactions respond to diphenhydramine (1–2 mg/kg IV) or benztropine (1–2 mg). Doses may be repeated in 20 min if necessary.

SALICYLATES   Poisoning with salicylates or other NSAIDs causes vomiting, tachycardia, hyperpnea, fever, tinnitus, lethargy, and confusion. Severe poisoning can result in seizures, coma, respiratory and cardiovascular failure, cerebral edema, and renal failure. Respiratory alkalosis is commonly coupled with metabolic acidosis (40–50%), but respiratory alkalosis (20%) and metabolic acidosis (20%) can occur separately. Lactic and other organic acids are responsible for the increased anion gap. PT may be prolonged. Salicylates in blood or urine can be detected by ferric chloride test.

Treatment includes GI decontamination then repeated administration of activated charcoal for up to 24 h. Forced alkaline diuresis (urine pH >8.0) increases excretion and decreases serum half-life. Seizures can be controlled with diazepam or phenobarbital. Hemodialysis should be considered in pts who fail conventional therapy or have cerebral edema or hepatic or renal failure.

STIMULANTS   Amphetamines; bronchodilators such as albuterol and metaproterenol; decongestants such as ephedrine, pseudoephedrine, phenylephrine, and phenylpropanolamines; and cocaine can cause nausea, vomiting, diarrhea, abdominal cramps, irritability, confusion, delirium, euphoria, auditory and visual hallucinations, tremors, hyperreflexia, seizures, palpitations, tachycardia, hypertension, arrhythmias, and cardiovascular collapse. Sympathomimetic symptoms include dilated pupils, dry mouth, pallor, flushing of skin, and tachypnea. Severe manifestations include hyperpyrexia, seizures, rhabdomyolysis, hypertensive crisis, intracranial hemorrhage, cardiac arrhythmias, and cardiovascular collapse. Rhabdomyolysis and intracranial hemorrhage can occur.

Treatment begins with gastric lavage followed by activated charcoal and a cathartic. Seizures are treated with benzodiazepines; hypertension with nitroprusside; fever with salicylates; and agitation with sedatives and, if necessary, paralyzing agents. Lidocaine and propranolol are useful for cardiac arrhythmias.

THALLIUM   Thallium is used as insecticide, in fireworks, in manufacturing, as an alloy, and in cardiac imaging, and epidemic poisoning has occurred with ingestion of grain contaminated with thallium. Acute manifestations include nausea and vomiting, abdominal pain, bloody diarrhea, and hematemesis. Subsequent manifestations include confusion, psychosis, choreoathetosis, organic brain syndrome, convulsions, coma, and sensory and motor neuropathy; autonomic nervous system effects include tachycardia, hypertension, and salivation. Optic neuritis, ophthalmoplegia, ptosis, strabismus, and cranial nerve palsies may occur. Late effects include diffuse hair loss, memory defects, ataxia, tremor, and foot drop.

Treatment includes gastrointestinal contamination by lavage or ipecac syrup and cathartics, forced diuresis with furosemide and KCl supplements, and either peritoneal dialysis, hemodialysis, or charcoal hemoperfusion.

THEOPHYLLINE   Vomiting, restlessness, irritability, agitation, tachypnea, tachycardia, and tremors are common. Coma and respiratory depression, generalized tonic-clonic and partial seizures, atrial arrhythmias, ventricular arrhythmias, and fibrillation can occur. Rhabdomyolysis with acute renal failure develops occasionally. Laboratory abnormalities include ketosis, metabolic acidosis, elevated amylase, hyperglycemia, and decreased potassium, calcium, and phosphorus.

Treatment requires prompt GI decontamination followed by administration of activated charcoal every 2–4 h for 12–24 h after ingestion. Metoclopramide and ondansetron may be given to control vomiting. Tachyarrhythmias are treated with propranolol and standard antiarrhythmics; hypotension requires volume expansion. Seizures are treated with benzodiazepines and barbiturates; phenytoin is ineffective. Indications for hemodialysis and hemoperfusion with acute ingestion include a serum level >500 μmol/L (>100 mg/L) and with chronic ingestion a serum level >200–300 μmol/L (>40–60 mg/L). Dialysis is also indicated in pts with lower serum levels who have refractory seizures or arrhythmias.

TRICYCLIC ANTIDEPRESSANTS These agents block reuptake of synaptic transmitters (norepinephrine, dopamine) and have central and peripheral anticholinergic activity. Manifestations include anticholinergic symptoms (fever, mydriasis, flushing of skin, urinary retention, decreased bowel motility). CNS manifestations include excitation, restlessness, myoclonus, hyperreflexia, disorientation, confusion, hallucinations, coma, and seizures. Cardiac effects include prolongation of the QRS complex, other AV blocks, and arrhythmias. QRS duration ≥0.10 ms is correlated with seizures and life-threatening cardiac arrhythmias. Serum levels >3300 nmol/L (>1000 ng/mL) indicate serious poisoning.

Treatment with ipecac is contraindicated. Gastric lavage is followed by activated charcoal every 2–4 h (with cathartics). Metabolic acidosis is treated with sodium bicarbonate; hypotension with volume expansion, norepinephrine, or high-dose dopamine; seizures with benzodiazepines and barbiturates; arrhythmias with sodium bicarbonate (0.5–1 mmol/kg), lidocaine, and bretyllium. Beta-adrenergic blockers and class 1A antiarrhythmics should be avoided. The efficacy of phenytoin is not established. Physostigmine reverses anticholinergic signs and may be given in mild poisoning. Hemodialysis and hemoperfusion have no benefit because of the large volume of distribution.

For a more detailed discussion, see Linden CH, Lovejoy FH Jr: Poisoning and Drug Overdosage, Chap. 391, p. 2523; and Hu H: Heavy Metal Poisoning, Chap. 397, p. 2564, in HPIM-14.

34

DIABETIC KETOACIDOSIS AND HYPEROSMOTIC COMA

DIABETIC KETOACIDOSIS (DKA)

DKA results from insulin deficiency with a relative or absolute increase in glucagon and may be caused by cessation of insulin therapy or by infection, surgery, or emotional stress. Anorexia, nausea and vomiting, and increased urine output are initial symptoms, and abdominal pain, altered consciousness, Kussmaul breathing, or frank coma may ensue. Volume depletion can lead to vascular collapse and renal shutdown. Leukocytosis is common. Body temperature is normal or decreased. Fever suggests infection, and a source must be sought.

Features infclude hyperglycemia and anion gap metabolic acidosis (with serum $HCO_3 < 10$ mmol/L) due to the elevated level of acetoacetate and β-hydroxybutyrate. Despite a normal or elevated serum potassium, total-body potassium is decreased by several hundred millimoles. Initial serum phosphorus also may be elevated despite depletion of body stores. Magnesium may be low. Serum sodium is decreased secondary to hyperglycemia.

Other causes of metabolic acidosis must be excluded: lactic acid acidosis, uremia, alcoholic ketoacidosis, and certain poisonings. If urine ketones are negative, another cause for acidosis is likely. If urine ketones are positive, plasma ketones should be measured; a strongly positive test in undiluted plasma may be due to starvation whereas a strongly positive reaction beyond a 1:1 dilution indicates ketoacidosis.

 TREATMENT

Diabetic ketoacidosis must be treated with insulin. Because insulin resistance cannot be identified prospectively, 25–50 U/h of regular insulin IV should be given until acidosis is reversed, and lesser amounts should be given for several hours thereafter [usually 0.1 (U/kg)/h]. Therapy also requires IV fluids; the usual fluid deficit is 3–5 L. 1–2 L isotonic saline is given initially, and additional amounts are determined by clinical assessment. When plasma glucose falls to about 17 mmol/L (300 mg/dL), 5% glucose solutions should be started, both as source of free water and to prevent late development of cerebral edema and hypoglycemia. Potassium should always be administered, but the timing of its administration varies. Potassium replacement (as potassium phosphate) should be initiated early if initial levels are normal or low. If initial levels are elevated, potassium replacement should begin as soon as the measured level begins to fall with correction of acidosis and shift of K^+ into intracellular water. Aggressive insulin and fluid therapy are not discontinued until plasma or urine ketones are negative for 4 h (correction of hyperglycemia is not an endpoint). Poor prognostic signs include hypotension, azotemia, deep coma, and associated illness. Bicarbonate should be given when acidosis is severe (pH $\leq$ 7.0), especially if hypotension is present. Most pts

Table 34-1

Complications of Diabetic Ketoacidosis

Complication	Clues
Acute gastric dilatation or erosive gastritis	Vomiting of blood or coffee-ground material
Cerebral edema	Obtundation or coma with or without neurologic signs, esp. if occurring after initial improvement
Hyperkalemia	Cardiac arrest
Hypoglycemia	Adrenergic or neurologic signs; rebound ketosis
Hypokalemia	Cardiac arrhythmias
Infection	Fever
Insulin resistance	Unremitting acidosis after 4–6 h of adequate therapy
Myocardial infarction	Chest pain, appearance of heart failure; appearance of hypotension despite adequate fluids
Mucormycosis	Facial pain, bloody nasal discharge, blackened nasal turbinates, blurred vision, proptosis
Respiratory distress syndrome	Hypoxemia in the absence of pneumonia, chronic pulmonary disease, or heart failure
Vascular thrombosis	Strokelike picture or signs of ischemia in nonnervous tissue

SOURCE: Adapted from DW Foster, in *Current Therapy in Endocrinology and Metabolism* 1985–1986, DT Krieger, CW Bardin (eds), Toronto/Philadelphia, Decker, 1985.

with diabetic ketoacidosis recover. Causes of death include MI and infection, particularly pneumonia. See Table 34-1 for complications of DKA.

HYPEROSMOLAR NONKETOTIC COMA

Sustained osmotic diuresis causes profound dehydration when pts are unable to drink sufficient water to replace urinary fluid losses. Commonly, an elderly diabetic develops a stroke or infection, which worsens hyperglycemia and prevents adequate water intake so that volume depletion causes prerenal azotemia. Seizures may occur. Other causes include tube feedings of high-protein formulas, peritoneal dialysis, high carbohydrate intake, and osmotic agents such as mannitol or urea.

Plasma glucose is generally around 55 mmol/L (1000 mg/dL). Mild metabolic acidosis may be present. Serum bicarbonate < 10 mmol/L and normal plasma ketones suggest lactic acidosis. The serum osmolality is high, but because of hyperglycemia serum Na may be normal. Serum osmolality can be estimated:

$$\text{Osmolality(mmol/kg)} = 2[\text{Na(mmol/L)} + \text{K(mmol/L)}]$$
$$+ \text{glucose(mmol/L)} + \text{BUN(mmol/L)}$$

The average fluid deficit is 10 L.

℞ TREATMENT

Sufficient IV fluids must be given to support circulation and urine flow. While free water is ultimately needed, 2–3 L isotonic saline should be given over first 1–2 h to restore intravascular volume. Subsequently, half-strength saline can be used. As plasma glucose approaches normal, 5% dextrose can be given as a vehicle for free water. Insulin should be given to control hyperglycemia. The mortality rate is > 50%.

For a more detailed discussion, see Foster DW: Diabetes Mellitus, Chap. 334, p. 2060, in HPIM-14.

35

HYPOGLYCEMIA

The brain uses glucose as its primary metabolic fuel and consequently is uniquely vulnerable to hypoglycemia. An effective counterregulatory response under the control of glucagon, catecholamines, cortisol, and growth hormone promotes hepatic glucose production and limits glucose utilization by nonvital tissues. Early symptoms of hypoglycemia (sweating, tachycardia, anxiety, and tremor) result from adrenergic stimulation, while symptoms of CNS dysfunction (dizziness, blurred vision, confusion, convulsions, syncope, and eventually coma) develop later. The fact that adrenergic symptoms can be blunted by beta-adrenergic blockade or by autonomic neuropathy makes such pts prone to serious neurologic consequences of hypoglycemia.

The diagnosis of hypoglycemia requires a plasma glucose <2.5–2.8 mmol/L (<45–50 mg/dL) in men and <1.9–2.2 mmol/L (<35–40 mg/dL) in women, hypoglycemic symptoms, and improvement of symptoms with the administration of glucose (Whipple's triad). When diagnosis is strongly suspected, glucose should be administered after drawing blood for diagnostic studies.

Postprandial (Reactive) Hypoglycemia

Hypoglycemia after eating occurs when gastrectomy, gastrojejunostomy, pyloroplasty, or vagotomy causes rapid gastric emptying, brisk absorption of glucose, and excessive insulin release. A more rapid decline in glucose than insulin levels results in hypoglycemia. Fructose intolerance, galactosemia, and leucine sensitivity are rare causes of postprandial hypoglycemia in children.

Fasting Hypoglycemia

Hypoglycemia after fasting is due to an imbalance between the production and utilization of glucose. Increased utilization (glucose demand of >10 g/h) usually results from hyperinsulinism (insulinoma, exogenous insulin, sulfonylurea ingestion, or insulin autoimmunity). Glucose overutilization with low plasma insulin can be due to extrapancreatic tumors (fibromas, sarcomas, hepatomas, carcinomas of GI tract, and adrenal tumors). Such tumors either produce insulin-like factors or utilize glucose directly. Hypoglycemia with low plasma insulin also may occur when free fatty acids are not available for oxidation, as in carnitine deficiency and carnitine palmitoyltransferase deficiency. Diminished glucose production occurs with adrenal or pituitary insufficiency or liver disease. Hepatic cirrhosis, hepatitis, or hepatic congestion are common causes of hypoglycemia, and ethanol ingestion, even at low levels, increases the NADH/NAD ratio and blocks gluconeogenesis and can cause fasting hypoglycemia (see Table 35-1).

DIAGNOSIS   Fasting hypoglycemia is established by the simultaneous measurement of serum glucose, insulin, cortisol, and C-peptide and urine sulfonylurea metabolites during an episode of symptoms consistent with hypoglycemia. If history is suggestive but fasting plasma glucose is normal, hospitalization for a 72-h fast is required; serial measurements of glucose and insulin are made until symptoms develop or fast is completed. Diagnosis of insulinoma requires a low plasma glucose and inappropriately high insulin. Exogenous insulin is excluded by the simultaneous measurement of C-peptide, while a screen for sulfonylureas eliminates the possibility of oral hypoglycemic agents. The presence of an extrapancreatic tumor is suggested by low glucose and insulin levels (see Table 35-2).

℞ TREATMENT
Initial rapid IV administration of 50–100 mL 50% glucose in water is followed by infusion of 10% glucose to keep plasma glucose >5.6 mmol/L (>100 mg/dL) in serious hypoglycemia. Pts with glucose overutilization may require >10 g glucose/h or pt can eat a diet containing >300 g carbohydrate/d. Glucagon (1 mg IM) is less desirable because its transient effects are blunted when hepatic glycogen is depleted. Hypoglycemia caused by sulfonylureas is often prolonged, and pts must be monitored for at least 24 h. Surgical excision is the treatment of choice for insulinoma. Localization should be attempted by CT scan, arteriography, or either preoperative or intraoperative ultrasonography. Medical therapy of insulinoma is indicated only in preparation for surgery or after failure to localize the tumor at surgery. Diazoxide IV or orally in doses of 300–1200 mg/d plus a diuretic may be used, or 150–450 μg/d octreotide is given SC in divided doses.

Treatment of other forms of hypoglycemia is dietary. Pts should avoid fasting and should ingest frequent small meals.

Table 35-1

Major Causes of Fasting Hypoglycemia

UNDERPRODUCTION OF GLUCOSE

Hormone deficiencies
  Hypopituitarism
  Adrenal insufficiency
  Catecholamine deficiency
  Glucagon deficiency
Enzyme defects
  Glucose-6-phosphatase
  Liver phosphorylase
  Pyruvate carboxylase
  Phosphoenolpyruvate carboxykinase
  Fructose-1,6-diphosphatase
  Glycogen synthetase
Substrate deficiency
  Ketotic hypoglycemia of infancy
  Severe malnutrition, muscle wasting
  Late pregnancy
Acquired liver disease
  Hepatic congestion
  Severe hepatitis
  Cirrhosis
  Uremia (probably multiple mechanisms)
  Hypothermia
Drugs
  Ethanol
  Propranolol
  Salicylates

OVERUTILIZATION OF GLUCOSE

Hyperinsulinism
  Insulinoma
  Exogenous insulin
  Sulfonylureas
  Immune disease with insulin or insulin receptor anti-
    bodies
  Drugs: quinine in falciparum malaria, disopyramide,
    pentamidine
  Endotoxic shock
Appropriate insulin levels
  Extrapancreatic tumors
  Systemic carnitine deficiency
  Deficiency in enzymes of fat oxidation
  3-Hydroxy-3-methylglutaryl-CoA lyase deficiency
  Cachexia with fat depletion

SOURCE: Foster DW, Rubenstein AH: HPIM-14, p. 2083.

Table 35-2

Differential Diagnosis of Insulinoma and Factitious Hyperinsulinism

Test	Insulinoma	Exogenous Insulin	Sulfonylurea
Plasma insulin	High	Very high*	High
Insulin/glucose ratio	High	Very high	High
Proinsulin	Increased	Normal or low	Normal
C-peptide	Increased	Normal or low[†]	Increased
Insulin antibodies	Absent	± Present[‡]	Absent
Plasma or urine sulfonylurea	Absent	Absent	Present

* Total plasma insulin in patients with insulinoma is rarely above 1435 pmol/L (200 μU/mL) in the basal state and often much lower. Values greater than 7175 pmol/L (100 μU/mL) are highly suggestive of exogenous insulin injection.
[†] C-peptide may be normal in absolute terms but low in relation to the increased insulin value. See text for C-peptide suppression test.
[‡] Insulin bodies may not be present if only a few injections have been given, especially with purified insulins.
SOURCE: Foster DW, Rubenstein AH: HPIM-14, p. 2086.

For a more detailed discussion, see Foster DW, Rubenstein AH: Hypoglycemia, Chap. 335, p. 2081, in HPIM-14.

ONCOLOGIC EMERGENCIES

Emergencies in the cancer pt may be classified into three categories: effects from tumor expansion, metabolic or hormonal effects mediated by tumor products, and treatment complications.

STRUCTURAL/OBSTRUCTIVE ONCOLOGIC EMERGENCIES

The most common problems are: superior vena cava syndrome; pericardial effusion/tamponade; spinal cord compression; seizures (see Chap. 175) and/or increased intracranial pressure (see Chap. 31); and intestinal, urinary, or biliary obstruction. The last three conditions are discussed in Chap. 104 in HPIM-14.

Superior Vena Cava Syndrome

Obstruction of the superior vena cava reduces venous return from the head, neck, and upper extremities. About 85% of cases are due to lung cancer; lymphoma and thrombosis of central venous catheters are also causes. Pts often present with facial swelling, dyspnea, and cough. In severe cases, the mediastinal mass lesion may cause tracheal obstruction. Dilated neck veins and increased collateral veins on anterior chest wall are noted on physical examination. CXR documents widening of the superior mediastinum; 25% of pts have a right-sided pleural effusion.

℞ TREATMENT

Radiation therapy is the treatment of choice for non-small cell lung cancer; addition of chemotherapy to radiation therapy is effective in small cell lung cancer and lymphoma. Clotted central catheters producing this syndrome should be withdrawn, and anticoagulation therapy initiated.

Pericardial Effusion/Tamponade

Accumulation of fluid in the pericardium impairs filling of the heart and decreases cardiac output. Most commonly seen in pts with lung or breast cancers, leukemias, or lymphomas, pericardial tamponade may also develop as a late complication of mediastinal radiation therapy. Common symptoms are dyspnea, cough, chest pain, orthopnea, and weakness. Pleural effusion, sinus tachycardia, jugular venous distention, hepatomegaly, and cyanosis are frequent physical findings. Paradoxical pulse, decreased heart sounds, pulsus alternans, and friction rub are less common with malignant than nonmalignant pericardial disease. Echocardiography is diagnostic; pericardiocentesis may show serous or bloody exudate, and cytology usually shows malignant cells.

℞ TREATMENT

Drainage of fluid from the pericardial sac may be lifesaving until a definitive surgical procedure can be performed.

Spinal Cord Compression

Primary spinal cord tumors occur rarely, and cord compression is most commonly due to epidural metastases from vertebral bodies involved with tumor, especially from prostate, lung, breast, and lymphoma primaries. Pts present with back pain, worse when recumbent, with local tenderness. Loss of bowel and bladder control may occur. On physical examination, pts have a loss of sensation below a horizontal line on the trunk, called a sensory level, that usually corresponds to one or two vertebrae below the site of compression. Weakness and spasticity of the legs and hyperactive reflexes with upgoing toes on Babinski testing are often noted. Spine radiographs may reveal erosion of the pedicles (winking owl sign), lytic or sclerotic vertebral body lesions, and vertebral collapse. Collapse alone is not a reliable indicator of tumor; it is a common manifestation of a more common disease, osteoporosis. MRI can visualize the cord throughout its length and define the extent of tumor involvement.

℞ TREATMENT

Radiation therapy plus dexamethasone, 4 mg IV or PO q4h, is successful in arresting and reversing symptoms in about 75% of pts who are diagnosed while still ambulatory. Only 10% of pts made paraplegic by the tumor recover the ability to ambulate.

EMERGENT PARANEOPLASTIC SYNDROMES

Most paraneoplastic syndromes have an insidious onset (see Chap. 66). Hypercalcemia, syndrome of inappropriate antidiuretic hormone (SIADH), and adrenal insufficiency may present as emergencies.

Hypercalcemia

The most common paraneoplastic syndrome, it occurs in about 10% of cancer pts, particularly those with lung, breast, head and neck, and kidney cancer and myeloma. Bone resorption mediated by parathormone-related protein is the most common mechanism; IL-1, IL-6, tumor necrosis factor, and transforming growth factor-β may act locally in tumor-involved bone. Pts usually present with nonspecific symptoms: fatigue, anorexia, constipation, weakness. Hypoalbuminemia associated with malignancy may make symptoms worse for any given serum calcium level because less calcium will be protein bound and more will be free.

℞ TREATMENT
Saline hydration, antiresorptive agents (such as pamidronate, 60–90 mg IV over 4 h), and glucocorticoids usually lower calcium levels significantly within 1–3 days. Treatment of the underlying malignancy is also important.

SIADH

Induced by the action of arginine vasopressin produced by certain tumors (especially small cell cancer of the lung), SIADH is characterized by hyponatremia, inappropriately concentrated urine, and high urine sodium excretion in the absence of volume depletion. Most pts with SIADH are asymptomatic. When serum sodium falls to <115 meq/L, pts may experience anorexia, depression, lethargy, irritability, confusion, weakness, and personality changes.

℞ TREATMENT
Water restriction controls mild forms. Demeclocycline (900–1200 mg PO bid) inhibits the effects of vasopressin on the renal tubule. Treatment of the underlying malignancy is also important.

Adrenal Insufficiency

The infiltration of the adrenals by tumor and their destruction by hemorrhage are the two most common causes. Symptoms such as nausea, vomiting, anorexia, and orthostatic hypotension may be attributed to progressive cancer or to treatment side effects. Certain treatments (e.g., ketoconazole, aminoglutethimide) may directly interfere with steroid synthesis in the adrenal.

℞ TREATMENT
In emergencies, a bolus of 100 mg IV hydrocortisone is followed by a continuous infusion of 10 mg/h. In nonemergent

but stressful circumstances, 100–200 mg/d oral hydrocortisone is the beginning dose, tapered to maintenance of 15–37.5 mg/d. Fludrocortisone (0.1 mg/d) may be required in the presence of hyperkalemia.

TREATMENT COMPLICATIONS

Complications from treatment may occur acutely or emerge only many years after treatment. Toxicity may be related either to the agents used to treat the cancer or from the response of the cancer to the treatment (e.g., leaving a perforation in a hollow viscus or causing metabolic complications such as the tumor lysis syndrome). Several treatment complications present as emergencies. Fever and neutropenia and tumor lysis syndrome will be discussed here; others are discussed in Chap. 104 in HPIM-14.

Fever and Neutropenia

Many cancer pts are treated with myelotoxic agents. When peripheral blood granulocyte counts are <1000/μL, the risk of infection is substantially increased (48 infections/100 pts). A neutropenic pt who develops a fever (>38°C) should undergo physical examination with special attention toward skin lesions, mucous membranes, IV catheter sites, and perirectal area. Two sets of blood cultures from different sites should be drawn, and a CXR performed, and any additional tests should be guided by findings from the history and physical examination. Any fluid collections should be tapped and urine and/or fluids should be examined under the microscope for evidence of infection.

℞ **TREATMENT**

After cultures are obtained, all pts should receive intravenous broad-spectrum antibiotics (e.g., ceftazidime 1 g q8h). If an obvious infectious site is found, the antibiotic regimen is designed to cover organisms that may cause the infection. Usually therapy should be started with an agent or agents that cover both gram-positive and -negative organisms. If the fever resolves, treatment should continue until neutropenia resolves. If the pt remains febrile and neutropenic after 7 days, amphotericin B should be added to the antibiotic regimen.

Tumor Lysis Syndrome

When rapidly growing tumors are treated with effective chemotherapy regimens, the rapid destruction of tumor cells can lead to the release of large amounts of nucleic acid breakdown products (chiefly uric acid), potassium, phosphate, and lactic acid. The phosphate elevations can lead to hypocalcemia. The increased uric acid, especially in the setting of acidosis, can precipitate in the renal tubules and lead to renal failure. The renal failure can exacerbate the hyperkalemia.

℞ TREATMENT

Prevention is the best approach. Maintain hydration with 3 L/d of saline, keep urine pH >7.0 with bicarbonate administration, and start allopurinol 300 (mg/m^2)/d 24 h before starting chemotherapy. Once chemotherapy is given, monitor serum electrolytes every 6 h. If serum potassium is above 6.0 meq/L and renal failure ensues, hemodialysis may be required. Maintain normal calcium levels.

For a more detailed discussion, see Finberg R: Infections in Patients with Cancer, Chap. 87, p. 537; and Gucalp R, Dutcher J: Oncologic Emergencies, Chap. 104, p. 627 in HPIM-14.

37

DRUG OVERDOSE

Drug overdose is a common medical emergency. Whereas iatrogenic drug toxicity is common, and serious intoxication can occur with any drug, the vast majority of ER treatments of drug overdose involve alcohol, other drugs of abuse (e.g., opioids, sedative-hypnotics, stimulants, hallucinogens) or drugs prescribed for psychiatric illness (antidepressants, antipsychotics, lithium). Psychiatric medications are common intoxicants both because they are potentially dangerous drugs and because of the suicidal proclivity of many pts taking such drugs. Diagnosis and treatment of drug overdose depend on recognizing the signs of specific drug effects. This chapter concerns the common drug overdose syndromes, except for that of alcohol, which is covered in Chap. 194. Drug dependence and withdrawal syndromes are covered in Chaps. 193 and 195.

CLINICAL APPROACH

The drug intoxications considered here are all metabolic encephalopathies and are thus associated with an altered mental state, either inhibition (from lethargy to coma) or excitation (from agitation to delirium). Structural lesions of the brain (e.g., mass lesion, stroke) can produce similar mental state changes but are usually distinguishable by other abnormalities such as an asymmetric neurologic exam, focal seizures, or impaired pupillary responses. Metabolic encephalopathies are generally associated with a symmetric neurologic exam and preserved pupillary responses. Other characteristics associated with metabolic encephalopathies that are uncommon with structural lesions include fluctuations in the level of consciousness, hyperthermia or hypothermia, multifocal seizures, and myoclonus or asterixis. Drug intoxications also need to be distinguished from metabolic encephalopathies arising from endogenous metabolic disturbances such as hypoglycemia, hepatic failure, hyperosmolar nonketotic hyperglycemia, and uremia, all of which can be diagnosed by appropriate laboratory studies. In addition, drug intoxications need to be distinguished from drug withdrawal syndromes, particularly those of alcohol and sedative-hypnotics, which also produce metabolic encephalopathies. Finally, meningitis, viral encephalitis, and subarachnoid hemorrhage may mimic drug intoxication.

In the ER, a pt with an altered mental state from whom a history of drug ingestion cannot be reliably obtained should be examined with particular attention to vital signs and meningeal signs. The neurologic exam should focus on the mental state, eye movement abnormalities (nystagmus, paralysis), pupillary abnormalities (miosis, mydriasis, impaired light reflex), ataxia and dysarthria, and any asymmetry of the motor, sensory, or reflex exam. Laboratory studies should include serum and urine toxicology screens which detect most common intoxicating agents. Tests of organ system failure (e.g., BUN and creatinine; LFT; PT/PTT; glucose), serum electrolytes (esp. Na and anion gap), serum osmolarity, and arterial blood gas are necessary to test for other metabolic encephalopathies. ECG is necessary to detect serious dysrhythmias that are frequent causes of morbidity and mortality with many drug overdoses. Head CT and/or lumbar puncture are indicated, especially in stuporous or comatose pts, to rule out a structural lesion, CNS infection, or subarachnoid hemorrhage.

SPECIFIC CLASSES OF DRUGS

Below are listed specific classes of drugs, signs of intoxication, and treatments.

OPIATES   Opioid drugs include heroin, morphine, methadone (Dolophine), codeine, meperidine (Demerol), hydromorphone (Dilaudid), oxycodon (Percodan), propoxyphene (Darvon), and pentazocine (Talwin).

Signs of Intoxication   The cardinal features of opiate overdose are drowsiness, pinpoint pupils, and respiratory depression. Other signs include nausea and vomiting, urinary retention, reduced GI mobility, noncardiogenic pulmonary edema, confusional states, and with more severe intoxication, stupor and coma. Seizures may occur with meperidine and propoxyphene overdoses.

℞ TREATMENT

Opiate overdose may require ventilatory support. Naloxone should be administered intravenously, 0.4–2 mg every 5 min, until evidence of clinical response or until 10 mg has been given. Pupillary dilation and, in the case of stuporous or comatose pts, full recovery of consciousness may occur promptly. With overdoses of long-acting narcotics such as methadone, the effects of naloxone may wear off before those of the opioid, and repeated doses of naloxone over 6–8 h may be required.

SEDATIVE-HYPNOTICS   This group includes barbiturates, nonbarbiturate sedatives, and the benzodiazepines. Barbiturates include phenobarbital (Luminal), amobarbital (Amytal), pentobarbital (Nembutal), and secobarbital (Seconal). Nonbarbiturate sedatives include meprobamate (Miltown), methaqualone (Quaalude), chloral hydrate (Noctec), ethchlorvynol (Placidyl), and glutethimide (Doriden). Benzodiazepines include diazepam (Valium), chlordiazepoxide (Librium), lorazepam (Ativan), alprazolam (Xanax), oxazepam (Serax), temazepam (Restoril), clorazepate (Tranxene), and triazolam (Halcion).

Signs of Intoxication   Hypotension, nystagmus or paralysis of eye movements, ataxia, dysarthria, hyporeflexia, respiratory depression, confusion, drowsiness, stupor and coma. Profound hypothermia (with an isoelectric EEG) is a common manifestation of severe overdose with barbiturates. Dilated pupils occur with glutethimide intoxication.

℞ TREATMENT

Respiratory and cardiovascular support are critical. Emesis should be induced only if pt is awake. Gastric lavage and administration of a cathartic and activated charcoal should be considered. Hemodialysis is effective for short-acting barbiturates, chloral hydrate, and ethchlorvynol, but its use is advised only for severely intoxicated pts. Renal elimination of phenobarbital is enhanced by administering sodium bicarbonate for alkalinization of the urine, but this is ineffectual for short-acting barbiturates and carries the risk of fluid overload.

STIMULANTS AND MONOAMINE OXIDASE (MAO) INHIBITORS

These two unrelated classes of drugs are listed together because signs of overdose are related to sympathomimetic effects for both. Stimulants include amphetamine (Benzedrine) and its derivatives, i.e., dextroamphetamine (Dexedrine), methamphetamine (Desoxyn, "speed"), and phenmetrazine (Preludin), as well as cocaine and its alkaloid derivative "crack". MAO inhibitors, a class of antidepressants, include phenelzine (Nardil), isocarboxazid (Marplan), and tranylcypromine (Parnate).

Signs of Intoxication   Overdose of any of these drugs can produce a confusional state consisting of elation, hyperactivity, and hypomania. If severe, there is extreme agitation, hallucinations, and schizophreniform paranoid psychosis. Physical signs include tachycardia, mydriasis, hyperthermia, hypertension, seizures, and coma. Morbidity and mortality as a result of cardiac dysrhythmias are common. Signs of MAO inhibitor overdose may be delayed by as much as 24 h after ingestion. Cerebral vasculitis has been reported in association with intravenous amphetamines. Myocardial infarction with cardiovascular collapse is being seen with increasing frequency in cocaine users.

℞ **TREATMENT**

There are no specific antidotes for any of these drugs. General life support measures are required in severe cases of intoxication. Amphetamine overdose requires treatment more often than cocaine overdose because of its longer duration of action. Parenteral administration of haloperidol may be used to treat the psychotic manifestations, and alpha-adrenergic blocking drugs such as clonidine may be used for severe hypertension.

HALLUCINOGENS

Among the hallucinogenic drugs, only phencyclidine (PCP) overdose is a common medical emergency. Lysergic acid diethylamide (LSD), mescaline, psilocybin, 2,5-dimethoxy-4-methylamhetamine (STP), *N,N*-dimethyltryptamine (DMT), and 3,4-methylenedioxyamphetamine (MDA, "ecstasy") may produce striking intoxication syndromes but they almost never cause life-threatening emergencies.

Signs of Intoxication   Common among signs of hallucinogenic drug overdose are nystagmus, ataxia, hypertonicity, hyperreflexia, and signs of sympathetic overactivity such as pupillary dilation, tachycardia, fever, and hypertension. Changes of mental state are variable and range from alterations in mood and affect; to cognitive changes with disorientation, amnesia, and feelings of detachment; to paranoia, visual and somatosensory hallucinations, and violent behavior. Intoxication with PCP can produce a striking degree of analgesia and at high doses can produce severe hypertension, catatonic states, malignant hyperthermia, status epilepticus, and coma.

℞ TREATMENT

Benzodiazepines may be useful for sedation. If antipsychotic therapy is required, butyrophenones (e.g., haloperidol) are preferable to phenothiazines because the latter tend to lower the seizure threshold. Otherwise, general supportive measures should be provided and severe hypertension, seizures, and malignant hyperthermia should be treated as they arise.

TRICYCLIC ANTIDEPRESSANTS AND ANTIPSYCHOTICS These two classes of drugs are listed together because the major manifestations of overdose of either class is due to prominent parasympatholytic (anticholinergic) effects. Tricyclic antidepressants include amitriptyline (Elavil), imipramine (Tofranil), doxepin (Sinequan), nortriptyline (Aventyl), and desipramine (Norpramin). Antipsychotics with prominent anticholinergic effects include chlorpromazine (Thorazine), thioridazine (Mellaril), perfenazine (Trilafon), fluphenazine (Prolixin), and trifluoperazine (Stelazine). There are many other anticholinergic medications which, in excess, can lead to similar overdose syndromes. These include atropine, scopolamine, trihexyphenidyl (Artane), benztropine (Cogentin), prochlorperazine (Compazine), hydroxyzine (Atarax, Vistaril), promethazine (Phenergan), and many over-the-counter H_1 antihistamines.

Signs of Intoxication Any of these agents can cause a confusional state characterized by an agitated delirium with hallucinations. Other common anticholinergic manifestations include fever, flushing, dry skin and mucous membranes, dilated pupils, and urinary retention. Cardiac dysrhythmias can be life-threatening. At higher doses, seizures and coma supervene.

℞ TREATMENT

There is no specific antidote for any of these medications, and treatment with cholinomimetic drugs, such as physostigmine, carry such high risks themselves that they are rarely used. For recent ingestions, gastric lavage, activated charcoal, and cathartics may be used. Otherwise, treatment is usually supportive unless serious cardiac dysrhythmia occurs.

LITHIUM Most cases of lithium intoxication occur gradually in pts on chronic therapy as serum levels rise, although acute intoxications also occur.

Signs of Intoxication With moderate intoxication, the altered mental state is characterized by confusion, anxiety, and delirium; more serious intoxications lead to stupor and coma. Other neurologic manifestations include tremor, ataxia, hyperreflexia, dystonic or choreiform movements, and seizures. Other physical signs include fever, hypotension, and cardiac dysrhythmias.

℞ TREATMENT

Hemodialysis is the treatment of choice to reduce lithium levels. Gastric lavage may be used for recent ingestions. It is critical to maintain sodium and water balance until the intoxication has cleared. Even with prompt treatment, some pts are left with permanent neurologic and renal damage.

For a more detailed discussion, see Lovejoy FH Jr, Linden CH: Poisoning and Drug Overdose, Chap. 391, p. 2523, in HPIM-14.

DROWNING AND NEAR-DROWNING

Pathophysiology

Approximately 90% of drowning victims aspirate fluid into lungs. Both freshwater and saltwater aspiration lead to severe hypoxemia due to ventilation/perfusion imbalance and significant pulmonary venous admixture, although mechanisms may differ between the two situations. In victims who do not aspirate, hypoxemia results from apnea. Contaminated water may pose additional risks, including obstruction of small bronchioles by particulate matter and infection by pathogens in the water.

Other physiologic changes occurring in drowning and near-drowning victims include changes in serum electrolytes and blood volume, although these are seen only rarely in persons successfully resuscitated. Hypotonicity may cause acute RBC lysis; however, this complication has been reported only rarely. Hypercarbia is less common than hypoxemia. Renal failure is uncommon, but when it does occur, it is secondary to hypoxemia, renal hypoperfusion, or, in extremely rare cases, significant hemoglobinuria.

℞ TREATMENT (See Fig. 38-1)

1. Remove victim from water as soon as possible and stabilize head and neck if trauma is suspected. The American Heart Association recommends that an abdominal thrust not be used routinely in victims of submersion as this maneuver can lead to regurgitation and aspiration of gastric contents.
2. Restore airway patency, breathing, and circulation immediately. Recall that hypothermia is protective of CNS function, and victims should not be presumed to have failed resuscitation until they have also been rewarmed.
3. Protect airway with endotracheal intubation if the patient is unconscious or obtunded. Correct hypoxemia with supplemental oxygen and mechanical ventilation with PEEP or CPAP if needed.
4. Establish venous access as soon as possible.
5. Monitor core body temperature and rewarm if necessary.
6. Monitor cardiac rhythm.
7. Measure and monitor serum electrolytes, renal function, ABGs. Bicarbonate administration for metabolic acidosis with a pH <7.20 is controversial but may be indicated in severe cases.

ANAPHYLAXIS AND TRANSFUSION REACTIONS

ANAPHYLAXIS

Definition

A life-threatening systemic hypersensitivity reaction to contact with an allergen; it may appear within minutes of exposure to the offending substance. Manifestations include respiratory distress; pruritus; urticaria; mucous membrane swelling; gastrointestinal disturbances including nausea, vomiting, pain, and diarrhea; and vascular collapse. Virtually any allergen may incite an anaphylactic reaction, but among the more common agents are proteins such as antisera, hormones, pollen extracts, *Hymenoptera* venom, foods; drugs (especially antibiotics); and diagnostic agents. Atopy does not seem to predispose to anaphylaxis from penicillin or venom exposures.

Clinical Presentation

Time to onset is variable but symptoms usually occur within seconds to minutes of exposure to the offending antigen:

* Respiratory: mucous membrane swelling, hoarseness, stridor, wheezing
* Cardiovascular: tachycardia, hypotension
* Cutaneous: pruritus, urticaria, angioedema

Diagnosis

Made by obtaining history of exposure to offending substance with subsequent development of characteristic complex of signs and symptoms.

℞ TREATMENT

Mild symptoms such as pruritus and urticaria can be controlled by administration of 0.2 to 0.5 mL of 1:1000 epinephrine solution SC, repeated at 20-min intervals as necessary.

An IV infusion should be initiated. Hypotension should be treated by IV administration of 2.5 mL of 1:50,000 epinephrine solution at 5 to 10-min intervals, volume expanders, e.g., as normal saline, and vasopressor agents, e.g., dopamine, if intractable hypotension occurs.

Epinephrine provides both alpha- and beta-adrenergic effects, resulting in vasoconstriction and bronchial smooth-muscle relaxation. Beta blockers are relatively contraindicated in persons at risk for anaphylactic reactions.

The following should also be used as necessary:

- Antihistamines such as diphenhydramine 50 to 80 mg IM or IV
- Aminophylline 0.25 to 0.5 g IV for bronchospasm
- Oxygen
- Glucocorticoids—IV; not useful for acute manifestations but may help control persistent hypotension or bronchospasm

Prevention

Avoidance of offending antigen, where possible; skin testing and desensitization to materials such as penicillin and *Hymenoptera* venom, if necessary.

TRANSFUSION REACTIONS

Transfusion reactions may be classified as immune or nonimmune.

Immunologically Mediated Reactions

Reaction may be directed against red or white blood cells, platelets, or IgA; in addition, other, less well-characterized reactions may occur.

ACUTE HEMOLYTIC TRANSFUSION REACTIONS Usually due to ABO incompatibility, although alloantibodies directed against other antigens may result in intravascular hemolysis; very rapid and massive hemolysis occurs. Symptoms and signs may include restlessness, anxiety, flushing, chest or back pain, tachypnea, tachycardia, nausea, shock, renal failure, coagulation disorders (including DIC).

DELAYED HEMOLYTIC TRANSFUSION REACTIONS Occur in pts previously sensitized to RBC alloantigens who have a negative alloantibody screen due to low antibody levels. When the pt is transfused an anamnestic alloantibody response occurs, leading to extravascular hemolysis of the transfused RBCs.

ALLERGIC REACTIONS Characterized by a pruritic rash, edema, headache, and dizziness. Related to plasma proteins found in transfused components.

ANAPHYLACTIC REACTIONS Severe reactions characterized by hypotension, difficulty breathing, bronchospasm, respiratory arrest, shock. Patients with IgA deficiency are at particular risk for severe reaction due to sensitization to IgA.

TRANSFUSION-RELATED ACUTE LUNG INJURY
Rare reaction that results from transfusion of donor plasma that contains high titer anti-HLA antibodies that bind to corresponding antigens on recipient leukocytes. Recipient develops respiratory compromise and signs of noncardiogenic pulmonary edema. Treatment is supportive; most pts recover without sequelae.

GRAFT-VERSUS-HOST DISEASE (GVH) Rare complication of transfusion mediated by donor T lymphocytes that recognize host HLA antigens as foreign and mount an immune response. Can occur when blood components that contain viable T lymphocytes are transfused into immunodeficient recipients or into immunocompetent recipients who share HLA antigens with the donor. Clinically, characterized by pancytopenia, cutaneous eruption, diarrhea, and liver function abnormalities. Transfusion GVH is notoriously resistant to treatment with immunosuppressive medications and is usually fatal. Transfusion-related GVH can be prevented by irradiation of cellular components before transfusion into pts at risk.

**LABORATORY INVESTIGATION
OF IMMUNE-MEDIATED REACTIONS**

- Careful check on identity of donor and recipient; samples of recipient blood to blood bank for analysis and further cross-matching
- Documentation of hemolysis—plasma and urine hemoglobin, haptoglobin, hematocrit, bilirubin
- Check renal status—urinalysis, BUN, creatinine
- Check coagulation status—platelet count, PT, PTT

℞ TREATMENT

- Avoid further transfusion unless absolutely necessary
- Management of shock and renal failure in intravascular hemolysis; osmotic diuresis and volume expansion may be indicated in certain cases; if renal failure ensues, adjust drug doses and closely monitor fluid/electrolyte status
- Factor replacement if needed to control coagulation abnormalities; platelet infusion if thrombocytopenia severe

Nonimmune Reactions

CIRCULATORY OVERLOAD Especially in infants and pts with renal or cardiac insufficiency. Effects of massive transfusion include hyperkalemia, ammonia and citrate toxicity, dilutional coagulopathy, thrombocytopenia.

TRANSMISSION OF INFECTION Hepatitis, syphilis, CMV, malaria, babesiosis, toxoplasmosis, brucellosis, and AIDS can all be transmitted by transfused blood.

IRON OVERLOAD With repeated transfusions; may require chelation therapy.

For a more detailed discussion, see Austen KF: Diseases of Immediate Type Hypersensitivity, Chap. 310, p. 1860; and Dzieczkowski JS, Anderson KC: Transfusion Biology and Therapy, Chap. 115, p. 718, in HPIM-14.

BITES, ENVENOMATIONS, STINGS, AND ECTOPARASITE INFESTATIONS

MAMMALIAN BITES

Between 1 and 2 million mammalian animal-bite wounds are sustained in the U.S. each year. The vast majority are from pet dogs and cats. A significant number result in infection, which may be life-threatening. The microbiology of bite-wound infections generally reflects the oropharyngeal flora of the biting animal, although organisms from the soil, the skin of the animal or victim, or the animal's feces may also be involved.

DOG BITES Dogs account for ~80% of bite wounds. Some 15–20% of dog-bite wounds become infected. Infection typically manifests 8–24 h after the bite, with increasing pain, soft tissue erythema and edema, and a purulent, sometimes foul-smelling discharge. Fever, lymphadenopathy, and lymphangitis may occur. If the dog's tooth penetrates synovium or bone, septic arthritis or osteomyelitis may develop. While infection usually remains localized, systemic spread (e.g., bacteremia, endocarditis, brain abscess) can take place. Dissemination is most likely in pts with poor lymphatic drainage of the affected area or with systemic immunocompromise.

The microbiology of dog-bite wound infections is usually mixed and includes staphylococci, alpha-hemolytic streptococci, *Pasteurella multocida*, *Eikenella corrodens*, and *Capnocytophaga canimorsus* (formerly designated DF-2). Anaerobes are often present as well. *C. canimorsus* infection can be fulminant, with sepsis syndrome, DIC, and renal failure, particularly in pts who have undergone splenectomy, who have hepatic dysfunction, or who are otherwise immunosuppressed. This fastidious, thin gram-negative rod is occasionally seen within PMNs on Wright-stained smears of peripheral blood from septic pts. In addition to bacterial infections, dog bites may transmit rabies (Chap. 99) and may lead to tetanus intoxication (Chap. 87).

CAT BITES   More than half of cat bites and scratches result in infection. Feline incisors are narrow and sharp and may penetrate deeply into tissues. Accordingly, cat bites are more likely than dog bites to cause septic arthritis or osteomyelitis, sequelae that are particularly likely following bites to the hand. Both cat-bite and cat-scratch wounds are typically infected by organisms originating in the feline oropharynx. *P. multocida* is the most important of these, causing infection that may manifest only a few hours after the bite, with pain, severe inflammation, and purulent or serosanguineous discharge. As in dog-bite wounds, a mixed bacterial flora is often present and dissemination may occur. The risk factors for systemic infection following cat bites are similar to those for dog bites. In addition, like dog bites, cat bites may transmit rabies or may lead to tetanus intoxication. Cat bites and scratches may also transmit *Bartonella henselae*, the agent of cat-scratch disease, which is a potential late sequela of these injuries (Chap. 86).

HUMAN BITES   Human bites are categorized as occlusional injuries, which are inflicted by actual biting, or clenched-fist injuries, which may result when the fist of one individual strikes the teeth of another. Human-bite wounds more frequently become infected than do bite wounds from other animals. Clenched-fist injuries are particularly prone to serious infection. Reflecting the human oral microflora, the flora of human-bite wounds is rich and diverse. Aerobic components include viridans streptococci, *Staphylococcus aureus*, *E. corrodens*, and *Haemophilus influenzae*. Anaerobic species, which are isolated from 50% of human-bite wounds, include *Fusobacterium nucleatum* as well as *Prevotella*, *Porphyromonas*, and *Peptostreptococcus* spp.

OTHER MAMMALIAN BITES   See Table 40-1.

R̄x̄ TREATMENT

Initial Assessment   Elicit a careful history including the type of animal responsible, whether or not the attack was provoked, and the time elapsed since the injury. Obtain details regarding possible antibiotic allergies, systemic immunosuppression, and immunization history. Contact public health authorities if rabies is a consideration. Consider domestic abuse if confronted with suspicious human-bite wounds. Assess the type of wound (e.g., puncture, laceration, crush injury, scratch), its depth, and the possibility of injury to joints, tendons, nerves, and/or bone. Look carefully for evidence of infection, including redness, exudate, foul odor, lymphangitis, lymphadenopathy, or fever. Because of their potentially debilitating consequences, hand injuries warrant consultation with a hand surgeon. Obtain radiographs if bony injury or retained tooth fragments are suspected. Stain and culture specimens from all infected wounds; include specimens for anaerobic culture if devitalized tissue, malodorous exudate, or frank abscess is present. Perform a WBC count and blood cultures if systemic infection is suspected. For bites of animals other than dogs or cats, culture samples from wounds whether infected or not, since the resident flora is unpredictable in those cases.

Wound Management   Wound closure is controversial in bite injuries. After thorough cleansing, facial wounds are usually sutured for cosmetic reasons and because the abundant facial blood supply and absence of dependent edema lessen the risk of infection there. For wounds elsewhere, many authorities do not attempt primary closure, preferring instead to irrigate copiously, debride devitalized tissue, remove foreign bodies, and approximate the margins. Delayed primary closure may be undertaken after the risk of infection has passed. Puncture wounds due to cat bites should not be sutured because of their high risk of infection.

Antibiotic Therapy   Antimicrobial prophylaxis for early bite wounds is controversial (Table 40-1). When given, prophylaxis should continue for 3–5 d. Antibiotics should certainly be used for all established bite-wound infections and should target likely pathogens (Table 40-1). Treatment is usually continued for 10–14 d (longer if osteomyelitis or septic arthritis develops). Elevation and immobilization of the site of injury are important adjunctive measures. Therapeutic response must be carefully monitored. If treatment fails, alternative diagnoses should be considered and surgical evaluation performed for possible drainage and debridement.

C. canimorsus sepsis requires a 2-week course of IV penicillin G (2×10^6 U q4h). Serious *P. multocida* infection should also be treated with IV penicillin. Alternative agents, albeit ones with which there is less clinical experience, include second- or third-generation cephalosporins and fluoroquinolones.

A tetanus booster immunization should be given for pts previously immunized but not boosted within 5 years. Patients not previously immunized should undergo primary immunization and should also receive tetanus immune globulin.

VENOMOUS SNAKEBITES

ETIOLOGY AND EPIDEMIOLOGY Venomous snakebites are rare in most developed countries (see Table 40-2). Worldwide, however, at least 30,000 to 40,000 people die from these injuries each year. Poisonous snakes indigenous to the U.S. include the rattlesnake, the copperhead, the coral snake, and the water moccasin. The mortality rate is <1% among U.S. victims who receive antivenin. Eastern and western diamondback rattlesnakes (*Crotalus adamanteus* and *C. atrox*, respectively) are responsible for most of these deaths. Snake venoms are molecularly complex mixtures; most can adversely affect multiple organs.

℞ **TREATMENT**

Field Management First aid should focus on delivering the victim to definitive care as soon as possible. The victim should be as inactive as is feasible in order to minimize systemic spread of the venom. After viperid bites, local suction to remove venom may be beneficial if applied within 3–5 min. A mechanical suction device should be used; mouth-to-wound suction should be avoided. Suction should be continued for at least 30 min. A proximal lymphatic-occlusive constriction band may also limit the spread of venom if applied within 30 min of the bite. *It should not be so tight as to interfere with arterial flow.* A bitten extremity should be splinted, if possible, and kept at heart level. Incisions into the bite wound, cooling, and electric shock should all be *avoided*.

Hospital Management The victim should be closely monitored (vital signs, cardiac rhythm, oxygen saturation). The level of erythema and swelling should be marked every 15 min. Intravenous access with a large-bore catheter should be established in an unaffected extremity. Blood work, including a complete blood count, an assessment of renal and hepatic function, coagulation studies, and typing and crossmatching, should be performed promptly, and the urine should

Table 40-1

Management of Wound Infections Following Animal Bites

Biting Species	Commonly Isolated Pathogens	Preferred Antibiotic(s)*
Dog	*Staphylococcus aureus, Pasteurella multocida,* anaerobes, *Capnocytophaga canimorsus*	Amoxicillin/clavulanic acid (250–500 mg PO tid); or ampicillin/sulbactam (1.5–3.0 g IV q6h)
Cat	*P. multocida, S. aureus,* anaerobes	Amoxicillin/clavulanic acid or ampicillin/sulbactam, as for dog bite
Human; occlusional bite	Viridans streptococci, *S. aureus, Haemophilus influenzae,* anaerobes	Amoxicillin/clavulanic acid or ampicillin/sulbactam, as for dog bite
Human; clenched-fist injury	As for occlusional bite plus *Eikenella corrodens*	Ampicillin/sulbactam, as for dog bite, or imipenem
Monkey	As for human bite	As for human bite
Rodent	*Streptobacillus moniliformis, Leptospira* spp., *P. multocida*	Penicillin VK (500 mg PO bid)
Snake	*Pseudomonas aeruginosa, Proteus* spp., *Bacteroides fragilis, Clostridium* spp.	Ampicillin/sulbactam, as for dog bite

* Antibiotic choices should be based on culture data, when available. These suggestions for empirical therapy need to be tailored to individual circumstances and local conditions. Intravenous regimens should be used for hospitalized pts. When the pt is to be discharged after initial management, a single IV dose of antibiotic may be given and followed by oral therapy. TMP-SMZ, trimethoprim-sulfamethoxazole.

Alternative Agent for Penicillin-Allergic Patient	Recommendation for Prophylaxis in Patients with Recent Uninfected Wounds	Other Considerations
Clindamycin (150–300 mg PO qid) plus either TMP-SMZ (1 double-strength tablet bid) or ciprofloxacin (500 mg PO bid)	Sometimes†	Consider rabies prophylaxis.
Clindamycin plus either TMP-SMZ or a fluoroquinolone	Usually, especially for hand wounds	Consider rabies prophylaxis; carefully evaluate for joint/bone penetration.
Erythromycin, fluoroquinolone	Always	—
Cefoxitin‡ (1.5 g IV q6h)	Always	Examine for tendon/nerve/joint involvement.
As for human bite	Always	For macaque monkeys, consider B virus prophylaxis with acyclovir.
Doxycycline (100 mg PO qd)	Sometimes†	—
Clindamycin plus either TMP-SMZ or a fluoroquinolone	Sometimes, especially for venomous snakebite	Use antivenin for venomous snakebite.

† Prophylactic antibiotics are suggested for severe or extensive wounds, facial wounds, or crush injuries; when bone or joint may be involved; or when comorbidity exists.

‡ Cefoxitin may be hazardous to pts with immediate-type hypersensitivity to penicillin.

SOURCE: Madoff LC: HPIM-14, p. 838.

Table 40-2

Venomous Snakes of the World

Family	Subfamily	Representative Species	Remarks
Viperidae	Crotalinae	Rattlesnakes (*Crotalus* and *Sistrurus* spp.); water moccasins and copperheads (*Agkistrodon* spp.), lancehead vipers (*Bothrops* spp.)	New World and Asian pit vipers
	Viperinae	Russell's viper (*Vipera russelli*), saw-scaled viper (*Echis carinatus*), puff adder (*Bitis arietans*)	European, Asian, African vipers
Elapidae		Cobras (*Naja* spp.), mambas (*Dendroaspis* spp.), taipan (*Oxyuranus scutellatus*)	Temperate and tropical New and Old World; all venomous terrestrial snakes of Australia
Hydrophiidae		Pelagic sea snake (*Pelamis platurus*)	Pacific and Indian Oceans
Atractaspididae		Burrowing asps (*Atractaspis* spp.)	Africa, Middle East
Colubridae		Boomslang (*Dispholidus typus*), twig snake (*Thelotornis kirtlandii*)	Rear-fanged snakes with toxic salivary secretions

SOURCE: Norris RL et al: HPIM-14, p. 2545.

be tested for blood or myoglobin. In severe cases, arterial blood gas studies, ECG, and CXR should also be undertaken. Laboratory values should be rechecked hourly until stability is assured. Shock should be treated initially with fluid resuscitation (normal saline or Ringer's lactate, up to 20–40 mL/kg of body weight). If hypotension persists, 5% albumin (10–20 mL/kg) should be tried next, followed by a dopamine infusion. Central hemodynamic monitoring may be helpful but must be instituted with great care if coagulopathy is present.

Attempts to locate an appropriate antivenin should begin early in all cases of known venomous snakebite. In the U.S., assistance in finding antivenin can be obtained 24 h a day from the University of Arizona Poison and Drug Information Center (520-626-6016). Rapidly progressive and severe local findings or manifestations of systemic toxicity (signs and symptoms or laboratory abnormalities) are indications for the administration of IV antivenin. Most antivenins are of equine origin and carry risks of anaphylactic, anaphylactoid, or delayed-hypersensitivity reactions. Patients should be premedicated with IV antihistamines (e.g., diphenhydramine, 1 mg/kg up to a maximum dose of 100 mg; plus cimetidine, 5–10 mg/kg up to a maximum dose of 300 mg). Intravascular volume expansion may also be helpful. Epinephrine should be immediately available. The antivenin should be administered slowly in dilute solution, with the physician at the bedside. In the absence of allergic phenomena, the rate can be increased such that the total dose runs in over 1–4 h. Additional doses may be necessary. The management of life-threatening envenomation in a victim apparently allergic to antivenin requires significant expertise but is often possible with intensive premedication.

The bite wound should be dressed with dry, sterile gauze, splinted, and elevated only when antivenin is available. Tetanus immunization should be updated. Antibiotic prophylaxis is controversial. The affected extremity should be watched closely for development of a muscle-compartment syndrome.

Whether or not antivenin is given, pts with signs of envenomation should be observed in the hospital for at least 24 h. Patients with apparently "dry" bites should be watched for at least 6–8 h (for up to 24 h for elapid or sea snake bites).

MARINE ENVENOMATIONS AND INFECTIONS

As with venomous snakebites, management of envenomations by marine creatures is mostly supportive.

INVERTEBRATES Hydroids, fire coral, jellyfish, Portuguese man-of-war, and sea anemones possess specialized stinging cells called nematocysts. The clinical consequences of envenomation by these species are similar but differ in severity. Prickling, burning, and throbbing pain; pruritus; and paresthesia usually develop immediately. Neurologic, cardiovascular, respiratory, rheumatologic, GI, renal, and ocular symptoms have been described.

℞ TREATMENT
The skin should be decontaminated immediately with a forceful jet of vinegar (5% acetic acid) or rubbing alcohol (40–70% isopropanol) to inactivate nematocysts. Shaving the skin may also be helpful. After decontamination, topical anesthetics, antihistamines, or steroids should be applied. Narcotics may be necessary for persistent pain. Muscle spasms may respond to 10% calcium gluconate (5–10 mL) or diazepam (5–10 mg) given IV. Contact with sea sponges, annelid worms (bristleworms), and sea urchins may also produce painful stings of varying severity.

VERTEBRATES *Envenomations* A number of marine vertebrates, including stingrays, scorpionfish, catfish, surgeonfish, and weever, are capable of envenomating humans. Clinical manifestations include immediate and intense pain, weakness, diaphoresis, nausea, vomiting, diarrhea, dysrhythmia, syncope, hypotension, muscle cramps, fasciculations, paralysis, and (in rare cases) death.

℞ TREATMENT
The management of most of these stings is similar. Except for stonefish and serious scorpionfish envenomations, no antivenin is available. The affected part should be immersed immediately in nonscalding hot water (113°F/45°C) for 30–90 min to inactivate venoms and relieve pain. Opiates or regional nerve block (with 1% lidocaine, 0.5% bupivacaine, and sodium bicarbonate mixed 5:5:1) may also help. After soaking and analgesia, the wound should be explored, debrided, and vigorously irrigated. Wounds should be left to heal by secondary intention. Tetanus immunization should be updated. Antibiotics should be considered for serious wounds or for wounds in immunocompromised hosts, targeting staphylococci and streptococci in normal hosts. If the host is compromised or if infection develops, *Vibrio* spp. should also be targeted.

Sources of Antivenins and Other Assistance

Antivenin for stonefish and severe scorpionfish envenomation is available in the U.S. through the pharmacies of Sharp Cabrillo Hospital Emergency Department, San Diego, CA (619-221-3429), and Community Hospital of Monterey Peninsula Emergency Department, Monterey, CA (408-625-4900). The latter also has sea snake antivenin. Divers Alert Network may also be a source of helpful information (24 h a day at 919-684-8111 or by Internet at http://www.dan.ycg.org).

Erysipelothrix rhusiopathiae Infection   This small gram-positive rod causes human infection after the skin is scratched or punctured during the handling of fish, shellfish, or organic material (e.g., soil) containing the organism. The infection, an occupational hazard for fish handlers, farmers, and veterinarians, manifests after 1–4 d as a purplish, painful pruritic area at the site of inoculation. A slowly spreading erythematous rash, pruritic vesicles, and papules follow. Although generally self-limited, the infection may disseminate or cause endocarditis. *Treatment* consists of penicillin VK (500 mg PO qid) or ciprofloxacin (500 mg PO bid).

ARTHROPOD BITES AND STINGS

SPIDER BITES   Only a small minority of all spider species defend themselves aggressively and have fangs capable of penetrating human skin. While most spider bites are painful but not otherwise harmful, envenomation by the brown or fiddle spiders (*Loxosceles* spp.), the widow spiders (*Latrodectus* spp.), and certain other spiders may be life-threatening. Identification of the offending spider should be attempted; specific treatments exist for bites of widow and brown recluse spiders.

Recluse Spider Bites and Necrotic Arachnidism   Severe necrosis of skin and subcutaneous tissue follows envenomation by *Loxosceles reclusa* (the brown recluse spider) and by several other varieties of spiders. Initially the bite is painless or produces a stinging sensation. Over the next few hours, the site becomes painful, pruritic, indurated, and surrounded by zones of ischemia and erythema. Lesions typically resolve without treatment in 2–3 d. In severe cases, erythema spreads and the lesion becomes hemorrhagic and necrotic with an overlying bulla. Local nerves may be injured and infection may develop. Fever, chills, headache, and other nonspecific systemic symptoms may develop within 3 d of the bite. Fatal complications are rare.

℞ TREATMENT

Initial management includes local cleansing, application of sterile dressings and cold compresses, elevation, and loose immobilization. Analgesics, antihistamines, antibiotics, and tetanus prophylaxis should be administered if indicated. Immediate surgical excision of the wound is detrimental. Dapsone administration within 48–72 h (50–100 mg PO bid after G6PD deficiency has been ruled out) may halt progression of necrotic lesions. Antivenin has not been approved for use in the U.S.

Widow Spider Bites   Female widow spiders are notorious for their potent neurotoxin. The black widow (*Latrodectus mactans*) has been found in every U.S. state except Alaska. The initial bite goes unnoticed or is perceived as a sharp pinprick. Two small red marks, mild erythema, and edema develop at the fang entrance site. Some persons experience no other symptoms. In others, painful cramps spread from the bite site to large muscles of the extremities and trunk within 30-60 min. Extreme abdominal muscular rigidity and pain may mimic peritonitis, but the abdomen is not tender to palpation. Other features include salivation, diaphoresis, vomiting, hypertension, tachycardia, labored breathing, anxiety, headache, weakness, fasciculations, paresthesia, hyperreflexia, urinary retention, uterine contractions, and premature labor. Death from respiratory arrest, cerebral hemorrhage, or cardiac failure may occur.

℞ TREATMENT

Treatment consists of local cleansing, application of ice packs, and tetanus prophylaxis. Analgesics and antispasmodics (e.g., benzodiazepines and methocarbamol) may mitigate hypertension. If not, specific antihypertensives should be given. Equine antivenin is widely available; administration of 1 or 2 vials IV rapidly relieves pain and can be lifesaving. Because of the risk of allergic reactions, however, the use of antivenin should be reserved for severe cases involving respiratory arrest, refractory hypertension, seizures, or pregnancy.

SCORPION STINGS   Scorpions are crablike arachnids. Painful but relatively harmless scorpion stings must be distinguished from the potentially lethal envenomations produced by about 30 of the ~1000 known scorpion species, which annually cause >5000 deaths worldwide. In the U.S., only the bark scorpion (*Centruroides sculpturatus* or *C. exilicauda*) is potentially lethal. This animal measures about 7 cm in length and is yellow-brown in color. *C. sculpturatus* envenomations are usually associated with little swelling, but pain, paresthesia, and hyperesthesia can be accentuated by tapping on the affected area. Dysfunction of cranial nerves and hyperexcitability of skeletal muscle develop within hours. Patients present with restlessness, blurred vision, abnormal eye movements, profuse salivation, lacrimation, rhinorrhea, slurred speech, diaphoresis, nausea, vomiting, and difficulty handling secretions. Complications include tachycardia, arrhythmias, hypertension, hyperthermia, rhabdomyolysis, and acidosis. Manifestations are maximal after about 5 h and may subside within a day or two.

℞ TREATMENT

Stings of nonlethal species require at most ice packs, analgesics, or antihistamines. For victims of dangerous envenomations who have cranial nerve or neuromuscular dysfunction, aggressive supportive care and judicious use of antivenin can reduce or eliminate mortality. Keep the pt calm and apply pressure dressings and cold packs. Avoid narcotics and sedatives in the setting of neuromuscular dysfunction unless endotracheal intubation is planned. Manage hypertension, pulmonary edema, and bradyarrhythmias. An investigational caprine *C. sculpturatus* antivenin available only in Arizona carries a risk of anaphylaxis or serum sickness.

HYMENOPTERA STINGS Stinging insects of the order Hymenoptera include apids (bees and bumblebees), vespids (wasps, hornets, and yellow jackets), and ants. About 50 deaths from hymenopteran stings occur annually in the U.S., nearly all from allergic reactions to venoms. Bees can sting only once; vespids can sting numerous times in succession. Uncomplicated stings cause immediate pain, a wheal-and-flare reaction, and local edema that subside within hours. Multiple stings can lead to vomiting, diarrhea, generalized edema, dyspnea, and hypotension. Death from envenomation has occurred in persons stung by honeybees 300–500 times in succession.

Large local reactions progressing over 1–2 d and resembling cellulitis are not uncommon and are caused by hypersensitivity. They are seldom accompanied by anaphylaxis. About 0.4–4% of the U.S. population exhibits immediate-type hypersensitivity to insect stings. Serious reactions include upper airway edema, bronchospasm, hypotension, and shock and may be rapidly fatal. Onset usually comes within 10 min of the sting.

℞ TREATMENT

Anaphylaxis is treated with epinephrine hydrochloride (0.3–0.5 mL of a 1:1000 solution SC q20–30 min as needed). For profound shock, epinephrine (2–5 mL of a 1:10,000 solution by slow IV push) is indicated. Parenteral antihistamines, fluid resuscitation, bronchodilators, oxygen, endotracheal intubation, and vasopressors may be required. Patients should be observed for 24 h until the risk of recurrence has passed. Adults with a history of anaphylaxis should undergo desensitization.

ECTOPARASITE INFESTATIONS

SCABIES *Pathogenesis* Gravid female *Sarcoptes scabiei* mites burrow beneath the stratum corneum to lay eggs. Sensitization to their deposited excreta causes pruritus. Person-to-person spread is facilitated by intimate contact. Crusted (or Norwegian) scabies is a hyperinfestation syndrome associated with certain immunodeficiencies and with neurologic or psychiatric illness.

Clinical Manifestations Scabies is characterized by intense itching that worsens at night and after a hot shower. Burrows appear as dark, wavy lines measuring 3–15 mm in length and ending in a pearly bleb. They generally develop on the volar wrists, between the fingers, on the elbows, and on the penis. The head, neck, palms, and soles are spared except in infants. Crusted scabies resembles psoriasis and usually is not pruritic.

Diagnosis Burrows are unroofed and scrapings examined for the mite, its eggs, or its excreta. A drop of mineral oil facilitates removal of the sample. In the absence of a positive scraping, the diagnosis is made clinically.

℞ **TREATMENT**

After bathing, 5% permethrin cream is applied thinly but thoroughly behind the ears and from the neck down; it is removed with soap and water after 8 h. Repeat treatments may be necessary. A single oral dose of ivermectin (200 μg/kg) effectively treats scabies in otherwise healthy persons. Two or more doses may be required for crusted scabies. Pruritus may persist for weeks or months.

PEDICULOSIS (LICE) *Pathogenesis* *Pediculus humanus* var. *capitis* infests the head; *P. humanus* var. *corporis*, the clothing; and *Phthirus pubis*, mainly the hair of the pubis. All feed on human blood daily. Eggs (nits) attach to hair and clothing. Transmission is facilitated by close contact, sharing of headgear and grooming implements, crowding, and failure to wash clothes or bedding. Lice transmit typhus, epidemic relapsing fever, and trench fever.

Clinical Manifestations Head lice cause pruritus of the scalp, neck, and shoulders, with oozing, crusting, and matting of hair. Pruritic lesions are particularly common around the neck line. Chronic infestations result in vagabonds' disease (postinflammatory hyperpigmentation and lichenification). Pubic lice cause intense pubic, axillary, and periocular pruritus. Blue macules, 2–3 mm in diameter, develop at the sites of bites.

Diagnosis Nits or adult lice can be identified on hair or in clothing.

℞ TREATMENT

Use of 1% permethrin cream rinse kills both lice and eggs. Thereafter, the hair should be combed with a fine-toothed nit comb to remove nits. Combs and brushes should be disinfected, as should clothing and bedding.

TICK INFESTATIONS AND TICK PARALYSIS In the U.S., hard ticks (Ixodidae) are now the most common carriers of vector-borne disease. Ticks attach and feed painlessly. Their secretions, however, may produce local reactions, febrile illness, or paralysis. Tick paralysis, a rare syndrome, is an ascending, symmetric, flaccid paralysis believed to be caused by a neurotoxin in tick saliva. Dog and wood ticks are the most common agents in the U.S. Manifestations begin 5–6 d after the tick's attachment. Diagnosis depends on finding the tick, which is often hidden beneath hair.

℞ TREATMENT

Removal of the tick results in prompt improvement and usually leads to full recovery. Ticks should be removed by firm traction with forceps placed near their point of attachment. The site should then be disinfected. Removal of ticks within the first 48 h of attachment prevents transmission of the agents of Lyme disease and babesiosis. In endemic areas, protective measures against ticks include avoidance of brushy vegetation, use of protective clothing sprayed with 0.5% permethrin (*not* for direct use on skin), and application of repellant containing N,N-diethyl-m-toluamide (DEET) to exposed skin. Trouser cuffs should be tucked inside socks, and the skin should be checked daily for ticks.

For a more detailed discussion, see Madoff LC: Infections from Bites, Scratches, and Burns, Chap. 135, p. 835; Norris RL, Oslund S, Auerbach PS: Disorders Caused by Reptile Bites and Marine Animal Envenomations, Chap. 392, p. 2544; and Maguire JH, Spielman A: Ectoparasite Infestations and Arthropod Bites and Stings, Chap. 393, p. 2548, in HPIM-14.

41

HYPOTHERMIA

Hypothermia is defined as a core body temperature of ≤35°C and is classified as mild (32–35°C), moderate (28–32°C), or severe (<28°C).

Epidemiology

Rates of hypothermia are difficult to estimate since mild hypothermia usually goes unreported. A total of 770 cases of fatal environmental hypothermia were reported between 1979 and 1991 in the U.S. Most cases occur during the winter in cold climates, but hypothermia may occur in mild climates at any season. Risk factors include extremes of age (especially old age), homelessness, alcohol use, poverty, mental illness, neuroleptic use, and hypothyroidism.

Pathogenesis

Hypothermia can have several causes and is usually multifactorial. Heat is generated in most tissues of the body and is lost by radiation, evaporation, conduction, and convection. Factors that impede heat generation and/or increase heat loss lead to hypothermia. Immersion in water results in hypothermia because of the high thermal conductivity of water. Extremely cold conditions alone can cause hypothermia in healthy individuals, but this condition rarely requires medical attention. Iatrogenic hypothermia may develop when obtunded pts are left uncovered in hospital rooms or during surgical procedures. Decreased heat production may result from malnutrition, sepsis, severe hypothyroidism, hepatic failure, hypoglycemia, and/or hypothalamic lesions. Drugs that may contribute to hypothermia include ethanol, phenothiazines, barbiturates, opiates, clonidine, lithium, and benzodiazepines.

Clinical Manifestations

Acute cold exposure causes tachycardia, increased cardiac output, peripheral vasoconstriction, and increased peripheral vascular resistance. As body temperature drops below 32°C, cardiac conduction becomes impaired and heart rate and cardiac output decrease. Atrial fibrillation with slow ventricular response is common. Other ECG changes include Osborn (J) waves. Additional manifestations of hypothermia include volume depletion, hypotension, increased blood viscosity (which can lead to thrombosis), coagulopathy, thrombocytopenia, DIC, acid-base disturbances, and bronchospasm. CNS abnormalities are diverse and can include ataxia, amnesia, hallucinations, delayed deep-tendon reflexes, and (in severe hypothermia) an isoelectric EEG.

Diagnosis

Since oral thermometers are usually calibrated only as low as 34.4°C, the exact temperature of a pt whose initial reading is <35°C should be determined with a thermometer reading down to 15°C or, ideally, with a rectal thermocouple probe inserted ≥15 cm.

℞ TREATMENT

Mild hypothermia is managed by passive external rewarming—i.e., by covering the pt with blankets in a warm environment and allowing endogenous heat production to restore normal body temperature. Moderate to severe hypothermia requires active rewarming, which may be either external (by application of heat sources such as heating blankets or by warm water immersion) or internal (by inspiration of heated, humidified O_2; by administration of IV fluids warmed to 40°C; or by peritoneal or pleural lavage with warm saline). The most efficient active internal rewarming techniques are extracorporeal rewarming by hemodialysis and cardiopulmonary bypass. External rewarming may cause a fall in blood pressure by relieving peripheral vasoconstriction. Volume should be repleted with warmed isotonic solutions; lactated Ringer's solution should be avoided because of impaired lactate metabolism in hypothermia. If sepsis is a possibility, empiric broad-spectrum antibiotics should be administered after blood is obtained for culture. Continuous cardiac monitoring is essential. Atrial arrhythmias usually require no specific treatment. Ventricular fibrillation is often refractory, and bretylium tosylate is the drug of choice for its treatment. Only a single attempt at electrical cardioversion should be made when the temperature is <30°C. Since it is sometimes difficult to distinguish profound hypothermia from death, cardiopulmonary resuscitation efforts and active internal rewarming should continue until the core temperature is >32°C or cardiovascular status has been stabilized.

For a more detailed discussion, see Petty KJ: Hypothermia, Chap. 19, p. 97, in HPIM-14.

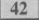

GENERAL EXAMINATION OF THE SKIN

As dermatologic evaluation relies heavily on the objective cutaneous appearance, physical examination is often performed prior to taking a complete history in pts presenting with a skin problem. A differential diagnosis can usually be generated on the basis of a thorough examination with precise descriptions of the skin lesion(s) and narrowed with pertinent facts from the history. Laboratory or diagnostic procedures are then used, when appropriate, to clarify the diagnosis.

PHYSICAL EXAMINATION

Examination of skin should take place in a well-illuminated room with pt completely disrobed. Helpful ancillary equipment includes a hand lens and a pocket flashlight to provide peripheral illumination of lesions. The examination often begins with an assessment of the entire skin viewed at a distance, which is then narrowed down to focus on the individual lesions.

Distribution

As illustrated in Fig. 42-1, the distribution of skin lesions can provide valuable clues to the identification of the disorder. Generalized (systemic diseases); sun-exposed (SLE, photoallergic, phototoxic, polymorphous light eruption, porphyria cutanea tarda); dermatomal (herpes zoster); extensor surfaces (elbows and knees in psoriasis); flexural surfaces (antecubital and popliteal fossae in atopic dermatitis).

Arrangement and Shape

Can describe individual or multiple lesions.

Linear [contact dermatitis such as poison ivy, lesions that appear at sites of local skin trauma (Koebner phenomenon)]; *annular*—"ring-shaped" lesion with an active border and central clearing (erythema chronicum migrans, erythema annulare centrificum, tinea corporis); *iris* or *target lesion*—two or three concentric circles of differing hue (erythema multiforme); *circinate*—circular lesion (urticaria, herald patch of pityriasis rosea); *nummular*—"coin-shaped" (nummular eczema); *guttate*—"droplike" (guttate psoriasis); *morbilliform*—"measles-like"

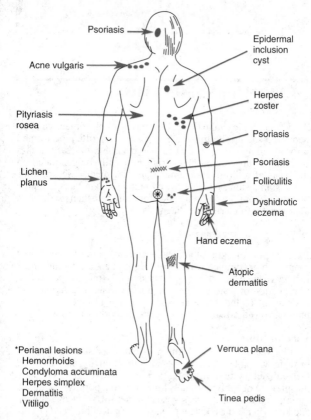

A

FIGURE 42-1A The distribution of some common dermatologic diseases and lesions.

with small confluent papules coalescing into unusual shapes (measles, drug eruption); *reticulated*—"netlike" (livedo reticularis); *herpetiform*—grouped vesicles, papules, or erosions (herpes simplex).

Primary Lesions

Cutaneous changes caused directly by disease process.

Macule—a flat circumscribed lesion of a different color,

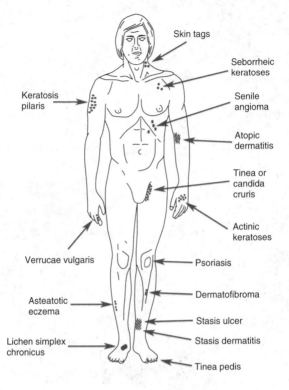

B

FIGURE 42-1B

allowing for differentiation from surrounding skin; *patch*—
macule >2 cm in diameter; *papule*—elevated, circumscribed
lesion of any color <1 cm in diameter, with the major portion
of lesion projecting above surrounding skin; *nodule*—palpable
lesion similar to a papule but >1 cm in diameter; *plaque*—an
elevated, flat-topped lesion >1 cm in diameter; *vesicle*—sharply
marginated elevated lesion <1 cm in diameter filled with clear
fluid; *bulla*—vesicular lesion >1 cm in diameter; *pustule*—a
well-marginated focal accumulation of inflammatory cells
within skin; *wheal*—a transient elevated lesion due to accumulation of fluid in upper dermis; *cyst*—lesion consisting of liquid

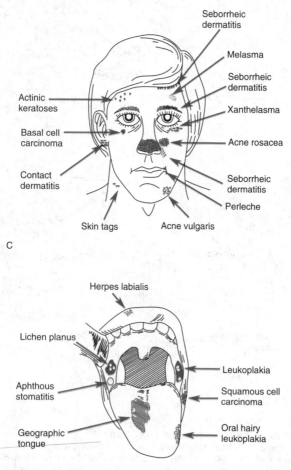

C

D

FIGURE 42-1C and 1D

or semisolid material contained within limits of cyst wall (true cyst).

Secondary Lesions

Changes in area of primary pathology often due to secondary events, e.g., scratching, secondary infection, bleeding.

Scale—a flaky accumulation of excess keratin that is partially adherent to skin; *crust*—a circumscribed collection of inflammatory cells and dried serum on skin surface; *excoriation*— linear, angular erosions caused by scratching; *erosion*—a circumscribed, usually depressed, moist lesion resulting from loss of overlying epidermis; *ulcer*—a deeper erosion involving epidermis plus underlying papillary dermis; may leave a scar on healing; *atrophy*: (1) epidermal—thinning of skin with loss of normal skin surface markings, (2) dermal—depression of skin surface due to loss of underlying collagen or dermal ground substance; *lichenification*—thickening of skin with accentuation of normal skin surface markings most commonly due to chronic rubbing; *scar*—collection of fibrous tissue replacing normal dermal constituents.

Other Descriptive Terms

Color e.g., violaceous, erythematous; physical characteristics e.g., warm, tender; sharpness of edge, surface contour—flat-topped, pedunculated (on a stalk), verrucous (wartlike), umbilicated (containing a central depression).

HISTORY

A complete history should be obtained, with special attention being paid to the following points:

1. Evolution of the lesion—site of onset, manner in which eruption progressed or spread, duration, periods of resolution or improvement in chronic eruptions
2. Symptoms associated with the eruption—itching, burning, pain, numbness, what has relieved symptoms, time of day when symptoms are most severe
3. Current or recent medications—both prescription and over-the-counter
4. Associated systemic symptoms (e.g., malaise, fatigue, arthralgias)
5. Ongoing or previous illnesses
6. History of allergies
7. Presence of photosensitivity
8. Review of systems

ADDITIONAL DIAGNOSTIC PROCEDURES

Potassium Hydroxide Preparation

Useful for detection of dermatophyte or yeast. Scale is collected from advancing edge of a scaling lesion by gently scraping with side of a microscope slide. Nail lesions are best sampled by trimming back nail and scraping subungual debris. A drop of 10–15% potassium hydroxide is added to slide, and cover slip is applied. The slide may be gently heated and examined under microscope. Positive preparations show translucent, septate branching hyphae among keratinocytes.

Tzanck Preparation

Useful for determining presence of herpes viruses. Optimal lesion to sample is an early vesicle. Lesion is gently unroofed with no. 15 scalpel blade, and base of vesicle is gently scraped with belly of blade (keep blade perpendicular to skin surface to prevent laceration). Scrapings are transferred to slide and stained with Wright's or Giemsa stain. A positive preparation has multinucleate giant cells.

Skin Biopsy

Minor surgical procedure. Choice of site very important.

Diascopy

Assesses whether a lesion blanches with pressure. Done by pressing a magnifying lens or microscope slide on lesion and observing changes in vascularity. For example, hemangiomas will usually blanch; purpuric lesions will not.

Wood's Light Examination

Useful for detecting bacterial or fungal infection or accentuating features of some skin lesions.

Patch Tests

To document cutaneous sensitivity to specific antigens.

For a more detailed discussion, see Lawley TJ, Yancey KB: Approach to the Patient with Skin Disorders, Chap. 54, p. 294 in HPIM-14.

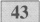

COMMON SKIN CONDITIONS

PAPULOSQUAMOUS DISORDERS

Disorders exhibiting papules and scale.

Psoriasis

A chronic, recurrent disorder. Classic lesion is a well-margin-ated, erythematous plaque with silvery-white surface scale. Distribution includes extensor surfaces (i.e., knees, elbows, and buttocks); may also involve palms and scalp (particularly anterior scalp margin). Associated findings include psoriatic arthritis (Chap. 156) and nail changes (onycholysis, pitting or thickening of nail plate with accumulation of subungual debris).

℞ TREATMENT

Maintain cutaneous hydration; topical glucocorticoids; coal tar ointment; topical vitamin D analogue (calcipotriol); UV light (PUVA when UV used in combination with psoralens); methotrexate for severe advanced disease.

Pityriasis Rosea

A self-limited condition lasting 3–8 weeks. Initially, there is a single 2–6 cm annular salmon-colored patch (herald patch) with a peripheral rim of scale, followed in days to weeks by a generalized eruption involving the trunk and proximal extremities. Individual lesions are similar to but smaller than the herald patch and are arranged in symmetric fashion with long axis of each individual lesion along skin lines of cleavage. Appearance may be similar to that of secondary syphilis.

℞ TREATMENT

Disorder is self-limited, so treatment is directed at symptoms; oral antihistamines for pruritus; topical glucocorticoids; UV-B phototherapy in some cases.

Lichen Planus

Disorder of unknown cause; can follow administration of certain drugs and in chronic graft-versus-host disease; lesions are pruritic, polygonal, flat-topped, and violaceous. Course is variable, but most pts have spontaneous remissions 6–24 months after onset of disease.

℞ **TREATMENT**
Topical glucocorticoids.

ECZEMATOUS DISORDERS

Eczema

Eczema, or dermatitis, is a reaction pattern that presents with variable clinical and histologic findings; it is the final common expression for a number of disorders.

Atopic Dermatitis

One aspect of atopic triad of hayfever, asthma, and eczema. Usually an intermittent, chronic, severely pruritic, eczematous dermatitis with scaly erythematous patches, vesiculation, crusting, and fissuring. Lesions are most commonly on flexures, with prominent involvement of antecubital and popliteal fossae; generalized erythroderma in severe cases. Most pts with atopic dermatitis are chronic carriers of *Staphylococcus aureus* in anterior nares and on skin.

℞ **TREATMENT**
Avoidance of irritants; cutaneous hydration; topical glucocorticoids; treatment of infected lesions. Systemic glucocorticoids only for severe exacerbations unresponsive to topical conservative therapy.

Allergic Contact Dermatitis

A delayed hypersensitivity reaction that occurs after cutaneous exposure to an antigenic substance. Lesions occur at site of contact and are vesicular, weeping, crusting; linear arrangement of vesicles is common. Most frequent allergens are resin from plants of the *Rhus* (or *Toxicodendron*) genus (poison ivy, oak, sumac), nickel, rubber, and cosmetics.

℞ **TREATMENT**
Avoidance of sensitizing agent; topical glucocorticoids; consideration of systemic glucocorticoids over 2–3 weeks for widespread disease or involvement of face or genitals.

Irritant Contact Dermatitis

Inflammation of the skin due to direct injury by an exogenous agent. The most frequent cause of hand eczema, where dermatitis is initiated or aggravated by chronic exposure to water and detergents. Features may include skin dryness, cracking, erythema, edema.

Rx TREATMENT
Avoidance of irritants; barriers (use of vinyl gloves); topical glucocorticoids; treatment of secondary bacterial or dermatophyte infection.

Seborrheic Dermatitis

A chronic noninfectious process characterized by erythematous patches with greasy yellowish scale. Lesions are generally on scalp, eyebrows, nasolabial folds, axillae, central chest, and posterior auricular area.

Rx TREATMENT
Nonfluorinated topical glucocorticoids; shampoos containing coal tar, salicylic acid, or selenium sulfide.

INFECTIONS AND INFESTATIONS

Impetigo

A superficial infection of skin secondary to either *S. aureus* or group A beta-hemolytic streptococci. The primary lesion is a superficial pustule that ruptures and forms a "honey-colored" crust. Tense bullae are associated with *S. aureus* infections (bullous impetigo). Lesions may occur anywhere but commonly involve the face.

Rx TREATMENT
Gentle debridement of adherent crusts with soaks and topical antibiotics; appropriate oral antibiotics depending on organism (see Chap. 69).

Erysipelas

Superficial cellulitis, most commonly on face, characterized by a bright red, sharply demarcated, intensely painful, warm plaque. Because of superficial location of infection and associated edema, surface of plaque may exhibit a *peau d'orange* (orange peel) appearance. Most commonly due to infection with group A beta-hemolytic streptococci, occurring at sites of trauma or other breaks in skin.

Rx TREATMENT
Appropriate antibiotics depending on organism (see Chap. 69).

Scabies

A common infestation of children and adults due to the mite *Sarcoptes scabiei*. Often presents as pruritus, commonly worse at night. Typical lesions include burrows (short linear lesions often in web spaces of fingers) and small vesiculopapular lesions in intertriginous areas. Excoriations often with bleeding may be prominent.

℞ TREATMENT

Topical permethrin; topical lindane (penetrates skin and has potential for CNS toxicity; should not be used in pregnant women or infants). To prevent reinfestation, clothing should be washed in hot water and close contacts treated simultaneously.

Herpes Simplex (See Chap. 94)

Recurrent eruption characterized by grouped vesicles on an erythematous base that progress to erosions; often secondarily infected with staphylococci or streptococci. Infections frequently involve mucocutaneous surfaces around the oral cavity, genitals, or anus. Can also cause severe visceral disease including esophagitis, pneumonitis, encephalitis, and disseminated herpes simplex virus infection. Tzanck preparation of an unroofed early vesicle reveals multinucleate giant cells.

℞ TREATMENT

Will differ based on disease manifestations and level of immune competence (see Chap. 94); appropriate antibiotics for secondary infections, depending on organism.

Herpes Zoster (See Chap. 94)

Eruption of grouped vesicles on an erythematous base usually limited to a single dermatome ("shingles"); disseminated lesions also can occur, especially in immunocompromised pts. Tzanck preparation reveals multinucleate giant cells; indistinguishable from herpes simplex except by culture. Postherpetic neuralgia, lasting months to years, may occur, especially in elderly.

℞ TREATMENT

Will differ based on disease manifestations and level of immune competence (see Chap. 94)

Dermatophyte Infection

Skin fungus, may involve any area of body; due to infection of stratum corneum, nail plate, or hair. Appearance may vary from mild scaliness to florid inflammatory dermatitis. Common sites of infection include the foot (tinea pedis), nails (tinea unguium), groin (tinea cruris), or scalp (tinea capitis). Classic lesion of tinea corporis ("ringworm") is an erythematous papulosquamous patch, often with central clearing and scale along peripheral advancing border. Hyphae are often seen on KOH preparation, although tinea capitis and tinea corporis may require culture or biopsy.

℞ TREATMENT

Depends on affected site and type of infection. Topical imidazoles, triazoles, and allylamines may be effective. Haloprogin, undecylenic acid, ciclopiroxolamine, and tolnaftate are also effective, but nystatin is not active against dermatophytes. Griseofulvin, 500 mg/d, if systemic therapy required.

Candidiasis

Fungal infection caused by a related group of yeasts. Manifestations may be localized to the skin or rarely systemic and life-threatening. Predisposing factors include diabetes mellitus, cellular immune deficiencies, and HIV (see Chap. 78). Frequent sites include the oral cavity, chronically wet macerated areas, around nails, intertriginous areas. Diagnosed by clinical pattern and demonstration of yeast on KOH preparation or culture.

℞ TREATMENT

(See Chap. 100) Removal of predisposing factors; topical nystatin or azoles; systemic therapy reserved for immunosuppressed patients, unresponsive chronic or recurrent disease.

Warts

Cutaneous neoplasms caused by human papilloma viruses (HPVs). Typically dome-shaped lesions with irregular filamentous surface. Propensity for the face, arms, and legs; often spread by shaving. HPVs are also associated with genital or perianal lesions and play a role in the development of neoplasia of the uterine cervix and external genitalia in females (see Chap. 75).

℞ TREATMENT

Cryotherapy with liquid nitrogen, keratinolytic agents (salicylic acid). For genital warts, application of podophyllin solution is effective but can be associated with marked local reactions.

ACNE

Acne Vulgaris

Usually a self-limited disorder of teenagers and young adults. Comedones (small cyst formed in hair follicle) are clinical hallmark; often accompanied by inflammatory lesions of papules, pustules, or nodules. May scar in severe cases.

℞ TREATMENT

Careful cleaning and removal of oils; oral tetracycline or erythromycin; topical antibacterials (e.g., benzoyl peroxide), topical retinoic acid. Systemic isotretinoin only for unresponsive severe nodulocystic acne (teratogenic—all females must be screened for pregnancy prior to drug initiation and maintain effective contraception during treatment course).

Acne Rosacea

Inflammatory disorder affecting predominantly the central face, rarely affecting patients <30 years of age. Tendency toward exaggerated flushing, with eventual superimposition of papules, pustules, and telangiectases. May lead to rhinophyma and ocular problems.

℞ TREATMENT

Oral tetracycline, 250–1500 mg/d; topical metronidazole and topical nonfluorinated glucocorticoids may be useful.

VASCULAR DISORDERS

Erythema Nodosum

Septal panniculitis characterized by erythematous, warm, tender subcutaneous nodular lesions typically over anterior tibia. Lesions are usually flush with skin surface but are indurated and have appearance of an erythematous/violaceous bruise. Lesions usually resolve spontaneously in 3–6 weeks without scarring. Commonly seen in sarcoidosis, treatment with some drugs (esp. sulfonamides, oral contraceptives, and estrogens), and a wide range of infections including streptococcus and tuberculosis; may be idiopathic.

℞ TREATMENT

Identification and treatment/removal of underlying cause. NSAID for severe or recurrent lesions, systemic glucocorticoids are effective but dangerous if underlying infection is not appreciated.

Erythema Multiforme

A reaction pattern of skin consisting of a variety of lesions but most commonly erythematous papules and bullae. "Target" or "iris" lesion is characteristic and consists of concentric circles of erythema and normal flesh-colored skin, often with a central vesicle or bulla. Distribution of lesions classically acral, esp. palms and soles. Three most common causes are drug reaction (particularly penicillins and sulfonamides) or concurrent herpetic or *Mycoplasma* infection. Can rarely affect mucosal surfaces and internal organs (erythema multiforme major or Stevens-Johnson syndrome).

℞ TREATMENT

Provocative agent should be sought and eliminated if drug-related. In mild cases limited to skin, only symptomatic treatment is needed (antihistamines, NSAID). For Stevens-Johnson, systemic glucocorticoids are controversial but often used; prevention of secondary infection and maintenance of nutrition and fluid/electrolyte balance are critical.

Urticaria

A common disorder, either acute or chronic, characterized by evanescent (individual lesions lasting <24 h), pruritic, edematous, pink to erythematous plaques with a whitish halo around margin of individual lesions. Lesions range in size from papules to giant coalescent lesions (10–20 cm in diameter). Often due to drugs, systemic infection, or foods (esp. shellfish). Food additives such as tartrazine dye (FD & C yellow no. 5), benzoate, or salicylates also have been implicated. If individual lesions last >24 h, consider diagnosis of urticarial vasculitis.

℞ TREATMENT
See Chap. 148.

Vasculitis

Palpable purpura (nonblanching, elevated lesions) is the cutaneous hallmark of vasculitis. Other lesions include petechiae (esp. early lesions), necrosis with ulceration, bullae, and urticarial lesions (urticarial vasculitis). Lesions usually most prominent on lower extremities. Associations include infections, collagen-vascular disease, primary systemic vasculitides, malignancy, hepatitis B, drugs (esp. thiazides), and inflammatory bowel disease. May occur as an idiopathic, predominantly cutaneous vasculitis.

Rx **TREATMENT**

Will differ based on cause. Pursue identification and treatment/elimination of an exogenous cause or underlying disease. If part of a systemic vasculitis, treat based on major organ threatening features (see Chap. 151). Immunosuppressive therapy should be avoided in idiopathic predominantly cutaneous vasculitis as disease frequently does not respond and rarely causes irreversible organ system dysfunction.

CUTANEOUS DRUG REACTIONS

Cutaneous reactions are among the most frequent medication toxicities. These can have a wide range of severity and manifestations including urticaria, photosensitivity, erythema multiforme, fixed drug reactions, erythema nodosum, vasculitis, lichenoid reactions, bullous drug reactions, and toxic epidermal necrolysis (TEN). Diagnosis is usually made by appearance and careful medication history.

Rx **TREATMENT**

Withdrawal of the medication. Treatment based on nature and severity of cutaneous pathology.

For a more detailed discussion, see Swerlick RA, Lawley TJ: Eczema, Psoriasis, Cutaneous Infections, Acne, and Other Common Skin Disorders, Chap. 55, p. 298; Wintroub BU, Stern RS: Cutaneous Drug Reactions, Chap. 56, p. 304; and Bologna JL, Braverman IM: Skin Manifestations of Internal Disease, Chap. 57, p. 310, in HPIM-14.

44

NUTRITIONAL REQUIREMENTS AND ASSESSMENT

Stability of body weight requires that energy intake and expenditure be balanced over time. In addition to energy the body requires 9 essential amino acids, 1 fatty acid, 13 vitamins, minerals, and water. Requirement of an essential nutrient is defined as the smallest amount that maintains normal body mass, chemical composition, morphology, and physical function. Since minimal requirements are hard to define, the clinical standard is the recommended dietary allowance (RDA), the amount of an essential nutrient judged by the Food and Nutrition Board of the National Research Council to be adequate to meet the nutrition needs of a healthy person.

Intake of an essential nutrient below a critical level causes disease, but intake of excess nutrients can also disturb body structure and function. Obesity, fluorosis, atherosclerosis, and hypervitaminoses A and D are usually consequences of excessive intake over long periods. Acute excess of nutrient intake can cause abdominal cramps, nausea, and diarrhea (food), hyponatremia (food), and arrhythmias (potassium). The healthy diet provides intake levels between the thresholds of minimal requirements and maximal tolerances and allows for variations in age, growth rate, physical activity, composition of the diet, variations in individual absorption, pregnancy and lactation, and coexisting disease states.

NUTRITIONAL REQUIREMENTS

Daily caloric requirements (kcal/d) can be estimated from calculation of basal energy expenditure (BEE) with appropriate adjustments for activity or illness-related energy expenditures and diet-induced thermogenesis:

$$BEE_{women} = 655 + (9.5 \times W) + (1.8 \times H) - (4.7 \times A)$$
$$BEE_{men} = 66 + (13.7 \times W) + (5 \times H) - (6.8 \times A)$$

where W is weight (kg), H is height (cm), and A is age (years).

Physical activity typically accounts for about one-third of total energy expenditure but may vary from 1.5 to 85 (kcal/kg body wt)/h. Diet-induced thermogenesis is the heat or energy production in excess of BEE caused by the ingestion of food.

Diet-induced energy expenditure increases energy expenditure by 6–10%. Other factors that increase energy expenditure include catabolic states (50–100%), burns or trauma (40–100%), and fever (13% per °C above normal). Even during the most severe illness, energy requirements rarely exceed 12,500 kJ/d (3000 kcal/d).

The usual water requirement in adults is 1.0–1.5 mL/kcal energy expenditure. Water requirement may increase with fluid loss from perspiration, diarrhea, hyperthermia, or urinary losses.

The adult RDA for protein is 0.6 g/kg body weight. Growth, pregnancy, lactation, and repletion after malnutrition enhance protein requirements, while liver or renal failure may diminish tolerance of dietary protein. The absolute requirement for fat is 1 g/d of linoleic acid for prostaglandin synthesis. The typical U.S. diet contains more than 35% calories from fat, 15% from protein, and the remainder from carbohydrate. RDAs for vitamins and minerals are published by the Food and Nutrition Board.

NUTRITIONAL ASSESSMENT

The three components of nutritional assessment are nutritional history, physical examination, and laboratory evaluation. Obesity and severe malnutrition can be recognized by history and physical examination, but subtle undernutrition is frequently overlooked, particularly in the presence of edema. Quantitative assessment of nutritional status (Table 44-1) can reveal life-threatening undernutrition and allow assessment of progress once repletion is begun. Objective indicators of nutritional status correlate with morbidity and mortality, but no single measurement is of predictive value in individual patients.

Nutritional History

This requires a chronological record of body weight and an estimation of dietary intake using a 24-h diet record. Significant weight changes suggest altered dietary intake or nutritional demand and should be investigated. Intake may be modified by medical factors such as illness, changes in taste perception, swallowing difficulty, gastrointestinal discomfort, drug intake, and psychosocial issues such as depression or financial problems. Nutritional demands are altered by illness, activity, rapid growth, pregnancy, and malabsorption.

Physical Examination

This includes the routine recording of weight and height during outpatient visits and of daily weight measurements in hospital-

Table 44-1

Suggested Weights at Ages 25 to 59 Based on Lowest Mortality*

Height		Small Frame, lb	Medium Frame, lb	Large Frame, lb
Feet	Inches			
MEN				
5	2	128–134	131–141	138–150
5	3	130–136	133–143	140–153
5	4	132–138	135–145	142–156
5	5	134–140	137–148	144–160
5	6	136–142	139–151	146–164
5	7	138–145	142–154	149–168
5	8	140–148	145–157	152–172
5	9	142–151	148–160	155–176
5	10	144–154	151–163	158–180
5	11	146–157	154–166	161–184
6	0	149–160	157–170	164–188
6	1	152–164	160–174	168–192
6	2	155–168	164–178	172–197
6	3	158–172	167–182	176–202
6	4	162–176	171–187	181–207
WOMEN				
4	10	102–111	109–121	118–131
4	11	103–113	111–123	120–134
5	0	104–115	113–126	122–137
5	1	106–118	115–129	125–140
5	2	108–121	118–132	128–143
5	3	111–124	121–135	131–147
5	4	114–127	124–138	134–151
5	5	117–130	127–141	137–155
5	6	120–133	130–144	140–159
5	7	123–136	133–147	143–163
5	8	126–139	136–150	146–167
5	9	129–142	139–153	149–170
5	10	132–145	142–156	152–173
5	11	135–148	145–159	155–176
6	0	138–151	148–162	158–179

* Assumes indoor clothing weighing 5 lb for men and 3 lb for women; shoes with 1-in. heels.

SOURCE: Metropolitan Life Insurance Co., 1983.

ized pts. As an example, weight loss of 0.4 kg/d implies total starvation. The body mass index [BMI = weight(kg)/height(m)^2] is useful for assessing nutrition. A BMI < 18.4 kg/m^2 is associated with an increased risk of protein-energy malnutrition, and a BMI > 25.0–27.0 kg/m^2 is associated with medical complications of obesity. Ideal body weight can be estimated from height, weight, and frame size using standardized tables (Table 44-1).

Measurements of fat and muscle mass are often useful in assessing energy balance. Anthropometric measurement of lean body mass requires only calipers and a tape measure. In the nondominant arm, triceps skinfold is pulled away from triceps muscle midway between the acromial and olecranon processes. Skinfold is then measured with calipers (mm).

Since creatinine excretion is a function of the amount of skeletal muscle, muscle mass can be estimated by comparing the ratio of urinary creatinine excretion (g/d) either to height (cm) or to ideal urinary creatinine excretion (23 mg/kg per day for men and 18 mg/kg per day for women).

Laboratory Assessment

At the simplest level, laboratory assessment involves measurement of serum levels of albumin, prealbumin, and transferrin. Low serum albumin in chronic illness is associated with longer hospital stays, frequent readmissions for poor wound healing and infection, and increased mortality. In acute illness, dehydration and fluid shifts cause early alterations in serum protein levels, and significant changes in synthesis and catabolism may be masked by very long half-lives of these proteins in serum. Transferrin (half-life of 8 d) provides a sensitive indicator of protein repletion after refeeding.

Estimation of nitrogen balance provides assessment of adequacy of nutritional support (see Table 44-2). After growth ceases, rates of anabolism and catabolism are normally in equilibrium (nitrogen balance of zero). Catabolic states (trauma, infection, burns) increase protein losses and cause negative nitrogen balance. Daily nitrogen balance can be estimated as follows:

$$N \text{ balance (g/d)} = \frac{\text{protein intake (g/d)}}{6.25} - [\text{urine urea nitrogen (g/d)} + 2.5 \text{ g/d}]$$

where 2.5 g/d is an estimate of nitrogen losses from stool and skin. Assessment of nitrogen balance provides insight into nutritional status during the periods of observation but not about

Table 44-2

Indices of Nutritional Status

	Normal	Malnutrition		
		Mild	Mod	Severe
Nitrogen balance (g/24 h): $\dfrac{\text{Protein intake (g)}}{6.25\ (\text{g protein per g N})} - [\text{24-h urine urea nitrogen (g)} + 2.5]$	0–3	−1	−2	−3
Body weight: $\dfrac{\text{Actual body weight}}{\text{Ideal body weight}} \times 100$	100	80	70–80	<70
Adipose tissue: Triceps skin fold (mm)	Men 8–23 Women 10–30			
24-h urinary creatinine/height index (mg/cm)	Men 10.5 Women 5.8	8.4–9.5 4.6–5.2	7.4–8.4 4.1–4.6	<7.4 <4.1
Visceral protein compartment: Serum transferrin	200–260	180–200	160–180	<160
Serum albumin (g/L)	40	35–39	25–30	<25
Immune function: Total lymphocyte count/μL	>1800	1500–1800	900–1500	<900
Skin test (mm induration) (Tuberculin/PPD, Candida, streptokinase/streptodornase, mumps)	>10	5–10	0–5	0

231

energy or protein stores, e.g., duration of malnutrition or overnutrition.

Immune competence requires normal protein nutrition (Table 44-2). Lymphocyte depletion and anergy to skin antigens (*Candida albicans*, mumps, streptokinase/streptodornase, and tuberculin/PPD) are associated with increase in morbidity and mortality. These parameters may revert to normal within weeks of initiating protein-energy repletion.

Once refeeding is initiated in the malnourished pt, weight, albumin, transferrin, creatinine excretion, midarm circumference, skin thickness, and immune function should be monitored weekly.

For a more detailed discussion, see Denke M, Wilson JD: Nutrition and Nutritional Requirements, Chap. 72, p. 445; Denke M, Wilson JD: Assessment of Nutritional Status, Chap. 73, p. 448; and Denke M, Wilson JD: Protein and Energy Malnutrition, Chap. 74, p. 452, in HPIM-14.

45

ANOREXIA NERVOSA AND BULIMIA

Anorexia nervosa and bulimia are eating disorders predominantly in young women who develop a paralyzing fear of becoming fat. In anorexia nervosa, this fear causes radical restriction of energy intake, the end result being emaciation. In bulimia, massive binge eating is followed by self-induced vomiting and laxative abuse. Separation of the two conditions is not always clearcut (Table 45-1).

ANOREXIA NERVOSA

This is a psychiatric disorder that involves destructive interpersonal relationships within the family and powerful cultural forces that result in an intense fear of becoming fat (Table 45-2).

Table 45-1

The Eating Disorders

	Anorexia Nervosa	Bulimia
Predominant sex	Female	Female
Method of weight control	Restriction of intake	Vomiting
Binge eating	Uncommon	Invariant
Weight at diagnosis	Markedly decreased	Near normal
Ritualized exercise	Usual	Rare
Amenorrhea	~100%	~50%
Antisocial behavior	Rare	Frequent
Cardiovascular changes (bradycardia, hypotension)	Common	Uncommon
Skin changes (hirsutism, dryness, carotenemia)	Usual	Rare
Hypothermia	Usual	Rare
Edema	+/−	+/−
Medical complications	Hypokalemia, cardiac arrhythmias	Hypokalemia, cardiac arrhythmias, aspiration of gastric contents, esophageal or gastric rupture

NOTE: These features are characteristic of pure anorexia nervosa and pure bulimia. Overlap syndromes occur, and anorexia may evolve to bulimia (the bulimia→ anorexia transformation is rare).
SOURCE: Foster DW: HPIM-14, p. 463.

The symptoms of anorexia nervosa usually become apparent before or shortly after puberty. Patients become emaciated but deny hunger, thinness, or fatigue. Body fat may be undetectable, but breast tissue is often preserved. Parotid gland enlargement and edema may be accompanied by anemia, leukopenia, hypokalemia, and hypoalbuminemia. Hypothalamic dysfunction is manifested by partial diabetes insipidus, abnormal thermoregulation, and hypogonadotropic hypogonadism with secondary amenorrhea. Menses usually return with weight gain.

Table 45-2

Diagnostic Criteria for Anorexia Nervosa

1. Refusal to maintain body weight at or above a minimally normal weight for age and height (e.g., weight loss leading to maintenance of body weight less than 85% of that expected; or failure to make expected weight gain during period of growth, leading to body weight less than 85% of that expected).
2. Intense fear of gaining weight or becoming fat, even though underweight.
3. Disturbance in the way in which one's body weight or shape is experienced, undue influence of body weight or shape on self-evaluation, or denial of the seriousness of the current body weight.
4. In postmenarchal females, amenorrhea, i.e., the absence of at least three consecutive menstrual cycles. [A woman is considered to have amenorrhea if her periods occur only following hormone (e.g., estrogen) administration.]

SOURCE: Foster DW: HPIM-14, after the American Psychiatric Association: Diagnostic and Statistical Manual of Mental Disorders, Fourth Edition. Washington, DC: American Psychiatric Association, 1994:554–555.

BULIMIA

Criteria for the diagnosis of bulimia are listed in Table 45-3. In bulimia, episodic ingestion of large amounts of food in binge pattern is associated with an awareness that the eating pattern is abnormal, a fear that the eating cannot be stopped voluntarily, and feelings of depression after the act. Eating episodes are followed by induced vomiting, with or without ingestion of laxatives. Secrecy about the eating/vomiting sequence is characteristic. Weight loss is not as profound as with anorexia so that functional manifestations such as amenorrhea are less common. Hypokalemia and metabolic alkalosis may be present.

COURSE

The course of anorexia and bulimia is variable. The mortality rate of 5–6% due to starvation and suicide is the highest of any psychiatric condition. Poor prognostic signs include onset after age 20, longer duration of illness, prominent vomiting, extreme weight loss, and significant depression.

Table 45-3

Diagnostic Criteria for Bulimia Nervosa

1. Recurrent episodes of binge-eating. An episode of binge-eating is characterized by both of the following:
   a. Eating, in a discrete period of time (e.g., within any 2-h period), an amount of food that is definitely larger than most people would eat during a similar period of time and under similar circumstances.
   b. A sense of lack of control over eating during the episode (e.g., a feeling that one cannot stop eating or control what or how much one is eating).
2. Recurrent inappropriate compensatory behavior to prevent weight gain, such as self-induced vomiting, misuse of laxatives, diuretics, or other medications; fasting; or excessive exercise.
3. The binge-eating and inappropriate compensatory behaviors both occur, on average, at least twice a week for 3 months.
4. Self-evaluation is unduly influenced by body shape and weight.
5. The disturbance does not occur exclusively during episodes of anorexia nervosa.

SOURCE: Foster DW: HPIM-14, after the American Psychiatric Association: Diagnostic and Statistical Manual of Mental Disorders, Fourth Edition. Washington, DC: American Psychiatric Association, 1994:549–550.

℞ **TREATMENT**
No specific therapy exists. Supportive treatment involves a combination of psychotherapy, family counseling, and hospitalization for nutritional support if malnutrition is severe or if hypokalemia, hypotension, or prerenal azotemia is present. Antidepressants such as fluoxetine have been used with some success. Treatment is long-term, often unsuccessful, and requires perseverance by patient, family, and physician.

For a more detailed discussion, see Foster DW: Anorexia Nervosa and Bulimia Nervosa, Chap. 76, p. 462, in HPIM-14.

46

OBESITY

Obesity is a chronic disease that is increasing in prevalence. The most widely used formula for assessing body weight is the body mass index [BMI is the body weight (kg)/height $(m)^2$]. A BMI between 20 and 25 kg/m^2 is considered an appropriate weight for most individuals. Overweight is defined as a BMI >27 kg/m^2, and obesity is defined as a BMI >30 kg/m^2. Mild obesity may not impart significant risk, but severe obesity poses a risk for increased mortality from diabetes mellitus, hypertension, cardiovascular disease, gall bladder disease, and certain forms of cancer.

PATHOGENESIS

Excess accumulation of body fat is the consequence of environmental and social forces and genetic factors. The common genetic susceptibility to obesity is polygenic in nature, and from 30–50% of the variability in total fat stores is believed to be genetically determined. Rare dysmorphic forms of human obesity in which genetics plays the major role include the Prader-Willi syndrome, Alstom's syndrome, the Laurence-Moon-Biedl syndrome, Cohen's syndrome, and Carpenter's syndrome. Animal models also exist in which a single-gene mutation causes obesity, but defects in the corresponding genes in humans appear to be very rare. Animal models of obesity make clear the central role of the adipocyte in the pathogenesis. In addition to storing fat, these cells secrete lipoprotein lipase, tumor necrosis factor, angiotensinogen, and leptin. Leptin is an important satiety signal that acts directly in the hypothalamus to reduce food intake.

Weight gain or loss in individuals is determined by the balance between energy (food) intake and energy expenditure. The strong correlation between energy expenditure and fat-free body mass indicates that heavier people must on average ingest more food to provide the excess energy for weight gain. Obese individuals tend to underreport food intake by 50% or more, and the obese individual who claims to eat sparingly is probably not reporting food intake accurately. Physiologic variables that promote weight gain in the absence of significant increase in food intake include low metabolic rate, enhanced oxidation of carbohydrate relative to lipid, and insulin resistance. Other factors that promote obesity include hypothalamic injury, hypothyroidism, Cushing's syndrome, and certain drugs (Table 46-1).

Table 46-1

Drugs That Enhance Appetite and Predispose to Obesity

Phenothiazines (chlorpromazine > thioridazine ≥ trifluoperazine > mesoridazine > promazine ≥ mepazine ≥ perphenazine ≥ prochlorperazine > haloperidol ≥ loxapine)
Antidepressants (amitriptyline > imipramine = doxepine = phenelzine ≥ amoxapine = desipramine = trazodone = tranylcypromine)
Antiepileptics (valproate; carbamazepine)
Steroids (glucocorticoids; megestrol acetate)
Antihypertensives (terazosin)

SOURCE: Bray GA; HPIM-14, p. 457.

ASSOCIATED RISKS

Increased mortality from obesity is primarily due to cardiovascular disease, hypertension, diabetes mellitus, and certain forms of cancer (Fig. 46-1). Cardiovascular mortality is linked to increased risk of sudden death from arrhythmias and the complications of atherosclerosis that are due to abnormal lipid profiles and elevated ratios of LDL cholesterol/HDL cholesterol. Hypertension is also common and is related to hyperinsulinemia and insulin resistance. Non-insulin-dependent diabetes mellitus occurs almost exclusively in individuals with a BMI >22 kg/m^2. The incidence of endometrial cancer and postmenopausal breast cancer in women, prostate cancer in men, and colorectal cancer in both men and women is increased with obesity. Sleep apnea in severely obese individuals poses potentially serious health risks.

Regional fat distribution may also influence the risks associated with obesity. Central obesity (high ratio of the circumference of the waist to the circumference of the hips) is associated with high triglyceride levels, low HDL cholesterol levels, and insulin resistance.

℞ TREATMENT

Obesity is a chronic disease that is increasing in prevalence. The etiology is uncertain, cure is unlikely, and palliation is the therapeutic aim. Treatment is important because of the associated health risks but is made difficult because few effective drugs have been available. Weight regain after weight loss is common with all forms of nonsurgical therapy.

The urgency and selection of treatment modalities should be based on the BMI and a risk assessment (Fig. 46-1). Associated risk factors such as age <40, family history of coronary artery disease or diabetes mellitus, or presence of a condition such as hypertension make treatment more urgent.

Low to Moderate Risk

Behavioral modifications of proven value in achieving extended weight loss should be initiated.

- Food-related behaviors should be monitored carefully (avoid cafeteria-style settings, eat small and frequent meals, eat breakfast)
- The diet should contain <25% of calories from fat.
- Physical activity should be increased. Exercise is not useful as a primary strategy to lose weight but helps to maintain weight loss.

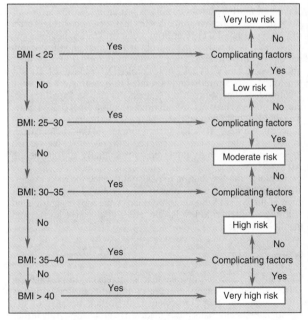

FIGURE 46-1 Algorithm for risk assessment of obesity. (From Bray GA, HPIM-14, p. 460.)

High Risk

Appetite-suppressing drugs such as fenfluramine and phentermine may result in greater weight loss than behavior modification alone; unfortunately, these drugs are associated with development of pulmonary hypertension and valvular heart disease and should be considered for use only in markedly obese patients who have significant comorbidity and who do not respond to other therapies.
* Surgery is also an option; weight regain and other medical problems are minimal with either a Roux-en-Y gastric bypass procedure or vertically-banded gastroplasty.

For a more detailed discussion, see Bray GA: Obesity, Chap. 75, p. 454, in HPIM-14.

47

DIET THERAPY

Nutritional intervention can be critical for prevention, management, or treatment of disease in both in- and outpatient settings. Diet prescription is essential for all hospitalized pts and for many outpatients (Table 47-1). However, people eat food rather than nutrients so that practical and psychological aspects of diet modification must be considered. A diet of approximately 105 kJ (25 kcal) per kilogram of body weight will usually suffice, but dietary intake and nutritional requirements can be altered by disease or therapy so that diet must frequently be modified to prevent malnutrition. To maintain a positive energy balance when energy expenditure is increased and to replete deficiency in malnourished pts, energy intake should be $1.5-2\times$ the average level.

In healthy adults recommended protein intake is 0.8 (g/kg body weight)/d, but under conditions of stress requirement may increase to 2–4 (g/kg)/d. Optimal ratio of kJ (kcal) to g protein intake in the healthy individual is 625:1 (150:1), and intermediate ratios may be appropriate in conditions of altered growth or repair needs.

Needs for special restrictions and/or additions to diet depend

Table 47-1

Principles of Diet Prescription

Assess energy and protein needs
Designate route of administration:
  oral intake, tube feeding, parenteral nutrition
Select texture and/or concentration
Specify frequency and/or rate of feeding
Designate special restrictions:
  Na^+, Ca^+, K^+, fluid, gastric irritants, fiber, residue, gluten, fat, carbohydrate, protein, purine, tyrosine, galactose, sucrose, oxalate, lactate
Designate special additions:
  fiber, medium chain triglycerides, vitamins, prepared nutritional supplements

---

on diagnosis (Table 47-1). Diet can be administered by oral intake, tube feeding, or parenterally. For oral intake, consistency can vary from clear liquid to pureed or soft to regular, and for tube feedings and parenteral formulas, concentration and osmolality must be specified.

TUBE FEEDING

When oral intake is inadequate, enteral feeding may be indicated. Such situations include anorexia, neurologic disorders such as dysphagia or cerebrovascular accidents, and malignancy. Enteral routes include nasogastric and nasoduodenal tubes, jejunostomy tubes, and gastrostomy tubes placed by percutaneous endoscopy. Small-bore Silastic or polyurethane tubes are associated with low rates of nasopharyngitis, rhinitis, otitis media, and stricture formation. The various preparations available for tube feeding vary from hospital to hospital but generally fall into two categories.

Clear Liquid Formulas

Such formulas are composed of di- and tripeptides and/or amino acids, glucose oligosaccharides, and vegetable oils or medium-chain triglycerides. Residue is minimal, and little digestion is required. Such formulas may be of use in pts with short bowel syndrome, partial small bowel obstruction, pancreatic insufficiency, inflammatory bowel disease, radiation enteritis, or bowel fistulas.

Full Liquid Formulas

These contain complex nutrients and can be used in most pts with a functional GI tract. To initiate bolus feeding, 50–100 mL of isotonic or slightly hypotonic liquid is given q3h. This may be increased by 50-mL increments, if tolerated, until the daily target is reached. Gastric residual should not exceed 100 mL 2 h after feeding. If this occurs, hold the next feeding and recheck residual in 1 h.

Continuous gastric infusion is initiated with half-strength diet at a rate of 25–50 mL/h. This can be advanced as tolerated to full strength and energy target. The head of the bed must be kept elevated. Single-nutrient modules for protein, carbohydrate, and fat can be used individually or combined to create formulas for specialized requirements, e.g., a high-energy, low-protein, low-sodium formula for a cachectic cirrhotic pt with ascites and encephalopathy.

Complications of enteral feeding include diarrhea, gastric distention/retention, aspiration, electrolyte imbalance (hyponatremia, hyperosmolality), warfarin resistance, sinusitis, and esophagitis.

PARENTERAL NUTRITION

Parenteral nutrition can either be partial for individuals capable of some oral intake that is inadequate for nutritional needs or total (TPN) for malnourished pts who cannot tolerate oral feedings. Additional indications for TPN include bowel rest for regional enteritis; well-nourished pts who require 10–14 d of abstinence from oral intake; prolonged coma when tube feeding is not possible; nutritional support in hypercatabolic states such as sepsis, burns, or trauma; pts receiving chemotherapy that precludes oral intake; and prophylactic use in malnourished pts undergoing surgery.

TPN should generally provide 140–170 kJ (32–40 kcal) per kg body weight and basal water intake of 0.3 mL/kJ (1.2 mL/kcal) per day (Table 47-2). To this should be added a volume equivalent to losses from diarrhea, stomal output, nasogastric suction, and fistula drainage. In oliguric pts a basal intake of 750–1000 mL fluid should be given, plus a volume equal to urine and other losses. In edematous states Na intake should be limited to 20–40 mmol/d.

Positive nitrogen balance can usually be achieved by infusing 0.5–1.0 g amino acids per kg of body weight per day, together with nonprotein energy. The protein-sparing effect of carbohydrate and fat is maximal at around 230–250 kJ (55–60 kcal) per kg ideal body weight per day. Carbohydrates and lipids can

Table 47-2

Representative Daily Protocols for TPN

Components	Fat Free	50% Lipid	85% Lipid
Amino acids, g	60	60	75
Glucose, g	750	375	187
Lipids, g	0	100	150
Electrolyte mix, mL	60	60	60
Trace element mix, mL	5	5	5
Vitamins, mL	10	10	10
Na^+, mg	125	125	132
K^+, mg	81	80	87
Total kcal*	2550	2375	2286
Total volume, mL	3075	2775	3075

* For kJ multiply kcal by 4.186.

be infused with amino acids to provide sufficient nonprotein calories using a Y connector. A mixture in which lipid provides half the energy simulates the normal diet, causes neither hyperinsulinemia nor hyperglycemia, and eliminates the need for exogenous insulin.

Complications related to catheter insertion include pneumothorax, thrombophlebitis, catheter embolism, and hyperglycemia (from hypertonic glucose infusions). Disseminated candidiasis may occur after prolonged nutritional support. Hypokalemia, hypomagnesemia, and hypophosphatemia may result in disorientation, convulsions, and coma. Hyperchloremic acidosis may occur with inadequate sodium acetate supplementation. Hypoglycemia may result from abrupt discontinuation of TPN secondary to relative insulin excess. The infusion rate should be tapered over 12 h, or a 10% dextrose infusion should be substituted for several hours.

SPECIFIC DIET THERAPIES

Cardiovascular Disease

Elevated levels of LDL cholesterol and triglyceride and low levels of HDL cholesterol are major risk factors for atherosclerosis that can sometimes be modified by dietary intervention. In individuals with moderate or high risk the intake of total and saturated fat should be reduced according to the Step 1 diet prepared by the National Cholesterol Education Program

Table 47-3

Diet Therapy for Diabetes Mellitus

1. Maintain as near-normal levels of blood glucose as possible by balancing food intake with medications (insulin or oral agents) and activity.
2. Achieve optimal serum lipid levels.
3. Provide calories to maintain or achieve reasonable weight for adults or to promote recovery from catabolic illness. Promote weight loss in obese patients.
4. Aim for protein intake of 10–20% and saturated fat of <10% of daily calories.
5. Distribute the remaining 60–70% of daily calories between carbohydrate and fat based on treatment goals for blood glucose and lipid levels. Emphasize monounsaturated fats over polyunsaturated fats.
6. Sucrose and other "simple sugars" may be substituted for other carbohydrates.
7. As in the general population, aim for 20–35 g/d of dietary fiber.
8. If hypertension is present, limit sodium to <2400 mg/d.
9. Limit alcoholic beverages to <2/d.
10. Vitamin and mineral supplementation is unnecessary for most patients.

SOURCE: Adapted from The American Diabetes Association, Inc., The American Dietetic Association, J Am Diet Assoc. 94:504, 1994.

(NCEP). The Step 2 diet is appropriate for those who do not respond to the Step 1 program.

Hypertension

Hypertension increases the risk of cardiovascular disease and stroke. Restriction of dietary sodium to 2 g/d and weight reduction in obese pts are useful nonpharmacologic adjuncts for management of hypertension.

Diabetes Mellitus

Dietary goals in pts with diabetes mellitus include: (1) maintenance of near-normal levels of blood glucose by balancing food intake with activity and medications; (2) achievement of optimal lipid levels; and (3) maintenance of a healthy body weight, including weight reduction for many pts. The diet recommended by the American Diabetes Association is similar to the NCEP Step 1 diet (Table 47-3).

Table 47-4

Dietary Modifications for Chronic Renal Failure

Dietary Factor	Predialysis	Hemodialysis	Peritoneal Dialysis
Protein	0.55–0.60 g/kg per day (0.35 g/kg per day high biologic value)	1.0–1.4 g/kg per day	1.2–1.4 g/kg per day
Calcium	1400–1600 mg/d	1400–1600 mg/d	1400–1600 mg/d
Phosphorus	5–10 mg/kg per day	≤17 mg/kg per day	≤17 mg/kg per day
Sodium	1000–3000 mg/d	1000–1500 mg/d	Remove excess with the dialysate
Potassium	Unnecessary unless hyperkalemic	1500–2700 mg/d	Rarely necessary

Chronic Renal Failure

Diet therapy is an important part of the management of all stages of renal disease and is particularly important in end-stage disease. Restriction of dietary protein to 0.55–0.60 g protein/kg per day may retard progression of renal disease (Table 47-4). Renal excretion of phosphorus, sodium, and potassium is decreased so amounts of these electrolytes should be restricted. 1,25-$(OH)_2$D and other vitamins may be depleted by dialysis, and appropriate vitamin supplementation may be appropriate.

Gastrointestinal Disease

Management of diarrhea requires volume repletion with isotonic saline, lactose restriction, and reduction of fat and fiber intake. Diets containing 2–3 times more fiber than in the standard diet are useful in managing constipation. Gastroesophageal reflux may also respond to dietary modification; foods to be avoided include chocolate, fatty foods, and peppermint, which lower esophageal sphincter pressure, and orange juice, tomato juice, and coffee, which act as direct mucosal irritants.

Liver Disease

In pts with hepatic necrosis and portal hypertension, large protein loads may precipitate encephalopathy, and overzealous protein restriction can cause malnutrition. The best approach is to start with about 0.5 g protein/kg per day and increase protein intake slowly to a goal of 1 g/kg per day while closely monitoring neurologic status.

Pulmonary Disease

Patients with chronic obstructive pulmonary disease (COPD) and weight loss have shorter survival than pts with stable weight. COPD increases caloric requirements because of the increased work of breathing, and improved nutrition enhances the strength of respiratory muscles and enhances pt endurance. Overfeeding with carbohydrate increases CO_2 production and may cause respiratory distress; high-fat diets are useful in this setting.

For a more detailed discussion, see Rock CL, Coulston AM, Ruffin MT IV: Diet Therapy, Chap. 77, p. 465; and Howard LJ: Enteral and Parenteral Nutrition Therapy, Chap. 78, p. 472, in HPIM-14.

48

EXAMINATION OF BLOOD SMEARS AND BONE MARROW

BLOOD SMEARS

Erythrocyte (RBC) Morphology

Normal: 7.5-μm diameter.

- *Reticulocytes* (Wright's stain)—large, grayish-blue, admixed with pink (polychromasia).
- *Anisocytosis*—variation in RBC size; large cells imply delay in erythroid precursor DNA synthesis caused by folate or B_{12} deficiency or drug effect; small cells imply a defect in hemoglobin synthesis caused by iron deficiency or abnormal hemoglobin genes.
- *Poikilocytosis*—abnormal RBC shapes; the following are examples:

  Acanthocytes (spur cells)—irregularly spiculated; abetalipoproteinemia, severe liver disease, rarely anorexia nervosa.

  Echinocytes (burr cells)—regularly shaped, uniformly distributed spiny projections; uremia, RBC volume loss.

  Elliptocytes—elliptical; hereditary elliptocytosis.

  Schistocytes (schizocytes)—fragmented cells of varying sizes and shapes; microangiopathic or macroangiopathic hemolytic anemia.

  Sickled cells—elongated, crescentic; sickle cell anemias.

  Spherocytes—small hyperchromic cells lacking normal central pallor; hereditary spherocytosis, extravascular hemolysis as in autoimmune hemolytic anemia, glucose-6-phosphate dehydrogenase (G6PD) deficiency.

  Target cells—central and outer rim staining with intervening ring of pallor; liver disease, thalassemia, hemoglobin C and sickle C diseases.

  Teardrop cells—myelofibrosis, other infiltrative processes of marrow (e.g., carcinoma).

  Rouleaux formation—alignment of RBCs in stacks; may be artifactual or due to paraproteinemia (e.g., multiple myeloma, macroglobulinemia).

RBC Inclusions

- *Howell-Jolly bodies*—1-μm diameter basophilic cytoplasmic inclusion that represents a residual nuclear fragment, usually single; asplenic pts.
- *Basophilic stippling*—multiple, punctate basophilic cytoplasmic inclusions composed of precipitated mitochondria and ribosomes; lead poisoning, thalassemia, myelofibrosis.
- *Pappenheimer (iron) bodies*—iron-containing granules usually composed of mitochondria and ribosomes resemble basophilic stippling but also stain with Prussian blue; lead poisoning, other sideroblastic anemias.
- *Heinz bodies*—spherical inclusions of precipitated hemoglobin seen only with supravital stains, such as crystal violet; G6PD deficiency (after oxidant stress such as infection, certain drugs), unstable hemoglobin variants.
- *Parasites*—characteristic intracytoplasmic inclusions; malaria, babesiosis.

Leukocyte Inclusions and Nuclear Contour Abnormalities

- *Toxic granulations*—dark cytoplasmic granules; bacterial infection.
- *Döhle bodies*—1- to 2-μm blue, oval cytoplasmic inclusions; bacterial infection, Chediak-Higashi anomaly.
- *Auer rods*—eosinophilic, rodlike cytoplasmic inclusions; acute myelogenous leukemia (some cases).
- *Hypersegmentation*—neutrophil nuclei contain more than the usual 2–4 lobes; usually >5% have ≥5 lobes or a single cell with 7 lobes is adequate to make the diagnosis; folate or B_{12} deficiency, drug effects.
- *Hyposegmentation*—neutrophil nuclei contain fewer lobes than normal, either one or two: Pelger-Hüet anomaly, pseudo-Pelger-Hüet or acquired Pelger-Hüet anomaly in acute leukemia.

Platelet Abnormalities

Platelet clumping—an in vitro artifact—is often readily detectable on smear; can lead to falsely low platelet count by automated cell counters.

BONE MARROW

Aspiration assesses cell morphology. *Biopsy* assesses overall marrow architecture, including degree of cellularity. Biopsy should precede aspiration to avoid bleeding artifacts.

Indications

ASPIRATION Hypoproliferative or unexplained anemia, leukopenia, or thrombocytopenia, suspected leukemia or myeloma, evaluation of iron stores, workup of some cases of fever of unknown origin.

Special Tests Histochemical staining (leukemias), cytogenetic studies (leukemias, lymphomas), microbiology (bacterial, mycobacterial, fungal cultures), Prussian blue (iron) stain (assess iron stores, diagnosis of sideroblastic anemias).

BIOPSY Performed in addition to aspiration for possible pancytopenia (rule out aplastic anemia), metastatic tumor, granulomatous infection (e.g., mycobacteria, brucellosis, histoplasmosis), myelofibrosis, lipid storage disease (e.g., Gaucher's, Niemann-Pick), any case with "dry tap" on aspiration.

Special Tests Histochemical staining (e.g., acid phosphatase for metastatic prostate carcinoma), immunoperoxidase staining (e.g., immunoglobulin detection in multiple myeloma, lysozyme detection in monocytic leukemia), reticulin staining (increased in myelofibrosis), microbiologic staining (e.g., acid-fast staining for mycobacteria).

Interpretation

CELLULARITY Decreases with age after age 65 years from about 50% to 25–30%.

ERYTHROID:GRANULOCYTIC (E:G) RATIO Normally about 1:2, the E:G ratio is decreased in acute and chronic infection, leukemoid reactions (e.g., chronic inflammation, metastatic tumor), acute and chronic myelogenous leukemia, myelodysplastic disorders ("preleukemia"), and pure red cell aplasia; increased in agranulocytosis, anemias with erythroid hyperplasia (megaloblastic, iron-deficiency, thalassemia, hemorrhage, hemolysis, sideroblastic), and erythrocytosis (excessive RBC production); normal in aplastic anemia (though marrow hypocellular), myelofibrosis (marrow hypocellular), multiple myeloma, lymphoma, anemia of chronic disease.

For a more detailed discussion, see Hillman RS: Anemia, Chap. 59, p. 334; and Holland SM, Gallin JI: Disorders of Granulocytes and Monocytes, Chap. 62, p. 351, in HPIM-14.

49

RED BLOOD CELL DISORDERS

ANEMIA

Blood hemoglobin (Hb) concentration <140 g/L (<14 g/dL) or hematocrit (Hct) <42% in adult males; Hb <120 g/L (<12 g/dL) or Hct <37% in adult females.

A physiologic approach to anemia diagnosis is based on the understanding that a decrease in circulating red blood cells (RBC) can be related to either inadequate production of RBC or increased RBC destruction or loss. Within the category of inadequate production, erythropoiesis can be either ineffective, due to an erythrocyte maturation defect (which usually results in RBC that are too small or too large), or hypoproliferative (which usually results in RBC of normal size, but too few of them).

Basic evaluations: (1) reticulocyte index (RI), (2) review of blood smear and RBC indices [particularly mean corpuscular volume (MCV)] (see Fig. 49-1).

The RI is a measure of RBC production. The reticulocyte count is corrected for the Hct level and for early release of marrow reticulocytes into the circulation, which leads to an increase in the life span of the circulating reticulocyte beyond the usual 1 day. Thus, RI = (% reticulocytes × patient Hct)/45% × (1/shift correction factor). The shift correction factor varies with the Hct: 1.5 for Hct = 35%, 2 for Hct = 25%, 2.5 for Hct = 15%. RI <2% implies inadequate RBC production; RI >2% implies excessive RBC destruction or loss.

If the anemia is associated with a low RI, RBC morphology helps distinguish ineffective erythropoiesis from hypoproliferative marrow states. Bone marrow examination is often helpful in the evaluation of anemia but is done most frequently to diagnose hypoproliferative marrow states.

HYPOPROLIFERATIVE ANEMIAS These are the most common anemias encountered in clinical practice. Usually the RBC morphology is normal and the RI is low. Marrow damage, early iron deficiency, and decreased erythropoietin production or action may produce anemia of this type.

Marrow damage may be caused by infiltration of the marrow with tumor or fibrosis that crowds out normal erythroid precursors or by the absence of erythroid precursors (aplastic anemia) as a consequence of exposure to drugs, radiation, chemicals, virsuses (e.g., hepatitis), or genetic factors, either hereditary (e.g., Fanconi's anemia) or acquired (e.g., paroxysmal nocturnal hemoglobinuria). Most cases of aplasia are idiopathic. The tumor or fibrosis that infiltrates the marrow may originate in the

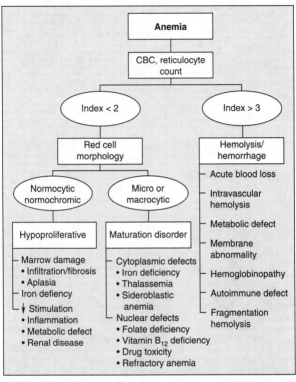

FIGURE 49-1   The classification of anemia. The complete blood count and reticulocyte index are used initially to classify an anemia as either hypoproliferative, a maturation disorder, or a hemolytic/hemorrhagic anemia. This provides a guide to the subsequent differential diagnosis of specific disease states within each category. The bone marrow examination and measurements of iron supply are very important in this differential.

marrow (as in leukemia or myelofibrosis) or be secondary to processes originating outside the marrow (as in metastatic cancer or myelophthisis).

Early iron-deficiency anemia (or iron-deficient erythropoiesis) is associated with a decrease in serum ferritin levels ($<15\mu$g/L), moderately elevated total iron-binding capacity, serum iron level <50 μg/dL, and an iron saturation of $<30\%$ but $>10\%$ (see Fig. 49-2). RBC morphology is generally normal until iron deficiency is severe (see below).

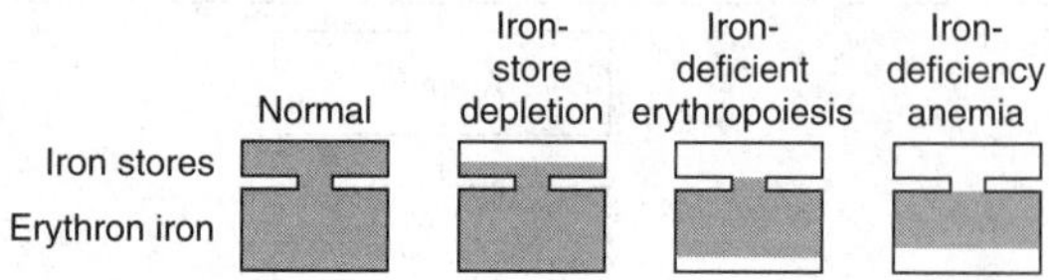

	Normal	Iron-store depletion	Iron-deficient erythropoiesis	Iron-deficiency anemia
Iron stores				
Erythron iron				
Marrow iron stores	1–3+	0–1+	0	0
Serum ferritin (μg/L)	50–200	<20	<15	<15
TIBC (μg/dL)	300–360	>360	>380	>400
SI (μg/dL)	50–150	NL	<50	<30
Saturation (%)	30–50	NL	<30	<10
Marrow sideroblasts (%)	40–60	NL	<10	<10
RBC protoporphyrin (μg/dL)	30–50	NL	>100	>200
RBC morphology	NL	NL	NL	Microcytic/hypochromic

FIGURE 49-2 Laboratory studies in the evolution of iron deficiency. Measurements of marrow iron stores, serum ferritin, and TIBC are sensitive to early iron-store depletion. Iron-deficient erythropoiesis is recognized from additional abnormalities in the SI, percent saturation of transferrin, the pattern of marrow sideroblasts, and the red blood cell protoporphyrin level. Finally, patients with iron-deficiency anemia demonstrate all of these same abnormalities plus an anemia characterized by microcytic hypochromic morphology. (From Hillman and Finch, with permission.)

Decreased stimulation of erythropoiesis can be a consequence of inadequate erythropoietin production [e.g., renal disease destroying the renal tubular cells that produce it or hypometabolic states (endocrine deficiency or protein starvation) in which insufficient erythropoietin is produced] or of inadequate erythropoietin action. The anemia of chronic disease is a common entity. It is multifactorial in pathogenesis: inhibition of erythropoietin production, inhibition of iron reutilization (which blocks the response to erythropoietin), and inhibition of erythroid colony proliferation by inflammatory cytokines (e.g., tumor necrosis factor, interferon). The laboratory tests shown in Table 49-1 may assist in the differential diagnosis of hypoproliferative anemias.

Table 49-1

Diagnosis of Hypoproliferative Anemias

Tests	Iron Deficiency	Inflammation	Renal Disease	Hypo-metabolic States
Anemia	Mild to severe	Mild	Mild to severe	Mild
MCV (fL)	70–90	80–90	90	90
Mor-phology	Normo-microcytic	Normocytic	Normo-cytic	Normo-cytic
SI	<30	<50	Normal	Normal
TIBC	>360	>300	Normal	Normal
Saturation (%)	<10	10–20	Normal	Normal
Serum ferri-tin (μg/L)	<15	30–200	115–150	Normal
Iron stores	0	2–4 +	1–4 +	Normal

NOTE: MCV, mean corpuscular volume.

MATURATION DISORDERS   These result from a defect in either hemoglobin synthesis, leading to cytoplasmic maturation defects and small red cells, or DNA replication, leading to nuclear maturation defects and large red cells. Defects in hemoglobin synthesis usually result from insufficient iron supply (iron deficiency), decreased globin production (thalassemia), or are idiopathic (sideroblastic anemia). Defects in DNA synthesis are usually due to nutritional (vitamin B_{12} and folate deficiency), toxic (methotrexate or other cancer chemotherapeutic agent exposure), or intrinsic defects (refractory anemia, myelodysplasia).

Laboratory tests useful in the differential diagnosis of the microcytic anemias are shown in Table 49-2. MCV is generally 60 to 80 fL. Increased lactic dehydrogenase (LDH) and indirect bilirubin levels favor a cause other than iron deficiency. Iron status is best assessed by measuring serum iron, total iron-binding capacity, and ferritin levels. Macrocytic MCVs are >94 fL. Folate status is best assessed by measuring red blood cell folate levels. Vitamin B_{12} status is best assessed by measuring serum B_{12}, homocysteine, and methylmalonic acid levels.

ANEMIA DUE TO RBC DESTRUCTION OR ACUTE BLOOD LOSS   *Blood Loss*   Trauma, GI hemorrhage (may be occult) are common causes; less common are genitourinary sources (menorrhagia, gross hematuria), internal—retroperito-

Table 49-2

Diagnosis of Microcytic Anemias

Tests	Iron Deficiency	Thalassemia	Sideroblastic Anemia
Smear	Micro/hypo	Micro/hypo with targeting	Variable
SI	Low	Normal to high	Normal to high
TIBC	High	Normal	Normal
Percent saturation	<10	30–80	30–80
Ferritin (μg/L)	<15	50–300	50–300
Hemoglobin pattern	Normal	Abnormal	Normal

neal, iliopsoas hemorrhage (e.g., in hip fractures). Acute bleeding is associated with manifestations of hypovolemia, reticulocytosis, macrocytosis; chronic bleeding is associated with iron deficiency, hypochromia, microcytosis.

Hemolysis Causes are listed in Table 49-3.

1. *Intracellular RBC abnormalities*—most are inherited enzyme defects [glucose-6-phosphate dehydrogenase deficiency (G6PD) Table 49-4), pyruvate kinase deficiency], hemoglobinopathies, sickle cell anemia and variants (Table 49-5), thalassemia, unstable hemoglobin variants.

G6PD deficiency leads to episodes of hemolysis precipitated by ingestion of drugs that induce oxidant stress on RBC. These include antimalarials (chloroquine), sulfonamides, analgesics (phenacetin), and other miscellaneous drugs.

Sickle cell anemia is characterized by a single amino acid change in β globin (valine for glutamic acid in the 6th residue) that produces a molecule of decreased solubility, especially in the absence of O_2. Although anemia and chronic hemolysis are present, the major disease manifestations relate to vasoocclusion from misshapen sickled RBC. Infarcts in lung, bone, spleen, retina, brain, and other organs lead to symptoms and dysfunction.

2. *Membrane abnormalities* (rare)—spur cell anemia (cirrhosis, anorexia nervosa), paroxysmal nocturnal hemoglobinuria, hereditary spherocytosis (increased RBC osmotic fragility,

Table 49-3

Classifications of Hemolytic Anemias

Intracorpuscular	1. Abnormalities of RBC interior
	  a. Enzyme defects
	  b. Hemoglobinopathies
	2. RBC membrane abnormalities
	  a. Hereditary spherocytosis, etc.
	  b. Paroxysmal nocturnal hemoglobinuria
	  c. Spur cell anemia
		Hereditary

Extracorpuscular	3. Extrinsic factors
	  a. Hypersplenism
	  b. Antibody: immune hemolysis
	  c. Microangiopathic hemolysis
	  d. Infections, toxins, etc.
		Acquired

spherocytes), hereditary elliptocytosis (causes mild hemolytic anemia).

3. *Immunohemolytic anemia* (positive Coombs' test, spherocytes). Two types: (a) *warm antibody* (usually IgG)—idiopathic, lymphoma, chronic lymphocytic leukemia, SLE, drugs (e.g., methyldopa, penicillins, quinine, quinidine, isoniazid, sulfonamides); and (b) *cold antibody*—cold agglutinin disease (IgM) due to *Mycoplasma* infection, infectious mononu-

Table 49-4

Drugs Causing Hemolysis in Subjects Deficient in G6PD

Antimalarials: Primaquine, pamaquine, dapsone
Sulfonamides: Sulfamethoxazole
Nitrofurantoin
Analgesics: Acetanilid
Miscellaneous: Vitamin K (water-soluble form),
  doxorubicin, methylene blue, nalidixic acid,
  furazolidone, niridazole, phenazopyridine

Table 49-5

Clinical Manifestations of Sickle Cell Anemia

```
Constitutional
  Impaired growth and development
  Increased susceptibility to infection ┐
Vasoocclusive                          ↓
  Microinfarcts ──→ │Painful crisis│
  Macroinfarcts ↘
                   ↘ Organ damage

Anemia
  Severe hemolysis
  Aplastic crises ←──────────────────┘
```

See Chap. 107, p. 648 in HPIM-14.

cleosis, lymphoma, idiopathic; paroxysmal cold hemoglobinuria (IgG) due to syphilis, viral infections.

4. *Mechanical trauma* (macro- and microangiopathic hemolytic anemias; schistocytes)—prosthetic heart valves, vasculitis, malignant hypertension, eclampsia, renal graft rejection, giant hemangioma, scleroderma, thrombotic thrombocytopenic purpura, hemolytic-uremic syndrome, DIC, march hemoglobinuria (e.g., marathon runners).

5. *Direct toxic effect*—infections (e.g., malaria, *Clostridium welchii* toxin, toxoplasmosis).

6. *Hypersplenism* (pancytopenia may be present).

Laboratory Abnormalities Elevated reticulocyte index, polychromasia and nucleated RBCs on smear; also spherocytes, elliptocytes, schistocytes, target, spur, or sickle cells may be present depending on disorder; elevated unconjugated serum bilirubin and LDH, elevated plasma hemoglobin, low or absent haptoglobin; urine hemosiderin present in intravascular but not extravascular hemolysis, Coombs' test (immunohemolytic anemias), osmotic fragility test (hereditary spherocytosis), hemoglobin electrophoresis (sickle cell anemia, thalassemia), G6PD assay (best performed after resolution of hemolytic episode to prevent false-negative result).

Rx TREATMENT

General Approaches The acuteness and severity determine whether transfusion therapy with packed RBCs is indicated. Rapid occurrence of severe anemia (e.g., after acute

GI hemorrhage resulting in Hct <25%, following volume repletion) is an indication for transfusion. For each unit of packed RBCs, Hct should increase 3 to 4% [Hb by 10 g/L (1 g/dL)], assuming no ongoing losses. Chronic anemia (e.g., B_{12} deficiency), even when severe, may not require transfusion therapy if the pt is compensated and specific therapy (e.g., parenteral B_{12}) is instituted.

Specific Disorders

1. *Iron deficiency:* treat cause of blood loss, oral iron (e.g., $FeSO_4$ 300 mg tid
2. *Folate deficiency:* common in malnourished, alcoholics; folic acid 1 mg PO qd (5 mg qd for pts with malabsorption)
3. *B_{12} deficiency:* parenteral B_{12} required in most cases (e.g., pernicious anemia—lack of intrinsic factor prevents dietary absorption), vitamin B_{12} 100 μg IM qd for 7 d, then 100 to 1000 μg IM per month
4. *Anemia of chronic disease:* treat underlying disease; in uremia use recombinant human erythropoietin, 50 to 150 U/kg tiw SC
5. *Sickle cell anemia:* hydroxyurea (antisickling), treat infections early, supplemental folic acid; painful crises treated with analgesics, hydration, and hypertransfusion; consider allogeneic bone marrow transplantation
6. β *thalassemia:* transfusion to maintain Hb >9 g/dL, folic acid, prevention of Fe overload with deferoximine chelation; consider splenectomy and allogeneic bone marrow transplantation
7. *Aplastic anemia:* antithymocyte globulin, bone marrow transplantation
8. *Autoimmune hemolysis:* glucocorticoids, sometimes immunosuppressive agents, danazol, plasmapheresis
9. *G6PD deficiency:* avoid agents known to precipitate hemolysis.

POLYCYTHEMIA (ERYTHROCYTOSIS)

This is an increase above the normal range of RBCs in the circulation. *Relative erythrocytosis*—due to plasma volume loss (e.g., severe dehydration, burns); does not represent a true increase in total RBC mass. *Absolute erythrocytosis*—increase in total RBC mass.

CAUSES Polycythemia vera (a clonal myeloproliferative disorder), erythropoietin-producing neoplasms (e.g., renal cancer, cerebellar hemangioma), chronic hypoxemia (e.g., high altitude, pulmonary disease), carboxyhemoglobin excess (e.g., smokers), high-affinity hemoglobin variants, Cushing's syndrome, androgen excess. Polycythemia vera is distinguished from secondary polycythemia by the presence of splenomegaly, leukocytosis, thrombocytosis, and elevated vitamin B_{12} levels, and by decreased erythropoietin levels.

COMPLICATIONS Hyperviscosity (with diminished O_2 delivery) with risk of ischemic organ injury.

TREATMENT
Phlebotomy recommended for Hct >55%, regardless of cause, to low-normal range.

For a more detailed discussion, see Hillman RS: Anemia, Chap. 59, p. 334; and Hillman RS, et al: Chaps. 106–111, pp. 638–679, in HPIM-14.

50

LEUKOCYTOSIS AND LEUKOPENIA

LEUKOCYTOSIS

Approach

Review smear (? abnormal cells present) and obtain differential count. The normal values for concentration of blood leukocytes are shown in Table 50-1.

Neutrophilia

Absolute neutrophil count (polys and bands) >10,000/μL. The pathophysiology of neutrophilia involves increased production, increased marrow mobilization, or decreased margination (adherence to vessel walls).

CAUSES (1) *Exercise, stress*; (2) *infections*—esp. bacterial; smear shows increased numbers of immature neutrophils ("left

Table 50-1

Normal Values for Leukocyte Concentration in Blood

Cell Type	Mean, cells/μL	95% Confidence Limits, cells/μL	Percent Total WBC
Neutrophil	3650	1830–7250	30–60
Lymphocyte	2500	1500–4000	20–50
Monocyte	430	200–950	2–10
Eosinophil	150	0–700	0.3–5
Basophil	30	0–150	0.6–1.8

shift"), toxic granulations, Döhle bodies; (3) *burns*; (4) *tissue necrosis* (e.g., myocardial, pulmonary, renal infarction); (5) *chronic inflammatory disorders* (e.g., gout, vasculitis); (6) *drugs* (e.g., glucocorticoids, epinephrine, lithium); (7) *cytokines* (e.g., G-CSF, GM-CSF); (8) *myeloproliferative disorders* (Chap. 54); (9) *metabolic* (e.g., ketoacidosis, uremia); (10) *other*—malignant neoplasms, acute hemorrhage or hemolysis, after splenectomy.

Leukemoid Reaction

Extreme elevation of leukocyte count (>50,000/μL) composed of mature and/or immature neutrophils.

CAUSES   (1) *Infection* (severe, chronic, e.g., tuberculosis), esp. in children; (2) *hemolysis* (severe); (3) *malignant neoplasms* (esp. carcinoma of the breast, lung, kidney); (4) *cytokines* (e.g., G-CSF, GM-CSF). May be distinguished from chronic myelogenous leukemia (CML) by measurement of the leukocyte alkaline phosphatase (LAP) level: elevated in leukemoid reactions, depressed in CML.

Leukoerythroblastic Reaction

Similar to leukemoid reaction with addition of nucleated RBCs and schistocytes on blood smear.

CAUSES   (1) *Myelophthisis*—invasion of the bone marrow by tumor, fibrosis, granulomatous processes; smear shows "teardrop" RBCs; (2) myelofibrosis—same pathophysiology as myelophthisis, but the fibrosis is a primary marrow disorder; (3) *hemorrhage* or *hemolysis* (rarely, in severe cases).

Lymphocytosis

Absolute lymphocyte count >5000/μL.

Causes (1) *Infection*—infectious mononucleosis, hepatitis, CMV, rubella, pertussis, tuberculosis, brucellosis, syphilis; (2) *endocrine*—thyrotoxicosis, adrenal insufficiency; (3) *neoplastic*—chronic lymphocytic leukemia (CLL), most common cause of lymphocyte count >10,000/μL.

Monocytosis

Absolute monocyte count >800/μL.

CAUSES (1) *Infection*—subacute bacterial endocarditis, tuberculosis, brucellosis, rickettsial diseases (e.g., Rocky Mountain spotted fever), malaria, leishmaniasis; (2) *granulomatous diseases*—sarcoidosis, Crohn's disease; (3) *collagen-vascular diseases*—rheumatoid arthritis, SLE, polyarteritis nodosa, polymyositis, temporal arteritis; (4) *hematologic*—leukemias, lymphoma, myeloproliferative and myelodysplastic syndromes, hemolytic anemia, chronic idiopathic neutropenia; (5) *malignant neoplasms*.

Eosinophilia

Absolute eosinophil count >500/μL.

CAUSES (1) *Drugs*, (2) *parasitic infections*, (3) *allergic diseases*, (4) *collagen-vascular diseases*, (5) *malignant neoplasms*, (6) *hypereosinophilic syndromes*.

Basophilia

Absolute basophil count >100/μL.

CAUSES (1) *Allergic diseases*, (2) *myeloproliferative disorders* (esp. CML), (3) *chronic inflammatory disorders* (rarely).

LEUKOPENIA

Definition

Total leukocyte count <4300/μL.

Neutropenia

Absolute neutrophil count <2500/μL (increased risk of bacterial infection with count<1000/μL). The pathophysiology of neutropenia involves decreased production or increased peripheral destruction.

CAUSES (1) *Drugs*—cancer chemotherapeutic agents are most common cause, also phenytoin, carbamazepine, indomethacin, chloramphenicol, penicillins, sulfonamides, cephalosporins, propylthiouracil, phenothiazines, captopril, methyldopa, procainamide, chlorpropamide, thiazides, cimetidine, allopurinol, colchicine, ethanol, penicillamine, and immunosuppressive agents; (2) *infections*—viral (e.g., influenza, hepatitis, infectious mononucleosis, human immunodeficiency virus), bacterial (e.g., typhoid fever, miliary tuberculosis, fulminant sepsis), malaria; (3) *nutritional*—B_{12}, folate deficiencies; (4) *benign*—mild neutropenia common in blacks, no associated risk of infection; (5) *hematologic*—cyclic neutropenia (q21d, with recurrent infections common), leukemia, myelodysplasia (preleukemia), aplastic anemia, bone marrow infiltration (uncommon cause), Chédiak-Higashi syndrome; (6) *hypersplenism*—e.g., Felty's syndrome, congestive splenomegaly, Gaucher's disease; (7) *autoimmune*—idiopathic, SLE, lymphoma (may see positive antineutrophil antibodies).

℞ **TREATMENT**

Of the Febrile, Neutropenic Patient (See Chap. 36)   In addition to usual sources of infection, consider paranasal sinuses, oral cavity (including teeth and gums), anorectal region; empirical therapy with broad-spectrum antibiotics is indicated after blood and other appropriate cultures are obtained. Prolonged febrile neutropenia (>7 d) leads to increased risk of disseminated fungal infections; requires addition of antifungal chemotherapy (e.g., amphotericin B). The duration of chemotherapy-induced neutropenia may be shortened by a few days by treatment with the cytokines GM-CSF or G-CSF.

Lymphopenia

Absolute lymphocyte count <1000/μL.

CAUSES (1) *Acute stressful illness*—e.g., myocardial infarction, pneumonia, sepsis; (2) *glucocorticoid therapy;* (3) *lymphoma* (esp. Hodgkin's disease); (4) *immune deficiency syndromes*—ataxia telangiectasia and Wiskott-Aldrich and DiGeorge's syndromes; (5) *immunosuppressive therapy*—e.g., antilymphocyte globulin, cyclophosphamide; (6) *after radiotherapy* (esp. for lymphoma); (7) *intestinal lymphangiectasia* (increased lymph loss); (8) *chronic illness*—e.g., CHF, uremia, SLE, disseminated malignancies; (9) *bone marrow failure/replacement*—e.g., aplastic anemia, miliary tuberculosis.

Monocytopenia

Absolute monocyte count <100/µL.

CAUSES   (1) *Acute stressful illness*, (2) *glucocorticoid therapy*, (3) *aplastic anemia*, (4) *leukemia* (certain types, e.g., hairy cell leukemia), (5) *chemotherapeutic and immunosuppressive agents*.

Eosinopenia

Absolute eosinophil count <50/µL.

CAUSES   (1) *Acute stressful illness*, (2) *glucocorticoid therapy*.

For a more detailed discussion, see Holland SM, Gallin JI: Disorders of Granulocytes and Monocytes, Chap. 62, p. 351; Castro-Malaspina H, O'Reilly RJ: Aplastic Anemia and Myelodysplasia, Chap. 110, p. 672; Spivak JL: Polycythemia Vera and Other Myeloproliferative Diseases, Chap. 111, p. 679, in HPIM-14.

BLEEDING AND THROMBOTIC DISORDERS

BLEEDING DISORDERS

Bleeding may result from abnormalities of (1) platelets, (2) blood vessel walls, or (3) coagulation. Platelet disorders characteristically produce petechial and purpuric skin lesions and bleeding from mucosal surfaces. Defective coagulation results in ecchymoses, hematomas, and mucosal and, in some disorders, recurrent joint bleeding (hemarthroses).

Platelet Disorders

THROMBOCYTOPENIA   Normal platelet count is 150,000–350,000/µL. Thrombocytopenia is defined as a platelet count <100,000/μL. Bleeding time, a measurement of platelet function, is abnormally increased if platelet count <100,000/μL; injury or surgery may provoke excess bleeding. Spontaneous bleeding is unusual unless count is <20,000/μL; platelet count <10,000/μL is often associated with serious hemorrhage. Bone marrow examination shows increased number of megakaryocytes in disorders associated with accelerated platelet destruction; decreased number in disorders of platelet production.

Causes: (1) Production defects such as marrow injury (e.g., drugs, irradiation), marrow failure (e.g., aplastic anemia), marrow invasion (e.g., carcinoma, leukemia, fibrosis); (2) sequestration due to splenomegaly; (3) accelerated destruction—causes include:

- *Drugs* such as chemotherapeutic agents, thiazides, ethanol, estrogens, sulfonamides, quinidine, quinine, methyldopa. *Heparin-induced* thrombocytopenia is seen in 5% of pts receiving >5 d of therapy and is due to in vivo platelet aggregation. Arterial and occasionally venous thromboses may result.
- *Autoimmune destruction* by an antibody mechanism; may be idiopathic or associated with SLE, lymphoma, HIV. *Idiopathic thrombocytopenic purpura* (ITP) has two forms: an acute, self-limited disorder of childhood requiring no specific therapy, and a chronic disorder of adults (esp. women 20–40 years of age). Chronic ITP may be due to autoantibodies to glycoprotein IIb-IIIa or glycoprotein Ib-IX complexes.
- *Disseminated intravascular coagulation* (DIC)—platelet consumption with coagulation factor depletion (prolonged PT, PTT) and stimulation of fibrinolysis (generation of fibrin split products, FSP). Blood smear shows microangiopathic hemolysis (schistocytes). *Causes*—infection (esp. meningococcal, pneumococcal, gram-negative bacteremias), extensive burns, trauma, or thrombosis; giant hemangioma, retained dead fetus, heat stroke, mismatched blood transfusion, metastatic carcinoma, acute promyelocytic leukemia.
- *Thrombotic thrombocytopenic purpura*—rare disorder characterized by microangiopathic hemolytic anemia, fever, thrombocytopenia, renal dysfunction (and/or hematuria), and neurologic dysfunction.
- Hemorrhage with extensive transfusion.

PSEUDOTHROMBOCYTOPENIA   Platelet clumping secondary to collection of blood in EDTA (0.3% of pts). Examination of blood smear establishes diagnosis.

THROMBOCYTOSIS   Platelet count >350,000/μL. Either primary (thrombocythemia; Chap. 54) or secondary (reactive);

latter secondary to severe hemorrhage, iron deficiency, surgery, after splenectomy (transient), malignant neoplasms (especially Hodgkin's disease), chronic inflammatory diseases (e.g., inflammatory bowel disease), recovery from acute infection, vitamin B_{12} deficiency, drugs (e.g., vincristine, epinephrine). Rebound thrombocytosis may occur after marrow recovery from cytotoxic agents, alcohol. Primary thrombocytosis may be complicated by bleeding and/or thrombosis; secondary rarely causes hemostatic problems.

DISORDERS OF PLATELET FUNCTION   Suggested by the finding of prolonged bleeding time with normal platelet count. Defect is in platelet adhesion, aggregation, or granule release. *Causes*: (1) Drugs—aspirin, other NSAIDs, dipyridamole, heparin, penicillins, esp. carbenicillin, ticarcillin; (2) uremia; (3) cirrhosis; (4) dysproteinemias; (5) myeloproliferative and myelodysplastic disorders; (6) von Willebrand's disease (see below); (7) cardiopulmonary bypass.

Hemostatic Disorders due to Blood Vessel Wall Defects

Causes: (1) Aging; (2) drugs—e.g., glucocorticoids (chronic therapy), penicillins, sulfonamides; (3) vitamin C deficiency; (4) thrombotic thrombocytopenic purpura (TTP); (5) hemolytic uremic syndrome; (6) Henoch-Schönlein purpura; (7) paraproteinemias; (8) hereditary hemorrhagic telangiectasia (Osler-Rendu-Weber disease).

Disorders of Blood Coagulation

CONGENITAL DISORDERS

1. *Hemophilia A*—incidence 1:10,000; sex-linked recessive deficiency of factor VIII (low plasma factor VIII coagulant activity, but normal amount of factor VIII–related antigen—von Willebrand's factor). *Laboratory features*: elevated PTT, normal PT.

2. *Hemophilia B* (Christmas disease)—incidence 1:100,000, sex-linked recessive, due to factor IX deficiency. Clinical and laboratory features similar to hemophilia A.

3. *von Willebrand's disease*—most common inherited coagulation disorder (1:800–1000), usually autosomal dominant; primary defect is reduced synthesis or chemically abnormal factor VIII–related antigen produced by platelets and endothelium, resulting in abnormal platelet function.

ACQUIRED DISORDERS

1. *Vitamin K deficiency*—impairs production of factors II (prothrombin), VII, IX, and X; vitamin K is a cofactor in the carboxylation of glutamate residues on prothrombin complex proteins; major source of vitamin K is dietary (esp. green vegetables), with minor production by gut bacteria. *Laboratory features*: elevated PT and PTT.

2. *Liver disease*—results in deficiencies of all clotting factors except VIII. Laboratory features: elevated PT, normal or elevated PTT.

3. *Other disorders*—DIC, fibrinogen deficiency (liver disease, L-asparaginase therapy, rattlesnake bites), other factor deficiencies, circulating anticoagulants (lymphoma, SLE, idiopathic), massive transfusion (dilutional coagulopathy).

℞ TREATMENT

Of Thrombocytopenia Caused by Drugs Includes discontinuation of possible offending agents; expect recovery in 7–10 d.

Of Heparin-Induced Thrombocytopenia Includes prompt discontinuation of heparin. Warfarin and/or a fibrinolytic agent (see below) should be used for treatment of thromboses.

Of Chronic ITP Prednisone, initially 1–2 (mg/kg)/d, then slow taper, to keep the platelet count >60,000/μL. Intravenous immunoglobulin to block phagocytic destruction may be useful. Splenectomy, danazol (androgen), or other agents (e.g., vincristine, cyclophosphamide) are indicated for pts requiring >5–10 mg prednisone daily.

Of DIC Control of underlying disease most important; platelets, fresh frozen plasma (FFP) to correct clotting parameters. Heparin may be beneficial in pts with acute promyelocytic leukemia.

Of Thrombotic Thrombocytopenic Purpura Plasmapheresis and FFP infusions, possibly intravenous IgG; recovery in two-thirds of cases.

Of Disorders of Platelet Function Remove or reverse underlying cause. Dialysis and/or cryoprecipitate infusions (10 bags/24 h) may be helpful for platelet dysfunction associated with uremia.

Of Hemostatic Disorders Withdraw offending drugs, replace vitamin C, plasmapheresis and plasma infusion for TTP.

Of Hemophilia A Factor VIII replacement for bleeding or before surgical procedure; degree and duration of replacement depends on severity of bleeding. Give factor VIII to obtain a 15% (for mild bleeding) to 50% (for severe bleeding) factor VIII level. The duration should range from a single dose of factor VIII to therapy bid for up to 2 weeks.

Of Hemophilia BH   FFP or factor IX concentrates (Proplex, Konyne).

Of von Willebrand's Disease   Cryoprecipitate (plasma product rich in factor VIII) or factor VIII concentrate (Humate-P, Koate HS); up to 10 bags bid for 48–72 h, depending on the severity of bleeding. Desmopressin (vasopressin analogue) may benefit some pts.

Of Vitamin K Deficiency   Vitamin K 10 mg SC or slow IV.

Of Liver Disease   Fresh frozen plasma.

THROMBOTIC DISORDERS

Hypercoagulable State

Consider in pts with recurrent episodes of venous thrombosis (i.e., deep venous thrombosis, DVT; pulmonary embolism). *Causes*: (1) Venous stasis (e.g., pregnancy, immobilization); (2) vasculitis; (3) myeloproliferative disorders; (4) oral contraceptives; (5) lupus anticoagulant—antibody to platelet phospholipid, stimulates coagulation; (6) heparin-induced thrombocytopenia; (7) deficiencies of endogenous anticoagulant factors—antithrombin III, protein C, protein S; (8) factor V Leiden—mutation in factor V (Arg $\to$ Glu at position 506) confers resistance to inactivation by protein C, accounts for 25% of cases of recurrent thrombosis; (9) other—paroxysmal nocturnal hemoglobinuria, dysfibrinogenemias (abnormal fibrinogen). *Treatment*: Correct underlying disorder whenever possible; long-term warfarin therapy is otherwise indicated.

℞ TREATMENT
Anticoagulant agents

1. *Heparin*—enhances activity of antithrombin III; parenteral agent of choice. In adults, 25,000–40,000 U continuous IV infusion over 24 h following initial IV bolus of 5000 U; monitor by following PTT, should be maintained between 1.5 and 2 times upper normal limit. Prophylactic anticoagulation to lower risk of venous thrombosis recommended in some pts (e.g., postoperative, immobilized); dosage is 5000 U SC q8–12h. Major complication of heparin therapy is hemorrhage—manage by discontinuing heparin; for severe bleeding, administer protamine (1 mg/100 U heparin); results in rapid neutralization.

2. *Warfarin* (Coumadin)—vitamin K antagonist, decreases levels of factors II, VII, IX, X and anticoagulant proteins C and S. Administered over 2–3 d; initial load of 5–10 mg PO qd followed by titration of daily dose to keep PT 1.5–2 times control PT or 2–3 if the International Normalized Ratio method is used. *Complications*—hemorrhage, warfarin-induced skin necrosis (rare, occurs in people deficient in protein C), teratogenic effects. Warfarin effect reversed by administration of vitamin K; FFP infused if urgent reversal necessary. Numerous drugs potentiate or antagonize warfarin effect. *Potentiating agents*—chlorpromazine, chloral hydrate, sulfonamides, chloramphenicol, other broad-spectrum antibiotics, allopurinol, cimetidine, tricyclic antidepressants, disulfiram, laxatives, high-dose salicylates, thyroxine, clofibrate. *Antagonizing agents*—vitamin K, barbiturates, rifampin, cholestyramine, oral contraceptives, thiazides.

In-hospital anticoagulation usually initiated with heparin, with subsequent maintenance on warfarin after an overlap of 3 d.

Fibrinolytic Agents

Tissue plasminogen activator (tPA, alteplase), streptokinase and urokinase; mediate clot lysis by activating plasmin, which degrades fibrin. *Indications*—treatment of DVT, with lower incidence of postphlebitic syndrome (chronic venous stasis, skin ulceration) than with heparin therapy; massive pulmonary embolism, arterial embolic occlusion of extremity, treatment of acute MI, unstable angina pectoris. Dosages for fibrinolytic agents: (1) *tPA*—for acute MI and massive PE (adult >65 kg), 10 mg IV bolus over 1–2 min, then 50 mg IV over 1 h and 40 mg IV over next 2 h (total dose = 100 mg). tPA is slightly more effective but more expensive than streptokinase for treatment of acute MI. (2) *Streptokinase*—for acute MI, 1.5 million IU IV over 60 min; or 20,000 IU as a bolus intracoronary (IC) infusion, followed by 2000 IU/min for 60 min IC. For pulmonary embolism or arterial or deep venous thrombosis, 250,000 IU over 30 min, then 100,000 IU/h for 24 h (pulmonary embolism) or 72 h (arterial or deep venous thrombosis). (3) *Urokinase*—for pulmonary embolism, 4400 IU/kg IV over 10 min, then 4400 (IU/kg)/h IV for 12 h.

Fibrinolytic therapy is usually followed by period of anticoagulant therapy with heparin. Fibrinolytic agents are contraindicated in pts with: (1) active internal bleeding; (2) recent (<2–3 months) cerebrovascular accident; (3) intracranial neoplasm, aneurysm, or recent head trauma.

Antiplatelet Agents

Aspirin (160–325 mg/d) with or without dipyridamole (50–100 mg qid) may be beneficial in lowering incidence of arterial thrombotic events (stroke, MI) in high-risk pts.

For a more detailed discussion, see Handin RI: Bleeding and Thrombosis, Chap. 60, p. 339; Disorders of the Platelet and Vessel Wall, Chap. 117, p. 730; Disorders of Coagulation and Thrombosis, Chap. 118, p. 736; and Anticoagulant, Fibrinolytic, and Antiplatelet Therapy, Chap. 119, p. 744, in HPIM-14.

TRANSFUSION AND PHERESIS THERAPY

TRANSFUSIONS

Whole Blood Transfusion

Indicated when acute blood loss is sufficient to produce hypovolemia, whole blood provides both oxygen-carrying capacity and volume expansion. In acute blood loss, hematocrit may not accurately reflect degree of blood loss for 48 h until fluid shifts occur.

Red Blood Cell Transfusion

Indicated for symptomatic anemia unresponsive to specific therapy or requiring urgent correction. Packed RBC transfusions may be indicated in patients who are symptomatic from cardiovascular or pulmonary disease when Hb is between 70 and 90 g/L (7 and 9 g/dL). Transfusion is usually necessary when Hb <70 g/L (<7 g/dL). One unit of packed RBCs raises the Hb by approximately 10 g/L (1 g/dL). If used instead of whole blood in the setting of acute hemorrhage, packed RBCs, fresh frozen plasma (FFP), and platelets in an approximate ratio of 3:1:10 units are an adequate replacement for whole blood. Removal of leukocytes reduces risk of alloimmunization and transmission of CMV. Washing to remove donor plasma reduces risk of allergic reactions. Irradiation prevents graft-versus-host disease in immunocompromised recipients.

OTHER INDICATIONS (1) *Hypertransfusion therapy* to block production of defective cells—e.g., thalassemia, sickle cell anemia; (2) *exchange transfusion*—hemolytic disease of newborn, sickle cell crisis; (3) *transplant recipients*—decreases rejection of cadaveric kidney transplants.

COMPLICATIONS (1) *Transfusion reaction*—immediate or delayed, seen in 1–4 per 100 transfusions; IgA-deficient pts at particular risk for severe reaction; (2) *infection*—bacterial (rare); hepatitis C, 1 in 103,000 transfusions; HIV transmission, 1 in 490,000; (3) *circulatory overload*; (4) *iron overload*—each unit contains 200–250 mg iron; hemachromatosis may develop after 100 U of RBCs (less in children), in absence of blood loss; iron chelation therapy with deferoxamine indicated; (5) graft-versus-host disease; (6) alloimmunization.

Autologous Transfusion

Use of pt's own stored blood avoids hazards of donor blood; also useful in pts with multiple RBC antibodies. Pace of autologous donation may be accelerated using erythropoietin (50–150 U/kg SC three times a week) in the setting of normal iron stores.

Platelet Transfusion

Prophylactic transfusions usually reserved for platelet count $<10,000/\mu L$ ($<20,000/\mu L$ in acute leukemia). One unit elevates the count by about $10,000/\mu L$ if no platelet antibodies are present as a result of prior transfusions. Efficacy assessed by 1-h and 24-h posttransfusion platelet counts. HLA-matched single-donor platelets may be required in pts with platelet alloantibodies.

Transfusion of Plasma Components

FFP is a source of coagulation factors, fibrinogen, antithrombin, and proteins C and S. It is used to correct coagulation factor deficiencies, rapidly reverse warfarin effects, and treat thrombotic thrombocytopenic purpura (TTP). Cryoprecipitate is a source of fibrinogen, factor VIII, and von Willebrand factor; it may be used when recombinant factor VIII or factor VIII concentrates are not available.

THERAPEUTIC HEMAPHERESIS

Hemapheresis is removal of a cellular or plasma constituent of blood; specific procedure referred to by the blood fraction removed.

Leukapheresis

Removal of WBCs; most often used in acute leukemia, esp. acute myelogenous leukemia (AML) in cases complicated by marked elevation ($>50,000/\mu L$) of the peripheral blast count, to lower risk of leukostasis (blast-mediated vasoocclusive events resulting in CNS or pulmonary infarction, hemorrhage). Leukapheresis is increasingly being used to harvest hematopoietic stem cells from the peripheral blood of cancer patients; such cells are then used to promote hematopoietic reconstitution following high-dose therapy.

Plateletpheresis

Used in some pts with thrombocytosis associated with myeloproliferative disorders with bleeding and/or thrombotic complications. Other treatments are generally used first. Also used to enhance platelet yield from blood donors.

Plasmapheresis

INDICATIONS (1) *Hyperviscosity states* (e.g., Waldenström's macroglobulinemia); (2) TTP; (3) *immune-complex* and *autoantibody disorders*—e.g., Goodpasture's syndrome, rapidly progressive glomerulonephritis, myasthenia gravis; possibly Guillain-Barré, SLE, idiopathic thrombocytopenic purpura; (4) cold agglutinin disease, cryoglobulinemia.

For a more detailed discussion, see Dzieczkowski JS, and Anderson KC: Transfusion Biology and Therapy, Chap. 115, p. 718, in HPIM-14.

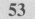

53

CANCER CHEMOTHERAPY

BIOLOGY OF TUMOR GROWTH

Two essential features of cancer cells are uncontrolled growth and the ability to metastasize. The malignant phenotype of a cell is the end result of a series of genetic changes that remove safeguards restricting cell growth and induce new features that enable the cell to metastasize, including surface receptors for binding to basement membranes, enzymes to poke holes in anatomic barriers, cytokines to facilitate mobility, and angiogenic factors to develop a new vascular lifeline for nutrients and oxygen. These genetic changes usually involve increased or abnormal expression or activity of certain genes known as proto-oncogenes (often growth factors or their receptors, enzymes in growth pathways, or transcription factors), deletion or inactivation of tumor suppressor genes, and defects in DNA repair enzymes. These genetic changes may occur by point mutation, gene amplification, gene rearrangement, or epigenetic changes such as altered gene methylation.

Once cells are malignant, their growth kinetics are similar to those of normal cells but lack regulation. For unclear reasons, tumor growth kinetics follow a Gompertzian curve: as the tumor mass increases, the fraction of dividing cells declines. Thus, by the time a cancer is large enough to be detected clinically, its growth fraction is often small. Unfortunately, tumor growth usually does not stop altogether before the tumor reaches a lethal tumor burden. Cancer cells proceed through the same cell-cycle stages as normal cycling cells: G_1 (period of preparation for DNA synthesis), S (DNA synthesis), G_2 (tetraploid phase preceding mitosis in which integrity of DNA replication is assessed), and M (mitosis). Some noncycling cells may remain in a G_0 or resting phase for long periods. Certain chemotherapeutic agents are specific for cells in certain phases of the cell cycle, a fact that is important in designing effective chemotherapeutic regimens.

DEVELOPMENT OF DRUG RESISTANCE

Drug resistance can be divided into de novo resistance or acquired resistance. De novo resistance refers to the tendency of many of the most common solid tumors to be unresponsive to chemotherapeutic agents. In acquired resistance, tumors initially responsive to chemotherapy develop resistance during treatment, usually because resistant clones appear within tumor cell populations. (See Table 53-1.)

Table 53-1

Response of Tumors to Chemotherapy

CURABLE BY CHEMOTHERAPY

Acute lymphocytic leukemia	Non-Hodgkin's lymphoma
Acute myelogenous leukemia	Burkitt's
Ewing's sarcoma	Diffuse large cell
Gestational trophoblastic carcinoma	Follicular mixed
Hodgkin's disease	Lymphoblastic
Testicular carcinoma	Rhabdomyosarcoma
Wilms' tumor	

CHEMOTHERAPY HAS SIGNIFICANT ACTIVITY

Anal carcinoma	Head and neck carcinoma
Bladder carcinoma	Lung (small cell) carcinoma
Breast carcinoma	Multiple myeloma
Chronic lymphocytic leukemia	Non-Hodgkin's lymphoma
Chronic myelogenous leukemia	Follicular lymphoma
Endometrial carcinoma	Ovarian carcinoma
Hairy cell leukemia	

CHEMOTHERAPY HAS MINOR ACTIVITY

Brain tumors (astrocytoma)	Lung (non-small cell carcinoma)
Cervical carcinoma	Melanoma
Colorectal carcinoma	Pancreatic carcinoma
Hepatocellular carcinoma	Prostate carcinoma
Kaposi's sarcoma	Renal cell carcinoma
	Soft tissue sarcoma

ADJUVANT CHEMOTHERAPY IS EFFECTIVE

Breast carcinoma (axillary lymph node positive)	Osteogenic sarcoma
Colorectal carcinoma (Dukes B2 or C)	Ovarian carcinoma (stage III)
	Testicular carcinoma

SOURCE: Slapak CA, Kufe DW, HPIM-14, p. 527.

Resistance can be to single drugs, because of defective transport of the drug, decreased activating enzymes, increased drug inactivation, increases in target enzyme levels, or alterations in target molecules. Multiple drug resistance occurs in cells overexpressing the P glycoprotein, a membrane glycoprotein responsible for enhanced efflux of drugs from cells, but there are other mechanisms as well.

CATEGORIES OF CHEMOTHERAPEUTIC AGENTS AND MAJOR TOXICITIES

(*Note*: List of toxicities is partial; some toxicities may apply only to certain members of a group of drugs.)

Alkylating agents	**Toxicity**
(add alkyl groups to N-7 or O-6 of guanine)	
Busulfan	Nausea and vomiting, bone
Chlorambucil	marrow depression,
Cyclophosphamide	pulmonary fibrosis, sterility,
Dacarbazine (DTIC)	hemorrhagic cystitis,
Mechlorethamine (nitrogen	secondary malignancies,
mustard)	alopecia
Nitrosoureas	
L-Phenylalanine mustard	
Thiotepa	

Antimetabolites	
(inhibit DNA or RNA synthesis)	
Azathioprine	Nausea and vomiting, bone
Chlorodeoxyadenosine	marrow depression, oral and
Cytarabine	GI ulceration, hepatic
Fludarabine	toxicity, alopecia, neurologic
Fluorouracil	defects
Hydroxyurea	
Methotrexate	
6-Mercaptopurine	
Pentostatin	
6-Thioguanine	

Tubulin poisons	
(block tubule polymerization or depolymerization)	
Docetaxel	Nausea and vomiting, local
Paclitaxel (Taxol)	pain upon extravasation,
Vinblastine	bone marrow depression,
	peripheral neuropathy,

Vincristine

alopecia, inappropriate ADH secretion, paralytic ileus, hypersensitivity reaction (taxanes)

Antibiotics
  (diverse antitumor
  mechanisms)
Bleomycin
Dactinomycin (actinomycin
  D)
Mithramycin
Mitomycin

Nausea and vomiting, bone marrow depression, cardiotoxicity, pulmonary fibrosis, hypocalcemia, alopecia, hypersensitivity reactions

Topoisomerase inhibitors
  (interfere with DNA
  unwinding)
9-Aminocamptothecin
Daunarubicin
Doxorubicin
Etoposide
Idarubicin
Mitoxantrone
Teniposide

Nausea, vomiting, tissue necrosis upon extravasation, myelosuppression, cardiac damage

Enzymes
L-Asparaginase

Nausea and vomiting, fever, anaphylaxis, CNS changes, pancreatitis, thrombosis, renal and hepatic damage

Miscellaneous agents
Interferon-α
Carboplatin
Cisplatin
Flutamide
Interleukin 2
Leuprolide
Procarbazine
Tamoxifen

Nausea and vomiting, bone marrow depression, fever, chills, renal damage, antiestrogen effects, gynecomastia, impotence, hot flashes

COMPLICATIONS OF THERAPY

While the effects of cancer chemotherapeutic agents may be exerted primarily on the malignant cell population, virtually all currently employed regimens have profound effects on normal tissues as well. Every side effect of treatment must be balanced against potential benefits expected, and pts must always be fully apprised of the toxicities they may encounter. While the duration of certain adverse effects may be short-lived, others, such as sterility and the risk of secondary malignancy, have long-term implications; consideration of these effects is of importance in the use of regimens as adjuvant therapy. The combined toxicity of regimens involving radiotherapy and chemotherapy is greater than that seen with each modality alone. Teratogenesis is a special concern in treating women of childbearing years with radiation or chemotherapy. The most serious late toxicities are sterility (common; from alkylating agents), secondary acute leukemia (rare; from alkylating agents and topoisomerase inhibitors), secondary solid tumors (0.5–1%/year risk for at least 25 years after treatment; from radiation therapy), premature atherosclerosis (3-fold increased risk of fatal MI; from radiation therapy), heart failure (rare; from anthracyclines), and pulmonary fibrosis (rare; from bleomycin).

For a more detailed discussion, see Slapak CA, Kufe DW: Principles of Cancer Therapy, Chap. 86, p. 523, in HPIM-14.

54

MYELOID LEUKEMIAS, MYELODYSPLASIA, AND MYELOPROLIFERATIVE SYNDROMES

ACUTE MYELOID LEUKEMIA

Acute myeloid leukemia (AML) is a clonal malignancy of myeloid bone marrow precursors in which poorly differentiated cells accumulate in the bone marrow and circulation. Signs and symptoms occur because of the absence of mature cells normally produced by the bone marrow including granulocytes (susceptibility to infection) and platelets (susceptibility to bleeding). In addition, if large numbers of immature malignant myeloblasts circulate, they may invade organs and rarely produce dysfunction. Distinct morphologic subtypes exist (see Table 54-1) that have largely overlapping clinical features. Of note is the propensity of pts with acute promyelocytic leukemia (APL) to develop

Table 54-1

The French-American-British (FAB) Classification of

FAB Subtype	% of Cases	Morphology
M0: Minimally differentiated leukemia	2–3	Immature morphology
M1: Myeloblastic leukemia without maturation	20	Few blasts with azurophilic granules, Auer rods, or both
M2: Myeloblastic leukemia with maturation	25–30	Azurophilic granules, Auer rods are often present Variant: M2Baso: blasts with basophil granules
M3: Hypergranular promyelocytic leukemia	8–15	Hypergranular promyelocytes with multiple Auer rods Variant: hypogranular
M4: Myelomonocytic leukemia	20–25	Granulocytic and monocytic blasts Variant: M4Eo: increase in abnormal marrow eosinophils
M5: Monocytic leukemia	20–25	M5a undifferentiated M5b differentiated
M6: Erythroleukemia (Di Guglielmo's disease)	5	Erythroblasts >50% of nucleated cells, myeloblasts >30% of nonerythroid cells
M7: Megakaryoblastic leukemia	1–2	Megakaryoblasts >30% of all nucleated cells

[a] Periodic acid Schiff staining is characteristic of the neoplastic erythroid precursors of M6.

[b] With fluoride inhibition.

[c] The antigens listed are the most commonly expressed in the given FAB subtype.

SOURCE: JM Bennett et al, Ann Intern Med 103:620, 1985; BD Cheson et al, J Clin Oncol 8:813, 1990.

AML

| Cytochemistry[a] | | Flow Cytometry[c] | Cytogenetic Association[d] |
Peroxidase/ Sudan Black	Nonspecific Esterase[b]		
−	−	CD13 or 33	
3% or more	−	CD13, 33, 34, HLA-DR +	
+	−	CD13, 15, 33, 34, HLA-DR +	t(8;21)(q22;q22)[e]
+	−	CD13, 15, 33, HLA-DR −	t(15;17) (q22;q11–12)
+/−	+	CD11b, 13, 14[f], 15, 33, HLA-DR +	M4Eo: inv(16) (pl3q22)
−	+	CD11b, 13, 14[f], 15, 33, HLA-DR +	11q23 translocations
+/−	−	CD33, HLA-DR +	
−	−	CD33,41	

[d] A subset of M2 and M5 demonstrate the listed cytogenetic abnormality.
[e] CD19 positivity is characteristically associated with t(8;21).
[f] CD14, if present, denotes monocytic lineage.

bleeding and DIC, especially during induction chemotherapy, because of the release of procoagulants from their cytoplasmic granules.

INCIDENCE AND ETIOLOGY About 7000 cases occur each year. AML accounts for about 80% of acute leukemias in adults. Etiology is unknown for the vast majority. Three environmental exposures increase the risk: chronic benzene exposure, radiation exposure, and prior treatment with alkylating agents and topoisomerase II inhibitors (e.g., doxorubicin and etoposide). Chronic myeloid leukemia, myelodysplasia, and myeloproliferative syndromes may all evolve into AML. Certain genetic abnormalities are associated with particular morphologic variants: t(15;17) with APL, inv(16) with eosinophilic leukemia; others occur in a number of types. Chromosome 11q23 abnormalities are often seen in leukemias developing after exposure to toposisomerase II inhibitors. The particular genetic abnormality has a strong influence on treatment outcome. Expression of MDR1 (multidrug resistance efflux pump) adversely affects prognosis.

CLINICAL AND LABORATORY FEATURES Initial symptoms of acute leukemia have usually been present for less than 3 months; a preleukemic syndrome may be present in some 25% of pts with AML. Signs of anemia, pallor, fatigue, weakness, palpitations, and dyspnea on exertion are most common. WBC may be low, normal, or markedly elevated; circulating blast cells may or may not be present; with WBC $>100 \times 10^9$ blasts per liter, leuko-stasis in lungs and brain may occur. Minor pyogenic infections of the skin are common. Thrombocytopenia leads to spontaneous bleeding, epistaxis, petechiae, conjunctival hemorrhage, gingival bleeding, bruising, especially with platelet count $<20 \times 10^9/L$. Anorexia and weight loss are common; fever may be present.

Bacterial and fungal infection are common; risk is heightened with total neutrophil count $<0.5 \times 10^9/L$, breakdown of mucosal and cutaneous barriers aggravates susceptibility; infections may be clinically occult in presence of severe leukopenia, and prompt recognition requires a high degree of clinical suspicion.

Hepatosplenomegaly occurs in about one-third of pts; leukemic meningitis may present with headache, nausea, seizures, papilledema, cranial nerve palsies.

Metabolic abnormalities may include hyponatremia, hypokalemia, elevated serum lactate dehydrogenase (LDH), hyperuricemia, and (rarely) lactic acidosis. With very high blast cell count in the blood, spurious hyperkalemia and hypoglycemia may occur.

℞ TREATMENT

Leukemic cell mass at time of presentation may be 10^{11}–10^{12} cells; when total leukemic cell numbers fall below approximately 10^9, they are no longer detectable in blood or bone marrow and pt appears to be in complete remission. Thus aggressive therapy must continue past the point when initial cell bulk is reduced if leukemia is to be eradicated. Typical phases of chemotherapy include remission induction, consolidation or early intensification, and maintenance with treatment lasting about 1 year.

Supportive care with transfusions of red cells and platelets (from CMV-seronegative donors, if pt is a candidate for bone marrow transplantation) is very important, as are aggressive prevention, diagnosis, and treatment of infections. Role of colony-stimulating factors is poorly defined. Febrile neutropenia should be treated with broad-spectrum antibiotics (e.g., ceftazidime 1 g q8h); if febrile neutropenia persists beyond 7 days, amphotericin B should be added.

60–80% of pts will achieve initial remission when treated with cytarabine (q12h for 3 d) and daunorubicin or idarubicin (daily for 7 d) followed by intensive consolidation and maintenance therapy; 10–30% of pts achieve 5-year disease-free survival and probable cure; duration of remission induced after relapse is short, and prognosis for pts who have relapsed is poor. In APL, addition of trans-retinoic acid (tretinoin) to chemotherapy induces differentiation of the leukemic cells and may improve outcome.

Bone marrow transplantation from identical twin or HLA-identical sibling is effective treatment for AML. Typical protocol uses high-dose chemotherapy ± total-body irradiation to ablate host marrow, followed by infusion of marrow from donor. Risks are substantial (unless marrow is from identical twin). Complications include graft-versus-host disease, interstitial pneumonitis, opportunistic infections (especially CMV). Up to 30% of otherwise end-stage pts with refractory leukemia achieve probable cure; results are better when transplant is performed during remission. Results are best for children and young adults.

CHRONIC MYELOID LEUKEMIA (CML)

CML is a clonal malignancy usually characterized by splenomegaly and production of increased numbers of granulocytes; course is initially indolent but eventuates in leukemic phase (blast crisis) that has a poorer prognosis than de novo AML; rate of progression to blast crisis is variable; overall survival averages 4 years from diagnosis.

INCIDENCE AND ETIOLOGY About 4000 cases occur each year. Over 90% of cases have a reciprocal translocation between chromosomes 9 and 22, creating the Philadelphia (Ph) chromosome and a fusion gene product called *bcr-abl* (*bcr* is from 9, *abl* from 22). The chromosome abnormality appears in all bone marrow–derived cells except T cells. The protein made by the chimeric gene is 210 kDa in chronic phase and 190 kDa in acute blast transformation. In some patients, the chronic phase is clinically silent and patients present with acute leukemia with the Ph chromosome.

CLINICAL AND LABORATORY FEATURES Symptoms develop gradually; easy fatigability, malaise, anorexia, abdominal discomfort and early satiety from the large spleen, excessive sweating. Occasional pts are found incidentally based upon elevated leukocyte count. WBC count is usually over 25 $\times$ $10^9/\mu L$ with granulocytes and their precursors back to the myelocyte stage; bands and mature forms predominate. Basophils may account for 10–15% of the cells in the blood. Platelet count is normal or increased. Anemia is often present. Neutrophil alkaline phosphatase score is low. Marrow is hypercellular with granulocytic hyperplasia. Marrow blast cell count is normal or slightly elevated. Serum levels of B_{12}, B_{12}-binding protein, and LDH are elevated in proportion to the WBC. With high blood counts, spurious hyperkalemia and hypoglycemia may be seen.

NATURAL HISTORY Chronic phase lasts 2–4 years. Accelerated phase is marked by anemia disproportionate to the disease activity or treatment. Platelet counts fall. Additional cytogenetic abnormalities appear. Blast cell counts increase. Usually within 6–8 months, overt blast crisis develops in which maturation ceases and blasts predominate. The clinical picture is that of acute leukemia. Half of the cases become AML, one-third have morphologic features of acute lymphocytic leukemia, 10% are erythroleukemia, and the rest are undifferentiated. Survival in blast crisis is often less than 4 months.

℞ **TREATMENT**
Chronic phase disease may be treated with interferon α (IFN) at 3 million units SC daily or tiw. The majority of pts obtain a hematologic response, and about 15% obtain cytogenetic remissions. Allopurinol, 300 mg/d, prevents urate nephropathy. The only curative therapy for the disease is HLA-matched allogeneic bone marrow transplantation. The optimal timing of transplantation is unclear, but transplantation in chronic phase is more effective than transplantation in accelerated

phase or blast crisis. Long-term disease-free survival may be obtained in 50–60% of pts. In pts without a matched donor, autologous transplantation may be helpful using peripheral blood stem cells. Treatment of pts in blast crisis is generally ineffective.

MYELODYSPLASTIC SYNDROMES (MDS)

These are clonal abnormalities of marrow cells characterized by varying degrees of cytopenias affecting one or more cell lines. These entities have been divided into five clinical syndromes (see Table 54-2). Other terms that have been used to describe one or more of the entities include *preleukemia* and *oligoblastic leukemia*.

INCIDENCE AND ETIOLOGY About 3000 cases occur each year, mainly in people over 50 years old. Like AML, exposure to benzene, radiation, and chemotherapeutic agents may lead to MDS. Chromosome abnormalities occur in up to 80% of cases, including deletion of part or all of chromosomes 5, 7, and 9 (20 or 21 less commonly) and addition of part or all of chromosome 8.

Table 54-2

French-American-British (FAB) Classification
of Myelodysplastic Syndromes

	FAB Types				
	RA	RARS	RAEB	CMML	RAEB-t
% Cases	28	24	23	16	9
% Blasts					
Marrow	<5	<5	5–20	1–20	20–30
Blood	<1	<1	<5	<5	>5
% Ringed Sideroblasts	<15	>15	<15	<15	<15
Monocytes	Rare	Rare	Rare	$>1 \times 10^9$/L	Variable
Dyspoiesis	+	+	+ +	+ +	+ +
% Leukemic transformation	11	5	23	20	2/8
Median survival, months	37	49	9	22	6

ABBREVIATIONS: RA, refractory anemia; RARS, refractory anemia with ringed sideroblasts; RAEB, refractory anemia with excess blasts; CMML, chronic myelomonocytic leukemia; RAEB-t, refractory anemia with excess blasts in transformation.

CLINICAL AND LABORATORY FEATURES Symptoms depend on the affected lineages. 85% of pts are anemic, 50% have neutropenia, and about one-third have thrombocytopenia. The pathologic features of MDS are a cellular marrow with varying degrees of cytologic atypia including delayed nuclear maturation, abnormal cytoplasmic maturation, accumulation of ringed sideroblasts (iron-laden mitochondria surrounding the nucleus), uni- or bilobed megakaryocytes, micromegakaryocytes, and increased myeloblasts. Table 54-2 lists features used to identify distinct entities.

℞ TREATMENT
Allogeneic bone marrow transplantation is the only curative therapy and may cure 60% of those so treated. However, the majority of pts with MDS are too old to receive transplantation. Chemotherapy has not clearly altered the natural history of disease. Patients with low erythropoietin levels may respond to erythropoietin, and a minority of pts with neutropenia respond to granulocyte colony stimulating factor. Supportive care is the cornerstone of treatment.

MYELOPROLIFERATIVE SYNDROMES

The three major myeloproliferative syndromes are polycythemia vera, idiopathic myelofibrosis, and essential thrombocytosis. All are clonal disorders of hematopoietic stem cells.

Polycythemia Vera

The most common myeloproliferative syndrome, this is characterized by an increase in RBC mass, massive splenomegaly, and clinical manifestations related to increased blood viscosity, including neurologic symptoms (vertigo, tinnitus, headache, visual disturbances) and thromboses (myocardial infarction, stroke, peripheral vascular disease; uncommonly, mesenteric and hepatic). It must be distinguished from other causes of increased RBC mass. This is most readily done by assaying serum erythropoietin levels. Polycythemia vera is associated with very low erythropoietin levels; in other causes of erythrocytosis, erythropoietin levels are high. Patients are effectively managed with phlebotomy. Some pts require splenectomy to control symptoms, and those with severe pruritus may benefit from psoralens and UV light. 20% develop myelofibrosis, <5% acute leukemia.

Idiopathic Myelofibrosis

This rare entity is characterized by marrow fibrosis, myeloid metaplasia with extramedullary hematopoiesis, and splenomegaly. Evaluation of a blood smear reveals tear-drop shaped RBC, nucleated RBC, and some early granulocytic forms including promyelocytes. However, many entities may lead to marrow fibrosis and extramedullary hematopoiesis, and the diagnosis of primary idiopathic myelofibrosis is made only when the many other potential causes are ruled out. The following diseases are in the differential diagnosis: CML, polycythemia vera, Hodgkin's disease, cancer metastatic to the marrow (especially from breast and prostate), infection (particularly granulomatous infections), and hairy cell leukemia. Supportive therapy is generally used; no specific therapy is known.

Essential Thrombocytosis

This is usually noted incidentally upon routine platelet count done in an asymptomatic person. Like myelofibrosis, many conditions can produce elevated platelet counts; thus, the diagnosis is one of exclusion. Platelet count must be >500,000/μL, and known causes of thrombocytosis must be ruled out including CML, iron deficiency, splenectomy, malignancy, infection, hemorrhage, polycythemia vera, myelodysplasia, and recovery from vitamin B_{12} deficiency. Although usually asymptomatic, pts should be treated if they develop migraine headache, transient ischemic attack, or other bleeding or thrombotic disease manifestations. Interferon α is effective therapy, as is oral hydroxyurea. Treatment should not be given just because the absolute platelet count is high in the absence of other symptoms.

For a more detailed discussion, see Castro-Malaspina H, O'Reilly RJ: Aplastic Anemia and Myelodysplasia, Chap. 110, p. 672; Spivak JL: Polycythemia Vera and Other Myeloproliferative Diseases, Chap. 111, p. 679; and Wetzler M, Bloomfield CD: Acute and Chronic Myeloid Leukemia, Chap. 112, p. 684, in HPIM-14.

55

LYMPHOID MALIGNANCIES

DEFINITION Neoplasms of lymphocytes usually represent malignant counterparts of cells at discrete stages of normal lymphocyte differentiation. When bone marrow and peripheral blood involvement dominate the clinical picture, the disease is classified as a *lymphoid leukemia*. When lymph nodes and/or other extranodal sites of disease are the dominant site(s) of involvement, the tumor is called a *lymphoma*. The distinction between lymphoma and leukemia is sometimes blurred; for example, small lymphocytic lymphoma and chronic lymphocytic leukemia are tumors of the same cell type and are distinguished arbitrarily on the basis of the absolute number of peripheral blood lymphocytes ($>5 \times 10^9$/L defines leukemia).

CLASSIFICATION Historically, lymphoid tumors have had separate pathologic classifications based on the clinical syndrome—lymphomas according to the Rappaport, Kiel, or Working Formulation systems, acute leukemias according to the French-American-British (FAB) system, Hodgkin's disease according to the Rye classification. Myelomas have generally not been subclassified by pathologic features of the neoplastic cells. Recently, the International Lymphoma Study Group has proposed a unifying classification system (revised European-American, or REAL, classification) that brings together all lymphoid neoplasms into a single framework. Although the new system codifies and standardizes the definitions of disease entities based upon histology, genetic abnormalities, and cell surface immunophenotype, its organization is based upon cell of origin (B cell vs. T cell) and maturation stage (precursor vs. mature) of the tumor, features that are of limited value to the clinician. Table 55-1 lists the disease entities according to a more clinically useful schema based upon the clinical manifestations and natural history of the diseases.

INCIDENCE Lymphoid tumors are increasing in incidence. Over 80,000 cases were diagnosed in 1997.

ETIOLOGY The cause(s) for the vast majority of lymphoid neoplasms is unknown. Like other cancers, the malignant cells are monoclonal and often contain numerous genetic abnormalities. Some genetic alterations are characteristic of particular histologic entities: t(8;14) in Burkitt's lymphoma, t(14;18) in follicular lymphoma, t(11;14) in mantle cell lymphoma, t(2;5) in anaplastic large cell lymphoma, translocations or mutations involving *bcl*-6 on 3q27 in diffuse large cell lymphoma, and others. In most cases, translocations involve insertion of a distant

Table 55-1

Clinical Schema of Lymphoid Neoplasms

Chronic lymphoid leukemias/lymphomas
    Chronic lymphocytic leukemia/small lymphocytic lymphoma (99% B cell, 1% T cell)
    Prolymphocytic leukemia (90% B cell, 10% T cell)
    Large granular lymphocyte leukemia (80% NK cell, 20% T cell)
    Hairy cell leukemia (99–100% B cell)
Indolent lymphoma
    Follicular center cell lymphoma, grades I and II (100% B cell)
    Lymphoplasmacytic lymphoma/Waldenström's macroglobulinemia (100% B cell)
    Marginal zone lymphoma (100% B cell)
        Extranodal [mucosa-associated lymphatic tissue (MALT) lymphoma]
        Nodal (monocytoid B cell lymphoma)
        Splenic marginal zone lymphoma
    Cutaneous T cell lymphoma (mycosis fungoides) (100% T cell)
Aggressive lymphoma
    Diffuse large cell lymphoma (85% B cell, 15% T cell), includes immunoblastic
    Follicular center cell lymphoma, grade III (100% B cell)
    Mantle cell lymphoma (100% B cell)
    Primary mediastinal (thymic) large B cell lymphoma (100% B cell)
    Burkitt-like lymphoma (100% B cell)
    Peripheral T cell lymphoma (100% T cell)
    Angioimmunoblastic lymphoma (100% T cell)
    Angiocentric lymphoma (80% T cell, 20% NK cell)
    Intestinal T cell lymphoma (100% T cell)
    Anaplastic large cell lymphoma (70% T cell, 30% null cell)
Acute lymphoid leukemias/lymphomas
    Precursor lymphoblastic leukemia/lymphoma (80% T cell, 20% B cell)
    Burkitt's leukemia/lymphoma (100% B cell)
    Adult T cell leukemia/lymphoma (100% T cell)
Plasma cell disorders (100% B cell)
    Monoclonal gammopathy of uncertain significance
    Solitary plasmacytoma
    Extramedullary plasmacytoma

(continued)

Table 55-1 (*Continued*)

Clinical Schema of Lymphoid Neoplasms

Multiple myeloma
Plasma cell leukemia
Hodgkin's disease (cell of origin uncertain and seemingly
heterogeneous)
  Lymphocyte predominant
  Nodular sclerosis
  Mixed cellularity
  Lymphocyte depleted

chromosome segment into the antigen receptor genes (either immunoglobulin or T cell receptor) during the rearrangement of the gene segments that form the receptors.

Two viruses, Epstein-Barr virus (a herpes family virus) and human T-lymphotropic virus type I (HTLV-I, a retrovirus) may cause some lymphoid tumors. EBV has been strongly associated with African Burkitt's lymphoma and the lymphomas that complicate immunodeficiencies (disease-related or iatrogenic). EBV has an uncertain relationship to mixed cellularity Hodgkin's disease and angiocentric lymphoma. HTLV-I is associated with adult T cell leukemia/lymphoma. Both the virus and the disease are endemic to southwestern Japan and the Caribbean. Gastric *Helicobacter pylori* infection is associated with gastric MALT lymphoma and perhaps gastric large cell lymphoma. Eradication of the infection produces durable remissions in about half of patients with gastric MALT lymphoma.

Inherited or acquired immunodeficiencies and autoimmune disorders predispose people to lymphoma. Lymphoma occurs with increased incidence in farmers and meat workers; Hodgkin's disease is increased in wood workers.

DIAGNOSIS AND STAGING   Excisional biopsy is the standard; adequate tissue must be obtained. Tissue undergoes three kinds of studies: (1) light microscopy to discern the pattern of growth and the morphologic features of the malignant cells, (2) flow cytometry for assessment of immunophenotype, and (3) genetic studies (cytogenetics, DNA extraction). Needle aspirates of nodal or extranodal masses are not adequate diagnostic procedures. Leukemia diagnosis and lymphoma staging include generous bilateral iliac crest bone marrow biopsies. Differential diagnosis of adenopathy is reviewed in Chap. 26.

Staging varies with the diagnosis. In Hodgkin's disease, defining the anatomic extent of disease is essential to define the optimal treatment approach. In acute leukemia, peripheral blood blast counts are most significant in assessing prognosis. In chronic leukemia, peripheral blood red blood cell and platelet counts are most significant in assessing prognosis. In indolent lymphoma, which is usually widespread at diagnosis, and in aggressive lymphoma, age, stage, lactate dehydrogenase (LDH) level, number of extranodal sites, and Karnofsky index predict outcome. In myeloma, serum levels of paraprotein, creatinine, and β_2-microglobulin predict survival.

CHRONIC LYMPHOID LEUKEMIAS/ LYMPHOMAS

Most of these entities have a natural history measured in years (prolymphocytic leukemia is very rare and can be very aggressive). Chronic lymphocytic leukemia is the most common entity in this group and the most common leukemia in the western world.

CHRONIC LYMPHOCYTIC LEUKEMIA (CLL) Usually presents as asymptomatic lymphocytosis in patients over age 60 years. The malignant cell is a CD5+ B cell that looks like a normal small lymphocyte. Trisomy 12 is the most common genetic abnormality. Prognosis is related to stage; stage is determined mainly by the degree to which the tumor cells crowd out normal hematopoietic elements from the marrow (see Table 55-2). Cells may infiltrate nodes and spleen as well as marrow. Nodal involvement may be related to the expression of an adhesion molecule that allows the cells to remain in the node rather than recirculate. Pts often have hypogammaglobulinemia. Up to 20% have autoimmune antibodies that may produce autoimmune hemolytic anemia, thrombocytopenia, or red cell aplasia. Death is from infection, marrow failure, or intercurrent illnesses. In 5%, the disease evolves to aggressive lymphoma (Richter's syndrome) that is refractory to treatment.

℞ **TREATMENT**

Supportive care is generally given until anemia or thrombocytopenia develop. At that time, tests are indicated to assess the cause of the anemia or thrombocytopenia. Decreased red blood cell and/or platelet counts related to peripheral destruction may be treated with splenectomy or glucocorticoids without cytotoxic therapy in many cases. If marrow replacement is the mechanism, cytotoxic therapy is indicated. Fludarabine 25 (mg/m^2)/d IV $\times$ 5 days every 4 weeks induces responses in about 75% of pts, complete responses in half. Glucocorticoids increase the risk of infection without adding a substan-

Table 55-2

Staging of B Cell CLL and Relation to Survival

Stage	Clinical Features	Median Survival, Years
RAI		
0	Lymphocytosis	12
I	Lymphocytosis + adenopathy	9
II	Lymphocytosis + splenomegaly	7
III	Anemia	1–2
IV	Thrombocytopenia	1–2
BINET		
A	No anemia/thrombocytopenia, <3 involved sites	>10
B	No anemia/thrombocytopenia, >3 involved sites	5
C	Anemia and/or thrombocytopenia	2

tial antitumor benefit. Monthly IV immunoglobulin significantly reduces risk of serious infection, but is expensive. Alkylating agents are also active against the tumor. Therapeutic intent is palliative in most pts. Young pts may be candidates for high-dose therapy and autologous or allogeneic hematopoietic cell transplantation; long-term disease-free survival has been noted.

See Chap. 113 in HPIM-14 for discussion of the rarer entities.

INDOLENT LYMPHOMAS

These entities have a natural history measured in years. Median survival is about 10 years. Follicular center lymphoma is the most common indolent lymphoma accounting for about one-third of all lymphoid malignancies.

FOLLICULAR CENTER LYMPHOMA Usually present with painless peripheral lymphadenopathy, often involving several nodal regions. "B symptoms" (fever, sweats, weight loss) occur in 10%, less common than with Hodgkin's disease. In about 25%, nodes wax and wane before the pt seeks medical attention. Median age is 55 years. Disease is widespread at diagnosis in 85%. Liver and bone marrow are commonly involved extranodal sites.

The tumor has a follicular growth pattern reflecting the follicular center origin of the malignant cell. The t(14;18) is present in 85% of cases, resulting in the overexpression of bcl-2 , a protein involved in prevention of programmed cell death. The normal follicular center B cell is undergoing active mutation of the immunoglobulin variable regions in an effort to generate antibody of higher affinity for the selecting antigen. Follicular center lymphoma cells also have a high rate of mutation that leads to the accumulation of genetic damage. Over time, follicular center lymphomas acquire sufficient genetic damage (e.g., mutated p53) to accelerate their growth and evolve into diffuse large cell lymphomas that are refractory to treatment. The majority of pts dying from follicular lymphoma have undergone histologic transformation.

℞ TREATMENT

Only 15% of pts have localized disease, but the majority of these pts are curable with radiation therapy. Although many forms of treatment induce tumor regression in advanced-stage pts, it is not clear that treatment of any kind alters the natural history of disease. No therapy, single-agent alkylators, nucleoside analogues (fludarabine, cladribine), combination chemotherapy, radiation therapy, and biologic agents (interferon-α, monoclonal antibodies) are all considered appropriate. Over 90% of pts are responsive to treatment; complete responses are seen in about half of pts treated aggressively. Younger pts are being treated experimentally with high-dose therapy and autologous hematopoietic stem cells. It is not yet clear whether this is curative. There is some evidence that combination chemotherapy with or without interferon maintenance may prolong survival and delay or prevent histologic progression.

See Chap. 113 in HPIM-14 for discussion of the other indolent lymphomas.

AGGRESSIVE LYMPHOMAS

A large number of pathologic entities share an aggressive natural history; survival untreated is 6–8 months, and nearly all untreated pts are dead within 1 year. Pts may present with asymptomatic adenopathy or symptoms referable to involvement of practically any nodal or extranodal site: mediastinal involvement may produce superior vena cava syndrome or pericardial tamponade; retroperitoneal nodes may obstruct ureters, abdominal masses may produce pain, ascites, or GI obstruction or perforation; CNS involvement may produce confusion, cranial nerve signs, headache, seizures, and/or spinal cord compression; bone involvement may produce pain or pathologic fracture. About 45% of pts have B symptoms.

Diffuse large cell lymphoma is the most common histologic diagnosis among the aggressive lymphomas, accounting for about 25% of all lymphomas. Aggressive lymphomas together account for about 55% of all lymphoid tumors. About 85% of aggressive lymphomas are of mature B cell origin; 15% are derived from peripheral (postthymic) T cells.

--- *Approach to the Patient* ---

Early diagnostic biospy is critical. Pt workup is directed by symptoms and known patterns of disease. Pts with Waldeyer's ring involvement should undergo careful evaluation of the GI tract. Pts with bone or bone marrow involvement should have a lumbar puncture to evaluate meningeal CNS involvement.

R_x TREATMENT

Localized aggressive lymphomas are usually treated with 4 cycles of CHOP (cyclophosphamide, doxorubicin, vincristine, prednisone) combination chemotherapy followed by involved-field radiation therapy. About 85% of these pts are cured. The specific therapy used for pts with more advanced disease is controversial. Treatment outcome with CHOP is influenced by tumor bulk (usually measured by LDH levels, stage, and number of extranodal sites) and physiologic reserve (usually measured by age and Karnofsky status). The influence of these factors on outcome is shown in Table 55-3. In most series, CHOP cures about one-third of pts. Some investigators have demonstrated cure rates about twice those achieved by CHOP using more aggressive combination chemotherapy regimens that do not require hematopoietic stem cell support. Furthermore, the use of a sequential high-dose chemotherapy regimen in pts with high-intermediate- and high-risk disease has yielded long-term survival in about 75% of pts.

About 30–45% of pts not cured with initial standard combination chemotherapy may be salvaged with high-dose therapy and autologous hematopoietic stem cell transplantation.

Specialized approaches are required for lymphomas involving certain sites (e.g., CNS, stomach) or under certain complicating clinical circumstances (e.g., concurrent illness, AIDS). Lymphomas occuring in iatrogenically immunosuppressed people may regress when immunosuppressive medication is withheld. Lymphomas occurring postallogeneic

Table 55-3

The International Index and Prognosis in Diffuse Aggressive Non-Hodgkin's Lymphoma

Risk Group (Patients of All Ages)	Risk Factors*	Distribution of Cases, %	Complete Response Rate, %	5-Year Survival Rate, %
Low	0, 1	35	87	73
Low-intermediate	2	27	67	51
High-intermediate	3	22	55	43
High	4, 5	16	44	26

*Age ($\leq$60 vs. >60); serum LDH (normal vs. >1 $\times$ normal); performance status (0 or 1 vs. 2–4) stage (I or II vs. III or IV); and extranodal involvement ($\geq$1 site vs. >1 site)

SOURCE: Adapted from Shipp.

marrow transplant may regress with infusions of donor leukocytes.

Pts with rapidly growing bulky aggressive lymphoma may experience tumor lysis syndrome when treated (see Chap. 36); prophylactic measures (hydration, urine alkalinization, allopurinol) may be lifesaving.

ACUTE LYMPHOID LEUKEMIAS/ LYMPHOMAS

ACUTE LYMPHOBLASTIC LEUKEMIA AND LYMPHOBLASTIC LYMPHOMA These are more common in children than adults. The majority of cases have tumor cells that appear to be of thymic origin, and pts may have mediastinal masses. Pts usually present with recent onset of signs of marrow failure (pallor, fatigue, bleeding, fever, infection). Hepatosplenomegaly and adenopathy are common. Males may have testicular enlargement reflecting leukemic involvement. Meningeal involvement may be present at diagnosis or develop later. Elevated LDH, hyponatremia, and hypokalemia may be present, in addition to anemia, thrombocytopenia, and high peripheral blood blast counts. The leukemic cells are more often FAB L2 in type in adults than in children, where L1 predominates. Leukemia diagnosis requires at least 30% lymphoblasts in the marrow. Prognosis is adversely affected by high presenting white count, age over 35 years, and the presence of t(9;22), t(1;19), and t(4;11) translocations.

TREATMENT

Successful treatment requires intensive induction phase, CNS prophylaxis, and maintenance chemotherapy that extends for about 2 years. Vincristine, L-asparaginase, cytarabine, daunorubicin, and prednisone are particularly effective agents. Intrathecal or high-dose systemic methotrexate is effective CNS prophylaxis. Long-term survival of 60–65% of pts may be achieved. The role and timing of bone marrow transplantation in primary therapy is debated, but up to 30% of relapsed pts may be cured with salvage transplantation.

BURKITT'S LYMPHOMA/LEUKEMIA   This is also more common in children. It is associated with translocations involving the c-*myc* gene on chromosome 8 rearranging with immunoglobulin heavy or light chain genes. Pts often have disseminated disease with large abdominal masses, hepatomegaly, and adenopathy. If a leukemic picture predominates, it is classified as FAB L3.

TREATMENT

Resection of large abdominal masses improves treatment outcome. Aggressive leukemia regimens that include vincristine, cyclophosphamide, 6-mercaptopurine, doxorubicin, and prednisone are active. Cure may be achieved in 50–60%. The need for maintenance therapy is unclear. Prophylaxis against tumor lysis syndrome is important (Chap. 36).

ADULT T-CELL LEUKEMIA/LYMPHOMA (ATL)   This is very rare, and only a small fraction of persons infected with HTLV-I go on to develop the disease. Some HTLV-I-infected pts develop spastic paraplegia from spinal cord involvement without developing cancer. The characteristic clinical syndrome of ATL includes high white count without severe anemia or thrombocytopenia, skin infiltration, hepatomegaly, pulmonary infiltrates, meningeal involvement, and opportunistic infections. The tumor cells are CD4+ T cells with cloven hoof–shaped nuclei. Hypercalcemia occurs in nearly all pts and is related to cytokines produced by the tumor cells.

TREATMENT

Aggressive therapy is associated with serious toxicity related to the underlying immunodeficiency. Glucocorticoids relieve hypercalcemia. The tumor is responsive to therapy, but responses are generally short-lived. Zidovudine and interferon may be palliative in some pts.

PLASMA CELL DISORDERS

The hallmark of plasma cell disorders is the production of immunoglobulin molecules or fragments from abnormal plasma cells. The intact immunoglobulin molecule, or the heavy chain or light chain produced by the abnormal plasma cell clone, is detectable in the serum and/or urine and is called the M (for monoclonal) component. The amount of the M component in any given pt reflects the tumor burden in that pt. In some, the presence of a clonal light chain in the urine (Bence Jones protein) is the only tumor product that is detectable. M components may be seen in pts with other lymphoid tumors, nonlymphoid cancers, and noncancerous conditions such as cirrhosis, sarcoidosis, parasitic infestations, and autoimmune diseases.

MULTIPLE MYELOMA A malignant proliferation of plasma cells in the bone marrow (notably not in lymph nodes). About 14,000 new cases are diagnosed each year. Disease manifestations result from tumor expansion, local and remote actions of tumor products, and the host response to the tumor. About 70% of pts have bone pain, usually involving the back and ribs, precipitated by movement. Bone lesions are multiple, lytic, and rarely accompanied by an osteoblastic response. Thus, bone scans are less useful than radiographs. The production of osteoclast-activating cytokines by tumor cells leads to substantial calcium mobilization, hypercalcemia, and symptoms related to it. Decreased synthesis and increased catabolism of normal immunoglobulins leads to hypogammaglobulinemia, and a poorly defined tumor product inhibits granulocyte migration. These changes create a susceptibility to bacterial infections, especially the pneumococcus, *Klebsiella pneumoniae,* and *Staphylococcus aureus* affecting the lung and *Escherichia coli* and other gram-negative pathogens affecting the urinary tract. Infections affect at least 75% of pts at some time in their course. Renal failure may affect 25% of pts; its pathogenesis is multifactorial—hypercalcemia, infection, toxic effects of light chains, urate nephropathy, dehydration. Neurologic symptoms may result from hyperviscosity, cryoglobulins, and rarely amyloid deposition in nerves. Anemia occurs in 80% related to myelophthisis and inhibition of erythropoiesis by tumor products. Clotting abnormalities may produce bleeding.

Diagnosis Marrow plasmacytosis >10%, lytic bone lesions, and a serum and/or urine M component are the classic triad. Monoclonal gammopathy of uncertain significance (MGUS) is much more common than myeloma; in general, MGUS is associated with a level of M component <20 g/L, low serum β_2-microglobulin, <10% marrow plasma cells, and no bone lesions. Lifetime risk of progression of MGUS to myeloma is about 11%.

Staging Disease stage influences survival (see Table 55-4).

℞ **TREATMENT**

About 10% of pts have very slowly progressive disease and do not require treatment until the paraprotein levels rise above 50 g/L or progressive bone disease occurs. Pts with solitary plasmacytoma and extramedullary plasmacytoma are usually cured with localized radiation therapy. Supportive care includes early treatment of infections; control of hypercalcemia with glucocorticoids, hydration, and natriuresis; chronic administration of bisphosphonates to antagonize skeletal destruction; and prophylaxis against urate nephropathy and dehydration. Therapy aimed at the tumor is usually palliative: melphalan 8 mg/m^2 orally for 4–7 days every 4–6 weeks plus prednisone. About 60% of pts have significant symptomatic improvement plus a 75% decline in the M component. Experimental approaches using sequential high-dose pulses of melphalan plus two successive autologous stem cell transplants have produced complete responses in about 50% of pts under the age of 65 years. Long-term follow-up is required to see whether survival is enhanced. Palliatively treated pts generally follow a chronic course for 2–5 years, followed by an acceleration characterized by organ infiltration with myeloma cells and marrow failure.

HODGKIN'S DISEASE

About 8000 new cases are diagnosed each year. Hodgkin's disease (HD) is a tumor of Reed-Sternberg cells, aneuploid cells of uncertain origin that usually express CD30 and CD15 but may also express other B or T cell markers. Most of the cells in an enlarged node are normal lymphoid, plasma cells, monocytes, and eosinophils. The etiology is unknown, but the incidence in both identical twins is 99-fold increased over the expected concordance, suggesting a genetic susceptibility. Distribution of histologic subtypes is 75% nodular sclerosis, 20% mixed cellularity, with lymphocyte predominant and lymphocyte depleted representing about 5%.

Clinical Manifestations Usually presents with asymptomatic lymph node enlargement or with adenopathy associated with fever, night sweats, weight loss, and sometimes pruritus. Mediastinal adenopathy (common in nodular sclerosing HD)

Table 55-4

Myeloma Staging System

Stage	Criteria	Estimated Tumor Burden, $\times 10^{12}$ cells/m^2

I	All the following:
	1. Hemoglobin >100 g/L (>10 g/dL)
	2. Serum calcium <3 mmol/L (<12 mg/dL)
	3. Normal bone x-ray or solitary lesion
	4. Low M-component production
	  a. IgG level <50 g/L (<5 g/dL)
	  b. IgA level <30 g/L (<3 g/dL)
	  c. Urine light chain <4 g/24 h
		<0.6 (low)

II	Fitting neither I nor III	0.6–1.20 (intermediate)

III	One or more of the following:
	1. Hemoglobin <85 g/L (<8.5 g/dL)
	2. Serum calcium >3 mmol/L (>12 mg/dL)
	3. Advanced lytic bone lesions
	4. High M-component production
	  a. IgG level >70 g/L (>7 g/dL)
	  b. IgA level >50 g/L (>5 g/dL)
	  c. Urine light chains >12 g/24 h
		>1.20 (high)

SUBCLASSIFICATION BASED ON SERUM CREATININE LEVELS

Level	Stage	Median Survival, Months
A < 177 μmol/L (≤2 mg/dL) B > 177 μmol/L (>2 mg/dL)	IA IIA, B IIIA IIIB	61 55 30 15

(*continued*)

Table 55-4 (*Continued*)

Myeloma Staging System

STAGING BASED ON SERUM β_2-MICROGLOBULIN LEVELS

Level	Stage	Median Survival, Months
<0.004 g/L ($\leq$4 μg/mL)	I	43
>0.004 g/L (>4 μg/mL)	II	12

may produce cough. Spread of disease tends to be to contiguous lymph node groups. SVC obstruction or spinal cord compression may be presenting manifestation. Involvement of bone marrow and liver is rare.

Differential Diagnosis

- Infection—mononucleosis, viral syndromes, toxoplasma, histoplasma, primary tuberculosis.
- Other malignancies—especially head and neck cancers.
- Sarcoidosis—mediastinal and hilar adenopathy.

Immunologic and Hematologic Abnormalities

- Defects in cell-mediated immunity (remains even after successful treatment of lymphoma); cutaneous anergy; diminished antibody production to capsular antigens of *Haemophilus* and pneumococcus.
- Anemia; elevated ESR; leukemoid reaction; eosinophilia; lymphocytopenia; fibrosis and granulomas in marrow.

Staging The Ann Arbor staging classification is shown in Table 55-5. It is important to determine extent of disease to guide choice of treatment; physical exam, CXR, thoracoabdominal CT, bone marrow biopsy; ultrasound examinations, lymphangiogram. Staging laparotomy should be used, especially to evaluate the spleen, if pt has early-stage disease and radiation therapy is being contemplated.

℞ TREATMENT

About 85% of pts are curable. Therapy should be performed by experienced clinicians in centers with appropriate facilities. Pts with stages I and II disease documented by negative laparotomy are treated with subtotal nodal radiation therapy. Those with stage III or IV disease receive six cycles of combi-

Table 55-5

Ann Arbor Staging System

Stage I	Involvement in single lymph node region or single extralymphatic site
Stage II	Involvement of two or more lymph node regions on the same side of diaphragm
	Localized contiguous involvement of only one extralymphatic site and lymph node region (stage IIE)
Stage III	Involvement of lymph node regions on both sides of diaphragm; may include spleen
Stage IV	Disseminated involvement of one or more extralymphatic organs with or without lymph node involvement

nation chemotherapy, usually either ABVD or MOPP-ABV hybrid therapy or MOPP/ABVD alternating therapy. Pts with any stage disease accompanied by a large mediastinal mass (>1/3 the greatest chest diameter) should receive combined modality therapy with MOPP/ABVD or MOPP-ABV hybrid followed by mantle field radiation therapy (radiation plus ABVD is too toxic to the lung). About two-thirds of pts not cured by their initial radiation therapy treatment are rescued by salvage combination chemotherapy. About two-thirds of pts not cured by their initial chemotherapy regimen may be rescued by high-dose therapy and autologous stem cell transplant.

With long-term follow-up, it has become clear that more pts are dying of late fatal toxicities related to radiation therapy (myocardial infarction, second cancers) than from HD. It may be possible to avoid radiation exposure by using combination chemotherapy in early-stage disease as well as in advanced-stage disease.

For a more detailed discussion, see Freedman AS, Nadler LM: Malignancies of Lymphoid Cells , Chap. 113, p. 695; and Longo DL: Plasma Cell Disorders, Chap. 114, p. 712, in HPIM-14.

56

SKIN CANCER

MALIGNANT MELANOMA

Most dangerous cutaneous malignancy; high metastatic potential; poor prognosis with metastatic spread.

Incidence

Melanoma is diagnosed in 38,300 people annually in the United States and causes 7,300 deaths.

Predisposing Factors

Fair complexion, sun exposure, family history of melanoma, dysplastic nevus syndrome (autosomal dominant disorder with multiple nevi of distinctive appearance and cutaneous melanoma, may be associated with 9p deletion), and presence of a giant congenital nevus. Blacks have a low incidence.

Types

1. *Superficial spreading melanoma:* Most common; begins with initial radial growth phase prior to invasion.
2. *Lentigo maligna melanoma:* Very long radial growth phase prior to invasion, lentigo maligna (Hutchinson's melanotic freckle) is precursor lesion, most common in elderly and in sun-exposed areas (esp. face).
3. *Acral lentiginous:* Most common form in darkly pigmented pts; occurs on palms and soles, mucosal surfaces, in nail beds and mucocutaneous junctions; similar to lentigo maligna melanoma but with more aggressive biologic behavior.
4. *Nodular:* Generally poor prognosis because of invasive growth from onset.

Clinical Appearance

Generally pigmented (rarely amelanotic); color of lesions varies, but red, white, and/or blue are common, in addition to brown and/or black. Suspicion should be raised by a pigmented skin lesion that is >6 mm in diameter, asymmetric, has an irregular surface or border, or has variation in color.

Prognosis

Best with thin lesions without evidence of metastatic spread; with increasing thickness or evidence of spread, prognosis worsens. Stage I and II (primary tumor without spread) have 85% 5-year survival. Stage III (palpable regional nodes with tumor) has a 50% 5-year survival when only one node is involved and 15–20% when 4 or more are involved. Stage IV (disseminated disease) has <5% 5-year survival.

℞ TREATMENT

Early recognition and wide local excision for localized disease is best; elective lymph node dissection is controversial, may be useful in a subset. Pts with stage III disease have improved survival with adjuvant interferon α (IFNα), 20 million units IV daily ×5 for 4 weeks, then 10 million units SC tiw for 11 months. Metastatic disease may be treated with chemotherapy or immunotherapy. Dacarbazine (250 mg/m^2 IV daily ×5 q3w) plus tamoxifen (20 mg/m^2 PO daily) may induce partial responses in 1/3 of patients. IFNα and interleukin 2 (IL-2) at maximum tolerated doses induce partial responses in 15% of pts. Rare long remissions occur with IL-2. No therapy for metastatic disease is curative.

BASAL CELL CARCINOMA

Most common form of skin cancer; most frequently on sun-exposed skin, esp. face.

Predisposing Factors

Fair complexion, chronic UV exposure, exposure to inorganic arsenic (i.e., Fowler's solution or insecticides such as Paris green), or exposure to ionizing radiation.

Types

Five general types: *noduloulcerative* (most common), *superficial* (mimics eczema), *pigmented* (may be mistaken for melanoma), *morpheaform* (plaquelike lesion with telangiectasia—with keratotic is most aggressive), *keratotic* (basosquamous carcinoma).

Clinical Appearance

Classically a pearly, translucent, smooth papule with rolled edges and surface telangiectasia.

℞ TREATMENT

Local removal with electrodesiccation and curettage, excision, cryosurgery, or radiation therapy; metastases are rare but may spread locally. Exceedingly unusual for BCC to cause death.

SQUAMOUS CELL CARCINOMA

Less common than basal cell but more likely to metastasize.

Predisposing Factors

Fair complexion, chronic UV exposure, previous burn or other scar (i.e., scar carcinoma), exposure to inorganic arsenic or ionizing radiation. Actinic keratosis is a premalignant lesion.

General Types

Most commonly occurs as an ulcerated nodule or a superficial erosion on the skin. Variants include:

1. *Bowen's disease:* Erythematous patch or plaque, often with scale; noninvasive; involvement limited to epidermis and epidermal appendages (i.e. SCC in situ).

2. *Scar carcinoma:* Suggested by sudden change in previously stable scar, esp. if ulceration or nodules appear.

3. *Verrucous carcinoma:* Most commonly on plantar aspect of foot; low-grade malignancy but may be mistaken for a common wart.

Clinical Appearance

Hyperkeratotic papule or nodule or erosion; nodule may be ulcerated.

℞ TREATMENT

Local excision and Moh's micrographic surgery are most common; radiation therapy in selected cases. Metastatic disease may be treated with radiation therapy or with combination biologic therapy; 13-*cis*-retinoic acid 1 mg/d PO plus IFNα 3 million units/d SC.

Prognosis

Favorable if secondary to UV exposure; less favorable if in sun-protected areas or associated with ionizing radiation.

SKIN CANCER PREVENTION

Most skin cancer is related to sun exposure. Encourage patients to avoid the sun and use sunscreen.

KAPOSI'S SARCOMA (See Chap. 78).

For a more detailed discussion, see Sober AJ, et al: Melanoma and Other Skin Cancers, Chap. 88, p. 543, in HPIM-14.

HEAD AND NECK CANCER

Epithelial cancers may arise from the mucosal surfaces of the head and neck including the sinuses, oral cavity, nasopharynx, oropharynx, hypopharynx, and larynx. These tumors are usually squamous cell cancers. Thyroid cancer is discussed in Chap. 162.

Incidence and Epidemiology

About 40,000 cases are diagnosed each year. Oral cavity, oropharynx, and larynx are the most frequent sites of primary lesions in the United States; nasopharyngeal primaries are more common in the Far East and Mediterranean countries. Alcohol and tobacco (including smokeless) abuse are risk factors.

Pathology

Nasopharyngeal cancer in the Far East has a distinct histology, nonkeratinizing undifferentiated carcinoma with infiltrating lymphocytes called *lymphoepithelioma*, and a distinct etiology, Epstein-Barr virus. Squamous cell head and neck cancer may develop from premalignant lesions (erythroplakia, leukoplakia), and the histologic grade affects prognosis. Pts who have survived head and neck cancer commonly develop a second cancer of the head and neck, lung, or esophagus, presumably reflecting the exposure of the upper aerodigestive mucosa to similar carcinogenic stimuli.

Genetic Alterations

Chromosomal deletions and mutations have been found in chromosomes 3p, 9p, 17p, 11q, and 13q; mutations in p53 have been reported. Cyclin D1 may be overexpressed.

Clinical Presentation

Most occur in people older than 50 years. Symptoms vary with the primary site. Nasopharynx lesions do not usually cause symptoms until late in the course and then cause unilateral serous otitis media or nasal obstruction or epistaxis. Oral cavity cancers present as nonhealing ulcers, sometimes painful. Oropharyngeal lesions also present late with sore throat or otalgia. Hoarseness may be an early sign of laryngeal cancer. Rare pts present with painless, rock-hard cervical or supraclavicular lymph node enlargement. Staging is based upon size of primary tumor and involvement of lymph nodes. Distant metastases occur in fewer than 10% of pts.

℞ TREATMENT

Three categories of disease are common: localized, locally or regionally advanced, and recurrent or metastatic. *Local disease* is treated with curative intent by surgery or radiation therapy. Radiation therapy is preferred for localized larynx cancer to preserve organ function; surgery is used more commonly for oral cavity lesions. *Locally advanced disease* is the most common presentation. Surgery followed by radiation therapy is standard; however, the disease is responsive to chemotherapy, and the use of three cycles of cisplatin (100 mg/m^2 IV day 1) plus 5-fluorouracil [1000 (mg/m^2)/d by 96- to 120-h continuous infusion] before or delivery of the same regimen during radiation therapy is as effective as (or more effective than) surgery plus radiation therapy. Head and neck cancer pts are frequently malnourished and often have intercurrent illness. Concomitant chemotherapy and radiation therapy shows a survival advantage, but mucositis is worse. Pts with *recurrent* or *metastatic disease* are treated palliatively with cisplatin plus 5-fluorouracil or paclitaxel (200–250 mg/m^2 with G-CSF support). Treatment outcome varies somewhat with primary site; in general, pts with localized disease have about 75% 5-year survival, those with locally advanced disease have about 35% 5-year survival, and those with metastatic disease have about 15% 5-year survival.

Prevention

Pts. with head and neck cancer who are rendered disease-free may benefit from chemopreventive therapy with *cis*-retinoic acid (3 months of 1.5 mg/kg/d followed by 9 months of 0.5 mg/kg/d PO).

For a more detailed discussion, see Vokes EE: Head and Neck Cancer, Chap. 89, p. 549, in HPIM-14.

LUNG CANCER

Incidence

Lung cancer is diagnosed in about 99,000 men and 78,000 women in the U.S. each year, and 86% of pts die within 5 years. Lung cancer, the leading cause of cancer death, accounts for 32% of all cancer deaths in men and 25% in women. Peak incidence occurs between ages 55 and 65 years.

Histologic Classification

Four major types account for 88% of primary lung cancers: epidermoid (squamous)—29%, adenocarcinoma (including bronchioloalveolar)—32%, large cell—9%, and small cell (or oat cell)—18%. Histology (small cell versus non-small cell types) is a major determinant of treatment approach. Small cell is usually widely disseminated at presentation, while non-small cell may be localized. Epidermoid and small cell typically present as central masses, while adenocarcinomas and large cell usually present as peripheral nodules or masses. Epidermoid and large cell cavitate in 20–30% of pts.

Etiology

The major cause of lung cancer is tobacco use, particularly cigarette smoking. Lung cancer cells may have 10 or more acquired genetic lesions, most commonly point mutations in *ras* oncogenes; amplification, rearrangement, or transcriptional activation of *myc* family oncogenes; overexpression of *bcl-2*, *Her-2/neu*, and telomerase; and deletions involving chromosomes 1p, 1q, 3p12-13, 3p14 (*FHIT* gene region), 3p21, 3p24–25, 3q, 5q, 9p (p16 and p15 cyclin-dependent kinase inhibitors), 11p13, 11p15, 13q14 (*rb* gene), 16q, and 17p13 (*p53* gene). Loss of 3p and 9p are the earliest events, detectable even in hyperplastic bronchial epithelium; *p53* abnormalities and *ras* point mutations are usually found only in invasive cancers.

Clinical Manifestations

Only 5–15% are detected while asymptomatic. Central endobronchial tumors cause cough, hemoptysis, wheeze, stridor, dyspnea, pneumonitis. Peripheral lesions cause pain, cough, dyspnea, symptoms of lung abscess resulting from cavitation. Metastatic spread of primary lung cancer may cause tracheal obstruction, dysphagia, hoarseness, Horner's syndrome. Other problems of regional spread include superior vena cava syndrome, pleural effusion, respiratory failure. Extrathoracic metastatic disease affects 50% of pts with epidermoid cancer, 80% with adenocarcinoma and large cell, and over 95% with small cell. Clinical problems result from brain metastases, pathologic fractures, liver invasion, and spinal cord compression. Paraneoplastic syndromes may be a presenting finding of lung cancer or first sign of recurrence. Systemic symptoms occur in 30% and include weight loss, anorexia, fever. Endocrine syndromes occur in 12% and include hypercalcemia (epidermoid), syndrome of inappropriate antidiuretic hormone secretion (small cell), gynecomastia (large cell). Skeletal connective tissue syndromes include clubbing in 30% (most often non-small cell) and hypertrophic pulmonary osteoarthropathy in 1–10% (most often adenocarcinomas), with clubbing, pain, and swelling.

Staging (See Table 58-1)

Two parts to staging are: (1) determination of location (anatomic staging) and (2) assessment of pt's ability to withstand antitumor treatment (physiologic staging). Non-small cell tumors are staged by the TNM/International Staging System (ISS). The T (tumor), N (regional node involvement), and M (presence or absence of distant metastasis) factors are taken together to define different stage groups. Small cell tumors are staged by two-stage system: limited stage disease—confined to one hemithorax and regional lymph nodes; extensive disease—involvement beyond this. General staging procedures include careful ENT examination, CXR, and chest CT scanning. CT scans may suggest mediastinal lymph node involvement and pleural extension in non-small cell lung cancer, but definitive evaluation of mediastinal spread requires histologic examination. Routine radionuclide scans are not obtained in asymptomatic pts. If mass lesion on CXR and no obvious contraindications to curative surgical approach, mediastinum should be investigated. Major contraindications to curative surgery include extrathoracic metastases, superior vena cava syndrome, vocal cord and phrenic nerve paralysis, malignant pleural effusions, metastases to contralateral lung, and histologic diagnosis of small cell cancer.

℞ TREATMENT   (See Table 58-2)

1. Surgery in pts with localized disease and non-small cell cancer; however, majority initially thought to have "curative" resection ultimately succumb to metastatic disease.

2. Solitary pulmonary nodule: factors suggesting resection include cigarette smoking, age ≥35, relatively large (>2 cm) lesion, lack of calcification, chest symptoms, and growth of lesion compared to old CXR.

Table 58-1

International TNM Staging System for Lung Cancer

Stage	TNM Descriptors	5-Year Survival, %
I	T1–2, N0, M0	60–80
II	T1–2, N1, M0	25–50
IIIA	T3, N0–1, M0	25–40
	T1-3, N2, M0	10–30
IIIB	Any T4 or N3, M0	<5
IV	Any M1	<5

PRIMARY TUMOR (T)

T1	Tumor <3 cm diameter
T2	Tumor >3 cm diameter or has associated atelecta-sis-obstructive pneumonitis extending to the hilar region
T3	Tumor with direct extension into the chest wall (including superior sulcus tumors), diaphragm, mediastinal pleura, or pericardium
T4	Tumor invades the mediastinum (heart, great vessels, trachea, esophagus, vertebral body, or carina) or the presence of a malignant pleural effusion

REGIONAL LYMPH NODES (N)

N0	No node involvement
N1	Metastasis to lymph nodes in the peribronchial and/or ipsilateral hilar region
N2	Metastasis to ipsilateral mediastinal or subcarinal lymph nodes
N3	Metastasis to contralateral mediastinal or hilar nodes, or any scalene or supraclavicular nodes

DISTANT METASTASIS (M)

M0	No known distant metastasis
M1	Distant metastasis present with site specified (e.g., brain)

SOURCE: Modified from Minna J, HPIM-14.

3. For unresectable non-small cell cancer, metastatic disease, or refusal of surgery: consider for radiation therapy; addition of chemotherapy may reduce death risk by 13% at 2 years.

4. Small cell cancer: combination chemotherapy is stan-

Table 58-2

Summary of Treatment Approach to Lung Cancer Patients

NON-SMALL CELL LUNG CANCER

   Resectable (stages I, II, IIIa, and selected T3, N2 lesions)
      Surgery
      Radiotherapy for "nonoperable" pts
      Postoperative radiotherapy for N2 disease
   Nonresectable (N2 and M1)
      Confined to chest: high-dose chest radiotherapy (RT) if
         possible plus chemotherapy (CT); consider neoadjuvant
         CT followed by surgery
      Extrathoracic: RT to symptomatic local sites; CT (for
         good-performance-status pts, with evaluable lesions)

SMALL CELL LUNG CANCER

   Limited stage (good performance status)
      CT + chest RT
   Extensive stage (good performance status)
      CT
   Complete tumor responders (all stages)
      Prophylactic cranial RT
   Poor-performance-status pts (all stages)
      Modified dose CT
      Palliative RT

ALL PATIENTS

   RT for brain metastases, spinal cord compression, weight-
   bearing lytic bony lesions, symptomatic local lesions (nerve
   paralyses, obstructed airway, hemoptysis in non-small cell
   lung cancer and in small cell cancer not responding to CT)
   Appropriate diagnosis and treatment of other medical problems and supportive care during CT
   Encouragement to stop smoking

SOURCE: Minna J, HPIM-14, p. 558.

dard mode of therapy; response after 6–12 weeks predicts
median and long-term survival

   5.   Laser obliteration of tumor through bronchoscopy in
presence of bronchial obstruction.

   6.   Radiotherapy for brain metastases, spinal cord compression, symptomatic masses, bone lesions.

   7.   Encourage cessation of smoking.

Prognosis

At time of diagnosis, only 20% of pts have localized disease. Overall 5-year survival is 30% for males and 50% for females with localized disease and 5% for pts with advanced disease.

For a more detailed discussion, see Minna JD: Neoplasms of the Lung, Chap. 90, p. 552, in HPIM-14.

BREAST CANCER

Incidence and Epidemiology

The most common tumor in women, 185,000 women in the U.S. are diagnosed and 46,000 die each year with breast cancer. Men also get breast cancer at a rate of 150:1. Breast cancer is hormone-dependent. Women with late menarche, early menopause, and first full-term pregnancy by age 18 have a significantly reduced risk. The average American woman has about a 1 in 9 lifetime risk of developing breast cancer. Dietary fat is a controversial risk factor. Oral contraceptives have little, if any, effect on risk. Estrogen replacement therapy may slightly increase the risk, but the beneficial effects of estrogen on quality of life, bone mineral density, and decreased risk of cardiovascular mortality appear to far outweigh the risk. Women who received therapeutic radiation before age 30 are at increased risk. Breast cancer risk is increased when a sister and mother also had the disease.

Genetics

Perhaps 8–10% of breast cancer is familial. BRCA-1 mutations account for about 5%. BRCA-1 maps to chromosome 17q21 and may be a transcription factor. Ashkenazi Jewish women have a 1% chance of having a common mutation. The BRCA-1 syndrome includes an increased risk of ovarian cancer in women and prostate cancer in men. BRCA-2 on chromosome 11 may account for 2–3% of breast cancer. Mutations are associated with an increased risk of breast cancer in men and women. Germline mutations in p53 (Li-Fraumeni syndrome) are very rare, but breast cancer, sarcomas, and other malignancies occur in such families. Sporadic breast cancers show many genetic alterations including overexpression of *HER-2/neu* in 25% of cases, p53 mutations in 40%, and loss of heterozygosity at other loci.

Diagnosis

Breast cancer is usually diagnosed by biopsy of a nodule detected by mammogram or by palpation. Women should be strongly encouraged to examine their breasts monthly. In premenopausal women, questionable or nonsuspicious (small) masses should be reexamined in 2–4 weeks. A mass in a premenopausal woman that persists throughout her cycle and any mass in a postmenopausal woman should be aspirated. If the mass is a cyst filled with non-bloody fluid that goes away with aspiration, the pt is returned to routine screening. If the cyst aspiration leaves a residual mass or reveals bloody fluid, the pt should have a mammogram and excisional biopsy. If the mass is solid, the pt should undergo a mammogram and excisional biopsy. Screening mammograms performed every other year beginning at age 50 have been shown to save lives. The controversy regarding screening mammograms beginning at age 40 relates to the following facts: (1) the disease is much less common in the 40- to 49-year age group; screening is generally less successful for less common problems; (2) workup of mammographic abnormalities in the 40- to 49-year age group less commonly diagnoses cancer; and (3) no clinical study has demonstrated the effectiveness of screening mammography beginning at age 40 to save lives. However, many believe in the value of screening mammography beginning at age 40.

Staging

Therapy and prognosis are dictated by stage of disease (see Table 59-1). Unless the breast mass is large or fixed to the chest wall, staging of the ipsilateral axilla is performed at the time of lumpectomy (see below). Within pts of a given stage, individual characteristics of the tumor may influence prognosis: expression of estrogen receptor improves prognosis, while overexpression of *HER-1/neu*, mutations in p53, high growth fraction, and aneuploidy worsen the prognosis. Breast cancer can spread almost anywhere but commonly goes to bone, lungs, liver, soft tissue, and brain.

Table 59-1

Staging of Breast Cancer*

PRIMARY TUMOR (T)

T0	No evidence of primary tumor
Tis	Carcinoma in situ
T1	Tumor ≤2 cm
T2	Tumor >2 cm but ≤5 cm
T3	Tumor >5 cm
T4	Extension to chest wall, inflammation

REGIONAL LYMPH NODES (N)

N0	No tumor in regional lymph nodes
N1	Metastasis to movable ipsilateral nodes
N2	Metastasis to matted or fixed ipsilateral nodes
N3	Metastasis to ipsilateral internal mammary nodes

DISTANT METASTASIS (M)

M0	No distant metastasis
M1	Distant metastasis (includes spread to ipsilateral supraclavicular nodes)

STAGE GROUPING

Stage 0	TIS	N0	M0
Stage 1	T1	N0	M0
Stage IIA	T0	N1	M0
	T1	N1	M0
	T2	N0	M0
Stage IIB	T2	N1	M0
	T3	N0	M0
Stage IIIA	T0	N2	M0
	T1	N2	M0
	T2	N2	M0
	T3	N1, N2	M0
Stage IIIB	T4	Any N	M0
	Any T	N3	M0
Stage IV	Any T	Any N	M1

* Modified from the TNM classification proposed by the American Joint Committee on Cancer, 1992.

Table 59-2

5-Year Survival Rate for Breast Cancer by Stage*

Stage	5-Year Survival (Percent of Patients)
0	99
I	92
IIA	82
IIB	65
IIIA	47
IIIB	44
IV	14

* Modified from data of the National Cancer Institute—Surveillance, Epidemiology, and End Results (SEER).

℞ TREATMENT

Five-year survival rate by stage is shown in Table 59-2. Outcome of primary therapy is the same with modified radical mastectomy or lumpectomy followed by breast radiation therapy. Women with tumors <1 cm and negative axillary nodes require no additional therapy beyond their primary lumpectomy and breast radiation. Adjuvant combination chemotherapy for 6 months appears to benefit premenopausal women with positive lymph nodes, pre- and postmenopausal women with negative lymph nodes but with large tumors or poor prognostic features, and postmenopausal women with positive lymph nodes whose tumors do not express estrogen receptors. Various regimens have been used. In women with up to three positive nodes, CMF (cyclophosphamide, 100 mg/m² PO days 1–14 or 600 mg/m² IV days 1 and 8; methotrexate, 40 mg/m² IV days 1 and 8; 5-fluorouracil, 600 mg/m² IV days 1 and 8) or CAF (cyclophosphamide, 500 mg/m² IV days 1 and 8; doxorubicin, 50 mg/m² IV days 1 and 8; 5-fluorouracil, 500 mg/m² IV days 1 and 8) are commonly given for six cycles. Women with 4–10 positive nodes may benefit from doxorubicin, 75 mg/m² IV q21d × 4 followed by CMF (same doses as above given on day 1 only, *not* days 1 and 8; cycles repeated q21d × 6). Tamoxifen adjuvant therapy (20 mg/d for 5 years) is used for postmenopausal women with tumors expressing estrogen receptors whose nodes are positive or whose nodes are negative but with large tumors or poor prognostic features. Breast cancer will recur in about half of pts with localized disease. Treatment for metastatic disease depends upon estrogen receptor status and treatment philosophy. No therapy is known to cure pts with metastatic disease, but many pts receive high-dose therapy with autologous stem cell transplantation, some of whom have excellent survival. Median survival is about 16 months with conventional treatment; tamoxifen for estrogen receptor–positive tumors, and combination chemotherapy for receptor-negative tumors.

For a more detailed discussion, see Lippman ME: Evaluation of Breast Masses in Men and Women, Chap. 64, p. 362, and Breast Cancer, Chap. 91, p. 562, in HPIM-14.

TUMORS OF THE GASTROINTESTINAL TRACT

ESOPHAGEAL CARCINOMA

In 1996 in the U.S., 12,300 cases and 11,200 deaths; less frequent in women than men. Highest incidence in focal regions of China, Iran, Afghanistan, Siberia, Mongolia. In U.S., blacks more frequently affected than whites; usually presents sixth decade or later; 5-year survival <5% because most pts present with advanced disease.

PATHOLOGY   85% squamous cell carcinoma, most commonly in upper two-thirds; <15% adenocarcinoma, usually in distal third, arising in region of columnar metaplasia (Barrett's esophagus), glandular tissue, or as direct extension of proximal gastric adenocarcinoma; lymphoma and melanoma rare.

RISK FACTORS   Major risk factors for squamous cell carcinoma: ethanol abuse, smoking (combination is synergistic); other risks: lye ingestion and esophageal stricture, radiation exposure, head and neck cancer, achalasia, smoked opiates, Plummer-Vinson syndrome, tylosis, chronic ingestion of extremely hot tea, deficiency of vitamin A, zinc, molybdenum. Barrett's esophagus is a risk for adenocarcinoma.

CLINICAL FEATURES Progressive dysphagia (first with solids, then liquids), rapid weight loss common, chest pain (from mediastinal spread), odynophagia, pulmonary aspiration (obstruction, tracheoesophageal fistula), hoarseness (laryngeal nerve palsy), hypercalcemia (parathyroid hormone–related peptide hypersecretion by squamous carcinomas); bleeding infrequent, occasionally severe; examination often unremarkable.

DIAGNOSIS Double-contrast barium swallow useful for screening; flexible esophagogastroscopy most sensitive and specific test; pathologic confirmation by combining endoscopic biopsy and cytologic examination of mucosal brushings (neither alone sufficiently sensitive); CT and endoscopic ultrasonography valuable to assess local and nodal spread.

℞ TREATMENT

Surgical resection feasible in only 40% of pts; associated with high complication rate (fistula, abscess, aspiration). *Squamous cell carcinoma:* Surgical resection after chemotherapy [5-fluorouracil (5-FU), cisplatin] prolongs survival and may provide improved cure rate. *Adenocarcinoma:* Curative resection rarely possible; fewer than one-fifth of pts with resectable tumors survive 5 years. Palliative measures include laser ablation, mechanical dilatation, radiotherapy, and a luminal prosthesis to bypass the tumor. Gastrostomy or jejunostomy are frequently required for nutritional support.

GASTRIC CARCINOMA

Highest incidence in Japan, China, Chile, Ireland; incidence decreasing worldwide, eightfold in U.S. over last 60 years; in 1996, 22,800 new cases and 14,000 deaths. Male:female = 2:1; peak incidence sixth and seventh decades; overall 5-year survival less than 15%.

RISK FACTORS Increased incidence in lower socioeconomic groups; environmental component is suggested by studies of migrants and their offspring. Several dietary factors correlated with increased incidence: nitrates, smoked foods, heavily salted foods; genetic component suggested by increased incidence in first-degree relatives of affected pts; other risk factors: atrophic gastritis, *Helicobacter pylori* infection; Billroth II gastrectomy, gastrojejunostomy, adenomatous gastric polyps, pernicious anemia, hyperplastic gastric polyps (latter two associated with atrophic gastritis). Ménétrier's disease; slight increased risk with blood group A.

PATHOLOGY Adenocarcinoma in 85%; usually focal (polypoid, ulcerative), two-thirds arising in antrum or lesser curvature, frequently ulcerative ("intestinal type"); less commonly diffuse infiltrative (linitis plastica) or superficial spreading (diffuse lesions more prevalent in younger pts; exhibit less geographic variation; have extremely poor prognosis); spreads primarily to local nodes, liver, peritoneum; systemic spread uncommon; lymphoma accounts for 15% (most frequent extranodal site in immunocompetent pts), either low-grade tumor of mucosa-associated lymphoid tissue (MALT) or aggressive diffuse large cell lymphoma; leiomyosarcoma is rare.

CLINICAL FEATURES Most commonly presents with progressive upper abdominal discomfort, frequently with weight loss, anorexia, nausea; acute or chronic GI bleeding (mucosal ulceration) common; dysphagia (location in cardia); vomiting (pyloric and widespread disease); early satiety; examination often unrevealing early in course; later, abdominal tenderness, pallor, and cachexia most common signs; palpable mass uncommon; metastatic spread may be manifest by hepatomegaly, ascites, left supraclavicular or scalene adenopathy, periumbilical, ovarian, or prerectal mass (Blummer's shelf), low-grade fever, skin abnormalities (nodules, dermatomyositis, acanthosis nigricans, or multiple seborrheic keratoses). Laboratory findings: iron-deficiency anemia in two-thirds of pts; fecal occult blood in 80%; rarely associated with pancytopenia and microangiopathic hemolytic anemia (from marrow infiltration), leukemoid reaction, migratory thrombophlebitis or acanthosis nigricans.

DIAGNOSIS Double-contrast barium swallow useful; gastroscopy most sensitive and specific test; pathologic confirmation by biopsy and cytologic examination of mucosal brushings; superficial biopsies less sensitive for lymphomas (frequently submucosal); important to differentiate benign from malignant gastric ulcers with multiple biopsies and follow-up examinations to demonstrate ulcer healing.

℞ **TREATMENT**

Adenocarcinoma: Gastrectomy offers only chance of cure; the rare tumors limited to mucosa are resectable for cure in 80%; deeper invasion, nodal metastases decrease 5-year survival to 20% of pts with resectable tumors in absence of obvious metastatic spread; CT and endoscopic ultrasonography may aid in determining tumor resectability. Palliative therapy for pain, obstruction, and bleeding includes surgery, endoscopic dilatation, radiation, chemotherapy. *Lymphoma:* Low-grade MALT lymphoma is caused by *Helicobacter py-*

lori infection, and eradication of the infection causes complete remissions in 50% of pts; rest are responsive to combination chemotherapy including cyclophosphamide, doxorubicin, vincristine, prednisone (CHOP). Diffuse large cell lymphoma may be treated with either combination chemotherapy alone or subtotal gastrectomy followed by chemotherapy; 50–60% 5-year survival. *Leiomyosarcoma:* Surgical resection curative in most pts.

BENIGN GASTRIC TUMORS

Much less common than malignant gastric tumors; hyperplastic polyps most common, with adenomas, hamartomas, and leiomyomas rare; 30% of adenomas and occasional hyperplastic polyps are associated with gastric malignancy; polyposis syndromes include Peutz-Jeghers and familial polyposis (hamartomas and adenomas), Gardner's (adenomas), and Cronkhite-Canada (cystic polyps). See ''Colonic Polyps,'' below.

CLINICAL FEATURES Usually asymptomatic; occasionally present with bleeding or vague epigastric discomfort.

R̲x̲ TREATMENT
Endoscopic or surgical excision.

SMALL BOWEL TUMORS

CLINICAL FEATURES Uncommon tumors (~5% of all GI neoplasms); usually present with bleeding, abdominal pain, weight loss, fever, or intestinal obstruction (intermittent or fixed); increased incidence of lymphomas in pts with gluten-sensitive enteropathy, Crohn's disease involving small bowel, AIDS, prior organ transplantation, autoimmune disorders.

PATHOLOGY Usually benign; most common are adenomas (usually duodenal), leiomyomas (intramural), and lipomas (usually ileal); 50% of malignant tumors are adenocarcinoma, usually in duodenum (at or near ampulla of Vater) or proximal jejunum, commonly coexisting with benign adenomas; primary intestinal lymphomas (non-Hodgkins) account for 25% and occur as focal mass (western type), which is usually a T cell lymphoma associated with prior celiac disease, or diffuse infiltration (Mediterranean type), which is usually immunoproliferative small-intestinal disease (IPSID; α-chain disease), a B cell lymphoma, which can present as intestinal malabsorption; carcinoid tumors (usually asymptomatic) occasionally produce bleeding or intussusception (see below).

DIAGNOSIS   Endoscopy and biopsy most useful for tumors of duodenum and proximal jejunum; otherwise barium x-ray examination best diagnostic test; direct small-bowel instillation of contrast (enteroclysis) occasionally reveals tumors not seen with routine small-bowel radiography; angiography (to detect plexus of tumor vessels) or laparotomy often required for diagnosis; CT useful to evaluate extent of tumor (esp. lymphomas).

℞ **TREATMENT**

Surgical excision; adjuvant chemotherapy appears helpful for focal lymphoma; IPSID appears to be curable with combination chemotherapy used in aggressive lymphoma plus oral antibiotics (e.g., tetracycline); no proven role for chemotherapy or radiation therapy for other small-bowel tumors.

COLONIC POLYPS

TUBULAR ADENOMAS   Present in ~30% of adults; pedunculated or sessile; usually asymptomatic; ~5% cause occult blood in stool; may cause obstruction; overall risk of malignant degeneration correlates with size (<2% if <1.5 cm diam; >10% if >2.5 cm diam) and is higher in sessile polyps; 65% found in rectosigmoid colon; diagnosis by barium enema, sigmoidoscopy, or colonoscopy. *Treatment:* Full colonoscopy to detect synchronous lesions (present in 30%); endoscopic resection (surgery if polyp large or inaccessible by colonoscopy); follow-up surveillance by colonoscopy every 2–3 years.

VILLOUS ADENOMAS   Generally larger than tubular adenomas at diagnosis; often sessile; high risk of malignancy (up to 30% when >2 cm); more prevalent in left colon; occasionally associated with potassium-rich secretory diarrhea. *Treatment:* As for tubular adenomas.

HYPERPLASTIC POLYPS   Asymptomatic; usually incidental finding at colonoscopy; rarely greater than 5 mm; no malignant potential. No treatment required.

HEREDITARY POLYPOSIS SYNDROMES

1.   *Familial polyposis coli* (FPC): Diffuse pancolonic adenomatous polyposis (up to several thousand polyps); autosomal dominant inheritance associated with deletion in adenomatous polyposis coli (*APC*) gene on chromosome 5; colon carcinoma from malignant degeneration of polyp in 100% by age 40. *Treatment:* Prophylactic total colectomy or subtotal colectomy with ileoproctostomy before age 30; subtotal resection avoids ileostomy but necessitates frequent proctoscopic surveillance;

periodic colonoscopic or annual radiologic screening of siblings and offspring of pts with FPC until age 35; preventive role of sulindac and other NSAIDs is under study.

2.   *Gardner's syndrome:* Variant of FPC with associated soft tissue tumors (epidermoid cysts, osteomas, lipomas, fibromas, desmoids); higher incidence of gastroduodenal polyps, ampullary adenocarcinoma. *Treatment:* As for FPC; surveillance for small-bowel disease with fecal occult blood testing after colectomy.

3.   *Turcot's syndrome:* Rare variant of FPC with associated malignant brain tumors. *Treatment:* As for FPC.

4.   *Nonpolyposis syndrome:* Familial syndrome with up to 50% risk of colon carcinoma; peak incidence in fifth decade; associated with multiple primary cancers (esp. endometrial); autosomal dominant; due to defective DNA repair.

5.   *Juvenile polyposis:* Multiple benign colonic and small-bowel hamartomas; intestinal bleeding common. Other symptoms: abdominal pain, diarrhea; occasional intussusception. Rarely recur after excision; low risk of colon cancer from malignant degeneration of interspersed adenomatous polyps. Prophylactic colectomy controversial.

6.   *Peutz-Jeghers syndrome:* Numerous hamartomatous polyps of entire GI tract, though denser in small bowel than colon; GI bleeding common; somewhat increased risk for the development of cancer at GI and non-GI sites. Prophylactic surgery not recommended.

COLORECTAL CANCER

Second most common internal cancer in humans; accounts for 20% of cancer-related deaths in U.S., incidence increases dramatically above age 50, approximately equal in men and women. In 1996, 133,500 new cases, 54,900 deaths.

ETIOLOGY AND RISK FACTORS   Most colon cancers arise from adenomatous polyps. Genetic steps from polyp to dysplasia to carcinoma in situ to invasive cancer have been defined, including: point mutation in K-*ras* proto-oncogene, hypomethylation of DNA leading to enhanced gene expression, allelic loss at the APC gene (a tumor suppressor), allelic loss at the *DCC* (deleted in colon cancer) gene on chromosome 18, and loss and mutation of p53 on chromosome 17. Hereditary nonpolyposis colon cancer arises from mutations in the *hMSH2* gene on chromosome 2 and the *hMLH1* gene on chromosome 3. These genes are involved in DNA repair. Mutations lead to colon and other cancers. Diagnosis requires three or more relatives with colon cancer, one of whom is a first-degree relative; one or more cases diagnosed before age 50; and involvement of at least two generations. Environmental factors also play a role; increased prevalence in developed countries, urban areas, advantaged socioeconomic groups; increased risk in pts with hypercholesterolemia, coronary artery disease; correlation of risk with low-fiber, high–animal fat diets, although direct effect of diet remains unproven; decreased risk with long-term dietary calcium supplementation and, possibly, daily aspirin ingestion; risk increased in first-degree relatives of pts, families with increased prevalence of cancer, and pts with history of breast or gynecologic cancer, familial polyposis syndromes, >10-year history of ulcerative colitis or Crohn's colitis, >15-year history of ureterosigmoidostomy. Tumors in pts with strong family history of malignancy are frequently located in right colon and commonly present before age 50; high prevalence in pts with *Streptococcus bovis* bacteremia.

PATHOLOGY Nearly always adenocarcinoma; 75% located distal to the splenic flexure (except in association with polyposis or hereditary cancer syndromes); may be polypoid, sessile, fungating, or constricting; subtype and degree of differentiation do not correlate with course. Degree of invasiveness at surgery (Dukes' classification) is single best predictor of prognosis: >90% 5-year survival for cancer confined to mucosa and submucosa (stage A); 70–85% with extension to muscularis (stage B1) or serosa (stage B2); (survival in these groups worse with tumor penetration of pericolic fat); 35–65% with regional lymph node involvement (stage C; survival in this group better with involvement of <5 lymph nodes); 5% with distant metastasis (e.g., liver, lung, bone; stage D). Rectosigmoid tumors may spread to lungs early because of systemic paravertebral venous drainage of this area. Other predictors of poor prognosis: preoperative serum carcinoembryonic antigen (CEA) >5 ng/mL (>5 μg/L), poorly differentiated histology, bowel perforation, venous invasion, adherence to adjacent organs, aneuploidy, specific deletions in chromosomes 5, 17, 18, and mutation of *ras* proto-oncogene. 15% have defects in DNA repair.

CLINICAL FEATURES Left-sided colon cancers present most commonly with rectal bleeding, altered bowel habits (narrowing, constipation, intermittent diarrhea, tenesmus), and abdominal or back pain; cecal and ascending colon cancers more frequently present with symptoms of anemia, occult blood in stool, or weight loss; other complications: perforation, fistula, volvulus, inguinal hernia; laboratory findings: anemia in 50% of right-sided lesions.

DIAGNOSIS Early diagnosis aided by screening asymptomatic persons with fecal occult blood testing (see below); more than half of all colon cancers are within reach of a 60-cm flexible sigmoidoscope; air-contrast barium enema will diagnose approximately 85% of colon cancers not within reach of sigmoidoscope; colonoscopy most sensitive and specific, permits tumor biopsy and removal of synchronous polyps (thus preventing neoplastic conversion), but incurs somewhat greater expense.

℞ TREATMENT

Local disease: Surgical resection of colonic segment containing tumor; preoperative evaluation to assess prognosis and surgical approach includes full colonoscopy, chest films, biochemical liver tests, plasma CEA level, and possible abdominal CT. Resection of isolated hepatic metastases possible in selected cases; adjuvant radiation therapy to pelvis (with or without concomitant chemotherapy) to decrease local recurrence rate of rectal carcinoma (no apparent effect on survival); radiotherapy without benefit on colon tumors; adjuvant chemotherapy (5-FU and levamisole) decreases recurrence rate and improves survival of stage C tumors; periodic determination of serum CEA level useful to follow therapy and assess recurrence. *Follow-up after curative resection:* Yearly liver tests, CBC, follow-up radiologic or colonoscopic evaluation at 1 year—if normal, repeat every 3 years, with routine screening interim (see below); if polyps detected, repeat 1 year after resection. *Advanced tumor* (locally unresectable or metastatic): Systemic chemotherapy (5-FU and folinic acid), intraarterial chemotherapy [floxuridine (FUDR)] and/or radiotherapy may palliate symptoms.

PREVENTION   Early detection of colon carcinoma may be facilitated by routine screening of stool for occult blood (Hemoccult II, Colo-Test, etc.); however, sensitivity only ~50% for carcinoma; specificity for tumor or polyp ~25–40%. False positives: ingestion of red meat, iron, aspirin; upper GI bleeding. False negatives: vitamin C ingestion, intermittent bleeding. Annual digital exam and fecal occult blood testing recommended for pts over age 40, screening flexible sigmoidoscopy every 3 years after age 50, earlier in pts at increased risk (see above); careful evaluation of all pts with positive fecal occult blood tests (flexible sigmoidoscopy and air-contrast barium enema or colonoscopy alone) reveals polyps in 20–40% and carcinoma in approximately 5%; screening of asymptomatic persons allows earlier detection of colon cancer (i.e., earlier Dukes' stage) and achieves greater resectability rate; decreased overall mortality from colon carcinoma seen only after 13 years of follow-up. More intensive evaluation of first-degree relatives of pts with colon carcinoma frequently includes screening air-contrast barium enema or colonoscopy after age 40.

ANAL CANCER

Accounts for 1–2% of large-bowel cancer; associated with chronic irritation, e.g., from condyloma accuminata, perianal fissures/fistulae, chronic hemorrhoids, leukoplakia, trauma from anal intercourse. Women are more commonly affected than men. Presents with bleeding, pain, and perianal mass. Radiation therapy plus chemotherapy leads to complete response in 80% when the primary lesion is <3cm. Abdominoperineal resection with permanent colostomy is reserved for those with large lesions or who recur after chemoradiotherapy.

BENIGN LIVER TUMORS

Hepatocellular adenomas occur most commonly in women in the third or fourth decades who take birth control pills. Most are found incidentally but may cause pain, and intratumoral hemorrhage may cause circulatory collapse. 10% may become malignant. Women with these adenomas should stop taking birth control pills. Large tumors near the liver surface may be resected. Focal nodular hyperplasia is also more common in women but seems not to be caused by birth control pills. Lesions are vascular on angiography and have septae and are usually asymptomatic.

HEPATOCELLULAR CARCINOMA

About 19,000 cases in the U.S. in 1996, but worldwide this may be the most common tumor. Male:female = 4:1; tumor usually develops in cirrhotic liver in persons in fifth or sixth decade. High incidence in Asia and Africa is related to etiologic relationship between this cancer and hepatitis B and C infections. Aflatoxin exposure contributes to etiology and leaves a molecular signature, a mutation in codon 249 of the gene for p53. Surgical resection or liver transplantation are therapeutic options but rarely successful. Screening populations at risk has given conflicting results. Hepatitis B vaccine prevents the disease. Interferon α may prevent liver cancer in people with chronic active hepatitis C disease.

PANCREATIC CANCER

In 1996 in the U.S., about 26,000 new cases and 27,800 deaths. The incidence is decreasing somewhat, but nearly all diagnosed cases are fatal. The tumors are ductal adenocarcinomas and are not usually detected until the disease has spread. About 70% of tumors are in the pancreatic head, 20% in the body, and 10% in the tail. Mutations in K-*ras* have been found in

85% of tumors, and the p16 cyclin-dependent kinase inhibitor on chromosome 9 may also be implicated. Long-standing diabetes, chronic pancreatitis, and smoking increase the risk; coffee-drinking, alcoholism, and cholelithiasis do not. Pts present with pain and weight loss, the pain often relieved by bending forward. Jaundice commonly complicates tumors of the head, due to biliary obstruction. Curative surgical resections are feasible in about 10%. Gemcitabine may palliate symptoms in pts with advanced disease.

ENDOCRINE TUMORS OF THE GI TRACT AND PANCREAS

CARCINOID TUMOR   Carcinoid tumor accounts for 75% of GI endocrine tumors; incidence is about 15 cases per million population. 90% originate in Kulchitsky cells of the GI tract, most commonly the appendix, ileum, and rectum. Carcinoid tumors of the small bowel and bronchus have a more malignant course than tumors of other sites. About 5% of pts with carcinoid tumors develop symptoms of the carcinoid syndrome, the classic triad being cutaneous flushing, diarrhea, and valvular heart disease. For tumors of GI tract origin, symptoms imply metastases to liver.

Diagnosis can be made by detecting the site of tumor or documenting production of more than 15 mg/d of the serotonin metabolite, 5-hydroxyindoleacetic acid (5-HIAA) in the urine. Octreotide scintigraphy identifies sites of primary and metastatic tumor in about 2/3 of cases.

℞ TREATMENT

Treatment includes surgical resection where feasible. Symptoms may be controlled with histamine blockers and octreotide, 150–1500 mg/d in three doses. Hepatic artery embolization and chemotherapy (5-FU plus streptozocin or doxorubicin) have been used for metastatic disease. Interferon α at 3–10 million units subcutaneously three times a week may relieve symptoms. Prognosis ranges from 95% 5-year survival for localized disease to 20% 5-year survival for those with liver meastases. Median survival of pts with carcinoid syndrome is 2.5 years from the first episode of flushing.

PANCREATIC ISLET-CELL TUMORS   Gastrinoma, insulinoma, VIPoma, glucagonoma, and somatostatinoma account for the vast majority of pancreatic islet-cell tumors; their characteristics are shown in Table 60-1. The tumors are named for the dominant hormone they produce. They are generally slow-growing and produce symptoms related to hormone production.

Table 60-1

Gastrointestinal Endocrine Tumor Syndromes

Syndrome	Cell Type	Clinical Features	Percentage Malignant	Major Products
Carcinoid syndrome	Enterochromaffin, enterochromaffin-like	Flushing, diarrhea, wheezing, hypotension	~100	Serotonin, histamine, miscellaneous peptides
Zollinger-Ellison, gastrinoma	Non-β islet cell, duodenal G cell	Peptic ulcers, diarrhea	~70	Gastrin
Insulinoma	Islet β cell	Hypoglycemia	~10	Insulin
VIPoma (Verner-Morrison, WDHA)	Islet D_1 cell	Diarrhea, hypokalemia, hypochlorhydria	~60	Vasoactive intestinal peptide
Glucagonoma	Islet A cell	Mild diabetes mellitus, erythema necrolytica migrans, glossitis	>75	Glucagon
Somatostatinoma	Islet D cell	Diabetes mellitus, diarrhea, steatorrhea, gallstones	~70	Somatostatin

Gastrinomas and peptic ulcer disease comprise the Zollinger-Ellison syndrome. Gastrinomas are rare (4 cases per 10 million population), and in 25–50%, the tumor is a component of a MEN I syndrome (see Chap. 167).

Insulinoma may present with Whipple's triad, fasting hypoglycemia, symptoms of hypoglycemia, and relief after intravenous glucose. Normal or elevated serum insulin levels in the presence of fasting hypoglycemia are diagnostic. Insulinomas may also be associated with MEN I.

Verner and Morrison described a syndrome of watery diarrhea, hypokalemia, achlorhydria, and renal failure associated with pancreatic islet tumors that produce vasoactive intestinal polypeptide (VIP). *VIPomas* are rare (1 case per 10 million) but often grow to a large size before producing symptoms.

Glucagonoma is associated with diabetes mellitus and necrolytic migratory erythema, a characteristic red, raised, scaly rash usually located on the face, abdomen, perineum, and distal extremities. Glucagon levels >1000 ng/L not suppressed by glucose are diagnostic.

The classic triad of *somatostatinoma* is diabetes mellitus, steatorrhea, and cholelithiasis.

Provocative tests may facilitate diagnosis of functional endocrine tumors: tolbutamide enhances somatostatin secretion by somatostatinomas; pentagastrin enhances calcitonin secretion from medullary thyroid (C cell) tumors; secretin enhances gastrin secretion from gastrinomas. If imaging techniques fail to detect tumor masses, angiography or selective venous sampling for hormone determination may reveal the site of tumor. Metastases to nodes and liver should be sought by CT or MRI.

℞ **TREATMENT**

Treatment is aimed at surgical removal of tumor, if possible. Octreotide inhibits hormone secretion in the majority of cases. Interferon α may reduce symptoms. Streptozocin plus doxorubicin combination chemotherapy may produce responses in 60–90% of cases. Embolization of hepatic metastases may be palliative.

For a more detailed discussion, see Mayer RJ: Gastrointestinal Tract Cancer, Chap. 92, p. 568; Isselbacher KI, Dienstag JL: Tumors of the Liver and Biliary Tract, Chap. 93, p. 578; Mayer RJ: Pancreatic Cancer, Chap. 94, p. 581; Kaplan LM: Endocrine Tumors of the Gastrointestinal Tract and Pancreas, Chap. 95, p. 584, in HPIM-14.

61

GENITOURINARY TRACT CANCER

BLADDER CANCER

INCIDENCE AND EPIDEMIOLOGY Annual incidence in the U.S. is about 52,900 cases with 11,700 deaths. Median age is 65 years. Smoking accounts for 50% of the risk. Exposure to polycyclic aromatic hydrocarbons increases the risk, especially in slow acetylators. Risk is increased in chimney sweeps, dry cleaners, and those involved in aluminum manufacturing. Chronic cyclophosphamide exposure increases risk 9-fold. *Schistosoma haematobium* infection also increases risk, especially of squamous histology.

ETIOLOGY Lesions involving chromosome 9q are an early event. Deletions in 17p (p53), 18q (the DCC locus), 13q (RB), 3p, and 5q are characteristic of invasive lesions. Overexpression of epidermal growth factor receptors and HER-2/neu receptors is common.

PATHOLOGY Over 90% of tumors are derived from transitional epithelium; 3% are squamous, 2% are adenocarcinomas, and <1% are neuroendocrine small cell tumors. Field effects are seen that place all sites lined by transitional epithelium at risk including the renal pelvis, ureter, bladder, and proximal 2/3 of the urethra. 90% of tumors are in the bladder, 8% in the renal pelvis, and 2% in the ureter or urethra. Histologic grade influences survival. Lesion recurrence is influenced by size, number, and growth pattern of the primary tumor.

CLINICAL PRESENTATION Hematuria is the initial sign in 80–90%; however, cystitis is a more common cause of hematuria (22% of all hematuria) than is bladder cancer (15%). Pts are initially staged and treated by endoscopy. Superficial tumors are removed at endoscopy; muscle invasion requires more extensive surgery.

℞ **TREATMENT**

Management is based on extent of disease: superficial, invasive, or metastatic. Frequency of presentation is 75% superficial, 20% invasive, and 5% metastatic. Superficial lesions are resected at endoscopy. Although complete resection is possible in 80%, 30–80% of cases recur; grade and stage progression occur in 30%. Intravesical instillation of bacille Calmette-Guérin (BCG) reduces the risk of recurrence by 40–45%. Recurrence is monitored every 3 months.

The standard management of muscle-invasive disease is

radical cystectomy. 5-year survival is 70% for those without invasion of perivesicular fat or lymph nodes, 50% for those with invasion of fat but not lymph nodes, 35% for those with one node involved, and 10% for those with six or more involved nodes. Pts who cannot withstand radical surgery may have 30–35% 5-year survival with 5000–7000 cGy external beam radiation therapy. Bladder sparing may be possible in up to 45% of pts with two cycles of chemotherapy with CMV (methotrexate 30 mg/m^2 days 1 and 8, vinblastine 4 mg/m^2 days 1 and 8, cisplatin 100 mg/m^2 day 2, q21 days) followed by 4000-cGy radiation therapy given concurrently with cisplatin.

Metastatic disease is treated with combination chemotherapy, either CMV (see above) or M-VAC (methotrexate 30 mg/m^2 days 1, 15, 22; vinblastine 3 mg/m^2 days 2, 15, 22; doxorubicin 30 mg/m^2 day 2; cisplatin 70 mg/m^2 day 2; q 28 days). About 70% of pts respond to treatment, and 20% have a complete response; 10–15% have long-term disease-free survival.

RENAL CANCER

INCIDENCE AND EPIDEMIOLOGY   Annual incidence in U.S. is about 30,600 cases with 12,000 deaths. Cigarette smoking accounts for 20–30% of cases. Risk is increased in acquired renal cystic disease. There are two familial forms: a rare autosomal dominant syndrome and von Hippel-Lindau disease. About 35% of pts with von Hippel-Lindau disease develop renal cancer. Incidence is also increased in tuberous sclerosis and polycystic kidney disease.

ETIOLOGY   Most cases are sporadic; however, the most frequent chromosomal abnormality (occurs in 60%) is deletion or rearrangement of 3p21-26. The von Hippel-Lindau gene has been mapped to that region and appears to have a novel activity, regulation of speed of transcription. It is unclear how lesions in the gene lead to cancer.

PATHOLOGY   Five variants are recognized: clear cell tumors (75%), chromophilic tumors (15%), chromophobic tumors (5%), oncocytic tumors (3%), and collecting duct tumors (2%). Clear cell tumors arise from cells of the proximal convoluted tubules. Chromophilic tumors tend to be bilateral and multifocal and often show trisomy 7 and/or trisomy 17. Chromophobic and eosinophilic tumors less frequently have chromosomal aberrations and follow a more indolent course.

CLINICAL PRESENTATION   The classic triad of hematuria, flank pain, and flank mass is seen in only 10–20% of pts; hematuria (40%), flank pain (40%), palpable mass (33%), weight loss (33%) are the most common individual symptoms. Paraneoplastic syndromes of erythrocytosis (3%), hypercalcemia (5%), and nonmetastatic hepatic dysfunction (Stauffers' syndrome) (15%) may also occur. Workup should include IV pyelography, renal ultrasonography, CT of abdomen and pelvis, CXR, urinalysis and urine cytology. Stage I is disease restricted to the kidney, stage II is disease contained within Gerota's fascia, stage III is locally invasive disease involving nodes and/ or inferior vena cava, stage IV is invasion of adjacent organs or metastatic sites. Prognosis is related to stage: 66% 5-year survival for I, 64% for II, 42% for III, and 11% for IV.

℞ TREATMENT

Radical nephrectomy is standard for stages I, II, and most stage III pts. Surgery may also be indicated in the setting of metastatic disease for intractable local symptoms (bleeding, pain). About 10–15% of pts with advanced stage disease may benefit from interleukin 2 and/or interferon α. Some remissions are durable.

TESTICULAR CANCER

INCIDENCE AND EPIDEMIOLOGY   Annual incidence is about 7400 cases with 370 deaths. Peak age incidence is 20–40. Occurs 4–5 times more frequently in white than black men. Cryptorchid testes are at increased risk. Early orchiopexy may protect against testis cancer. Risk is also increased in testicular femininization syndromes, and Klinefelter's syndrome is associated with mediastinal germ cell tumor.

ETIOLOGY   The cause is unknown. Disease is associated with a characteristic cytogenetic defect, isochromosome 12p.

PATHOLOGY   Two main subtypes are noted; seminoma and nonseminoma. Each account for about 50% of cases. Seminoma has a more indolent natural history and is highly sensitive to radiation therapy. Four subtypes of nonseminoma are defined; embryonal carcinoma, teratoma, choriocarcinoma, and endodermal sinus (yolk sac) tumor.

CLINICAL PRESENTATION   Painless testicular mass is the classic initial sign. In the presence of pain, differential diagnosis includes epididymitis or orchitis; a brief trial of antibiotics may be undertaken. Staging evaluation includes measurement of serum tumor markers alphafetoprotein (AFP) and β human chorionic gonadotropin (hCG), CXR, and CT scan of abdomen and pelvis. Lymph nodes are staged at resection of the primary tumor through an inguinal approach. Stage I disease is limited to the testis, epididymis, or spermatic cord; stage II involves retroperitoneal nodes; and stage III is disease outside the retroperitoneum. Among seminoma pts, 70% are stage I, 20% are stage II, and 10% are stage III. Among nonseminoma germ cell tumor pts, 33% are found in each stage. hCG may be elevated in either seminoma or nonseminoma, but AFP is elevated only in nonseminoma. 95% of pts are cured if treated appropriately.

℞ **TREATMENT**

For stages I and II seminoma, inguinal orchiectomy followed by retroperitoneal radiation therapy to 2500–3000 cGy is effective. For stages I and II nonseminoma germ cell tumors, inguinal orchiectomy followed by retroperitoneal lymph node dissection is effective. For pts of either histology with bulky nodes or stage III disease, chemotherapy is given. Cisplatin (20 mg/m^2 days 1–5), etoposide (100 mg/m^2 days 1–5), and bleomycin (30 U days 2, 9, 16) given every 21 d for four cycles is the standard therapy. If tumor markers return to zero, residual masses are resected. Most are necrotic debris or teratomas. Salvage therapy rescues about 25% of those not cured with primary therapy.

For more detailed discussion, see Scher HI, Motzer RJ: Bladder and Renal Cell Cancer, Chap. 96, p. 592; Motzer RJ, Bosl GL: Testicular Cancer, Chap. 98, p. 602, in HPIM-14.

62

GYNECOLOGIC CANCER

OVARIAN CANCER

INCIDENCE AND EPIDEMIOLOGY Annually in the U.S., about 27,000 new cases are found and nearly 15,000 women die of ovarian cancer. Incidence begins to rise in the fifth decade, peaking in the eighth decade. Risk is increased in nulliparous women and reduced by pregnancy (risk decreased about 10% per pregnancy) and oral contraceptives. About 5% of cases are familial.

GENETICS Mutations in *BRCA-1* predispose women to both breast and ovarian cancer. Cytogenetic analysis of epithelial ovarian cancers that are not familial often reveals complex karyotypic abnormalities including structural lesions on chromosomes 1 and 11 and loss of heterozygosity for loci on chromosomes 3q, 6q, 11q, 13q, and 17. C-*myc*, H-*ras*, K-*ras*, and *HER2/neu* are often mutated or overexpressed.

CLINICAL PRESENTATION Most pts present with abdominal pain, bloating, urinary symptoms, and weight gain indicative of disease spread beyond the true pelvis. Localized ovarian cancer is usually asymptomatic and detected on routine pelvic examination as a palpable nontender adnexal mass. Most ovarian masses detected incidentally in ovulating women are ovarian cysts that resolve over one to three menstrual cycles. Adnexal masses in postmenopausal women are more often pathologic and should be surgically removed. CA-125 serum levels are ≥35 U/mL in 80–85% of women with ovarian cancer, but other conditions may also cause elevations. Screening is not effective outside of high risk families.

PATHOLOGY Half of ovarian tumors are benign, one-third are malignant, and the rest are tumors of low malignant potential. These borderline lesions have cytologic features of malignancy but do not invade. Malignant epithelial tumors may be of five different types: serous (50%), mucinous (25%), endometrioid (15%), clear cell (5%), and Brenner tumors (1%, derived from urothelial or transitional epithelium). The remaining 4% of ovarian tumors are stromal or germ cell tumors, which are managed like testicular cancer in men (see Chap. 61). Histologic grade is an important prognostic factor for the epithelial varieties.

STAGING Extent of disease is ascertained by a surgical procedure that permits visual and manual inspection of all peritoneal surfaces and the diaphragm. Total abdominal hysterectomy, bilateral salpingo-oopherectomy, partial omentectomy, pelvic and paraaortic lymph node sampling, and peritoneal washings should be performed. The staging system and its influence on survival is shown in Table 62-1.

℞ **TREATMENT**

Pts with stage I disease, no residual tumor after surgery, and well- or moderately differentiated tumors need no further treatment after surgery and have a 5-year survival over 95%. For stage II pts totally resected and stage I pts with poor histologic grade, adjuvant therapy with total abdominal radiation therapy, single-agent cisplatin, or cisplatin plus paclitaxel produces 5-year survival of 80%. Advanced-stage pts should receive paclitaxel, 135 mg/m^2 by 24-h infusion, followed by cisplatin, 75 mg/m^2 every 3 or 4 weeks.

ENDOMETRIAL CANCER

INCIDENCE AND EPIDEMIOLOGY   The most common gynecologic cancer, 34,000 cases are diagnosed in the U.S. and 6000 pts die annually. It is primarily a disease of postmenopausal women. Obesity, altered menstrual cycles, infertility, late menopause, and postmenopausal bleeding are commonly encountered in women with endometrial cancer. Women taking tamoxifen to prevent breast cancer recurrence and those taking estrogen replacement therapy are at a modestly increased risk. Peak incidence is in the sixth and seventh decades.

CLINICAL PRESENTATION   Abnormal vaginal discharge (90%), abnormal vaginal bleeding (80%), and leukorrhea (10%) are the most common symptoms.

PATHOLOGY   Endometrial cancers are adenocarcinomas in 75–80% of cases. The remaining cases include mucinous carcinoma, papillary serous carcinoma, and secretory, ciliated, and clear cell varieties. Prognosis depends on stage, histologic grade, and degree of myometrial invasion.

STAGING   Total abdominal hysterectomy and bilateral salpingo-oopherectomy is both the staging procedure and the treatment of choice. The staging scheme and its influence on prognosis are shown in Table 62-1.

℞ **TREATMENT**

In women with poor histologic grade, deep myometrial invasion, or extensive involvement of the lower uterine segment or cervix, intracavitary or external beam radiation therapy is given. If cervical invasion is deep, preoperative radiation

Table 62-1

Staging and Survival in Gynecologic Malignancies

Stage	Ovarian	5-Year Survival, %	Endometrial	5-Year Survival, %	Cervix	5-Year Survival, %
0	—		—		Carcinoma in situ	100
I	Confined to ovary	90	Confined to corpus	89	Confined to uterus	85
II	Confined to pelvis	70	Involves corpus and cervix	80	Invades beyond uterus but not to pelvic wall	60
III	Intraabdominal spread	15–20	Extends outside the uterus but not outside the true pelvis	30	Extends to pelvic wall and/or lower third of vagina, or hydronephrosis	33
IV	Spread outside abdomen	1–5	Extends outside the true pelvis or involves the bladder or rectum	9	Invades mucosa of bladder or rectum or extends beyond the true pelvis	7

therapy may improve the resectability of the tumor. Stage III disease is managed with surgery and radiation therapy. Stage IV disease is usually treated palliatively. Progestational agents such as hydroxyprogesterone or megastrol and the antiestrogen tamoxifen may produce responses in 20% of pts. Doxorubicin, 60 mg/m^2 IV day 1, and cisplatin, 50 mg/m^2 IV day 1, every 3 weeks for 8 cycles produces a 45% response rate.

CERVIX CANCER

INCIDENCE AND EPIDEMIOLOGY In the U.S. about 16,000 cases of invasive cervical cancer are diagnosed each year and 50,000 cases of carcinoma in situ are detected by Pap smear. Cervical cancer kills 4900 women a year, 85% of whom never had a Pap smear. It is a major cause of disease in underdeveloped countries and is more common in lower socioeconomic groups, women with early sexual activity, multiple sexual partners, and in smokers. Human papilloma virus (HPV) types 16 and 18 are the major types associated with cervical cancer. The virus attacks the G1 checkpoint of the cell cycle; its E7 protein binds and inactivates Rb protein, and E6 induces the degradation of p53.

SCREENING Women should begin screening when they begin sexual activity or at age 20. After two consecutive negative annual Pap smears, the test should be repeated every 3 years. Abnormal smears dictate the need for a cervical biopsy, usually under colposcopy, with the cervix painted with 3% acetic acid, which shows abnormal areas as white patches. If there is evidence of carcinoma in situ, a cone biopsy is performed, which is therapeutic.

CLINICAL PRESENTATION Pts present with abnormal bleeding or postcoital spotting or menometrorrhagia or intermenstrual bleeding. Vaginal discharge, low back pain, and urinary symptoms may also be present.

STAGING Staging is clinical and consists of a pelvic exam under anesthesia with cystoscopy and proctoscopy. CXR, IV pyelography, and abdominal CT are used to search for metastases. The staging system and its influence on prognosis are shown in Table 62-1.

℞ **TREATMENT**

Carcinoma in situ is cured with cone biopsy. Stage I disease may be treated with radical hysterectomy or radiation therapy. Stages II–IV disease are usually treated with radiation therapy, often with both brachytherapy and teletherapy. Pelvic exenteration is used uncommonly to control the disease. The role of chemotherapy is to act as a radiosensitizer. Hydroxyurea, 5-fluorouracil (5-FU), and cisplatin have all shown promising results given concurrently with radiation therapy. Cisplatin, 100 mg/m^2 IV day 1, and 5-FU, 1000 mg/m^2 24-h infusion days 1–5, is an effective radiosensitizing regimen.

For a more detailed discussion, see Young RC: Gynecologic Malignancies, Chap. 99, p. 605, in HPIM-14.

PROSTATE HYPERPLASIA AND CARCINOMA

PROSTATE HYPERPLASIA

Enlargement of the prostate is nearly universal in aging men. Hyperplasia usually begins by age 45 years, occurs in the area of the prostate gland surrounding the urethra, and produces urinary outflow obstruction. Symptoms develop on average by age 65 in whites and 60 in blacks. Symptoms develop late because hypertrophy of the bladder detrusor compensates for ureteral compression. As obstruction progresses, urinary stream caliber and force diminish, hesitancy in stream initiation develops, and postvoid dribbling occurs. Dysuria and urgency are signs of bladder irritation (perhaps due to inflammation or tumor) and are usually not seen in prostate hyperplasia. As the postvoid residual increases, nocturia and overflow incontinence may develop. Common medications such as tranquilizing drugs and decongestants, infections, or alcohol may precipitate urinary retention. Because of the prevalence of hyperplasia, the relationship to neoplasia is unclear.

On digital rectal exam (DRE), a hyperplastic prostate is smooth, firm, and rubbery in consistency; the median groove may be lost. Prostate-specific antigen (PSA) levels may be elevated but are ≤10 ng/mL unless cancer is also present (see below).

TREATMENT

Asymptomatic pts do not require treatment, and those with complications of urethral obstruction such as inability to urinate, renal failure, recurrent UTI, hematuria, or bladder stones clearly require surgical extirpation of the prostate, usually by transurethral resection (TURP). However, the approach to the remaining pts should be based on the degree of incapacity or discomfort from the disease and the likely side effects of any intervention. If the pt has only mild symptoms, watchful waiting is not harmful and permits an assessment of the rate of symptom progression. If therapy is desired by the pt, two medical approaches may be helpful: terazosin (1 mg at bedtime, titrated to symptoms up to 20 mg/d), an alpha$_1$-adrenergic blocker, relaxes the smooth muscle of the bladder neck and increases urine flow; finasteride (5 mg/d), an inhibitor of 5α-reductase, blocks the conversion of testosterone to dihydrotestosterone and causes an average decrease in prostate size of about 24%. TURP has the greatest success rate but also the greatest risk of complications.

PROSTATE CARCINOMA

The most common malignancy in humans, prostate cancer was diagnosed in 317,000 men in 1996 in the U.S. The major increase in detection appears related to the early diagnosis of cancers in mildly symptomatic men found on screening to have elevated serum levels of PSA. Like most other cancers, incidence is age-related. The disease is more common in blacks than whites. Symptoms are generally similar to and indistinguishable from those of prostate hyperplasia, but those with cancer more often have dysuria and back or hip pain. On histology, 95% are adenocarcinomas. Biologic behavior is affected by histologic grade (Gleason score).

In contrast to hyperplasia, prostate cancer generally originates in the periphery of the gland and may be detectable on DRE as one or more nodules on the posterior surface of the gland, hard in consistency and irregular in shape. An approach to diagnosis is shown in Fig. 63-1. Those with a negative DRE and PSA ≤ 4 ng/mL may be followed annually. Those with an abnormal DRE or a PSA > 10 ng/mL should undergo transrectal ultrasound-guided biopsy (TRUS). Those with normal DRE and PSA of 4.1–10 ng/mL may be handled differently in different centers. Some would perform transrectal ultrasound and biopsy any abnormality or follow if no abnormality is found. Some would repeat the PSA in a year and biopsy if the increase over that period was >0.75 ng/mL. Other methods of using PSA to distinguish early cancer from hyperplasia include quantitating

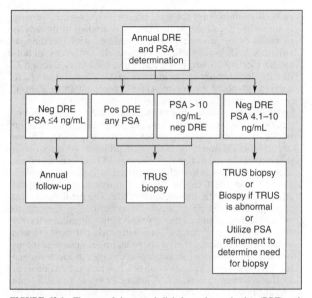

FIGURE 63-1 The use of the annual digital rectal examination (DRE) and measurement of prostate-specific antigen (PSA) as guides for deciding which men should have transrectal prostate biopsy under sonography (TRUS). There are at least three schools of thought about what to do if the DRE is negative and the PSA is equivocal (4.1 to 10 ng/mL).

bound and free PSA and relating the PSA to the size of the prostate (PSA density). Perhaps 1/3 of persons with prostate cancer do not have PSA elevations.

Lymphatic spread is assessed surgically; it is present in only 10% of those with Gleason grade 5 or lower and in 70% of those with grade 9 or 10. PSA level also correlates with spread; only 10% of those with PSA < 10 ng/mL have lymphatic spread. Bone is the most common site of distant metastasis. Whitmore-Jewett staging includes A: tumor not palpable but detected at TURP; B: palpable tumor in one (B1) or both (B2) lobes; C: palpable tumor outside capsule; and D: metastatic disease.

℞ TREATMENT

For pts with stages A through C disease, surgery (radical retropubic prostatectomy) and radiation therapy are said to have similar outcomes; however, most pts are treated surgically. Both modalities are associated with impotence. Surgery is more likely to lead to incontinence. Radiation therapy is more likely to produce proctitis, perhaps with bleeding or stricture. Addition of radiation therapy, chemotherapy, or hormonal therapy to surgical treatment of stage A through C disease does not appear to improve results. Stage A pts have survival identical to age-matched controls without cancer. Stage B and C pts have a 10-year survival of 82% and 42%, respectively. For pts with metastatic disease, androgen deprivation is the treatment of choice. Surgical castration is effective, but most pts prefer to take leuprolide, 7.5 mg depot form IM monthly (to inhibit pituitary gonadotrophin production), plus flutamide, 250 mg PO tid (an androgen receptor blocker). Alternative approaches include adrenalectomy, hypophysectomy, estrogen administration, and medical adrenalectomy with aminoglutethimide. The median survival of stage D pts is 33 months. Pts occasionally respond to withdrawal of hormonal therapy with tumor shrinkage. Rarely a second hormonal manipulation will work, but most pts who progress on hormonal therapy have androgen-independent tumors, often associated with genetic changes in the androgen receptor and new expression of bcl-2, which may contribute to chemotherapy resistance. Chemotherapy is generally not useful in prostate cancer. Bone pain from metastases may be palliated with strontium-89.

For a more detailed discussion, see Sagalowsky AI, Wilson JD: Chap. 97, Hyperplasia and Carcinoma of the Prostate, p. 596, in HPIM-14.

64

CANCER OF UNKNOWN PRIMARY SITE

Cancer of unknown primary site (CUPS) is defined as follows: biopsy-proven malignancy; primary site unapparent after history, physical exam, CXR, abdominal and pelvic CT, CBC, chemistry survey, mammography (women), β human chorionic gonadotropin (hCG) levels (men), alpha-fetoprotein (AFP) levels (men), and prostate-specific antigen (PSA) levels (men); and histologic evaluation not consistent with a primary tumor at the biopsy site. CUPS incidence is declining, probably because of better pathology diagnostic criteria; they account for about 3% of all cancers today, down from 10–15% 10 years ago. Most pts are over age 60. Cell lines derived from such tumors frequently have abnormalities in chromosome 1.

CLINICAL PRESENTATION Pts may present with fatigue, weight loss, pain, bleeding, abdominal swelling, subcutaneous masses, and lymphadenopathy. Once metastatic malignancy is confirmed, diagnostic efforts should be confined to evaluating the presence of potentially curable tumors, such as lymphoma, Hodgkin's disease, germ cell tumor, ovarian cancer, head and neck cancer, and primitive neuroectodermal tumor, or tumors for which therapy may be of significant palliative value such as breast cancer or prostate cancer. In general, efforts to evaluate the presence of these tumor types depends more on the pathologist than on expensive clinical diagnostic testing. Localizing symptoms, a history of carcinogen exposure, or a history of fulguration of skin lesion may direct some clinical testing; however, the careful light microscopic, ultrastructural, immunologic, karyotypic, and molecular biologic examination of adequate volumes of tumor tissue is the most important feature of the diagnostic workup in the absence of suspicious findings on history and physical exam (see Table 64-1).

HISTOLOGY About 60% of CUPS tumors are adenocarcinomas, 10–20% are squamous cell carcinomas, and 20-30% are poorly differentiated neoplasms not further classified on light microscopy.

PROGNOSIS Pts with squamous cell carcinoma have a median survival of 9 months; those with adenocarcinoma or unclassifiable tumors have a median survival of 4-6 months. Pts in whom a primary site is identified usually have a better prognosis. Limited sites of involvement and neuroendocrine histology are favorable prognostic factors. Patients without a primary diagnosis should be treated palliatively with radiation therapy to symptomatic lesions. All-purpose chemotherapy regimens rarely pro-

Table 64-1

Possible Pathologic Evaluation of Biopsy Specimens from Patients with Metastatic Cancer of Unknown Primary Site

Evluation/Findings	Suggested Primary Site or Neoplasm
HISTOLOGY (HEMATOXYLIN AND EOSIN STAINING)	
Psammoma bodies, papillary configuration	Ovary, thyroid
Signet ring cells	Stomach
IMMUNOHISTOLOGY	
Leukocyte common antigen (LCA, CD45)	Lymphoid neoplasm
Leu-M1	Hodgkin's disease
Epithelial membrane antigen	Carcinoma
Cytokeratin intermediate filaments	Carcinoma
CEA	Carcinoma
HMB45	Melanoma
Desmin	Sarcoma
Thyroglobulin	Thyroid carcinoma
Calcitonin	Medullary carcinoma of the thyroid
Myoglobin	Rhabdomyosarcoma
PSA/prostatic acid phosphatase	Prostate
AFP	Liver, stomach, germ cell
Placental alkaline phosphatase	Germ cell
B, T cell markers	Lymphoid neoplasm
S-100 protein	Neuroendocrine tumor, melanoma
Gross cystic fluid protein	Breast, sweat gland
Factor VIII	Kaposi's sarcoma, angiosarcoma
FLOW CYTOMETRY	
B, T cell markers	Lymphoid neoplasm
ULTRASTRUCTURE	
Actin-myosin filaments	Rhabdomyosarcoma
Secretory granules	Neuroendocrine tumors
Desmosomes	Carcinoma
Premelanosomes	Melanoma

(*continued*)

Table 64-1 (*Continued*)

Possible Pathologic Evaluation of Biopsy Specimens from Patients with Metastatic Cancer of Unknown Primary Site

Evluation/Findings	Suggested Primary Site or Neoplasm
CYTOGENETICS	
Isochromosome 12p; 12q($-$)	Germ cell
t(11;22)	Ewing's sarcoma, primitive neuroectodermal tumor
t(8;14)*	Lymphoid neoplasm
3p($-$)	Small cell lung carcinoma; renal cell carcinoma, mesothelioma
t(X;18)	Synovial sarcoma
t(12;16)	Myxoid liposarcoma
t(12;22)	Clear cell sarcoma (melanoma of soft parts)
t(2;13)	Alveolar rhabdomyosarcoma
1p($-$)	Neuroblastoma
RECEPTOR ANALYSIS	
Estrogen/progesterone receptor	Breast
MOLECULAR BIOLOGIC STUDIES	
Immunoglobulin, *bcl-2*, T-cell receptor gene rearrangement	Lymphoid neoplasm

* Or any other rearrangement involving an antigen-receptor gene.

duce responses but always produce toxicity. Certain clinical features may permit individualized therapy.

Syndrome of Unrecognized Extragonadal Germ Cell Cancer

In pts < 50 years old with tumor involving midline structures, lung parenchyma, or lymph nodes and evidence of rapid tumor growth, germ cell tumor is a possible diagnosis. Serum tumor markers may or may not be elevated. Cisplatin, etoposide, and bleomycin (see Chap. 61) chemotherapy may induce complete responses in 25% or more, and about 15% may be cured. A trial of such therapy should probably also be undertaken in pts whose tumors have abnormalities in chromosome 12.

Peritoneal Carcinomatosis in Women

Women who present with pelvic mass or pain and an adenocarcinoma diffusely throughout the peritoneal cavity, but without a clear site of origin, have primary peritoneal papillary serous carcinoma. The presence of psammoma bodies in the tumor or elevated CA-125 levels may favor ovarian origin. Such pts should undergo debulking surgery followed by paclitaxel plus cisplatin combination chemotherapy (see Chap. 62). About 20% of pts will respond, and 10% will survive at least 2 years.

Carcinoma in an Axillary Lymph Node in Women

Such women should receive adjuvant breast cancer therapy appropriate for their menopausal status even in the absence of a breast mass on physical examination or mammography and undetermined or negative estrogen and progesterone receptors on the tumor (see Chap. 59). Unless the ipsilateral breast is radiated, up to 50% of these pts will later develop a breast mass. Although this is a rare clinical situation, long-term survival similar to women with stage II breast cancer is possible.

Osteoblastic Bone Metastases in Men

The probability of prostate cancer is high; a trial of empirical hormonal therapy (leuprolide and flutamide) is warranted (see Chap. 63).

Cervical Lymph Node Metastases

Even if panendoscopy fails to reveal a head and neck primary, treatment of such pts with cisplatin and 5-fluorouracil chemotherapy may produce a response; some responses are long-lived (see Chap. 57).

For a more detailed discussion, see Stone RM: Metastatic Cancer of Unknown Primary Site, Chap. 101, p. 614, in HPIM-14.

65

SARCOMAS OF BONE AND SOFT TISSUES

SOFT TISSUE SARCOMAS

INCIDENCE AND ETIOLOGY   About 6400 cases are diagnosed each year in the U.S. 60% arise in extremities, lower:upper = 3:1; 30% on the the trunk, often the retroperitoneum; 10% in the head and neck region. Although malignant nerve sheath tumors may develop from neurofibromas, nearly all other sarcomas arise de novo and are not malignant transformations of benign tumors. Sarcomas occur with increased frequency in persons who have undergone radiation therapy (usually within the treatment port), who are immunosuppressed (congenital or acquired), or who have been exposed to chemical carcinogens such as polycyclic hydrocarbons, asbestos, and dioxin. Sarcomas may rarely develop within a scar from a prior operation, burn, injury, or foreign body implantation. Kaposi's sarcoma is associated with human herpes virus 8 infection. Individuals with germline mutations in the p53 gene (Li-Fraumeni syndrome) are at increased risk for these and other malignancies. Those who have survived congenital retinoblastoma (germline mutations in the *Rb* gene) are at risk of developing sarcomas.

PATHOLOGY AND CLINICAL FEATURES   A common presentation is with an asymptomatic mass. Local symptoms may be related to pressure, traction, or entrapment of nerves. The tumor spreads hematogenously; lung is the most common site. About 20 different types of sarcomas are recognized, based upon the normal tissue from which they derive (e.g., fibrous tissue, skeletal muscle, smooth muscle, blood vessels, fat). Diagnosis is based upon an incisional biopsy placed so that it can be encompassed by a subsequent definitive surgical procedure. Imaging of the primary tumor is best with plain radiographs and MRI for extremity or head and neck lesions and by CT for truncal primaries.

STAGING   The only routine staging test is the CXR. Other tests should be done only when indicated by signs and symptoms. Two staging systems exist: American Joint Commission on Cancer (AJCC) and Musculoskeletal Tumor Society. Both are predominantly based upon the histologic grade of the tumor. The AJCC system classifies grade 1 (well differentiated) tumors as stage I, grade 2 (intermediate differentiation) as stage II, and grade 3 (poorly differentiated) as stage III. Tumors are also classified on the basis of size: A, <5cm; B, ≥5cm. Pts with metastatic disease are stage IV. Prognosis is related to stage:

75% 5-year survival for stage I; 55% for stage II; 29% for stage III; <20% for stage IV.

℞ TREATMENT

Radical excision with documented histologic negative margins is the treatment of choice. Although some histologies behave differently (e.g., chondrosarcoma and GI leiomyosarcomas are refractory to chemotherapy), soft tissue sarcomas are generally lumped together for treatment. Adjuvant radiation therapy and/or chemotherapy improve local control and permit the use of a limb-sparing surgical procedure. Several doxorubicin-based combination chemotherapy programs are similar in efficacy and improve disease-free survival. Impact on overall survival is less consistent. Combination chemotherapy with doxorubicin and ifosfamide is used in the setting of metastatic disease and may cure 10–15% of pts.

BONE SARCOMAS

INCIDENCE AND ETIOLOGY   Multiple myeloma is the most common neoplasm of bone (see Chap 55). Osteosarcoma, chondrosarcoma, Ewing's sarcoma, and malignant fibrous histiocytoma are the major sarcomas involving bone. About 2500 new cases occur each year. Benign bone tumors such as enchondromas and osteochondromas may transform into chondrosarcoma, and fibrous dysplasia and Paget's disease of bone may transform into osteosarcoma or malignant fibrous histiocytoma.

OSTEOSARCOMA   Osteosarcoma accounts for about 45% of bone sarcomas; 60% of osteosarcomas occur in children and adolescents. Males are affected 1.5–2 times more frequently than females. Osteosarcoma has a predilection for the metaphyses of long bones, especially the distal femur and proximal tibia and humerus. Malignant fibrous histiocytoma is considered part of the spectrum of osteosarcoma. Pts present with pain and swelling of the affected area. Plain radiograph reveals a destructive lesion with a "moth-eaten" appearance, a spiculated periosteal reaction ("sunburst" appearance), and a cuff of periosteal new bone formation at the margin of the soft tissue mass (known as Codman's triangle). It spreads hematogenously to the lungs. The most important prognostic factor is response to chemotherapy. Preoperative chemotherapy with doxorubicin, ifosfamide, cisplatin, and high-dose methotrexate followed by limb-sparing surgery and postoperative chemotherapy is the standard treatment approach. The disease is radioresistant. Long-term survival of extremity primaries is 60–70%. Resection of pulmonary metastases may lead to long-term survival in pts with metastatic disease.

CHONDROSARCOMA Chondrosarcoma accounts for about 25% of bone sarcomas; peak incidence is in the fourth to sixth decades of life. It has a predilection for flat bones, especially the shoulder and pelvis. The disease has an indolent natural history, presenting with pain and swelling. On radiography, lesions may appear lobular with mottled, punctate, or annular calcification. Chondrosarcomas are difficult to distinguish from benign cartilage tumors radiographically; clinical signs of progressive tumor growth and inflammation favor the malignant diagnosis. This neoplasm is resistant to chemotherapy. Surgery is the treatment of choice.

EWING'S SARCOMA Ewing's sarcoma comprises 10–15% of bone sarcomas; peak incidence is in teenagers. It has a predilection for the diaphyses of long bones and for flat bones. Radiographs show a characteristic "onion peel" periosteal reaction with a soft tissue mass. The tumor consists of sheets of small, round, blue-staining cells that may be confused with lymphoma, small cell lung cancer, or embryonal rhabdomyosarcoma. The diagnosis is confirmed by detecting p30/32, the product of the *mic-2* gene on the cell surface. Ewing's sarcoma is a member of a family of tumors called *peripheral primitive neuroectodermal tumors* (PNETs), most of which occur in soft tissues. The characteristic chromosomal translocation associated with PNETs including Ewing's sarcoma is t(11;22), which creates a chimeric gene product with components from the *fli-1* gene on chromosome 11 and *ews* on 22. The disease commonly spreads to lungs, other bones, and bone marrow. Systemic chemotherapy with doxorubicin, ifosfamide, etoposide, and vincristine is effective treatment and usually employed before limb-sparing surgery. Peripheral primary lesions (below the elbow and mid-calf) have a 5-year survival of 80%. Even with metastatic disease, 25–40% are curable with high-dose therapy and stem cell transplantation.

For a more detailed discussion, see Patel SR, Benjamin RS: Sarcomas of Soft Tissue and Bone, Chap. 100, p. 611, in HPIM-14.

PARANEOPLASTIC SYNDROMES

ENDOCRINE SYNDROMES

Both benign and malignant tumors of nonendocrine tissue can secrete a variety of hormones, principally peptide hormones, and many tumors produce more than one hormone (Table 66-1). At the clinical level, ectopic hormone production is important for two reasons.

First, endocrine syndromes that result may either be the presenting manifestations of the neoplasm or occur late in the course. The endocrine manifestations in some instances are of greater significance than the tumor itself, as in patients with benign or slowly growing malignancies that secrete corticotropin-releasing hormone and cause fulminant Cushing's syndrome. The frequency with which ectopic hormone production is recognized varies with the criteria used for diagnosis. The most common syndromes of clinical import are those of ACTH hypersecretion, hypercalcemia, and hypoglycemia. Indeed, ectopic ACTH secretion is responsible for 15–20% of pts with Cushing's syndrome, and approximately half of pts with persistent hypercalcemia have a malignancy rather than hyperparathyroidism. Because of the rapidity of development of hormone secretion in some rapidly growing tumors, diagnosis may require a high index of suspicion, and hormone levels may be elevated out of proportion to the manifestations.

Second, ectopic hormones serve as valuable peripheral markers for neoplasia. Because of the broad spectrum of ectopic hormone secretion, screening measurements of plasma hormone levels for diagnostic purposes are not cost-effective. However, in pts with malignancies that are known to secrete hormones, serial measurements of circulating hormone levels can serve as markers for completeness of tumor excision and for effectiveness of radiation or chemotherapy. Likewise, tumor recurrence may be heralded by reappearance of elevated plasma hormone levels before mass effects of the tumor are evident. However, some tumors at recurrence do not secrete hormones, so that hormone measurements cannot be relied on as the sole evidence of tumor activity.

 TREATMENT

Therapy of ectopic hormone-secreting tumors should be directed when possible toward removal of the tumor. When the tumor cannot be removed or is incurable, specific therapy can be directed toward inhibiting hormone secretion (octreotide

Table 66-1

Common Paraneoplastic Endocrine Syndromes

Syndrome	Proteins	Tumors Typically Associated with Syndrome
Hypercalcemia of malignancy	Parathyroid hormone-related peptide (PTHrP) Parathyroid hormone (PTH)	Non-small cell lung cancer Breast cancer Renal cell carcinoma Head and neck cancer Bladder cancer Myeloma
Syndrome of inappropriate vasopressin secretion (SIADH)	Arginine vasopressin (AVP) Atrial natriuretic peptide	Small cell lung cancer Head and neck cancer Non-small cell lung cancer
Cushing's syndrome	Adrenocorticotropic hormone (ACTH) Corticotropin-releasing hormone (CRH)	Small cell lung cancer Carcinoid tumors
Acromegaly	Growth hormone–releasing hormone (GHRH) Growth hormone (GH)	Carcinoid Small cell lung cancer Pancreatic islet cell tumors
Gynecomastia	Human chorionic gonadotropin (hCG)	Testicular cancer Lung cancer Carcinoid tumors of the lung and gastrointestinal tract
Non-islet cell tumor hypoglycemia	Insulin-like growth factor-2 (IGF-2)	Sarcomas

for ectopic acromegaly or mitotane to inhibit adrenal steroidogenesis in the ectopic ACTH syndrome) or blocking the action of the hormone at the tissue level (demeclocycline for inappropriate vasopressin secretion).

Hypercalcemia

The most common paraneoplastic syndrome, hypercalcemia of malignancy accounts for 40% of all hypercalcemia. 80% of cancer pts with hypercalcemia have humoral hypercalcemia mediated by parathyroid hormone–related peptide; 20% have local osteolytic hypercalcemia mediated by cytokines such as interleukin and tumor necrosis factor. Many tumor types may produce hypercalcemia (Table 66-1). Pts may have malaise, fatigue, confusion, anorexia, bone pain, polyuria, weakness, constipation, nausea, and vomiting. At high calcium levels, confusion, lethargy, coma, and death may ensue. Median survival of hypercalcemic cancer pts is 1–3 months. Treatment with saline hydration, furosemide diuresis, and pamidronate (60–90 mg IV) controls calcium levels within 7 days in 80% of cases.

Hyponatremia

Most commonly discovered in asymptomatic individuals as a result of serum electrolyte measurements, hyponatremia is usually due to tumor secretion of arginine vasopressin and is called syndrome of inappropriate antidiuretic hormone (SIADH). Atrial natriuretic hormone may also produce hyponatremia. SIADH occurs most commonly in small cell lung cancer (15%) and head and neck cancer (3%). A number of drugs may produce the syndrome. Symptoms of fatigue, poor attention span, nausea, weakness, anorexia, and headache may be controlled by restricting fluid intake to 500 mL/d or blocking the effects of the hormone with 600–1200 mg demeclocycline a day.

Ectopic ACTH Syndrome

When pro-opiomelanocortin mRNA in the tumor is processed into ACTH, excessive secretion of glucocorticoids and mineralocorticoids may ensue. Pts develop Cushing's syndrome with hypokalemic alkalosis, weakness, hypertension, and hyperglycemia. About half the cases occur in small cell lung cancer. ACTH production adversely affects prognosis. Ketoconazole (400–1200 mg/d) or metyrapone (1–4 g/d) may be used to inhibit adrenal steroid synthesis.

For a more detailed discussion, see Johnson BE: Paraneoplastic Syndromes, Chap. 102, p. 618, in HPIM-14.

67

NEUROLOGIC MANIFESTATIONS OF SYSTEMIC NEOPLASIA

Varied neurologic disorders occur in pts with systemic neoplasia (Table 67-1). Paraneoplastic syndromes are those related to a remotely located neoplasm; they often evolve over days to weeks and may precede detection of neoplasm by months or even years. Recognition of a distinctive paraneoplastic syndrome should prompt a search for cancer, although these disorders also occur without cancer (idiopathic). Diagnosis is based upon the clinical pattern (Table 67-2), exclusion of other cancer-related disorders, confirmatory serum or CSF antibodies (Table 67-3), or electrodiagnostic testing. Tumors most often associated are cancers of lung, stomach, breast, ovary, colon, but neurologic disorders occur with 1 in 6 ovarian tumors and 1 in 7 lung tumors. One postulated mechanism is an autoimmune response directed against common antigenic determinants expressed by tumor and neural cells; demonstrated in Lambert-Eaton myasthenic syndrome (antibodies to presynaptic calcium channels and associated proteins) and myasthenia gravis (antibodies to postsynaptic acetylcholine receptors). Known auto-

Table 67-1

Effects of Malignancy on the Nervous System

Direct invasion
Metastatic invasion
  Parenchymatous
  Vascular neoplastic angioendotheliosis
  Meningeal (meningeal carcinomatosis)
Opportunistic infections
  Bacterial (e.g., listeriosis)
  Nonbacterial
    Typical and atypical viral (e.g., progressive multifo-
      cal leukoencephalopathy)
    Fungal (e.g., cryptococcosis)
Complications of antineoplastic therapy
  Complications of radiation therapy (e.g., radiation
    necrosis)
  Complications of chemotherapy (e.g., vincristine
    neuropathy)
Metabolic complications
  Nutritional deficiency
  Ectopic hormone production
Paraneoplastic syndromes

Table 67-2

Paraneoplastic Neurologic Syndromes

Site	Evolution	Clinical Features
BRAIN, BRAINSTEM, CEREBELLUM		
Photoreceptor retinal degeneration	Weeks to months	Painless visual loss, progressing to blindness
Limbic encephalitis	Weeks to months	Agitated, confusional state, memory loss followed by dementia
Brainstem encephalitis	Days to weeks	Nystagmus, diplopia, vertigo, ataxia, dysarthria, dysphagia
Subacute cortical cerebellar degeneration	Weeks to months	Cerebellar ataxia, dysarthria
Opsoclonus-myoclonus	Weeks	Dancing eyes and feet, cerebellar ataxia, and possibly encephalopathy in adults
SPINAL CORD		
Necrotizing myelopathy	Hours, days, or weeks	Para- or quadriplegia, areflexia, sensory loss, bladder dysfunction
Subacute motor neuropathy	Weeks or months	Flaccid weakness and muscle atrophy; legs affected > arms
PERIPHERAL NERVE		
Acute demyelinating polyneuropathy (Guillain-Barré syndrome)	Hours to days	Ascending paralysis, areflexia, ascending sensory loss, high spinal fluid protein
Chronic demyelinating polyneuropathy	Weeks to months	Chronic progressive or relapsing weakness, sensory loss, elevated spinal fluid protein
Neuropathy with paraproteinemia	Weeks to months	Chronic; sensory or motor
Subacute sensory neuronopathy	Weeks to months	Severe sensory loss, areflexia, ataxia; paresthesia, pain

Cancer	Pathology
SCLC, rarely cervical cancer	Loss of rods and cones, infiltration of retina with mononuclear cells
SCLC	Neuronal loss in medial temporal lobe and limbic system; perivascular and meningeal lymphocytic infiltration
SCLC	Neuronal loss in brainstem, inflammatory
SCLC; ovarian, breast cancer; Hodgkin's disease	Loss of Purkinje cells
Neuroblastoma, bronchial carcinoma	In adults, degeneration of dentate nuclei
SCLC, lymphoma	Severe necrosis of gray and white matter
Non-Hodgkin's lymphoma	Inflammation of ventral horns, loss of anterior horn cells
Hodgkin's disease	Segmental demyelination, inflammation of peripheral nerves
Lymphoma, myeloma; rarely lung, breast, or gastric cancer	As in acute demyelinating polyneuropathy
Myeloma, osteosclerotic myeloma	As in acute demyelinating polyneuropathy
SCLC and other lung tumors	Inflammation and neuronal degeneration in dorsal root ganglia; secondary axon loss

(*continued*)

Table 67-2 (*Continued*)

Paraneoplastic Neurologic Syndromes

Site	Evolution	Clinical Features
Sensorimotor neuropathy	Weeks to months	Distal motor and sensory loss
NEUROMUSCULAR JUNCTION		
Lambert-Eaton myasthenic syndrome	Weeks to months	Proximal weakness, fatigability, dry mouth
Myasthenia gravis	Weeks to months	Weakness, fatigability, ptosis, diplopia
MUSCLE		
Polymyositis	Months to years	Proximal weakness, myalgias, high CPK, cardiomyopathy
Necrotizing myopathy	Days to weeks	Rapidly progressive proximal weakness, +/− dysphagia, dyspnea

antibodies are associated with a number of paraneoplastic syndromes (Table 67-3). Treatment is difficult, usually unsuccessful. Resection of underlying tumor is usually ineffective, but isolated reports of improvement exist. Immunosuppression is generally without benefit, although plasma exchange or immunosuppression has been used successfully to treat Lambert-Eaton syndrome or myasthenia gravis.

Cancer	Pathology
SCLC	Axonopathy, some segmental loss of myelin
SCLC; breast, prostate, stomach cancer	Disruption of active zones on pre-synaptic terminals
Thymoma	Disruption of postsynaptic junctional membrane folds
Association with breast, ovary, lung, tumors; lymphoma	Lymphocytic inflammation of muscle interstitium; myofiber necrosis, phagocytosis
Bronchial carcinoma, SCLC	Severe myonecrosis with minimal inflammation or phagocytosis

NOTE: SCLC, small cell lung carcinoma.

Table 67-3

Defined Antibodies Associated with Paraneoplastic Neurologic Syndromes*

Antibody	Paraneoplastic Syndrome	Tumor	Antigen
Anti-CAR	Retinopathy	SCLC	Recoverin, 25-kDa cone Ca^{2+} binding protein
Anti-Hu	Encephalo-myelitis, sensory neu-ronopathy	Mainly SCLC	35- to 40-kDa nuclear RNA-binding pro-teins
Anti-Yo	Cerebellar de-generation	Gyneco-logic tumors, breast cancer	34- and 62-kDa leucine zipper proteins
Anti-Ri	Opsoclonus-myoclonus	Breast cancer	55-kDa RNA-binding pro-tein in motor system neurons
Anti-MAG	Demyelinat-ing neu-ropathy	Myeloma	Myelin-associated glycoprotein
LEMS Ab	Lambert-Eaton myasthenic syndrome	SCLC	Voltage-sensitive calcium channel and associated proteins
MG Ab	Myasthenia gravis	Thymoma	Acetylcholine receptor subunit

* Other patterns of reactivity have also been described for some of these antigens.
NOTE: SCLC, small cell lung carcinoma.

For a more detailed discussion, see Johnson BE: Paraneoplastic Neurologic Syndromes, Chap. 103, p. 622, in HPIM-14.

68

DIAGNOSIS

The laboratory diagnosis of infection requires the demonstration, either directly or indirectly, of viral, bacterial, mycotic, or parasitic agents of disease in tissues, fluids, or excreta of the host. The traditional detection methods of microscopy and/or culture are increasingly being complemented by more rapid and sensitive techniques, including serology, nucleic acid probing, and polymerase chain reaction (PCR).

DIRECT DETECTION

MICROSCOPY *Wet Mounts* The wet mount is the simplest method for microscopic evaluation, involving no fixation of the specimen prior to examination. In general, it is used for certain large and/or motile organisms that can be visualized without staining. Wet mounts of duodenal aspirates may show pathogenic protozoans (e.g., giardial trophozoites), while mounts of fresh stool may reveal protozoans or helminths (e.g., amebic cysts, *Strongyloides* larvae, ascarid or schistosome eggs). Mounts of fresh blood may reveal microfilariae (in brugian or bancroftian filariasis or loiasis) or spirochetes (in relapsing fever). Motile trichomonads may be found in cervical secretions. Wet mounts with dark-field illumination are used to detect *Treponema* in spirochetal genital lesions. To detect fungal elements in skin scrapings or hair, 10% KOH preparations may be used. For certain wet-mount applications, staining is used to enhance detection or visualization of morphologic elements (e.g., India ink to visualize encapsulated cryptococci in CSF, lactophenol cotton blue for fungal speciation).

Gram's Stain Gram's stain enhances detection of bacteria and polymorphonuclear leukocytes (PMNs) and differentiates bacteria with thick peptidoglycan cell walls (gram-positive; purple) from those with alcohol- or acetone-labile outer membranes (gram-negative; pink). In a properly decolorized slide, the nuclei of PMNs appear pink. Purulent respiratory secretions will have >25 PMNs and <10 epithelial cells per low-power field; the presence of >10 epithelial cells per low-power field reflects contamination of the specimen by saliva. A bacterial content of >10^4/mL in a specimen from a normally sterile site should be detectable by Gram's stain. Specimens may be concentrated by centrifugation to promote the detection of rare organisms.

Acid-Fast Stain The acid-fast stains detect organisms, such as *Mycobacterium* spp., that are capable of retaining carbol fuchsin dye after acid/organic solvation (e.g., 3% HCl in 95% ethanol). The modified acid-fast stains detect weakly acid-fast organisms, such as *Nocardia* and *Cryptosporidium,* which retain the dye on treatment with dilute acid (e.g., 1% HCl) but not acid-alcohol. Acid-fast organisms appear pink or red against the blue background of the counterstain. Because mycobacteria may be sparse in clinical specimens, the more sensitive auramine-rhodamine combination fluorescent dye technique was developed.

Other Stains for Light Microscopy Giemsa or Wright's stain of peripheral blood may reveal certain bacteria and intra- or extracellular parasites (e.g., *Borrelia recurrentis, Plasmodium, Babesia,* or *Trypanosoma*). Other commonly used stains include toluidine blue (for *Pneumocystis carinii*) and methenamine silver (for *P. carinii* and for fungal hyphae in tissue sections).

Immunofluorescent Stains Immunofluorescent stains can be used to detect viruses within cultured cells or tissue specimens (e.g., herpesviruses, rabies virus) or to reveal difficult-to-grow bacterial agents within clinical specimens (e.g., *Legionella pneumophila*). Direct immunofluorescent antibody (DFA) stains use antibodies directed at the agent of interest coupled to a fluorescent compound such as fluorescein, which directly labels the target. Indirect immunofluorescent antibody (IFA) stains use an unlabeled primary antibody to the target antigen followed by a labeled secondary antibody to the primary antibody. Since a single primary antibody molecule is bound by many secondary antibody molecules, the fluorescent signal is amplified with the indirect approach. In either case, the stained specimen is examined under UV light, and visible light is emitted.

OTHER METHODS ***Macroscopic Antigen Detection*** Latex agglutination assays and enzyme immunoassays (EIAs) are rapid and inexpensive methods for identifying bacteria, viruses, or extracellular bacterial toxins by means of their protein or polysaccharide antigens. These assays can be performed either directly on clinical specimens, or after growth of organisms in the laboratory. Conditions that may be diagnosed by these means include cryptococcosis, histoplasmosis, legionellosis, hepatitis B and D, and HIV infection.

Detection of Nucleic Acids Techniques to detect pathogen-specific DNA or RNA sequences in clinical specimens have become powerful tools for microbiologic diagnosis. All such techniques capitalize on the great specificity of Watson-Crick base pairing. Probes are available to detect a number of pathogens directly in clinical specimens (e.g., *L. pneumophila, C. trachomatis, N. gonorrhoeae,* group A *Streptococcus, G. vaginalis, T. vaginalis,* and *Candida* spp.). Other probes are available for confirmation of culture results. The sensitivity and specificity of probe assays are comparable to those of culture or EIA. Nucleic acid amplification strategies have also entered the clinical arena. PCR is the best known of these and is far more sensitive than traditional detection methods. It is, however, susceptible to false-positives from even low levels of contamination. Amplification assays are currently available to detect *M. tuberculosis* and *C. trachomatis.*

DETECTION BY CULTURE

The success or failure of efforts to culture bacterial, mycotic, or viral pathogens depends critically on the nature of the sample provided and the means by which it is collected and transported. Table 68-1 lists procedures for collection and transport of common clinical specimens. Physicians in doubt about the procedure appropriate for a particular situation should seek advice from the microbiology laboratory before obtaining the specimen.

DETECTION BY SEROLOGIC METHODS

Measurement of serum antibody to a specific agent provides indirect evidence of past or current infection. Serologic methods are used to detect many viral infections and have applications in other areas of microbiologic diagnosis as well. Detection systems include agglutination reactions, immunofluorescence, EIA, hemagglutination inhibition, and complement fixation. Serologic methods may be used to establish the existence of immunity by documenting that antibody quantity exceeds the protective level (e.g., for rubella, rubeola, or varicella-zoster virus) or to detect current infection by demonstrating a rise in antibody titer between acute- and convalescent-phase samples collected 10–14 d apart (e.g., for arboviral infections, brucellosis, legionellosis, or ehrlichiosis).

Table 68-1

Instructions for Collection and Transport of Specimens

Type of Culture (Synonyms)	Specimen	Minimum Volume
BLOOD		
Blood, routine (blood culture for aerobes, anaerobes, and yeasts)	Whole blood	10 mL in each of 2 bottles for adults and children; 5 mL, if possible, in each of 2 bottles for infants; less for neonates
Blood for fungi/ *Mycobacterium* spp.	Whole blood	10 mL in each of 2 bottles, as for routine blood cultures, or in Isolator tube requested from laboratory
Blood, Isolator (lysis centrifugation)	Whole blood	10 mL
RESPIRATORY TRACT		
Nose	Swab from nares	1 swab
Throat	Swab of posterior pharynx, ulcerations, or areas of suspected purulence	1 swab
Sputum	Fresh sputum (not saliva)	2 mL

for Culture

Container	Other Considerations
See below.[a]	See below.[b]
Same as for routine blood culture	Specify "hold for extended incubation," since fungal agents may require 4 weeks or more to grow.
Isolator tubes	Use mainly for isolation of fungi, *Mycobacterium,* or other fastidious aerobes and for elimination of antibiotics from cultured blood in which organisms are concentrated by centrifugation.
Sterile culturette or similar transport system containing holding medium	Swabs made of calcium alginate may be used.
Sterile culturette or similar swab specimen collection system containing holding medium	See below.[c]
Commercially available sputum collection system or similar sterile container with screw cap	*Cause for rejection:* Care must be taken to ensure that the specimen is sputum and not saliva. Examination of Gram's stain, with number of epithelial cells and PMNs noted, can be an important part of the evaluation process. Induced sputum specimens should not be rejected.

(*continued*)

Table 68-1 (*Continued*)

Instructions for Collection and Transport of Specimens

Type of Culture (Synonyms)	Specimen	Minimum Volume
Bronchial aspirates	Transtracheal aspirate, bronchoscopy specimen, or bronchial aspirate	1 mL of aspirate or brush in transport medium

STOOL

Stool for routine culture; stool for *Salmonella, Shigella,* and *Campylobacter*	Rectal swab or (preferably) fresh, randomly collected stool	1 g of stool or 2 rectal swabs
Stool for *Yersinia, E. coli* O157	Fresh, randomly collected stool	1 g
Stool for *Aeromonas* and *Plesiomonas*	Fresh, randomly collected stool	1 g

UROGENITAL TRACT

Urine	Clean-voided urine specimen or urine collected by catheter	0.5 mL
Urogenital secretions	Vaginal or urethral secretions, cervical swabs, uterine fluid, prostatic fluid, etc.	1 swab or 0.5 mL of fluid

BODY FLUIDS, ASPIRATES, AND TISSUES

Cerebrospinal fluid (lumbar puncture)	Spinal fluid	1 mL for routine cultures; ≥5 mL for *Mycobacterium*
Body fluids	Aseptically aspirated body fluids	1 mL for routine cultures

for Culture

Container	Other Considerations
Sterile aspirate or bronchoscopy tube, bronchoscopy brush in a separate sterile container	Special precautions may be required, depending on diagnostic considerations (e.g., *Pneumocystis*).
Plastic-coated cardboard cup or plastic cup with tight-fitting lid. Other leak-proof containers are also acceptable.	If *Vibrio* spp. are suspected, the laboratory must be notified, and appropriate collection/transport methods should be used.
Plastic-coated cardboard cup or plastic cup with tight-fitting lid	*Limitations:* Procedure requires enrichment techniques.
Plastic-coated cardboard cup or plastic cup with tight-fitting lid	*Limitations:* Stool should not be cultured for these organisms unless also cultured for other enteric pathogens.
Sterile, leak-proof container with screw cap or special urine transfer tube	See below.[d]
Transwab containing Amies transport medium or similar system containing holding medium for *Neisseria gonorrhoeae;* modified Todd-Hewitt broth for group B *Streptococcus* surveillance cultures	Vaginal swab samples for "routine culture" should be discouraged whenever possible unless a particular pathogen is suspected. For detection of multiple organisms (e.g., group B *Streptococcus, Trichomonas, Chlamydia,* or *Candida* spp.), 1 swab per test should be obtained.
Sterile tube with tight-fitting cap	Do not refrigerate; transfer to laboratory as soon as possible.
Sterile tube with tight-fitting cap. Specimen may be left in syringe used for collection if the syringe is capped before transport.	For some body fluids (e.g., peritoneal lavage samples), increased volumes enhance detection of rare bacteria.

(continued)

Table 68-1 (*Continued*)

Instructions for Collection and Transport of Specimens

Type of Culture (Synonyms)	Specimen	Minimum Volume
Biopsy and aspirated materials	Tissue removed at surgery, bone, anticoagulated bone marrow, biopsy samples, or other specimens from normally sterile areas	1 mL of fluid or a 1-g piece of tissue
Wounds	Purulent material or abscess contents obtained from wound or abscess without contamination by normal microflora	2 swabs or 0.5 mL of aspirated pus

SPECIAL RECOMMENDATIONS

Fungi	Specimen types listed above may be used. When urine or sputum is cultured for fungi, a first morning specimen is usually preferred.	1 mL or as specified above for individual listing of specimens. Large volumes may be useful for urinary fungi.
Mycobacterium (acid-fast bacilli)	Sputum, tissue, urine, body fluids	10 mL of fluid or small piece of tissue. Swabs should not be used.
Legionella	Pleural fluid, lung biopsy, bronchoalveolar lavage fluid, bronchial/ transbronchial biopsy. Rapid transport to laboratory is critical.	1 mL of fluid; any size tissue sample, although a 0.5-g sample should be obtained when possible

Container	Other Considerations
Sterile ''culturette''-type swab or similar transport system containing holding medium. Sterile bottle or jar should be used for tissue specimens.	Accurate identification of specimen and source is critical. Enough tissue should be collected for both microbiologic and histopathologic evaluations.
Culturette swab or similar transport system or sterile tube with tight-fitting screw cap. For simultaneous anaerobic cultures, send specimen in anaerobic transport device or closed syringe.	*Collection:* Abscess contents or other fluids should be collected in a syringe (see above) when possible to provide an adequate sample volume and an anaerobic environment.
Sterile, leak-proof container with tight-fitting cap	*Collection:* Specimen should be transported to microbiology laboratory within 1 h of collection. Contamination with normal flora from skin, rectum, vaginal tract, or other body surfaces should be avoided.
Sterile container with tight-fitting cap	Detection of *Mycobacterium* spp. is improved by use of concentration techniques. Smears and cultures of pleural, peritoneal, and pericardial fluids often have low yields. Multiple cultures from the same patient are encouraged. Culturing in liquid media shortens the time to detection.
—	

(*continued*)

Table 68-1 (*Continued*)

Instructions for Collection and Transport of Specimens

Type of Culture (Synonyms)	Specimen	Minimum Volume
Anaerobic organisms	Aspirated specimens from abscesses or body fluids	1 mL of aspirated fluid or 2 swabs
Viruses[f]	Respiratory secretions, wash aspirates from respiratory tract, nasal swabs, blood samples (including buffy coats), vaginal and rectal swabs, swab specimens from suspicious skin lesions, stool samples (in some cases)	1 mL of fluid, 1 swab, or 1 g of stool in each appropriate transport medium

[a]For samples from adults and children, two bottles (smaller for pediatric samples) should be used; one with dextrose phosphate, tryptic soy, or another appropriate broth and the other with thioglycollate or another broth containing reducing agents appropriate for isolation of obligate anaerobes. For special situations (e.g., suspected fungal infection, culture-negative endocarditis, or mycobacteremia), different blood collection systems may be used (Isolator systems; see table).

[b]*Collection:* An appropriate disinfecting technique should be used on both the bottle septum and the patient. Do not allow air bubbles to get into anaerobic broth bottles. *Special considerations:* There is no more important clinical microbiology test than the detection of blood-borne pathogens. The rapid identification of bacterial and fungal agents is a major determinant of patients' survival. Bacteria may be present in blood either continuously (as in endocarditis, overwhelming sepsis, and the early stages of salmonellosis and brucellosis) or intermittently (as in most other bacterial infections, in which bacteria are shed into the blood on a sporadic basis). Most blood culture systems employ two separate bottles containing broth medium: one that is vented in the laboratory for the growth of facultative and aerobic organisms and a second that is maintained under anaerobic conditions. In cases of suspected continuous bacteremia/fungemia, two or three samples should be drawn before the start of therapy, with additional sets obtained if fastidious organisms are thought to be involved. For intermittent bacteremia, two or three samples should be obtained at least 1 h apart during the first 24 h.

[c]Normal microflora includes alpha-hemolytic streptococci, saprophytic *Neisseria* spp., diphtheroids, and *Staphylococcus* spp. Aerobic culture of the throat ("routine") includes screening for and identification of beta-hemolytic *Streptococcus* spp. and other potentially pathogenic organisms. Although considered components of the normal microflora, organisms such as *Staphylococcus aureus, Haemophilus*

for Culture

for Container	Other Considerations
An appropriate anaerobic transport device is required.[e]	Specimens cultured for obligate anaerobes should be cultured for facultative bacteria as well.
Fluid or stool samples in sterile containers or swab samples in viral culturette devices (kept on ice but not frozen) are generally suitable. Plasma samples and buffy coats in sterile collection tubes should be kept at 4 to 8°C. If specimens are to be shipped or kept for a long time, freezing at −80°C is usually adequate.	Most samples for culture are transported in holding medium containing antibiotics to prevent bacterial overgrowth and viral inactivation. Many specimens should be kept cool but not frozen, provided they are transported promptly to the laboratory. Procedures and transport media vary with the agent to be cultured and the duration of transport.

influenzae, and *Streptococcus pneumoniae* will be identified by most laboratories, if requested. When *Neisseria gonorrhoeae* or *Corynebacterium diphtheriae* is suspected, a special culture request is recommended.

[d](1) Clean-voided specimens, midvoid specimens, and Foley or indwelling catheter specimens that yield ≥50,000 organisms/mL and from which no more than three species are isolated should have organisms identified. (2) Straight-catheterized, bladder-tap, and similar urine specimens should undergo a complete workup (identification and susceptibility testing) for all potentially pathogenic organisms, regardless of colony count. (3) Certain clinical problems (e.g., acute dysuria in women) may warrant identification and susceptibility testing of isolates present at concentrations of <50,000 organisms/mL.

[e]Aspirated specimens in capped syringes or other transport devices designed to limit oxygen exposure are suitable for the cultivation of obligate anaerobes. A variety of commercially available transport devices may be used. Contamination of specimens with normal microflora from the skin, rectum, vaginal vault, or another body site should be avoided. Collection containers for aerobic culture (such as dry swabs) and inappropriate specimens (such as refrigerated samples; expectorated sputum; stool; gastric aspirates; and vaginal, throat, nose, and rectal swabs) should be rejected as unsuitable.

[f] Laboratories generally use diverse methods to detect viral agents, and the specific requirements for each specimen should be checked before a sample is sent.

SOURCE: Appendix B, HPIM-14, p. A-9.

For a more detailed discussion, see Onderdonk AB: Laboratory Diagnosis of Infectious Diseases, Chap. 121, p. 754, in HPIM-14.

69

ANTIMICROBIAL THERAPY

Antimicrobial agents represent one of the twentieth century's major contributions to human longevity and quality of life. They are among the most commonly prescribed drugs and may be lifesaving. Used inappropriately, however, they can drive up the cost of health care, cause drug interactions and other adverse events, and foster the emergence of resistant pathogens.

Adherence to several guiding principles will promote the most effective use of antimicrobial agents. (1) Whenever possible, material for diagnostic purposes (culture, stains, and special studies) should be obtained before the initiation of therapy so that the pathogen can be identified and its antimicrobial susceptibility determined; (2) once the pathogen and its susceptibility are known, the antimicrobial therapy chosen should have the narrowest possible spectrum so that the emergence of resistance and the perturbation of the normal flora are minimized; (3) the choice of antimicrobial agent should be guided by the pharmacokinetic and adverse-reaction profile of active compounds, the site of infection, the immune status of the host, and evidence of efficacy from appropriate, well-designed clinical trials; and (4) if other factors are equal, the least expensive regimen should be used.

ANTIBACTERIAL THERAPY
See Table 69-1.

ANTIVIRAL THERAPY
See Chaps. 94 through 99.

ANTIFUNGAL THERAPY
See Chap. 100.

DRUGS FOR PARASITIC INFECTIONS
See Chaps. 102 and 103.

For a more detailed discussion, see Archer GL, Polk RE: Treatment and Prophylaxis of Bacterial Infections, Chap. 140, p. 856; Wright PW, Wallace RJ Jr: Antimycobacterial Agents, Chap. 170, p. 997; Dolin R: Antiviral Chemotherapy, Chap. 183, p. 1072; Bennett JE: Diagnosis and Treatment of Fungal Infections, Chap. 202, p. 1148; and Liu LX, Weller PF: Therapy for Parasitic Infections, Chap. 214, p. 1171, in HPIM-14.

Table 69-1

Major Antibacterial Agents

Drug	Organisms	Dosage Range	Routes of Administration	Dose Reduction for Renal Insufficiency	Major Toxicities
PENICILLINS					
Penicillin G	*Streptococcus, Listeria, Neisseria meningitidis, Actinomyces, Clostridium* (but not *difficile*), *Treponema pallidum*	1,200,000 to 24,000,000 U/d IV divided q4h	IV, IM	Moderate	Hypersensitivity (rash, fever, anaphylaxis 1:10,000)
Penicillin V	*Streptococcus*	0.25–0.5 g qid	PO	None	Same as penicillin G
Oxacillin	*Staphylococcus aureus* [but not methicillin-resistant strains (MRSA)], *Streptococcus*	1–2 g q4h IV	IV, IM, PO	None	Hypersensitivity (rash, fever), hepatitis
Ampicillin	*Streptococcus, Enterococcus, Listeria, N. meningitidis, Salmonella, Shigella, Proteus*	1–2 g q4h IV	IV, IM	Minor	Diarrhea, rash, urticarial rash (not allergy) in infectious mononucleosis

(continued)

363

Table 69-1 (*Continued*)

Major Antibacterial Agents

Drug	Organisms	Dosage Range	Routes of Administration	Dose Reduction for Renal Insufficiency	Major Toxicities
Piperacillin	Most gram-negative bacilli (including *Pseudomonas aeruginosa*), anaerobes, *Streptococcus*, *Enterococcus faecalis*	3–4 g q4–6h	IV	Minor	Hypersensitivity (rash, fever)
Ampicillin/ sulbactam	Most gram-negative bacilli (not *P. aeruginosa*), *Streptococcus*, *S. aureus* (not MRSA), anaerobes	1.5–3.0 g q6h IV	IV, IM	Minor	Same as for ampicillin
CEPHALOSPORINS					
Cefazolin	*Streptococcus*, *S. aureus* (not MRSA), *Escherichia coli*, *Klebsiella*	1–2 g q8h IV	IV, IM	Moderate	↑Alkaline phosphatase

Cefuroxime	*Streptococcus, S. aureus* (not MRSA), *Neisseria gonorrhoeae, N. meningitidis, Haemophilus influenzae, E. coli, Klebsiella, Salmonella, Shigella*	750 mg to 1.5 g q8h, 125–250 mg PO (cefuroxime axetil)	IV, IM, PO	Moderate	Phlebitis, hypersensitivity (eosinophilia), ↑SGOT, ↑alkaline phosphatase
Cefoxitin	As for cefuroxime (not *H. influenzae*) plus anaerobes	1 g q8h to 2 g q4h	IV, IM	Moderate	Hypersensitivity, false ↑creatinine
Cefotetan	As for cefoxitin (but not as active against *Bacteroides* other than *B. fragilis*)	1–3 g q12h	IV, IM	Moderate	Bleeding (check PT before and during therapy; consider alternatives in cases of preexisting coagulopathy). ↑LFTs
Ceftizoxime	*Streptococcus, S. aureus* (not MRSA and not as active as cefazolin), gram-negative organisms except *Stenotrophomonas maltophilia* and *Legionella*; anaerobes controversial	1 g q12h to 4 g q8h	IV, IM	Moderate	Phlebitis, hypersensitivity (rash, eosinophilia, ↑SGOT

(continued)

Table 69-1 (*Continued*)

Major Antibacterial Agents

Drug	Organisms	Dosage Range	Routes of Administration	Dose Reduction for Renal Insufficiency	Major Toxicities
Ceftriaxone	As for ceftizoxime (but not active against *P. aeruginosa* or anaerobes)	1–2 g q24h (or q12h)	IV, IM	None	As for ceftizoxime; sludge in gallbladder on US with symptomatic cholelithiasis in 9%
Ceftazidime	As for ceftizoxime except active against most strains of *P. aeruginosa* (but not against anaerobes)	1–2 g q8h	IV, IM	Moderate	As for ceftizoxime
CARBAPENEMS					
Imipenem/ cilastatin	Gram-positive cocci (but not *Enterococcus faecium* or MRSA), gram-negative organisms (but not *S. maltophilia*), anaerobes	500 mg to 1 g q6h	IV, IM (requires dose reduction and lidocaine)	Moderate	Phlebitis, hypersensitivity, seizures (especially in patients with renal dysfunction), nausea, vomiting, diarrhea

MONOBACTAMS

| Aztreonam | Only gram-negative aerobes | 1 g q8h to 2 g q6h | IV | Moderate | Phlebitis, hypersensitivity (but no cross-reaction with penicillins), ↑SGOT |

AMINOGLYCOSIDES

Gentamicin	Gram-negative aerobes; synergistic with penicillins against *Enterococcus*	3–5 (mg/kg)/d divided q8h	IV, IM	Major	Nephrotoxicity, ototoxicity; peak and trough levels should be monitored
Tobramycin	Same as gentamicin but more active against *P. aeruginosa*	Same as gentamicin	IV, IM	Major	Same as gentamicin
Amikacin	Same as gentamicin but more active against gentamicin-resistant organisms	15 (mg/kg)/d divided q8–12h	IV, IM	Major	Same as gentamicin

(continued)

Table 69-1 (*Continued*)

Major Antibacterial Agents

Drug	Organisms	Dosage Range	Routes of Administration	Dose Reduction for Renal Insufficiency	Major Toxicities
TETRACYCLINES					
Doxycycline	*Francisella tularensis, Brucella, Vibrio vulnificus, Chlamydia, Mycoplasma pneumoniae, Rickettsia*	100 mg q12h	IV, PO	Minor	Nausea, erosive esophagitis; phototoxicity and tooth deposition less than with tetracycline
MACROLIDES					
Erythromycin	*Streptococcus, M. pneumoniae, Legionella*	250 mg to 1 g q6h	IV, PO	None	Nausea, vomiting, cramps, ↑SGOT, cholestatic jaundice (especially with estolate), phlebitis, transient deafness

Clarithromycin	As for erythromycin but also active against *H. influenzae, Mycobacterium avium* complex	500 mg bid	PO	Minor	Adverse GI effects less prominent than with erythromycin
Azithromycin	As for erythromycin but more active against *M. avium* complex, *H. influenzae, Chlamydia* (FDA-approved for urethritis/cervicitis)	500 mg qd	PO	Minor	As with clarithromycin, adverse GI effects less prominent than with erythromycin
QUINOLONES					
Ciprofloxacin	Gram-positive cocci (but not serious pneumococcal or enterococcal infections or MRSA), gram-negative organisms (but not *Burkholderia cepacia*), not active against anaerobes; only some staphylococcal strains known to be sensitive	500 or 750 mg bid PO; 200–400 mg q12h IV	IV, PO	Minor	Adverse GI effects, including nausea, diarrhea, vomiting; not to be used for children or pregnant women because of effects on cartilage

(continued)

Table 69-1 (*Continued*)

Major Antibacterial Agents

Drug	Organisms	Dosage Range	Routes of Administration	Dose Reduction for Renal Insufficiency	Major Toxicities
Ofloxacin	Same as ciprofloxacin but may have slightly greater gram-positive activity	200 or 400 mg bid PO; 200–400 mg q12h IV	IV, PO	Moderate	Nausea, diarrhea, insomnia, headache
OTHER					
Vancomycin	Gram-positive organisms	1g q12h IV; 125–500 mg q6h PO	IV, PO (for *C. difficile* colitis only)	Major	Phlebitis, "red man" syndrome, ototoxicity, +/− nephrotoxicity; may be increased when given with aminoglycosides (trough levels should be <10 mg/mL)

Clindamycin	Streptococcus, S. aureus (not MRSA), anaerobes	600–900 mg q8h IV; 150–450 mg q6h PO	IV, IM, PO	None	Diarrhea, C. difficile colitis, rash
Metronidazole	Anaerobes	500 mg q6–8h	IV, PO	None	Nausea, vomiting, metallic taste, headache, disulfiram-like reaction with alcohol; dose must be reduced in severe liver disease
Trimethoprim-sulfamethoxazole	Gram-negative aerobes, including Moraxella catarrhalis and H. influenzae, Salmonella, Shigella; Streptococcus (if sensitive)	8 (mg/kg)/d TMP component divided q6h up to 15–20 (mg/kg)/d; for Pneumocystis pneumonia, 1–2 DS tabs PO bid	IV, PO	Moderate	Rash, nausea, vomiting, diarrhea, neutropenia

SOURCE: Adapted from Archer GL, Polk RE: Treatment and Prophylaxis of Bacterial Infections, Chap. 140, p. 856, in HPIM-14; and Sanford JP, Gilbert DN, Sande M: Guide to Antimicrobial Therapy. Dallas, Antimicrobial Therapy, Inc., 1996.

70

IMMUNIZATION AND ADVICE TO TRAVELERS

IMMUNIZATION

Vaccination against infectious diseases is one of the most potent and effective tools of medicine. Through immunization, many once-prevalent infectious diseases (e.g., smallpox, polio, measles, *Haemophilus influenzae* infection) have been eliminated or drastically curtailed. Yet complacency and socioeconomic barriers have impeded the attainment of universal and appropriate immunization. Adults in particular often fail to receive indicated immunizations, such as pneumococcal vaccination, influenza vaccination, and tetanus-diphtheria boosters.

Active immunization refers to administration of a vaccine or a toxoid in order to elicit long-lasting protection. Live vaccines are usually contraindicated for pts who are immunosuppressed, febrile, or pregnant (see Tables 70-1 and 70-2). *Passive* immunization refers to the provision of temporary immunity by administration of exogenously produced immune substances such as antibodies (see Table 70-3).

ADVICE TO TRAVELERS

Persons anticipating travel, particularly to developing countries, often seek assistance in preventing the acquisition of infectious diseases. During a pretravel evaluation, the practitioner obtains a careful medical history and a detailed itinerary of the planned trip. The traveler is then provided with recommendations for disease avoidance as well as specific medications and vaccinations. Current information can be obtained by internet or telephone from the Centers for Disease Control and Prevention (http://www.cdc.gov; 404-332-4559). Complicated travel problems, including those involving children, pregnant women, and immunocompromised pts and situations in which yellow fever vaccine is recommended, require referral to a travel medicine specialist or center.

MALARIA Prevention of malaria, a major cause of life-threatening illness in travelers, should stress avoidance of mosquitoes by staying indoors and use of DEET-containing mosquito repellents. Most travelers to malaria-endemic areas should receive weekly chemoprophylaxis with mefloquine (250 mg PO weekly) or—in the limited areas where drug-resistant *Plasmodium falciparum* is not found—with chloroquine (300 mg of

Table 70-1

Active Immunization of Normal Adults

Vaccine and Type	Administration and Target Group
Diphtheria and tetanus toxoids (Td)	IM at least q10 years; also after tetanus-prone wounds if >5 years since last Td.

Comment: Lower dose of diphtheria toxoid in Td than in DTP for children. Give previously unimmunized adults passive immunization plus Td at time of injury.

Influenza, inactivated vaccine	IM or SC yearly in autumn. For all adults >65 years old or with chronic disease (see Table 70-2).

Comment: Acute febrile illness is a contraindication. Most pts with egg allergy can be immunized with special precautions.

Pneumococcal 23-valent polysaccharide vaccine	SC once. For all adults >65 years old or with increased risk of severe infection (see Table 70-2).

Comment: May be given simultaneously with influenza vaccine at separate sites.

Measles, mumps, rubella live attenuated vaccine (MMR)	SC once. For all adults born after 1956 without history of infection or immunization. Second dose may be required in some work or school settings.

Comment: Serologic testing for immunity is not necessary since previous infection or immunization is not a contraindication for revaccination. Pregnancy is a contraindication. Women should prevent pregnancy for 3 months after receiving vaccine.

Hepatitis A, inactivated vaccine	IM twice (6–12 months apart) for individuals requiring long-term protection.

Comment: For individuals at risk.

Hepatitis B, recombinant protein vaccine	IM in 3 doses at 0, 1, and 6 months.

Comment: For individuals at risk.

(continued)

Table 70-1 *(Continued)*

Active Immunization of Normal Adults

Vaccine and Type	Administration and Target Group
Varicella-zoster virus, live attenuated vaccine	SC twice (1–2 months apart) for individuals ≥13 years of age who have not had chickenpox.

Comment: Avoid during pregnancy or in immunocompromised persons.

SOURCE: Modified from Keusch GT, Bart KJ: HPIM-14.

Table 70-2

Active Immunization of Individuals at High Risk of Acquiring or Developing Severe Infections

Vaccine and Type	Administration and Target Group
Influenza, inactivated vaccine	IM or SC yearly. For pts with chronic cardiac, pulmonary, renal, metabolic (e.g., diabetes) diseases; severe anemia; immunosuppression (including AIDS); for personnel caring for these pts; and for residents of institutions housing these pts.

Comment: To reduce morbidity and mortality in these pts at risk for complications of influenza. Children should only be given "split-virus" vaccine.

| Pneumococcal 23-valent polysaccharide vaccine | IM or SC once. Same population as for influenza vaccine and pts with cirrhosis, alcoholism, functional/anatomic asplenia (e.g., sickle cell), myeloma, nephrotic syndrome, CSF leaks, immunosuppression (e.g., from HIV infection). |

(continued)

Table 70-2 *(Continued)*

Active Immunization of Individuals at High Risk of Acquiring or Developing Severe Infections

Vaccine and Type	Administration and Target Group

Comment: See also Table 70-1. Revaccination indicated after 6 years for high-risk individuals (e.g., asplenia) and after 3–5 years for pts with nephrotic syndrome or renal failure and for transplant recipients.

Vaccine and Type	Administration and Target Group
Hepatitis B, inactivated or recombinant sub-unit vaccine	3 doses IM in deltoid at 0, 1, and 6 months. For health care personnel exposed to blood products, household and sexual contacts of carriers, clients and staff of institutions for mentally handicapped, pts receiving hemodialysis or clotting factors, pts with multiple sexual partners, IV drug abusers, prisoners, groups with highly endemic infection, infants of HBsAg-positive mothers. For all children, 3 doses IM between birth and 18 months.

Comment: Pregnancy is not a contraindication for vaccination in women at high risk of acquiring hepatitis B virus infection.

Vaccine and Type	Administration and Target Group
Meningococcal 4-valent polysaccharide vaccine	SC once. For control of epidemics and as adjunct to chemoprophylaxis of household contacts; for pts with functional/anatomic asplenia (e.g., sickle cell), defects in terminal complement components.

Comment: No vaccine against type B infection, which is most common. Give rifampin to contacts as well as cases.

Vaccine and Type	Administration and Target Group
Haemophilus influenzae type b conjugate vaccine (Hib)	For all children. Given IM on a 3- or 4-dose schedule between 2 and 15 months of age, depending on type of vaccine used. Also for high-risk adults.

(continued)

Table 70-2 (*Continued*)

Active Immunization of Individuals at High Risk of Acquiring or Developing Severe Infections

Vaccine and Type	Administration and Target Group
Varicella-zoster virus, live attenuated vaccine	For all children, single SC dose. For susceptible adults, 2 doses 1–2 months apart.

Comment: Avoid during pregnancy or immunocompromise.

Adenovirus, bivalent live attenuated vaccine	PO once. For military recruits only.
Rabies, human diploid cell vaccine (HDCV)	Preexposure prophylaxis: 3 IM doses at 0, 7, and 28 d. Postexposure prophylaxis: 5 IM doses at 0, 3, 7, 14, and 28 d with HRIG (see Table 70-3).

Comment: Preexposure prophylaxis for individuals with a high risk of exposure (veterinarians, laboratory workers).

Polio

Live attenuated vaccine (OPV)	4 oral doses at 0, 1–2, 3–4, and 9–16 months. For unimmunized adults at immediate risk of exposure.

Comment: Routine immunization of adults against polio is not recommended in U.S.

Inactivated vaccine (IPV-e)	3 SC doses at 0, 1–2, and 6–12 months. For unimmunized pts with immunosuppression and their household contacts, health care providers, and travelers to high-risk areas.

Comment: For rapid protection, give 2 doses 4 weeks apart. For immediate protection (including in pregnancy), administer OPV. Now used for initial immunization (first 2 doses) of all children to decrease small risk of paralytic disease from OPV.

Hepatitis A	2 doses IM. For travelers or persons living in high-risk areas.
Typhoid, live oral vaccine (Ty21a)	4 oral doses; 1 qod. For international travelers.

(*continued*)

Table 70-2 (*Continued*)

Active Immunization of Individuals at High Risk of Acquiring or Developing Severe Infections

Vaccine and Type	Administration and Target Group

Comment: Avoid during pregnancy or immunocompromise.

Typhoid, polysaccharide Vi vaccine	Single dose IM. For international travelers.

Comment: Reimmunization suggested every 2 years for repeated or continuous exposure.

BCG, live attenuated vaccine (tuberculosis)	SC or intradermally once. For groups with high endemic infection and personnel caring for such pts.

Comment: Immunodeficiency (e.g., HIV infection) is a contraindication.

Yellow fever, live attenuated vaccine	SC once every 10 years, administered at WHO-registered vaccination centers. For international travelers.

Comment: Contraindicated for immunosuppressed or pregnant pts and for infants <6 months old.

Cholera, killed bacillus vaccine	SC every 6 months. Only for travelers to countries requiring vaccination for entry.

Comment: Infection is more effectively prevented by taking precautions in handling food and drink.

Japanese B encephalitis, inactivated virus vaccine	For travelers to rural areas of the Far East, including China and Korea.

Comment: Routinely given to children in endemic areas.

SOURCE: Modified from Keusch GT, Bart KJ: HPIM-14.

base PO weekly), beginning 2 weeks before departure and continuing until 4 weeks after return.

DIARRHEA Traveler's diarrhea, which is usually caused by enterotoxigenic *Escherichia coli* but may also be caused by many other pathogens, can often be avoided by consuming only well-cooked hot foods, peeled or cooked fruits and vegetables, and bottled or boiled beverages. When diarrhea occurs without fever or bloody stool, it can be self-treated with an antibiotic

Table 70-3

Passive Immunization

Disease	Preparation of Choice	Target Group and Schedule
PROPHYLAXIS		
Hepatitis A	Standard human immune globulin	Contacts in day care centers, households, and custodial institutions. 0.02–0.04 mL/kg IM.

Comment: Up to 0.06 mL/kg IM for preexposure prophylaxis for foreign travel or every 5 months for continuous exposure.

Hepatitis B	Hepatitis B immune globulin (HBIG)	1. Infants of HbsAg-positive mothers. 0.5 mL IM. 2. Persons with percutaneous or mucous-membrane contact with a hepatitis B–infected person or with infected blood or serum. 0.06 mL/kg IM.

Comment: Usually given with appropriate doses of hepatitis B vaccine.

Varicella	Varicella-zoster immune globulin (VZIG)	1. Exposed infants and children at high risk of severe infection, including perinatally exposed newborns. 2. Exposed susceptible adults. 125 units (1 vial)/10 kg IM (minimum, 125; maximum, 625).
Tetanus	Tetanus immune globulin (TIG)	Pts with wounds (other than clean minor wounds) and without a clear history of full, up-to-date tetanus immunization. 250–500 units IM, with part of dose infiltrated around wound.

Comment: Tetanus with diphtheria toxoids (Td) normally given as well.

(continued)

Table 70-3 (*Continued*)

Passive Immunization

Disease	Preparation of Choice	Target Group and Schedule
Rabies	Human rabies immune globulin (HRIG)	Individuals thought to have had significant exposure to a rabid or potentially rabid animal; 20 IU/kg, half infiltrated around wound and half IM. Pts known to be immune and/or fully immunized against rabies require not HRIG but rather 2 doses of rabies vaccine on days 0 and 3.

Comment: Give early and follow with a 5-dose course of rabies vaccine on days 0, 3, 7, 14, and 28.

Measles	Standard human immune globulin	Susceptible household and close contacts, within 6 d of exposure, particularly immunosuppressed individuals (including those with HIV infection) and infants. 0.25–0.5 mL/kg IM. Maximum, 15 mL.

Comment: Routine measles vaccination should be postponed until 3–6 months after immune globulin administration.

Cytomegalovirus	CMV immune globulin (CMVIG)	Prophylaxis for liver, kidney, and possibly bone marrow transplant recipients.
Respiratory syncytial virus	RSV immune globulin	Infants at high risk for complications of RSV infection.
Rubella	Standard human immune globulin	Pregnant women exposed in early pregnancy, where termination is not an option. 0.55 mL/kg IM.

Comment: Efficacy is unreliable. Passive immunization does not ensure protection of the fetus.

(continued)

Table 70-3 (*Continued*)

Passive Immunization

Disease	Preparation of Choice	Target Group and Schedule

TREATMENT OF ESTABLISHED DISEASE

Botulism	Equine trivalent antitoxin*	Pts with food-borne or wound botulism.
Comment: Not used to treat infant botulism.		
Diphtheria	Equine diphtheria antitoxin*	Pts with clinical diagnosis of diphtheria.
Comment: Probably of no value in cutaneous diphtheria.		
Cytomegalovirus	CMV immune globulin (CMVIG)	Pts with bone marrow transplants and CMV pneumonia.
Comment: Used with antiviral agents.		
Tetanus	Tetanus immune globulin (TIG)	Pts with clinical diagnosis of tetanus.

*Tests for sensitivity and, if necessary, desensitization should be undertaken for these products.
SOURCE: Modified from Keush GT, Bart KJ: HPIM-14.

such as trimethoprim-sulfamethoxazole or ciprofloxacin and an antimotility agent such as loperamide.

VACCINE-PREVENTABLE ILLNESSES The use of vaccines by travelers (Table 70-2) depends upon the location of travel and international requirements. Yellow fever vaccine is recommended for travelers to endemic areas and is the only vaccine currently required by law for entry into some countries. It must be obtained at a center sanctioned by the World Health Organization (WHO). Active or passive immunization against hepatitis A should be offered to most travelers to developing countries. Other vaccines to be considered in some circumstances include typhoid, meningococcal polysaccharide, varicella, cholera, rabies, and Japanese encephalitis.

For a more detailed discussion, see Keusch GT, Bart KJ: Immunization Principles and Vaccine Use, Chap. 122, p. 758; and Keystone JS, Kozarsky PE: Health Risks to Travelers, Chap. 123, p. 772, in HPIM-14.

71

SEPSIS AND SEPTIC SHOCK

Definitions

The systemic inflammatory response syndrome (SIRS), recently defined by critical-care specialists, incorporates clinical criteria (fever or hypothermia, tachypnea, tachycardia, and abnormal WBC count) that may be manifestations of microbial infection or conditions of other etiologies. When the syndrome is caused by microbial infection, it is called *sepsis*. *Septic shock* refers to the overwhelming of host homeostatic mechanisms by sepsis, which results in hypotension and organ dysfunction. These and related terms are defined in Table 71-1.

Epidemiology/Etiology/Pathogenesis

There are 300,000–500,000 cases of sepsis annually in the U.S., and sepsis contributes to more than 100,000 deaths. Approximately two-thirds of cases occur in hospitalized pts. Moreover, 30–60% of pts with sepsis and 60-80% of pts with septic shock have positive blood cultures. Two-thirds of cultures yield gram-negative bacteria; 10–20%, gram-positive cocci; and 2–5%, fungi. Risk factors for gram-negative rod bacteremia include diabetes, lymphoproliferative disease, cirrhosis, burns, invasive procedures or devices, and neutropenia. Risk factors for gram-positive bacteremia include the presence of intravascular catheters or mechanical devices, burns, and IV drug injection. The incidence of sepsis appears to be increasing, probably because of an increase in the size of the population with risk factors. Sepsis results from complex host reactions to microbial signal molecules: lipopolysaccharide (LPS, also called endotoxin), peptidoglycan, and lipoteichoic acid of gram-positive bacteria as well as various extracellular enzymes and toxins. The host response is mediated by leukocytes, humoral factors (cytokines, prostaglandins, coagulation factors), and the vascular endothelium.

Clinical Manifestations

Signs of sepsis include the abrupt onset of fever, chills, tachycardia, tachypnea, altered mental status, and/or hypotension, particularly in a pt with localized infection. However, the septic response may develop gradually, and many or all of these signs may be absent. Hyperventilation, disorientation, and confusion are diagnostically useful early signs. Hypotension and DIC may develop. Cutaneous signs are frequent and include cyanosis and ischemic necrosis of peripheral tissue, cellulitis, pustules, bullae, and hemorrhagic lesions. Some skin lesions suggest specific

Table 71-1

Definitions Often Used to Describe the Condition of Septic Patients

Bacteremia (fungemia)	Presence of viable bacteria (fungi) in the blood, as evidenced by positive blood cultures
Septicemia	Systemic illness caused by the spread of microbes or their toxins via the bloodstream
Systemic inflammatory response syndrome (SIRS)*	At least 2 of the following 4 conditions: (1) oral temperature of >38°C or <36°C; (2) respiratory rate of >20 breaths/min or Pa_{CO_2} of <32 mmHg; (3) heart rate of >90 beats/min; (4) leukocyte count of >12,000/μL or <4,000/μL or >10% bands
Sepsis*	SIRS that has a proven or suspected microbial etiology
Severe sepsis* (similar to "sepsis syndrome")	Sepsis with one or more signs of organ dysfunction, hypoperfusion, or hypotension, such as metabolic acidosis, acute alteration in mental status, oliguria, or adult respiratory distress syndrome
Hypotension*	Systolic blood pressure <90 mmHg—or 40 mmHg less than patient's baseline blood pressure—in the absence of other reasons for hypotension
Septic shock*	Sepsis with hypotension that is unresponsive to fluid resuscitation plus organ dysfunction or perfusion abnormalities as listed above for severe sepsis
Refractory septic shock	Septic shock that lasts for >1 h and does not respond to fluid and pressor administration
Multiple-organ dysfunction syndrome (MODS)*	Dysfunction of more than one organ, requiring intervention to maintain homeostasis

SOURCE: Munford RS: HPIM-14, p. 776.

* Term preferred by the American College of Chest Physicians/Society of Critical Care Medicine Consensus Conference, 1992.

pathogens: petechial or purpuric lesions suggest meningococcemia or Rocky Mountain spotted fever; a bullous lesion surrounded by edema with central hemorrhage and necrosis (ecthyma gangrenosum) suggests *Pseudomonas* sepsis; generalized erythroderma in a septic pt suggests toxic shock syndrome; bullous lesions in a pt who has eaten raw oysters suggest *Vibrio vulnificus* sepsis; and the same lesions in a pt after a dog bite suggest *Capnocytophaga* sepsis. GI manifestations include nausea, vomiting, diarrhea, ileus, gastric ulceration with bleeding, and cholestatic jaundice.

Complications

ARDS ("shock lung"), mediated by pulmonary capillary microvascular injury, develops in 20–50% of pts with sepsis and causes diffuse pulmonary infiltrates and hypoxemia. Septic shock usually results from a severe decrease in systemic vascular resistance (with normal or elevated cardiac output) and functional hypovolemia due to diffuse capillary leak. Oliguria, azotemia, proteinuria, and nonspecific renal casts are frequent. Renal failure is usually caused by acute tubular necrosis. Thrombocytopenia occurs in 10–30% of cases. Profound thrombocytopenia (<50,000 platelets/μL) usually reflects DIC. Dysfunction of multiple organs usually indicates widespread endovascular injury and is associated with high fatality rates.

Diagnosis

There is no reliable laboratory test for the early diagnosis of sepsis. Clinical manifestations (listed above) are variably present and nonspecific. Laboratory findings may include leukocytosis with a left shift, thrombocytopenia, hyperbilirubinemia, and proteinuria. Leukopenia may also develop. Active hemolysis may occur in clostridial bacteremia, malaria, or DIC. In DIC there may be evidence of microangiopathic changes on peripheral smear. Early, hyperventilation-induced respiratory alkalosis may be followed by metabolic acidosis and hypoxemia. CXR may reveal ARDS or underlying pneumonia. Definitive diagnosis requires isolation of microorganisms from the blood or from a local site of infection. At least two blood samples should be obtained for culture from different venipuncture sites. If blood cultures are negative (as they are in around 30% of cases), the diagnosis depends on Gram's stain and culture of the primary site of infection or of secondarily infected cutaneous tissue. With overwhelming bacteremia, smears of peripheral-blood buffy coat may reveal microorganisms.

R̲x̲ **TREATMENT**

Sepsis is a medical emergency that requires immediate action to treat the local site of infection, to provide hemodynamic and respiratory support, and to eliminate the offending microorganism. Antibiotics should be given as soon as samples of blood and other sites have been obtained for culture. Empirical therapy should be based on information about the pt and about antimicrobial susceptibility patterns in the community and the hospital. Pending culture results, therapy including agents active against both gram-negative and gram-positive bacteria should be given. Suggested empirical regimens in different populations of pts are listed in Table 71-2. Removal or drainage of any focal site of infection is essential (indwelling IV or urinary catheters; paranasal sinuses; abdominal, perinephric, or pelvic collections). Hemodynamic support should restore oxygen delivery to tissue. IV fluid, typically 1–2 L of normal saline over 1–2 h, should be administered to restore effective intravascular volume. Monitoring of pulmonary capillary wedge pressure (target range, 14–18 mmHg) is essential in pts with refractory shock or underlying cardiac or renal disease. Dopamine [4–20 (μg/kg)/min] may be used to restore a mean arterial blood pressure of >60 mmHg and a cardiac index of $\geq$2.2 (L/min)/m^2. Higher doses may cause peripheral vasoconstriction with ischemia. Norepinephrine may be used when pts are refractory to dopamine, with dosing carefully titrated to maintain mean blood pressure at >60 mmHg (dose range, 2–20 μg/min). Ventilatory support is indicated for progressive hypoxemia, hypercapnia, neurologic deterioration, or respiratory muscle failure. Intubation can ensure adequate oxygenation, divert blood flow from the muscles of respiration, and reduce afterload. Glucocorticoid supplementation (hydrocortisone, 50 mg IV q6h) is indicated only in the rare instance of adrenal insufficiency, which should be suspected in cases of refractory hypotension, fulminant *Neisseria meningitidis* bacteremia, disseminated tuberculosis, prior glucocorticoid use, or AIDS.

Despite early diagnosis and prompt and aggressive management, approximately 25–35% of pts with sepsis and 40–55% of pts with septic shock die. Prognosis is affected by the prior clinical condition of the pt and the rate at which complications develop and is less affected by the etiologic agent. Prevention offers the best opportunity to reduce morbidity and mortality from sepsis. Preventive measures include minimizing the number of invasive procedures, limiting the use and duration of indwelling vascular and bladder catheters, reducing the incidence and duration of profound neutropenia, aggressively treating localized infection, and immunizing pts against specific pathogens.

Table 71-2

Initial Antimicrobial Therapy for Severe Sepsis with No Obvious Source in Adults with Normal Renal Function

Type of Patient	Antimicrobial Regimens*
Immunocompetent adult	The many acceptable regimens include (1) ticarcillin-clavulanate *or* piperacillin-tazobactam (6.2 and 7.5 g q6h, respectively) *plus* gentamicin or tobramycin (1.5 mg/kg q8h); (2) ampicillin (30 mg/kg q4h) *plus* gentamicin (1.5 mg/kg q8h) *plus* clindamycin (900 mg q8h); and (3) imipenem-cilastatin (0.5 g q6h). If the patient is allergic to β-lactam agents, ciprofloxacin (400 mg q12h) *or* aztreonam (2 g q8h) should be substituted for ampicillin in regimen 2.
Neutropenic patient (<500 neutrophils/μL)	Regimens include (1) ticarcillin, mezlocillin, or piperacillin (3 g q4h) *or* ceftazidime (2 g q8h) *plus* tobramycin (1.5 mg/kg q8h) and (2) imipenem-cilastatin (0.5 g q6h) *or* ceftazidime. If the patient is allergic to β-lactam agents, aztreonam or ciprofloxacin should be used with tobramycin. If the patient has an infected vascular catheter or if the involvement of staphylococci is suspected, vancomycin (15 mg/kg q12h) should be added.

(*continued*)

Table 71-2 (*Continued*)

Initial Antimicrobial Therapy for Severe Sepsis with No Obvious Source in Adults with Normal Renal Function

Type of Patient	Antimicrobial Regimens*
Splenectomized patient	Cefotaxime (2 g q4h) *or* ceftriaxone (2 g q12h) should be used. If the local prevalence of cephalosporin-resistant pneumococci is high, vancomycin can be added. If the patient is allergic to β-lactam drugs, vancomycin (15 mg/kg q12h) *plus* ciprofloxacin (400 mg q12h) *or* aztreonam (2 g q8h) should be used.
Intravenous drug user	Nafcillin *or* oxacillin (2 g q4h) *plus* gentamicin (1.5 mg/kg q8h) should be used. If the local prevalence of methicillin-resistant *Staphylococcus aureus* is high or if the patient is allergic to β-lactam drugs, vancomycin (15 mg/kg q12h) with gentamicin should be used.
AIDS patient	Ticarcillin-clavulanate (3 g q4h) *plus* tobramycin (1.5 mg/kg q8h) should be used. If the patient is allergic to β-lactam drugs, ciprofloxacin (400 mg q12h) *plus* vancomycin (15 mg/kg q12h) *plus* tobramycin should be used.

SOURCE: Munford RS: HPIM-14, p. 779.

* All administered intravenously.

For a more detailed discussion, see Munford RS: Sepsis and Septic Shock, Chap. 124, p. 776, in HPIM-14.

72

INFECTIVE ENDOCARDITIS

The term *infective endocarditis* denotes infection of the endocardium, an invariably fatal condition if untreated. While valvular endocardium is most commonly involved, endocarditis may also develop on a septal defect or the mural endocardium. Endocarditis may be classified by *tempo* (acute vs. subacute disease) or by *substrate* (native valve, prosthetic valve, injection drug use). Particular types of microorganisms are associated with each subgroup (Table 72-1). In general, organisms of greater virulence are likely to be the cause if disease presents acutely and if it involves anatomically normal cardiac valves. Regardless of subgroup, males are more commonly affected than females.

Epidemiology

NATIVE VALVE ENDOCARDITIS Most pts are >50 years old. 60–80% have a predisposing cardiac lesion, such as rheumatic valvular disease (30%; affecting the mitral valve most commonly and the aortic valve next most commonly), congenital heart disease (10–20%; including bicuspid aortic valve, patent ductus arteriosus, ventricular septal defect, tetralogy of Fallot, coarctation of the aorta, and pulmonic stenosis), or mitral valve prolapse (10–33%). Degenerative heart disease also predisposes to endocarditis, particularly calcific aortic stenosis in the elderly. Unusual predisposing lesions include asymmetric septal hypertrophy, Marfan's syndrome, and syphilitic aortic valve. In 20–40% of patients, no underlying lesion is found.

ENDOCARDITIS IN INJECTION DRUG USERS The typical injection drug user with endocarditis is a young man without a predisposing cardiac lesion. The etiologic agent usually derives from the skin flora; *Staphylococcus aureus* is especially common. The tricuspid valve is most frequently involved.

PROSTHETIC VALVE ENDOCARDITIS Prosthetic valve infections now account for 10–20% of cases of endocarditis, are most common in men >60 years old, and are particularly difficult to eradicate. Aortic valvular prostheses are more often involved than mitral ones; infection is usually centered along the suture line. The incidence of endocarditis is 1–2% within the first postoperative year and about 0.5% per year thereafter. Valvular contamination at surgery accounts for most cases of early-onset endocarditis (symptoms beginning within 60 d of surgery), while late-onset disease (onset of symptoms >60 d

Table 72-1

Etiology of Infective Endocarditis, by Epidemiologic Subgroup

Epidemiologic Subgroup	Organisms	Frequency, %
Native valve endocarditis	Streptococci	55
	(Viridans streptococci)	(41)
	(*S. bovis*)	(11)
	(Other streptococci)	(2–3)
	Staphylococci	30
	(*S. aureus*)	(25–27)
	(Other staphylococci)	(3–5)
	Enterococci	6
	HACEK group*	—
Prosthetic valve endocarditis Early onset (<2 months)	Staphylococci (commonly coagulase-negative)	50
	Gram-negative bacilli	15
	Fungi (commonly *Candida* spp.)	10
Late onset (>2 months)	Streptococci (mainly viridans group)	40
	Staphylococci (commonly coagulase-negative)	33
Endocarditis in injection drug users	Staphylococci (mainly *S. aureus*)	>50
	Streptococci and enterococci	20
	Gram-negative bacilli (especially *Pseudomonas* spp.)	6
	Fungi (especially *Candida* spp.)	6

Haemophilus, Actinobacillus, Cardiobacterium, Eikenella, and *Kingella.*

after surgery) results either from indolent organisms introduced at surgery or from transient intercurrent bacteremia unrelated to surgery.

Pathogenesis

Sterile collections of platelets and fibrin (nonbacterial thrombotic endocarditis) form over areas of endothelial trauma, vascular turbulence, or scarring or in the setting of systemic wasting disease such as malignancy. Bacteria transiently present in the blood, particularly if they are intrinsically adherent, may colonize these "vegetations," thereby initiating infection. The clinical manifestations of endocarditis result directly from the presence of the vegetations (embolization, valvular occlusion), from valvular destruction (valvular incompetence, late stenosis), from tissue invasion (conduction abnormalities, ventricular septal rupture), and from the immune response to the infection (immune complex–mediated glomerulonephritis, arthritis, mucocutaneous vasculitis).

Clinical Manifestations

ACUTE ENDOCARDITIS   By definition, the onset of acute endocarditis is rapid; the pt typically has high fever and systemic toxicity. A new or changing cardiac murmur may be noted. Arthralgias and myalgias are common. Early and potentially catastrophic complications include systemic emboli (to the CNS; the renal, mesenteric, or coronary arteries; or the extremities), sudden valvular incompetence, heart block, and overwhelming sepsis. In right-sided endocarditis, emboli travel to the lungs. With the exception of Janeway lesions, the peripheral stigmata of endocarditis are less common in acute than in subacute disease.

SUBACUTE ENDOCARDITIS   The onset of subacute endocarditis is gradual, with low-grade fever and malaise. In disease of long standing, significant cachexia may be evident. Subacute endocarditis is a classic cause of fever of unknown origin. Cardiac murmurs are common; splenomegaly and petechiae (frequently found on conjunctivae, palate, buccal mucosa, and upper extremities) occur in about 30% of cases. Peripheral stigmata of endocarditis, *all of which are nonspecific findings,* include splinter hemorrhages (subungual, dark-red linear streaks; 10–30% of pts), Roth's spots (oval retinal hemorrhages with a clear pale center; <5%), Osler's nodes (small tender nodules developing especially often on finger or toe pads; 10–25%), and Janeway lesions (small hemorrhages on the palms or soles with slight nodularity; <5%). As in acute disease, emboli may occur at any time before, during, or after therapy; the risk of their occurrence diminishes as treatment progresses.

Neurologic Complications

Neurologic complications have an overall incidence of 20–40%, may occur in acute or subacute disease, and are more common with left-sided than with right-sided disease. They include cerebral emboli (~20% of pts), encephalopathy from microemboli (~10%), leakage of a mycotic aneurysm (<5%), and meningitis or macroscopic brain abscess (<5%, mostly in the setting of acute endocarditis due to *S. aureus*). Heart failure may occur during endocarditis or long after its cure. Contributing factors include valvular destruction, myocarditis, coronary arterial emboli with infarction, and myocardial abscesses.

Diagnosis

Endocarditis should be suspected in any pt with a heart murmur and unexplained fever lasting ≥7 d and in any febrile injection drug user even in the absence of a murmur. Well-defined clinical criteria for the diagnosis of infective endocarditis have recently been introduced (Table 72-2). Blood cultures are positive in >95% of cases, and bacteremia is usually continuous. Blood cultures may be negative in infections due to fastidious organisms (e.g., those of the HACEK group), in fungal endocarditis, and in endocarditis in pts recently given antimicrobial chemotherapy. For suspected acute disease, therapy should be delayed no more than 2–3 h while culture results are awaited. Ancillary laboratory findings include normochromic normocytic anemia, elevated sedimentation rate, proteinuria, and microscopic hematuria. Rheumatoid factor is present in 50% of pts symptomatic for >6 weeks. Transesophageal echocardiography has substantially better resolution than transthoracic echocardiography and is particularly useful for detecting prosthetic valvular vegetations and myocardial abscesses.

℞ **TREATMENT**

Antibiotic regimens for use in various therapeutic situations are detailed in Table 72-3. Surgery should be considered for pts with persistent or recurrent positive blood cultures, with fever lasting >1 week despite appropriate antibiotic therapy, with severe CHF, with recurrent emboli in spite of treatment, or with evidence of myocardial or valve ring abscess (e.g., conduction defects or arrhythmias) and when effective antimicrobial therapy is not available. Less definitive indications for surgery include the presence of large vegetations and a fungal etiology.

Table 72-2

Clinical Diagnosis of Infective Endocarditis

I. *Definite infective endocarditis:* Two major criteria *or* one major and three minor criteria *or* five minor criteria

   A. Major criteria

   1. Isolation of viridans streptococci, *S. bovis,* HACEK-group organisms, or (in the absence of a primary focus) community-acquired *S. aureus* or *Enterococcus* from two separate blood cultures *or* isolation of a microorganism consistent with endocarditis in (1) blood cultures ≥12 h apart or (2) all of three or most of four or more blood cultures, with first and last at least 1 h apart

   2. Evidence of endocardial involvement on echocardiography: oscillating intracardiac mass or abscess *or* new partial dehiscence of prosthetic valve *or* new valvular regurgitation

   B. Minor criteria

   1. Predisposing lesion or intravenous drug use
   2. Fever of ≥38.0°C
   3. Major arterial emboli, septic pulmonary infarcts, mycotic aneurysm, intracranial hemorrhage, conjunctival hemorrhages, Janeway lesions
   4. Glomerulonephritis, Osler's nodes, Roth's spots, rheumatoid factor
   5. Positive blood cultures not meeting the major criterion (excluding single cultures positive for organisms that do not typically cause endocarditis) *or* serologic evidence of active infection with an organism that causes endocarditis
   6. Echocardiogram consistent with endocarditis but not meeting the major criterion

II. *Possible infective endocarditis:* Findings that fall short of "definite" but do not fall into the "rejected" category

III. *Rejected:* Alternative diagnosis *or* resolution of syndrome *or* no evidence of infective endocarditis at surgery or autopsy with ≤4 d of antibiotic therapy

SOURCE: Kaye D: HPIM-14, p. 788.

Table 72-3

Therapy for Infective Endocarditis

STREPTOCOCCI WITH PENICILLIN G MICs of ≤0.1 μg/mL

Regimen A	Penicillin G, 12–18 million units/d IV in divided doses q4h × 4 weeks
Regimen B	Penicillin as in regimen A plus gentamicin, 1 mg/kg IV q8h, both × 2 weeks
Regimen C	Ceftriaxone, 2 g IV or IM once daily × 4 weeks
Regimen D	Vancomycin, 15 mg/kg IV q12h × 4 weeks

STREPTOCOCCI WITH PENICILLIN G MICs OF >0.1 BUT <0.5 μg/mL

Regimen E	Penicillin G, 18 million units/d IV in divided doses q4h × 4 weeks, plus gentamicin, 1 mg/kg IV q8h for the first 2 weeks; or regimen D if patient is allergic to penicillin

ENTEROCOCCI OR STREPTOCOCCI WITH PENICILLIN G MICs of ≥0.5 μg/mL OR NUTRITIONALLY VARIANT VIRIDANS STREPTOCOCCI

Regimen F	Penicillin G, 18–30 million units/d IV, or ampicillin, 12 g/d IV, in divided doses q4h, plus gentamicin, 1 mg/kg IV q8h, both × 4–6 weeks
Regimen G	Vancomycin, 15 mg/kg IV q12h, plus gentamicin as in regimen F, both × 4–6 weeks

METHICILLIN-SUSCEPTIBLE STAPHYLOCOCCI ON A NATIVE VALVE

Regimen H	Nafcillin or oxacillin, 2 g IV q4h × 4–6 weeks, with or without gentamicin, 1 mg/kg IV q8h × the first 3–5 d
Regimen I	Cefazolin*, 2 g IV q8h × 4–6 weeks, with or without gentamicin as in regimen H
Regimen J	Vancomycin, 15 mg/kg IV q12h × 4–6 weeks, with or without gentamicin as in regimen H

(*continued*)

Table 72-3 (*Continued*)

Therapy for Infective Endocarditis

METHICILLIN-RESISTANT STAPHYLOCOCCI OR
CORYNEBACTERIUM SPP. ON A NATIVE VALVE

Regimen K   Vancomycin as in regimen J, with or without gentamicin as in regimen H, for staphylococci; continue gentamicin × 4–6 weeks for *Corynebacterium* spp.

THE ABOVE ORGANISMS ON A PROSTHETIC VALVE

Streptococci or enterococci: Regimen F or G. Streptococci: Penicillin or vancomycin × 6 weeks, with gentamicin × the first 2 weeks or longer. Enterococci: Penicillin or vancomycin plus an aminoglycoside × 6–8 weeks
Methicillin-susceptible staphylococci: Regimen H, I, or J × 6–8 weeks, with gentamicin × the first 2 weeks and rifampin (300 mg orally q8h) for the entire course
Methicillin-resistant staphylococci: Regimen J × 6–8 weeks, with gentamicin × the first 2 weeks and rifampin (300 mg orally q8h) for the entire course

HACEK BACTERIA

Regimen L   Use regimen C

*Another first-generation cephalosporin may be used instead of cefazolin.

NOTE: Serum concentrations of gentamicin should be about 3 μg/mL 1 h after a 20- to 30-min IV infusion or IM injection. Streptomycin may be substituted for gentamicin in regimens B, E, F, and G at 7.5 mg/kg IM every 12 h; serum concentrations should be about 20 μg/mL 1 h after injection. The maximal dose of vancomycin is 1 g every 12 h; serum concentrations of vancomycin 1 h after completion of the infusion should be 30–45 μg/mL.

SOURCE: Kaye D: HPIM-14, p. 789.

Outpatient/Home Care Considerations

Home therapy is cost-effective and has been used successfully for clinically stable pts who are not injection drug users, do not live alone, are highly motivated, and are able to administer therapy to themselves. Regimen C or D has been used most frequently for streptococcal disease and regimen J for staphylococcal disease (Table 72-3).

Table 72-4

Antimicrobial Prophylaxis against Infective Endocarditis

DENTAL, ORAL, NASAL, OR OTHER PROCEDURES INVOLVING
OR PASSING THROUGH THE OROPHARYNX

Low-risk pts:	
Recommended:	Amoxicillin 3 g PO 1 h before and 1.5 g PO 6 h after
Penicillin allergy:	Erythromycin 1 g PO 2 h before and 0.5 g 6 h after
Alternative:	Clindamycin 300 mg PO 1 h before and 150 mg PO 6 h after
High-risk pts:	
Recommended:	Ampicillin 2 g IV or IM and gentamicin 1.5 mg/kg IM or IV, both 30 min before; and amoxicillin 1.5 g PO 6 h after
Penicillin allergy:	Vancomycin 1 g IV over 1 h starting 1 h before

GASTROINTESTINAL OR GENITOURINARY PROCEDURES
(GENERALLY NOT INDICATED FOR COLONOSCOPY OR
BARIUM ENEMA)

Recommended:	Ampicillin 2 g IV or IM and gentamicin 1.5 mg/kg IM or IV, both 30 min before; and amoxicillin 1.5 g PO 6 h after
Penicillin allergy:	Vancomycin 1 g IV over 1 h starting 1 h before and gentamicin 1.5 mg/kg IV or IM 1 h before
Low-risk pts with minor procedure:	
Recommended:	Amoxicillin 3 g PO 1 h before and 1.5 g 6 h after

(continued)

Table 72-4 (*Continued*)

Antimicrobial Prophylaxis against Infective Endocarditis

CARDIAC SURGERY (NOT INDICATED FOR PTS UNDERGOING
CARDIAC CATHETERIZATION)

Recommended:	Cefazolin 2 g IV and gentamicin 1.5 mg/kg IV starting immediately preoperatively; repeat doses q8h × 2
Alternative:	Vancomycin 15 mg/kg IV over 1 h beginning 1 h before and gentamicin 1.5 mg/kg IV before, then gentamicin q8h × 2, then vancomycin 10 mg/kg at end of operation, then vancomycin 7.5 mg/kg q6h × 3 doses

SOURCE: Modified from Chap. 80, p. 368, in HPIM-13 *Companion Handbook.*

Prophylaxis

Antibiotic prophylaxis against endocarditis is recommended for pts with predisposing cardiac lesions who are undergoing procedures known to cause bacteremia (Table 72-4). The highest-risk pts are those with prosthetic valves. Other predisposing factors include valvular or congenital heart disease (except uncomplicated atrial septal defect), asymmetric septal hypertrophy, and previous endocarditis. Pts with mitral valve prolapse generally receive prophylaxis only if they have mitral regurgitation or echocardiographically demonstrable thickening and redundancy of mitral valvular leaflets.

For a more detailed discussion, see Kaye D: Infective Endocarditis, Chap. 126, p. 785, in HPIM-14.

73

INTRAABDOMINAL INFECTIONS

PERITONITIS

PATHOGENESIS Intraperitoneal infections generally arise when a normal anatomic barrier is disrupted and the usually sterile peritoneal space becomes seeded with microorganisms. Peritonitis is either *primary* (without an apparent inciting event) or *secondary*. In adults, primary or spontaneous bacterial peritonitis (SBP) is most common among pts with cirrhosis of the liver due to alcoholism. PTS with preexisting ascites are predisposed to infection at this site. The pathogenic mechanism is presumed to be seeding of ascites when the diseased liver with altered portal circulation is unable to perform its usual filtration function. A single bacterial species usually causes SBP, and accompanying bacteremia is common. Secondary peritonitis develops when bacteria contaminate the peritoneum as a result of spillage from a ruptured viscus. Mixed aerobic and anaerobic bacteria are the rule in secondary peritonitis.

CLINICAL MANIFESTATIONS *SBP* Fever, the most common presenting symptom, is documented in 80% of cases of SBP. Abdominal pain, acute onset of symptoms, and peritoneal signs on physical exam are diagnostically helpful, but absence of these findings does not exclude this subtle diagnosis. Ascites virtually always predates infection.

Secondary Peritonitis Localized symptoms, if present, depend on the inciting event. In cases of perforated gastric ulcer, epigastric pain is evident. In appendicitis, initial symptoms may be vague and may include nausea or periumbilical discomfort gradually localizing to the RLQ. Symptoms of secondary peritonitis include abdominal pain that increases with motion, coughing, or sneezing. Pts often lie with knees drawn up to avoid stretching peritoneal nerve fibers. Findings on abdominal exam include voluntary and involuntary guarding, tenderness, and, at a later stage, rebound tenderness.

DIAGNOSIS To diagnose SBP, a tap of the ascites is essential in every febrile cirrhotic pt. Peritoneal fluid should be placed in a blood culture bottle to increase yield. Blood should be cultured. For secondary peritonitis, diagnosis should focus on identifying the inciting event; a tap of peritoneal fluid is rarely needed.

℞ TREATMENT
Therapy for SBP should be directed at the organism recovered. Empirical therapy should include coverage for gram-negative

aerobic bacilli and gram-positive cocci. Third-generation cephalosporins, carbapenems, or broad-spectrum penicillin/ β-lactamase inhibitor combinations are reasonable options. If mixed flora (particularly anaerobes) are recovered in suspected SBP, the pt should be evaluated for secondary peritonitis. Treatment for secondary peritonitis includes antibiotics directed at aerobic gram-negative bacilli and at anaerobes as well as surgical intervention for the inciting process.

INTRAPERITONEAL ABSCESSES

PATHOGENESIS Intraperitoneal abscesses represent both a disease process and a host response. Anaerobic organisms, particularly *Bacteroides fragilis*, are critical in the development of these abscesses. The most important virulence factor of this organism is the capsular polysaccharide, which is responsible for the development of abscesses. Several host factors, including peritoneal macrophages, PMNs, and T cells, also appear to interact and stimulate abscess formation.

CLINICAL MANIFESTATIONS Intraabdominal abscesses can be either intraperitoneal or retroperitoneal and are associated with no specific organ in 74% of cases. Infections of the female genital tract and pancreatitis are common causative events. Fever is the most common presenting symptom. As in secondary peritonitis, localizing symptoms depend on the inciting process. In psoas abscess, back or abdominal pain is common and associated osteomyelitis is found frequently.

VISCERAL ABSCESSES *Liver Abscesses* The liver is the intraabdominal organ in which abscesses develop most often. Fever is the most common presenting symptom. Only 50% of pts have signs or symptoms that direct attention to the RUQ, including hepatomegaly, tenderness, or jaundice.

Splenic Abscesses These frequently are diagnosed only at autopsy. Generally, abscesses in the spleen arise from hematogenous spread. Bacterial endocarditis is the most common associated infection. Abdominal pain is reported in 50% of cases but is localized to the LUQ in only half of these instances. Fever is common; splenomegaly is documented in about 50% of cases.

Perinephric and Renal Abscesses These generally arise from an initial urinary tract infection, often in association with nephrolithiasis. The clinical presentation is nonspecific. Pts may have flank and abdominal pain; 50% have fever. Pain may be referred to the groin or leg.

DIAGNOSIS Scanning procedures generally are diagnostic; CT is most useful. Ultrasonography is particularly helpful for the RUQ, kidneys, and pelvis. Gallium- and indium-labeled WBCs localize in abscesses and may be useful in finding a collection. If one study is negative, a second study is sometimes revealing.

℞ TREATMENT

Treatment of intraabdominal infections involves establishment of an initial focus of infection, administration of antibiotics targeted at likely organisms, and performance of a drainage procedure if one or more definitive abscesses are found. Antibiotic treatment is adjunctive to drainage (percutaneous or surgical) and usually is directed at organisms involved in the inciting infection, which generally include aerobic gram-negative bacilli and anaerobes. Against gram-negative aerobic and facultative bacteria, aminoglycosides, third-generation cephalosporins, and the quinolones are the most widely tested agents, but they must be used in combination with another antibiotic active against anaerobes (e.g., metronidazole) when the latter organisms are likely to be involved in the process.

For a more detailed discussion, see Zaleznik DF, Kasper DL: Intraabdominal Infections and Abscesses, Chap. 127, p. 792, in HPIM-14; and Anaerobic Infections, Chap. 87, p. 495 in the Companion.

74

INFECTIOUS DIARRHEAS

Etiology and Pathogenesis

Infectious diarrhea may be caused by a wide variety of microorganisms and may be mediated by toxins and/or by direct invasion of the GI mucosa. It is useful to categorize diarrheal diseases according to whether the responsible pathogens cause inflammatory or noninflammatory intestinal changes. Infections with pathogens that induce acute inflammation (e.g., *Shigella* species and *Entamoeba histolytica*) tend to involve the lower GI tract; cause small, purulent or bloody stools; and are accompanied by fever. Infections due to noninflammatory pathogens (e.g., enterotoxigenic *Escherichia coli*, *Giardia lamblia*) tend to involve the upper GI tract and cause more voluminous but nonbloody stools that do not contain PMNs.

—————— *Approach to the Patient* ——————

The history should include inquiries about fever, abdominal pain, nausea/vomiting, character of stools (whether watery or bloody; volume), food recently ingested (seafood; a possible common source, such as a picnic or restaurant), travel (exact location, duration, and nature of trip), sexual exposures, and general medical history (especially other illnesses and therapy with immunosuppressive drugs, antibiotics, or gastric-acid inhibitors). A complete physical exam should be performed, with particular attention to abdominal findings. Stool specimens should be examined grossly for consistency and the presence of blood and microscopically for the presence of PMNs. Stool should be cultured for *Salmonella*, *Shigella*, and *Campylobacter* if the diarrhea is inflammatory. The other diagnostic tests selected will depend on the clinical circumstances and may include an assay for *Clostridium difficile* cytotoxin (in the setting of recent use of antibiotics), an examination for ova and parasites (travel), and cultures for vibrios (seafood ingestion) and for *Yersinia* and enterohemorrhagic *E. coli*.

NONINFLAMMATORY DIARRHEA

ENTEROTOXIGENIC *E. COLI* ETEC causes most cases of traveler's diarrhea. The illness presents after 24–72 h of incubation as watery diarrhea, which is usually mild and is only occasionally accompanied by fever or vomiting. This diarrhea is usually self-limited (3–6 d in duration) and may be treated with oral fluid replacement (commercial or homemade solution consisting of 3.5 g of sodium chloride, 2.5 g of sodium bicarbonate, 1.5 g of potassium chloride, and 20 g of glucose per liter of water) or antimotility agents (e.g., loperamide, 4 mg at onset and 2 mg after each loose stool; up to 16 mg/d). Antibiotic therapy reduces the duration of illness to 24–36 h. Bismuth subsalicylate, which has both antimicrobial and anti-inflammatory properties, has only a minimal effect on the normal GI flora. It may be taken as 2 tablets (525 mg) every 30–60 min for up to 8 doses. TMP-SMZ (160/800 mg bid), doxycycline (100 mg bid), or ciprofloxacin (500 mg bid; for adults only) also may be used, each for a 3-d course.

CLOSTRIDIUM PERFRINGENS *C. perfringens* produces a preformed toxin in food that causes illness 8–14 h after ingestion of contaminated meat, poultry, or legumes. The illness is manifest by diarrhea and crampy abdominal pain and rarely lasts more than 24 h. It is treated by fluid replacement, if necessary, and does not require antibiotics.

STAPHYLOCOCCUS AUREUS Ingestion of *S. aureus* preformed enterotoxin causes a rapid onset (within 2–6 h) of vomiting and diarrhea. Staphylococcal food poisoning is associated epidemiologically with institutional outbreaks and high attack rates. The illness is of short duration (<10 h) and requires, at most, fluid replacement for treatment.

BACILLUS CEREUS *B. cereus* produces two clinical syndromes. An emetic form, caused by a staphylococcal type of enterotoxin, resembles staphylococcal food poisoning and is epidemiologically associated with contaminated fried rice. A diarrheal form, caused by an *E. coli* LT–like enterotoxin, presents commonly in conjunction with abdominal cramps.

VIBRIO CHOLERAE Caused by toxin-producing *V. cholerae*, cholera occurs principally in the Ganges delta, Southeast Asia, and Africa. An ongoing epidemic in South and Central America began in 1991. The disease occurs sporadically in coastal Texas and Louisiana. Clinical signs developing after an incubation period of 12–48 h include profuse watery diarrhea, vomiting, and dehydration. Cholera is diagnosed by culture of stool on special medium. *Treatment* consists primarily of fluid replacement (IV or oral) and tetracycline administration (2 g as a single oral dose in adults). Ciprofloxacin (30 mg/kg as a single oral dose, not to exceed 1 g) may be used for strains resistant to tetracycline. Erythromycin (40 mg/kg daily, given tid for 3 d) is the preferred treatment for children.

ROTAVIRUS The most important cause of severe dehydrating diarrhea in children under 3 years of age worldwide, rotavirus infection presents as vomiting of <24 h duration, diarrhea, and low-grade fever. It occurs more commonly in colder months and is treated by fluid replacement.

NORWALK-LIKE VIRUSES These food- and waterborne agents cause one-third of epidemics of nonbacterial diarrhea in developed countries. Disease occurs year-round, mainly affecting older children and adults. The illness is usually mild and does not require treatment.

G. LAMBLIA AND *CRYPTOSPORIDIUM* See Chap. 102.

INFLAMMATORY DIARRHEA

CAMPYLOBACTER *Campylobacter jejuni* is a leading cause of food-borne diarrhea in the U.S. and is also associated with exposure to infected (often asymptomatic) animals and with travel to developing countries. After an incubation period of 2–6 d, the illness presents as fever, crampy abdominal pain, and diarrhea. It is generally self-limited but may persist for days or up to 3–4 weeks. Similar disease may be caused by related species of *Campylobacter* (e.g., *C. coli*, *C. upsaliensis*). Diagnosis requires culture of the pathogen from stool on special medium at 42°C. *Treatment* consists of erythromycin (250 mg PO qid for 5–7 d). *Campylobacter fetus* is an occasional agent of diarrhea that causes septicemia in compromised hosts.

SHIGELLA Shigellosis is caused most often by *Shigella sonnei* in the U.S. and by *Shigella flexneri* and *Shigella dysenteriae* in the developing world. Person-to-person transmission is common, and 20–40% of household contacts develop disease. The prevalence is greatest among children and homosexual men. Although referred to as bacillary dysentery, shigellosis has clinical manifestations ranging from mild watery diarrhea to severe dysentery, often accompanied by fever, with onset after an incubation period of 1–7 d. Without treatment, fever persists for 3–4 d and diarrhea for 1–2 weeks. Hemolytic-uremic syndrome is a rare but serious complication of shigellosis. The diagnosis of shigellosis is based on the finding of fecal leukocytes and the culture of the organism from stool. *Treatment* includes fluid replacement and antibiotic administration. Resistance to ampicillin is now common among shigellae, and resistance to TMP-SMZ is increasing in frequency. Susceptible isolates may still be treated with one of these agents (ampicillin, 500 mg qid; TMP-SMZ, 160/800 mg bid) or with ciprofloxacin (500 mg bid; for adults only) or IV ceftriaxone (50 mg/kg daily for 5 d).

ENTEROHEMORRHAGIC *E. COLI* Certain *E. coli*, particularly serotype O157:H7, produce a Shiga-like toxin and cause a syndrome of bloody diarrhea. Outbreaks are frequently food-borne. Hemolytic-uremic syndrome is a rare but serious complication of infection with EHEC. The diagnosis may be made by identification of the organism in stool cultured on special medium.

CLOSTRIDIUM DIFFICILE Infection with the cytotoxin-producing anaerobe *C. difficile* is commonly associated with antibiotic use and classically causes pseudomembranous colitis. Clinical manifestations include fever, elevated WBC count, and diarrhea. The infection is diagnosed by the detection of cytotoxin in stool specimens. *Treatment* should include the discontinuation of any offending antibiotics and the administration of metronidazole (250 mg PO qid) or vancomycin (125 mg PO qid) for 7–10 d.

VIBRIO PARAHAEMOLYTICUS Present in coastal waters throughout the world, *V. parahaemolyticus* causes disease most frequently in association with the consumption of raw or undercooked seafood. It most commonly produces acute watery diarrhea accompanied by abdominal cramps, nausea, and vomiting and sometimes by fever and chills after an incubation period of 4 h to 4 d. The diagnosis is made by culture of the organism on special medium and must be suspected on the basis of exposure to seafood or the sea. *Treatment* of severe cases consists of fluid repletion and antibiotic administration (tetracycline, 500 mg qid).

E. HISTOLYTICA See Chap. 102.

SALMONELLA Salmonellae are acquired by consumption of contaminated food or drink, most commonly from eggs or poultry, and may cause clinical illness ranging from gastroenteritis to enteric fever. *S. typhimurium*, *S. enteritidis*, *S. heidelberg*, and *S. newport* cause most cases of human disease in the U.S. Pts at increased risk for salmonellosis include those using antacids, antibiotics, antimotility drugs, or immunosuppressive agents and those with HIV infection or sickle cell disease. Gastroenteritis is the most common manifestation. After an incubation period of 24–48 h, diarrhea develops and may be accompanied by cramps, nausea, vomiting, and fever. Stools may show fecal leukocytes and are sometimes frankly dysenteric. Illness is usually mild and self-limited but may become severe in elderly pts or neonates. Blood cultures may become positive, especially as gastroenteritis resolves. The diagnosis is based on culture of stool or blood.

Bacteremia/Enteric Fevers Prolonged *Salmonella*-positive blood cultures with sepsis (sometimes found in conjunction with schistosomiasis) generally are not preceded by diarrhea. This illness is similar to typhoid fever (see below) but may be more acute and is not associated with classic manifestations of typhoid such as rose spots, leukopenia, and relative bradycardia. This syndrome, frequently associated with *Salmonella choleraesuis* or *Salmonella dublin*, is serious and carries a high mortality. Pts with HIV infection have a high risk of *Salmonella* (particularly *S. typhimurium*) bacteremia, which may be refractory to treatment.

Localization of Systemic Infection Bloodborne salmonellae, usually present following GI infection, can invade any tissue or organ. Arterial infection may occur in preexisting arteriosclerotic aortic aneurysms, especially in men over age 50. Osteomyelitis (associated with sickle cell disease), hepatobiliary infection, splenic abscess, and UTI are all examples of localized *Salmonella* infection.

Typhoid Fever This form of enteric fever, caused by the exclusively human pathogen *Salmonella typhi* (and less commonly by *Salmonella paratyphi*), is linked epidemiologically to the ingestion of contaminated food, water, or milk and occurs most frequently in travelers. The risk of infection is increased by antibiotic use, malnutrition, and HIV infection. After an average incubation period of 10 d (range, 3–60 d), clinical manifestations include the insidious onset of headache, malaise, anorexia, an altered sensorium, and fever (which lasts 4–8 weeks and may then abate). Findings on physical exam include rose spots (erythematous macules of 2–4 mm on the upper abdomen), relative bradycardia, and hepatosplenomegaly. Complications include intestinal perforation and localized infection (meningitis, hepatitis, cholecystitis, nephritis, myocarditis, pneumonia, parotitis, orchitis). Chronic carriage develops in 3–5% and relapse in 20% of treated pts. Diagnosis depends on isolation of the organism from blood (with a 90% positivity rate in the first week and a decline thereafter) or stool (75% positivity by the third week). Serologic (Widal) testing is less reliable.

R̲x̲ **TREATMENT**

Uncomplicated *Salmonella* gastroenteritis does not require treatment and may prolong carriage except in pts with fever of long duration, aneurysms or vascular prostheses, or underlying immunosuppression (HIV disease, lymphoma, malignancy, sickle cell disease). Alternatives for the treatment of these pts include chloramphenicol (3 g/d), a third-generation cephalosporin (e.g., ceftriaxone, 1–2 g q12h), ciprofloxacin (500 mg bid), or ampicillin (6–12 g/d), each of which is also effective for bacteremia and localized infection. Many strains of *Salmonella* are resistant to ampicillin, chloramphenicol, and TMP-SMZ. Typhoid fever caused by sensitive strains may be treated with chloramphenicol (3–4 g/d PO) for 2 weeks; the dose may be reduced to 2 g/d when the pt becomes afebrile. Other agents effective against sensitive typhoid include amoxicillin (1–1.5 g PO qid), TMP-SMZ (160/800 mg PO qid), and ciprofloxacin (500 mg PO bid), each for 2 weeks. Alternatively, ceftriaxone (3–4 g/d IV) for as few as 3 d may be used. Glucocorticoids (dexamethasone, loading dose of 3 mg/kg followed by 1 mg/kg q6h for 24–48 h) may have an adjunctive role in severe typhoid.

For a more detailed discussion, see Butterton JR, Calderwood SB: Acute Infectious Diarrheal Diseases and Bacterial Food Poisoning, Chap. 128, p. 796; Kasper DL, Zaleznik DF: Gas Gangrene, Antibiotic-Associated Colitis, and Other Clostridial Infections, Chap. 148, p. 906; Keusch GT: Salmonellosis, Chap. 158, p. 950; Keusch GT: Shigellosis, Chap. 159, p. 957; Blaser MJ: Infections Due to *Campylobacter* and Related Species, Chap. 160, p. 960; Keusch GT, Deresiewicz RL: Cholera and Other Vibrioses, Chap. 161, p. 962; and Greenberg HB: Viral Gastroenteritis, Chap. 194, p. 1116, in HPIM-14.

75

SEXUALLY TRANSMITTED DISEASES

See Table 75-1 for a list of sexually transmitted pathogens and Table 75-2 for pathogens associated with clinical syndromes.

GONOCOCCAL INFECTIONS

ETIOLOGY   Gonorrhea, an infection of columnar and transitional epithelium, is caused by *Neisseria gonorrhoeae*, a gram-negative coccus found in pairs.

EPIDEMIOLOGY   Gonorrhea is the most common reportable communicable disease in the U.S. Its incidence has decreased from a peak of 473 cases per 100,000 in 1975 to 150 cases per 100,000 in 1995. Incidence and prevalence rates are related to age, gender, sexual preference, race, socioeconomic status, marital status, area of residence (urban, suburban, rural), and level of education. The incidence is higher among men, while the prevalence is higher among women. Gonorrhea is usually spread by asymptomatic carriers.

Table 75-1

Predominantly Sexually Transmitted Pathogens

Bacteria	Viruses	Other
Neisseria gonorrhoeae	Human immunodeficiency viruses	*Trichomonas vaginalis*
Chlamydia trachomatis	Human T-cell lymphotropic virus type I	*Phthirus pubis*
Treponema pallidum	Herpes simplex virus type 2	
Haemophilus ducreyi	Human papillomavirus	
Calymmatobacterium granulomatis	Hepatitis B virus*	
Ureaplasma urealyticum	Cytomegalovirus	
	Molluscum contagiosum virus	

* Among U.S. patients for whom a risk factor can be ascertained, most hepatitis B infections are sexually transmitted.

SOURCE: Modified from Holmes KK, Handsfield HH: HPIM-14, p. 802.

Table 75-2

Etiologic Agents of Common STD Syndromes

Syndrome	Primary Sexually Transmitted Agents*
Urethritis: males	*N. gonorrhoeae, C. trachomatis, U. urealyticum,* HSV
Epididymitis	*C. trachomatis, N. gonorrhoeae*
Lower genital tract infections: female	
Cystitis/urethritis	*C. trachomatis, N. gonorrhoeae,* HSV
Mucopurulent cervicitis	*C. trachomatis, N. gonorrhoeae*
Vulvovaginitis	*C. albicans, T. vaginalis*
Bacterial vaginosis	*Gardnerella vaginalis,* anaerobes, mycoplasmas
Acute pelvic inflammatory disease	*N. gonorrhoeae, C. trachomatis,* bacterial vaginosis–associated bacteria
Ulcerative genital lesions	HSV-2, *T. pallidum, H. ducreyi, C. trachomatis* (LGV strains), *C. granulomatis*
Proctitis	*C. trachomatis, N. gonorrhoeae,* HSV, *T. pallidum*
Acute arthritis	*N. gonorrhoeae* (e.g., DGI), *C. trachomatis* (e.g., Reiter's syndrome), HBV, HIV
Genital and anal warts	Human papillomavirus

* Some of these syndromes may also be caused by agents that are not sexually transmitted.

SOURCE: Modified from Holmes KK, Handsfield HH: HPIM-14, p. 803.

CLINICAL MANIFESTATIONS *Males* Urethritis develops 2–7 d after exposure, with symptoms of purulent urethral discharge (90–95%), dysuria, and meatal erythema. In the antibiotic era, complications due to *N. gonorrhoeae* (e.g., epididymitis, prostatitis, inguinal lymphadenitis) are rare. In homosexual men, rectal gonorrhea may produce anorectal pain, pruritus, tenesmus, or a bloody, mucopurulent rectal discharge. Pharyngeal infection may produce exudative tonsillitis in males or females but is frequently asymptomatic.

Females Gonococcal infection in the female involves (in descending order of frequency) the endocervix, urethra, anal canal, and pharynx. Up to one-half of women infected with *N. gonorrhoeae*, or perhaps an even larger portion, never develop symptoms. Acute uncomplicated gonorrhea produces mucopurulent (yellow) endocervical discharge and causes easily induced cervical bleeding; dysuria (due to urethritis) and anorectal discomfort (due to proctitis) are common. Extension of infection from the endocervix to the fallopian tubes occurs shortly after acquisition or during menstruation in at least 15% of cases, resulting in acute endometritis followed by acute salpingitis, the major complication of gonorrhea. Spread of infection to the upper abdomen may cause perihepatitis (Fitz-Hugh–Curtis syndrome), with right-sided or bilateral upper quadrant abdominal pain, tenderness, and occasionally a hepatic friction rub. Unilateral acute Bartholin's gland inflammation frequently is due to gonorrhea.

Children During delivery, the gonococcus may infect the conjunctivae, pharynx, respiratory tract, or anal canal of the infant. The risk of infection increases with prolonged rupture of membranes. Prophylaxis against gonococcal ophthalmia neonatorum is given routinely and consists of 1% silver nitrate eyedrops or an erythromycin-containing ophthalmic preparation.

Disseminated Gonococcal Infection (DGI) Two-thirds of patients with DGI are women; symptoms of bacteremia often begin during menses. Most women or men with DGI do not have symptoms of urogenital, anorectal, or pharyngeal gonorrhea. Pts present either with manifestations of gonococcemia (fever, polyarthralgias, and the appearance—usually on the distal extremities—of 3–20 papular, petechial, pustular, hemorrhagic, or necrotic skin lesions) or with purulent oligoarthritis. Initial joint manifestations are characteristically limited to tenosynovitis involving several joints asymmetrically, most commonly the wrists, fingers, knees, and ankles. Septic arthritis may ensue, often without prior fever, polyarthralgia, or skin lesions, and usually causes pain and swelling of a single joint.

DIAGNOSIS The presence of intracellular diplococci on Gram's stain of urethral or endocervical exudate is grounds for a presumptive diagnosis of gonorrhea. The organism is cultured on Thayer-Martin selective medium in a humidified, CO_2-enriched atmosphere. Acceptable specimens may be obtained with swabs of the urethra, endocervix, anorectum, and pharynx. Endocervical culture is positive in 80–90% of cases of gonorrhea in women; the yield can be increased by concomitant rectal, urethral, and pharyngeal cultures. All pts with gonorrhea should be serologically tested for syphilis and should be offered HIV testing.

℞ TREATMENT

(See Table 75-3) Treatment failures with the combination of ceftriaxone and doxycycline are rare. Pts do not routinely require follow-up cultures but should be evaluated if symptoms persist or recur after treatment. Reevaluation should include consideration of gonococcal reinfection or concomitant chlamydial infection.

CHLAMYDIAL INFECTIONS

Chlamydia trachomatis Genital Infections

EPIDEMIOLOGY An estimated 4 million cases of *C. trachomatis* genital infection occur each year, making these infections the most common bacterial STDs in the U.S. *C. trachomatis* and *N. gonorrhoeae* often coinfect women with cervicitis and heterosexual men with urethritis.

CLINICAL MANIFESTATIONS *Nongonococcal and Postgonococcal Urethritis* These terms refer, respectively, to pts with symptomatic urethritis who do not have gonococcal infection and those who become symptomatic 2–3 weeks after single-dose treatment for gonococcal infection. *C. trachomatis* accounts for 20–40% of cases of symptomatic urethritis among heterosexual men but is a less common cause among homosexual men.

Epididymitis *C. trachomatis* is the major cause of epididymitis in heterosexual men <35 years old in the U.S., accounting for 70% of cases. Men typically present with unilateral scrotal pain, fever, and epididymal tenderness or swelling. Testicular torsion should be excluded.

Reiter's Syndrome This syndrome consists of conjunctivitis, urethritis (in males) or cervicitis (in females), arthritis, and characteristic mucocutaneous lesions. *C. trachomatis* may be recovered from the urethra of up to 70% of men with nondiarrheal Reiter's syndrome and associated urethritis.

Proctitis Cases occur in people of either sex who practice receptive anal intercourse. Pts present with mild rectal pain, mucous discharge, tenesmus, and (occasionally) bleeding.

Mucopurulent Cervicitis (MPC) MPC, an inflammation of the columnar epithelium and subepithelium of the endocervix,

Table 75-3

Recommended Treatment for Gonococcal Infection: 1993 Guidelines of the Centers for Disease Control and Prevention

Diagnosis	Treatment of Choice
Uncomplicated infection of urethra, cervix, rectum, or pharynx	
Standard regimens	Ceftriaxone, 125-mg single IM dose
	or
	Cefixime, 400-mg single PO dose
	or
	Ciprofloxacin, 500-mg single PO dose
	or
	Ofloxacin, 400-mg single PO dose
	plus
	Doxycycline, 100 mg PO bid × 7 d
	or
	Azithromycin, 1-g single PO dose
Alternative regimens	Spectinomycin, 2-g single IM dose
	Ceftizoxime, 500-mg single IM dose
	Cefotaxime, 500-mg single IM dose
Gonorrhea in pregnancy	Ceftriaxone, 125-mg single IM dose
	or
	Spectinomycin, 2-g single IM dose
	plus
	Erythromycin base or stearate, 500 mg PO qid × 7 d
	or
	Erythromycin ethylsuccinate, 800 mg PO qid × 7 d

(continued)

Table 75-3 (*Continued*)

Recommended Treatment for Gonococcal Infection: 1993 Guidelines of the Centers for Disease Control and Prevention

Diagnosis	Treatment of Choice
DGI	
Initial therapy*	Ceftriaxone, 1 g IV or IM q24h
	or
	Cefotaxime or ceftizoxime, 1 g IV q8h
	or†
	Spectinomycin, 2 g IM q12h
	until 24–48 h after symptoms resolve
Subsequent therapy§	Cefixime, 400 mg PO bid
	or
	Ciprofloxacin, 500 mg PO bid
	to complete a 7- to 10-d course

* Hospitalization is recommended to exclude endocarditis, meningitis, and other diagnoses.
† Spectinomycin is given if the pt is allergic to β-lactam agents.
§ For pts without endocarditis or meningitis whose compliance is reliable.
SOURCE: Modified from Holmes KK, Morse SA: HPIM-14, p. 920.

is the most common major STD syndrome in women and can be a harbinger of pelvic inflammatory disease (PID). *C. trachomatis* is its most common cause, although *N. gonorrhoeae* is often responsible. Although many females with *C. trachomatis* infection of the cervix have no signs or symptoms, a careful speculum examination will reveal MPC in 30–50% of cases.

DIAGNOSIS The gold standard for diagnosis is isolation of *C. trachomatis* by cell culture techniques, which generally are available only at larger medical centers and have a sensitivity of 60–80%. Since the organism is an intracellular pathogen, specimens for culture must include epithelial cells. Antigen detection methods, nucleic acid hybridization tests, and tests based on DNA amplification have also been developed.

℞ TREATMENT
For uncomplicated genital infection, doxycycline (100 mg bid PO) or tetracycline (500 mg qid PO) can be given for 7 d.

For complicated infections (e.g., epididymitis, PID), a 14-d course is recommended. Azithromycin (1 g PO in a single dose) is effective in uncomplicated chlamydial infection and has appeal when follow-up care may not be possible. Ofloxacin (300 mg bid PO for 7 d) is also effective. These agents, however, are expensive. For pregnant pts, erythromycin base (500 mg qid PO for 10–14 d) is recommended. Sexual partners should be screened and treated whether or not they are symptomatic.

Lymphogranuloma Venereum

ETIOLOGY   Lymphogranuloma venereum (LGV) is a sexually transmitted infection caused by the L serovars of *C. trachomatis*.

CLINICAL MANIFESTATIONS   A primary genital lesion is noted in fewer than one-third of heterosexual men with LGV and in only a few women with this infection. When present, this lesion is small and painless and usually heals in a few days without scarring. Primary anal or rectal infection can develop after receptive anal intercourse; in women, it may also arise via contiguous perineal spread of infected vaginal secretions. Lymphadenitis results from spread from the primary site to regional nodes. The inguinal syndrome is the most common presentation in heterosexual men and is characterized by painful inguinal adenopathy beginning 2–6 weeks after exposure. In two-thirds of cases, the adenopathy is unilateral. Lymph nodes become matted, fluctuant, and suppurative. The overlying skin becomes inflamed, and draining fistulas may develop. Constitutional symptoms are common. LGV proctitis may present as anorectal pain; mucopurulent, bloody rectal discharge; and tenesmus. Symptoms accompanying regional lymphadenopathy include fever, chills, headache, meningismus, anorexia, myalgias, and arthralgias. Systemic complications are infrequent but may include arthritis with sterile effusion, aseptic meningitis, meningoencephalitis, conjunctivitis, hepatitis, and erythema nodosum.

DIAGNOSIS   LGV strains can be isolated from lymph nodes or the rectum and rarely from the urethra or cervix. Serologic testing is more useful diagnostically for LGV than for other *C. trachomatis* infections.

℞ TREATMENT
Fluctuant buboes should be aspirated through normal-appearing skin. The recommended antibiotic is tetracycline (500 mg qid PO) for a minimum of 14 d.

PELVIC INFLAMMATORY DISEASE

ETIOLOGY First episodes of acute PID generally are caused by the agents of sexually transmitted cervicitis—namely, *N. gonorrhoeae* and/or *C. trachomatis*. These pathogens are less often implicated in recurrent bouts of acute PID and in episodes in pts with intrauterine devices (IUDs).

EPIDEMIOLOGY The annual incidence of PID in the U.S. has declined since the mid-1970s. Risk factors for the development of PID include a history of salpingitis, a recent history of vaginal douching, and the use of an IUD.

CLINICAL MANIFESTATIONS *Nontuberculous Salpingitis* Symptoms evolve by stage of infection, which proceeds from cervicitis (mucopurulent vaginal discharge) to endometritis (midline abdominal pain and abnormal vaginal bleeding) to salpingitis (bilateral lower abdominal and pelvic pain) to peritonitis (nausea, vomiting, and increased abdominal tenderness). Abnormal uterine bleeding precedes or coincides with abdominal pain in 40% of women with PID; symptoms of urethritis (dysuria) occur in 20%. Symptoms of proctitis (anorectal pain, tenesmus, and rectal discharge or bleeding) are seen occasionally in pts with gonococcal or chlamydial infection. On speculum examination, MPC is found in the majority of pts with either of these infections. On bimanual examination, cervical motion tenderness, uterine fundal tenderness, and abnormal adnexal tenderness are found. The onset of salpingitis coincides with menses in pts with gonococcal or chlamydial infection. IUD-associated PID tends to be relatively indolent.

Tuberculous Salpingitis Unlike nontuberculous salpingitis, tuberculous salpingitis is found more often in older women, with 50% of cases documented after menopause. Common presenting symptoms include abnormal vaginal bleeding, pain, and infertility.

Perihepatitis Symptoms occur in 3–10% of pts with acute PID and include pleuritic upper abdominal pain and tenderness, usually localized to the RUQ. Perihepatitis or Fitz-Hugh–Curtis syndrome historically was attributed exclusively to gonococcal PID; most cases are now associated with chlamydial salpingitis.

Periappendicitis Appendiceal serositis without involvement of the intestinal mucosa can develop as a complication of gonococcal or chlamydial salpingitis.

Influence of HIV Infection HIV-infected women with PID are more likely than women without HIV infection to present with tuboovarian abscess, to require hospitalization, and to require surgery for PID.

DIAGNOSIS   Laparoscopy is the most specific method for diagnosis of acute salpingitis and yields culture specimens that can be used for bacteriologic diagnosis. Endometrial biopsy with the finding of tuberculous granulomas confirms the diagnosis of tuberculous salpingitis.

℞ TREATMENT

Two inpatient regimens have been used extensively: (1) doxycycline (100 mg IV q12h) plus cefoxitin (2 g IV q6h) or cefotetan (2 g IV q12h); and (2) clindamycin (900 mg IV q8h) plus gentamicin (1.5 mg/kg IV q8h after a loading dose of 2 mg/kg IV). Parenteral therapy should be continued until at least 48 h after the pt's condition improves, at which time doxycycline (100 mg PO bid) should be given to complete a 14-d course. For pts treated with regimen 2, clindamycin (450 mg qid) is an alternative oral agent; its enhanced anaerobic spectrum is particularly useful in cases with tuboovarian abscess. For pts who are not hospitalized, one reasonable outpatient regimen is ceftriaxone (a single dose of 250 mg IM) followed by doxycycline (100 mg PO bid for 14 d). An alternative outpatient regimen that provides good coverage of the major pathogens is ofloxacin (400 mg PO bid) plus metronidazole (500 mg PO bid) or clindamycin (450 mg PO qid) for 14. d. Sexual partners of pts with acute PID should be evaluated for STDs and promptly treated with a regimen effective against uncomplicated gonococcal and chlamydial infection.

SYPHILIS

ETIOLOGY   Syphilis is a chronic systemic infection caused by the spirochete *Treponema pallidum*.

EPIDEMIOLOGY   Nearly all cases of syphilis follow sexual contact with infectious lesions; less common modes of transmission include nonsexual personal contact, in utero exposure, and blood transfusion. A rather steady increase since 1956 in the number of new cases of infectious syphilis in the U.S. has been punctuated by four cycles of 7–10 years, each with a rapid rise and fall in incidence. Since the most recent peak in 1990, the number of cases reported annually has again declined by more than 50%. During the early part of the AIDS epidemic, about half of all pts with early syphilis were homosexual and bisexual men. Because of changes in sexual practices due to the epidemic, this proportion has decreased. The most recent epidemic of syphilis predominantly involved black heterosexual men and women and occurred largely in urban areas. The incidence of congenital syphilis parallels that of infectious syphilis in women.

CLINICAL MANIFESTATIONS   Syphilis is characterized by episodes of active disease interrupted by periods of latency and conventionally is divided into stages.

Primary Syphilis   The typical primary chancre usually begins as a single painless papule that rapidly becomes eroded and usually becomes indurated. Atypical primary lesions are common. In heterosexual men, the chancre is most often located on the penis. In homosexual men it can be found in the anal canal or rectum, in the mouth, or on the external genitalia, while in women common sites are the cervix and labia. Consequently, primary syphilis is less often recognized in women and homosexual men than in heterosexual men. Regional lymphadenopathy usually appears within 1 week of the primary lesion. The nodes are firm, nonsuppurative, and painless. The chancre generally heals within 4–6 weeks, but lymphadenopathy may persist for months.

Secondary Syphilis   Manifestations of secondary syphilis vary widely but include skin lesions, lymphadenopathy, and constitutional symptoms. The skin rash begins as pale, pink or red macules that may go unnoticed; proceeds to papules; and may progress to lesions that resemble pustules. The palms and soles are involved frequently. In intertriginous areas, papules enlarge to form moist pink or gray-white lesions called *condylomata lata*, which are highly infectious. During relapses of secondary syphilis, these lesions are particularly prominent. Mucous patches, which are superficial mucosal erosions, occur in 10–15% of cases. Constitutional symptoms may precede or accompany other manifestations and include sore throat (15–30%), fever (5–8%), weight loss (2–20%), malaise (25%), anorexia (2–10%), headache (10%), and meningismus (5%). Acute meningitis develops in only 1–2% of cases, but protein levels or WBC counts may be elevated in the CSF in ≥30%. Less common complications of secondary syphilis include hepatitis, nephropathy, GI involvement, arthritis, periostitis, and iridocyclitis.

Latent Syphilis   Positive reaginic and specific treponemal antibody tests for syphilis in a pt with a normal CSF examination and no clinical manifestations of syphilis indicate a diagnosis of latent syphilis. *Early latent syphilis* refers to latency during the first year after infection, whereas *late latent syphilis* refers to latency that has persisted longer. Untreated latent syphilis progresses to late syphilis in 30% of cases but may persist throughout life; it rarely if ever resolves without treatment.

Late Syphilis (Tertiary Stage)

1. *Neurosyphilis:* The spectrum of symptomatic neurosyphilis includes meningeal syphilis (occurring 2–20 months after infection, usually within the first year), meningovascular syphilis (on average, 7 years after infection), general paresis (after about 20 years), and tabes dorsalis (after about 25–30 years). Symptoms of meningeal syphilis include headache, nausea, vomiting, neck stiffness, cranial nerve palsies, seizures, and changes in mental status. Meningovascular syphilis presents most commonly as a stroke syndrome in the middle cerebral artery distribution, often preceded by a subacute encephalitic syndrome (headaches, vertigo, insomnia, psychological abnormalities). General paresis includes abnormalities of the personality, affect, reflexes (hyperactive), eye, sensorium, intellect, and speech. Tabes dorsalis presents as symptoms and signs of demyelination of the posterior columns, dorsal roots, and dorsal root ganglia (e.g., ataxic wide-based gait; footslap; paresthesias; bladder disturbances; impotence; areflexia; and loss of position, deep pain, and temperature sensation reflecting demyelination of the posterior columns). Trophic joint degeneration (Charcot's joints) results from loss of pain sensation. The small, irregular Argyll Robertson pupil, a feature of both general paresis and tabes dorsalis, reacts to accommodation but not to light.

2. *Cardiovascular syphilis:* Cardiovascular manifestations occur in ~10% of pts with untreated late latent disease and include aortitis, aortic regurgitation, saccular aneurysm (particularly in the ascending and transverse segments of the aortic arch), and coronary ostial stenosis. Symptoms appear 10–40 years after infection. Syphilitic aneurysms rarely dissect.

3. *Gummas:* Gummas are granulomatous inflammatory lesions that range from microscopic size to several centimeters in diameter. The most commonly involved sites are skin, bones, mouth, upper respiratory tract, larynx, liver, and stomach. The rapid healing of gummas after penicillin treatment may be diagnostically helpful.

DIAGNOSIS   Syphilis is most often diagnosed serologically. Nontreponemal tests, including the VDRL and the RPR, are used for initial screening; titers usually become negative with treatment. Specific treponemal tests, including the FTA-ABS and MHA-TP, confirm syphilis (when positive), identify false-positive nontreponemal tests (when negative), and remain positive even after therapy. Dark-field examination is used to evaluate suspicious moist cutaneous lesions. For the test to be considered truly negative, the results should be negative on 3 successive days. Direct immunofluorescence and PCR-based techniques are being developed. Evaluation for neurosyphilis is essential for any seropositive pt with neurologic signs, is recommended for all pts with untreated syphilis of unknown or >1 year's duration, and should be considered in pts whose VDRL or RPR tests remain positive 1 year after treatment. CSF should be examined; the most common findings are pleocytosis and an elevated protein level. The CSF VDRL is a highly specific but relatively insensitive diagnostic test. All pts with newly diagnosed syphilis should undergo HIV testing. Conversely, pts with newly diagnosed HIV infection should be tested for syphilis. Syphilis may be especially likely to progress to neurosyphilis in HIV-infected pts. Some authorities recommend CSF evaluation for all HIV-infected pts with syphilis. Serologic testing after treatment is important in all pts, particularly those also infected with HIV.

℞ TREATMENT

(See Table 75-4) Therapy for syphilis should be administered to both pregnant and nonpregnant pts according to the stage of the disease. The Jarisch-Herxheimer reaction to treatment for syphilis and certain other spirochetal infections consists of fever, chills, myalgias, headache, tachycardia, increased respiratory rate, increased circulating neutrophil count, and vasodilatation with mild hypotension. This reaction is self-limited and of undefined pathogenesis. It occurs in about 50% of pts treated for primary syphilis, 90% treated for secondary syphilis, and 25% treated for early latent syphilis. The onset usually comes within 2 h of the initiation of treatment, with resolution in 12–24 h. In neurosyphilis, the reaction is more delayed, peaking after about 12–14 h. For neurosyphilis and syphilis in pregnancy, penicillin is the drug of choice regardless of penicillin allergy history. With such a history, skin testing should be performed; if the allergy is confirmed, desensitization should precede penicillin therapy. For HIV-infected pts with syphilis, some authorities recommend treatment like that for neurosyphilis, whatever the stage of the syphilitic infection. The response of early syphilis to treatment should be determined by monitoring the quantitative VDRL or RPR titer 1, 3, 6, and 12 months after treatment (more frequently in HIV-infected pts). If the titer fails to fall by fourfold, if it rises, or if symptoms persist or recur, the pt should be re-treated. After treatment for neurosyphilis, CSF cell counts should be determined every 3–6 months for 3 years or until findings normalize.

Table 75-4

Recommendations for the Treatment of Syphilis*

Stage of Syphilis	Nonpenicillin Allergic	Penicillin Allergic
Primary, secondary, or early latent	Penicillin G benzathine (single dose of 2.4 million units IM, 1.2 million units in each buttock)	Tetracycline hydrochloride (500 mg PO qid) or doxycycline (100 mg PO bid) for 2 weeks
Late latent (or latent of uncertain duration), cardiovascular, or benign tertiary	Lumbar puncture CSF normal: Penicillin G benzathine (2.4 million units IM weekly for 3 weeks) CSF abnormal: treat as neurosyphilis	Lumbar puncture CSF normal: tetracycline hydrochloride (500 mg PO qid) or doxycycline (100 mg PO bid) for 4 weeks CSF abnormal: treat as neurosyphilis
Neurosyphilis† (asymptomatic or symptomatic)	Aqueous penicillin G (12–24 million units/d IV, given in divided doses every 4 h) for 10–14 days *or* Aqueous penicillin G procaine (2.4 million units/d IM) plus oral probenecid (500 mg qid), both for 10–14 days	Desensitization and treatment with penicillin if allergy is confirmed by skin testing
Syphilis in pregnancy	According to stage	Desensitization and treatment with penicillin if allergy is confirmed by skin testing

* See text for discussion of syphilis therapy in HIV-infected individuals.
† Some authorities recommend following these regimens with three doses of 2.4 million units of penicillin G benzathine, given IM 1 week apart. Penicillin G benzathine alone has given inferior results when used for the treatment of neurosyphilis. Drugs other than penicillin are not recommended.

SOURCE: Modified from Lukehart SA, Holmes KK: HPIM-14, p. 1031.

Table 75-5

Treatment of Genital Herpesvirus Infections

Indication	Therapy
First-episode infection	Acyclovir (200 mg PO 5×/d or 400 mg PO tid), valacyclovir (1000 mg PO bid), or famciclovir (250 mg PO bid) is administered for 10–14 d.
Severe disease or neurologic complication	Acyclovir (5 mg/kg IV) is given for 5 d.
Symptomatic recurrent infection	Acyclovir (200 mg PO 5×/d), valacyclovir (500 mg PO bid), or famciclovir (125 mg PO bid) for 5 d shortens durations of lesions and viral excretion.
Suppression of recurrences	Acyclovir (200 mg PO bid or tid, 400 mg PO bid, or 800 mg PO qd), valacyclovir (500 mg PO bid or 1000 mg PO qd), or famciclovir (250 mg PO bid) prevents symptomatic reactivation.

HERPES SIMPLEX VIRUS (HSV) INFECTIONS
(See also Chap. 94)

CLINICAL MANIFESTATIONS Fever, headache, malaise, and myalgias, along with local symptoms of pain, itching, dysuria, vaginal and urethral discharge, and tender inguinal lymphadenopathy, characterize primary genital infection with HSV. Lesions include vesicles, pustules, or painful erythematous ulcers. More than 80% of women have cervical or urethral involvement in first-episode infection. Recurrence rates within 12 months are about 90% for HSV-2 and 55% for HSV-1. HSV-1 and HSV-2 can cause rectal and perianal infections.

DIAGNOSIS The diagnosis can be made clinically with support from a positive Tzanck preparation showing multinucleated giant cells. The definitive diagnosis is made by isolation of the virus in tissue culture.

℞ **TREATMENT**
See Table 75-5.

CHANCROID

EPIDEMIOLOGY Chancroid, genital ulceration and inguinal adenitis caused by *Haemophilus ducreyi*, occurs throughout the world and is a significant health problem in developing countries. Although less common in the U.S., its incidence has increased dramatically in recent years.

CLINICAL MANIFESTATIONS Chancroid causes painful genital ulcers with ragged edges and minimal induration that bleed easily. About half of pts develop enlarged, tender inguinal lymph nodes that become fluctuant and may rupture.

DIAGNOSIS An accurate diagnosis of chancroid relies on cultures of *H. ducreyi* from the lesion. Selective, nutritionally rich medium is necessary.

R̲x̲ **TREATMENT**
Effective regimens include ceftriaxone, 250 mg IM as a single dose; erythromycin, 500 mg PO qid for 7 d; TMP-SMZ, one double-strength tablet PO bid for 7 d (in regions where resistant strains are not prevalent); and ciprofloxacin, 500 mg PO bid for 3 d.

DONOVANOSIS (GRANULOMA INGUINALE)

EPIDEMIOLOGY Donovanosis, of which the bacterial agent is *Calymmatobacterium granulomatis*, is a rare cause of genital ulcers in the U.S.

CLINICAL MANIFESTATIONS Most lesions appear within 30 d of sexual exposure. The process begins as a papule that ulcerates and develops into a painless, elevated zone of clean, beefy-red, friable granulation tissue. When secondary anaerobic infection occurs, pain and a foul-smelling exudate may be found. The disease is usually chronic; delays of months in seeking treatment are common. The inguinal region can be affected; diffuse intradermal and subcutaneous swelling creates a pseudobubo, so named because underlying lymph nodes are minimally involved.

DIAGNOSIS The diagnosis is best made by examination of impression smears prepared from specimens obtained by punch biopsy of granulation tissue from the periphery of a lesion. The specimen is ultimately stained with Wright-Giemsa. Donovan bodies appear as rounded coccobacilli of 1 by 2 μm lying within cystic spaces in the cytoplasm of large mononuclear cells.

℞ TREATMENT

Commonly used antibiotics include tetracycline (500 mg PO q6h), erythromycin (500 mg PO q6h), or TMP-SMZ (160/800 mg PO q12h). The newer quinolones, gentamicin, and chloramphenicol are also effective. Treatment is usually continued until the lesion has healed completely.

HUMAN PAPILLOMAVIRUS (HPV) INFECTIONS

ETIOLOGY   HPVs are nonenveloped viruses of the Papovaviridae family that infect the epithelium of the skin or mucous membranes.

CLINICAL MANIFESTATIONS   The incubation period of HPV disease is usually 3–4 months, with a range of 1 month to 2 years. Infections may be asymptomatic, produce warts, or be associated with a variety of benign and malignant neoplasms. Anogenital warts (condylomata acuminata) are sexually transmitted and occur on skin and mucosal surfaces of external genitalia and perianal areas. HPV has been associated strongly with dysplasia and carcinoma of the uterine cervix as well as with squamous carcinomas and dysplasias of the penis, anus, vagina, and vulva. HPV types 6 and 11 are most commonly associated with condylomata acuminata, whereas types 16 and 18 are most frequently detected in dysplasias and carcinomas of the genital tract.

DIAGNOSIS   Most visible genital warts can be diagnosed clinically. Colposcopy is invaluable in assessing vaginal and cervical lesions. Papanicolaou smears from cervical specimens may reveal cytologic evidence of HPV. Histologic examination of biopsy specimens is useful for persistent or atypical lesions. PCR can be used to detect HPV nucleic acids and to identify specific virus types.

℞ TREATMENT

Available modes of treatment are not completely effective, and some have significant side effects. Moreover, lesions may resolve spontaneously. Frequently used therapies include cryosurgery, application of caustic agents, electrodesiccation, surgical excision, and laser ablation. Topical 5-fluorouracil has also been used. Various interferon preparations have been employed with modest success; a topically applied interferon inducer, imiquimod, appears to be of benefit.

For a more detailed discussion, see Holmes KK, Handsfield HH: Sexually Transmitted Diseases: Overview and Clinical Approach, Chap. 129, p. 801; Holmes KK: Pelvic Inflammatory Disease, Chap. 130, p. 812; Holmes KK, Morse SA: Gonococcal Infections, Chap. 150, p. 915; Murphy TF, Kasper DL: Infections Due to *Haemophilus influenzae*, Other *Haemophilus* Species, the HACEK Group, and Other Gram-Negative Bacilli, Chap. 152, p. 924; Holmes KK: Donovanosis (Granuloma Inguinale), Chap. 166, p. 986; Lukehart SA, Holmes KK: Syphilis, Chap. 174, p. 1023; Stamm WE: Chlamydial Infections, Chap. 181, p. 1055; Corey L: Herpes Simplex Viruses, Chap. 184, p. 1080; and Reichman RC: Human Papillomavirus Infections, Chap. 190, p. 1098, in HPIM-14.

76

INFECTIONS OF SKIN, SOFT TISSUES, JOINTS, AND BONES

SKIN AND SOFT TISSUE INFECTIONS

The etiologic agents of several types of skin and soft tissue infections are listed in Table 76-1.

Erysipelas

Erysipelas, or lymphangitis of the dermis, features a fiery red, intensely painful, demarcated swelling of the face or extremities. Classic erysipelas is due to *Streptococcus pyogenes* and may be treated with penicillin. If the condition's appearance is not sufficiently distinctive to exclude cellulitis, it is prudent to broaden coverage as described below for cellulitis.

Cellulitis

Cellulitis is an acute inflammatory condition of the skin caused either by indigenous flora colonizing the skin or by a wide

Table 76-1

Skin and Soft Tissue Infections

Lesion, Clinical Syndrome	Infectious Agent	HPIM-14 Chapter
Vesicles		
Smallpox	Variola virus	188
Chickenpox	Varicella-zoster virus	185
Shingles (herpes zoster)	Varicella-zoster virus	185
Cold sores, herpetic whitlow, herpes gladiatorum	Herpes simplex virus	184
Hand-foot-and-mouth disease	Coxsackievirus A16	195
Orf	Parapoxvirus	188
Molluscum contagiosum	Pox-like virus	188
Bullae		
Staphylococcal scalded-skin syndrome	*Staphylococcus aureus*	142
Necrotizing fasciitis	*Streptococcus pyogenes, Clostridium* spp., mixed aerobes and anaerobes	169
Gas gangrene	*Clostridium* spp.	148
Halophilic vibrio	*Vibrio vulnificus*	161
Crusted lesions		
Bullous impetigo	*S. aureus*	142
Impetigo contagiosa	*S. pyogenes*	143
Ringworm	Superficial dermatophyte fungi	210
Sporotrichosis	*Sporothrix schenckii*	210
Histoplasmosis	*Histoplasma capsulatum*	203
Coccidioidomycosis	*Coccidioides immitis*	204
Blastomycosis	*Blastomyces dermatitidis*	205
Cutaneous leishmaniasis	*Leishmania* spp.	216
Cutaneous tuberculosis	*Mycobacterium tuberculosis*	171
Nocardiosis	*Nocardia asteroides*	167

(continued)

Table 76-1 (*Continued*)

Skin and Soft Tissue Infections

Lesion, Clinical Syndrome	Infectious Agent	HPIM-14 Chapter
Folliculitis		
Furunculosis	*S. aureus*	142
Hot-tub folliculitis	*Pseudomonas aeruginosa*	157
Swimmer's itch	*Schistosoma* spp.	224
Acne vulgaris	*Propionibacterium acnes*	55
Ulcers with or without eschars		
Anthrax	*Bacillus anthracis*	144
Ulceroglandular tularemia	*Francisella tularensis*	163
Bubonic plague	*Yersinia pestis*	164
Buruli ulcer	*Mycobacterium ulcerans*	173
Leprosy	*Mycobacterium leprae*	172
Cutaneous tuberculosis	*M. tuberculosis*	171
Erysipelas	*S. pyogenes*	143
Necrotizing fasciitis		
Streptococcal gangrene	*S. pyogenes*	143
Fournier's gangrene	Mixed aerobic and anaerobic bacteria	169
Myositis and myonecrosis		
Pyomyositis	*S. aureus*	142
Streptococcal necrotizing myositis	*S. pyogenes*	143
Gas gangrene	*Clostridium* spp.	148
Nonclostridial (crepitant) myositis	Mixed aerobic and anaerobic bacteria	169
Synergistic nonclostridial anaerobic myonecrosis	Mixed aerobic and anaerobic bacteria	169

SOURCE: Stevens DL: HPIM-14, p. 828.

variety of exogenous bacteria. These organisms can (1) be inoculated through small breaks in the skin (*S. pyogenes*) or via bites (*Pasteurella, Eikenella,* anaerobes); (2) originate in wounds, ulcers, or abscesses (*Staphylococcus aureus*); (3) be associated with sinusitis (*Haemophilus influenzae*); or (4) gain entry during immersion in water (*Aeromonas, Vibrio vulnificus*). Cellulitis is characterized by localized pain, erythema, swelling, and heat.

℞ TREATMENT

If an etiologic agent is suggested by the patient's history, treatment is directed at a specific pathogen or group of pathogens. Both blood and any abscess, open wound, or drainage should be cultured. In the absence of a specific etiology, treatment is directed at gram-positive pathogens. IV therapy with oxacillin (2 g q6h) or cefazolin (2 g q8h) is administered until signs of systemic toxicity have resolved and acute inflammation has improved substantially; oral treatment is then given to complete a 2-week course.

Impetigo

Impetigo begins as multiple pruritic erythematous lesions that evolve into yellow crusts. This infection may be caused by *S. pyogenes* (*impetigo contagiosa*) or *S. aureus* (*bullous impetigo*). It is important to recognize impetigo caused by *S. pyogenes* because of the risk of poststreptococcal glomerulonephritis. *Treatment* consists of dicloxacillin (500 mg PO qid), cephalexin (500 mg PO qid), or topical mupirocin ointment.

Necrotizing Fasciitis

This life-threatening infection of the fascia and soft tissues investing the muscles of the trunk or extremities may be caused by group A streptococci (often from apparent or inapparent infection via the skin), *Clostridium perfringens* (accompanying gas gangrene), or mixed aerobic and anaerobic bacteria (usually of GI origin). The infection presents acutely as pain, fever, and systemic toxicity, often with a paucity of cutaneous findings. Necrotizing fasciitis can extend to cutaneous structures, causing thrombosis, skin discoloration, crepitus, anesthesia, and bulla formation. As the infection extends rapidly along fascial planes and via veins and lymphatics, cutaneous and fascial necrosis and shock occur (e.g., streptococcal toxic shock syndrome). Early surgical exploration is critical to both diagnosis and therapy.

℞ TREATMENT

Antibiotic therapy is directed at the offending pathogen; for group A streptococci and clostridia, experimental data suggest that clindamycin (600–900 mg IV q8h) may be superior to penicillin. When polymicrobial infection is suspected, therapy consists of either a three-drug combination of metronidazole (750 mg q6h) plus ampicillin (2–3 g IV q6h) plus gentamicin (1–1.5 mg/kg q8h) or ampicillin/sulbactam (3 g IV q6h). Hyperbaric oxygen therapy may be useful in clostridial disease.

Myositis

Myositis can arise spontaneously (*S. aureus, S. pyogenes*) or after penetrating trauma (*Clostridium*). Streptococcal necrotizing myositis can accompany necrotizing fasciitis and can cause a systemic toxic shock syndrome.

BONE AND JOINT INFECTIONS

Infectious Arthritis

Acute bacterial arthritis is a common medical problem affecting individuals of all ages and requiring prompt recognition and treatment.

ETIOLOGY AND PATHOGENESIS Approximately 75% of nongonococcal pyarthroses are due to gram-positive cocci. *S. aureus* is the most common pathogen; next most common are streptococci of groups A and G, viridans streptococci, pneumococci, and—in neonates—group B streptococci. Gram-negative bacilli account for 20% of infections, typically affecting pts with risk factors for gram-negative bacteremia. Gonococcal infection is another common cause of septic arthritis (see Chap. 75). Infection usually occurs via hematogenous seeding of the synovium. Predisposing factors include infancy, immunosuppressive illness or therapy, alcoholism, IV drug use, and prior joint damage. Direct seeding of the joint may be attributable to trauma, arthroscopy, or surgery. An extraarticular focus of infection is identified in 25% of cases. Prosthetic joint infections are usually due to staphylococci (either coagulase-negative staphylococci or *S. aureus*) and occur in 1–4% of prosthetic joints over a 10-year period, with an increased rate in joints that have undergone revision. Other causes of acute infectious arthritis include rubella virus, hepatitis B virus, mumps virus, coxsackievirus, adenovirus, and parvovirus. *Borrelia burgdorferi* and *Treponema pallidum* may cause a more chronic, slowly progressive arthritis, as do *Mycobacterium tuberculosis* and fungal agents such as *Coccidioides, Sporothrix,* and *Histoplasma. Candida* and *Blastomyces* may cause acute or chronic arthritis.

CLINICAL MANIFESTATIONS Acute bacterial arthritis presents as a monarticular process involving the large joints (most commonly the knee and hip; next most commonly the ankle, wrist, elbow, and shoulder and the sternoclavicular and sacroiliac joints). Infection due to gram-positive cocci usually presents as an acute onset of swelling, pain, warmth, and limitation of movement. In the hip, effusion may be difficult to detect, and pain may be minimal or referred to the groin, buttock, lateral thigh, or anterior knee. Gram-negative infections tend to be more indolent, and pts typically present after 3 weeks of illness, frequently with coexistent osteomyelitis. Infections of prosthetic joints are even more indolent, with presenting symptoms so mild that diagnosis may be delayed by several months; there is always accompanying osteomyelitis.

DIAGNOSIS Analysis of aspirated synovial fluid is necessary for the diagnosis of bacterial joint infection. The fluid is usually turbid, with >25,000 WBCs/μL (typically >100,000/μL, with >90% neutrophils). Gram's staining identifies the pathogen in 75% of gram-positive and 30–50% of gram-negative infections. Cultures of joint fluid are usually positive. Blood should also be cultured. In gonococcal infection, Gram's staining rarely gives a positive result and synovial fluid culture is positive in only 40% of cases. Culture of skin and mucosal lesions on special medium and PCR-based assays of synovial fluid will improve the diagnostic yield. Prosthetic joint infections are generally diagnosed by the finding of loosening of the implant or of osteomyelitis on radiographs; the diagnosis is confirmed by needle aspiration of the joint. The ESR is usually elevated.

R︀X︀ **TREATMENT**
Optimal management requires IV antibiotic administration, drainage (usually by repeated daily aspiration), and immobilization of the joint. Open surgical drainage should be considered when the hip, shoulder, or sternoclavicular joint is infected; when fluid loculations occur; when cultures are persistently positive; or when effusion persists for >7 d. Prosthetic joints should be removed and replaced after antibiotic therapy. The choice of antibiotics is based initially on Gram's stain and then on culture. Staphylococcal infections are initially treated IV with oxacillin (2 g q4h), cefazolin (2 g q8h), or vancomycin (1 g q12h) for 4 weeks. Streptococcal arthritis is treated with penicillin G (2 million U q4h) for 2

weeks. Gram-negative septic arthritis is treated with a second- or third-generation cephalosporin (e.g., cefuroxime, 1.5 g IV q8h; or ceftriaxone, 1–2 g IV q12–24h) for 3–4 weeks. Infection due to *Pseudomonas aeruginosa* is treated for at least 3 weeks with a combination of an extended-spectrum penicillin (e.g., mezlocillin, 3 g IV q4h) and an aminoglycoside (e.g., tobramycin, 1.7 mg/kg IV q8h). If tolerated, this regimen is continued for an additional 2–3 weeks; alternatively, oral ciprofloxacin (750 mg bid) may be substituted for the aminoglycoside. Gonococcal arthritis is treated initially with ceftriaxone (1 g IV/IM q24h). After signs of local and systemic inflammation begin to resolve, therapy may be switched to an oral agent (cefixime, 400 mg bid; or ciprofloxacin, 500 mg bid) to complete a 7- to 10-d course. Amoxicillin (500 mg PO tid) may be used to complete therapy against penicillin-susceptible isolates.

Osteomyelitis

ETIOLOGY AND PATHOGENESIS   Microorganisms enter the bone by hematogenous spread or directly via a wound or from an adjacent site of infection. The metaphyses of long bones (tibia, femur, humerus) and the vertebrae are the most frequently involved sites. *S. aureus* and coagulase-negative staphylococci are the most common pathogens; gram-negative bacillary (*Pseudomonas, Serratia, Salmonella, Escherichia coli*), anaerobic, and polymicrobial infections occur in certain situations (e.g., diabetic foot ulcers). Tuberculosis, brucellosis, histoplasmosis, coccidioidomycosis, and blastomycosis are less frequent causes of osteomyelitis.

CLINICAL MANIFESTATIONS   Half of pts with osteomyelitis present with vague pain in the affected limb or the back (or in vertebral osteomyelitis, with pain due to nerve root irritation) of 1–3 months' duration with little or no fever. Children may experience an acute onset of fever, irritability, and lethargy, with local inflammation of <3 weeks' duration. Findings on physical exam may include point tenderness, muscle spasm, and draining sinus (especially with chronic osteomyelitis or an infected prosthetic joint).

DIAGNOSIS   Osteomyelitis is diagnosed by culture of appropriate specimens. If blood cultures are negative, pus obtained by needle aspiration from bone or bone biopsy should be cultured. Cultures from superficial sites are not reliable. Findings on plain films do not become positive for at least 10 d, and lytic lesions may not be visible for 2–6 weeks. Radionuclide bone scan may become positive within 2 d of infection. CT or MRI may become positive early and may aid in the localization of lesions and the demonstration of sequestra. The ESR is usually elevated but falls in response to therapy.

℞ TREATMENT

With prompt treatment, fewer than 5% of pts with acute hematogenous osteomyelitis develop chronic disease. Antibiotics should be given only after appropriate specimens have been obtained for culture. For acute hematogenous osteomyelitis, IV antibiotics active against the organisms identified should be given for 4–6 weeks. Surgical debridement should be considered if there is a poor response to therapy in the first 48 h or if there is undrained pus or septic arthritis. Appropriate therapy for *S. aureus* or empirical therapy in the absence of a positive culture includes oxacillin (2 g IV q4h) or cefazolin (2 g IV q8h). Treatment of gram-negative osteomyelitis must be based on identification of the organism and determination of its susceptibility. Because *Pseudomonas* and *Enterobacter* show a propensity to develop resistance during therapy, osteomyelitis due to these organisms should be treated with a combination of an aminoglycoside (e.g., tobramycin for *Pseudomonas* infection and gentamicin for *Enterobacter* at doses of 1.7 mg/kg q8h) and a β-lactam antibiotic (e.g., mezlocillin, 3 g q4h). A quinolone (e.g., ciprofloxacin, 400 mg IV q12h) may be substituted for the β-lactam antibiotic against *Pseudomonas* or used alone against *Enterobacter*. For other gram-negative bacillary infections of bone, treatment is based on susceptibility of the organism and ordinarily consists of a single agent, such as a cephalosporin (e.g., cefazolin, 2 g IV q8h; or ceftriaxone, 1 g IV q12h) or a fluoroquinolone (e.g., ciprofloxacin, 400 mg IV q8h). When sensitivity of the organism allows, oral ciprofloxacin (750 mg q12h) may be given after or instead of IV therapy. Chronic osteomyelitis requires complete drainage, debridement of sequestra, and removal of any prosthetic material as well as a 4- to 6-week course of antibiotics whose selection is based on culture of the bone. Skin flaps and bone grafts may facilitate healing. If the identity of the infecting organism(s) is known, antibiotic therapy should begin several days before surgery.

For a more detailed discussion, see Maguire JH: Osteomyelitis, Chap. 132, p. 824; Stevens DL: Infections of the Skin, Muscle, and Soft Tissues, Chap. 133, p. 827; Wessels MR: Streptococcal and Enterococcal Infections, Chap. 143, p. 885; and Thaler SJ, Maguire JH: Infectious Arthritis, Chap. 324, p. 1944, in HPIM-14.

INFECTIONS IN THE IMMUNOCOMPROMISED HOST

The immunocompromised pt is at increased risk for infection with both common and opportunistic pathogens and may have a blunted clinical response that challenges diagnosis. A person's immunity may be lowered by an inborn immune defect, acquired disease, loss of physical barriers, chemotherapy, or organ or marrow transplantation. The type of immune deficit and the anticipated infection (Tables 77-1 and 77-2) should guide therapy. The severely immunocompromised pt in whom infection is suspected should receive prompt, empiric antimicrobial therapy and undergo a thorough clinical evaluation. In life-threatening infection, treatment aimed at correction of the immune defect (e.g., immunoglobulin replacement or cytokine infusion) may improve outcome. See also Chap. 36.

For a more detailed discussion, see Finberg R: Infections in Patients with Cancer, Chap. 87, p. 537; and Finberg R, Fingeroth J: Infections in Transplant Recipients, Chap. 136, p. 840, in HPIM-14.

Table 77-1

Infections Associated with Common Defects in

Host Defect	Disease or Therapy Associated with Defect
NONSPECIFIC IMMUNITY	
Impaired cough	Rib fracture, neuromuscular dysfunction
Loss of gastric acidity	Achlorhydria, histamine blockade
Loss of cutaneous integrity	Penetrating trauma, athlete's foot
	Burn
	Intravenous catheter
Implantable device	Heart valve
	Artificial joint
Loss of normal bacterial flora	Antibiotic use
Impaired clearance	
Poor drainage	Urinary tract infection
Abnormal secretions	Cystic fibrosis
INFLAMMATORY RESPONSE	
Neutropenia	Hematologic malignancy, cytotoxic chemotherapy, aplastic anemia, HIV infection
Chemotaxis	Chédiak-Higashi syndrome, Job's syndrome, protein-calorie malnutrition
Phagocytosis (cellular)	Systemic lupus erythematosus, chronic myelogenous leukemia, megaloblastic anemia
Splenectomy	—
Microbicidal defect	Chronic granulomatous disease
	Chédiak-Higashi syndrome
	Interferon γ-receptor defect

Inflammatory or Immunologic Response

Common Etiologic Agent of Infection

Bacteria causing pneumonia, aerobic and anaerobic oral flora

Salmonella spp., enteric pathogens
Staphylococcus spp., *Streptococcus* spp.
Pseudomonas aeruginosa
Staphylococcus spp., *Streptococcus* spp., gram-negative rods,
  coagulase-negative staphylococci
Streptococcus spp., coagulase-negative staphylococci,
  Staphylococcus aureus
Staphylococcus spp., *Streptococcus* spp., gram-negative rods
Clostridium difficile, *Candida* spp.

Escherichia coli
Chronic pulmonary infection with *P. aeruginosa*

Gram-negative enteric bacilli, *Pseudomonas* spp., *Staphylococcus*
  spp., *Candida* spp.

S. aureus, Streptococcus pyogenes, Haemophilus influenzae,
  gram-negative bacilli

Streptococcus pneumoniae, H. influenzae

H. influenzae, S. pneumoniae, other streptococci,
  Capnocytophaga spp., *Babesia microti, Salmonella* spp.
Catalase-positive bacteria and fungi: staphylococci, *E. coli*,
  Klebsiella spp., *P. aeruginosa, Aspergillus* spp., *Nocardia* spp.
S. aureus, S. pyogenes
Mycobacterium spp., *Salmonella* spp.

(*continued*)

Table 77-1 (*Continued*)

Infections Associated with Common Defects in

Host Defect	Disease or Therapy Associated with Defect
COMPLEMENT SYSTEM	
C3	Congenital liver disease, systemic lupus erythematosus, nephrotic syndrome
C5	Congenital
C6, C7, C8	Congenital, systemic lupus erythematosus
Alternative pathway	Sickle cell disease
IMMUNE RESPONSE	
T lymphocyte deficiency/ dysfunction	Thymic aplasia, thymic hypoplasia, Hodgkin's disease, sarcoidosis, lepromatous leprosy AIDS
	Mucocutaneous candidiasis
	Purine nucleoside phosphorylase deficiency
B cell deficiency/ dysfunction	Bruton's X-linked agammaglobulinemia
	Agammaglobulinemia, chronic lymphocytic leukemia, multiple myeloma, dysglobulinemia
	Selective IgM deficiency
	Selective IgA deficiency
Mixed T and B cell deficiency/dysfunction	Common variable hypogammaglobulinemia
	Ataxia-telangiectasia
	Severe combined immunodeficiency
	Wiskott-Aldrich syndrome

SOURCE: Madoff LC, Kasper DL: HPIM-14, p. 750 (as adapted from Masur H, Fauci A: HPIM-13, p. 497).

Inflammatory or Immunologic Response

Common Etiologic Agent of Infection

S. aureus, S. pneumoniae, Pseudomonas spp., *Proteus* spp.

Neisseria spp., gram-negative rods
Neisseria meningitidis, Neisseria gonorrhoeae

S. pneumoniae, Salmonella spp.

Listeria monocytogenes, Mycobacterium spp., *Candida* spp.,
  Aspergillus spp., *Cryptococcus neoformans,* herpes simplex
  virus, varicella-zoster virus
Pneumocystis carinii, cytomegalovirus, herpes simplex virus,
  Mycobacterium avium-intracellulare, C. neoformans, Candida
  spp.
Candida spp.
Fungi, viruses

S. pneumoniae, other streptococci

H. influenzae, N. meningitidis, S. aureus, Klebsiella pneumoniae,
  E. coli, Giardia lamblia, P. carinii, enteroviruses

S. pneumoniae, H. influenzae, E. coli
G. lamblia, hepatitis virus, *S. pneumoniae, H. influenzae*
P. carinii, cytomegalovirus, *S. pneumoniae, H. influenzae,*
  various other bacteria
S. pneumoniae, H. influenzae, S. aureus, rubella virus, *G.*
  lamblia
S. aureus, S. pneumoniae, H. influenzae, Candida albicans, P.
  carinii, varicella-zoster virus, rubella virus, cytomegalovirus
Agents of infections associated with T and B cell abnormalities

Table 77-2

Infections and Cancer

Cancer	Underlying Immune Abnormality	Organisms Causing Infection
Multiple myeloma	Hypogammaglobulinemia	*Streptococcus pneumoniae, Haemophilus influenzae, Neisseria meningitidis*
Chronic lymphocytic leukemia	Hypogammaglobulinemia	*S. pneumoniae, H. influenzae, N. meningitidis*
Acute myelocytic or lymphocytic leukemia	Granulocytopenia, skin and mucous-membrane lesions	Extracellular gram-positive and -negative bacteria, fungi
Hodgkin's disease	Abnormal T cell function	Intracellular pathogens (*Mycobacterium tuberculosis, Listeria, Salmonella, Cryptococcus, Mycobacterium avium*) *Pneumocystis carinii*
Non-Hodgkin's lymphoma and acute lymphocytic leukemia	Steroid chemotherapy, T and B cell dysfunction	
Colon and rectal tumors	Local abnormalities*	*Streptococcus bovis* (bacteremia)
Hairy cell leukemia	Abnormal T cell function	Intracellular pathogens (*M. tuberculosis, Listeria, Cryptococcus, M. avium*)

*The reason for this association is not well defined.
SOURCE: Finberg R: HPIM-14, p. 539.

434

78

HIV INFECTION AND AIDS

Definition

AIDS (acquired immunodeficiency syndrome), was originally defined empirically by the Centers for Disease Control and Prevention (CDC) as "the presence of a reliably diagnosed disease that is at least moderately indicative of an underlying defect in cell-mediated immunity." Following the recognition of the causative virus, HIV (formerly called HTLV-III/LAV), and the development of sensitive and specific tests for HIV infection, the definition of AIDS has undergone substantial revision. The current surveillance definition categorizes HIV-infected persons on the basis of clinical conditions associated with HIV infection and CD4 + T lymphocyte counts (see Tables 308-1 and 308-2, p.1792, in HPIM-14). From a practical standpoint, the clinician should view HIV infection as a spectrum of disorders ranging from primary infection, with or without the acute HIV syndrome, to the asymptomatic infected state to advanced disease.

Etiology

AIDS is caused by infection with the human retroviruses HIV-1 or HIV-2. HIV-1 is the most common cause worldwide; HIV-2 has about 40% sequence homology with HIV-1, is more closely related to simian immunodeficiency viruses, and has been identified predominantly in western Africa. HIV-2 infection has now, however, been reported in Europe, South America, Canada, and the United States. These viruses are passed through sexual contact; through contact with blood, blood products, or other bodily fluids (as in drug abusers who share contaminated intravenous needles); intrapartum or perinatally from mother to infant; or via breast milk. There is no evidence that the virus can be passed through casual or family contact or by insects such as mosquitoes. There is a definite, though small, occupational risk of infection for health care workers and laboratory personnel who work with HIV-infected specimens. The risk of transmission of HIV from an infected health care worker to his or her pts through invasive procedures is extremely low.

Epidemiology

By January 1, 1997, a cumulative total of approximately 570,000 cases of AIDS had been reported in the United States; approximately 60% of those had died. It has been estimated that there are between 630,000 and 897,000 HIV-infected people in the

U.S. Major risk groups continue to be men who have had sex with men and men and women injection drug users (IDUs); however, the numbers of cases that are transmitted heterosexually, particularly among women, are increasing rapidly (see Table 308-4 and Fig. 308-10, p.1800, in HPIM-14). These women also transmit the infection to their children. As the majority of IDU-associated cases are among inner-city minority populations, the burden of HIV infection and AIDS falls increasingly and disproportionately on minorities, especially in the cities of the Northeast and Southeast U.S. Cases of AIDS are still being found among individuals who have received contaminated blood products in the past, although the risk of acquiring new infection through this route is extremely small in the U.S. HIV infection/AIDS is a global pandemic, especially in developing countries. The World Health Organization estimates that by the year 2000 there will be 40 to 100 million HIV-infected people worldwide.

Pathophysiology and Immunopathogenesis

The hallmark of HIV disease is a profound immunodeficiency resulting from a progressive quantitative and qualitative deficiency of the subset of T lymphocytes referred to as helper or inducer T cells. This subset of T cells is defined phenotypically by the expression on the cell surface of the CD4 molecule, which serves as the primary cellular receptor for HIV. Recently, it has been demonstrated that a coreceptor must be present with CD4 for efficient entry of HIV-1 into target cells. These coreceptors belong to the seven-transmembrane-domain G protein–coupled family of receptors. The molecule termed CXCR4, or *fusin*, is the coreceptor for T cell–tropic strains of HIV-1, and the β-chemokine receptor CCR-5 is the coreceptor for macrophage-tropic strains of HIV-1. Although the CD4+ T lymphocyte and CD4+ monocyte lineage are the principal cellular targets of HIV, virtually any cell that expresses CD4 along with one of the coreceptors can potentially be infected by HIV.

PRIMARY INFECTION   Following initial transmission, the virus infects CD4+ cells, probably T lymphocytes, monocytes, or bone marrow–derived dendritic cells. Both during this initial stage and later in infection, the lymphoid system is a major site for the establishment and propagation of HIV infection. Initially, lymph node architecture is preserved, but ultimately it is completely disrupted and the efficiency of the node in trapping virions declines, leading to equilibration of the viral burden between peripheral blood cells and lymph node cells.

Most pts undergo a viremic stage during primary infection,

in some pts associated with the "acute retroviral syndrome," a mononucleosis-like illness. This phase is important in disseminating virus to lymphoid and other organs throughout the body, and it is ultimately contained partially by the development of an HIV-specific immune response and the trapping of virions in lymphoid tissue.

ESTABLISHMENT OF CHRONIC AND PERSISTENT INFECTION   Despite the robust immune response that is mounted following primary infection, the virus, with very few exceptions, is not cleared from the body. Instead, a chronic infection develops that persists for a median time of 10 years before the patient becomes clinically ill. During this period of clinical latency, the number of CD4 + T cells gradually declines but few, if any, clinical findings are evident; however, active viral replication can almost always be detected by measurable plasma viremia and the demonstration of virus replication in lymphoid tissue. The level of steady-state viremia (referred to as the viral *set point*) at approximately 1 year postinfection has important prognostic implications for the progression of HIV disease; individuals with a low viral set point at 6 months to 1 year after infection progress to AIDS more slowly than those whose set point is very high at this time.

ADVANCED HIV DISEASE   After some period of time (often years), CD4 + T cell counts will fall below some critical level (approximately 200 cells/μL) and patients become highly susceptible to opportunistic disease.

Immune Abnormalities in HIV Disease

A broad range of immune abnormalities has been documented in HIV-infected pts. These include both quantitative and qualitative defects in lymphocyte, monocyte/macrophage, and natural killer (NK) cell function, as well as the development of autoimmune phenomena.

Immune Response to HIV Infection

Both humoral and cellular immune responses to HIV develop soon after primary infection (see summary in Table 308-9 and Fig. 308-17, p. 1813, in HPIM-14). Humoral responses include antibodies with HIV binding and neutralizing activity, as well as antibodies participating in antibody-dependent cellular cytotoxicity (ADCC). Cellular immune responses include the generation of HIV-specific CD4 + and CD8 + T lymphocytes, as well as NK cells and mononuclear cells mediating ADCC. CD8 + T lymphocytes may also suppress HIV replication in a noncytolytic, non-MHC restricted manner. This effect is mediated by soluble factors such as the β-chemokines RANTES, MIP-1α, and MIP-1β as well as other as yet unidentified factors secreted by CD8 + T lymphocytes.

Diagnosis of HIV Infection

Laboratory diagnosis of HIV infection depends on the demonstration of anti-HIV antibodies and/or the detection of HIV or one of its components.

The standard screening test for HIV infection is the detection of anti-HIV antibodies using ELISA (enzyme-linked immunosorbent assay). This test is highly sensitive (>99.5%) and is quite specific. Western blot is the most commonly used confirmatory test and detects antibodies to HIV antigens of specific molecular weights. Antibodies to HIV begin to appear within 2 weeks of infection, and the period of time between initial infection and the development of detectable antibodies is rarely longer than 3 months. The HIV p24 antigen can be measured using a capture assay, an ELISA-type assay. Plasma p24 antigen levels rise during the first few weeks following infection, prior to the appearance of anti-HIV antibodies. HIV can be cultured directly from tissue, peripheral blood cells, or plasma, but this is most commonly done in a research setting. HIV genetic material can be detected using PCR. This is a useful test in pts with a positive or indeterminate ELISA and an indeterminate western blot or in pts in whom serologic testing may be unreliable (such as those with hypogammaglobulinemia).

Laboratory Monitoring of Patients with HIV Infection

Measurement of the CD4 + T cell count and level of plasma HIV RNA are important parts of the routine evaluation and monitoring of HIV-infected individuals. The CD4 + T cell count is a generally accepted indicator of the immunologic competence of the patient with HIV infection, and there is a close relationship between the CD4 + T cell count and the clinical manifestations of AIDS. Pts with CD4 + T cell counts below 200/μL are at high risk of infection with *Pneumocystis carinii,* while pts with CD4 + T cell counts below 100/μL are at high risk for developing CMV disease and infection with *Mycobacterium avium-intracellulare.* While the CD4 + T cell count provides information on the current immunologic status of the pt, the HIV RNA level predicts what will happen to the CD4 + T cell count in the near future and hence predicts the clinical prognosis. Measurement of plasma HIV RNA is also useful in making therapeutic decisions. A level of HIV RNA >20,000 copies/mL is felt by many experts to be an indication for initiation of antiretroviral therapy regardless of the CD4 + T cell count (see below).

Clinical Manifestations of HIV Infection

A complete discussion is beyond the scope of this chapter. Several classes of infected pts have been described, as defined in the CDC classification:

Group I   Acute HIV syndrome (acute retroviral syndrome)
Group II   Asymptomatic infection
Group III   Persistent generalized adenopathy
Group IV   Other diseases:
    Subgroup A: Constitutional disease (e.g., fever, weight loss, diarrhea)
    Subgroup B: Neurologic disease
    Subgroup C: Secondary infectious diseases
    Subgroup D: Secondary neoplasms
    Subgroup E: Other conditions

Characteristics of each of these groups are summarized below.

Group I—Acute HIV (Retroviral) Syndrome Approximately 50 to 70% of infected individuals experience an acute syndrome following primary infection. Acute syndrome follows infection by 3 to 6 weeks. Characterized by fevers, rigors, arthralgias, myalgias, maculopapular rash, urticaria, abdominal cramps, diarrhea, and aseptic meningitis; lasts 1 to 2 weeks and resolves spontaneously as immune response to HIV develops. Most pts will then enter a phase of clinical latency, although an occasional pt will experience progressive immunologic and clinical deterioration.

Group II—Asymptomatic Infection Length of time between infection and development of disease varies greatly, but the median is estimated to be 10 years. HIV disease with active viral replication usually progresses during this asymptomatic period, and CD4 + T-cell counts fall. The rate of disease progression is directly correlated with plasma HIV RNA levels. Pts with high levels of HIV RNA progress to symptomatic disease faster than do those with low levels of HIV RNA.

Group III—Persistent Generalized Lymphadenopathy Palpable adenopathy at two or more extrainguinal sites that persists for more than 3 months without explanation other than HIV infection. Many pts will go on to disease progression.

Group IV—Other Diseases

- *Subgroup A—constitutional symptoms:* Fever persisting for more than 1 month, involuntary weight loss of more than

10% of baseline, diarrhea for longer than 1 month in absence of explainable cause.

- *Subgroup B— neurologic disease:* Most common is HIV encephalopathy (AIDS dementia complex); other neurologic complications include opportunistic infections, primary CNS lymphoma, CNS Kaposi's sarcoma, aseptic meningitis, myelopathy, peripheral neuropathy and myopathy.
- *Subgroup C—secondary infectious diseases:* (for complete list of clinical manifestations and treatment, see Table 308-21, p.1826, in HPIM-14). *P. carinii* pneumonia is most common opportunistic infection, occurring in approximately 80% of individuals during the course of their illness. Other common pathogens include CMV (chorioretinitis, colitis, pneumonitis, adrenalitis), *Candida albicans* (oral thrush, esophagitis), *M. avium-intracellulare* (localized or disseminated infection), *M. tuberculosis, Cryptococcus neoformans* (meningitis, disseminated disease), *Toxoplasma gondii* (encephalitis, intracerebral mass lesion), herpes simplex virus (severe mucocutaneous lesions, esophagitis), diarrhea due to *Cryptosporidium* spp. or *Isospora belli,* bacterial pathogens (especially in pediatric cases).
- *Subgroup D—secondary neoplasms:* Kaposi's sarcoma (cutaneous and visceral, more fulminant course than in non-HIV-infected patients), lymphoid neoplasms (especially B cell lymphomas of brain, marrow, GI tract).
- *Subgroup E—other diseases:* A variety of organ-specific syndromes can be seen in HIV-infected patients, either as primary manifestations of the HIV infection or as complications of treatment.

[Rx] **TREATMENT**   (See HPIM-14, Chap. 308, p. 1845)
General principles of pt management include counseling, psychosocial support, and screening for infections and require comprehensive knowledge of the disease processes associated with HIV infection.

Antiretroviral Therapy (See Table 308-26 p. 1847, in HPIM-14)

The cornerstone of medical management of HIV infection is antiretroviral therapy. Suppression of HIV replication is an important component in prolonging life as well as in improving the quality of life of pts with HIV infection. The drugs that are currently licensed for the treatment of HIV infection are listed below.

   Nucleoside Analogues   These should only be used in combination with other antiretroviral agents. The most common usage is together with another nucleoside analogue and a protease inhibitior (see below). *Zidovudine* (AZT, 3′-azido-2′,3′-dideoxythymidine) is the prototype of these agents. The only indication for zidovudine monotherapy is the prophylaxis of maternal-fetal transmission of HIV when the mother herself does not require antiretroviral therapy based on the stage of her disease. Major toxicities are due to bone marrow suppression, especially anemia. Standard dose is 200 mg 3 times daily.

Didanosine (ddI, 2′,3′-dideoxyinosine) is the second drug to be approved for anti-HIV therapy. At present it is FDA-approved for any HIV pt who has received prolonged zidovudine therapy or as initial therapy in pts with fewer than 500 CD4 + T cells/μL. However, a more common practice is to use didanosine as part of a combination regimen (see below). Major toxicities include painful sensory peripheral neuropathy and pancreatitis. Standard dose is 200 mg bid, for pts weighing more than 60 kg; 100 mg bid, for pts weighing less than 60 kg.

Zalcitabine (ddC, 2′,3′-dideoxycytidine) is currently licensed for use in combination therapy with zidovudine. Toxicities similar to didanosine, although pancreatitis not seen as frequently. Standard dose is 0.75 mg tid.

Stavudine (d4T, 2′,3′-didehydro-3′-deoxythymidine) is currently licensed for pts who are unable to take either zidovudine or didanosine because of intolerance or clinical failure. However, stavudine is more commonly used as part of a combination regimen (see below). Stavudine is antagonistic with zidovudine in vitro and possibly in vivo; hence, this combination should be avoided. The standard dose of stavudine is 40 mg bid, for patients weighing more than 60 kg; 30 mg bid, for patients weighing less than 60 kg. Peripheral neuropathy is the predominant toxicity seen with this drug.

Lamivudine (3TC, 2′,3′-dideoxy-3′-thiacytidine), a cytidine analogue, is licensed for use only in combination with zidovudine. However, it is often used as part of other combinations (see Table 308-26, p. 1847, in HPIM-14). The combination of lamivudine and zidovudine in vitro is the most potent nucleoside combination studied to date. Many experts feel that this combination, together with a protease inhibitor (see below), is the preferred initial therapeutic regimen for treating HIV infection. The standard dose of lamivudine is 150 mg bid. Although the main toxicities of lamivudine are peripheral neuropathy and pancreatitis, it is among the best tolerated of the nucleoside analogues.

Nonnucleoside Reverse Transcriptase Inhibitors These agents interfere with the function of HIV-1 reverse transcriptase by binding to regions outside the active site and causing conformational changes in the enzyme that render it inactive. These agents are very potent; however, when they are used as monotherapy, they induce rapid emergence of drug-resistant mutants. Two members of this class, *nevirapine* and *delavirdine* are currently available for clinical use. Both drugs are licensed for use in combination with other antiretrovirals. The main toxicities of these drugs are maculopaplar rash, which usually resolves without the need for discontinuing therapy, and elevations in hepatic enzymes levels. The usual dose of delavirdine is 400 mg tid; and for nevirapine is 200 mg/d × 1 week, then 200 mg bid.

Protease Inhibitors These drugs are potent and selective inhibitors of the HIV-1 protease enzyme, are active in the nanomolar range, and, thus far, have been associated with considerably less toxicity than the reverse transcriptase inhibitors. Unfortunately, as in the case of the nonnucleoside reverse transcriptase inhibitiors, this potency is accompanied by the rapid emergence of resistant isolates when these drugs are used as monotherapy. Thus, the protease inhibitors should be used only in combination with other antiretroviral drugs.

Saquinavir was the first protease inhibitor licensed; it is one of the better tolerated protease inhibitors, but it appears to be the least potent. HIV resistance to protease inhibitors is quite complex, but it seems that strains of HIV resistant to saquinavir are generally not resistant to either ritonavir or indinavir (see below), suggesting that combination therapy with different protease inhibitors may be of value. This must be approached with caution, since saquinavir is metabolized by the cytochrome P450 system and ritonavir therapy results in inhibition of the P450 system. Thus, the use of both drugs together has the potential to result in unpredictable increases in saquinavir levels. The usual dose of saquinavir is 600 mg q8h.

Ritonavir is the first protease inhibitor for which clinical efficacy was demonstrated. Strains of HIV resistant to ritonavir are also resistant to indinivir. The main side effects of ritonavir are nausea, abdominal pain, diarrhea, and circumoral paresthesias. These side effects can be reduced somewhat by initiating therapy at 300 mg bid and then rapidly escalating the dose over 5 to 7 days to the full dose of 600 mg bid. Ritonavir has a high affinity for certain isoforms of cytochrome P450, and thus it can produce large increases in the plasma levels of drugs that are metabolized by this enzyme. Among the agents affected in this manner are saquinavir, macrolide antibiotics, terfenadine, astemizole, warfarin, ondansetron, rifampin, most calcium channel blockers, glucocorticoids, sedative-hypnotics (alprazolam, diazepam, flurazepam, midazolam, and triazolam), and analgesics (fentanyl citrate, hydrocodone, oxycodone, methadone). Great care should be taken when prescribing additional drugs to pts receiving ritonavir.

Indinavir was the third protease inhibitor licensed. The usual dose is 800 mg q8h. HIV isolates that are resistant to indinavir show cross-resistance to ritonavir and varying degrees of cross-resistance to saquinavir. The main side effects of indinavir are nephrolithiasis and asymptomatic indirect hyperbilirubinemia. Indinavir is also metabolized by cytochrome P450 and coadministration of indinavir with any of the antihistamines, sedative-hypnotics, and analgesics listed above should be avoided. Levels of indinavir are decreased during concurrent therapy with rifampin and nevirapine and increased during concurrent therapy with ketoconazole and delaviridine. Dosages of indinavir should be appropriately modified in these situations. Rifampin should not be administered concurrently with indinavir or the other currently available protease inhibitors. Concurrent administration of indinavir with rifabutin results in a twofold increase in rifabutin levels; thus, the rifabutin dose should be decreased by one-half if given with indinavir.

Nelfinavir was approved in March, 1997, for the treatment of adult or pediatric HIV infection when antiretroviral therapy is warranted. At present, limited clinical data are available for this drug. Mild diarrhea, seen in approximately 20% of pts is the main side effect noted to date. The usual dose is 750 mg tid.

Choice of Antiretroviral Treatment Strategy

The large number of available antiretroviral agents coupled with a relative paucity of clinical end-point studies make the subject of antiretroviral therapy one of the more controversial in the management of HIV-infected pts. The current goal of antiretroviral therapy is to suppress viral replication to as a low a level as possible (preferrably below the level of detection by currently available assays) and for as long a period as possible to halt the progression of immunodeficiency and allow the residual or regenerated immune system to protect the pt from opportunistic infections. To achieve this goal with the currently available antiretroviral drugs will require the use of multidrug combinations given for an extended period of time. However, it is unclear whether currently available drugs are either potent enough or safe enough to achieve prolonged suppression of viral replication. In an attempt to provide a range of potential approaches to therapy of the HIV-

Table 78-1

Different Antiviral Treatment Strategies*

	Aggressive	Conservative
When to start	Time of diagnosis	CD4 + T cell count <500/μL
What to start with	AZT plus lamivudine plus protease inhibitor	Didanosine AZT plus zalcitabine AZT plus didanosine AZT plus lamivudine
When to change	0.5-log increase in HIV RNA or 10% decrease in CD4 + T cell count	CD4 + T cell count <200/μL
What to change to	Two new nucleosides (or a new nucleoside and a nonnucleoside) plus a new protease inhibitor	Two new nucleosides plus a protease inhibitor

See Chap. 308, HPIM-14 for current approach of the authors.

infected individual, we present a conservative approach, an aggressive approach, and our preferred approach. The reader should bear in mind that the field of HIV therapeutics is evolving so rapidly that new drugs and new information on the use of currently available drugs may call for substantial modifications of these recommendations.

The *conservative approach* is outlined in Table 78-1 and uses only those strategies that have been shown to be of clinical benefit; it would generally involve withholding antiretroviral therapy until the CD4 + T cell count falls below 500/μL. The *aggressive approach* would involve using combination therapy from the time of diagnosis of HIV infection (Table 78-1). The *author's current approach* falls between these two options and is influenced by the fact that the median time from infection to clinical disease is 10 years and that some pts may do extremely well without therapy for extended periods of time. For the asymptomatic pt with a stable CD4 + T cell count of >500/μL and a plasma virus level of <20,000 copies of HIV per milliliter, we would not treat but would perform repeat evaluations every 6 months. We would initiate antiretroviral therapy if one or more of the following occurs: plasma HIV RNA levels rise to >20,000 copies/mL; the

CD4 + T cell count falls below 500/μL; the pt becomes symptomatic; or if there is indication of progressive disease. Our preferred initial therapeutic regimen consists of two nucleosides and a protease inhibitor. The goal of therapy, once begun, is to decrease plasma viremia to as low as possible for as long as possible. We would monitor the patient every 3 to 4 months. If the plasma HIV level rose above the baseline by 0.5 log or the CD4 + T cell count fell by more than 25%, therapy would be modified to replace the current regimen with two new nucleosides or one new nucleoside and a nonnucleoside in combination with one or two different protease inhibitors. The same approach would be used for a new pt whose care we assume and who is already receiving antiretroviral therapy. In the rare setting of diagnosing a pt with the acute retroviral syndrome, we would treat with two nucleosides and a protease inhibitor. This regimen would be continued for at least 1 year; many experts would continue treatment indefinitely. Definitive recommendations await the results of clinical trials.

Treatment of Secondary Infections and Neoplasms

Specific for each infection and neoplasm (see Table 308-21, pp. 1826–1828, in HPIM-14).

Prophylaxis against Secondary Infections   Primary prophylaxis is clearly indicated for *P. carinii* pneumonia (especially when CD4 + T cell counts fall below 200 cells/μL), *M. avium* complex infections, and *M. tuberculosis* infections in pts with a positive PPD or anergy if at high risk of TB. Vaccination with pneumococcal polysaccharide and *H. influenzae* type b vaccines is recommended. Secondary prophylaxis, when available, is indicated for virtually every infection experienced by HIV-infected pts.

HIV and the Health Care Worker

There is a small but definite risk to health care workers of acquiring HIV infection via needle stick exposures, large mucosal surface exposures, or exposure of open wounds to HIV-infected secretions or blood products. The risk of HIV transmission after a skin puncture by an object contaminated with blood from a person with documented HIV infection is approximately 0.3%, compared to 20 to 30% risk for hepatitis B infection from a similar incident. The role of antiretroviral agents in postexposure prophylaxis is still controversial. However, a U.S. Public Health Service working group has recommended that chemoprophylaxis be given as soon as possible after occupational exposure. While the precise regimen remains a subject of debate, we currently recommend a combination of zidovudine, lamivudine, and indinavir. These drugs should be begun as soon as possible after exposure.

Prevention of exposure is the best strategy and includes following universal precautions and proper handling of needles and other potentially contaminated objects.

Transmission of tuberculosis is another potential risk for all health care workers, including those dealing with HIV-infected pts. All workers should know their PPD status, which should be checked yearly.

Vaccines

Development of a safe and effective HIV vaccine is the object of active investigation at present. Extensive animal work is ongoing, and clinical trials of candidate vaccines have begun in humans.

Prevention

Education, counseling, and behavior modification remain the cornerstones of HIV prevention efforts. While abstinence is an absolute way to prevent sexual transmission, other strategies include "safe sex" practices such as use of condoms together with the spermatocide nonoxynol-9. Avoidance of shared needle use by IDUs is critical. If possible, breast feeding should be avoided by HIV-positive women, as the virus can be transmitted to infants via this route.

For a more detailed discussion, see Fauci AS, Lane HC: Human Immunodeficiency Virus (HIV) Disease: AIDS and Related Disorders, Chap. 308, p.1791, in HPIM-14.

79

HOSPITAL-ACQUIRED INFECTIONS

Nosocomial infections are acquired during or as a result of hospitalization and generally manifest after 48 h of hospitalization.

Epidemiology

It is estimated that 3–5% of pts admitted to an acute-care hospital in the U.S. acquire a new infection; this estimate translates into about 2 million nosocomial infections per year, with an annual cost in excess of $2 billion. The most common type of hospital-acquired infection is UTI (40–45%); next in frequency are surgical wound infection (25–30%), pneumonia (15–20%), and bacteremia (5–7%).

Risk factors for the development of UTI include female sex, prolonged urinary catheterization, absence of systemic antibiotics, and inappropriate catheter care. Risk factors for surgical wound infection include presence of a drain, longer preoperative hospital stay, preoperative shaving of the field, longer duration of surgery, presence of an untreated remote infection, and higher-risk surgeon. An index for assessing the risk of wound infection has been developed, with risk factors including abdominal surgery, surgery lasting >2 h, contaminated or dirty-infected surgery (according to the classic classification system), and three or more diagnoses for one pt.

Risk factors for pneumonia include ICU stay, intubation, altered level of consciousness (especially with a nasogastric tube in place), old age, chronic lung disease, prior surgery, and use of H_2 blockers or antacids. The use of sucralfate (a medication that heals ulcers without altering gastric pH), unlike the use of antacids or H_2 blockers, does not appear to increase the risk of pneumonia in intubated pts. The major risk factors for the development of primary bacteremia are the presence of an indwelling intravascular device and hyperalimentation.

Clinical Manifestations and Diagnosis

DIFFERENTIAL DIAGNOSIS OF FEVER　Important infectious sources of new fever in a hospitalized pt include antibiotic-associated diarrhea caused by *Clostridium difficile,* decubitus ulcers, and sinusitis. Noninfectious sources of fever to consider include drugs (drug fever may occur with or without eosinophilia or rash), thrombophlebitis, and pulmonary embolism.

WORKUP FOR NEW FEVER　The workup of a hospitalized pt with new fever should include a thorough history directed at symptoms such as headache, cough, abdominal pain, diarrhea, flank pain, dysuria, urinary frequency, and leg pain. Features of the hospitalization, such as the presence of IV devices, use of a urinary catheter, performance of surgical procedures, and use of new medications, are all important items. The physical exam should pay particular attention to skin, lungs, abdomen (especially the RUQ), costovertebral angles, surgical wounds, calves, and current or old IV sites. Laboratory tests for all febrile hospitalized pts should include CBC with differential, CXR, and blood and urine cultures. Other diagnostic tests to consider include LFTs; abdominal studies; routine aerobic cultures of sputum, stool, or other relevant body fluids; and testing of stool for *C. difficile* toxin in cases of diarrhea.

URINARY TRACT INFECTION Fever, dysuria, frequency, leukocytosis, and flank pain or costovertebral angle tenderness correlate well with bladder infection or pyelonephritis in pts who have had urinary catheters in place. In pts with fever alone, the finding of WBCs without epithelial cells in the urinary sediment or the detection of leukocyte esterase or nitrite on urinalysis is suggestive of UTI. A urine culture positive for a single organism in an asymptomatic hospitalized pt is not diagnostic of UTI.

SURGICAL WOUND INFECTION Erythema extending >2 cm beyond the margin of the wound, localized tenderness and induration, fluctuance, drainage of purulent material, and dehiscence of sutures are all findings suggestive of a wound infection. In pts with sternal wounds, ongoing fever or the development of rocking or instability of the sternum may indicate the need for surgical exploration of the wound.

PNEUMONIA In pts outside the ICU, pneumonia should be suspected in the setting of a new infiltrate on CXR, a new cough, fever, leukocytosis, and sputum production. In pts receiving intensive care, especially those who are intubated, signs may be more subtle; purulent sputum and abnormal CXRs are common. A change in character or quantity of sputum in an intubated pt with fever, with or without accompanying CXR changes, is significant. Organisms of concern in nosocomial pneumonia are gram-negative aerobic bacilli—particularly *Pseudomonas aeruginosa, Klebsiella pneumoniae,* and *Enterobacter* spp.— and *Staphylococcus aureus.* Viruses such as respiratory syncytial virus and adenovirus are also important. Depending on the institution, pathogens such as methicillin-resistant *S. aureus, Xanthomonas* spp., *Flavobacterium* spp., and even *Legionella* spp. may be of special concern.

BACTEREMIA AND INTRAVASCULAR DEVICE–RE-LATED INFECTION The only presenting symptom may be fever. The exit site of an existing or previous IV line should be evaluated for erythema, induration, tenderness, and/or purulent drainage. Organisms of particular concern include coagulase-negative staphylococci, *Candida* spp., *S. aureus,* and entero-cocci.

℞ **TREATMENT**

Therapy should be directed at the most likely cause of infection and, when possible, should be chosen on the basis of culture results. When an infection is known to be related to an intravascular device or when no other source of infection is apparent, the device should usually be removed and the catheter tip sent for quantitative culture. Whenever feasible, a new intravascular device should be inserted at a different site.

Hospital Infection Control

Infection control departments determine the general and specific measures used to control infections. Cross-infection is particularly important, and hand washing is the single most important preventive measure in hospitals. Minimizing invasive procedures and vascular and bladder catheterizations to those that are absolutely necessary will also reduce rates of nosocomial infection. Category-specific isolation measures include strict isolation (e.g., for chickenpox), contact isolation (e.g., for staphylococcal wound infections), respiratory isolation (e.g., for untreated meningitis), acid-fast bacillus isolation (e.g., for suspected tuberculosis, with fulfillment of specific ventilation requirements), enteric precautions (e.g., for *C. difficile* diarrhea), and drainage/secretion precautions (e.g., for minor wound infections). Universal precautions have largely replaced blood and body fluid precautions.

For a more detailed discussion, see Zaleznik DF: Hospital-Acquired and Intravascular Device–Related Infections, Chap. 137, p. 846; and Weinstein RA: Infection Control in the Hospital, Chap. 138, p. 849, in HPIM-14.

80

PNEUMOCOCCAL INFECTIONS

The pneumococcus (*Streptococcus pneumoniae*) is a gram-positive encapsulated coccus that colonizes the oropharynx and causes serious illness, including pneumonia, meningitis, and otitis media.

EPIDEMIOLOGY AND PATHOGENESIS

Pneumococci colonize the oropharynx of 5–10% of healthy adults and 20–40% of children. After colonization, protection is afforded by nonspecific immune mechanisms until type-specific antibody is produced. Otitis media, a common childhood illness, develops when inflamed mucosal surfaces impede clearance of the organisms from the inner ear. Pneumococci cause 40–50% of otitis media cases in which a causative agent is identified. Any perturbation in the normal defenses of the lower respiratory tract (e.g., depressed cough, alcohol intoxication, impaired ciliary activity, viral infection) may allow infection of the lungs with pneumococci. Impaired production of specific antibody by any mechanism (e.g., multiple myeloma, HIV infection) also predisposes to infection. Pneumococcal pneumonia occurs at an annual rate of 20 cases per 100,000 young adults and 280 cases per 100,000 individuals >70 years of age. Epidemic pneumococcal pneumonia may occur in crowded living conditions such as prisons or military barracks but does not generally occur in schools or workplaces. Of all cases of pneumococcal pneumonia, 20–25% result in bacteremia. Among children under age 2, pneumococcal bacteremia develops at an annual rate of 160 cases per 100,000 and is often unassociated with pneumonia. Bacteremia, with or without pneumonia, leads to pneumococcal infection at other sites, such as the joints, the meninges, or the cardiac valves.

PNEUMONIA

Pts frequently present with a preexisting respiratory illness that has worsened. Often the temperature rises to 38.9–39.4°C (102–103°F) and sputum production becomes prominent. The "classic" presentation with coryza, followed by the abrupt onset of a shaking chill and fever and subsequent severe pleuritic chest pain, is not common. In the elderly the onset may be insidious. On physical exam, pts usually appear ill and anxious. Dullness to percussion is frequently found, and tubular breath sounds and fine crepitant rales may be heard. Without treatment, high fever and cough persist for 7–10 d, with subsequent defervescence. Most pts defervesce within 12–36 h of the initiation of therapy, but some take up to 4 d. The physical exam yields normal findings within 2–4 weeks, but the CXR may remain abnormal for 8–18 weeks. Pleural effusions, which are found in up to 50% of cases, are usually sterile, but empyema may occur in 2% of treated cases. Empyema can cause extensive pleural scarring if the fluid is not drained. Many pts develop abdominal distention, herpes labialis, and abnormal LFTs or frank jaundice. Rare complications include pericarditis, arthritis (especially in children), endocarditis (see below), and paralytic ileus.

Gram's stain of sputum shows PMNs and slightly elongated gram-positive cocci in pairs and chains. Culture is less sensitive than Gram's stain. Blood cultures are positive in 20–25% of pts. The WBC count is usually >12,000/μL but may be low in overwhelming infection. In pts with asplenia or multiple myeloma and rarely in immunocompetent hosts, pneumococci may be seen in Wright's-stained buffy coat. CXR usually shows homogeneous density in an involved lobe or segment, but abnormalities may be multilobar or atypical, especially with underlying pulmonary disease.

EXTRAPULMONARY INFECTION

MENINGITIS The pneumococcus is the leading cause of bacterial meningitis in adults (except during outbreaks due to the meningococcus). Because of the success of the *Haemophilus influenzae* vaccine, the pneumococcus is now the leading cause in children (except for neonates) as well. Pneumococcal meningitis may present as a primary disease; as a complication of pneumonia; by extension from otitis, mastoiditis, or sinusitis; or subsequent to a skull fracture with CSF leak. The CSF is a secondary site of infection in pneumococcal endocarditis. Pts present with sudden onset of fever, headache, and stiff neck, with progression to obtundation over 24–48 h in the absence of treatment. Physical exam reveals an acutely ill pt with nuchal rigidity. LP should be performed immediately except in cases with papilledema or focal neurologic findings. If LP is deferred for any reason, treatment should be started immediately. CSF findings include increased pressure, cloudiness, increased protein level, and decreased glucose level. The Gram's stain is usually positive for bacteria; latex agglutination or counterimmunoelectrophoresis is positive in 80% of culture-positive cases and may be positive when culture is negative (e.g., in the presence of antibiotics). With appropriate therapy, 70% of pts recover.

ENDOCARDITIS Endocarditis is a rare complication of pneumococcal pneumonia. The clinical picture is one of acute bacterial endocarditis with fever, splenomegaly, loud murmurs, metastatic infections, and rapid destruction of previously normal heart valves (particularly the aortic valve), sometimes with the development of CHF. Blood cultures are uniformly positive in the absence of antibiotics.

PERITONITIS Pneumococcal peritonitis is a rare complication of transient pneumococcal bacteremia. Infection via the vagina and fallopian tubes may account for an increased incidence among adolescent girls and among women using intrauterine devices. The disease is also associated with cirrhosis, carcinoma of the liver, and nephrotic syndrome. Diagnosis is based on an elevated cell count and a positive culture of ascitic fluid. Blood cultures are often positive.

R̲x̲ **TREATMENT**

In the past, pneumococcal infection was uniformly susceptible to penicillin. During the past several years, however, resistance to penicillin as well as to many other antibiotics has emerged; by 1995 in the U.S., 15–20% of isolates showed intermediate levels of resistance to penicillin and 2–5% showed high-level resistance. Susceptibility testing should thus be routinely performed on all pneumococcal isolates, and empiric treatment should be guided by local patterns of susceptibility.

Pneumonia Pts with pneumococcal pneumonia should generally be hospitalized, particularly if they are elderly, have undergone splenectomy, appear acutely ill, exhibit oxygen desaturation or confusion, or have underlying chronic conditions such as heart failure, renal failure, lung disease, or cirrhosis. Admission to an ICU should be considered for pts with hypotension, substantial hypoxemia, hypercarbia, multilobar pneumonia, or a WBC count of <6000/μl. Treatment with 1 million units of penicillin G IV q6h should be effective for both sensitive and intermediately resistant isolates. Alternatives include cefazolin (1 g IV q8h) and procaine penicillin (2.4 million units IM initially, followed by 1.2 million units q12h). For outpatient treatment, amoxicillin (500 mg initially, followed by 250 mg PO q8h) may be used. Clindamycin (300 mg PO q8h) is active against most strains that are susceptible or intermediately susceptible to penicillin. For the pt with the life-threatening markers mentioned above and perhaps for all hospitalized pts, an empiric regimen active against resistant pneumococci should be considered. This regimen can consist of cefotaxime (1 g IV q6h), ceftriaxone (1 g IV q12h), or imipenem (500 mg IV q6h). If resistance to these antibiotics becomes common, vancomycin (1 g IV q12h) should be used. The optimal duration of therapy has not been established by controlled trial, but 3–5 d of observed therapy with IV antibiotics followed by oral antibiotics for a total duration of 5 afebrile days appears reasonable.

Meningitis Because this pneumococcal infection is the most life-threatening, empiric therapy should include vancomycin (1 g IV q12h) *and* a third-generation cephalosporin—either ceftriaxone (1 g IV q12h) or cefotaxime (2 g IV q6h)—pending the availability of susceptibility data. For isolates shown to be penicillin susceptible, treatment may continue with penicillin (4 million units IV q4h). For isolates with intermediate susceptibility to penicillin but susceptibility to the third-generation cephalosporins, vancomycin may be discontinued. The total duration of therapy is 10–14 d. The use of adjunctive glucocorticoids remains controversial. Pts with pneumococcal meningitis should be cared for initially in an ICU.

Endocarditis Treatment with vancomycin (1 g IV q12h) should be begun pending susceptibility information. Treatment may continue with a β-lactam antibiotic should the isolate prove susceptible. Pts with pneumococcal endocarditis should be cared for initially in an ICU. Surgical intervention may be mandated by valvular injury or myocardial abscess.

Empyema All pleural effusions should be aspirated for diagnosis and as a guide to therapy. Drainage by chest tube is indicated if pleural fluid has a pH <7.1, contains frank pus, or contains bacteria visible on Gram's stain. Complete drainage should be confirmed by CT. Empyema complicates about 2% of pneumonia cases.

PREVENTION

The 23-valent pneumococcal vaccine (0.5 mL IM) should be given to all persons over 65 years of age; those with cardiac, pulmonary, hepatic, or renal disease; those with diabetes, malignancy, asplenia, CSF leak, or HIV infection; and those >2 years of age with sickle cell disease. Revaccination is recommended after 5–7 years (after 3 years in pts with nephrotic syndrome, renal failure, or immunosuppression).

For a more detailed discussion, see Musher DM: Pneumococcal Infections, Chap. 141, p. 869, in HPIM-14.

81

STAPHYLOCOCCAL INFECTIONS

The staphylococci are hardy and ubiquitous colonizers of human skin and mucous membranes. They cause a variety of syndromes, including superficial and deep pyogenic infections, systemic intoxications, and UTIs. Staphylococci are nonmotile, nonsporulating gram-positive cocci, 0.5–1.5 μm in diameter, that occur singly and in pairs, short chains, and irregular three-dimensional clusters. The more virulent staphylococci clot plasma ("coagulase-positive"), while the less virulent ones do not ("coagulase-negative"). Of coagulase-positive staphylococci, *S. aureus* is the only important human pathogen. Coagulase-negative staphylococci, especially *S. epidermidis,* adhere avidly to prosthetic materials and are increasingly important nosocomial pathogens. *S. saprophyticus,* another coagulase-negative species, is a common cause of UTIs.

STAPHYLOCOCCUS AUREUS

Epidemiology and Pathogenesis

Humans constitute the major reservoir of *S. aureus* in nature; the cross-sectional carriage rate in adults is 15–40%. The mucous membranes of the anterior nasopharynx are the principal site of carriage.

   S. aureus causes two types of syndromes: *intoxications* and *infections.* In intoxications, the manifestations of illness are attributable solely to the action of one or a few toxins. Infections involve bacterial proliferation, invasion or destruction of host tissues, and, in most cases, local and systemic host responses. No single product is responsible for all manifestations of infection, whose histologic hallmark is the pyogenic abscess. Hosts at particular risk for staphylococcal infection include those with frequent or chronic disruptions in epithelial integrity, disordered leukocyte chemotaxis, phagocytes defective in oxidative killing, or indwelling foreign bodies.

STAPHYLOCOCCAL INTOXICATIONS *Toxic Shock Syndrome* TSS is an acute, life-threatening intoxication characterized by fever, hypotension, rash, multiorgan dysfunction, and desquamation during the early convalescent period. Overt infection with *S. aureus* is not required; mere colonization with a toxigenic strain may suffice. TSS toxin 1 and staphylococcal enterotoxin B are responsible for virtually all cases. The reported incidence of TSS among menstruating women is 1 case per 100,000. About half of all cases are nonmenstrual and occur in individuals of both sexes and all ages. Nonmenstrual TSS is characterized by complicated skin lesions of many types, including chemical or thermal burns, insect bites, varicella infections, and surgical wounds. Mortality is about 2.5% for menstrual TSS and 6.4% for nonmenstrual TSS.

TSS is a clinically defined syndrome whose differential diagnosis is that of a severe febrile exanthem with hypotension. Other diagnoses to consider include streptococcal TSS, staphylococcal scalded skin syndrome, Kawasaki syndrome, Rocky Mountain spotted fever, leptospirosis, meningococcemia, gram-negative sepsis, exanthematous viral syndromes, and severe drug reactions. Staphylococcal and streptococcal TSS can be clinically indistinguishable.

℞ TREATMENT

Treatment of TSS involves decontamination of the toxin production site, aggressive fluid resuscitation, and administration of antibiotics. Recent surgical wounds should be explored and irrigated. Pressors should be used for hypotension unresponsive to fluids. Electrolyte abnormalities must be corrected. Clindamycin (900 mg IV q8h) should be given either alone or with a β-lactam antibiotic or vancomycin. A 14-d course of therapy is reasonable, some of which may be oral. For severe illness or an undrainable focus of infection, immunoglobulin (a single dose of 400 mg/kg IV) should be given. The risk of recurrent menstrual illness can be assessed by testing for seroconversion to TSST-1: women who do not seroconvert after acute illness should refrain indefinitely from using tampons or barrier contraceptives.

Staphylococcal Scalded Skin Syndrome SSSS encompasses a range of cutaneous diseases of varying severity caused by exfoliative toxin–producing strains of *S. aureus*. The most severe form is termed *Ritter's disease* in newborns and *toxic epidermal necrolysis* (TEN) in older subjects. TEN or Ritter's disease often begins with a nonspecific prodrome. The acute phase starts with an erythematous rash beginning in the periorbital and perioral areas and spreading to the trunk and limbs. The skin has a sandpaper texture and is often tender. Periorbital edema is common. In infants and children, fever and irritability or lethargy are common, but systemic toxicity is not. Within hours or days, wrinkling and sloughing of the epidermis begin; Nikolsky's sign is present. The denuded areas are red and glistening but not purulent. Exfoliation may continue in large sheets or in ragged snippets of tissue. Large flaccid bullae may develop. Significant fluid and electrolyte loss and secondary infection can occur at this stage. Within ~48 h, exfoliated areas dry and secondary desquamation begins. The entire illness resolves within about 10 d. Mortality (from hypovolemia or sepsis) is about 3% in children but up to 50% in adults.

℞ TREATMENT

Treatment includes antistaphylococcal antibiotics, fluid and electrolyte management, and local care of denuded skin.

Staphylococcal Food Poisoning Staphylococcal food poisoning, caused by the ingestion of any of the enterotoxins produced by *S. aureus* in contaminated food before it is eaten, has a high attack rate and is most common during summer. This brief illness begins abruptly 2–6 h after ingestion of contaminated food, with nausea, vomiting, crampy abdominal pain, and diarrhea. The diarrhea is usually noninflammatory and is of lower volume than that in cholera or toxigenic *Escherichia coli* infection. Fever and rash are absent, and the pt is neurologically normal.

℞ TREATMENT

The majority of cases are self-limited and require no specific treatment.

STAPHYLOCOCCAL INFECTIONS *Skin and Soft Tissue Infections* *S. aureus* is the most common etiologic agent of skin and soft tissue infections. Staphylococcal infections originating in hair follicles range in severity from trivial to life-threatening. *Folliculitis*, denoting infection of follicular ostia, presents as domed, yellow pustules with a narrow red margin. Infection is often self-limited, although healing may be hastened by topical antiseptics and more severe cases may benefit from topical or systemic antibiotics. A *furuncle* ("boil") reflects deep-seated, necrotic infection of a hair follicle, most often located on the buttocks, face, or neck. Furuncles are painful and tender and are often accompanied by fever and constitutional symptoms. Surgical drainage and systemic antibiotics are frequently required. *Carbuncles* denote deep infection of a group of contiguous follicles. These painful, necrotic lesions, often accompanied by high fever and malaise, occur most often on the back of the neck, shoulders, hips, and thighs, typically in middle-aged or elderly men. Surrounding and underlying connective tissue is intensely inflamed; bacteremia may be present. Surgical drainage and systemic antibiotics are indicated.

Cellulitis, a spreading infection of subcutaneous tissue, is occasionally caused by *S. aureus*. Although β-hemolytic streptococci are much more commonly responsible, secondary infection of surgical and traumatic wounds is more likely to be staphylococcal, and empiric treatment directed against both *S. aureus* and streptococci is reasonable.

Respiratory Tract Infections Staphylococcal pneumonia is a relatively uncommon but severe infection characterized clinically by chest pain, systemic toxicity, and dyspnea and pathologically by intense neutrophilic infiltration, necrosis, and abscess formation. It is typical in tracheally intubated hospitalized pts and after viral respiratory infection. The diagnosis is often readily established by Gram's staining of expectorated sputum.

Hematogenous seeding of the lungs with *S. aureus* follows embolization from an intravascular nidus of infection. Common settings for septic pulmonary embolization are right-sided endocarditis, which is especially common among injection drug users, and septic thrombophlebitis, which is usually a complication of indwelling venous catheterization. CXR typically shows multiple nodular infiltrates. *Empyema* is a common sequela of staphylococcal pneumonia and increases the already considerable morbidity of this infection.

Infections of the CNS *S. aureus* is a major cause of *brain abscess,* especially as a result of embolization during left-sided endocarditis. Brain abscess can also develop by direct extension from frontoethmoid or sphenoid sinuses or from soft tissue.

S. aureus is the most common cause of *spinal epidural abscess,* most often in association with vertebral osteomyelitis or diskitis. While the diagnosis is suggested by fever, back pain, radicular pain, lower extremity weakness, bowel or bladder dysfunction, and leukocytosis, the presentation is often subtle (e.g., difficulty walking in the absence of objective findings). The principal danger is spinal cord necrosis, which must be recognized early if sequelae are to be averted. Spinal MRI detects an epidural collection, and needle aspiration or open drainage confirms the infectious etiology. Prompt surgical decompression is often required, although a trial of antibiotics alone may be considered if focal neurologic deficits are absent.

Endovascular Infections *S. aureus* is the most common cause of acute bacterial *endocarditis* of both native and prosthetic valves. Staphylococcal endocarditis presents as an acute febrile illness, rarely of more than a few weeks' duration; complications include meningitis, brain or visceral abscess, peripheral embolization, valvular incompetence with heart failure, myocardial abscess, and purulent pericarditis. The diagnosis is suggested by a heart murmur and conjunctival hemorrhages, subungual petechiae, or purpuric lesions on the distal extremities. It is confirmed by multiple positive blood cultures and valvular vegetations on echocardiography. Evaluation for metastatic infection is often warranted. Staphylococcal endocarditis carries a mortality rate of 40–60% and mandates prompt antimicrobial therapy. Indications for valve replacement are the same as for endocarditis caused by other organisms. Early consultation with a cardiothoracic surgeon is advisable; about half of pts require valve replacement—many urgently. Once removal of an infected valve is indicated, nothing is gained and much may be lost by delaying surgery.

Right-sided endocarditis, most often a complication of injection drug use or venous catheterization, is frequently complicated in turn by septic pulmonary emboli but otherwise has a lower rate of serious complications than left-sided disease. Short-course parenteral therapy (2 weeks) may be curative, and the prognosis is relatively good. Surgery is rarely required. In contrast, *S. aureus* infection of a prosthetic valve almost always requires surgery.

S. aureus is the major cause of endovascular infections other than endocarditis. Vascular infection may follow hematogenous seeding of damaged vessels, resulting in development of a "mycotic aneurysm"; spread from a contiguous focus of infection, often resulting in an infected pseudoaneurysm; or contamination of an intravascular device, resulting in "septic phlebitis." Staphylococcal infection of an atherosclerotic artery, which may be aneurysmal to begin with, is potentially catastrophic. Such infections are associated with high-grade bacteremia, may result in rupture and massive hemorrhage, and are almost never curable without surgical resection and bypass of the infected vessel. Septic phlebitis is also associated with high-grade bacteremia and systemic toxicity but is less likely than arteritis to result in rupture. Persistent bacteremia suggests the need for surgical removal of infected thrombus or vein, but the technical difficulty of surgery may warrant an attempt at cure with antibiotics and anticoagulants alone.

Several criteria increase the probability that a pt has endocarditis as opposed to simple bacteremia: community-acquired (vs. nosocomial) infection, absence of an identifiable primary site of infection, and evidence of metastatic infection.

Musculoskeletal Infections *S. aureus* is the most common cause of *acute osteomyelitis* in adults and one of the leading causes in children. Acute osteomyelitis results from either hematogenous seeding of bone, especially damaged bone, or direct extension from a contiguous focus of infection. The most common site of hematogenous staphylococcal osteomyelitis in adults is the vertebral bodies; in children, it is the highly vascular metaphyses of long bones. Acute osteomyelitis in adults usually presents with constitutional symptoms and pain over the affected area, often developing over weeks or months. The diagnosis may be subtle; leukocytosis and an elevated ESR are laboratory clues. Bacteremia may or may not be demonstrable. Cure usually follows 4–6 weeks of parenteral antibiotics.

S. aureus is also a major cause of *chronic osteomyelitis,* which develops at sites of previous surgery, trauma, or devascularization.

A special form of osteomyelitis is that associated with prosthetic joints or orthopedic fixation devices. Pain, fever, swelling, and decreased range of motion are cardinal features of an infected prosthesis. A plain film may suggest loosening of the prosthesis, often as radiolucency at the interface between bone and cement. Cure with antibiotics alone is rare.

S. aureus is a prominent cause of *septic arthritis* in adults. Predisposing factors include injection drug use, rheumatoid arthritis, use of systemic or intraarticular steroids, penetrating trauma, and previous damage to joints. In addition to parenteral antibiotics, cure requires either repeated joint aspirations or open or arthroscopic debridement and drainage. Failure to drain joints adequately risks permanent loss of function.

S. aureus infections of muscle (*pyomyositis*) are relatively uncommon in the U.S. *Psoas abscess,* the major exception, is easily diagnosed by abdominal CT or MRI.

Diagnosis

S. aureus infection generally is readily diagnosed by isolation of the organism from purulent material or normally sterile body fluid. Gram's staining of purulent material from a staphylococcal abscess invariably reveals abundant neutrophils and intra- and extracellular cocci—singly or in pairs, short chains, tetrads, or clusters. *S. aureus* grows readily on standard laboratory media. Rarely, if ever, should *S. aureus* growing from even a single blood culture be considered a contaminant. The diagnosis of staphylococcal intoxications (e.g., TSS) may be more difficult and may rely entirely on clinical data.

℞ TREATMENT

The essential elements of therapy for staphylococcal infections are drainage of purulent collections of pus, debridement of necrotic tissue, removal of foreign bodies, and administration of antibiotics. The importance of adequate drainage cannot be overemphasized. In skin and soft tissue infections, surgical drainage alone is occasionally curative. It is almost impossible to eradicate *S. aureus* infection in the presence of a foreign body.

Antimicrobial Resistance   Today, >95% of *S. aureus* strains are resistant to penicillin. In some tertiary care institutions, >40% of *S. aureus* isolates are now methicillin resistant as well. In 1997 a few reports of *S. aureus* with intermediate resistance to vancomycin appeared.

Selection of Antibiotics   Nafcillin or oxacillin, β-lactamase-resistant penicillins, are the drugs of choice for parenteral treatment of serious staphylococcal infections. Penicillin remains the drug of choice for infections caused by susceptible organisms. Combinations of a penicillin plus a β-lactamase inhibitor are also effective but are best reserved for mixed infections. Penicillin-allergic pts can usually be treated with a cephalosporin, although caution is essential if the adverse reaction to penicillin was anaphylaxis; first-generation agents (e.g., cefazolin) are preferred. The best alternative for parenteral administration is vancomycin. Dicloxacillin and cephalexin are recommended for oral administration for minor infections or for continuation therapy. Several other agents are available to treat susceptible strains.

There is usually no significant benefit to treating *S. aureus* infections with more than a single drug to which the organism is susceptible. An aminoglycoside/β-lactam combination hastens the sterilization of blood in endocarditis and is often used for the first 5–7 d of therapy for *S. aureus* bacteremia. Thereafter, the added toxicity of an aminoglycoside outweighs its benefit. Use of rifampin with a β-lactam antibiotic (or vancomycin) occasionally results in sterilization in otherwise refractory infections, particularly those involving foreign bodies or avascular tissue. Rifampin should never be administered as monotherapy because resistance emerges rapidly.

Route and Duration of Therapy   To minimize seeding of secondary sites, bacteremic infections should be treated with high doses of antibiotics (e.g., 2 g of nafcillin IV q4h). For infections requiring high serum antibiotic levels for adequate tissue levels (e.g., endocarditis, osteomyelitis, infections of the CNS), parenteral therapy should be used for the duration. Oral agents may suffice for treatment of nonbacteremic infections in which high antibiotic levels are not requisite, such as skin, soft tissue, or upper respiratory tract infections.

Except for bacteremia and osteomyelitis, duration of therapy for *S. aureus* infections can be tailored to the severity of illness, the immunologic status of the host, and the response to therapy. Acute osteomyelitis in adults requires 4–6 weeks of parenteral therapy, with the actual duration depending on vascular supply at the site of infection and response to treatment. Chronic osteomyelitis is occasionally treated parenterally for 6–8 weeks and then orally for several months. Acute endocarditis and other endovascular infections should be treated with parenteral antibiotics for 4 weeks (6 weeks for prosthetic valves). Simple bacteremia requires shorter therapy, but a 2-week course of *parenteral* therapy is recommended *for all patients* with *S. aureus* bacteremia. A challenge in treating staphylococcal bacteremia is deciding whether to administer parenteral therapy for 2 or 4 weeks. A conservative approach supported by numerous studies dictates that *4 weeks* should be standard unless specific criteria are met (Table 81-1).

Table 81-1

Criteria for the Selection of Short-Course (2-Week) Parenteral Antibiotic Therapy for Patients with *S. aureus* Bacteremia

Subjects with *S. aureus* bacteremia who meet *all* criteria may be treated with parenteral antibiotics for 2 rather than 4 weeks.

1. No serious underlying condition, such as hematologic malignancy, poorly controlled diabetes, cirrhosis, severe malnutrition, rheumatoid arthritis, or AIDS
2. No hemodynamically significant valvular dysfunction
3. No "seedable sites," such as prosthetic heart valve, aortic aneurysm, necrotic bone, transvenous pacemaker, or prosthetic joint
4. A primary focus of infection that is readily apparent and amenable to removal (e.g., intravenous catheter) or surgical drainage
5. A short interval between the presumed onset of bacteremia and initiation of therapy (e.g., removal of catheter and start of antibiotics)
6. A staphylococcal isolate that proves to be susceptible to antibiotic(s) chosen initially
7. A prompt response to removal of the catheter and initiation of antibiotic treatment: defervescence within 72 h, negative blood cultures after catheter removal
8. No suppurative phlebitis at the catheter entry site
9. No evidence of metastatic foci of infection during the first 2 weeks of therapy

SOURCE: Deresiewicz RL, Parsonnet J: HPIM-14, p. 883.

Prevention and Control

Pts with exposed wounds and those with nasal colonization are important reservoirs of *S. aureus,* whose transmission can be reduced most effectively by meticulous hand washing before and after pt contact. More stringent infection control measures must be taken to prevent the nosocomial spread of resistant strains (MRSA).

COAGULASE-NEGATIVE STAPHYLOCOCCI

Coagulase-negative staphylococci are a major cause of nosocomial infection and are the organisms most frequently isolated from the blood of hospitalized patients. Most such infections are indolent, are caused by strains resistant to multiple antibiotics, and are associated with a medical device of some kind, removal of which is usually required to effect cure.

CLINICAL SYNDROMES   Coagulase-negative staphylococci are the most common pathogens complicating the use of IV catheters, hemodialysis shunts and grafts, CSF shunts, peritoneal dialysis catheters, pacemaker wires and electrodes, prosthetic joints, vascular grafts, and prosthetic valves. Coagulase-negative staphylococcal infection of IV catheters may be accompanied by signs of inflammation at the site of insertion, and the degree of systemic toxicity (including fever) ranges from minimal to considerable. The diagnosis is established by culture of blood drawn from the catheter and by venipuncture. Infection of CSF shunts usually becomes evident within several weeks of implantation; malfunction of the shunt may be the only manifestation of infection. Infection of a prosthetic joint often becomes evident long after implantation.

Coagulase-negative staphylococci are a prominent cause of *bacteremia* in immunosuppressed pts. Those with neutropenia may have high-grade bacteremia resulting in significant systemic toxicity. A serious consequence of bacteremia is seeding of a secondary foreign body.

Coagulase-negative staphylococci are the foremost cause of *prosthetic valve endocarditis,* accounting for the majority of infections occurring within several months of implantation and for many late infections. They also cause <5% of cases of *native valve endocarditis,* usually affecting abnormal valves.

S. saprophyticus is a major cause of UTI, especially among sexually active young women. The syndrome, which is indistinguishable from that caused by other etiologic agents, is amenable to therapy with most drugs commonly used to treat UTIs.

DIAGNOSIS Although coagulase-negative staphylococci are the most common cause of nosocomial bacteremia, they are also the most common contaminant of blood cultures. "True positives" are more likely when a clinical illness suggests infection, when an indwelling catheter or some other risk factor is involved, and when multiple cultures of blood drawn from separate sites yield organisms similar in phenotype and antimicrobial susceptibility pattern.

℞ TREATMENT

When coagulase-negative staphylococcal infection is related to a foreign body, removing the foreign body often constitutes adequate therapy. Most such infections require this measure, but cures of such infections with antibiotics alone have been reported. Infections of peritoneal dialysis catheters are cured often enough with antibiotics alone that an attempt should be made to do so. Coagulase-negative staphylococcal infections of central venous catheters are also amenable to medical therapy, although relapses are common. Persistent bacteremia during therapy is an absolute indication for removing a catheter, and bacteremia after a catheter's removal suggests seeding of a secondary site.

Most strains of coagulase-negative staphylococci isolated from pts in U.S. hospitals are resistant not only to penicillin but also to penicillinase-resistant penicillins and cephalosporins. Nosocomial isolates are usually resistant to other classes of antibiotics as well. Vancomycin, to which coagulase-negative staphylococci remain uniformly susceptible, is by necessity the drug of choice for *empiric* treatment of serious infections caused by these organisms. Strains proven to be susceptible to nafcillin (oxacillin) or penicillin should be treated with one of these agents or with a first-generation cephalosporin.

Synergistic antibiotic combinations are often useful. Rifampin plays a unique and important role by virtue of its potency against most staphylococci, its excellent penetration into tissues (including those that are poorly vascularized), and its high levels within human cells. Unfortunately, rifampin must be used with other antibiotics because of frequent and rapid emergence of microbial resistance during therapy. The concomitant use of a β-lactam antibiotic to which the organism is susceptible plus rifampin (300 mg PO bid) plus an aminoglycoside (usually gentamicin) affords the best chance for eradication of infection of a medical device without its removal. Vancomycin is substituted for the β-lactam if so dictated by an organism's susceptibility pattern or a pt's drug allergy.

For a more detailed discussion, see Deresiewicz RL, Parsonnet J: Staphylococcal Infections, Chap. 142, p. 875, in HPIM-14.

82

STREPTOCOCCAL AND ENTEROCOCCAL INFECTIONS AND DIPHTHERIA

STREPTOCOCCAL INFECTIONS

Group A *Streptococcus* (*S. pyogenes*)

Streptococci of group A commonly cause pharyngitis as well as skin and soft tissue infection; they less often cause pneumonia, puerperal sepsis, and the postinfectious complications of acute rheumatic fever (ARF) and acute glomerulonephritis (AGN). Streptococci possess many virulence factors, including antiphagocytic M proteins and a hyaluronic acid capsule, as well as a variety of extracellular toxins and enzymes, including pyrogenic toxins, streptolysins, streptokinase, and DNases.

PHARYNGITIS Streptococcal pharyngitis is a common infection among children over age 3; streptococci account for 20–40% of all cases of exudative pharyngitis in children. This infection usually spreads from person to person via respiratory droplets but also can be food-borne. After an incubation period of 1–4 d, pts develop sore throat, fever, chills, and malaise and sometimes abdominal symptoms and vomiting. Both symptoms and signs are quite variable, ranging from mild with minimal findings to severe with markedly enlarged tonsils; a purulent exudate over the tonsils and posterior pharyngeal wall; and tender, enlarged cervical lymph nodes. The usual course of uncomplicated streptococcal pharyngitis lasts 3–5 d. Suppurative complications, uncommon since the widespread use of antibiotics, include acute otitis media, sinusitis, cervical lymphadenitis, peritonsillar or retropharyngeal abscess, meningitis, pneumonia, bacteremia, and endocarditis. Scarlet fever, a group A streptococcal infection, usually takes the form of pharyngitis accompanied by a characteristic rash. In the past this infection was thought to occur in hosts who were not immune to one of the streptococcal pyrogenic exotoxins (A, B, or C). More recent studies suggest that the rash may be due to a hypersensitivity reaction requiring prior exposure to the toxin. The rash typically develops within 2 d of the sore throat; it begins on the neck, upper chest, and back and then spreads over the remainder of the body, sparing the palms and soles. This diffuse, blanching erythema with 1- to 2-mm punctate elevations has a "sandpaper" texture and is most intense along skin folds (Pastia's lines). Circumoral pallor and a "strawberry tongue" (enlarged papillae on a coated tongue, which later becomes denuded) frequently accompany the rash. The rash subsides after 6–9 d and is followed by desquamation of the palms and soles. The most feared complications of streptococcal pharyngitis are the late nonsuppurative complications. ARF is a rare but serious disease that follows streptococcal pharyngitis. AGN (see Chap. 132) may follow either pharyngitis or skin infection.

Diagnosis   Clinical criteria alone are unreliable for the diagnosis of streptococcal pharyngitis. Throat culture remains the gold standard. Rapid diagnostic kits are useful if the result is positive; however, because of low sensitivity, a negative result must be confirmed with a throat culture. Serologic tests such as antistreptolysin O confirm past infection in pts with suspected ARF or AGN but are not useful for the diagnosis of pharyngitis.

℞ TREATMENT

Treatment is given mainly to prevent ARF and must be started within 9 d of onset (Table 82-1).

SKIN AND SOFT TISSUE INFECTION   ***Impetigo (pyoderma)***   Impetigo is a localized purulent skin infection that occurs predominantly in children 2–6 years of age in warm climates and affects especially the face and lower extremities. While it is usually due to group A streptococci, it may occasionally be caused by other streptococci or by *Staphylococcus aureus*. Papules become vesicular, with surrounding erythema, and form thick, honey-like crusts over 4–6 d. This infection, which is more common in conditions of poor hygiene and may follow minor trauma, is diagnosed by culture of the base of the lesion. Impetigo is not associated with ARF but frequently precedes AGN.

Table 82-1

Treatment of Group A Streptococcal Infections

Infection	Treatment*
Pharyngitis	Benzathine penicillin G, 1.2 million units IM; or penicillin V, 250 mg PO qid × 10 d (Children <27 kg: Benzathine penicillin G, 600,000 units IM; or penicillin V, 125 mg PO qid × 10 d)
Impetigo	Same as pharyngitis
Erysipelas/ cellulitis	Severe: Penicillin G, 1–2 million units IV q4h Mild to moderate: Procaine penicillin, 1.2 million units IM bid
Necrotizing fasciitis/ myositis	Surgical debridement plus penicillin G, 2–4 million units IV q4h
Pneumonia/ empyema	Penicillin G, 2–4 million units IV q4h, plus drainage of empyema

*Penicillin allergy: Erythromycin (10 mg/kg PO qid up to a maximum of 250 mg/dose) may be substituted for oral penicillin. Alternative agents for parenteral therapy include first-generation cephalosporins—if the penicillin allergy does not manifest as immediate hypersensitivity (anaphylaxis or urticaria) or as another potentially life-threatening reaction (e.g., severe rash and fever)—and vancomycin.
SOURCE: Wessels MR: HPIM-14, p. 886.

℞ TREATMENT

Agents active against both streptococci and *S. aureus* provide the most reliable therapy for impetigo. These drugs include dicloxacillin (500 mg PO qid), cephalexin (500 mg PO qid), and topical mupirocin ointment. If the infection is known to be due to group A streptococci, the regimens used for pharyngitis (Table 82-1) are cheaper and equally effective.

Cellulitis Cellulitis, an infection of the skin and subcutaneous tissue, is caused by group A streptococci or *S. aureus*. The involved area is red, warm, and tender; fever and systemic symptoms often develop, and regional lymphadenopathy may be documented. Erysipelas is a form of cellulitis caused almost exclusively by group A streptococci and typically involving the face or lower extremities. There is an acute onset of pain and of a raised plateau of redness (formed by engorgement of lymphatic tissue) that is sharply demarcated from normal skin. Erysipelas may be associated with high fever and bacteremia.

R̲x̲ TREATMENT

Agents active against both streptococci and *S. aureus* provide the most reliable therapy for cellulitis. Therapy is initiated with oxacillin (2 g IV q4h) or cefazolin (2 g IV q8h); if the pt is allergic to penicillin or if methicillin-resistant *S. aureus* infection is suspected, vancomycin (1 g IV q12h) is used. If the infection is known to be due to group A streptococci, penicillin is preferred (Table 82-1).

Necrotizing fasciitis A rapidly life-threatening infection of the superficial or deep fascia, necrotizing fasciitis is caused by group A streptococci in 60% of cases. (Other cases, particularly those related to an abdominal or peritoneal process or surgery, are caused by bowel flora.) The onset of symptoms is acute and is marked by severe pain at the site of infection, malaise, fever, chills, and a toxic appearance. As the process evolves (often quite rapidly), skin changes become increasingly apparent, with dusky or mottled erythema; edema and anesthesia of the involved area may be noted. Surgical exploration is required both for confirmation of the diagnosis and for treatment. While antibiotic therapy (Table 82-1) is adjunctive, surgical debridement and resection are lifesaving.

PNEUMONIA AND EMPYEMA Group A streptococci occasionally cause pneumonia, generally in previously healthy individuals. Pleuritic chest pain, fever, chills, and dyspnea are characteristic presenting symptoms, with either an abrupt or a gradual onset. Streptococcal pneumonia is accompanied by pleural effusion in 50% of cases, and the effusion is almost always infected. *Treatment* should include antibiotics and early drainage of the empyema (Table 82-1).

BACTEREMIA, PUERPERAL SEPSIS, AND STREPTO-COCCAL TOXIC SHOCK–LIKE SYNDROME Bacteremia may complicate an identifiable local infection, particularly cellulitis, pneumonia, or necrotizing fasciitis. In the absence of a focus, evaluation for endocarditis, abscess, or osteomyelitis should be pursued. Occasionally, group A streptococci still cause endometritis and bacteremia complicating childbirth. Outbreaks of these infections have been associated with asymptomatic carriage of group A streptococci by delivery room personnel.

A toxic shock–like syndrome has been described in association with group A streptococcal infections, especially necrotizing fasciitis, cellulitis, myositis, and pneumonia. This syndrome manifests as fever, hypotension, and multisystem organ failure and is associated with 30% mortality. In contrast to staphylococcal toxic shock syndrome, the streptococcal syndrome is usually characterized by the lack of a rash and by positive blood cultures.

℞ TREATMENT

Treatment of these infections requires aggressive supportive care, surgical debridement of involved local sites, and antibiotic administration. Data from experimental animals suggest that clindamycin (600 mg IV q6h) might be more effective than β-lactam antibiotics; however, there are currently no data on the treatment of humans with this regimen. Likewise, IV administration of immune globulin preparations has been used adjunctively in the treatment of streptococcal toxic shock syndrome, but no relevant controlled trials have been performed.

Group B *Streptococcus* (GBS)

NEONATAL INFECTIONS GBS is the most frequent cause of neonatal sepsis and meningitis, with an incidence of 2 per 1000 births. (*Escherichia coli* is the second most frequent cause.) Early-onset infections become evident within 7 d of birth, with signs often present at birth. The infants involved most often present with respiratory distress, lethargy, and hypotension. Almost all are bacteremic, half have pneumonia or respiratory distress syndrome, and one-third have meningitis. Late-onset disease occurs between 1 week and 3 months after birth; generally presents as bacteremia with or without meningitis, occasionally with other focal infections; and is associated with a lower mortality rate than early-onset disease. Many meningitis survivors have neurologic sequelae. Infants with suspected neonatal sepsis should be treated with high-dose penicillin and gentamicin; penicillin may be given alone once GBS has been identified as the causative organism. Between 5 and 40% of women are identified by antenatal culture as carriers of GBS in the vagina or rectum. The CDC has suggested a strategy for prevention of GBS infection in neonates: Women should be screened for colonization by swab culture of the lower vagina and rectum at 35–37 weeks of gestation. Intrapartum chemoprophylaxis (penicillin G, 5 million units IV followed by 2.5 million units q4h until delivery, with clindamycin or erythromycin substituted when women are allergic to penicillin) should be *offered* to all carriers and is *recommended* for women with the following risk factors: preterm delivery, early rupture of membranes (>24 h before delivery), prolonged labor, fever, chorioamnionitis, multiple gestation, or prior birth of an infant with GBS infection.

ADULT INFECTIONS   Peripartum infections are the most common GBS infections in adults. The organism may cause puerperal sepsis or chorioamnionitis. Bacteremic cases may be complicated by meningitis or endocarditis. Other adult infections involve the elderly or those with other underlying conditions, such as diabetes mellitus, cirrhosis, HIV infection, or malignancy. These GBS infections include UTIs, diabetic skin ulcers, pneumonia, endocarditis, septic arthritis, intraabdominal abscesses, and osteomyelitis.

℞ TREATMENT
Appropriate treatment consists of penicillin G (12 million U/d). Meningitis and endocarditis should be treated with even higher doses (18–24 million U/d). Vancomycin (1 g q12h) may be substituted for penicillin in cases of allergy.

Group D *Streptococcus*

S. bovis is the main human pathogen among group D streptococci. Endocarditis due to *S. bovis* is associated with neoplasms and other lesions of the GI tract. In contrast to enterococci, *S. bovis* is highly susceptible to penicillin, which is the drug of choice for the infections it causes.

Groups C and G Streptococci

Streptococci of groups C and G cause infections similar to those caused by group A streptococci, including pharyngitis, bacteremia, pneumonia, cellulitis, soft tissue infection, septic arthritis, and endocarditis. Bacteremia involving these organisms tends to occur in elderly, debilitated, or chronically ill pts.

℞ TREATMENT
Appropriate therapy for adult infection consists of high-dose penicillin (18 million U/d) and aspiration or open debridement of infected joint spaces; for endocarditis or septic arthritis, gentamicin (1 mg/kg q8h) is added for synergy.

Viridans Streptococci

The viridans streptococci include multiple species of alpha-hemolytic streptococci. These organisms are part of the normal mouth flora and are the most frequent causative agents of bacterial endocarditis. Viridans streptococcal endocarditis may be treated with penicillin (12 million U/d). Occasional isolates characterized as nutritional variants require vitamin B_6 for growth; against these isolates, gentamicin (1 mg/kg q8h) should be added for optimal coverage. The *S. milleri* or *S. intermedius* group (*S. intermedius, S. anginosus,* and *S. constellatus*) are usually considered viridans streptococci but may be beta-hemolytic and often cause suppurative infections such as intraabdominal or brain abscesses. These organisms are sensitive to penicillin, which is the drug of choice for treatment of the infections they cause. Viridans streptococcal bacteremia occurs with relatively high frequency among neutropenic pts with cancer and may cause a sepsis syndrome with high fever and shock. Risk factors include profound neutropenia, antibiotic prophylaxis with TMP-SMZ or fluoroquinolones, mucositis, and antacid/histamine antagonist therapy. In this setting, viridans streptococci are more commonly resistant to penicillin, and the infections they cause should be treated empirically with vancomycin (1 g IV q12h) pending susceptibility testing.

ENTEROCOCCAL INFECTIONS

Previously classified as group D streptococci, enterococci are now recognized as a separate genus. Enterococcal infections tend to occur in pts who are elderly or debilitated or whose mucosal or skin barriers have been disrupted. Enterococci also cause superinfections in antibiotic-treated pts. Enterococcal infections most commonly involve the urinary tract, particularly in pts with anatomic abnormalities and in those who have undergone instrumentation. Enterococci account for 10–20% of cases of bacterial endocarditis. The presentation of enterococcal endocarditis is usually subacute but may also be acute with valvular destruction. Enterococci are frequently isolated from the biliary tract and may cause infections related to biliary surgery. Moreover, these organisms are often recovered in mixed infections from intraabdominal abscesses, surgical wounds, and diabetic foot ulcers.

℞ TREATMENT

While it is not always necessary to direct antimicrobial therapy at enterococci in mixed infections, these organisms should be covered by treatment when they are predominant or when they are present in blood cultures. Ampicillin (2 g IV q4h) is usually sufficient for the treatment of uncomplicated UTI. However, other types of enterococcal infection require the addition of an aminoglycoside, usually gentamicin (1 mg/kg

IV q8h with normal renal function), for synergy. Vancomycin (1 g q12h) may be substituted for penicillin in penicillin-allergic pts. Because of the increasing incidence of antibiotic resistance in enterococci (especially *E. faecium*), susceptibility testing should be performed for all isolates causing serious infections. Strains with high-level gentamicin resistance may be susceptible to other aminoglycosides or may respond to ampicillin alone. Infections due to enterococci that are resistant to penicillins on the basis of β-lactamase production may be treated with vancomycin, ampicillin/sulbactam, amoxicillin/clavulanate, or imipenem in combination with an aminoglycoside. Moderately resistant enterococci (MIC of penicillin and ampicillin, 16–64 μg/mL) may be susceptible to high-dose penicillin or ampicillin in combination with gentamicin, but strains with MICs of ≥200 μg/mL require treatment with vancomycin and gentamicin. Vancomycin-resistant enterococci have recently emerged as relatively common pathogens in some hospitals. For isolates resistant to both vancomycin and β-lactam antibiotics, there are no established therapies. Chloramphenicol or tetracycline may be used if there is in vitro evidence of susceptibility. Anecdotal and experimental data indicate some success with combination therapies such as ciprofloxacin/rifampin/gentamicin or ampicillin/vancomycin. Teicoplanin, an agent not currently available in the U.S., is effective against some vancomycin-resistant enterococci.

DIPHTHERIA

Diphtheria is a localized infection of mucous membranes or skin caused by *Corynebacterium diphtheriae*. Its incidence is increased among alcoholics, persons in lower socioeconomic groups, and Native Americans as well as under conditions of crowding. Its usual method of spread is by droplet. After an incubation period of 2–5 d, the illness manifests as low-grade fever and oropharyngeal pain, with the development of a thick gray membrane that covers the tonsils and pharynx and may extend over the larynx and cause airway obstruction. Dislodging of the membrane usually causes bleeding. The major toxic manifestations of diphtheria—myocarditis and peripheral neuritis—manifest as listlessness, pallor, and tachycardia progressing to vascular collapse and are most often associated with mucous membrane disease. Cutaneous diphtheria may involve preexisting wounds, burns, or abrasions. A diagnosis is made by Gram's staining of the lesion, which reveals characteristic club-shaped, gram-positive rods in palisades or a "Chinese character" configuration, or by culture of the organism on selective tellurite medium.

℞ TREATMENT

Treatment requires antitoxin, which must be administered in the following doses as early as possible after the diagnosis is suspected: for mild or early (<48 h) pharyngeal or laryngeal disease, 20,000–40,000 U; for nasopharyngeal involvement, 40,000–60,000 U; and for disease that is extensive, of ≥3 d duration, or accompanied by diffuse swelling of the neck, 80,000–100,000 U. Some authorities recommend 20,000 U of antitoxin for cutaneous diphtheria. The pt should first be tested for hypersensitivity to horse serum, and the antiserum should then be administered IV in saline over 60 min. In addition, erythromycin (500 mg PO/IV qid for 14 d) or procaine penicillin G (600,000 units IM q12h) should be given for eradication of the organism in acute respiratory illness. Pts with cutaneous diphtheria and carriers can be treated with erythromycin (500 mg PO qid) or rifampin (600 mg PO qd) for a 7-d course. Diphtheria is preventable by immunization with DTP in childhood (at 2, 4, 6, and 12–18 months and 5 years of age) and reimmunization with Td every 10 years in adulthood.

OUTPATIENT/HOME CARE CONSIDERATIONS

Persons with group A streptococcal pharyngitis and impetigo may be treated as outpatients with oral antibiotics. More serious infections, including cellulitis, mandate hospitalization and parenteral antibiotic therapy. Pts who exhibit a good response to parenteral antibiotic therapy (including resolution of signs of acute inflammation) may be switched to an oral regimen and complete their therapy as outpatients. Once their condition has stabilized, their fever has resolved, and their bacteremia has cleared, pts with viridans streptococcal endocarditis who show no signs of complications (such as embolization, heart block, or valvular failure) may complete their parenteral antibiotic therapy at home when this alternative is logistically feasible.

For a more detailed discussion, see Wessels MR: Streptococcal and Enterococcal Infections, Chap. 143, p. 885; and Holmes RK: Diphtheria, Other Corynebacterial Infections, and Anthrax, Chap. 144, p. 892, in HPIM-14.

83

MENINGOCOCCAL AND LISTERIAL INFECTIONS

MENINGOCOCCAL INFECTIONS

EPIDEMIOLOGY AND PATHOGENESIS *Neisseria meningitidis*, an encapsulated gram-negative coccus, is a commensal of the human oropharynx that can cause rapidly fatal bacteremia and meningitis. Humans are the only host for the organism, and transmission is from person to person but only rarely leads to disease. Most infections occur in children 6–36 months of age. Disease develops with increased frequency in winter and early spring. Epidemics may take place, particularly in economically deprived segments of the population. The risk is increased for household contacts of individuals with disease, for alcoholics, for military recruits, and for persons with terminal complement deficiencies or asplenia. Meningococcal infections occur at increased frequency in areas of sub-Saharan Africa, the Middle East, and Asia. Of all meningococcal infections, 99% are caused by serogroups A, B, C, 29E, W-135, and Y. Endemic disease in the U.S. is caused most often by serogroup B. Serogroup C strains have caused more infections in older age groups, and serogroup B strains have been especially common among very young children. The rate of nasopharyngeal carriage is approximately 10% but may increase to 60–80% in closed populations such as those at military camps or schools. Nasopharyngeal carriage is thought to lead to the development of protective antibodies; it is in the first few days of colonization, prior to the development of antibody, that the risk of invasive infection is greatest.

CLINICAL MANIFESTATIONS *Meningococcemia* Between 30 and 40% of pts who develop meningococcal disease have bacteremia without meningitis. Meningococcemia sometimes presents as a prodromal syndrome of sore throat, rhinorrhea, cough, and headache. Manifestations of meningococcemia include a sudden onset of spiking fever, chills, nausea, vomiting, rash, arthralgias, and myalgias. Pts are acutely ill, with high fever (though some with fulminant disease may be afebrile or hypothermic), tachycardia, and tachypnea; 75% of pts have a rash, which may be maculopapular, petechial, or ecchymotic and may be sparsely distributed on the trunk and extremities. In fulminant disease (previously called Waterhouse-Friderichsen syndrome, 10–20% of cases), shock, DIC, and multiple-organ failure supervene, and petechiae and purpuric lesions expand rapidly. Mortality ranges from 10% for uncomplicated meningococcemia to 50–60% for fulminant disease.

Meningitis Frequently associated with meningococcemia and most common among children from 6 months to 10 years of age, meningitis presents as an abrupt onset of symptoms in approximately 25% of pts. However, most pts have URI symptoms followed by progressive fever, vomiting, headache, and confusion over several days; 20–40% have meningitis without accompanying meningococcemia. Sequelae include seizures or deafness, peripheral neuropathies, and cranial nerve palsies and are uncommon. Most sequelae clear after several months.

Other manifestations Chronic meningococcemia (1–2% of all cases) presents as recurrent fever, maculopapular or petechial rash, and arthralgias lasting for weeks to months. During afebrile intervals the pt may appear well. Arthritis, most commonly involving the large joints, occurs in 5–10% of pts with meningococcemia and is usually immune mediated. Rare manifestations of meningococcal infection include sinusitis, conjunctivitis, pneumonia (primary or postviral, associated with serogroup Y), endocarditis, urethritis, endometritis, and endophthalmitis.

DIAGNOSIS Early recognition of meningococcal disease depends on distinguishing it from other acute illnesses since it resembles common viral infections. The detection of mottled erythema or a faint maculopapular rash (like rose spots of typhoid) should raise diagnostic suspicion. Diagnosis depends on culture of the organism from blood, spinal fluid, or petechial scraping. Growth of the organism in blood culture may be inhibited by the common additive sodium polyanetholesulfonate. Meningococcal capsular polysaccharide antigen can be detected in blood, urine, or synovial or spinal fluid by latex agglutination or CIE. Gram's stain of spinal fluid reveals gram-negative diplococci in half of meningitis pts. Altogether, the findings on Gram's stain, culture, and immunoassay detect 95% of cases. PCR of spinal fluid may detect 90% of meningitis cases. Other findings, such as elevated peripheral or CSF WBC count, reduced CSF glucose level, and elevated CSF protein level, are not specific.

℞ TREATMENT

Primary therapy is with penicillin G (200,000–300,000 units/kg q6h, with a maximum daily dose of 24 million units) for 7 d. Alternatives include chloramphenicol [75–100 (mg/kg)/d divided q6h; maximum, 4 g/d]. Ceftriaxone and cefotaxime are also effective and are often used initially when the etiology of meningitis is unknown. Supportive care is required for fulminant disease with shock.

PREVENTION   Meningococcal disease in persons at high risk (e.g., household contacts) can be prevented with rifampin (10 mg/kg, up to 600 mg, q12h for 2 d). A single oral dose of ciprofloxacin (500 mg) or ofloxacin (400 mg) is an acceptable alternative in nonpregnant adults but not in children or pregnant women. A single dose of 250 mg of ceftriaxone IM is recommended for pregnant contacts. A vaccine active against serogroups A, C, Y, and W-135 is used to prevent infections in military recruits, persons with functional or anatomic asplenia, persons with complement deficiencies, and travelers to areas with epidemic disease and to prevent late infections in close contacts of cases.

LISTERIAL INFECTIONS

EPIDEMIOLOGY AND PATHOGENESIS   *Listeria monocytogenes*, a motile gram-positive bacillus, is responsible for food-borne invasive infections, primarily sepsis and meningitis. Cases may occur sporadically or in outbreaks associated with particular foods. Implicated foods have included Mexican-style and other soft cheeses, coleslaw, pasteurized milk, and food from delicatessens. At highest risk are pregnant women and persons immunocompromised by disease (HIV, renal, or hepatic disease, lymphomas) or drugs (glucocorticoids, cyclosporine, cytotoxic agents), although infection occasionally occurs in immunocompetent hosts.

CLINICAL MANIFESTATIONS   Listeriosis not associated with pregnancy generally occurs in immunocompromised persons or the elderly. Cases of bacteremia and meningitis due to *Listeria* cannot be distinguished clinically from those caused by other organisms. Pregnancy-associated listeriosis develops most often in the third trimester but may occur at any time; 33–50% of pregnant women have a mild illness, with fever, myalgias, malaise, and occasional GI complaints. Transplacental spread of infection can lead to chorioamnionitis, premature labor, fetal demise, or neonatal infection. Neonatal infection may be of early (<7 d) or late onset. Early-onset infection usually occurs within the first 2 d of life, with sepsis, respiratory distress, skin lesions, or disseminated abscesses involving multiple organs. Infants with late-onset infection are more likely to have meningitis. Recent studies of common-source outbreaks have indicated that *Listeria* is an occasional cause of an acute diarrhea syndrome in immunocompetent persons. *Listeria* may also cause encephalitis, cerebritis, intracranial abscesses, and (rarely) endocarditis and other focal infections.

DIAGNOSIS   Listeriosis is diagnosed by culture of the organism from a normally sterile body site (e.g., CSF or blood).

Culture from stool or vagina is not reliable because approximately 5% of healthy individuals carry the organism.

℞ TREATMENT

Nonpregnant adults with listeriosis should be treated with ampicillin (2 g IV q4h) or penicillin G (15–20 million units/d in 6 divided doses); immunosuppressed pts can also receive gentamicin for synergy (1.3 mg/kg IV q8h). Penicillin-allergic pts can receive TMP-SMZ (15/75 mg/kg daily in 3 divided doses). Listeriosis in pregnancy is treated with ampicillin (1–1.5 g IV q6h for 2 weeks); erythromycin may be used as an alternative in the penicillin-allergic pt during the last month of pregnancy. For neonatal listeriosis, treatment consists of a 2-week course of ampicillin. In infants weighing <2000 g, the dose is 100 mg/kg daily in 2 divided doses during the first week of life and 150 mg/kg daily during the second week. Infants weighing ≥2000 g should receive 150 (mg/kg)/d in 3 equal doses during the first week of life and 200 (mg/kg)/d during the second week. Gentamicin can be added for neonatal listeriosis at 5 mg/kg daily in 2 divided doses during the first week of life and 7.5 (mg/kg)/d in 3 divided doses during the second week. Therapy for meningitis in an immunocompetent pt should continue for 2–3 weeks following defervescence. Immunosuppressed pts should probably receive 4–6 weeks of therapy.

PREVENTION Prevention of listeriosis requires dietary counseling of those at high risk of disease and measures to reduce the contamination of food sources.

For a more detailed discussion, see Solberg CO: Meningococcal Infections, Chap. 149, p. 910; and Schuchat A, Broome CV: Infections Caused by *Listeria monocytogenes*, Chap. 145, p. 899, in HPIM-14.

84

INFECTIONS CAUSED BY *HAEMOPHILUS, BORDETELLA, MORAXELLA,* AND HACEK GROUP ORGANISMS

HAEMOPHILUS INFLUENZAE

ETIOLOGY   *H. influenzae* is a small pleomorphic coccobacillary gram-negative pathogen that often stains only faintly with phenosafranin and therefore can easily be overlooked. The six capsular polysaccharide–based serotypes are designated a through f. *H. influenzae* type b (Hib) and unencapsulated strains, termed *nontypable H. influenzae* (NTHi), are the most frequently isolated pathogens.

PATHOGENESIS   *H. influenzae* is part of the normal oropharyngeal flora and causes systemic disease by invasion and hematogenous spread to distant sites such as the meninges, bones, and joints. The type b capsular polysaccharide is an antiphagocytic barrier, while *H. influenzae* endotoxin (LPS) can damage mucosal cells and cause CNS inflammation and the sepsis syndrome. NTHi strains cause disease by local invasion of mucosal surfaces. The incidence of invasive disease caused by nontypable strains is low but increasing.

EPIDEMIOLOGY   Since 1991, vaccines of type b capsular polysaccharide conjugated to carrier proteins have greatly reduced rates of Hib meningitis among children. The rate of nasopharyngeal colonization by Hib strains has similarly decreased. Where vaccination is not practiced, 20–50 cases occur per 100,000 children from 6 months to 2 years of age. In adults, half of invasive infections are due to NTHi; risk factors include female gender, pregnancy, HIV infection, and malignancy.

CLINICAL MANIFESTATIONS   *H. influenzae* causes community-acquired pneumonia, especially in elderly adults with chronic lung disease or prolonged tobacco use and in pts with HIV infection. More than 80% of isolates from cases of pneumonia are nontypable. NTHi is one of the three most common causes of otitis media in children (the other two being *Streptococcus pneumoniae* and *Moraxella catarrhalis*). Obstetric infections caused by NTHi are severe, with maternal-fetal transmission of the organism, premature birth, and high infant mortality. Epiglottitis in adults may feature fever, sore throat, respiratory distress, and hoarseness or drooling; mortality from airway obstruction is 7%.

DIAGNOSIS *H. influenzae* is isolated from 80–90% of blood cultures in pneumonia and epiglottitis. Counterimmunoelectrophoresis detects antigen in CSF, blood, and urine.

℞ TREATMENT

All isolates from seriously infected pts should be considered resistant to β-lactam antibiotics until proven otherwise, and non-β-lactam agents should be used. When an isolate is shown to be sensitive, therapy should be changed to ampicillin 200–400 (mg/kg)/d (up to 6 g). Third-generation cephalosporins (e.g., ceftriaxone, cefotaxime) that reach therapeutic levels in CSF are effective for the treatment of meningitis. Early administration of glucocorticoids (dexamethasone, 0.6 mg/kg qd) protects against hearing loss in children with Hib meningitis. Approximately 25% of NTHi strains produce β-lactamase and are resistant to ampicillin. Infections caused by ampicillin-resistant strains can be treated with trimethoprim-sulfamethoxazole (TMP-SMZ), erythromycin/sulfisoxazole, amoxicillin/clavulanic acid, various extended-spectrum cephalosporins, fluoroquinolones, and clarithromycin. Preschool contacts of children infected with type b strains should receive prophylaxis with rifampin, 20 (mg/kg)/d (up to 600 mg) for 4 d. Epiglottitis may require intubation for airway protection.

BORDETELLA PERTUSSIS

ETIOLOGY Humans are the sole host for the gram-negative coccobacillus *B. pertussis,* which grows slowly on selective media.

PATHOGENESIS *B. pertussis* colonizes the respiratory tract, adhering to respiratory epithelium via pili, filamentous hemagglutinin, and pertactin. The organism elaborates pertussis toxin, which exerts a number of biologic effects and probably plays a role in producing the pertussis clinical syndrome.

EPIDEMIOLOGY Pertussis (whooping cough) is probably underdiagnosed. Rates of communicability to nonimmune household contacts of pertussis pts are 90–100%. In the U.S., two-thirds of children with pertussis are not adequately vaccinated; 11% of pts are ≥20 years of age. The case-fatality rate is 0.2% overall but is 10.6% under 6 months of age.

CLINICAL MANIFESTATIONS Pertussis infection incubates for 7–10 d. The three stages of illness are *catarrhal* (1–2 weeks), *paroxysmal* (2–4 weeks), and *convalescent* (2–3 weeks). Coughing is distinctive: 10–30 coughs per spasm, 10–25 paroxysms per 24 h, with a posttussive whoop in 40–60%

of cases. Adolescents and adults have cough with or without whooping for 1–2 weeks. Lymphocytosis is more common among children than adults. Complications include cyanosis, apnea, and pneumonia.

DIAGNOSIS The presentation of prolonged paroxysmal cough accompanied by whoops and lymphocytosis is highly specific. For the isolation of *B. pertussis,* a nasopharyngeal swab specimen is immediately inoculated onto selective media. The sensitivity of culture is 70–80% in the first 2 weeks of illness. Polymerase chain reaction of nasopharyngeal specimens may increase the yield and is helpful in pts treated with antibiotics.

℞ TREATMENT
B. pertussis should be eradicated from the airway with erythromycin (preferably estolate), 50 (mg/kg)/d (maximum, 2 g/d) in two to four divided doses for 14 d. Household and other close contacts should be treated with the same regimen, regardless of age and immunization status. Efficacy rates for whole-cell vaccine are 80–90% initially and decline over time. New acellular vaccines cause fewer adverse effects and reportedly are more efficacious than whole-cell vaccines.

MORAXELLA CATARRHALIS

ETIOLOGY *Moraxella (Branhamella),* a gram-negative diplococcus, produces β-lactamase.

EPIDEMIOLOGY *M. catarrhalis* colonizes the upper airway of 50% of healthy schoolchildren and 7% of adults. The incidence of infections peaks in late winter/early spring.

CLINICAL MANIFESTATIONS *M. catarrhalis* causes otitis media, tracheobronchitis, pneumonia, and rare cases of empyema, bacteremia, septic arthritis, meningitis, and endocarditis. Respiratory infections occur in patients over 50 years of age with chronic pulmonary disease.

DIAGNOSIS Gram's staining of sputum reveals gram-negative diplococci.

℞ TREATMENT
Amoxicillin/clavulanate (250–500 mg PO tid), a second- or third-generation cephalosporin, or erythromycin is effective.

HACEK GROUP ORGANISMS

ETIOLOGY *Haemophilus aphrophilus, H. paraphrophilus, H. parainfluenzae, Actinobacillus actinomycetemcomitans, Cardiobacterium hominis, Eikenella corrodens,* and *Kingella kingae* are fastidious, CO_2-requiring pathogens.

PATHOGENESIS All HACEK organisms cause endocarditis of abnormal valves.

CLINICAL MANIFESTATIONS Endocarditis due to HACEK organisms can be insidious or complicated, with embolization in 60% of cases and mortality as high as 30% with *Haemophilus*. Sources of infection include human bites, periodontitis, meningitis, septic arthritis, and osteomyelitis.

DIAGNOSIS Blood cultures should be observed for at least 7 d.

℞ TREATMENT
For endocarditis, ampicillin (9–12 g/d) plus an aminoglycoside [3 (mg/kg)/d] should be administered for 6 weeks. Sensitivity testing should be done.

For a more detailed discussion, see Murphy TF, Kasper DL: Infections Due to *Haemophilus influenzae,* Other *Haemophilus* Species, the HACEK Group, and Other Gram-Negative Bacilli, Chap. 152, p. 924; Musher DM: *Moraxella (Branhamella) catarrhalis,* Other *Moraxella* Species, and *Kingella,* Chap. 151, p. 922; and Siber GR, Samore MH: Pertussis, Chap. 154, p. 933, in HPIM-14.

85

DISEASES CAUSED BY GRAM-NEGATIVE ENTERIC BACTERIA, *PSEUDOMONAS*, AND *LEGIONELLA*

GRAM-NEGATIVE ENTERIC BACILLI

The gram-negative enteric bacilli are a diverse group of bacteria that reside in the human colon. Collectively, they account for about one-third of septicemia isolates, two-thirds of bacterial gastroenteritis isolates, and three-quarters of UTI isolates.

Escherichia coli

PATHOGENESIS AND CLINICAL SYNDROMES *E. coli* is a major cause of enteric infections and UTIs, a common component of polymicrobial intraabdominal infections, and an occasional cause (either alone or in combination with other pathogens) of a variety of other infections, including pneumonia, osteomyelitis, septic arthritis, and sinusitis. Hosts compromised by neutropenia, vascular disease, diabetes mellitus, or traumatic injury are at added risk for invasive infections. Bacteremia and sepsis syndrome are serious potential consequences of *E. coli* infections. Strains bearing the K1 capsular serotype are important agents of neonatal meningitis and bacteremia.

Strains producing enteric infections are classified as enterotoxigenic (ETEC), enteropathogenic (EPEC), enteroinvasive (EIEC), or enterohemorragic (EHEC). ETEC strains are common agents of traveler's diarrhea, producing watery, noninflammatory diarrheal syndromes. EPEC strains are causes of childhood diarrhea, especially in developing countries. EIEC strains cause dysentery syndromes similar to that caused by *Shigella* species. EHEC strains, typically of serotype O157:H7, cause colitis in which stools lack inflammatory cells but may be grossly bloody. A minority of pts subsequently develop the hemolytic-uremic syndrome (HUS), in which Shiga-like cytotoxins are involved.

Acute UTIs usually occur in sexually active females; bacteria colonize the periurethral region and ascend the urethra. Sequelae may include asymptomatic bacteriuria, urethritis, cystitis, pyelitis, and pyelonephritis. Polymicrobial intraabdominal infections typically follow fecal spillage into the peritoneum; *E. coli* and other facultative enteric gram-negative organisms are responsible for the early peritonitis and sepsis syndrome that often follows such catastrophes. *E. coli* bacteremia usually originates from the bowel, biliary tree, or urinary tract.

Table 85-1

Antibiotics Used in the Treatment of Infections with Enterobacteriaceae

Antibiotic Class	Representative Antibiotics	Properties to Consider
Early penicillins	Ampicillin (parenteral), amoxicillin (oral)	Resistance (30%) among bacteria causing urinary infections in the U.S.; inexpensive; bactericidal
Extended-spectrum penicillins	Ticarcillin, piperacillin	Useful in some infections with resistant *Enterobacter* spp. when combined with an aminoglycoside; useful in some polymicrobial infections (e.g., diabetic foot infections) when combined with a β-lactamase inhibitor
First-generation cephalosporins	Cephalothin, cefazolin	Inexpensive; bactericidal; useful in many infections with *E. coli* and in some infections with *Klebsiella* spp. and *Proteus mirabilis*
Third-generation cephalosporins	Ceftriaxone, cefotaxime, ceftizoxime, cefpodoxime (oral)	Broad-spectrum; bactericidal; IV forms excellent for treating meningitis; resistance in many *Enterobacter* spp.; oral agents useful in uncomplicated UTI caused by susceptible bacteria (most *E. coli, K. pneumoniae*)

Carbacephems	Loracarbef (oral)	Similar to oral third-generation cephalosporins, with activity against common urinary tract pathogens but not *Enterobacter* spp.
Carbapenems	Imipenem/cilastatin	Broad-spectrum; may cause seizures in pts with renal failure or CNS lesions; useful in infections with resistant *Enterobacter* spp.
Sulfonamides	Trimethoprim-sulfamethoxazole	Inexpensive; useful in UTI; IV form useful in serious infections (meningitis) caused by *Enterobacter* spp.
Monobactams	Aztreonam	Useful in pts allergic to penicillin; may be used in pregnant pts
Quinolones	Ciprofloxacin, ofloxacin, norfloxacin, lomefloxacin, enoxacin	Useful in pts traveler's diarrhea, UTI, osteomyelitis, and infections with resistant *Enterobacter* spp.; should not be used by pregnant pts
Aminoglycosides	Gentamicin, tobramycin, amikacin	Once-daily dosing may reduce toxicity; should not be used by pts with renal dysfunction and diabetes mellitus unless absolutely necessary; prolonged therapy to be avoided; useful in infections with resistant *Enterobacter* spp.

SOURCE: Eisenstein BI, Watkins V: HPIM-14, p. 939.

DIAGNOSIS The diagnosis of *E. coli* infection rests on the combination of suspicious clinical findings and laboratory isolation of the organism. Specific identification is generally made biochemically. Growth of *E. coli* from a normally sterile site (e.g., blood, CSF, pleural fluid) should be considered diagnostic of infection at that site. In contrast, isolation from a normally nonsterile site (e.g., the GI tract) must be interpreted thoughtfully. Gram's staining is not specific for *E. coli*. Screening for *E. coli* O157:H7 infection is conducted on sorbitol-MacConkey agar.

℞ TREATMENT

Traveler's diarrhea is often self-limited but may be treated with oral TMP-SMZ or a fluoroquinolone. EHEC infections are managed supportively; signs of HUS should be sought for 1 week after onset of diarrhea. Uncomplicated cystitis in healthy, nonpregnant women is treated for 3 d with TMP-SMZ. A fluoroquinolone may be substituted in pts allergic to sulfonamides. Cystitis in a diabetic or pregnant pt requires 7 d of treatment. For the pregnant pt, the choice of agents is limited to amoxicillin, macrocrystalline nitrofurantoin, or cefpodoxime proxetil. Uncomplicated, mild pyelonephritis can be treated with oral TMP-SMZ or a fluoroquinolone for 10–14 d. Pregnant pts with pyelonephritis—and any pt with severe pyelonephritis—should be hospitalized initially and given IV antibiotics; choices include ceftriaxone, ciprofloxacin (not for pregnant pts), an extended-spectrum penicillin, or gentamicin, which may be given with or without a cell wall–active agent. Treatment (the latter part of which may be oral) should be continued for 14–21 d. In many circumstances, therapy for *E. coli* infections must be individualized; several weeks of treatment may be required for serious or deep-seated infections. Considerations in choosing antibiotic therapy are presented in Table 85-1.

Klebsiella, Enterobacter, Serratia

ETIOLOGY These genera, lactose-fermenting members of the tribe Klebsielleae, are opportunistic and nosocomial pathogens.

CLINICAL MANIFESTATIONS *K. pneumoniae* causes community-acquired lobar pneumonia, typically in alcoholic men over 40 years of age with comorbid conditions (e.g., diabetes, chronic obstructive pulmonary disease). The disease mimics pneumococcal pneumonia except that lung abscess and empyema are more frequent sequelae. Bulging fissures, a nonspecific radiographic finding, may occur. In the hospital, the Klebsielleae are major causes of infections of the urinary tract, lower respiratory tract, biliary tract, surgical wounds, and bloodstream.

DIAGNOSIS Diagnostic considerations discussed above for *E. coli* apply to the Klebsielleae as well. Their isolation from the respiratory secretions of a hospitalized pt must be interpreted in the context of the overall clinical situation: the clinical likelihood of pneumonia, the appearance of the CXR, *and the presence or absence of PMNs on sputum smears.* On Gram's stain, *K. pneumoniae* may appear as short, plump gram-negative rods; a large nonstaining capsule may be evident.

℞ **TREATMENT**

Treatment must be individualized (Table 85-1). Empiric antibiotic coverage should be chosen according to the severity of the illness, the underlying status of the host, and the prevalence of antibacterial resistance in a given institution. A variety of resistance mechanisms are prevalent among the Klebsielleae, including an inducible chromosomal cephalosporinase (whose presence may be missed on routine sensitivity testing) in *Serratia* and *Enterobacter* spp. Combination therapy is often prudent—e.g., with ceftriaxone (1–2 g IV q12h) or mezlocillin (3 g IV q4–6h) plus gentamicin (3–5 mg/kg IV qd).

Proteus, Morganella, Providencia

ETIOLOGY *Proteus, Morganella,* and *Providencia,* of the tribe Proteeae, are actively motile bacteria that do not ferment lactose. *P. mirabilis* causes most *Proteus* infections; almost all strains are indole negative. Virtually all other strains in the tribe are indole positive.

CLINICAL MANIFESTATIONS *P. mirabilis* causes acute UTI in healthy adults but otherwise rarely causes primary disease in normal hosts. *Proteus* is an important cause of chronic UTI; its urease activity alkalinizes the urine and promotes formation of struvite stones. Like other gram-negative bacteria, *Proteus* may contaminate surgical wounds, burns, and decubitus ulcers. These organisms have been associated with posttraumatic corneal ulcers and with destructive chronic mastoid or middle-ear infections that sometimes progress to involve the CNS. The urinary tract serves as the portal of entry in most cases of *Proteus* bacteremia.

DIAGNOSIS Microbiologic isolation from a normally sterile site is necessary for diagnosis. *P. mirabilis* swarms on moist agar.

R̲x̲ **TREATMENT**
Most strains of *P. mirabilis* are sensitive to most β-lactams and aminoglycosides. Treatment for uncomplicated cystitis consists of ampicillin (0.5–1 g IV q6h); that for severe infections consists of either ampicillin (2–3 g IV q6h) plus gentamicin (3–5 mg/kg IV qd) or a third-generation cephalosporin such as ceftriaxone (1–2 g IV q12h). Infected struvite stones must often be removed. The indole-positive Proteeae tend to be more resistant to antibiotics than are most *P. mirabilis* strains.

PSEUDOMONAS AND RELATED ORGANISMS

ETIOLOGY   *Pseudomonas* spp. and phylogenetically related organisms are ubiquitous, free-living, opportunistic gram-negative pathogens. Of this group, *P. aeruginosa* is the most common agent of human disease. A small aerobic rod, it is widespread in nature and has a predilection for moist environments. *Burkholderia cepacia* and *Stenotrophomonas maltophilia* are occasional nosocomial pathogens. *B. pseudomallei* causes melioidosis; *B. mallei* causes glanders.

PATHOGENESIS   *P. aeruginosa* infections occur after normal cutaneous or mucosal barriers are breached, immunologic defenses are compromised, or the normal flora is eradicated by broad-spectrum antibiotics. Glanders is associated with close contact with horses and other equines.

EPIDEMIOLOGY   *P. aeruginosa* causes hospital-acquired infections. Individuals with cystic fibrosis, diabetes mellitus, IV drug use, neutropenia, wounds, burns, and urinary catheterization are predisposed to infection. *B. cepacia* causes infection in similar circumstances. Melioidosis is endemic to Southeast Asia.

CLINICAL MANIFESTATIONS   *P. aeruginosa* causes pneumonia, bacteremia with ecthyma gangrenosum, endocarditis, sinusitis, "swimmer's ear," malignant otitis externa (in diabetics), contact lens–associated keratitis, septic arthritis and osteomyelitis, UTI, pyoderma, burn wound infection, and hot-tub folliculitis. Melioidosis and glanders present as acute or chronic pulmonary or nonpulmonary suppurative diseases or as acute septicemia.

DIAGNOSIS   *P. aeruginosa* can be identified by Gram's staining and culture. Its blue-green pigment and fruity odor are distinctive. *B. pseudomallei* has a characteristic bipolar "safety-pin" appearance on staining with methylene blue. In addition to culture, serologic methods are available for diagnosis of *B. pseudomallei* and *B. mallei* infections.

℞ TREATMENT

Agents with antipseudomonal activity include aminoglycosides, selected third-generation cephalosporins (e.g., ceftazidime, cefoperazone), selected extended-spectrum penicillins (e.g., ticarcillin, ticarcillin/clavulanate, mezlocillin, piperacillin, piperacillin/tazobactam, azlocillin), carbapenems (e.g., imipenem, meropenem), monobactams (e.g., aztreonam), and fluoroquinolones (e.g., ciprofloxacin, ofloxacin). Local patterns of antimicrobial susceptibility should influence the choice of initial empiric therapy, while the susceptibility profile of the isolate from a particular case should dictate definitive therapy. For most severe infections, two agents are used in combination for synergy—e.g., a β-lactam antibiotic such as ceftazidime (1–2 g) plus an aminoglycoside such as gentamicin (1–1.5 mg/kg) IV q8h. Uncomplicated lower UTIs due to *P. aeruginosa* may be amenable to short-course treatment with a single agent. Surgical intervention is necessary for drainage and debridement of pus and necrotic material and for removal of infected foreign bodies. For left-sided *P. aeruginosa* endocarditis, valve replacement should be performed early. Chronic lung infection in cystic fibrosis requires frequent pulmonary toileting; antibiotics should be given for acute exacerbations. Delivery by the aerosolized route has been used successfully in some instances. Nonmalignant external otitis and *Pseudomonas* dermatitis associated with exposure to contaminated water are self-limited and usually require no specific therapy.

LEGIONELLA INFECTIONS

ETIOLOGY Legionellae are aerobic, gram-negative bacilli whose natural habitats are fresh-water aquatic environments. They may multiply in man-made aquatic reservoirs. *L. pneumophila* causes 80–90% of human *Legionella* infections.

PATHOGENESIS The modes of transmission of *Legionella* to humans include aerosolization, aspiration, and direct instillation into the lung during respiratory tract manipulations. Direct human-to-human transmission is thought not to occur.

EPIDEMIOLOGY *Legionella* infections account for ~3–15% of community-acquired pneumonias and for 10–50% of nosocomial pneumonias when a hospital's water supply is colonized with the organisms. Most sporadic cases probably go

Table 85-2

Clinical Clues Suggestive of Legionnaires' Disease

Diarrhea
High fever (>40°C)
Numerous neutrophils but no organisms revealed by Gram's staining of respiratory secretions
Hyponatremia (serum sodium level of <131 meq/L)
Failure to respond to β-lactam drugs (penicillins or cephalosporins) and aminoglycoside antibiotics
Occurrence of illness in an environment in which the potable water supply is known to be contaminated with *Legionella*
Onset of symptoms within 10 days after discharge from the hospital

SOURCE: Mulazimoglu L, Yu VL: HPIM-14, p. 930.

undiagnosed. Host-specific risk factors include cigarette smoking, chronic lung disease, advanced age, and immunosuppression. Pontiac fever occurs in epidemics reflecting airborne transmission.

CLINICAL MANIFESTATIONS *Legionella* pneumonia (Legionnaires' disease) features high fever, nonproductive cough, and GI symptoms. Shortness of breath and confusion are not uncommon. Clues to the diagnosis of Legionnaires' disease are presented in Table 85-2. Chest examination reveals rales early in the course and evidence of consolidation as the disease progresses. Abnormalities on CXR are virtually uniformly evident on presentation but are nonspecific. Pleural effusion is evident in one-third of cases. Pontiac fever, another disease syndrome linked to legionellae, is an acute, self-limited, flulike illness characterized by malaise, fatigue, myalgias, fever, and headache. Pneumonia does not develop. Extrapulmonary legionellosis may occur; the heart is the site most commonly involved.

DIAGNOSIS The utilities of special tests for the diagnosis of Legionnaires' disease are presented in Table 85-3.

℞ TREATMENT
High-dose erythromycin (4 g/d divided q6h) has been the traditional regimen of choice for *Legionella* infections but is associated with potential problems of excessive volume load, GI intolerance, and ototoxicity. Newer macrolides (e.g., azithromycin, clarithromycin) display superior in vitro activ-

Table 85-3

Utility of Special Laboratory Tests for the Diagnosis of Legionnaires' Disease

Test	Sensitivity, %	Specificity, %
Culture		
Sputum*	80	100
Transtracheal aspirate	90	100
DFA staining of sputum	50–70	96–99
Urinary antigen testing†	70	100
Antibody serology‡	40–60	96–99

*Use of multiple selective media with dyes.

†Serogroup 1 only.

‡IgG and IgM testing of both acute- and convalescent-phase sera. A single titer of ≥1:128 is considered presumptive, while a single titer of ≥1:256 or fourfold seroconversion is considered definitive.

SOURCE: Mulazimoglu L, Yu VL: HPIM-14, p. 931.

ity against legionellae and greater intracellular and lung tissue penetration and may soon become the agents of choice. Quinolones are also highly active against *Legionella* in vitro. For severely ill pts, rifampin (600 mg PO or IV q12h) is combined with erythromycin (1 g IV q6h) or ciprofloxacin (400 mg IV q8h) for initial therapy. A clinical response usually occurs within 3–5 d, after which the pt may be switched to oral therapy—e.g., erythromycin (500 mg PO q6h) or azithromycin (500 mg PO q24h)—to complete a 10- to 14-d course. Immunosuppressed pts with advanced disease should be given a 3-week course. Tetracyclines and TMP-SMZ are alternative agents. Pontiac fever is treated supportively, without antibiotics.

For a more detailed discussion, see Eisenstein BI, Watkins V: Diseases Caused by Gram-Negative Enteric Bacilli, Chap. 155, p. 936; Pollack M: Infections Due to *Pseudomonas* Species and Related Organisms, Chap. 157, p. 943; and Mulazimoglu L, Yu VL: *Legionella* Infection, Chap. 153, p. 928, in HPIM-14.

86

DISEASES CAUSED BY OTHER GRAM-NEGATIVE BACTERIA

BRUCELLOSIS

EPIDEMIOLOGY   Brucellosis is a zoonosis caused by four species of aerobic gram-negative bacilli. *Brucella melitensis*, the most common cause, is acquired from goats, sheep, and camels. *B. suis* is acquired from hogs, *B. abortus* from cattle, and *B. canis* from dogs. Humans become infected by exposure to animal tissues (e.g., slaughterhouse workers, butchers) or by ingestion of untreated milk or milk products or raw meat.

CLINICAL MANIFESTATIONS   The acute illness presents after a 7- to 21-d incubation period, with the onset of fever, chills, fatigue, anorexia, weight loss, and sweats. Other common symptoms include headaches, myalgias, low back pain, constipation, sore throat, and dry cough. Localized infections may occur as well, including osteomyelitis (especially of the lumbosacral vertebrae), arthritis, splenic abscess, epididymoorchitis, CNS infection, and endocarditis. Finally, brucellosis may present chronically, with generalized ill health for >1 year following onset of the disease.

DIAGNOSIS   Most cases are diagnosed on the basis of potential exposure, compatible clinical features, and elevated levels of *Brucella* agglutinins (usually detected by a standard tube agglutination test). A titer of ≥1:160 is considered positive, and IgM assays are positive in early infection. The most definitive evidence of infection is isolation of the organism from blood (optimally with special culture techniques), bone marrow, lymph nodes, or granuloma. Cultures are positive in 50–70% of cases. Samples in which the presence of *Brucella* is suspected should be so labeled to alert the laboratory to use special culture techniques and to be aware of the hazard posed by this material to laboratory personnel.

℞ TREATMENT

Optimal treatment consists of doxycycline (100 mg bid) plus an aminoglycoside (with netilmicin preferred and given at a dose of 2 mg/kg IV or IM q12h) for 4 weeks followed by a combination of doxycycline and rifampin (600–900 mg PO qd) for 4–8 weeks. Young children and pregnant women may be treated with trimethoprim-sulfamethoxazole and rifampin for 8–12 weeks. Blood cultures clear and IgG levels fall with successful treatment.

TULAREMIA

EPIDEMIOLOGY *Francisella tularensis* is transmitted to humans by skin contact, inhalation, or ingestion of material from multiple species of wild animals. In the U.S., transmission takes place primarily through skin contact with infected wild rabbits or by tick or deerfly bite. Tularemia is common in Arkansas, Oklahoma, and Missouri; these three states account for more than 50% of U.S. cases. Cases have been reported with increasing frequency from Scandinavia, eastern Europe, and Siberia.

CLINICAL MANIFESTATIONS Tularemia presents as several different clinical syndromes, most of which are associated with fever, chills, headache, and myalgias, after a 2- to 10-d incubation period. Ulceroglandular tularemia (75–85% of cases) follows skin inoculation of *F. tularensis*; a papule forms and evolves into a punched-out-appearing ulcer with a necrotic base. Large, tender regional lymph nodes develop. Oculoglandular disease develops after inoculation into the eye and presents as purulent conjunctivitis and regional lymphadenopathy. Pulmonary tularemia, which has a high mortality rate and may complicate other forms of the disease or follow inhalation of the organism, presents as nonproductive cough and bilateral patchy infiltrates. The typhoidal form, which is now thought to be rare in the U.S., presents as fever without skin lesions or adenopathy.

DIAGNOSIS Cultures are usually negative, and diagnosis is based on serologic agglutination tests. A fourfold rise in titer over 2–3 weeks is diagnostic of acute infection. A single titer of ≥1:160 constitutes presumptive evidence of infection. Gram's staining of material usually yields negative results, although special stains and fluorescent antibody may be revealing. Culture and isolation of *F. tularensis* are difficult, pose a major risk to laboratory personnel, and should be attempted only in laboratories with adequate isolation techniques and experienced personnel.

℞ TREATMENT

The treatment of choice is streptomycin (7.5–10 mg/kg IM q12h) for 7–10 d; in severe infections, 15 mg/kg q12h may be used for the first 48–72 h. Gentamicin (1.7 mg/kg IV or IM q8h) also may be used. Chloramphenicol and tetracycline have been used to treat tularemia, with good initial response rates but unacceptable relapse rates.

PLAGUE

EPIDEMIOLOGY *Yersinia pestis* causes sporadic cases of human disease that are transmitted by the bite of the rodent flea, predominantly in the southwestern U.S. Plague occurs sporadically both in rural areas throughout the world and in a few urban areas of southern Asia. In its pulmonic form, plague can be transmitted from person to person.

CLINICAL MANIFESTATIONS Bubonic plague is characterized by fever, myalgias, arthralgias, and painful lymphadenopathy (the bubo) following a 2- to 6-d incubation period. Insect contact often is not recalled, but an eschar, papule, pustule, scab, or ulcer may indicate the point of inoculation. If left untreated, bubonic plague may progress to sepsis, hypotension, DIC, and death within 2–10 d. Secondary pneumonia develops in 10–20% of pts, characteristically with initially diffuse interstitial pneumonitis in which sputum production is scant. Primary *Y. pestis* pneumonia develops after an incubation period of 1–4 d, with acute onset of fever, chills, myalgia, headache, cough, and dyspnea (often accompanied by hemoptysis); CXR shows involvement of a single lobe progressing to multilobar involvement. The illness is fulminant, and death occurs within 2–6 d in the absence of treatment. Meningitis is a serious but unusual manifestation of plague.

DIAGNOSIS The diagnosis is usually based on stains and cultures of blood, sputum, an aspirated bubo, or CSF. Stains reveal characteristic bipolar "safety-pin" forms. Culture is usually positive but requires 48–72 h. Serology may serve to confirm cases.

℞ TREATMENT

The drug of choice for plague is streptomycin (1 g IM q12h for 10 d; 15 mg/kg q12h in children). Gentamicin (1.5 mg/kg IV q8h) and tetracycline (500 mg PO or IV q6h) are alternatives. Pts with pneumonic plague should be placed in respiratory isolation, and contacts should receive prophylactic tetracycline (250–500 mg PO qid).

BARTONELLOSIS

Bartonella henselae

CLINICAL MANIFESTATIONS *Cat-Scratch Disease* Cat-scratch disease follows a primary skin inoculation by the lick, scratch, or bite of a cat. *B. henselae*, a tiny gram-negative rod, is now thought to be the only causative agent of cat-scratch disease. Frequently, a skin lesion (papule or pustule) develops after 2–5 d at the primary site of inoculation. Tender lymphadenopathy occurs after 1–2 weeks (often after resolution of the skin lesion) and persists for 3–6 weeks or longer. Dissemination of infection is rare in normal hosts and causes meningoencephalitis, osteomyelitis, or hepatitis.

Disease in Immunocompromised Hosts In immunocompromised hosts, especially those with HIV infection, *B. henselae* may disseminate to involve virtually any organ system, causing a lobular proliferation of new blood vessels. On the skin, this condition is recognized as cutaneous bacillary angiomatosis (also called epithelioid angiomatosis). Characteristically, the lesions are red or purple, resembling Kaposi's sarcoma; they develop anywhere on the skin or mucous membranes. Disseminated bacillary angiomatosis may involve the liver, spleen, bone marrow, lymph nodes, and/or CNS. Dissemination causes persistent fever, abdominal pain, weight loss, and malaise. When the disease involves the liver or spleen, it produces bacillary peliosis hepatis, which may cause abdominal pain and the appearance of nodular lesions on CT or MRI of the organ.

DIAGNOSIS *B. henselae* may be identified in tissue by Warthin-Starry silver stain. In addition, in cases involving immunocompromised hosts, the bacteria may be isolated from cultures of blood and other sites, although lengthy incubation is required. Serology is usually positive in cat-scratch disease, but its usefulness in bacillary angiomatosis has not been established.

℞ TREATMENT

Cat-scratch disease is generally self-limited and resolves spontaneously. Cutaneous bacillary angiomatosis usually responds to treatment with erythromycin (500 mg PO qid) or doxycycline (100 mg PO bid) for 3 weeks. Disseminated disease is usually treated initially with erythromycin (2 g IV qd) or ciprofloxacin (800 mg IV qd) and then with a prolonged course of an oral antibiotic.

Bartonella bacilliformis

EPIDEMIOLOGY *Bartonella bacilliformis* is a tiny gram-negative bacillus that causes Oroya fever and, in its chronic form, skin lesions called *verruga peruana*. These diseases occur almost exclusively in the Andes Mountains of Peru, Ecuador, and Colombia.

CLINICAL MANIFESTATIONS Oroya fever is characterized by fever, chills, malaise, headache, altered mentation, and muscle and joint pains that may begin insidiously or acutely approximately 3 weeks after the bite of the sandfly vector. Profound anemia results from parasitization of erythrocytes, which are then phagocytosed and destroyed by the host. Red or purple cutaneous lesions called *verrugas* may develop during the convalescent phase.

℞ TREATMENT

Oroya fever is usually treated with chloramphenicol.

OTHER GRAM-NEGATIVE RODS ASSOCIATED WITH ANIMAL INJURIES

Pasteurella multocida

This small gram-negative coccobacillus is transmitted by bites or scratches from animals, particularly cats and dogs. Infections are characterized by the rapid development of intense inflammation and purulent drainage. There is a high risk of deep tissue infections, including osteomyelitis, tendon sheath involvement, or septic arthritis. *Treatment* consists of ampicillin/sulbactam (1.5–3.0 g IV q6h), amoxicillin/clavulanic acid (500/125 mg PO tid), or—in the penicillin-allergic pt—TMP-SMZ (160/800 mg PO or IV q12h).

Capnocytophaga canimorsus

This gram-negative rod (formerly designated DF-2) is associated with septicemia following dog bites, particularly in immunocompromised alcoholics or splenectomized pts. Pts present with fever that is sometimes accompanied by meningitis or endocarditis. In splenectomized pts, DIC, gangrene, adrenal hemorrhage, pulmonary hemorrhage, and fulminant sepsis may occur. The organism may be identified on Gram's or Wright's stain of buffy coat of blood from splenectomized individuals. *Treatment* of *C. canimorsus* sepsis consists of penicillin G (2 million units IV q4h for 14 d). Alternatives for use in the penicillin-allergic pt include cephalosporins and fluoroquinolones.

For a more detailed discussion, see Madoff LC: Infections from Bites, Scratches, and Burns, Chap. 135, p. 835; Madkour MM: Brucellosis, Chap. 162, p. 969; Jacobs RF: Tularemia, Chap. 163, p. 971; Campbell GL, Dennis DT: Plague and Other *Yersinia* Infections, Chap. 164, p. 975; and Tompkins LS: *Bartonella* Infections, Including Cat-Scratch Disease, Chap. 165, p. 983, in HPIM-14.

87

ANAEROBIC INFECTIONS

TETANUS

EPIDEMIOLOGY   Tetanus, while preventable by immunization, has a worldwide distribution. In the U.S., most disease occurs in elderly unimmunized or incompletely immunized pts and follows an acute injury such as a puncture wound, abrasion, or laceration with exposure to soil.

PATHOGENESIS   Under conditions of low oxidation-reduction potential, germination and toxin production follow contamination of a wound with spores of *Clostridium tetani*. The toxin tetanospasmin is transported to the nerve cell body and migrates across the synapse to presynaptic terminals, blocking the release of inhibitory neurotransmitters. Rigidity results from increases in the resting firing rate of the alpha motor neuron with diminished inhibition.

CLINICAL MANIFESTATIONS   The median incubation period after injury is 7 d. The first symptoms are increased tone in the masseter muscles (trismus or lockjaw) followed by dysphagia, stiffness, or pain in the neck, shoulder, and back muscles. Contraction of facial muscles produces risus sardonicus, and contraction of back muscles causes an arched back (opisthotonos). Muscle spasms may be violent, may be provoked by even the slightest stimulation, and may threaten ventilation. Fever may or may not develop; mentation is unimpaired. Autonomic dysfunction commonly complicates severe cases. Complications can include pneumonia, fractures, muscle rupture, deep vein thrombophlebitis, pulmonary emboli, decubitus ulcer, and rhabdomyolysis. Neonatal tetanus develops in children born to unimmunized mothers after unsterile treatment of the umbilical cord stump.

DIAGNOSIS   The diagnosis of tetanus is made clinically. The organism frequently cannot be recovered from wounds of pts with tetanus and may be recovered from wounds of pts without tetanus.

 TREATMENT

Goals of treatment are to eliminate the source of toxin, neutralize unbound toxin, prevent muscle spasms, and provide support (especially respiratory) until after recovery. Pts should be admitted to a quiet room in intensive care. Antibiotic therapy is given to eradicate vegetative cells, the source of toxin. Although of unproven value, the use of penicillin G

(10–12 million units qd IV for 10 d) has been recommended; metronidazole (500 mg q6h or 1 g q12h IV) is preferred by some experts on the basis of the latter drug's excellent antimicrobial activity and a survival rate higher than that obtained with penicillin in one nonrandomized trial. Additional specific antimicrobial therapy should be given for active infection with other organisms. Human tetanus immune globulin (TIG) at a dose of 3000–6000 units IM should be given promptly to neutralize circulating and unbound toxin. Pooled IV immunoglobulin may be an alternative to TIG. Equine tetanus antitoxin can be given at a dose of 10,000 units IM but commonly elicits hypersensitivity and has a shorter half-life than TIG. Diazepam is used to treat muscle spasms; mechanical ventilation and therapeutic paralysis with a nondepolarizing neuromuscular blocking agent may be required for severe spasms or laryngospasm. However, because prolonged paralysis after discontinuation of therapy with such agents has been described, both the need for continued therapeutic paralysis and the occurrence of complications should be assessed daily. Optimal therapy for sympathetic overactivity is not clear; labetalol, esmolol, clonidine, morphine sulfate, parenteral magnesium sulfate, and continuous spinal or epidural anesthesia have been used.

Pts must be actively immunized against tetanus, since natural disease does not induce immunity. The preventive regimen for adults is three doses of tetanus and diphtheria toxoids (Td), with the first and second doses administered IM 4–8 weeks apart and the third dose 6–12 months after the second. A booster dose is required every 10 years. For any wound, Td should be given if (1) the pt's immunization status is unknown, (2) fewer than three doses have been given in the past, or (3) more than 10 years have elapsed since the administration of three doses. For contaminated or severe wounds, a booster is given if more than 5 years have elapsed since immunization. In addition, TIG (250 mg IM) should be administered for all but clean, minor wounds if the pt's immunization status is incomplete or unknown.

BOTULISM

EPIDEMIOLOGY Human botulism occurs worldwide. *Food-borne botulism* is acquired from ingestion of food contaminated with preformed toxin—most commonly, home-canned food. *Wound botulism* develops when wounds, including those contaminated by soil, those of chronic drug abusers, and those related to cesarean delivery, are contaminated with *C. botuli-*

num. Infant botulism occurs when an infant ingests spores and toxin is elaborated in the intestine. Botulism of undetermined classification is produced in older children and adults by a mechanism similar to that described for infant botulism.

CLINICAL MANIFESTATIONS *Food-borne Botulism* The incubation period for botulism is usually 18–36 h after ingestion of food containing toxin. Cranial nerve involvement marks the onset of symptoms, which usually consist of diplopia, dysarthria, and/or dysphagia. Paralysis is symmetric and descending and can lead to respiratory failure and death. Nausea, vomiting, and abdominal pain may precede or follow the onset of paralysis. Dizziness, blurred vision, dry mouth, and dry or sore throat are common. Fever usually is not documented. Ptosis is common; fixed or dilated pupils are noted in 50% of cases. The gag reflex can be suppressed, and deep tendon reflexes can be either normal or decreased. Paralytic ileus, severe constipation, and urinary retention are common.

Wound Botulism The presentation of wound botulism is similar to that of food-borne disease except that the incubation period is longer (about 10 d) and no GI symptoms develop.

DIAGNOSIS The diagnosis of botulism must be suspected on clinical grounds in the context of an appropriate history. Conditions often confused with botulism include myasthenia gravis and Guillain-Barré syndrome. Definitive diagnosis is made by the demonstration of toxin in serum; however, the test may be negative despite infection and cannot be conducted in all laboratories. Other fluids that may yield toxin are vomitus, gastric fluid, and stool. Isolation of the organism from food is not diagnostic.

℞ TREATMENT

Pts should be monitored carefully, particularly for signs of respiratory failure. In food-borne illness, trivalent equine antitoxin (types A, B, and E) should be administered as soon as possible after laboratory specimens are collected. The dose is two vials (either both vials IV or one vial IV and one IM). A repeat dose is probably not necessary but may be given after 2–4 h. Cathartics may be used unless there is ileus. Antibiotics are of unproven value. Wound botulism is treated with exploration and debridement of the wound and the administration of penicillin (to eradicate the organism) and equine antitoxin. Supportive treatment is undertaken for infant botulism.

OTHER CLOSTRIDIAL INFECTIONS

PATHOGENESIS   Despite the isolation of clostridial species from many severe traumatic wounds, the incidence of severe infections due to these organisms is low. Tissue necrosis and a low oxidation-reduction potential appear to be essential to the development of serious disease. Clostridial disease is mediated by toxins.

CLINICAL MANIFESTATIONS *Food poisoning C. perfringens* is the second or third most common cause of food poisoning in the U.S. Primary sources are recooked meats, meat products, and poultry. Symptoms develop 8–24 h after ingestion and include epigastric pain, nausea, and watery diarrhea lasting for 12-24 h. Fever and vomiting are uncommon.

Antibiotic-Associated Colitis   Strains of *C. difficile* that produce toxins detectable in the stool have been identified as the major cause of colitis in pts with antibiotic-associated diarrhea. Any antibiotic (including metronidazole and vancomycin, which are used to treat the infection) can cause this syndrome, which is defined as diarrhea that has no other cause and that develops during antibiotic treatment or within 4 weeks of its discontinuation. Diarrhea is usually watery, voluminous, and without gross blood or mucus. Most pts have abdominal cramps and tenderness, fever, and leukocytosis. Four categories of diarrhea have been based on the appearance of the colon: (1) normal colonic mucosa; (2) mild erythema with some edema; (3) granular, friable, or hemorrhagic mucosa; and (4) pseudomembrane formation.

Suppurative Deep-Tissue Infection   Clostridia are recovered, with or without other organisms, in a variety of conditions with severe local inflammation but usually without systemic signs attributable to toxins. These conditions include intraabdominal sepsis, empyema, pelvic abscess, subcutaneous abscess, frostbite with gas gangrene, infection of stumps in amputees, brain abscess, prostatic abscess, perianal abscess, conjunctivitis, and infection of aortic grafts. At least 50% of cases of emphysematous cholecystitis are caused by clostridial species.

Skin and Soft Tissue Infections   Localized infections Localized clostridial infections of skin and soft tissues tend to be indolent and devoid of systemic signs of toxicity, pain, and edema. Typical examples include cellulitis, perirectal abscesses, and diabetic foot ulcers. Gas may be present in the wound and the immediate surrounding tissues but is not present intramuscularly. A form of suppurative myositis is found in heroin addicts.

Spreading cellulitis and fasciitis This syndrome is abrupt in onset, with rapid spread of suppuration and gas through fascial planes. Myonecrosis is absent, but overwhelming toxemia develops and can be fatal. On examination, crepitance is prominent, but there is little localized pain. This syndrome is most common among pts with carcinoma, especially of the sigmoid and cecum.

Clostridial myonecrosis (gas gangrene) Clostridial myonecrosis occurs in deep necrotic wounds, often following trauma or surgery. The incubation period is short—always <3 d, often <24 h. In contrast to spreading cellulitis, gas gangrene begins with sudden pain in the region of the wound. Local swelling and edema follow, accompanied by a thin hemorrhagic exudate. Toxemia, hypotension, renal failure, and crepitance ensue; the pt often has a heightened awareness of surroundings before death.

Clostridial bacteremia and septicemia Clostridial bacteremia may occur transiently without septicemia. Clostridial septicemia is uncommon but is almost always fatal and follows clostridial infections of the uterus (esp. after septic abortion), colon, or biliary tract. Pts develop sepsis 1–3 d after abortion, with fever, chills, malaise, headache, severe myalgias, abdominal pain, nausea, vomiting, and (occasionally) diarrhea. Oliguria, hypotension, jaundice, and hemoglobinuria secondary to hemolysis develop rapidly. Like those with gas gangrene, pts with clostridial septicemia exhibit increased alertness and apprehension. In cases with bowel or biliary-tree sources, localized infection may not develop. Pts have chills and fever, and 50% have intravascular hemolysis. In pts with malignancy, *C. septicum* causes rapidly fatal septicemia with fever, tachycardia, hypotension, abdominal pain, nausea, and vomiting. Only 20–30% of these pts develop hemolysis; death may occur within 12 h.

DIAGNOSIS The diagnosis of clostridial infection must be based primarily on clinical findings because the mere presence of clostridia in a wound does not necessarily indicate severe disease. The detection of gas by radiography provides a clue, but gas is sometimes documented in mixed anaerobic-aerobic infections as well. Clostridial myonecrosis can be diagnosed by examination of a frozen section of muscle. Pts may have hemolytic anemia, hemoglobinuria, and disseminated intravascular hemolysis. *C. difficile*–associated colitis can be diagnosed by identification of toxin in stool by tissue culture, with appropriate neutralization by antitoxin.

Rx TREATMENT

Until recently, penicillin G (20 million units qd) was the antibiotic of choice for clostridial infections of tissues. Studies in experimental models of infection demonstrated that protein synthesis inhibitors may be preferable to cell wall–active drugs. In these studies clindamycin treatment enhanced survival more than penicillin therapy, and the combination of clindamycin and penicillin was superior to penicillin alone. For severe clostridial sepsis, clindamycin may be used at a dose of 600 mg q6h in combination with high-dose penicillin. A number of other antibiotics can be considered in the case of penicillin allergy, but the sensitivity of the infecting strain to these alternative drugs should be evaluated. Drainage of infected sites or surgery is a mainstay of therapy for clostridial myonecrosis. Amputation may be required for rapidly spreading infection in a limb; repeated debridement is necessary for abdominal wall myonecrosis; and hysterectomy must be performed for uterine myonecrosis. *C. difficile* enterocolitis is treated by discontinuation of the offending antibiotic. Treatment with metronidazole (250 mg qid or 500 mg tid PO) or vancomycin (125 mg qid PO) for 7–10 d shortens the duration of symptoms. The dose of vancomycin may be increased to 500 mg qid PO in severe cases. Strategies such as adding rifampin to vancomycin, tapering doses of vancomycin, switching from metronidazole to vancomycin or vice versa, and administering cholestyramine have all been tried in refractory or relapsing cases.

MIXED ANAEROBIC INFECTIONS

CLINICAL MANIFESTATIONS *Head and Neck* Infections of the head and neck that involve anaerobes include gingivitis, pharyngeal infections (including Ludwig's angina), fascial infections in which oropharyngeal organisms from mucous membranes or sites of dental manipulation spread to potential spaces in the head and neck, sinusitis, and otitis. Complications of these infections include osteomyelitis of the skull or mandible, intracranial infection (such as brain abscess), mediastinitis, or pleuropulmonary infection.

Central Nervous System When sought by optimal bacteriologic methods, anaerobes are found in 85% of brain abscesses. Anaerobic gram-positive cocci predominate; fusobacteria and *Bacteroides* spp. are next most common.

Pleuropulmonary Sites Four clinical syndromes are associated with anaerobic pleuropulmonary infection produced by aspiration: aspiration pneumonia, necrotizing pneumonia, lung abscess, and empyema. Aspiration pneumonia generally develops slowly, with low-grade fever, malaise, and sputum production, in pts with a predisposition for aspirating. Pts with lung abscess typically present with a syndrome of fever, chills, malaise, weight loss, and foul-smelling sputum developing over a period of weeks. Empyema is a manifestation of long-standing anaerobic pulmonary infection and has a clinical presentation similar to that of lung abscess. Pts may also have pleuritic chest pain and chest wall tenderness. Empyema can result from subdiaphragmatic extension.

Intraabdominal Sites (See Chap. 73)

Pelvic Sites Anaerobes are encountered frequently in tuboovarian abscess, septic abortion, pelvic abscess, endometritis, and postoperative wound infection, especially after hysterectomy.

Skin and Soft Tissue Anaerobes are sometimes isolated in cases of crepitant cellulitis, synergistic cellulitis, gangrene, necrotizing fasciitis, cutaneous abscess, rectal abscess, and axillary sweat gland infection. Synergistic (Meleney's) gangrene is a progressive, exquisitely painful skin process, with erythema, swelling, induration, and a central zone of necrosis. Anaerobic cocci and *Staphylococcus aureus* are common pathogens. While necrotizing fasciitis is usually attributed to group A streptococci, it can be caused by anaerobes, including *Peptostreptococcus* and *Bacteroides* spp.

Bones and Joints Anaerobic osteomyelitis usually develops by extension of a soft tissue infection. Septic arthritis often is not polymicrobial and can arise from hematogenous seeding.

Bacteremia *Bacteroides fragilis* is the most common anaerobic isolate from the blood. While the clinical presentation of anaerobic bacteremia may be quite similar to that of sepsis due to aerobic gram-negative bacilli, septic thrombophlebitis and septic shock are uncommon.

DIAGNOSIS When infections develop in proximity to mucosal surfaces normally harboring an anaerobic flora, anaerobes should be considered as potential etiologic agents. Cultures need to be processed for anaerobes, usually in a transport medium. Since laboratory isolation of the pathogen(s) can be time-consuming, diagnosis must sometimes be presumptive.

℞ TREATMENT
Successful therapy for anaerobic infection involves a combination of appropriate antibiotics, surgical resection, and drain-

age. If anaerobic infection is suspected, effective empirical treatment can nearly always be administered, since patterns of antimicrobial susceptibility are usually predictable. Despite an increasing number of reports of penicillin resistance, penicillin remains the drug of choice for empirical therapy of most anaerobic infections of oral origin. Clindamycin appears to be superior for the treatment of lung abscess. As therapy for infections involving *B. fragilis*, metronidazole is the drug of choice, but clindamycin, cefoxitin, imipenem, ampicillin/sulbactam, and ticarcillin/clavulanic acid are all active as well. Anaerobic infections that have failed to respond to treatment should be reassessed, with a consideration of antibiotic resistance, of the need for additional drainage, and of superinfection with aerobic organisms. Since most infections involving anaerobes are bacteriologically mixed and involve aerobic bacteria, therapy must also be directed at those organisms.

For a more detailed discussion, see Abrutyn E: Tetanus, Chap. 146, p. 901; Abrutyn E: Botulism, Chap. 147, p. 904; Kasper DL, Zaleznik DF: Gas Gangrene, Antibiotic-Associated Colitis, and Other Clostridial Infections, Chap. 148, p. 906; and Kasper DL: Infections due to Mixed Anaerobic Organisms, Chap. 169, p. 991, in HPIM-14.

NOCARDIOSIS AND ACTINOMYCOSIS

NOCARDIOSIS

The term *nocardiosis* refers to invasive disease due to *Nocardia* species, aerobic actinomycetes that cause several characteristic syndromes. The two most common syndromes—pneumonia and disseminated infection— may follow inhalation of fragmented nocardial mycelia. Three other syndromes may follow transcutaneous inoculation: cellulitis, a lymphocutaneous syndrome, and actinomycetoma. Finally, nocardial keratitis may result from corneal trauma and nocardial inoculation.

EPIDEMIOLOGY Nocardiae are common inhabitants of soil worldwide. Of the approximately 1000 cases of nocardiosis that occur annually in the U.S., 85% are either pulmonary or systemic. The risk of pulmonary or systemic disease is increased in persons with impaired cell-mediated immunity, especially those who have lymphoma or AIDS or have undergone solid organ or bone marrow transplantation. Nocardiosis is also associated with pulmonary alveolar proteinosis, tuberculosis, and chronic granulomatous disease.

CLINICAL MANIFESTATIONS *Pulmonary Disease* Nocardial pneumonia is typically subacute. Cough is prominent and productive of scant, thick, purulent, nonmalodorous sputum. Fever, anorexia, weight loss, and malaise are common. Nodular pulmonary infiltrates and cavitation are frequently evident on radiographs. In half of all cases of pulmonary nocardiosis, extrapulmonary disease is also evident.

Extrapulmonary Dissemination Disseminated nocardiosis typically manifests as abscesses presenting subacutely. The most common site of dissemination is the CNS, where one or more abscesses—usually supratentorial and often multiloculated—may be found. Other common sites of dissemination include skin and supporting structures, kidneys, bone, and muscle. Around 80% of pts with disseminated nocardiosis have demonstrable concurrent pulmonary involvement.

Disease Following Transcutaneous Inoculation After transcutaneous inoculation, disease may take one of three forms: (1) cellulitis, a subacute illness characterized by painful, firm, warm, nonfluctuant, erythematous lesions; (2) a lymphocutaneous sporotrichoid form; and (3) actinomycetoma, a chronic, deforming, locally invasive entity with minimal systemic manifestations.

Keratitis *Nocardia* spp. are uncommon causes of keratitis. Nocardial keratitis develops subacutely after eye trauma.

DIAGNOSIS The diagnosis of nocardiosis is suggested by the finding of beaded, branching, gram-positive, weakly acid-fast organisms on stains of sputum or pus. Cultural confirmation usually requires selective media and may take 2–4 weeks.

℞ TREATMENT

Sulfonamides are the drugs of choice for the treatment of nocardiosis. For initial management, sulfadiazine or sulfisoxazole (1.5–2 g PO qid) is given. Once disease is controlled, the dose may be decreased to 1 g qid. For refractory cases, the dose should be adjusted to maintain serum sulfonamide levels at 100–150 μg/mL. Trimethoprim-sulfamethoxazole (TMP-SMZ) may also be used (5–10 mg/kg of the TMP component PO bid for initial management, 2.5 mg/kg PO bid once control is achieved). Minocycline (100–200 mg PO bid) is a well-established alternative to the sulfonamides. If parenteral administration is desirable, amikacin (5–7.5 mg/kg IV q12h) can be given, as can TMP-SMZ (in the same dosage used for oral treatment). Combination therapy with two or more agents has often been used; whether combinations are more effective than monotherapy is unknown. Nocardiosis typically requires a protracted course of treatment. The exact duration is somewhat arbitrary and depends both on the condition being treated and on the immune status of the host (Table 88-1). Nocardial abscesses that are large and surgically accessible should be drained.

ACTINOMYCOSIS

Actinomycosis is an indolent bacterial infection caused by any of several gram-positive, non-spore-forming anaerobic or microaerophilic rods, most but not all of which are in the genus *Actinomyces*. Characteristic features of actinomycosis include the violation of normal tissue plane barriers by the spreading infection, the formation of draining sinus tracts, and the presence of actinomycotic "sulfur granules" (yellow aggregates of organisms) in drainage or pus. In certain circumstances, actinomycosis may be easily mistaken for malignancy.

EPIDEMIOLOGY AND PATHOGENESIS The agents of actinomycosis are members of the normal oral flora and may also be found in the bronchi, GI tract, and female genital tract. A critical step in the development of actinomycosis is disruption of the mucosal barrier, which allows actinomycetes to invade

Table 88-1

Recommended Durations of Therapy for Various Nocardial Syndromes

Syndrome	Duration of Treatment*
IMMUNOCOMPETENT HOSTS	
CNS nocardiosis	12 months
Pulmonary or systemic nocardiosis sparing the CNS	6–12 months
Cellulitis or lymphocutaneous syndrome	
Without bony involvement	2 months
With bony involvement	4 months
Actinomycetoma	6–12 months after apparent clinical cure
Keratitis†	2–4 months after apparent clinical cure
IMMUNOSUPPRESSED HOSTS‡	
CNS nocardiosis	At least 12 months
Pulmonary or systemic nocardiosis sparing the CNS	12 months

*The durations listed are guidelines only. If nocardial disease is unusually extensive or if the response to therapy is slow, the recommended durations should be exceeded. Nocardiosis is particularly tenacious and likely to relapse in pts with chronic granulomatous disease.

†Keratitis should be treated with both oral and topical sulfonamides until clinical cure is achieved and then with oral sulfonamides alone for an additional 2–4 months.

‡If necessary, immunosuppressive therapy may be continued for the treatment of underlying disease or the prevention of allograft rejection. Certain AIDS pts with nocardiosis have required the indefinite continuation of an antinocardial regimen.

beyond their endogenous habitat. Local infection, subsequent extension, and (in rare cases) hematogenous seeding may ensue. Actinomycosis is associated with poor dental hygiene, with the use of intrauterine contraceptive devices, and with HIV infection.

CLINICAL MANIFESTATIONS Actinomycosis occurs most frequently at an oral, cervical, or facial site and should be considered in the differential diagnosis of any mass lesion or relapsing infection of the head and neck. "Woody" induration is a common finding. Other common presentations include thoracic, abdominal, pelvic, and musculoskeletal disease. CNS infection and disseminated disease are both rare.

DIAGNOSIS The finding of macro- or microscopic actinomycotic sulfur granules in drainage or purulent material is highly suggestive of actinomycosis. The isolation of an actinomycete from granules or from a normally sterile site confirms the diagnosis but takes from 5 days to 4 weeks.

℞ TREATMENT

Like nocardiosis, actinomycosis typically requires protracted treatment. For extensive or serious infection, a reasonable regimen is IV penicillin G (3–4 million units q4h) for 2–6 weeks followed by oral penicillin or amoxicillin for 6–12 months. For limited disease, less intensive therapy may suffice. Extending treatment beyond the resolution of demonstrable disease minimizes the likelihood of relapse. Tetracycline, erythromycin, minocycline, and clindamycin are alternative agents for the penicillin-allergic pt. Adjunctive surgical treatment is warranted for pts critically ill with actinomycosis and for those infected at a critical site (e.g., the CNS). The role of surgery in other circumstances is uncertain.

For a more detailed discussion, see Filice GA: Nocardiosis, Chap. 167, p. 987; and Russo TA: Actinomycosis, Chap. 168, p. 989, in HPIM-14.

89

TUBERCULOSIS AND OTHER MYCOBACTERIAL INFECTIONS

Mycobacteria are distinguished by their surface lipids, which cause them to be acid-fast in the laboratory. They may be divided into several groups: the *M. tuberculosis* complex (*M. tuberculosis, M. bovis,* and *M. africanum*), members of which cause tuberculosis (TB); *M. leprae,* which causes leprosy; and the nontuberculous mycobacteria (*M. avium* and others), a heterogeneous group that causes disseminated disease in immunocompromised hosts and a variety of local infectious syndromes in both immunocompromised and immunocompetent individuals. The vast majority of TB cases are caused by *M. tuberculosis.*

TUBERCULOSIS

EPIDEMIOLOGY In the U.S. in 1995, a total of 22,813 cases of TB were reported. This figure represents an increase of 2.8% over the lowest-ever number of cases reported (22,201 in 1985). Factors implicated in the increasing rates of TB in the U.S. include the AIDS epidemic, immigration from high-prevalence areas of the world, and social problems such as poverty, homelessness, and drug abuse. Accordingly, in this country, TB tends to be a disease of the elderly, of young adults with HIV infection, of immigrants, and of the economically disadvantaged. In certain developing areas of the world, the HIV epidemic is responsible for the doubling or even tripling of the numbers of TB cases reported over the past decade; if the worldwide TB control situation remains as it is, some 90 million new cases and 30 million deaths will occur in the 1990s. *M. tuberculosis* is transmitted from person to person via the respiratory route. The infectivity of a given case correlates with the concentration of organisms in expectorated sputum, the extent of pulmonary disease, and the frequency of cough.

PATHOGENESIS After entry into the lungs in aerosolized droplets, tubercle bacilli are ingested by macrophages and transported to regional lymph nodes. From there, they disseminate widely. Whether in the lung, lymph nodes, or sites of dissemination, lesions are contained by a delayed-type hypersensitivity response (DTH; the *tissue-damaging response*) and by the cell-mediated *macrophage-activating response.* The development of host immunity and DTH to *M. tuberculosis* is evidenced by acquisition of skin-test reactivity to tuberculin purified protein derivative (PPD). The PPD skin test is the only test that reliably detects *M. tuberculosis* infection in asymptomatic persons. With the development of specific immunity and the accumulation of large numbers of activated macrophages at the sites of infection, granulomatous lesions (tubercles) form. The organisms survive within macrophages or necrotic material but do not spread further; reactivation (postprimary disease) may occur at a later time. In some cases, the immune response is inadequate to contain the infection, and symptomatic, progressive primary disease develops.

CLINICAL MANIFESTATIONS   TB is usually classified as pulmonary or extrapulmonary. In the absence of HIV infection, more than 80% of cases involve the lungs only. In the presence of HIV, up to two-thirds of pts with TB have either extrapulmonary disease alone or both pulmonary and extrapulmonary disease.

Pulmonary TB   Pulmonary tuberculous disease may be categorized as primary or postprimary.

- *Primary disease* is often seen in children and is frequently localized to the middle and lower lung zones. In the majority of cases, the lesion heals spontaneously; the Ghon lesion is the small calcific nodular remnant. In children with impaired immunity (e.g., malnutrition, AIDS), primary disease may progress rapidly and may evolve in different ways (pleural effusion, acute cavitation, bronchial compression by enlarging lymph nodes, miliary TB, or tuberculous meningitis).
- *Postprimary disease* results from endogenous reactivation of latent infection and is usually localized to the apical and posterior segments of the upper lobes; in addition, the superior segments of the lower lobes are frequently involved. The extent of parenchymal involvement varies greatly, from the development of small infiltrates to extensive cavitary disease. Massive involvement and coalescence of lesions may produce tuberculous pneumonia; up to one-third of untreated pts succumb within a few weeks or months, others experience spontaneous remission, and still others have disease that follows a chronic, progressively debilitating course ("consumption"). Early signs and symptoms are often nonspecific and insidious (fever, night sweats, malaise, weight loss). Cough and blood-streaked sputum eventually develop in the majority of cases. Massive hemoptysis may occur. Physical findings are of limited diagnostic utility. The classic tuberculous amphoric breath sounds may be heard over areas with large cavities.

Extrapulmonary TB   The extrapulmonary sites most commonly involved are the lymph nodes, pleura, genitourinary (GU) tract, bones and joints, meninges, and peritoneum. Virtually any organ system may be affected.

- *Pleural involvement* is common during primary TB and results from DTH to bacilli in the pleural space; these organisms are typically few in number. Fever, pleuritic chest pain, and dyspnea may be present. The pleural fluid is straw-colored, with a protein content that is >50% of the serum value, a normal or low glucose level, a pH of <7.2, and detectable WBCs (usually 500–2500/μL). This form of pleural TB responds well to chemotherapy and may resolve spontaneously. Tuberculous empyema is less common, results from rupture of a tuberculous cavity into the pleura, and may lead to severe pleural fibrosis and restrictive lung disease.
- *Tuberculous lymphadenitis* occurs in more than 25% of cases of extrapulmonary TB and is particularly common among HIV-infected pts. Involved nodes are swollen, discrete, and painless. Fistulous drainage of caseous debris may occur. Systemic symptoms usually develop only in HIV-infected pts. Concomitant pulmonary disease may or may not exist.
- *Genitourinary TB* accounts for 15% of extrapulmonary cases, may involve any part of the GU tract, and is usually due to hematogenous seeding following primary infection. Local symptoms predominate. In women, genital TB (fallopian tubes, endometrium) may cause infertility or menstrual irregularities. Men may develop epididymitis, orchitis, or prostatitis. These infections at GU sites respond well to chemotherapy.
- *Skeletal TB,* formerly responsible for 8–9% of extrapulmonary cases, is now infrequent. Weight-bearing joints (spine, hips, knees) are affected most often. Spinal TB (Pott's disease) often involves adjacent vertebral bodies and destroys the intervertebral disk. Spinal cord compression by a tuberculous abscess or lesion is a medical emergency. In advanced Pott's disease, vertebral collapse may lead to kyphosis. Skeletal TB responds to chemotherapy, although severe cases may require surgery.
- *Gastrointestinal TB* may affect any portion of the GI tract. The terminal ileum and cecum are the sites most commonly involved. Cases with intestinal-wall ulcerations and fistulae may simulate Crohn's disease. Surgical intervention is required in most cases. *Tuberculous peritonitis* presents as fever, abdominal pain, and ascites; ascitic fluid is exudative, with an elevated protein level and—in most cases—lymphocytic pleocytosis.
- *Central nervous system TB* accounts for 5% of extrapulmo-

nary cases and occurs most often in young children and in HIV-infected pts. Tuberculous meningitis results either from hematogenous spread or from rupture of a subependymal tubercle into the subarachnoid space. The disease may present acutely or subacutely. Cranial nerve palsies (particularly of ocular nerves) and hydrocephalus are common. CSF examination reveals lymphocytic pleocytosis (with PMNs sometimes predominating early on), an elevated protein level (100–800 mg/dL), and hypoglycorrhachia. Repeated CSF examinations increase the diagnostic yield; CSF culture is positive in up to 80% of cases. While the disease responds to chemotherapy, neurologic sequelae are common. Glucocorticoids are a useful therapeutic adjunct.

- *Miliary TB* is due to hematogenous spread and may represent either newly acquired infection or reactivation of latent disease. Clinical manifestations are nonspecific and protean. Fever, night sweats, anorexia, weakness, and weight loss characterize the majority of cases. Hepatomegaly, splenomegaly, lymphadenopathy, and choroidal (ocular) tubercles may occur. A high index of suspicion is required for the diagnosis; PPD results may be negative in up to 50% of untreated cases.

HIV-Associated TB   TB is an important opportunistic infection among HIV-infected persons worldwide. As of mid-1996, some 8.5 million persons in developing countries were coinfected with HIV and tubercle bacilli. In certain areas, such as New York City, some 50% of pts with TB also carry HIV. The manifestations of TB in HIV carriers vary with the stage of the HIV infection. When cell-mediated immunity is only partly compromised, pulmonary TB presents as typical upper-lobe cavitary disease. In late HIV infection, a primary TB-like pattern may be evident, with diffuse interstitial or miliary infiltrates, little or no cavitation, and intrathoracic lymphadenopathy. Extrapulmonary TB occurs frequently in HIV-infected pts (at a rate of 40–60% in some series). Common syndromes include lymph nodal, disseminated, pleural, and pericardial TB as well as mycobacteremia and tuberculous meningitis. The diagnosis may be rendered difficult by atypical radiographic and histologic manifestations and PPD anergy.

DIAGNOSIS   Initial suspicion of pulmonary TB is often based on abnormal CXR findings in a symptomatic pt. The classic picture is that of upper lobe infiltrates and cavitary disease; however, virtually any pattern may be seen. A diagnosis of active infection is established by the demonstration of acid-fast organisms in sputum, bodily fluids, or tissues. The fluorescent auramine-rhodamine stain is used by most modern laboratories. Traditional acid-fast stains are also useful but are more time-consuming. Primary isolation in culture may require 4–8 weeks. Radiometric growth detection and nucleic acid probe identification make it possible to isolate the infecting organism and identify it to the species level within 2–3 weeks. Sputum induction or bronchoalveolar lavage increases the diagnostic yield over that obtained with expectorated sputum alone; similarly, sampling of bodily fluids (pleural, pericardial, peritoneal, cerebrospinal) or tissue biopsy (of pleura, pericardium, peritoneum, liver, or bone marrow) is appropriate for suspected extrapulmonary or disseminated disease. Blood from HIV-infected pts with suspected TB should be cultured for the organism. In the future, PCR-based diagnostic methods may become standard. The PPD skin test is useful in screening for prior mycobacterial infection. The Mantoux method is most reliable and should be read at 48–72 h as the transverse diameter of induration (*not* erythema) in millimeters. Recommendations for isoniazid (INH) prophylaxis, based on the PPD result, are given in Table 89-1.

℞ TREATMENT

Recommendations for treatment are summarized in Tables 89-2 and 89-3. Symptoms are alleviated in most cases within 2–3 weeks, but sputum conversion may take 3 months. Drug resistance is a serious problem and may be either primary (i.e., infection caused by a strain that is resistant before the start of treatment) or acquired (i.e., resistance arising during treatment because the regimen is inadequate or the pt is noncompliant). Strains resistant to both INH and rifampin (so-called multidrug-resistant, or MDR, strains) are being seen with increasing frequency in the U.S., especially in New York City. Immigrants with TB acquired in certain developing areas (e.g., Haiti, Southeast Asia, and many parts of Latin America) commonly have MDR disease. A high index of suspicion, prescription of adequate chemotherapeutic regimens, education of pts, direct observation of therapy, and close and careful follow-up of pts are all crucial in maximizing cure rates and minimizing the spread of MDR strains.

LEPROSY

ETIOLOGY Leprosy (Hansen's disease), which is caused by *M. leprae,* is a chronic granulomatous infection that attacks skin and peripheral nerves.

EPIDEMIOLOGY There are currently about 1.8 million pts with leprosy worldwide. The disease most often affects the rural poor; cases in India, Brazil, Bangladesh, Indonesia, and

Table 89-1

Recommendations for Isoniazid Prophylaxis

Risk Group	Tuberculin Reaction, mm	Duration of Treatment, Months
HIV-infected persons	≥5*	12
Close contacts of tuberculosis pts	≥5†	6 (9 for children)
Persons with fibrotic lesions on CXR	≥5	12
Recently infected persons	≥10	6
Persons with high-risk medical conditions‡	≥10	6–12
High-risk group, <35 years of age§	≥10	6
Low-risk group, <35 years of age	≥15	6

*Anergic HIV-infected persons with an estimated risk of *M. tuberculosis* infection of 10% may also be considered candidates.

†Tuberculin-negative contacts, especially children, should receive prophylaxis for 2 or 3 months after contact ends and should then be retested with PPD. Those whose results remain negative should discontinue prophylaxis.

‡Includes diabetes mellitus, prolonged therapy with systemic glucocorticoids, other immunosuppressive therapy, some hematologic and reticuloendothelial diseases, injection drug use (with HIV seronegativity), end-stage renal disease, and clinical situations associated with rapid weight loss.

§Includes persons born in high-prevalence countries, members of medically underserved low-income populations, and residents of long-term-care facilities.

NOTE: INH prophylaxis is administered at a dose of 5 mg/kg qd (maximum, 300 mg) or 15 mg/kg twice weekly (maximum, 900 mg). The principal contraindication is active liver disease.

SOURCE: Raviglione MC, O'Brien RJ: HPIM-14, p. 1013; based on recommendations of the American Thoracic Society and the Centers for Disease Control and Prevention, 1994.

Myanmar represent about three-quarters of the total. About 150 new infections are diagnosed in the U.S. each year. Leprosy can present at any age but is most common in childhood. Person-to-person transmission is believed to be responsible for most cases. The incubation period is usually 3–5 years.

CLINICAL MANIFESTATIONS The wide spectrum of clinical and histologic manifestations of leprosy is attributable

Table 89-2

Recommended Drugs and Dosages for the Initial Treatment of Tuberculosis in Adults*

Drug	Dosage	
	Daily	Thrice Weekly†
Isoniazid	5 mg/kg, max. 300 mg	15 mg/kg, max. 900 mg
Rifampin	10 mg/kg, max. 600 mg	10 mg/kg, max. 600 mg
Pyrazinamide	15–30 mg/kg, max. 2 g	50–70 mg/kg, max. 3 g
Ethambutol	15–25 mg/kg	25–30 mg/kg
Streptomycin	15 mg/kg, max. 1 g	25–30 mg/kg, max. 1.5 g

*Dosages for children are similar, except that some authorities recommend higher doses of isoniazid (10–20 mg/kg daily; 20–40 mg/kg intermittent) and rifampin (10–20 mg/kg).

†Dosages for twice-weekly administration are the same except for pyrazinamide (maximum, 4 g/d) and ethambutol (50 mg/kg).

SOURCE: Raviglione MC, O'Brien RJ: HPIM-14, p. 1010; based on recommendations of the American Thoracic Society and the Centers for Disease Control and Prevention, 1994.

to the variability of the immune response to *M. leprae*. The two "poles" of clinical disease are tuberculoid leprosy and lepromatous leprosy.

Early or Indeterminate Leprosy   The pt may notice only an anesthetic or paresthetic patch on the skin. The lesions are subtle. One or more hypo- or hyperpigmented macules or plaques may be seen. Sensation is often relatively preserved in early lesions.

Tuberculoid Leprosy   The hallmark of this disease is one or a few hypopigmented, sharply demarcated macular lesions that enlarge by peripheral spread, are densely anesthetic, and have lost sweat glands and hair follicles. Nerves become involved early and may be palpable. Neuritic pain may be prominent. On histologic section, bacilli are frequently absent or difficult to detect.

Lepromatous Leprosy   Cutaneous involvement is extensive and symmetric across the midline. Individual lesions are highly variable and may include macules, nodules, plaques, or

Table 89-3

Recommended Regimens for the Treatment of Tuberculosis

Indication	Initial Phase		Continuation Phase	
	Duration, Months	Drugs	Duration, Months	Drugs
New smear- or culture-positive case	2	HRZE*	4	HR*
New culture-negative case	2	HRZE*	2	HR*
Intolerance to H	2	RZE	7	RE
Intolerance to R	2	HES (±Z)	16	HE
Intolerance to Z	2	HRE	7	HR
Pregnancy	2	HRE	7	HR
Failure and relapse†	—	—	—	—
Standard retreatment (susceptibility testing unavailable)	3	HRZES‡	5	HRE

Resistance to H + R	Throughout (12–18)	ZE + O + S (or another injectable agent§)	—	—
Resistance to all first-line drugs	Throughout (24)	1 injectable agent§ + 3 of these 4: ethionamide, cycloserine, PAS, O	—	—

*All drugs can be given daily or intermittently (three times weekly throughout or twice weekly after the initial phase of daily therapy).

†Regimen is tailored according to the results of drug susceptibility tests.

‡Streptomycin treatment should be discontinued after 2 months.

§Amikacin, kanamycin, or capreomycin. Treatment with all of these agents should be discontinued after 2–6 months, depending upon the pt's tolerance and response.

NOTE: Pyridoxine (10–25 mg/d) should be added to the regimen given to persons at high risk for vitamin deficiency. H, isoniazid; R, rifampin; Z, pyrazinamide; E, ethambutol; S, streptomycin; O, ofloxacin; PAS, para–aminosalicylic acids.

SOURCE: Raviglione MC, O'Brien RJ: HPIM-14, p. 1011.

papules, all with ill-defined borders. There is diffuse infiltration of the dermis between discrete lesions, and apparently normal skin usually contains demonstrable bacilli. Sites of predilection include the face, ears, wrists, elbows, buttocks, and knees. Nasal stuffiness, epistaxis, and obstructed breathing are common early symptoms. Involvement of major nerve trunks is less common than in the tuberculoid form, but diffuse hypesthesia is common in advanced disease.

Borderline Leprosy   The borderline portion of the leprosy spectrum lies between the tuberculoid and lepromatous poles and is usually subdivided into borderline tuberculoid, borderline (or dimorphous), and borderline lepromatous types. Classification is less precise within the borderline region of the spectrum than at the poles. Skin lesions tend to increase in number and heterogeneity but decrease in size as the lepromatous pole is approached. Involvement of multiple peripheral nerve trunks is more common in borderline tuberculoid than in polar tuberculoid disease. The histopathology of the granulomas in borderline leprosy changes from an epithelioid cell predominance in borderline tuberculoid disease to a macrophage predominance as the lepromatous pole is approached. Bacilli are found in large numbers in the skin granulomas of pts with borderline, borderline lepromatous, and polar lepromatous disease (multibacillary leprosy), while few bacilli are found in the skin granulomas of pts with polar tuberculoid, borderline tuberculoid, and indeterminate disease (paucibacillary leprosy). In contrast to the polar states, the borderline states are unstable.

DIAGNOSIS   The diagnosis is suggested by the demonstration of acid-fast bacilli in skin smears made by the scraped-incision method and is confirmed by skin biopsy, which should be interpreted by a pathologist with experience in leprosy.

℞ TREATMENT

In addition to drug administration, the treatment of leprosy entails a broad multidisciplinary approach, including orthopedics, ophthalmology, and physical therapy. The drugs used in leprosy include dapsone, rifampin, and clofazimine. Second-line and novel agents are also available for problematic cases. Because resistance can emerge during dapsone monotherapy, multidrug regimens are currently favored. Therapy for multibacillary disease should consist of all three drugs: dapsone, 50–100 mg/d PO; rifampin, 600 mg/d PO; and clofazimine, 50–200 mg/d PO. Clofazimine should not be given in pregnancy. If the organism is known to be dapsone-sensitive, dapsone plus rifampin may be given for borderline or borderline lepromatous cases. For lepromatous cases, a third drug should be added. The optimal duration of therapy is unknown, but a minimum of 2 years is recommended by WHO. For paucibacillary disease, two drugs (usually dapsone plus rifampin) are adequate. WHO recommends a 6-month course.

OTHER MYCOBACTERIAL INFECTIONS

Mycobacteria other than members of the *M. tuberculosis* complex and *M. leprae* are termed *atypical mycobacteria, mycobacteria other than tuberculosis* (MOTT), or *nontuberculous mycobacteria* (NTM). In contrast to *M. tuberculosis,* NTM are ubiquitous in the environment.

Disseminated NTM Infections in AIDS and Other Immunodeficiencies

ETIOLOGY   The *M. avium* complex (MAC, consisting of *M. avium* and *M. intracellulare*) is a microbiologic designation retained in clinical practice but rendered obsolete by modern molecular diagnostic methods. The majority of mycobacterial infections in immunocompromised hosts in the U.S., including essentially all those formerly attributed to MAC, are caused by *M. avium. M. genavense* is an occasional cause of similar infections.

EPIDEMIOLOGY AND HOST FACTORS   Infection is probably acquired by the oral route. There is no evidence for nosocomial person-to-person spread. Disseminated infections with NTM almost exclusively affect severely immunosuppressed pts, usually those with AIDS. Rare cases occur in transplant recipients and in pts with leukemia (especially hairy cell leukemia), lymphoma, or certain congenital immunodeficiencies. In pts with AIDS, NTM infection is a late event: AIDS pts whose CD4 cell counts have been <10/μL for 1 year have a 40% probability of having a blood culture positive for NTM.

CLINICAL MANIFESTATIONS   No distinctive diagnostic features exist. Disseminated NTM infection should be suspected on the basis of prolonged fever and weight loss. Abdominal lymphadenopathy and/or hepatosplenomegaly may be evident either clinically or radiographically; diarrhea and abdominal pain may also be present. Anemia and leukopenia are frequent concomitants and may or may not be etiologically related to NTM. Suspicion of the diagnosis should prompt the performance of blood cultures.

DIAGNOSIS   Blood cultures on special media are the cornerstone for the diagnosis of NTM infection. Two or three such cultures are usually sufficient. With the liquid Bactec system, positive results may be obtained within 7–14 d; the detection of *M. genavense* may require much longer. Acid-fast stains of liver or bone marrow biopsy material may permit a more rapid presumptive diagnosis. The yield of liver biopsy approaches 50% in pts with unequivocally abnormal LFTs but is much lower in pts with negative blood cultures and normal or nearly normal LFTs.

℞ TREATMENT

The agents most active against MAC are the macrolides clarithromycin and azithromycin. Monotherapy may lead to resistance and should therefore be avoided. For the initial period of treatment, a three-drug regimen is used: (1) clarithromycin (500 mg bid) or azithromycin (500 mg/d); (2) ethambutol (15–25 mg/kg qd); and (3) rifabutin (300 mg/d), clofazimine (100 mg/d), rifampin (600 mg/d), or ciprofloxacin (500 mg bid). After 3 months, therapy can be cut back to a two-drug regimen (usually clarithromycin plus ethambutol). Many experts recommend lifelong therapy. Data on the potential roles of adjunctive cytokine administration and liposomal drug encapsulation are accumulating. Anti-MAC prophylaxis should be considered for AIDS pts with a CD4 cell count of <100/μL. Rifabutin (300 mg/d), clarithromycin (500 mg qd or bid), or azithromycin (1200 mg weekly) is a reasonable choice.

Localized Infections due to NTM

PULMONARY DISEASE   Preexisting lung disease (e.g., chronic obstructive pulmonary disease, cancer, previous TB, bronchiectasis, cystic fibrosis, or silicosis) is the main predisposing factor for NTM pulmonary disease. The organisms most frequently involved are *M. intracellulare, M. avium,* and *M. kansasii.* Accurate identification to the species level is important; both clinical significance and therapeutic strategies differ with the organism. *M. avium* rarely causes significant pulmonary disease in pts with AIDS. Its isolation from sputum in the absence of radiographic changes is usually without significance. On the other hand, the isolation of *M. kansasii,* which causes a pulmonary TB-like illness, is clinically significant. Most pts with NTM lung infection present with chronic cough, low-grade fever, and malaise. Hemoptysis may develop. Minimal diagnostic criteria include a pulmonary infiltrate of indeterminate cause and the repeated isolation from sputum of multiple colonies of the same strain of NTM.

R̽ **TREATMENT**

Pts with minimal disease do not need treatment. Likewise, solitary nodular NTM disease identified upon surgical resection requires no further treatment. Most other pts with pulmonary NTM disease are treated with antimicrobial agents; they may require surgery as well. The regimens used in therapy for disseminated MAC infection are preferred for the treatment of localized infection with *M. avium* or *M. intracellulare* as well. Infection with *M. kansasii* is treated with INH (300 mg/d), rifampin (600 mg/d), and ethambutol (15–25 mg/kg daily). Most pts are treated for 18–24 months.

LYMPHADENITIS   This disease occurs most often in children 1–5 years old and is characterized by painless swelling of one or a group of nodes, with fistulas to the skin. The anterior cervical chain is often affected. *M. scrofulaceum* and MAC organisms are the most common agents. Once TB has been excluded, the treatment of choice is surgical excision.

SKIN DISEASES   *Swimming-Pool and Fish-Tank Granuloma*   The causative organism is almost always *M. marinum,* and the usual incubation period is 2–3 weeks. After contact with a contaminated tropical fish tank, swimming pool, or saltwater fish, a small violet nodule or pustule appears at a site of minor trauma. The lesion may evolve into a crusted ulcer or small abscess. Dissemination may occur. In cases of persistence or dissemination, rifampin (300–600 mg/d) in combination with ethambutol (15–25 mg/kg qd), TMP-SMZ (160/800 mg bid), or minocycline (100 mg/d) may be tried for at least 3 months.

Buruli Ulcer   This entity occurs in the tropics and is due to *M. ulcerans.* Disease begins as a pruritic nodule, which then ulcerates; the course is prolonged. Excision constitutes the usual therapy.

INFECTIONS LINKED TO INJECTIONS AND SURGERY   Occasionally, mycobacteria are isolated from nodular skin lesions of hospitalized pts, particularly those who are immunosuppressed. Many cases are linked to injections (e.g., in diabetic pts) or follow surgery (e.g., in ophthalmologic or cardiac pts). These infections are usually due to the rapidly growing and notoriously resistant *M. fortuitum* complex (*M. fortuitum, M. chelonae,* or *M. abscessus*). Debridement is best combined with the administration of two or three antimicrobial agents (selected from amikacin, ciprofloxacin, sulfonamides, clofazimine, and clarithromycin).

For a more detailed discussion, see Raviglione MC, O'Brien RJ: Tuberculosis, Chap. 171, p. 1004; Miller RA: Leprosy (Hansen's Disease), Chap. 172, p. 1014; Hirschel B: Infections due to Nontuberculous Mycobacteria, Chap. 173, p. 1019; and Friedland GH, Selwyn PA: Infections (Excluding AIDS) in Injection Drug Users, Chap. 134, p. 831, in HPIM-14.

90

LYME DISEASE AND OTHER SPIROCHETAL INFECTIONS

LYME BORRELIOSIS

ETIOLOGY *Borrelia burgdorferi,* a fastidious spirochete, is the causative agent of Lyme disease. Three groups of *B. burgdorferi* organisms exist and are generally responsible for causing diseases with different manifestations in different parts of the world.

EPIDEMIOLOGY Lyme disease is a tick-transmitted illness; the distribution parallels the geographic range of certain ixodid ticks. The major areas of disease include the northeastern U.S. and Wisconsin and Minnesota in the Midwest. The principal vector in these regions is *Ixodes dammini;* >20% of these ticks are infected with *B. burgdorferi* in these areas. Lyme disease also occurs in the western U.S., Europe, Asia, and Australia. The ticks have different animal hosts; the host of the immature *I. dammini* is the white-footed mouse, while that of the mature tick is the white-tailed deer. The incidence of disease peaks during the summer. More than 50,000 cases have been reported to the CDC during the past 10 years.

CLINICAL MANIFESTATIONS *Early Infection: Stage 1 (Localized Infection)* The principal site of stage 1 infection is the skin. After a 3- to 32-d incubation period, erythema migrans (EM) appears in around 75% of cases. Usually beginning as a red macule or papule at the site of the tick bite, EM expands to form a large annular lesion, often with a bright-red outer border and partial central clearing. Ixodid ticks are so small that most pts do not notice the initial tick bite. The lesion is warm but not usually painful. About 25% of pts do not have EM.

Early Infection: Stage 2 (Disseminated Infection) Within days of the onset of EM, *B. burgdorferi* can spread hematogenously to many sites. Secondary annular skin lesions are similar in appearance to the primary lesion and are frequently accompanied by severe headache, mild neck stiffness, fever, chills, migratory musculoskeletal pain, arthralgias, and profound malaise and fatigue. These early symptoms usually resolve in several weeks, even without treatment. After several weeks or months, about 15% of pts develop neurologic abnormalities, including meningitis, subtle encephalitis, cranial neuritis (including facial palsy), motor or sensory radiculoneuropathy, mononeuritis multiplex, chorea, and/or myelitis. The CSF shows lymphocytic pleocytosis (about 100 cells/mL), often with an elevated protein level and a normal or slightly low glucose level. Early neurologic abnormalities resolve completely in months, but chronic neurologic disease may occur later. Cardiac abnormalities develop in about 8% of pts within several weeks of onset of illness. The most common finding is fluctuating degrees of atrioventricular block. Some pts have myopericarditis. Like early neurologic findings, cardiac involvement usually resolves but may recur. Musculoskeletal pain is common during stage 2, with migratory pain in joints, tendons, bursae, muscles, or bones without joint swelling.

Late Infection: Stage 3 (Persistent Infection) Months after the initial infection, about 60% of untreated pts in the U.S. develop arthritis, typically intermittent attacks of oligoarticular arthritis in large joints (especially the knees) lasting for weeks or months. Most pts have fewer recurrent attacks each year, but a few develop chronic arthritis of one or both knees, with erosion of cartilage and bone. Less commonly, chronic neurologic or skin involvement may develop months or years after initial infection.

DIAGNOSIS Lyme disease is diagnosed by the recognition of a characteristic clinical picture with serologic confirmation. Several weeks after infection, most pts develop an antibody response to *B. burgdorferi* that is detectable by ELISA. Western blotting in cases with equivocal or positive results is recommended to identify false-positive ELISAs. The persistence of serologic positivity in pts who have had Lyme disease is common and may cause confusion if another illness with similar manifestations develops. About 20–30% of acute-phase serum samples are positive. IgM- and IgG-specific assays are recommended in the first month of illness; thereafter, only IgG assays are of value. PCR is being evaluated as a diagnostic tool.

℞ TREATMENT
See Fig. 90-1.

YAWS

CLINICAL MANIFESTATIONS Yaws is a chronic infectious disease of childhood caused by *Treponema pallidum* ssp. *pertenue*. The disease is characterized by one or more initial skin lesions (often a papule on the leg) followed by relapsing, nondestructive secondary lesions of skin and bone. In the late stages, destructive lesions of skin, bone, and joints develop.

DIAGNOSIS Serologic tests are required for diagnosis, since clinical features have become less distinctive with the decreasing prevalence of disease.

℞ TREATMENT
Therapy with IM benzathine penicillin G (2.4 million units for adults and 1.2 million units for children) leads to rapid resolution of lesions and prevents recurrence. Tetracycline (500 mg qid PO for 14 d) may be used in penicillin-allergic pts. Contacts of infected pts should be treated with antibiotics in areas where <5% of the population has active disease.

PINTA

CLINICAL MANIFESTATIONS Pinta, an infectious disease of the skin, is caused by *Treponema carateum*. The initial lesion is a small papule, located most often on the extremities, face, neck, or buttocks, that increases in size by peripheral extension and is accompanied by regional lymphadenopathy. Secondary lesions without adenopathy appear 1 month to 1 year after the initial lesion. The lesions become pigmented upon exposure to the sun.

DIAGNOSIS Seroconversion takes about four times longer in pinta than in venereal syphilis.

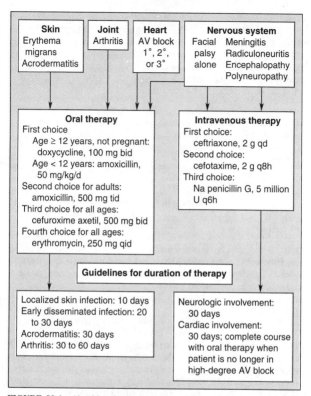

FIGURE 90-1 Algorithm for the treatment of the various acute or chronic manifestations of Lyme borreliosis. Relapse may occur with any of these regimens, and a second course of treatment may be necessary. AV, atrioventricular. (From Steere AC: HPIM-14,.p. 1044.)

℞ TREATMENT

The treatment for pinta is the same as that for yaws.

LEPTOSPIROSIS

EPIDEMIOLOGY Leptospirosis is thought to be the most widespread zoonosis in the world, affecting at least 160 mammalian species. Infection in humans occurs mainly in hot weather; it is acquired through incidental contact with contaminated water (two-thirds of cases) or through contact with urine or tissues of infected animals. Leptospires enter through abraded skin or mucous membranes. Certain occupational groups are at especially high risk; included are veterinarians, agricultural workers, and sewage workers. Recreational waters are also a source of exposure to leptospires.

PATHOGENESIS   Like other spirochetal diseases, leptospirosis begins with spirochetemia, which develops soon after the entry of organisms and disseminates widely. Cellular and humoral immune responses abort spirochetemia, but organisms persist in immunologically protected sites such as the kidney.

CLINICAL MANIFESTATIONS   The incubation period averages 10 d. Leptospirosis typically is a biphasic illness in which an acute leptospiremic phase is followed by an "immune" leptospiruric phase. The initial phase of leptospiremia is characterized by an abrupt onset of headache (usually frontal), severe muscle aches (most prominent in the thighs and the lumbar area), cutaneous hyperesthesia, chills, and a rapidly rising temperature (>38.9°C). Symptoms usually last for 4–9 d. Anorexia, nausea, and vomiting occur in more than 50% of cases. Physical findings include relative bradycardia, normal blood pressure, and conjunctival suffusion, which appears on the third or fourth day of illness. Less common findings include pharyngeal injection, cutaneous hemorrhages, and skin rashes. The "immune" phase follows an asymptomatic period of 1–3 d and coincides with the appearance of IgM antibodies. Symptoms vary but include earlier symptoms plus meningismus. Even in the absence of meningeal signs, CSF pleocytosis is evident after the seventh day in 50–90% of cases. Though often transient or absent in the second phase, fevers can recur; they usually last only 1–3 d, and temperatures rarely exceed 38.9°C. *Weil's syndrome*— severe leptospirosis with jaundice, usually accompanied by azotemia, hemorrhages, anemia, altered consciousness, and continued fever—occurs in 1–6% of cases. Leptospirosis occasionally causes aseptic meningitis and myocarditis.

DIAGNOSIS   The diagnosis is made by culture or serology. Leptospires can be cultured in special semisolid medium from blood or CSF during the initial phase or from urine during the second phase. Shedding in the urine may continue for up to 11 months. Antibodies to the organism appear between day 6 and day 12 of illness, and the antibody titer can rise by fourfold over the course of the illness. Pts with hepatic involvement typically have elevated serum levels of bilirubin and alkaline

Table 90-1

Treatment and Chemoprophylaxis of Leptospirosis

Purpose of Drug Administration	Regimen
Treatment	
Mild leptospirosis	Doxycycline, 100 mg PO bid *or* Ampicillin, 500–750 mg PO qid *or* Amoxicillin, 500 mg PO qid
Moderate/severe leptospirosis	Penicillin G, 1.5 million units IV qid *or* Ampicillin, 1 g IV qid *or* Amoxicillin, 1 g IV qid *or* Erythromycin, 500 mg IV qid
Chemoprophylaxis	Doxycycline, 200 mg PO once a week

NOTE: All regimens used for treatment are administered for 7 days.

SOURCE: From Speelman P: HPIM-14, p. 1038.

phosphatase as well as mild increases in serum levels of aminotransferases.

Rx TREATMENT
See Table 90-1.

RELAPSING FEVER

EPIDEMIOLOGY   Two types of relapsing fever are caused by *Borrelia* species: louse-borne and tick-borne. Louse-borne disease is endemic in Central and East Africa. Tick-borne relapsing fever has a worldwide distribution.

CLINICAL MANIFESTATIONS   Louse-borne relapsing fever has a more severe clinical course than tick-borne disease. The illness begins with an abrupt onset of rigors and fevers, headache, arthralgias, and myalgias. Abdominal pain, nausea, vomiting, and mental confusion are common, as are epistaxis (10–40%), jaundice (15–45%), petechiae or ecchymoses (60%),

Table 90-2

Antibiotic Treatment of Louse-Borne and Tick-Borne Relapsing Fever in Adults

Medication	Louse-Borne Relapsing Fever (Single Dose)	Tick-Borne Relapsing Fever (7-Day Schedule)
Oral		
Erythromycin	500 mg	500 mg q 6 h
Tetracycline	500 mg	500 mg q 6 h
Doxycycline	100 mg	100 mg q 12 h
Chloramphenicol	500 mg	500 mg q 6 h
Parenteral*		
Erythromycin	500 mg	500 mg q 6 h
Tetracycline	250 mg	250 mg q 6 h
Doxycycline	100 mg	100 mg q 12 h
Chloramphenicol	500 mg	500 mg q 6 h
Penicillin G (procaine)	600,000 IU	600,000 IU daily

* For tick-borne relapsing fever, parenteral therapy is used only until oral treatment is tolerated.

SOURCE: From Dennis DT, Campbell GL: HPIM-14, p. 1041.

and meningismus (40%). The first attack lasts 3–6 d and ends in a crisis that may be fatal; survivors have relapses after 5-10 d of feeling relatively well. In tick-borne relapsing fever, neurologic sequelae are more common.

DIAGNOSIS A definitive diagnosis is made by the demonstration of borreliae in peripheral blood films.

℞ TREATMENT
See Table 90-2.

For a more detailed discussion, see Perine PL: Endemic Treponematoses, Chap. 175, p. 1033; Speelman P: Leptospirosis, Chap. 176, p. 1036; Dennis DT, Campbell GL: Relapsing Fever, Chap. 177, p. 1038; and Steere AC: Lyme Borreliosis, Chap. 178, p. 1042, in HPIM-14.

91

RICKETTSIAL INFECTIONS

The rickettsiae are obligate intracellular parasites about the size of bacteria. The majority of rickettsiae are maintained in nature by a cycle that involves an insect vector and an animal reservoir. Except for louse-borne typhus, humans are incidental hosts. Only *Coxiella burnetii* (the agent of Q fever) can survive for an extended period outside the mammalian reservoir or the insect vector.

TICK- AND MITE-BORNE SPOTTED FEVERS

Rocky Mountain Spotted Fever (RMSF)

EPIDEMIOLOGY RMSF, so called because the first cases were described in Idaho and Montana, has now been documented in 48 states and in Canada, Mexico, Costa Rica, Panama, Colombia, and Brazil. In the U.S., two types of ticks may transmit *Rickettsia rickettsii* to humans: the wood tick (*Dermacentor andersoni*) and the dog tick (*D. variabilis*). The likelihood that an individual tick carries *R. rickettsii* is slight. From 1986 to 1992, approximately 600 cases of RMSF were reported annually. The mortality rate (20–25% in the preantibiotic era) is now about 5%.

CLINICAL MANIFESTATIONS Fever, headache, malaise, myalgia, nausea, vomiting, and anorexia are frequent but nonspecific manifestations during the first 3 d of clinical illness. Rash usually appears between the third and fifth febrile days, beginning as pink macules on the wrists and ankles. Lesions spread centripetally, convert to maculopapules that blanch on compression, and eventually become nonblanching and petechial. While diagnostically helpful when present, the rash does not appear until day 6 or later in 20% of cases; 10% of pts, including some with fatal cases, never develop a rash. Severe manifestations begin by the second week: widespread microvascular damage leads to increased vascular permeability, resulting in edema, hypovolemia, hypoalbuminemia, prerenal azotemia, and/or noncardiogenic pulmonary edema. Mechanical ventilation may be required—a poor prognostic sign. Encephalitis due to vascular injury is apparent in 25% of cases, often presenting as confusion and lethargy; stupor, delirium, ataxia, coma, and seizures are signs of more severe involvement. CSF pleocytosis, typically mononuclear, occurs in one-third of cases. The CSF protein concentration may be elevated, but the CSF glucose level is usually normal. Nonspecific GI disturbances are common, as are mildly or moderately elevated serum aminotransferase concentrations (38%) and heme-positive vomitus or stools (10%); hepatic failure does not occur. In ultimately fatal untreated cases, the pt usually dies within 2 weeks after the onset of illness.

DIAGNOSIS The diagnosis of RMSF during the acute stage is often difficult; early on, clinical and epidemiologic considerations (exposure within 12 d of onset to a potentially tick-infested environment during a season of possible tick activity) are more important than laboratory confirmation. During the acute phase, the only potentially diagnostic test is immunohistologic examination of a biopsy of involved skin. Serologic tests for RMSF are usually negative at presentation. Treatment should not be delayed while serologic results are pending. The most common confirmatory test is the indirect immunofluorescence assay, which is usually positive (titer, ≥64) by day 7–10. Moreover, latex agglutination is usually positive (titer, ≥128) at 1 week. Both tests are sensitive and highly specific. A solid-state enzyme immunoassay is also available. The Weil-Felix test is unreliable and should no longer be ordered.

℞ **TREATMENT**

Therapy is most effective when given early. The treatment of choice for nonpregnant adults with RMSF is doxycycline (100 mg PO or IV q12h). The oral route should be used unless precluded by the pt's condition. Tetracycline (25–50 mg/kg PO qd, divided q6h) is an equivalent alternative. For children <9 years of age and for pregnant women, chloramphenicol (50–75 mg/kg qd, divided q6h) can be used. ICU support may be necessary.

Mediterranean Spotted Fever (Boutonneuse Fever) and Other Spotted Fevers

EPIDEMIOLOGY AND CLINICAL MANIFESTATIONS A number of tick-borne rickettsial infections occur in the eastern hemisphere. *Mediterranean spotted fever (boutonneuse fever), Kenya tick typhus, Indian tick typhus, Israeli spotted fever,* and *Astrakhan spotted fever* are regional synonyms for the disease produced by *Rickettsia conorii,* which is prevalent in southern Europe, all of Africa, and southwestern and south-central Asia. High fever, rash, and—in most locales—an inoculation eschar at the site of the tick bite are characteristic. *R. africae* is prevalent in central, eastern, and southern Africa and causes *African tick-bite fever,* an illness milder than Mediterranean spotted fever. *R. japonica* causes *Japanese (Oriental)* *spotted fever. R. australis* causes *Queensland tick typhus,* an Australian illness characterized by maculopapular or vesicular rash and an inoculation eschar.

DIAGNOSIS AND TREATMENT Table 91-1 summarizes the laboratory diagnosis and treatment of the above tick-borne spotted fevers and other rickettsial diseases. The spotted fevers are diagnosed presumptively on clinical and epidemiologic grounds, and the diagnosis is generally confirmed serologically. In an endemic area, pts presenting with fever, rash, and an inoculation eschar (a black, necrotic area or crust with surrounding erythema) should be considered to have one of the rickettsial spotted fevers.

Rickettsialpox

EPIDEMIOLOGY *Rickettsia akari,* the etiologic agent of rickettsialpox, infects mice and their mites and is transmitted to humans by mite bites. While formerly not uncommon in the northeastern U.S., the disease is now rarely diagnosed.

CLINICAL MANIFESTATIONS The lesion at the site of the mite bite evolves from papular to vesicular and then to a painless black eschar with an erythematous halo. Regional lymphadenopathy is common. After a 10-d incubation period, malaise, chills, fever, headache, and myalgia begin. Rash begins 2–6 d later, evolving from papules to vesicles to crusts that heal without scarring. Without treatment, the illness lasts for 6–10 d and is self-limited.

DIAGNOSIS AND TREATMENT See Table 91-1.

FLEA- AND LOUSE-BORNE RICKETTSIAL DISEASES

Endemic (Murine) Typhus (Flea-Borne)

EPIDEMIOLOGY Murine typhus is a global disease caused by two rickettsial species, *R. typhi* and *R. felis*. *R. typhi* is classically maintained in rats and is transmitted to humans by the Oriental rat flea (*Xenopsylla cheopis*). *R. felis* has been characterized more recently and is maintained in a cycle involving opossums and cat fleas (*Ctenocephalides felis*). The fewer than 100 cases of endemic typhus reported annually in the U.S. occur year-round, mainly in warm areas.

CLINICAL MANIFESTATIONS The incubation period is 8–16 d. Prodromal symptoms of headache, myalgia, arthralgia, nausea, and malaise may occur. The onset of acute illness is characterized by the abrupt onset of chills and fever; nausea

Table 91-1

Laboratory Diagnosis and Treatment of Selected

Disease(s)	Laboratory Diagnosis
Mediterranean spotted fever Japanese or Oriental spotted fever Queensland tick typhus Flinders Island spotted fever	Isolation of rickettsiae, shell-vial culture; serology, IFA* (IgM, ≥1:64; or IgG, ≥1:128); PCR amplification of DNA from tissue specimens (especially for *R. japonica*)
Rickettsialpox	IFA: seroconversion to a titer of ≥1:64 or a single titer of ≥1:128; cross-absorption to eliminate antibodies to shared antigens necessary for a specific diagnosis of the spotted fever rickettsial species
Endemic (murine) typhus	IFA: fourfold rise to a titer of ≥1:64 or a single titer of ≥1:128; immunohistology: skin biopsy; PCR amplification of *R. typhi* or *R. felis* DNA from blood; dot ELISA* and immunoperoxidase methods also available
Epidemic typhus	IFA: titer of ≥1:128; necessary to use clinical and epidemiologic data to distinguish among louse-borne epidemic typhus, flying-squirrel typhus, and Brill-Zinsser disease
Scrub typhus	IFA: titer of ≥1:200; PCR amplification of *Orientia tsutsugamushi* DNA from blood of febrile pts

*IFA, indirect immunofluorescence assay; ELISA, enzyme-linked immunosorbent assay.

†Not approved by the Food and Drug Administration.
SOURCE: Walker D et al: HPIM-14, p. 1048.

Rickettsial Diseases

Treatment

Doxycycline (100 mg bid PO for 1–5 d)
or
Ciprofloxacin (750 mg bid PO for 5 d)
or
Chloramphenicol (500 mg qid PO for 7–10 d)
or (in pregnancy)
Josamycin† (3 g/d PO for 5 d)

Doxycycline (100 mg bid PO for 1–5 d)
or
Ciprofloxacin (750 mg bid PO for 5 d)
or
Chloramphenicol (500 mg qid PO for 7–10 d)
or (in pregnancy)
Josamycin† (3 g/d PO for 5 d)

Doxycycline (100 mg bid PO for 7–15 d)
or
Chloramphenicol (500 mg qid for 7–15 d)

Doxycycline (200 mg PO as a single dose or until pt is afebrile for 24 h)

Doxycycline (100 mg bid PO for 7–15 d) or chloramphenicol (500 mg qid PO for 7–15 d; for children, 150 mg/kg qd for 5 d); azithromycin more effective than doxycycline in vitro against both doxycycline-susceptible and -resistant strains of *O. tsutsugamushi*

and vomiting are nearly universal. Rash occurs in somewhat more than half of pts. It most often appears about the sixth day of the illness, and, in contrast to the rash of RMSF, is mostly confined to the trunk, with sparse involvement of the extremities, palms, soles, and face. Early lesions are macular and are hidden in the axillae and inner surfaces of the arms; later, a more generalized, discrete maculopapular rash involves the upper part of the abdomen, shoulders, chest, arms, and thighs. A hacking, nonproductive cough is a frequent finding. CXRs are abnormal in about 25% of cases. Headache is the most common neurologic finding and may dominate the clinical picture. Without treatment, the illness lasts an average of 12 d. Pts recover rapidly after defervescing; mortality was <1% even before the introduction of antibiotic therapy.

DIAGNOSIS AND TREATMENT   See Table 91-1.

Epidemic Typhus (Louse-Borne)

EPIDEMIOLOGY   Epidemic typhus is caused by *R. prowazekii* and is transmitted to humans by the body louse (*Pediculus humanus corporis*), infestation which is associated with poor hygiene. Lice pass the infection from person to person. Epidemic typhus is associated with poverty, war, cold weather, and natural disasters. In the U.S., sporadic cases result from transmission by the fleas of flying squirrels. *Brill-Zinsser disease* is a recrudescent, mild form of epidemic typhus occurring years after the acute disease; *R. prowazekii* can remain dormant for years and reactivate if immunity wanes.

CLINICAL MANIFESTATIONS   Epidemic typhus resembles murine typhus but is more severe. The incubation period is about 7 d. Disease onset is abrupt, with prostration, severe headache, and rapidly mounting fever. Rash appears by the fifth febrile day. It is initially macular and confined to the axillary folds but later involves the trunk and extremities and may become petechial and confluent. Photophobia, conjunctival injection, and ocular pain are frequent. In untreated cases, up to 40% of which are fatal, azotemia, multivisceral involvement, and digital gangrene may occur; 12% of such cases have prominent neurologic manifestations. Sporadic North American cases are much milder than epidemic cases. Brill-Zinsser disease resembles epidemic typhus. While it is not always mild, recovery is the rule.

DIAGNOSIS AND TREATMENT   See Table 91-1.

CHIGGER-BORNE SCRUB TYPHUS

EPIDEMIOLOGY   Scrub typhus is caused by *Orientia tsutsugamushi* and is transmitted to humans by the bites of infected trombiculid mite larvae (genus *Leptotrombidium*). The disease occurs in areas of heavy scrub vegetation, typically during the wet season when mites lay their eggs. It is endemic in eastern and southern Asia, in northern Australia, and in islands of the western Pacific.

CLINICAL MANIFESTATIONS Scrub typhus varies in severity from mild to fatal. After an incubation period of 6–21 d, the illness begins with fever, headache, myalgia, cough, and GI symptoms. Classic but infrequently observed signs include an inoculation eschar, regional lymphadenopathy, and a maculopapular rash. In severe cases, vascular injury may lead to encephalitis and interstitial pneumonia.

DIAGNOSIS AND TREATMENT See Table 91-1.

EHRLICHIOSIS

Human infection with *Ehrlichia* species is an emerging cause of life-threatening disease in the U.S. Two forms of human ehrlichiosis are known: human monocytic ehrlichiosis, caused by *E. chaffeensis,* and human granulocytic ehrlichiosis, the agent of which is as yet unnamed but is virtually indistinguishable from *E. equi.* Ehrlichiae are small, gram-negative, obligately intracellular bacteria that grow as microcolonies in phagosomes. Visible vacuolar clusters of ehrlichiae within phagocytes are termed *morulae.*

Human Monocytic Ehrlichiosis (HME)

EPIDEMIOLOGY The major vector for *E. chaffeensis* infection is the Lone Star tick (*Amblyomma americanum*); the white-tailed deer is an important reservoir host. Most U.S. cases have occurred in the south-central, southeastern, and mid-Atlantic regions. Cases have also been documented in Africa and Europe. Disease acquisition is most common in summer months and in rural areas.

CLINICAL MANIFESTATIONS Clinical illness occurs in about one-third of persons who seroconvert. The median incubation period is 9 d, and the median duration of clinical illness is 23 d. Manifestations are nonspecific and include (in order of decreasing frequency) fever, headache, myalgia, anorexia, nausea, vomiting, rash, cough, pharyngitis, diarrhea, lymphadenopathy, abdominal pain, and confusion. Severe cases can include respiratory insufficiency, neurologic involvement, acute renal failure, GI bleeding, and/or opportunistic viral or fungal infection. The mortality rate is 2–3%. Laboratory findings suggestive of the diagnosis include thrombocytopenia, leukopenia, and elevated serum levels of aminotransferases. Ehrlichial morular inclusions are seldom seen in peripheral blood but may be found in macrophages in CSF, bone marrow, and various solid organs.

DIAGNOSIS Clinical suspicion of HME should be triggered by fever and a history of tick exposure in an endemic area within the previous 3 weeks. PCR of peripheral blood may be positive for *E. chaffeensis* DNA during acute illness. Antibodies to the organism may be detected by indirect immunofluorescence during convalescence. A titer of ≥64 is considered positive.

℞ TREATMENT

Once HME has been presumptively identified, treatment should be initiated promptly. Tetracyclines (e.g., doxycycline, 100 mg q12h) shorten the course of illness. Chloramphenicol appears to have been effective in some cases but is not uniformly so.

Human Granulocytic Ehrlichiosis (HGE)

EPIDEMIOLOGY Most U.S. cases of HGE occur in the upper Midwest and in the Northeast, in the summer, and in a distribution similar to that of Lyme disease. *Ixodes* ticks—particularly *I. scapularis (dammini)* but also the southern-type *I. scapularis* as well as *I. pacificus* and *I. ricinus*—are probable vectors. Mammalian reservoir hosts are incompletely defined. HGE predominantly affects males and older persons.

CLINICAL MANIFESTATIONS The median incubation period is 8 d. HGE presents as a flulike illness, with fever, chills, malaise, headache, nausea, and vomiting and sometimes with cough or confusion. Rash is rare. Thrombocytopenia, leukopenia, anemia, and elevated serum aminotransferase levels are common. Untreated illness lasts for 3–11 weeks. The mortality rate is 5%. As in HME, opportunistic fungal infections may occur. The possibility of coinfection with *Borrelia burgdorferi* (Lyme disease) or *Babesia microti* (babesiosis) should be entertained in all HGE cases, since the *I. scapularis (dammini)* vector is shared by all three agents.

DIAGNOSIS HGE should be suspected in a pt with fever and flulike symptoms who has been exposed to an environment infested with the appropriate ticks, especially if thrombocytopenia is detected. Ehrlichial morulae within PMNs may be evident in peripheral blood. PCR may also be useful acutely. Serodiagnosis by indirect immunofluorescence assay may provide retrospective confirmation.

℞ TREATMENT
Doxycycline is therapeutically effective.

Q FEVER

EPIDEMIOLOGY   Q fever is a zoonosis caused by *C. burnetii,* an organism with a global distribution. The primary sources of human infection are infected cattle, sheep, and goats. In the infected female mammal, *C. burnetii* localizes to the uterus and mammary glands, reaches high concentrations in the placenta, and is dispersed as an aerosol at parturition. Infection follows inhalation of aerosolized organisms, ingestion of infected milk, or transfusion of infected blood. Abattoir workers and veterinarians are at particular risk. Rare cases of person-to-person transmission have followed delivery of an infant to an infected woman or autopsy of an infected cadaver.

CLINICAL MANIFESTATIONS   *Acute Q Fever*   With an incubation period of 3–30 d, Q fever may present in a variety of ways. Recognized syndromes include a flulike illness, prolonged fever, pneumonia, hepatitis, pericarditis, myocarditis, meningo-encephalitis, and infection during pregnancy. Symptoms are nonspecific; fever, extreme fatigue, and severe headache are common. Chills, sweats, nausea, vomiting, diarrhea, and cough may also occur. Neurologic manifestations are infrequent. Thrombocytopenia is noted in about 25% of cases during the acute phase. Multiple rounded opacities on CXR are common and are highly suggestive of Q fever pneumonia in the appropriate epidemiologic setting.

Chronic Q Fever   Chronic Q fever almost always implies endocarditis. This infection occurs in pts with previous valvular heart disease, immunosuppression, or chronic renal insufficiency. Nonspecific symptoms may exist for up to 1 year before diagnosis. Fever is absent or low-grade. Hepatomegaly and/or splenomegaly is usually detectable. The diagnosis should be considered in all pts with valvular heart disease, unexplained purpura, renal insufficiency, stroke, and/or progressive heart failure. A positive rheumatoid factor titer, an elevated ESR or C-reactive protein level, and/or an elevated gamma globulin concentration also suggests this diagnosis.

DIAGNOSIS   Serology (CF, ELISA, or indirect immuno-fluorescence) is the diagnostic tool of choice. Indirect immuno-fluorescence is sensitive and specific and can be used to diagnose both acute and chronic Q fever. PCR can be used to amplify *C. burnetii* DNA from tissue specimens. Culture of the organism is possible but potentially dangerous.

℞ TREATMENT

Acute Q fever is treated with doxycycline (100 mg q12h for 14 d) or a quinolone. Chronic Q fever is treated with at least two active agents—e.g., doxycycline (100 mg q12h) plus rifampin (300 mg/d). A minimum treatment duration of 3 years is recommended. An alternative regimen—doxycycline plus hydroxychloroquine (600 mg/d)—is under investigation.

For a more detailed discussion, see Walker D, Raoult D, Brouqui P, Marrie T: Rickettsial Diseases, Chap. 179, p. 1045, in HPIM-14.

92

MYCOPLASMA INFECTIONS

Mycoplasmas, which are ubiquitous in nature, are the smallest free-living microorganisms and lack rigid cell walls.

MYCOPLASMA PNEUMONIAE

EPIDEMIOLOGY   A common cause of respiratory tract infection, *M. pneumoniae* is the most important pathogen of the *Mycoplasma* group. Approximately 10–20% of all cases of pneumonia are due to *M. pneumoniae*. This organism is believed to spread by large droplets and spreads easily in closed settings such as households, institutions, and dormitories. With an incubation period of 1–3 weeks, *M. pneumoniae* infection is most common among children and young adults but may occur at any age.

CLINICAL MANIFESTATIONS   The most common clinical syndrome is acute or subacute tracheobronchitis accompanied by upper respiratory tract symptoms. Pneumonitis is also common. Symptoms generally include headache, malaise, feverishness, sore throat, and dry paroxysmal cough that later becomes productive. Complications or associated infections can include otitis media, bullous myringitis, maculopapular rashes, erythema multiforme, and occasionally Stevens-Johnson syndrome. Small pleural effusions develop in up to 20% of cases. Rare complications include meningoencephalitis, cerebellar ataxia, radiculopathies, monarticular arthritis, myocarditis, pericarditis, coagulopathies, hemolytic anemia, pulmonary edema, and hepatitis.

DIAGNOSIS Clinical, radiologic, and laboratory findings in *M. pneumoniae* infection are not sufficiently distinctive for diagnostic purposes. Definitive diagnosis is difficult during acute infection, since most clinical laboratories do not have the capability to isolate the organism. Cold agglutinin responses are detected in <50% of cases. Serologic tests are confirmatory when seroconversion is evident from paired sera taken 2–4 weeks apart. The ELISA is the preferred serologic method. A fourfold rise in complement fixation titer between paired sera is diagnostic. Leukocytosis or left shift of the differential count is unusual; the ESR is elevated.

℞ TREATMENT

The disease generally resolves spontaneously in 2–4 weeks without therapy, but appropriate antibiotic treatment shortens the course. Oral erythromycin (500 mg qid), tetracycline (250 mg qid), or doxycycline (100 mg bid) for 10–14 d is recommended for adults. For severely ill pts, IV erythromycin (500 mg q6h) can be used. For children under the age of 8–10 years, erythromycin 30–50 (mg/kg)/d PO for 14 d is recommended. Tetracyclines should be reserved for older pts. Newer macrolides such as clarithromycin and azithromycin are active against *Mycoplasma* but have not been shown to be superior to erythromycin.

OTHER MYCOPLASMAL INFECTIONS

ETIOLOGY Other mycoplasmal infections are usually caused by *M. hominis* or *Ureaplasma urealyticum* and involve genitourinary syndromes or perinatal infection.

CLINICAL MANIFESTATIONS Manifestations include urethritis, salpingitis, amnionitis, pyelonephritis, postpartum sepsis, and neonatal pneumonia or meningitis. Occasionally, arthritis or abscesses may be encountered in immunocompromised pts. Infection with *M. hominis* has been documented in surgical wounds, at sites of trauma, and on prosthetic heart valves. Pts with agammaglobulinemia develop joint inflammation that can be due to *Mycoplasma*.

DIAGNOSIS Diagnosis by culture usually requires that the specimen be sent to a reference laboratory, although *M. hominis* can be recovered in some routine blood culture systems.

 TREATMENT

Treatment for *M. hominis* infection consists of tetracycline (250 mg PO qid) or clindamycin (150 mg PO qid); erythromycin is not effective. Up to 40% of *M. hominis* strains may now be resistant to tetracycline. For *Ureaplasma* infections, erythromycin or tetracycline may be used.

For a more detailed discussion, see Cassell GH, Gray GC, Waites KB: *Mycoplasma* Infections, Chap. 180, p. 1052, in HPIM-14.

93

CHLAMYDIAL INFECTIONS

The genus *Chlamydia* contains three species: *C. psittaci, C. trachomatis,* and *C. pneumoniae* (formerly called TWAR). Chlamydiae are obligate intracellular parasites. Different serovars are associated with different clinical syndromes. Chlamydiae cause conjunctival, genital, and respiratory infections.

C. TRACHOMATIS GENITAL INFECTIONS AND LYMPHOGRANULOMA VENEREUM

See Chap. 75.

TRACHOMA AND ADULT INCLUSION CONJUNCTIVITIS

EPIDEMIOLOGY In trachoma-endemic areas, *C. trachomatis* (usually serovar A, B, Ba, or C) is the major preventable cause of blindness. Transmission is from eye to eye via hands, flies, or fomites. In nonendemic areas, disease is usually confined to inclusion conjunctivitis and is caused by serovars D–K, which are transmitted from the genital tract to the eye.

CLINICAL MANIFESTATIONS Endemic trachoma usually begins as conjunctivitis with small lymphoid follicles in children <2 years old. It progresses to corneal involvement with inflammatory leukocytic infiltrations and superficial vascularization (pannus formation). Conjunctival scarring leads to distortion of the eyelids, inturned lashes that abrade and ulcerate the corneal epithelium, and subsequently corneal scarring and blindness. Eye infection with genital strains usually causes an acute onset of unilateral follicular conjunctivitis and preauricular lymphadenopathy in sexually active young adults.

DIAGNOSIS Classic trachoma is usually diagnosed clinically if two of the following signs are present: (1) lymphoid follicles on the upper tarsal conjunctiva, (2) typical conjunctival scarring, (3) vascular pannus, and (4) limbal follicles. The most sensitive laboratory tests are isolation of the organism in cell culture, newer antigen detection tests, and chlamydial polymerase chain reaction. Intracytoplasmic inclusions on Giemsa-stained conjunctival smears are diagnostic but are less sensitive. For adult inclusion conjunctivitis, culture or Giemsa or immunofluorescent staining of conjunctival smears is used and should be accompanied by genital examinations and cultures. Serum antibody tests are not diagnostic.

℞ TREATMENT

Therapy includes the topical application of tetracycline or erythromycin ointment for 21–60 d. Alternatively, tetracycline or erythromycin (500 mg qid PO for 3 weeks) may be used in adults and erythromycin (50 mg/kg PO daily for 3 weeks) in children. Treatment of sexual partners is important in genitally acquired infection. Topical therapy is not necessary if oral antibiotics are used.

PSITTACOSIS

EPIDEMIOLOGY Psittacosis (infection with *C. psittaci*) is transmitted via the respiratory route from many avian species, including psittacine birds (parrots, parakeets), pigeons, ducks, turkeys, chickens, and other birds. Infected birds may not manifest symptoms. The incubation period is 7–14 d or longer.

CLINICAL MANIFESTATIONS Prominent headache, fevers increasing over a 3- to 4-d period, and a dry hacking cough occurring as late as 5 d after fevers begin are the most common manifestations. Pulmonary symptoms are usually more prominent than signs. Other symptoms may include myalgias, lethargy, mental depression, agitation progressing to stupor or coma in severe cases, and GI symptoms such as abdominal pain, vomiting, and diarrhea. Splenomegaly is found in 10–70% of cases. Psittacosis should be considered strongly in pts with acute pneumonitis and splenomegaly.

DIAGNOSIS CXRs usually show diffuse, patchy infiltrates but may yield a variety of findings. The WBC count, ESR, and LFTs usually are normal. The diagnosis can be made only by isolating the organism or by demonstrating a fourfold rise in CF antibody. Early antibiotic treatment may delay the convalescent antibody response by weeks or months.

℞ TREATMENT

Tetracycline (500 mg qid) usually leads to defervescence and improvement in symptoms in 24–48 h. Treatment should be continued for 7–14 d after fever abates to avoid relapse. Erythromycin can be used for pts allergic to or intolerant of tetracycline.

C. PNEUMONIAE INFECTIONS

EPIDEMIOLOGY Serologic studies indicate that *C. pneumoniae* infections are ubiquitous. Seroprevalence rates in adult populations exceed 40%. The route of transmission appears to be from person to person. Primary infection seems to occur in young adults, with less severe reinfection episodes in older adults. Epidemiologic studies have demonstrated an association between serologic evidence of *C. pneumoniae* infection and atherosclerotic disease of the coronary and other arteries. *C. pneumoniae* has been identified in atherosclerotic plaques by several techniques. The clinical significance of these findings is not yet clear.

CLINICAL MANIFESTATIONS The clinical spectrum includes acute pharyngitis, sinusitis, bronchitis, and pneumonitis. Upper respiratory tract symptoms usually precede fever and nonproductive cough. The pneumonitis often resembles *Mycoplasma pneumoniae* pneumonia. Pulmonary findings generally are minimal. Leukocytosis is typically absent. CXRs generally show small segmental infiltrates.

DIAGNOSIS Diagnosis is difficult because culture and antigen detection techniques are not available. A rise in CF antibody between acute- and convalescent-phase serum samples can allow a retrospective diagnosis but does not distinguish *C. pneumoniae* from *C. trachomatis* and *C. psittaci*.

℞ **TREATMENT**

The recommended therapy consists of erythromycin or tetracycline (500 mg qid PO) for 10–14 d.

For a more detailed discussion, see Stamm WE: Chlamydial Infections, Chap. 181, p. 1055, in HPIM-14.

94

HERPESVIRUS INFECTIONS

HERPES SIMPLEX VIRUSES

The genome of herpes simplex virus is a linear, double-stranded DNA molecule that encodes for more than 70 gene products. Overall DNA sequence homology between HSV-1 and HSV-2 is about 50%. HSV infection of some neuronal cells does not result in cell death; viral genomes are maintained by the cell in a repressed state known as *latency*. The process of activation of the viral genome that leads to viral replication and causes recurrent lesions is known as *reactivation*.

PATHOGENESIS   Exposure of mucosal surfaces or abraded skin to virus permits entry of the virus and initiation of its replication in epidermal and dermal cells. Sensory or autonomic nerve endings may become infected whether or not clinically apparent lesions develop. Initially, virus replicates in ganglia and contiguous neural tissue; spread occurs via peripheral sensory nerves. While the mechanism of reactivation is not known, stimuli such as UV light, immunosuppression, and trauma to skin or ganglia are associated with reactivation.

EPIDEMIOLOGY   Infection with HSV-1 is acquired more frequently and at an earlier age than infection with HSV-2. By the fifth decade of life, more than 90% of adults have antibodies to HSV-1. Antibodies to HSV-2 are not routinely detected until puberty; their prevalence varies with the population studied. In obstetric and family planning clinic populations, 25% of women have antibody to HSV-2, although only 10% give a history of genital lesions. In adults attending STD clinics, the prevalence of antibody to HSV-2 is 50%. The incubation period for HSV infection ranges from 1 to 26 d (median, 6–8 d). HSV can be transmitted by contact with active lesions or with an asymptomatic person excreting the virus; the efficiency of transmission is greater from active lesions.

CLINICAL MANIFESTATIONS   *Oral-Facial Infections*
Gingivostomatitis and pharyngitis are the most common clinical manifestations of first-episode HSV-1 infection and are most prevalent among children and young adults. Clinical symptoms and signs include fever, malaise, myalgias, inability to eat, irritability, and cervical adenopathy that may last 3–14 d. Lesions may involve the hard and soft palates, gingiva, tongue, lips, and facial area. Reactivation may lead to asymptomatic excretion, intraoral mucosal ulcerations, or herpetic ulcerations of the vermilion border of the lip or external facial skin. In immunosuppressed pts, including those with AIDS, severe mucositis due to HSV can develop. Pts with eczema may develop severe oral-facial lesions (eczema herpeticum) with occasional visceral dissemination. HSV-1 has recently been implicated as a cause of Bell's palsy. Erythema multiforme is often associated with HSV infection.

Rectal and Perianal Infections   HSV-1 and HSV-2 can cause rectal and perianal infections. Symptoms of HSV proctitis include anorectal pain, discharge, tenesmus, and constipation, with ulcerative lesions of the distal 10 cm of rectal mucosa.

Genital Infections   See Chap. 75.

Herpetic Whitlow   Clinical symptoms of herpetic whitlow include an abrupt onset of edema, erythema, and localized tenderness of the infected finger after direct inoculation. Vesicular or pustular lesions, fever, and lymphadenitis make this infection clinically indistinguishable from a pyogenic infection. Surgical debridement may exacerbate the condition.

Herpes Gladiatorum   Mucocutaneous HSV infections of the thorax, ears, face, and hands have been described among wrestlers.

Herpetic Eye Infections   HSV infection is the most common cause of corneal blindness in the U.S. Herpetic keratitis presents as an acute onset of pain, blurring of vision, chemosis, conjunctivitis, and characteristic dendritic lesions of the cornea. Chorioretinitis occurs in neonates or HIV-infected pts, usually as a manifestation of disseminated infection. Acute necrotizing retinitis is a rare but serious manifestation of HSV infection.

Central and Peripheral Nervous System Infections   HSV is the most common cause of acute sporadic viral encephalitis in the U.S., accounting for 10–20% of cases. HSV-1 causes more than 95% of cases, with peaks at 5–30 years and >50 years of age. Clinical manifestations include an acute onset of fever and focal neurologic (especially temporal lobe) symptoms. The diagnosis can be made by brain biopsy; the most sensitive early noninvasive method is demonstration of HSV DNA in the CSF by PCR. Treatment with IV acyclovir is started for a presumptive diagnosis. HSV meningitis, usually seen in association with primary genital HSV infection, is a self-limited disease, with headache, fever, and mild photophobia but no neurologic sequelae. Autonomic nervous system dysfunction, especially of the sacral region, is associated with both HSV and varicella-zoster virus (VZV) infections. Symptoms include numbness, tingling of the buttock or perineal areas, urinary retention, constipation, CSF pleocytosis, and (in males) impotence; these symptoms resolve slowly over days or weeks. In rare instances, HSV infection is associated with transverse myelitis, with rapidly progressive, symmetric lower-extremity paralysis or Guillain-Barré syndrome. Peripheral nervous system involvement includes Bell's palsy or cranial polyneuritis related to reactivation of HSV-1 infection.

Visceral Infections Visceral HSV infection commonly involves multiple organs and results from viremia. HSV esophagitis presents as odynophagia, dysphagia, substernal pain, weight loss, and multiple oval ulcerations on an erythematous base with or without a patchy white pseudomembrane. The distal esophagus is most frequently involved. The diagnosis can be made only by endoscopic biopsy with cytology and culture. HSV pneumonitis mainly affects severely immunocompromised pts. Focal necrotizing pneumonitis results from the extension of herpetic tracheobronchitis. Hematogenous dissemination from mucocutaneous disease causes bilateral interstitial pneumonitis. HSV is an uncommon cause of hepatitis. The presentation includes fever, abrupt elevations of serum levels of bilirubin and aminotransferases, and leukopenia. DIC may be present. Other rare disseminated manifestations include monarticular arthritis, adrenal necrosis, idiopathic thrombocytopenia, and glomerulonephritis. In immunocompromised pts, rare sites of organ involvement can include the adrenal glands, pancreas, small and large intestines, and bone marrow.

Neonatal Infections Infants <6 weeks of age have the highest frequency of visceral and/or CNS infection due to HSV. Without treatment, more than 70% of neonatal cases disseminate or develop into CNS infection. Neonatal cases almost always result from contact with infected genital secretions at delivery; 70% of cases are caused by HSV-2.

DIAGNOSIS A clinical diagnosis can be made by scraping the base of lesions and demonstrating multinucleated giant cells by Tzanck preparation or characteristic giant cells or intranuclear inclusions by cytology. Cultures become positive in 48–96 h. Methods such as immunofluorescence assay, ELISA, and some DNA hybridization techniques are almost as sensitive as viral isolation from lesions; PCR may be more sensitive. Restriction endonuclease analysis of viral DNA can differentiate HSV-1 from HSV-2. Seroconversion can be used to document primary infections.

℞ TREATMENT
See Table 94-1.

VARICELLA-ZOSTER VIRUS

VZV is a herpesvirus that causes two distinct clinical entities: varicella, or chickenpox, and herpes zoster, or shingles. Only enveloped virions are infectious.

PATHOGENESIS Primary infection occurs via the respiratory route and is followed by viremia. Reactivation results in herpes zoster by mechanisms that are unknown. It is presumed that VZV infects the dorsal root ganglia during chickenpox and remains latent at that site until reactivated.

EPIDEMIOLOGY Attack rates for chickenpox are 90% among susceptible pts. Cases occur throughout the year, but the disease is epidemic during the late winter and early spring in temperate climates. Children 5–9 years of age account for 50% of cases. The incubation period ranges between 10 and 21 d but is usually 14–17 d. Pts are infectious 48 h before vesicles erupt, during vesicle formation (usually 4–5 d), and until all vesicles are crusted. The incidence of herpes zoster is highest in the sixth through eighth decades of life, but the disease can occur at any age. Most pts with herpes zoster have no exposure to other persons infected with VZV.

CLINICAL MANIFESTATIONS *Chickenpox* Low-grade fever and malaise may precede the exanthem by 24–48 h. Fever and lassitude generally last 3–5 d in immunocompetent hosts. The rash consists of maculopapules, vesicles, and scabs in various stages of evolution. Characteristic lesions are vesicles described as "dewdrops on a rose petal." Crops of lesions develop over 2–4 d. Lesions may be found on the pharyngeal or vaginal mucosa. Younger pts tend to have fewer lesions overall than older individuals. Lesions of immunocompromised pts, especially those with leukemia, may be more numerous, may

Table 94-1

Antiviral Chemotherapy for HSV Infection

Mucocutaneous HSV infections
Infections in immunosuppressed pts
Acute symptomatic first or recurrent episodes: IV acyclovir (5 mg/kg q8h) or oral acyclovir (400 mg qid for 7–10 d) relieves pain and speeds healing. With localized external lesions, 5% topical acyclovir ointment applied 4–6 times/d may be beneficial.
Suppression of reactivation disease: IV acyclovir (5 mg/kg q8h) or oral acyclovir (400 mg 3–5 times/d) prevents recurrences during high-risk periods, e.g., the immediate posttransplantation period. In HIV-infected persons, oral famciclovir (500 mg bid) reduces rates of HSV-1 and HSV-2 reactivation.
Genital herpes
First episodes: Oral acyclovir (200 mg 5 times/d or 400 mg tid) is given. Oral valacyclovir (1000 mg bid) or famciclovir (250 mg bid) for 10–14 d is effective. IV acyclovir (5 mg/kg q8h for 5 d) is given for severe disease or neurologic complications such as aseptic meningitis.
Symptomatic recurrent genital herpes: Oral acyclovir (200 mg 5 times/d for 5 d), valacyclovir (500 mg bid), or famciclovir (125 mg bid) is effective in shortening lesion duration and viral excretion time.
Suppression of recurrent genital herpes: Oral acyclovir (200-mg capsules bid or tid, 400 mg bid, or 800 mg qd), famciclovir (250 mg bid), or valacyclovir (500 mg bid, 250 mg bid, or 1000 mg qd) prevents symptomatic reactivation.
Oral-labial HSV infections
First episode: Oral acyclovir (200 mg) is given 4 or 5 times/d.
Recurrent episodes: Topical penciclovir cream is effective in speeding the healing of oral-labial HSV. Topical acyclovir cream is licensed in Europe. The ointment formulation of acyclovir available in the U.S. has no clinical benefit. Oral acyclovir has minimal benefit.
Suppression of reactivation of oral-labial HSV: Oral acyclovir (400 mg bid), if started before exposure and continued for the duration of exposure (usually 5–10 d), will prevent reactivation of recurrent oral-labial HSV infection associated with severe sun exposure.

(continued)

Table 94-1 (*Continued*)

Antiviral Chemotherapy for HSV Infection

Herpetic whitlow: Oral acyclovir (200 mg) is given 5 times/d for 7–10 d.

HSV proctitis: Oral acyclovir (400 mg 5 times/d) is useful in shortening the course of infection. In immunosuppressed pts or in pts with severe infection, IV acyclovir (5 mg/kg q8h) may be useful.

Herpetic eye infections: In acute keratitis, topical trifluorothymidine, vidarabine, idoxuridine, acyclovir, and interferon are all beneficial. Debridement may be required; topical steroids may worsen disease.

CNS HSV infections

HSV encephalitis: Intravenous acyclovir (10 mg/kg q8h; 30 (mg/kg)/d) for 10 d is preferred.

HSV aseptic meningitis: No studies of systemic antiviral chemotherapy exist. If therapy is to be given IV, acyclovir (15–30 (mg/kg)/d) should be used.

Autonomic radiculopathy: No studies are available.

Neonatal HSV infections: Acyclovir (45–60 (mg/kg)/d) is given. Neonates appear to tolerate this high dose of acyclovir. The recommended duration of treatment is 21 d.

Visceral HSV infections

HSV esophagitis: Systemic acyclovir (15 (mg/kg)/d) should be considered. In some pts with milder forms of immunosuppression, oral therapy with valacyclovir or famciclovir is effective.

HSV pneumonitis: No controlled studies exist. Systemic acyclovir (15 (mg/kg)/d) should be considered.

Disseminated HSV infections: No controlled studies exist. IV acyclovir nevertheless should be tried. No definite evidence indicates that therapy will decrease the risk of death.

Erythema multiforme associated with HSV: Anecdotal observations suggest that oral acyclovir (400 mg bid or tid) will suppress erythema multiforme.

Infections due to acyclovir-resistant HSV: Foscarnet (40 mg/kg IV q8h) should be given until lesions heal. The optimal duration of therapy and the usefulness of its continuation to suppress lesions are unclear. Some pts may benefit from cutaneous application of trifluorothymidine or 5% cidofovir gel. Trials of systemic cidofovir are under way.

SOURCE: Corey L: HPIM-14, p. 1085.

be hemorrhagic, and may take longer to resolve; these pts may be at greater risk of visceral complications. The most common complication of varicella is bacterial superinfection of the skin, usually caused by *Streptococcus pyogenes* or *Staphylococcus aureus*. In children, CNS involvement is the most common extracutaneous manifestation. A syndrome of cerebellar ataxia and meningeal irritation generally develops about 21 d after the onset of rash, is usually self-limited, and does not require hospitalization. Other CNS manifestations include aseptic meningitis, encephalitis, transverse myelitis, Guillain-Barré syndrome, and Reye's syndrome. Varicella pneumonia is the most common serious complication of chickenpox, occurring more commonly among adults (in up to 20% of cases) than among children. Usually developing 3–5 d into the illness, varicella pneumonia is associated with tachypnea, cough, dyspnea, and fever. CXR findings include nodular infiltrates and interstitial pneumonitis. Other complications include myocarditis, corneal lesions, nephritis, arthritis, bleeding diatheses, acute glomerulonephritis, and hepatitis. Hepatic involvement distinct from Reye's syndrome is common, is usually characterized by elevation of serum aminotransferase levels, and is generally asymptomatic. Perinatal varicella is most severe when maternal disease develops within 5 d before and 48 h after delivery. Congenital varicella is extremely uncommon.

Herpes Zoster   Herpes zoster is characterized by a unilateral vesicular eruption within a dermatome accompanied by severe local pain. Pain heralds infection and may precede the development of lesions by 48–72 h. Erythematous maculopapules evolve rapidly into vesicles. The most debilitating consequences of herpes zoster are acute neuritis and postherpetic neuralgia, both of which are more common among adults than among children and the latter of which is increasingly common with advancing age. Zoster ophthalmicus is an infection involving the ophthalmic division of the trigeminal nerve. Ramsay Hunt syndrome occurs with involvement of the sensory branch of the facial nerve and is characterized by lesions on the ear canal, ipsilateral facial palsy, and loss of taste in the anterior two-thirds of the tongue. CNS involvement includes asymptomatic CSF pleocytosis; symptomatic meningoencephalitis with headache, fever, photophobia, meningitis, and vomiting; and, in rare instances, granulomatous angiitis with contralateral hemiplegia. Transverse myelitis with or without paralysis may also develop. In immunocompromised pts, especially those with Hodgkin's or non-Hodgkin's lymphoma, the clinical syndrome is more severe and the risk of disseminated skin lesions—or even visceral dissemination—is greater. Cutaneous dissemination occurs in about 40% of these pts. Visceral dissemination, including pneumonitis, meningoencephalitis, and hepatitis, occurs in 5–10% of pts with cutaneous dissemination. Even disseminated infection is rarely fatal.

DIAGNOSIS The diagnosis of both chickenpox and herpes zoster can be made clinically on the basis of the epidemiology, appearance, and distribution of lesions. Results obtained with a Tzanck preparation are positive but do not distinguish VZV from HSV infection. Serologic tests include fluorescent antibody to membrane antigen (FAMA) and ELISA. Confirmation is possible with viral isolation in tissue culture. VZV takes longer to isolate than HSV.

℞ **TREATMENT**

For chickenpox of ≤24 h duration in adolescents or adults, acyclovir (800 mg PO 5 times daily for 5–7 d) is recommended. When initiated early, therapy with acyclovir at a dose of 20 mg/kg q6h also may be of benefit to children <12 years old. Aspirin should not be administered to children because of its association with Reye's syndrome. Palliative measures are directed at the control of itching and drying lesions. For herpes zoster, acyclovir (800 mg PO 5 times daily for 7–10 d) speeds the healing of skin lesions and decreases acute pain but does not alter the incidence of postherpetic neuralgia. Pts with zoster ophthalmicus should see an ophthalmologist in addition to receiving acyclovir. Postherpetic neuralgia is extremely difficult to treat; analgesics, amitriptyline hydrochloride, and fluphenazine hydrochloride are used. For immunocompromised pts with either chickenpox or herpes zoster, IV acyclovir is recommended at a dose of 10–12.5 mg/kg q8h for 7 d; oral therapy should not be used. Susceptible pts with significant exposure to VZV can be given varicella-zoster immune globulin (VZIG) prophylactically within 96 h (preferably <72 h) after exposure. Candidates for VZIG include immunodeficient pts <15 years old with a negative or unknown history of chickenpox, neonates born to mothers who develop chickenpox 5 d before delivery or within 48 h post partum, pregnant women with a negative history or negative serology for chickenpox, and premature infants born at ≥28 weeks of gestation to mothers who have not had chickenpox or at ≤28 weeks to any mother. It is recommended that serologic status be determined before administration of VZIG to normal adolescents or adults with significant exposure. A live attenuated vaccine is now available for the prevention of VZV infection and is recommended for routine immunization of children and for vaccination of susceptible adults.

HUMAN HERPESVIRUS TYPES 6, 7, AND 8

HHV-6 is a T-lymphotropic virus that causes exanthem subitum (roseola), a common childhood illness characterized by fever and subsequent rash. HHV-6 has also been associated with febrile seizures (without rash) during infancy and, in older age groups, with mononucleosis syndromes and focal encephalitis. It causes pneumonitis and disseminated disease in immunocompromised hosts. HHV-7 is frequently acquired during childhood and is present in saliva but has not been definitively linked with any known disease. HHV-8 has been assigned a putative etiologic role in Kaposi's sarcoma.

For a more detailed discussion, see Corey L: Herpes Simplex Viruses, Chap. 184, p. 1080; Whitley RJ: Varicella-Zoster Virus Infections, Chap. 185, p. 1086; and Hirsch MS: Cytomegalovirus and Human Herpesvirus Types 6, 7, and 8, Chap. 187, p. 1092, in HPIM-14.

95

CYTOMEGALOVIRUS AND EPSTEIN-BARR VIRUS INFECTIONS

CYTOMEGALOVIRUS (CMV) INFECTIONS

CMV is a member of the beta herpesvirus group, containing double-stranded DNA, a protein capsid, and a lipoprotein envelope.

EPIDEMIOLOGY   CMV has a worldwide distribution, with infection common in the perinatal and childhood periods. In the U.S., about 1% of newborns are infected. Spread does not occur casually but rather takes place through repeated or prolonged intimate exposure. Transmission occurs in day-care centers, through sexual contact, and after transfusion of blood products (at a frequency of 0.14–10% per unit transfused). When an infected child introduces CMV into a household, the conversion rate is 50% among susceptible household contacts within 6 months.

PATHOGENESIS   Once acquired during asymptomatic or symptomatic primary infection, CMV persists indefinitely in latent form in tissues. If T cell function of the host becomes compromised, the virus can be reactivated to cause a variety of syndromes.

CLINICAL MANIFESTATIONS   *Congenital CMV Infection*   Most congenital CMV infections are not apparent at birth; 5–25% of asymptomatically infected infants develop psychomotor, hearing, ocular, or dental abnormalities over the next several years. Cytomegalic inclusion disease develops in about 5% of infected fetuses, almost exclusively in those whose mothers have acquired primary infection during pregnancy. Petechiae, hepatosplenomegaly, and jaundice are the most common signs (60–80% of cases). Microcephaly (with or without cerebral calcifications), intrauterine growth retardation, and prematurity are seen in 30–50% of cases. Mortality rates are as high as 20–30% among the most severely affected infants.

Perinatal Infection   The majority of infants infected at or after delivery remain asymptomatic. Infection is contracted by passage through an infected birth canal or, after birth, via maternal milk. CMV causes rare cases of protracted interstitial pneumonia in premature infants.

CMV Mononucleosis   Heterophile-negative mononucleosis is the most common manifestation of CMV infection in normal hosts beyond the neonatal period. The incubation period is 20–60 d, with clinical illness generally lasting 2–6 weeks. CMV mononucleosis is characterized by prolonged high fevers, sometimes with chills, fatigue, and malaise. While myalgias, headache, and splenomegaly are frequent, exudative pharyngitis and cervical lymphadenopathy are rare (in contrast to Epstein-Barr virus mononucleosis, in which these findings are prominent). The major laboratory finding is relative peripheral lymphocytosis with >10% atypical lymphocytes. Moderately elevated serum levels of aminotransferases and alkaline phosphatase are common; jaundice is rare.

CMV Infection in the Immunocompromised Host   CMV is the most common and important viral pathogen affecting organ transplant recipients. Infections in these hosts include fever and leukopenia, hepatitis, pneumonitis, esophagitis, gastritis, colitis, and retinitis. The period of maximal risk is 1–4 months after transplantation. The greatest risk of disease appears to follow primary infection. The transplanted organ seems to be particularly susceptible, with CMV hepatitis common in liver transplant recipients and CMV pneumonitis in lung transplant recipients. CMV pneumonitis also occurs in 15–20% of bone marrow transplant recipients, most frequently 5–13 weeks after transplantation; the case-fatality rate is 84–88%. CMV is a significant pathogen in AIDS pts, generally causing clinical syndromes at CD4 cell counts of <100/μL. CMV retinitis is a prominent cause of blindness in AIDS; disseminated CMV infection is likewise common. GI involvement, including esophageal ulcers and colitis, also occurs in AIDS pts.

DIAGNOSIS Diagnosis requires the isolation of CMV in tissue culture, which may take only a few days if the titer of virus is high but may also take several weeks. To expedite this process, many laboratories use a shell-vial technique on overnight tissue cultures, which employs monoclonal antibodies and immunocytochemical detection of early antigens. Viral isolation from urine or saliva does not confirm infection, since shedding may continue for months or even years after infection; detection of CMV viremia by culture or early-antigen testing of peripheral blood leukocytes is a better predictor of infection. While a fourfold rise in antibody titer can confirm a primary infection, antibody rises may take up to 4 weeks, and titers may remain high for years.

R̲x̲ TREATMENT

Ganciclovir has produced response rates of 70–90% among AIDS pts treated for CMV retinitis or colitis. The induction dose of ganciclovir (5 mg/kg bid IV for 14–21 d) is followed by maintenance therapy (5 mg/kg qd IV, 6 mg/kg IV 5 d/week, or 3 g/d PO). Neutropenia, the major toxic effect, can be lessened by the use of colony-stimulating factors. In bone marrow transplant recipients, ganciclovir plus CMV immune globulin have elicited a favorable clinical response in 50–70% of episodes of CMV pneumonitis. For ganciclovir-resistant strains, foscarnet is active and compares favorably with ganciclovir in the treatment of CMV retinitis in AIDS. The induction dose of foscarnet (60 mg/kg q8h or 90 mg/kg q12h for 14–21 d) is followed by maintenance infusions of 90–120 mg/kg qd. Foscarnet exerts considerable toxicity: renal dysfunction, hypomagnesemia, hypokalemia, hypocalcemia, seizures, fever, and rash are each seen in more than 5% of pts.

EPSTEIN-BARR VIRUS (EBV) INFECTIONS

EBV is a human herpesvirus that consists of a linear double-stranded DNA core surrounded by an icosahedral nucleocapsid and a glycoprotein-containing envelope. It is cytotropic for B lymphocytes.

EPIDEMIOLOGY EBV is transmitted primarily in saliva and occasionally by blood transfusion and is not highly contagious. Primary infection tends to occur at an early age in lower socioeconomic groups and in developing countries. Primary EBV infection among adolescents and young adults accounts for most cases of infectious mononucleosis (IM). By adulthood, more than 90% of individuals are seropositive for EBV. The virus is shed from the oropharynx for up to 18 months after primary infection and intermittently thereafter in the absence of clinical illness.

CLINICAL MANIFESTATIONS *Infection in Infants and Young Children* EBV infection in this group is generally asymptomatic or presents as mild pharyngitis with or without tonsillitis.

Infectious Mononucleosis The incubation period for IM is 4–6 weeks. Prodromal symptoms of malaise, anorexia, and myalgia frequently precede the onset of pharyngitis, fever, and lymphadenopathy by a few days. Severe pharyngitis usually prompts the pt to seek medical attention. Fever develops in 90% of pts, and temperatures may reach 39–40C°. Findings on physical exam include diffuse pharyngitis with exudate in one-third of pts, posterior and/or anterior cervical lymphadenopathy in more than 90%, splenomegaly in about 50% during the second or third week of illness, and rash in 5%. After ampicillin administration, most pts with IM develop a pruritic maculopapular eruption that is not predictive of future penicillin allergy. The clinical course of the illness encompasses pharyngitis that is maximal for 5–7 d and resolves over the next 7–10 d, fevers that last 7–14 d or occasionally longer, lymphadenopathy that usually resolves within 3 weeks, and malaise that may persist for months. Complications are infrequent but may be dramatic and include autoimmune hemolytic anemia, thrombocytopenia, granulocytopenia, splenic rupture, cranial nerve palsies, encephalitis, hepatitis, pericarditis, myocarditis, coronary artery spasm, and airway obstruction from pharyngeal or paratracheal adenopathy.

Other Diseases Associated with EBV Infection EBV-associated lymphoproliferative disease occurs in pts with congenital or acquired immunodeficiency, including AIDS, ataxia-telangiectasia, severe combined immunodeficiency, and transplantation. Pts present with fever and lymphadenopathy or GI symptoms. X-linked lymphoproliferative syndrome (Duncan's syndrome), a disorder in immune responsiveness to EBV, permits overwhelming EBV infection in young boys. Oral hairy leukoplakia, an early feature in pts with HIV infection that is characterized by raised white corrugated tongue lesions, is caused by EBV. A rare chronic form of EBV infection (distinct from chronic fatigue syndrome) is characterized by multiple organ involvement, including hepatosplenomegaly, lymphadenopathy, and pneumonitis, uveitis, or neurologic disease.

EBV-Associated Malignancy   First described in association with 90% of cases of African Burkitt's lymphoma, EBV has been associated with American Burkitt's lymphoma (15% of cases), anaplastic nasopharyngeal carcinoma, and B cell lymphomas, especially in pts immunosuppressed as a result of organ allografts, ataxia-telangiectasia, and AIDS.

DIAGNOSIS   A relative and absolute lymphocytosis is detected in about 75% of pts with IM and peaks in the second and third weeks of illness. Heterophile antibodies (antibodies to sheep, horse, or cow erythrocytes, which can be removed by absorption with guinea pig kidney cells) are present in 40% of pts with IM during the first week and in 80–90% during the third week. Monospot tests may be slightly more sensitive than heterophile titers. While more specific EBV antibodies can be measured, these studies are rarely required for the diagnosis of IM except in heterophile-negative or atypical cases. IgM antibodies to viral capsid antigen (VCA) are diagnostic of primary EBV infection and persist for only 2 months; IgG antibodies to VCA develop early in infection and persist for life. Antibodies to Epstein-Barr nuclear antigen (EBNA) appear at about 6–8 weeks and persist for life. The presence of IgM antibody to VCA and seroconversion to EBNA are diagnostic of primary EBV infection.

Rx **TREATMENT**

The treatment of IM is supportive. Excessive physical activity (e.g., contact sports) should be avoided for 6–8 weeks to avert splenic rupture. Glucocorticoids are indicated for airway obstruction and severe hemolytic anemia or thrombocytopenia. Occasional pts with protracted illness also may benefit from a short course of prednisone, but routine steroid use is not advised.

For a more detailed discussion, see Cohen JI: Epstein-Barr Virus Infections, Including Infectious Mononucleosis, Chap. 186, p. 1089; and Hirsch MS: Cytomegalovirus and Human Herpesvirus Types 6, 7, and 8, Chap. 187, p. 1092, in HPIM-14.

96

INFLUENZA AND OTHER VIRAL RESPIRATORY DISEASES

INFLUENZA

ETIOLOGY Influenza viruses, members of the Orthomyxoviridae family, include types A, B, and C. Strains are designated according to the site of origin, isolate number, year of isolation, and (for influenza A virus) subtype, which is based on surface hemagglutinin (H) and neuraminidase (N) antigens. The genome of influenza A virus is segmented, consisting of eight single-stranded segments of RNA; this characteristic leads to a high frequency of gene reassortment.

EPIDEMIOLOGY Outbreaks of influenza occur virtually every year, although their extent and severity vary widely. Localized outbreaks take place at variable intervals, usually every 1–3 years, while global epidemics or pandemics have occurred approximately every 10–15 years since the 1918–1919 pandemic. The most extensive and severe outbreaks are caused by influenza A virus because of the propensity of its antigens to undergo variation. Major antigenic variations, referred to as *antigenic shifts,* likely arise from genome segment reassortment between viral strains, which results in the expression of a different H and/or N antigen. Minor variations, referred to as *antigenic drifts,* probably arise from point mutations. In human infections, three major H antigens (H1, H2, and H3) and two N antigens (N1 and N2) have been recognized. Epidemics of influenza A begin abruptly, peak over 2–3 weeks, generally last 2–3 months, and often subside rapidly. These epidemics take place almost exclusively during the winter months in the northern and southern hemispheres. Outbreaks of influenza B are generally less extensive and less severe. The H and N antigens of influenza B virus undergo less frequent and less extensive variation. Influenza B outbreaks are most common in schools and military camps. Influenza C virus appears to cause subclinical infection; the prevalence of antibody is high in the general population, but the virus is infrequently associated with human disease.

CLINICAL MANIFESTATIONS Influenza is an acute respiratory illness characterized by the abrupt onset of headache, fevers, chills, myalgia, malaise, cough, and sore throat. In uncomplicated influenza, the acute illness generally resolves over 2–5 d, and most pts largely recover within 1 week.

The major problem posed by influenza consists of its complications, the most common of which is pneumonia—primary influenza viral pneumonia, secondary bacterial pneumonia, or mixed viral and bacterial pneumonia. Primary influenza pneumonia is less common but more severe than secondary bacterial pneumonia. Pts fail to defervesce and develop progressive dyspnea and cough with scant sputum. Cyanosis eventually may ensue. CXR reveals diffuse interstitial infiltrates and/or acute respiratory distress syndrome. Pts with cardiac disease, especially mitral stenosis, appear to have a predilection for developing influenza pneumonia.

The hallmark of secondary bacterial pneumonia is the reappearance of fever, accompanied by productive cough and physical signs of consolidation, in a pt whose condition has improved for 2–3 d following acute influenza. *Streptococcus pneumoniae, Staphylococcus aureus,* and *Haemophilus influenzae* are common pathogens. Pts at particular risk for this complication include elderly individuals or persons with chronic pulmonary or cardiac disease.

Mixed viral and bacterial pneumonia may be the most common pneumonic complication and has clinical features of both primary and secondary pneumonia.

Extrapulmonary complications include Reye's syndrome, myositis, rhabdomyolysis, and myoglobinuria. Encephalitis, transverse myelitis, and Guillain-Barré syndrome have been associated with influenza, but an etiologic role for influenza virus has not been established in these conditions. Reye's syndrome occurs in children 2–16 years of age as a serious complication of influenza B or—less often—of influenza A or varicella-zoster virus infection. The syndrome begins with 1–2 d of nausea and vomiting followed by CNS symptoms, including changes in mental status that range from lethargy to coma and can encompass delirium and seizures. Elevated serum aminotransferase levels, elevated serum ammonia concentrations, and hepatomegaly are common; serum bilirubin levels are usually normal. An epidemiologic association of Reye's syndrome with the ingestion of aspirin has been noted, and the incidence of Reye's syndrome has declined markedly with widespread warnings about aspirin use in children with viral infections.

DIAGNOSIS Influenza can be diagnosed during its acute phase by isolation of virus from throat swabs, nasopharyngeal washes, or sputum in tissue culture within 48–72 h after inoculation. Viral antigens may be detected somewhat earlier by immunodiagnostic techniques in tissue culture or in exfoliated nasopharyngeal cells obtained by washings, although these techniques are less sensitive than viral isolation. Acute infection can be diagnosed retrospectively by fourfold or greater rises in titers of hemagglutination inhibition or complement fixation antibody or by significant rises in ELISA antibody between the acute illness and 10–14 d after onset.

R̲ TREATMENT

Treatment for uncomplicated influenza is for relief of symptoms only. Salicylates should be avoided in children (<18 years old) because of the association of their use with Reye's syndrome. Amantadine (200 mg/d PO for 3–7 d) reduces the duration of systemic and respiratory symptoms by 50% if given within 48 h of onset. Amantadine is active only against influenza A virus and causes mild CNS side effects (jitteriness, anxiety, insomnia, difficulty concentrating) in 5–10% of pts. Rimantadine, given at the same dose as amantadine, appears to be equally efficacious and less frequently causes CNS side effects. Both agents are given at a reduced dose of 100 mg/d to the elderly and to persons with renal insufficiency. Ribavirin has been reported to be effective against both type A and type B viruses when administered as an aerosol but is relatively ineffective when administered orally. It is not known whether these antiviral agents are effective in the treatment of complications such as influenza pneumonia. Antibacterial therapy should be reserved for bacterial complications of influenza, such as bacterial pneumonia.

PROPHYLAXIS The most common preventive measure is yearly vaccination against influenza A and B; an inactivated vaccine derived from strains circulating the previous year is used. Individuals for whom vaccination is recommended include pts >6 months of age with chronic pulmonary or cardiovascular disorders, residents of nursing homes or chronic care facilities, pts >65 years old, health care providers, and pts with diabetes, renal disease, hemoglobinopathies, or immunosuppression. Individuals who care for high-risk pts or who come into frequent contact with them (including household members) should also be vaccinated to reduce the risk of transmission. Since the vaccine is "killed," it may be administered to immunosuppressed pts. Live attenuated ("cold-adapted") influenza A vaccines for intranasal administration appear promising in ongoing trials in adults and children. Amantadine and rimantadine are also effective for prophylaxis of influenza A but must be administered daily. Amantadine (200 mg/d PO) is used most frequently during outbreaks that are more severe than anticipated; the drug can be given simultaneously with vaccine and subsequently until antibody to the vaccine has been made. In addition, amantadine can be used during an outbreak caused by a strain of influenza A virus not included in or not well covered by the yearly vaccine.

OUTPATIENT AND HOME CARE CONSIDERATIONS
Most pts with acute influenza can be cared for at home. Hospitalization is generally reserved for those who develop complications such as primary or secondary pneumonia.

OTHER VIRAL RESPIRATORY INFECTIONS

Acute viral respiratory illnesses are among the most common of human diseases, accounting for one-half or more of all acute illnesses.

Rhinovirus

Rhinoviruses, members of the Picornaviridae family, are small and nonenveloped and have a single-stranded RNA genome. One hundred distinct serotypes of rhinovirus have been recognized.

EPIDEMIOLOGY Rhinoviruses are a prominent cause of the common cold, with seasonal peaks in the early fall and spring. Infection rates are highest among infants and young children and decrease with age. The infection is spread by contact with infected secretions or respiratory droplets or by hand-to-hand contact, with autoinoculation of the conjunctival or nasal mucosa.

CLINICAL MANIFESTATIONS After an incubation period of 1–2 d, pts develop rhinorrhea, sneezing, nasal congestion, and sore throat. Systemic symptoms, including fever, are unusual. The illness generally lasts 4–9 d and resolves spontaneously. Although bronchitis, bronchiolitis, and bronchopneumonia have been reported in children, rhinoviruses are not a major cause of pediatric lower respiratory tract disease. Rhinoviruses may cause exacerbations of asthma and chronic pulmonary disease in adults.

DIAGNOSIS Because of the mild nature and short duration of the illness, a specific diagnosis is not commonly needed; however, viral cultures can be performed.

℞ TREATMENT
Treatment is not usually required, and no specific antiviral therapy is available.

Coronavirus

Coronaviruses are pleomorphic, single-stranded RNA viruses.

EPIDEMIOLOGY   Coronaviruses account for 10–20% of common colds. They are most active in late fall, winter, and early spring—a period when rhinovirus is relatively inactive.

CLINICAL MANIFESTATIONS   Symptoms are similar to those of rhinovirus infections, but the incubation period is longer (3 d). The illness usually lasts 6–7 d.

Respiratory Syncytial Virus

Respiratory syncytial virus (RSV) is an enveloped virus of the Paramyxoviridae family with a single-stranded RNA genome. Two distinct subtypes, A and B, have been described.

EPIDEMIOLOGY   RSV is the major respiratory pathogen of young children and is the foremost cause of lower respiratory disease in infants. Rates of illness peak at 2–3 months of age, when attack rates among susceptible individuals approach 100%. RSV accounts for 20–25% of hospital admissions of infants and young children for pneumonia and for up to 75% of cases of bronchiolitis in this age group. This virus is an important nosocomial pathogen in both children and adults. It is transmitted by close contact with contaminated fingers or fomites as well as through coarse (not fine) aerosols produced by coughing or sneezing. The incubation period is 4–6 d; viral shedding by children may last 2 weeks or longer and that by adults for shorter periods.

CLINICAL MANIFESTATIONS   In infants, RSV disease begins with rhinorrhea, low-grade fever, and mild systemic symptoms, often accompanied by cough and wheezing; 25–40% of cases include lower respiratory tract involvement. RSV illness is especially severe in pts with congenital cardiac disease; the mortality rate for RSV pneumonia among these pts is 37%. In adults, the symptoms of RSV infection are usually the same as those of the common cold. RSV can cause severe pneumonia in immunocompromised or elderly adults.

DIAGNOSIS   RSV can be isolated in tissue cultures. Immunofluorescence microscopy of nasal washings or scrapings provides a rapid diagnosis.

℞ TREATMENT

Treatment with aerosolized ribavirin has demonstrated benefit in infants with RSV infection. No data exist for treatment in adults.

PROPHYLAXIS Prophylactic administration of immuno-globulins with high titers of RSV antibodies has been shown to reduce the incidence and severity of lower respiratory disease in high-risk infants. No data exist for prophylaxis in adults.

Parainfluenza Virus

Parainfluenza viruses are single-stranded RNA viruses of the Paramyxoviridae family.

EPIDEMIOLOGY In the U.S., parainfluenza viruses cause 4–22% of respiratory illnesses in children. Parainfluenza virus is an important cause of mild illnesses and of croup (laryngotra-cheobronchitis), bronchiolitis, and pneumonia. In young children, parainfluenza virus ranks second only to RSV as a cause of lower respiratory infection. In adults, parainfluenza infections are generally mild and account for <5% of respiratory illnesses.

CLINICAL MANIFESTATIONS In adults and older children, parainfluenza virus infection presents as a mild common cold or hoarseness with cough. In young children, it may present as an acute febrile illness with coryza, sore throat, hoarseness, and cough. The brassy or barking cough of croup may progress to frank stridor. Most children recover in 1–2 d, but progressive airway obstruction and hypoxia occasionally ensue, and bronchiolitis or pneumonia may develop. Severe or even fatal infection has been reported in both children and adults with profound immunosuppression.

DIAGNOSIS The diagnosis is established by isolation of the virus from respiratory tract secretions, throat swabs, or nasopharyngeal washings or by immunofluorescence microscopy of exfoliated respiratory cells.

℞ TREATMENT
In mild illness, treatment is symptom-based. Mild croup may be treated with moisturized air from a vaporizer. More severe cases require hospitalization and close observation for development of respiratory distress. No specific antiviral treatment is available.

Adenovirus

Adenoviruses are complex DNA viruses.

EPIDEMIOLOGY Infections with adenovirus occur most frequently in infants and children, with a seasonal distribution of fall to spring. Certain serotypes are associated with outbreaks of acute respiratory disease in military recruits. Transmission can take place via the inhalation of aerosolized virus, through the inoculation of the conjunctival sacs, and probably by the fecal-oral route.

CLINICAL MANIFESTATIONS   The spectrum of clinical symptoms in children includes rhinitis, pharyngoconjunctival fever (bilateral conjunctivitis, low-grade fever, rhinitis, sore throat, and cervical adenopathy), and occasional cases of bronchiolitis and pneumonia. In adults, the most frequent syndrome is the acute respiratory disease seen in military recruits, with prominent sore throat, fever on the second or third day of illness, cough, coryza, and regional lymphadenopathy. Adenoviruses also have been associated with pneumonia in immunosuppressed pts (including pts with AIDS) and with diseases outside the respiratory tract, including acute diarrhea in young children, hemorrhagic cystitis, and epidemic keratoconjunctivitis.

DIAGNOSIS AND TREATMENT   The diagnosis is established by isolation of the virus. No specific antiviral therapy is available. A live oral vaccine is available and used widely to prevent outbreaks among military recruits. Purified subunit vaccines are under investigation.

For a more detailed discussion, see Dolin R: Influenza, Chap. 193, p. 1112; and Dolin R: Common Viral Respiratory Infections, Chap. 191, p. 1100, in HPIM-14.

97

RUBEOLA, RUBELLA, MUMPS, AND PARVOVIRUS INFECTIONS

MEASLES (RUBEOLA)

Measles is a highly contagious acute respiratory disease with a characteristic clinical picture and a pathognomonic enanthem. Measles virus is a member of the family Paramyxoviridae.

EPIDEMIOLOGY   Measles has a worldwide distribution. The disease is transmitted by direct transfer of nasopharyngeal secretions or in airborne droplets. It is highly contagious: an infected individual can transmit the virus during a period from 5 d after exposure to 5 d after the appearance of skin lesions. In the U.S., the number of cases decreased progressively after the advent of routine childhood vaccination, but in the recent past, the number of cases again increased substantially (particularly in 1990, when 28,000 cases occurred). However, by 1993, the disease was once again brought under control, with only 312 cases reported to the CDC in 1993. Outbreaks have involved not only unvaccinated infants and preschool children but also high school and college students with vaccination rates of >95%.

CLINICAL MANIFESTATIONS   The incubation period for measles is 8–12 d. Pts first experience 3–4 d of prodromal symptoms, including malaise, irritability, fever, conjunctivitis with excessive lacrimation, edema of the eyelids, photophobia, hacking cough, and nasal discharge. Koplik's spots, which are pathognomonic for measles, appear 1–2 d before the onset of rash and are small, red, irregular lesions with blue-white centers found on mucous membranes, especially opposite the second molars. The rash of measles appears first on the forehead and spreads downward over the face, neck, trunk, and feet. The lesions are erythematous maculopapules that coalesce over the face and upper trunk. Most other symptoms resolve within 1–2 d of the appearance of rash, but cough may persist.

Measles is usually a self-limited disease, but a number of complications may ensue. Important complications include croup, bronchitis, and bronchiolitis; rare instances of interstitial giant cell pneumonia in immunocompromised children; conjunctivitis with progression to corneal ulceration, keratitis, and blindness; myocarditis; hepatitis; transient acute glomerulonephritis; bacterial pneumonia; and encephalomyelitis. This last complication, with headache, high fever, drowsiness, and coma, occurs in 1 of every 1000 pts 4–7 d after the appearance of rash; the mortality rate is 10%. An extremely rare condition, subacute sclerosing panencephalitis, is a late complication of measles.

Atypical measles can develop in pts who have received formalin-inactivated measles vaccine and can present with a variety of rashes; pneumonia and high fever are common. Despite the severity of atypical measles, pts invariably recover after a convalescence that may be prolonged.

DIAGNOSIS Lymphopenia and neutropenia are common in measles; leukocytosis may herald a bacterial superinfection. Measles virus can be isolated by inoculation of sputum, nasal secretions, or urine onto cell cultures. Immunofluorescent antibody staining of infected respiratory or urinary epithelial cells can detect measles antigen. Serologic tests include complement fixation, enzyme immunoassay, immunofluorescence, and hemagglutination inhibition assays. Specific IgM antibodies are detectable within 1–2 d after the appearance of a rash, and IgG titers rise significantly after 10 d.

℞ TREATMENT
No therapy is indicated for uncomplicated measles. Clinical trials suggest benefit from high doses of vitamin A in severe or potentially severe measles, especially in children <2 years of age; a dose of 200,000 IU is used for children >1 year of age. Ribavirin is effective against measles virus in vitro and may be considered for use in immunocompromised individuals.

PREVENTION Measles should be controlled by vaccination. Live attenuated measles vaccine is given as part of the measles-mumps-rubella (MMR) vaccine at 12–15 months of age and again at either 4–5 years of age (CDC) or 12 years of age (American Academy of Pediatrics). Vaccine can also be given as prophylaxis within 3 d of exposure. Pts who received killed measles vaccine between 1963 and 1967 should be considered unprotected and are at risk for atypical measles. Pts infected with HIV who are susceptible should be vaccinated against measles; actively immunosuppressed pts should not receive live vaccine. Gamma globulin (0.25 mL/kg, not to exceed 15 mL) modifies or prevents acquisition of measles if given within 6 d of exposure.

RUBELLA (GERMAN MEASLES)

Rubella is an acute viral infection that characteristically includes rash, fever, and lymphadenopathy and has a broad spectrum of other possible manifestations. Rubella virus, a togavirus, is closely related to the alphaviruses.

CLINICAL MANIFESTATIONS The time from exposure to appearance of the rash is 14–21 d. In adults, a prodrome of malaise, headache, fever, mild conjunctivitis, and lymphadenopathy may precede the rash by 1–7 d; children may present with a rash before these other symptoms develop. Subclinical infection is common. The distribution of the rash in rubella is the same as that in measles, but lesions are lighter in hue in rubella and are usually discrete. Enlarged, tender lymph nodes become apparent before onset of the rash and are most impressive during the eruptive phase; postauricular and suboccipital nodes are strikingly involved. Arthralgias and slight swelling of the joints sometimes accompany rubella, especially in young women, and may persist for 1–14 d after other manifestations have disappeared. Recurrences of joint symptoms for a year or more have been reported.

The most important factor in the pathogenicity of rubella virus for the fetus is gestational age at the time of infection. Maternal infection in the first trimester is most dangerous, leading to fetal infection in about half of cases. The congenital rubella syndrome consists of heart malformations (patent ductus arteriosus, interventricular septal defect, or pulmonic stenosis), eye lesions (corneal clouding, cataracts, chorioretinitis, and microphthalmia), microcephaly, and deafness. The "expanded" rubella syndrome was defined after an American epidemic in 1964 and includes mental retardation, thrombocytopenic purpura, hepatosplenomegaly, intrauterine growth retardation, interstitial pneumonia, myocarditis or myocardial necrosis, and metaphyseal bone lesions as well as the previously described manifestations.

DIAGNOSIS The diagnosis is made by isolation of virus or changes in antibody titers. The most commonly used test is an ELISA for IgG and IgM antibodies. Rubella antibodies may be detectable by the second day of rash and increase in titer over the next 10–21 d. Biopsied tissues and/or blood and CSF have also been used for demonstrating rubella antigens with monoclonal antibodies and for detection of rubella RNA by in situ hybridization and polymerase chain reaction.

TREATMENT AND PREVENTION Rubella is a mild illness that does not require treatment. It is prevented by vaccination, the goal of which is the elimination of congenital infection. Live attenuated rubella vaccine is given as part of the MMR vaccine. Vaccination is contraindicated in immunosuppressed pts but is given to children with HIV infection. Although no cases of congenital rubella syndrome have occurred in women inadvertently vaccinated during pregnancy, the vaccine should not be administered to pregnant women or to women who might become pregnant within 3 months.

MUMPS

Mumps is an acute, systemic, communicable viral infection whose most distinctive feature is a swelling of one or both parotid glands. The etiologic agent is a paramyxovirus.

ETIOLOGY AND EPIDEMIOLOGY Humans are the only reservoir for mumps virus. In 1968 (before widespread immunization), 152,209 cases of mumps were reported in the U.S. The 1537 cases reported in 1994 represent a reduction in the number of cases by >99% from prevaccine levels. The incubation period for mumps is generally 14–18 d. Infection tends to occur in the spring, with an especially high frequency in April and May. The virus is transmitted in infected salivary secretions but may be spread via urine as well. Infectivity is greatest from 1 or 2 d before the onset of parotitis to 5 d after the appearance of glandular enlargement; pts generally are no longer contagious 9 d after the onset of parotid swelling.

CLINICAL MANIFESTATIONS *Salivary Adenitis* There is frequently a prodrome of fever, myalgia, malaise, and anorexia. The onset of parotitis is usually sudden and in many cases is the first sign of illness. Pain and tenderness are generally marked; warmth and erythema are unusual. In two-thirds of cases, swelling is bilateral, although the onset on the two sides may not be synchronous. The submaxillary and sublingual glands are involved less often than the parotid glands and are almost never involved alone.

Epididymoorchitis Orchitis is a complication of mumps in 20–30% of postpubertal males. Testicular involvement, which is bilateral in 3–17% of cases, usually appears 7–10 d after the onset of parotitis but may precede it or develop simultaneously. Occasionally, mumps orchitis occurs without parotitis. The testicle becomes swollen to several times its normal size and is acutely painful, with accompanying high fevers, shaking chills, malaise, and headache. In 50% of cases, orchitis is followed by atrophy; even with bilateral involvement, sterility is rare in the absence of atrophy. Oophoritis in women is far less common than orchitis in men.

Pancreatitis Pts with pancreatic involvement develop abdominal pain and tenderness; shock and pseudocyst formation are rare. While serum amylase levels are elevated in parotitis as well as in mumps pancreatitis, serum lipase levels are increased only in the latter.

CNS Involvement About 60% of pts with clinical mumps have lymphocytic pleocytosis of the CSF, with up to 1000 cells/μL; 10% have symptoms of meningitis (headache, stiff neck, drowsiness). CNS symptoms tend to occur 3–10 d after onset of parotitis; in 30–40% of laboratory-proven cases, parotitis is absent. True encephalitis is unusual. Mumps can produce mild paralytic poliomyelitis and, in rare cases, transverse myelitis, cerebellar ataxia, or Guillain-Barré syndrome.

Other Manifestations Mumps virus can cause subacute thyroiditis, ocular manifestations (dacryoadenitis, optic neuritis, keratitis, iritis, conjunctivitis, and episcleritis), myocarditis, hepatitis (without jaundice), thrombocytopenic purpura, interstitial pneumonia (in young children), polyarthritis, and acute hemorrhagic glomerulonephritis.

DIAGNOSIS In uncomplicated parotitis, there may be mild leukopenia with relative lymphocytosis. When orchitis develops, WBC counts rise markedly, with a left shift. Definitive diagnosis depends on isolation of the virus from blood, throat swabs, or secretions from Stensen's duct, CSF, or urine. Rapid diagnosis can be made by immunofluorescence assay for viral antigen in oropharyngeal cells. The best serologic test is the ELISA. Acute mumps can be diagnosed either by examination of acute- and convalescent-phase sera for an increase in antibody titer or by demonstration of specific IgM in one serum specimen.

℞ **TREATMENT**

No treatment is generally needed. While its effectiveness has not been demonstrated in controlled studies, prednisone (60 mg qd tapered over 7–10 d) has been used in orchitis. Anecdotal information on a small number of pts with orchitis suggests that the administration of interferon α may be helpful.

PREVENTION Live attenuated mumps vaccine is administered at 15 months of age as part of the MMR vaccine. Vaccination is contraindicated for pts with a febrile illness or malignancy and for pregnant women. Children with HIV infection can be safely immunized against mumps.

PARVOVIRUS

ETIOLOGY One parvovirus, designated B19, is known to be a human pathogen. It is a small, nonenveloped, single-stranded DNA virus.

EPIDEMIOLOGY Outbreaks of erythema infectiosum occur in schools during winter and spring months. Symptomatic infection occurs in 20–60% of children in outbreaks; 10% of infections are asymptomatic. Pts with transient aplastic crisis are highly infectious. The route of transmission of parvovirus B19 is unknown but may be respiratory or through direct contact.

CLINICAL MANIFESTATIONS *Erythema Infectiosum*
Erythema infectiosum, or fifth disease, is the most common manifestation of parvovirus B19 infection and is seen predominantly in children. The typical presentation is a facial rash with a "slapped cheek" appearance, sometimes preceded by low-grade fever. The rash also develops on the arms and legs, with a lacy, reticular, erythematous appearance. Arthralgias and arthritis are uncommon in children but common in adults; rash is often absent or nonspecific in adults.

Arthropathy Parvovirus B19 infection in adults most often involves arthralgias and arthritis, sometimes accompanied by rash. Wrists, hands, and knees are most frequently involved in symmetric, nondestructive arthritis. Symptoms usually last about 3 weeks but may persist for months (or even years) in a small percentage of cases.

Transient Aplastic Crisis This syndrome develops in pts with chronic hemolytic disease, including sickle cell disease, erythrocyte enzyme deficiencies, hereditary spherocytosis, thalassemias, paroxysmal nocturnal hemoglobinuria, and autoimmune hemolysis. Pts develop sudden, severe anemia that can be life-threatening and can be accompanied by weakness, lethargy, and pallor. Bone marrow examination reveals an absence of erythrocyte precursors despite a normal myeloid series. Reticulocytopenia usually lasts for 7–10 d. Unlike pts with fifth disease or arthritis, these pts are viremic and infectious.

Chronic Anemia Immunodeficient pts—e.g., those with HIV infection, congenital immunodeficiencies, or acute lymphocytic leukemia (during maintenance chemotherapy)—and recipients of bone marrow transplants may develop chronic, transfusion-dependent anemia due to parvovirus B19 infection, with destruction of erythroid precursors in the bone marrow.

Fetal Infection Maternal infection usually does not adversely affect the fetus. Parents should be counseled as to the relatively low risk of infection to the fetus. Fewer than 10% of maternal B19 infections lead to fetal death; when fetal death occurs, the cause is nonimmune hydrops fetalis. There is no evidence that B19 infection causes congenital anomalies. Exposure of a pregnant woman to a child with fifth disease is unlikely to result in maternal infection, since the infectious stage of illness is probably over by the time the rash develops. Pregnant women with known exposure to B19 virus should have their serum monitored for IgM antibodies to the virus and for alpha-fetoprotein levels, and ultrasonic examinations of the fetus for hydrops should be conducted. Some hydropic fetuses survive B19 infection and appear normal at delivery.

DIAGNOSIS Diagnosis relies on measurements of parvovirus B19–specific IgM and IgG antibodies. Pts with transient aplastic crisis may have IgM antibodies but nevertheless usually have high titers of virus and viral DNA in serum. Immunodeficient pts with chronic anemia lack antibody but have viral particles and viral DNA in serum. Viral DNA may be detected in amniotic fluid or fetal blood in cases of hydrops fetalis. Fetal infection may be recognized by hydrops fetalis and the presence of B19 DNA in amniotic fluid or fetal blood in association with maternal IgM antibodies to B19 virus.

℞ **TREATMENT**
Erythema infectiosum requires no treatment; arthritis can be treated with NSAIDs. Transient aplastic crisis is usually treated with erythrocyte transfusions. Anemia in immunodeficient pts appears to respond to treatment with commercial IV gamma globulin.

PREVENTION Prophylaxis of B19 infection with immunoglobulin should be considered for pts with chronic hemolysis or immunodeficiency and for pregnant women. Pts hospitalized with transient aplastic crisis or chronic anemia that is suspected of being related to parvovirus B19 should be put in private rooms and managed with contact and respiratory isolation precautions.

For a more detailed discussion, see Gershon A: Measles (Rubeola), Chap. 196, p. 1123; Rubella (German Measles), Chap. 197, p. 1125; and Mumps, Chap. 198, p. 1127; Blacklow NR: Parvovirus, Chap. 189, p. 1096, in HPIM-14.

98

ENTEROVIRAL INFECTIONS

Enteroviruses belong to the family of small, nonenveloped viruses with single-stranded RNA called *picornaviruses.* Their stability allows these viruses to survive in the presence of acid and standard disinfectants and to persist for days at room temperature. Enteroviruses include polioviruses, coxsackieviruses, echoviruses, and recently discovered agents so far designated simply as enteroviruses. Nearly 70 serotypes are known to infect humans via intestinal tract epithelium and lymphoid tissue. Although enteroviruses are shed in stool, the clinical syndromes they cause are not gastrointestinal.

EPIDEMIOLOGY Enteroviruses are distributed worldwide and commonly cause asymptomatic infection. In temperate climates, most infections occur in the late summer and fall. The common mode of transmission is via direct or indirect fecal-oral spread. Incubation periods can be 2–14 d long but generally last for <1 week. More is known about poliovirus than about other enteroviruses. Poliovirus can persist in the oropharynx for up to 3 weeks after infection and can be shed in stool for up to 8 weeks; shedding by immunocompromised pts can persist for much longer.

POLIOVIRUS INFECTIONS

PATHOGENESIS After ingestion, poliovirus is thought to infect epithelial cells in the mucosa of the GI tract and then to spread to submucosal lymphoid tissue. After spread to regional lymph nodes, the first (minor) viremic phase occurs, with replication in organs of the reticuloendothelial system. In some cases a secondary (major) viremic phase occurs. Virus enters the CNS either during viremia or via peripheral nerves.

CLINICAL MANIFESTATIONS Most poliovirus infections are mild or asymptomatic. Disease falls into three classes: (1) abortive poliomyelitis, a nonspecific febrile illness of 2–3 days' duration with no signs of CNS localization; (2) nonparalytic poliomyelitis, aseptic meningitis with complete recovery in a few days (about 1% of pts); and (3) paralytic poliomyelitis, the least common presentation. After one or several days, signs of aseptic meningitis are followed by severe back, neck, and muscle pain and by the development of motor weakness. In some cases the disease appears to be biphasic, with a period of apparent recovery following the aseptic meningitis. Weakness is generally asymmetric and may involve the legs, the arms, or the abdominal, thoracic, or bulbar muscles. Paralytic disease is more common among older individuals, pregnant women, and persons with muscle trauma (including that incurred by strenuous exercise) at the time of CNS symptoms. Paralysis develops during the febrile phase of the illness, and many pts recover some or all function. Findings include weakness, fasciculations, and absent or decreased deep-tendon reflexes; sensation is intact. Postpolio syndrome consists of progressive muscle weakness beginning 20–30 years after the original infection and is thought not to involve persistent or reactivated infection.

COXSACKIEVIRUS, ECHOVIRUS, AND OTHER ENTEROVIRAL INFECTIONS

Between 5 and 10 million symptomatic enteroviral infections occur in the U.S. each year, with different serotypes accounting for different types of disease.

CLINICAL MANIFESTATIONS *Nonspecific Febrile Illness* In contrast to other respiratory viral infections, enteroviral febrile illness generally occurs in the summer. After an incubation period of 3–6 d, pts present with an acute onset of fever, malaise, and headache, often accompanied by upper respiratory symptoms and sometimes by nausea and vomiting. Symptoms generally persist for 3–4 d; most resolve within a week.

Aseptic Meningitis Enteroviruses cause up to 90% of the cases of aseptic meningitis in children and young adults in which an etiology is identified. Pts present with fever, headache, photophobia, and stiff neck and may have signs of meningeal irritation and drowsiness or irritability but no localizing neurologic findings. CSF analysis shows pleocytosis, with an early predominance of PMNs sometimes making it difficult to exclude a diagnosis of bacterial meningitis (particularly if the infection has been partially treated). In enteroviral meningitis, a shift to lymphocyte predominance occurs within 24 h of presentation, and the total WBC count is generally <1000/μl. The CSF glucose level is usually normal, and the CSF protein concentration is normal or only slightly elevated. Symptoms generally resolve within a week, but CSF abnormalities may persist for several weeks. Enteroviral encephalitis occurs less commonly and generally carries a good prognosis except in immunocompromised pts, who may develop chronic meningitis or encephalitis.

Acute Myocarditis/Pericarditis Enteroviruses, most commonly coxsackievirus B, cause an estimated one-third of cases of acute myocarditis/pericarditis.

Generalized Disease of the Newborn Enteroviral infection of the heart, liver, adrenals, brain, and other organs may resemble bacterial sepsis and is highly lethal. Most disease occurs during the first week of life, although cases may occur up to 3 months of age.

Herpangina Usually caused by coxsackievirus A serotypes, herpangina involves mucous membranes and is characterized by the acute onset of fever and sore throat and the appearance of small white papules or vesicles over the posterior half of the palate.

Pleurodynia (Bornholm Disease) An acute onset of fever and intense lower thoracic or abdominal pain aggravated by breathing or movement characterizes this syndrome, which is usually caused by coxsackievirus B.

Hand-Foot-and-Mouth Disease This illness, often caused by coxsackievirus A16, is characterized by fever, anorexia, and malaise followed by the development of vesicular lesions in the oral cavity and on the dorsum or palm of the hands.

Other Illnesses Enteroviruses commonly cause exanthems in children in summer and early fall. A sudden onset of severe eye pain, blurred vision, photophobia, and watery discharge from the eye characterizes acute hemorrhagic enteroviral conjunctivitis, which is often caused by enterovirus 70 and coxsackievirus A24. Enteroviruses are uncommon causes of childhood pneumonia and the common cold.

DIAGNOSIS Enteroviral infections are most often diagnosed by isolation of virus from throat swabs, stool, or rectal swabs. However, isolation of virus from these sites does not prove an association with disease since many pts with subclinical infections are colonized. Isolation of virus from normally sterile body fluids (CSF, pleural or pericardial fluid) or from tissues is less common but diagnostic. PCR of CSF is highly sensitive and specific and is more rapid than culture. Serologic testing is usually reserved for critical cases or epidemiologic studies since the large number of serotypes makes it expensive and cumbersome.

TREATMENT AND PREVENTION *Treatment* is supportive and directed at symptoms. Glucocorticoids are contraindicated. For polio, prevention is key. Two vaccines are licensed in the U.S.—inactivated and live, oral, attenuated. Oral polio vaccine (OPV) offers several advantages, including ease of administration, low cost, high efficacy, and induction of intestinal immunity. However, vaccine-associated paralytic poliomyelitis occurs at a rate of about 1 case per 2.6 million doses of

OPV (a figure accounting for all cases of paralytic polio in the U.S.), and OPV must be avoided in immunosuppressed pts, including those infected with HIV and their family members. Inactivated vaccine (IPV-e) is administered subcutaneously and is recommended for adults and immunocompromised individuals. In 1996, the CDC recommended that children receive a sequential schedule of two doses of IPV-e followed by two doses of OPV. This strategy is expected to reduce the number of vaccine-associated poliomyelitis cases by 50–75%. A four-dose regimen of either vaccine is also considered acceptable and may be preferable in some circumstances.

For a more detailed discussion, see Cohen JI: Enteroviruses and Reoviruses, Chap. 195, p. 1118, in HPIM-14.

99

INSECT- AND ANIMAL-BORNE VIRAL INFECTIONS

RABIES

Rabies virus is an enveloped, single-stranded RNA virus belonging to the rhabdovirus group. The binding of viral glycoproteins to acetylcholine receptors contributes to neurovirulence.

EPIDEMIOLOGY   Rabies is rare in the U.S. and usually arises from an animal bite inflicted in another country. Southeast Asia, the Philippines, Africa, the Indian subcontinent, and tropical South America are areas in which rabies is common. In the U.S., 85% of cases of animal rabies occur in wildlife, especially raccoons, bats, skunks, and foxes; 3% of cases occur in domestic cats and 2% in domestic dogs. Cat rabies is now reported more frequently than dog rabies. A few cases of person-to-person rabies transmission via corneal transplantation have been reported. The virus generally is transmitted in saliva. The incubation time for rabies is variable, probably depending on the amount of virus introduced, the distance of the inoculation from the CNS, and the host's defense status. The mean incubation time is 1–2 months, but the range is 10 d to >1 year.

CLINICAL MANIFESTATIONS A *prodromal* period of 1-4 d is marked by fever, headache, malaise, myalgias, increased fatigability, anorexia, nausea and vomiting, sore throat, and nonproductive cough. Paresthesia and/or fasciculations at or near the site of viral inoculation are found in 50–80% of cases in the prodromal stage and constitute the only symptom suggestive of rabies. An *encephalitic* phase follows, with periods of excessive motor activity, excitation, and agitation. Confusion, combativeness, aberrations of thought, muscle spasms, seizures, focal paralysis, and fever are interspersed with shortening periods of lucidity. Hyperesthesia and autonomic dysfunction, with manifestations including dilated irregular pupils, increased lacrimation, salivation, perspiration, and postural hypotension, are common. *Brainstem dysfunction* becomes apparent shortly after the encephalitic phase begins. Manifestations include cranial nerve involvement (diplopia, facial palsies, optic neuritis, and difficulty with deglutition, which, combined with excessive salivation, produces characteristic "foaming at the mouth"); hydrophobia; painful violent involuntary contractions of the diaphragm and of accessory respiratory, pharyngeal, and laryngeal muscles initiated by swallowing liquids (seen in 50% of pts); priapism; and spontaneous ejaculation. The prominence of early brainstem dysfunction distinguishes rabies from other viral encephalitides. The median period of survival after the onset of symptoms is 4 d. With respiratory support, late complications may appear, including inappropriate secretion of vasopressin, diabetes insipidus, cardiac arrhythmias, vascular instability, ARDS, GI bleeding, thrombocytopenia, and paralytic ileus. Recovery is extremely rare.

DIAGNOSIS The specific diagnosis of rabies can be made by several techniques, including (1) isolation of the virus from saliva or brain tissue by mouse inoculation; (2) demonstration of viral antigen in infected tissue samples, such as corneal impression smears, skin biopsies, or brain biopsies, by fluorescent antibody (FA) staining; (3) a fourfold rise in neutralizing antibody titers; (4) histologic and/or electron-microscopic examination for Negri bodies; or (5) detection of rabies virus RNA by reverse transcription PCR. Pts receiving postexposure rabies prophylaxis usually have serum and CSF antibody titers of <1:64, whereas in human rabies, CSF antibody titers are generally >1:200.

TREATMENT AND PREVENTION A number of factors guide the decision to administer postexposure rabies prophylaxis. When an individual is exposed to saliva or another bodily fluid from an animal that might have rabies, the animal should be captured if possible. If the animal is wild, ill, unvaccinated, or a stray, it should be destroyed humanely and the brain submitted for FA examination. If the result is positive, the exposed party should receive globulin and vaccine. If the animal escapes and is of a species that is capable of carrying rabies (e.g., a bat, raccoon, skunk, or fox), the exposed individual should receive treatment. A healthy domestic animal that has inflicted a bite should be confined for 10 d of observation. If any illness or abnormal behavior develops in the animal, the brain should be subjected to FA examination; if the animal remains healthy, the bite is unlikely to have transmitted rabies.

Postexposure prophylaxis includes local wound treatment (careful washing with soap and water, administration of tetanus toxoid and antibiotics), passive immunization [human rabies immune globulin (HRIG), 20 U/kg, with 50% of the dose given by local infiltration into the wound and 50% injected into the gluteal region], and active immunization [human diploid cell vaccine (HDCV), five 1-mL doses IM on days 0, 3, 7, 14, and 28, respectively, after exposure]. An equine antiserum is also available for passive immunization at a dose of 40 U/kg but is more likely than human antiserum to result in serum sickness. Preexposure prophylaxis should be given to individuals at high risk of exposure, such as veterinarians, cave explorers, laboratory workers, and animal handlers. Three doses of HDCV (1 mL IM or 0.1 mL intradermally) are given on days 0, 7, and 28, respectively. Serologic testing should be conducted after the series and then every 2–6 years, depending on risk. When antibody titers fall below 1:5, a booster dose of HDCV (1 mL IM or 0.1 mL intradermally) should be given. Postexposure prophylaxis for those who have received preexposure prophylaxis consists of two doses of HDCV (1 mL IM) on days 0 and 3, respectively.

INFECTIONS CAUSED BY ARTHROPOD- AND RODENT-BORNE VIRUSES

Arthropod- and rodent-borne viruses are transmitted by a variety of vectors. Table 99-1 lists the syndromes and major viruses causing human disease in this category.

Viruses Causing Fever, Myalgia, and Rash

Fever, myalgia, and rash constitute the syndrome most commonly associated with zoonotic virus infection. The syndrome is caused by many agents belonging to the seven major families of zoonotic viruses. Typically, the syndrome begins with the

Table 99-1

Syndromes and Major Viruses Transmitted by Arthropods and Rodents

Syndrome	Virus
Fever and myalgia	Lymphocytic choriomeningitis
	Bunyamwera
	Group C
	Tahyna
	Oropouche
	Sandfly fever
	Toscana
	Punta Toro
	Dengue
	Colorado tick fever
	Orbivirus
	Vesicular stomatitis
Encephalitis	La Crosse
	St. Louis encephalitis
	Japanese encephalitis
	West Nile
	Central European tick-borne encephalitis
	Russian spring-summer encephalitis
	Powassan
	Eastern equine encephalitis
	Western equine encephalitis
	Venezuelan equine encephalitis

(*continued*)

abrupt onset of fever, chills, intense myalgia, and malaise. Arthralgias are frequent, but arthritis is not. Anorexia is characteristic and is frequently associated with nausea and vomiting. Headache may be severe. Some viruses cause a maculopapular rash and others aseptic meningitis. Most pts recover completely with only supportive therapy.

LYMPHOCYTIC CHORIOMENINGITIS (LCM) *Epidemiology* Mice are the primary host for LCM, which is worldwide in distribution. Human infections are secondary to contact with an infected rodent, with transmission thought to be via airborne spread or contact with infected excrement.

Table 99-1 (*Continued*)

Syndromes and Major Viruses Transmitted by Arthropods and Rodents

Syndrome	Virus
Arthritis and rash	Sindbis
	Chikungunya
	Mayaro
	Ross River
Hemorrhagic fever (HF)	Lassa
	South American HF
	Rift Valley fever
	Crimean Congo HF
	Hantavirus
	Hantaan
	Puumala
	Marburg
	Ebola
	Yellow fever
	Kyasanur Forest

Clinical Manifestations The most common clinical pattern is an influenza-like illness. In some pts the illness may be biphasic with subsequent aseptic meningitis or encephalitis. Fever develops in all cases. Malaise, weakness, myalgia (especially lumbar), retroorbital headache, photophobia, anorexia, nausea, and light-headedness are found in >50% of pts. Physical findings may include skin rash, pharyngeal injection without exudate, mild cervical or axillary lymphadenopathy, alopecia, or meningeal signs. Testicular pain or frank orchitis, usually unilateral, and parotid pain can lead to a misdiagnosis of mumps. Pts with aseptic meningitis generally recover without sequelae; 25–30% of pts with encephalitis have neurologic residua. In pregnant women, LCM virus infection may lead to congenital hydrocephalus and fetal chorioretinitis.

Diagnosis Leukopenia and thrombocytopenia are observed during the first week of illness. The CSF of pts with meningeal signs usually contains several hundred cells per microliter, with a lymphocytic predominance. In some series, 50% of pts have had CSF cell counts of >1000/μL. The CSF protein level is usually slightly elevated; unlike other viral meningitides, LCM tends to be associated with low CSF glucose levels (27%

of pts). Recovery of LCM virus from blood or spinal fluid requires a biosafety level 3 facility. The most direct method for the diagnosis of LCM, therefore, is IgM-capture ELISA of serum or CSF; recently, reverse transcription (RT)-PCR assays have been developed for application to CSF.

℞ TREATMENT
There is no specific treatment for LCM.

DENGUE Dengue viruses are flaviviruses. Four serotypes have been identified.

Epidemiology Dengue is transmitted by *Aedes* mosquitoes and is endemic over large areas of the tropics and subtropics, Asia, Oceania, Africa, Australia, and the Americas, including the Caribbean. Classic dengue, also known as breakbone fever, usually occurs in nonimmune individuals, children, and adults who do not reside in an indigenous area. Dengue hemorrhagic fever occurs almost exclusively in indigenous populations and is thought to be immunologically mediated.

Clinical Manifestations Dengue viruses frequently produce inapparent infection. When symptoms develop, three clinical patterns are seen: classic dengue, a mild atypical form, and hemorrhagic fever.

1. *Classic dengue:* After an incubation period of 5–8 d, a short prodrome of mild conjunctivitis or coryza may precede by a few hours the abrupt onset of severe headache, retroorbital pain, backache (especially lumbar), and leg and joint pains. Ocular soreness, anorexia, and weakness are common; cough is rare. Skin rashes that vary in appearance are common, as is lymphadenopathy. The fever may follow a diphasic course. The febrile illness usually lasts for 5–6 d and terminates abruptly.

2. *Atypical dengue:* Symptoms of mild atypical illness include fever, anorexia, headache, and myalgia. An evanescent rash may develop; lymphadenopathy is absent. Symptoms usually last for <72 h.

3. *Dengue hemorrhagic fever (DHF):* Illness begins abruptly with a relatively mild stage (2–4 d) consisting of fever, cough, pharyngitis, headache, anorexia, nausea, vomiting, and abdominal pain, which may be severe. Myalgia, arthralgia, and bone pain, which are common in classic dengue, are unusual in DHF. Hemorrhagic manifestations include a positive tourniquet test, petechiae, purpura, ecchymoses, epistaxis, bleeding gums, hematemesis, melena, enlargement of the liver, thrombocytopenia, hemoconcentration, and hematocrit increased by ≥20%.

Dengue shock syndrome is diagnosed when there is a rapid, weak pulse with narrowing of the pulse pressure to ≤20 mmHg or hypotension with cold, clammy skin and restlessness.

Diagnosis Primary viral isolation may be accomplished by inoculation of blood obtained in the first 3–5 d of illness into mosquitoes or mosquito tissue cell cultures. Serologic diagnosis can be made by IgM ELISA or testing of paired serum specimens during recovery or by antigen-detection ELISA or RT-PCR during the acute phase.

℞ TREATMENT

Treatment is supportive. Glucocorticoids are not effective. The use of heparin in DIC is controversial. Interferon was tried in Cuba with some indication of efficacy.

Arboviruses Causing Encephalitis

EPIDEMIOLOGY Since arboviruses causing encephalitis are transmitted by mosquitoes, infections occur during peak mosquito season (late spring to early fall). Table 99-2 lists features of the four predominant types of arboviral encephalitis in the U.S.

CLINICAL MANIFESTATIONS Features of arboviral encephalitis differ among age groups and depend on the specific infecting virus. In infants <1 year of age, the only consistent symptom is a sudden onset of fever, often accompanied by focal or generalized convulsions. Bulging fontanelles, rigidity of the extremities, and abnormal reflexes may also be seen. In children of 5–14 years, headache, fever, and drowsiness often precede by 2–3 d nausea, vomiting, muscular pain, photophobia, and (less frequently) convulsions. The children generally are acutely ill, are lethargic, and often have nuchal rigidity and intention tremors. In adults, initial symptoms include abrupt onset of fever, nausea with vomiting, and severe headache (usually frontal), followed in the next 24 h by confusion and disorientation. Disturbances in mentation are the most prominent neurologic findings, ranging from subtle abnormalities detected by cerebral function tests to coma. Other findings include tremor (most common among pts >40 years old), cranial nerve abnormalities, and reflex abnormalities (exaggerated palmomental reflexes and suck and snout reflexes). Fever and neurologic symptoms and signs vary in duration from several days to a month but usually last 4–14 d. Once fevers subside, clinical improvement usually follows within several days unless irreversible anatomic changes have occurred.

Table 99-2

Arboviral Encephalitides Common in the United States

Disease	Area of Predominance in the U.S.	Urban/Rural	Age, Years	Sex	Unique Clinical Features	Mortality, %	Residua
California encephalitis	Midwest	Rural	5–10	M	Seizures	2	Seizures (one-fourth in acute phase), behavioral problems (15%)
Eastern equine encephalitis	Eastern seaboard	Both	<5 >55	=	CSF may have >1000 WBCs/μL	50	Emotional lability, retardation, convulsions in children <10 years old
St. Louis encephalitis	East and Midwest	Both	>35	=	Dysuria	2–12	Ataxia, speech difficulties (5%)
Western equine encephalitis	Entire	Both	<1 >55	=	None	3	Behavioral problems, convulsions in children <3 months old

SOURCE: Modified from Sanford JP: HPIM-13, p. 843.

DIAGNOSIS CSF findings include pleocytosis (usually several hundred cells per microliter, but occasionally >1000 cells/μL), with an initial neutrophil predominance shifting after several days to a lymphocyte predominance. The CSF protein level is usually slightly elevated and may increase with time; the CSF glucose concentration is normal. A specific diagnosis rests on isolation of the virus or a rise in antibody level between acute- and convalescent-phase sera.

℞ TREATMENT
Treatment is supportive.

Alphaviruses Causing Arthritis and Rash

True arthritis is a common accompaniment of several viral diseases, such as rubella, parvovirus B19 infection, and hepatitis B. In addition, the alphaviruses cause true arthritis and a maculopapular rash.

SINDBIS VIRUS INFECTION *Epidemiology* Sindbis virus is transmitted among birds by mosquitoes. Infections with the northern European and genetically related southern African strains are particularly likely to cause an arthritis-rash syndrome.

Clinical Manifestations The incubation period is <1 week. Clinical symptoms begin with rash and arthralgia. The rash lasts about a week and spreads from the trunk to the extremities, evolving from macules to papules that frequently vesiculate. The arthritis is multiarticular, migratory, and incapacitating.

℞ TREATMENT
There is no specific therapy.

CHIKUNGUNYA VIRUS INFECTION *Epidemiology* Chikungunya virus is transmitted among humans by *Aedes* mosquitoes. The virus is endemic in rural Africa and is intermittently epidemic in towns and cities of Africa and Asia.

Clinical Manifestations The incubation period is 2–3 d. Fever and severe arthralgia are accompanied by chills and constitutional symptoms such as headache, photophobia, conjunctival injection, anorexia, nausea, and abdominal pain. Migratory arthritis primarily affects small joints.

R̲x̲ TREATMENT
No specific therapy is available.

EPIDEMIC POLYARTHRITIS   *Epidemiology*   Ross River virus causes epidemics of distinctive disease in Australia, New Guinea, and the eastern Pacific islands. This virus is transmitted among humans by *Aedes* mosquitoes.

Clinical Manifestations   The incubation period is 7–11 d, and the onset of illness is sudden, with joint pain usually ushering in the disease. The rash develops around the same time. Most pts are incapacitated for considerable periods by joint involvement. Joint fluid contains 1000–60,000 mononuclear cells/μL. The detection of IgM antibodies is diagnostic.

R̲x̲ TREATMENT
No specific therapy is available.

Viruses Causing Hemorrhagic Fevers

LASSA FEVER   *Epidemiology*   Lassa fever is a highly contagious arenavirus first described in Lassa, a town in northeastern Nigeria, in 1969 and subsequently found in Sierra Leone, Guinea, and Liberia. The virus is carried in a species of rat that is widespread in Africa. Spread takes place through small-particle aerosols, but person-to-person transmission also occurs.

Clinical Manifestations   The incubation period is 7–18 d. The onset of illness is insidious, with fevers, rigors, headache, malaise, and myalgia. After 4–9 d, anorexia, nausea, vomiting, headache, nonproductive cough (two-thirds of pts), and pharyngitis develop. Physical findings can include flushing of the face and neck, a whitish exudate on the palatine arches that occasionally coalesces into a pseudomembrane, oral ulcerations (50%), and generalized nontender lymphadenopathy (50%). Pts who ultimately recover defervesce in the second week of illness, while pts who die develop signs of shock, clouding of the sensorium, rales, signs of pleural effusion, agitation, and occasionally grand mal seizures. In outbreaks, mortality has ranged from 8 to 52%. The fetal death rate is 92% in the last trimester.

Diagnosis   The diagnosis can be made by the demonstration of a fourfold rise in antibody titer between acute- and convalescent-phase sera. The diagnosis is unlikely if IgM antibodies are absent by day 14 of illness.

TREATMENT

Ribavirin appears to be effective in reducing mortality rates. The drug should be given by slow IV infusion in a dose of 32 mg/kg; this dose should be followed by 16 mg/kg q6h for 4 d and then by 8 mg/kg q8h for 6 d. As a precaution against nosocomial spread, pts should be isolated.

Hantavirus Pulmonary Syndrome *Epidemiology* The causative agents of hantavirus pulmonary syndrome are hantaviruses associated with the rodent subfamily Sigmodontinae. Sin Nombre virus chronically infects the deer mouse and is the most important virus causing hantavirus pulmonary syndrome in the U.S.

Clinical Manifestations The disease begins with a prodrome of 3–4 d comprising fever, myalgia, malaise, and (in many cases) GI disturbances. Pts usually present as the pulmonary phase begins. Typical findings include slightly lowered blood pressure, tachycardia, tachypnea, mild hypoxemia, and early pulmonary edema. Over several hours, decompensation progresses rapidly to respiratory failure.

Diagnosis A specific diagnosis is made by IgM testing of acute-phase serum. RT-PCR is usually positive when used to test blood clots in the first 7–9 d of illness.

TREATMENT

Appropriate management during the first few hours after presentation is critical. The goal is to prevent severe hypoxemia with oxygen therapy and, if needed, intubation and intensive respiratory management. Mortality remains at about 40% with good management. Ribavirin inhibits the virus in vitro but did not have a marked clinical effect on pts in an open-label study.

MARBURG AND EBOLA VIRUSES

EPIDEMIOLOGY Marburg and Ebola viruses are Filoviridae. Marburg virus was first identified in Germany. Of the 25 cases of primary Marburg infection, 7 ended in death. Isolated cases have been reported in Africa. In 1976, epidemics of severe hemorrhagic fever due to Ebola virus occurred simultaneously in Zaire and Sudan. Among 550 cases, there were more than 470 deaths. The virus was spread by close person-to-person contact and reuse of needles for injections. In 1995, another Ebola epidemic occurred in Zaire, with 250 cases and 80% mortality. Strict quarantine measures arrested this epidemic. The reservoirs for the filoviruses are unknown.

CLINICAL MANIFESTATIONS After an incubation period of 3–9 d, pts develop frontal and temporal headache, malaise, myalgias, nausea, and vomiting. Fever of around 40°C is characteristic, and about half of pts develop conjunctivitis. Between 1 and 3 d after onset, watery diarrhea, lethargy, and a change in mentation are noted. A nonpruritic maculopapular rash begins on the fifth to seventh day and usually spreads from the face and neck to the extremities. The rash desquamates around the tenth day. Hemorrhagic manifestations (including GI, renal, and/or conjunctival manifestations) develop at about this time. The temperature response is frequently biphasic, with lysis after the first week and a recurrence around the end of the second week.

DIAGNOSIS Leukopenia and thrombocytopenia are typical, and pts with fatal cases develop DIC. A characteristic clinical course and compatible epidemiologic features form the basis for diagnosis. A specific diagnosis requires isolation of the virus or detection of serologic evidence of infection in paired serum samples. Attempts to isolate the virus must be made only in specialized high-security laboratories.

℞ TREATMENT
Supportive care is all that can currently be offered.

For a more detailed discussion, see Corey L: Rabies Virus and Other Rhabdoviruses, Chap. 199, p. 1128; Peters CJ: Infections Caused by Arthropod- and Rodent-Borne Viruses, Chap. 200, p. 1132; and Corey L: Marburg and Ebola Viruses (Filoviridae), Chap. 201, p. 1146, in HPIM-14.

FUNGAL INFECTIONS

CRYPTOCOCCOSIS

EPIDEMIOLOGY/PATHOGENESIS The yeastlike fungus *Cryptococcus neoformans* elaborates a large polysaccharide capsule. Humans become infected by inhalation of the fungus. Pulmonary infection is frequently asymptomatic. Dissemination, including to the CNS, occurs via the bloodstream. Pts with late-stage HIV infection are at substantial risk for this infection (as of 1993, 6.2% of AIDS pts had developed cryptococcosis), as are pts who have undergone solid organ transplantation, those with sarcoidosis, and those receiving glucocorticoid therapy.

CLINICAL MANIFESTATIONS *Meningoencephalitis* Headache, nausea, staggering gait, dementia, irritability, confusion, and blurred vision are common early symptoms. One-third of pts have papilledema at diagnosis. Fever and nuchal rigidity are often mild or lacking. Cranial nerve palsies, typically asymmetric, occur in about one-fourth of cases. With progression of the infection, deepening coma and signs of brainstem compression appear.

Pulmonary Infection Chest pain occurs in 40% of cases, cough in 20%. CXRs commonly show one or more dense infiltrates, which are often well circumscribed.

Disseminated Infection Some 10% of pts with cryptococcosis have skin lesions, and the vast majority of those who do also have disseminated infection. Cutaneous findings begin with one or more papular lesions, which tend eventually to ulcerate. Rare manifestations of disseminated disease include prostatitis, osteomyelitis, endophthalmitis, hepatitis, pericarditis, endocarditis, and renal abscess.

DIAGNOSIS LP is the single most useful diagnostic test for cryptococcal meningitis. The India ink smear is positive in >50% of cases. Among non-AIDS pts, hypoglycorrhachia is present half of the time and elevated CSF protein levels and lymphocytic pleocytosis are also common. Among AIDS pts, CSF abnormalities are less pronounced but the India ink smear is more often positive. A CSF or serum latex agglutination test is positive in 90% of cases of cryptococcal meningitis. Fungemia develops in 10–30% and is particularly common among persons with AIDS. For the diagnosis of pulmonary or disseminated cryptococcosis, biopsy (with culture) is usually required. Sputum culture is positive in only 10% of cases of cryptococcal pneumonia and serum latex agglutination in only one-third.

℞ TREATMENT

In non-AIDS pts, cryptococcosis may be treated with amphotericin B alone (0.5–0.7 mg/kg IV qd) or with amphotericin (0.3–0.5 mg/kg IV qd) plus flucytosine (25–37.5 mg/kg q6h). In cases of abnormal renal function, the flucytosine dose should be adjusted downward to maintain serum levels of 50–100 μg/mL. The duration of therapy is based on the results of serial CSF examinations; at least 6 weeks of treatment should be given. For pts with AIDS and cryptococcosis, therapy begins with IV amphotericin B (with or without flucytosine) and continues with oral fluconazole (400 mg/d) during active infection. After infection is controlled, suppressive therapy with oral fluconazole (200 mg/d) is continued indefinitely. Surgical excision of a solitary lesion, without systemic therapy, may be appropriate for selected immunocompetent pts with no cryptococci in blood, CSF, or urine.

CANDIDIASIS

ETIOLOGY/PATHOGENESIS *Candida* spp., common commensals of humans, are found most often in the mouth, stool, and vagina. Candidiasis is often preceded by expansion of the commensal population as a result of broad-spectrum antibiotic therapy. Additional host factors, both local and systemic, favor infection. Examples include diabetes mellitus, HIV infection, and denture wear, all of which favor the development of oropharyngeal thrush; macerated skin (regardless of etiology), which favors the development of cutaneous candidiasis; and the third trimester of pregnancy, during which vulvovaginal candidiasis is especially common. *Candida* can pass from colonized surfaces to deep tissues when the integrity of the mucosa or skin is violated (as a consequence, for example, of GI perforation by trauma or surgery, use of an indwelling catheter, or mucosal damage from cytotoxic chemotherapy). Hosts who are particularly susceptible to *Candida* once it has traversed the integumentary barrier include neonates of very low birth weight, people with neutropenia, and pts who are using or have recently used high-dose glucocorticoids. Hematogenous seeding is particularly evident in the retinas, kidneys, spleen, and liver.

CLINICAL MANIFESTATIONS *Oral thrush* presents as discrete adherent white plaques in the mouth and on the tongue. *Cutaneous candidiasis* presents as redness and maceration in intertriginous areas. *Vulvovaginal thrush* causes pruritus and discharge and is sometimes responsible for dyspareunia or dysuria. Oral and vaginal thrush, circumscribed hyperkeratotic skin lesions, dystrophic nails, and partial alopecia characterize *chronic mucocutaneous candidiasis.* A variety of defects in T cell function have been described in pts with this condition, who may also exhibit hypofunction of the parathyroid, adrenal, or thyroid gland. Dysphagia or substernal chest pain occurs in *esophageal candidiasis,* the most common type of GI candidiasis. Endoscopic findings include areas of redness and edema, focal white patches, and/or ulcers. *Hematogenous dissemination* presents with varied severity, ranging from fever alone to septic shock. Other findings may include retinal lesions, multiple small hepatosplenic abscesses, nodular pulmonary infiltrates, endocarditis, chronic meningitis or arthritis, and (in rare cases) focal manifestations such as osteomyelitis, pustular skin lesions, myositis, and brain abscess.

DIAGNOSIS Demonstration of pseudohyphae on wet smear with confirmation by culture is the procedure of choice for diagnosing superficial candidiasis. Deeper lesions due to *Candida* may be diagnosed by histologic section of biopsy specimens or by culture of blood, CSF, joint fluid, or surgical specimens. Serologic tests for antibody or antigen are not useful.

℞ **TREATMENT**
For cutaneous candidiasis, nystatin powder or a cream containing ciclopirox or an azole is applied topically. For vulvovaginal candidiasis, vaginal azole formulations are therapeutically superior to nystatin suppositories. A single oral dose of fluconazole (150 mg) is a convenient alternative but is more likely to cause adverse effects. Oral or esophageal candidiasis responds better to clotrimazole troches taken five times a day than to nystatin suspension swished and swallowed. Ketoconazole (200–400 mg/d), itraconazole (200 mg/d), or fluconazole (100–200 mg/d) is effective for esophageal candidiasis; fluconazole is the initial agent of choice for oral or esophageal candidiasis in the setting of AIDS. For AIDS pts with azole-resistant disease, amphotericin B (0.3–0.5 mg/kg IV qd) may be used. Bladder thrush responds to bladder irrigation with amphotericin B (50 mg/L for 5 d); oral fluconazole may be substituted in the treatment of noncatheterized pts with candiduria. For disseminated disease, amphotericin B (0.5–0.7 mg/kg qd) is the treatment of choice. In pts without a contraindication to its use, flucytosine (100–150 mg/kg qd) may be added and the amphotericin B dose reduced to 0.3–0.5 mg/kg qd. All pts from whose peripheral blood *Candida* is cultured should receive IV amphotericin B for the treatment of acute infection and the prevention of late sequelae. Oral

fluconazole (400 mg/d) is used prophylactically against invasive candidiasis in recipients of allogeneic bone marrow transplants.

ASPERGILLOSIS

EPIDEMIOLOGY/PATHOGENESIS   *Aspergillus* species are ubiquitous in the environment and cause several syndromes, including allergic bronchopulmonary aspergillosis, aspergilloma, and invasive aspergillosis. Invasive disease originates in the lung after inhalation of *Aspergillus* spores and is confined almost entirely to immunosuppressed hosts. In roughly 90% of such cases, two of the following risk factors are present: neutropenia (granulocyte count <500/μL), history of high-dose glucocorticoid therapy, or history of treatment with cytotoxic drugs. Invasive infection, which may also complicate AIDS, is characterized by hyphal invasion of blood vessels, thrombosis, necrosis, and hemorrhagic infarction.

CLINICAL MANIFESTATIONS   *Allergic bronchial aspergillosis* presents in pts with preexisting asthma as eosinophilia, fleeting pulmonary infiltrates, and demonstrable IgE antibody to *Aspergillus*. *Endobronchial pulmonary aspergillosis* presents as chronic productive cough, often with hemoptysis, in pts with prior chronic lung disease. The term *aspergilloma* refers to a ball of hyphae that forms within a preexisting pulmonary cyst or cavity, usually in an upper lobe. *Invasive aspergillosis* presents as an acute, rapidly progressive, densely consolidated pulmonary infiltrate. In the pt recovering from neutropenia, cavitation is a classic occurrence. Infection may spread hematogenously or by direct extension.

DIAGNOSIS   The repeated isolation of *Aspergillus* from sputum implies colonization or infection. The diagnosis of invasive aspergillosis is suggested by even a single isolation of *Aspergillus* from the sputum of a neutropenic pt with pneumonia. A biopsy and culture are usually required for definitive diagnosis, the latter for confirmation and speciation. Blood cultures are rarely positive. A fungus ball in the lung is usually detectable by CXR. Serum IgG antibodies to *Aspergillus* are often found in pts colonized with the organism and are nearly universally present in those with aspergilloma.

℞ **TREATMENT**

Pts with pulmonary aspergilloma and severe hemoptysis may benefit from lobectomy. Systemic therapy is of no value in endobronchial or endocavitary aspergillosis. Treatment with

IV amphotericin B (1.0–1.5 mg/kg qd) has resulted in the arrest or cure of invasive aspergillosis when immunosuppression is not severe. Itraconazole (200 mg bid) may be used judiciously by pts who are not severely immunosuppressed and who have indolent or slowly progressive invasive infection.

HISTOPLASMOSIS

EPIDEMIOLOGY/PATHOGENESIS   *Histoplasma capsulatum* is found in moist surface soil, particularly soil enriched by droppings of certain birds and bats. In the U.S., infection is most common in the southeastern, mid-Atlantic, and central states. Case clusters have occurred among groups of people exposed to dust (e.g., while raking, cleaning dirt-floored chicken coops, bulldozing, or spelunking). Infection follows inhalation of the organism and is usually a self-limited condition.

CLINICAL MANIFESTATIONS   In the vast majority of cases, *acute pulmonary histoplasmosis* is either asymptomatic or mild. Symptoms and signs may include cough, fever, malaise, and CXR findings of hilar adenopathy, with or without areas of pneumonitis. Erythema nodosum and erythema multiforme have been reported in a few outbreaks. *Chronic pulmonary histoplasmosis* is characterized by subacute onset of productive cough, weight loss, and night sweats. CXRs show uni- or bilateral fibronodular apical infiltrates. In one-third of pts, the disease stabilizes or improves spontaneously. In the remainder, it progresses insidiously and may terminate in death from cor pulmonale, bacterial pneumonia, or histoplasmosis itself. The findings in *acute disseminated histoplasmosis,* which resemble those in miliary tuberculosis, include fever, hepatosplenomegaly, lymphadenopathy, jaundice, and pancytopenia. Indurated ulcers of the mouth, tongue, nose, or larynx occur in about one-fourth of cases. AIDS pts may develop disseminated disease years after exposure in an endemic area. CXRs are abnormal in 50% of cases, showing discrete nodules or a miliary pattern. *Ocular histoplasmosis syndrome* is a distinct form of uveitis in which a positive histoplasmin skin test is required for diagnosis and active histoplasmosis is absent.

DIAGNOSIS   Culture of *H. capsulatum* is the preferred diagnostic method but is often difficult. Blood should be cultured by the lysis-centrifugation technique and plates held at 30°C for at least 2 weeks. Cultures of bone marrow, mucosal lesions, liver, and bronchoalveolar lavage fluid are useful in disseminated disease. Sputum culture is preferred for suspected chronic pulmonary histoplasmosis, but visible growth requires 2–4 weeks. Histologic diagnosis is possible but requires considerable expertise. A radioactive assay for *Histoplasma* antigen in blood or urine is available and is useful for diagnosis and monitoring of AIDS pts with disseminated infection. Serology is of limited value, and histoplasmin skin testing is of no clinical utility.

℞ TREATMENT

Acute pulmonary histoplasmosis does not require therapy. Pts with disseminated or chronic pulmonary histoplasmosis should receive chemotherapy. Amphotericin B (0.6 mg/kg qd) is the agent of choice for pts who are severely ill, who are immunosuppressed, or whose infection involves the CNS. The regimen can be changed to itraconazole (200 mg bid) once improvement becomes evident. Immunocompetent pts with mild or moderate disease can immediately be given itraconazole (200 mg bid) and are generally treated for 6–12 months. Ketoconazole (400–800 mg/d) is an alternative for these pts if CNS disease is absent. A third alternative for immunocompetent pts is amphotericin B (0.5 mg/kg qd). Maintenance therapy with itraconazole (200 mg once or twice daily, to maintain blood levels of ≥2 μg/mL) is continued for life in AIDS pts.

BLASTOMYCOSIS

EPIDEMIOLOGY/PATHOGENESIS   Blastomycosis is acquired by inhalation of *Blastomyces dermatitidis* from soil, decomposed vegetation, or rotting wood. The disease is uncommon in any locality; the majority of cases occur in the southeastern, central, and mid-Atlantic areas of the U.S.

CLINICAL MANIFESTATIONS   A minority of pts have acute, self-limited pneumonia. Most cases, however, have an indolent onset and a chronically progressive course. Fever, cough, weight loss, lassitude, chest ache, and skin lesions are common. The skin lesions enlarge over many weeks from pimples to verrucous, crusted, or ulcerated forms. CXR findings are abnormal in two-thirds of cases, revealing one or more nodular or pneumonic infiltrates. Infection may spread to the brain or meninges. Osteolytic lesions, which may be found in nearly any bone, present as cold abscesses or draining sinuses. Prostatic and epididymal lesions resemble those of tuberculosis.

DIAGNOSIS   The diagnosis is made by culture of *B. dermatitidis* from sputum, pus, or urine or by wet smear or histology.

℞ TREATMENT

Every pt should receive chemotherapy. As with histoplasmosis, severe disease should be treated with amphotericin B. Skin and noncavitary lung lesions should be treated for 8–10 weeks (cumulative dose, 2.0 g). Cavitary lung disease and disease extending beyond the lungs and skin should be treated for 10–12 weeks (total dose, 2.5 g). Itraconazole (200 mg bid) is the drug of choice for indolent, nonmeningeal blastomycosis of mild to moderate severity in compliant pts. Ketoconazole (400–800 mg/d) is an effective alternative. Itraconazole or ketoconazole should be given for 6–12 months.

COCCIDIOIDOMYCOSIS

EPIDEMIOLOGY/PATHOGENESIS *Coccidioides immitis* is a soil saprophyte found in certain arid regions of the U.S., Mexico, and Central and South America. Infection results from inhalation of windborne arthrospores from soil. Within the U.S., most cases are acquired in California, Arizona, and western Texas.

CLINICAL MANIFESTATIONS *Primary pulmonary coccidioidomycosis* is symptomatic in about 40% of cases. When present, symptoms include fever, cough, chest pain, and malaise. Hypersensitivity reactions (e.g., erythema nodosum, erythema multiforme, toxic erythema) sometimes occur. CXRs may show an infiltrate, hilar adenopathy, or pleural effusion. Mild peripheral eosinophilia may be present. Recovery usually begins after several days to 2 weeks of illness and is usually complete. *Chronic progressive pulmonary coccidioidomycosis* causes cough, sputum production, variable degrees of fever, and weight loss. *Disseminated coccidioidomycosis* is characterized by malaise, fever, and hilar or paratracheal lymphadenopathy, with serologic evidence of abnormal fungal persistence. With time, lesions appear in bone, skin, subcutaneous tissue, meninges, joints, and other sites.

DIAGNOSIS The diagnosis is made by wet smear and culture of sputum, urine, or pus. The suspicion of coccidioidomycosis should be clearly indicated on the requisition to ensure that laboratory personnel exercise appropriate caution. Serology is also helpful; a positive CF test of unconcentrated CSF is diagnostic of coccidioidal meningitis. Seroconversion may be delayed for up to 8 weeks, however. Skin test conversion occurs 3–21 d after the onset of symptoms, but skin testing for the diagnosis of acute infection is of limited utility since results remain positive after remote exposure and may be negative in thin-walled pulmonary cavitary or disseminated disease.

℞ TREATMENT

Pts with disseminated disease should be treated. Pts with severe or rapidly progressive disseminated cases should receive amphotericin B (0.5–0.7 mg/kg qd). Once improvement occurs or when an infection is relatively indolent, ketoconazole (400 mg/d), itraconazole (200 mg bid), or fluconazole (400–600 mg/d) may be given. Oral therapy is continued for years. Coccidioidal meningitis is treated with fluconazole (400–800 mg/d) but may also require intrathecal amphotericin B. Single, thin-walled pulmonary cavities are poorly responsive to chemotherapy but tend to close spontaneously.

PARACOCCIDIOIDOMYCOSIS

EPIDEMIOLOGY   Paracoccidioidomycosis, formerly called South American blastomycosis, follows inhalation of spores of *Paracoccidioides brasiliensis*. Infection is acquired only in South or Central America or in Mexico.

CLINICAL MANIFESTATIONS   Signs include indurated ulcers of the mouth, oropharynx, larynx, and nose; enlarged and draining lymph nodes; lesions of the skin (particularly that of the genitalia); productive cough, dyspnea, and weight loss; and, in some cases, fever. CXRs most frequently show bilateral patchy infiltrates.

DIAGNOSIS   Cultures of sputum, pus, or mucosal lesions are often diagnostic. Serology may provide an initial clue to the diagnosis.

℞ TREATMENT

Mild cases may be cured by 1 year of oral ketoconazole or itraconazole (200–400 mg/d). More advanced cases are treated with IV amphotericin B followed by an oral agent.

MUCORMYCOSIS

EPIDEMIOLOGY/PATHOGENESIS   *Mucormycosis* refers to infection by any of several fungal genera, the most common of which in human disease are *Rhizopus, Rhizomucor,* and *Cunninghamella.* The organisms are ubiquitous in nature; person-to-person spread does not take place. The disease is largely confined to pts with serious preexisting conditions. Mucormycosis originating in the paranasal sinuses and nose (*rhinocerebral mucormycosis*) classically occurs in pts with poorly controlled diabetes mellitus. Pts who have undergone organ transplantation, who have a hematologic malignancy, or who have received long-term deferoxamine therapy are predisposed to *sinus* or *pulmonary mucormycosis*. *Gastrointestinal mucormycosis* may occur in a variety of settings, including uremia, severe malnutrition, and diarrheal disease. Regardless of the anatomic location of the infection, vascular hyphal invasion is prominent and leads to hemorrhagic or ischemic necrosis.

CLINICAL MANIFESTATIONS Disease arising in the nose and paranasal sinuses produces the characteristic clinical picture of low-grade fever, dull sinus pain, and sometimes a thin bloody nasal discharge; following in a few days are double vision, increasing fever, and obtundation. On examination, a unilateral generalized reduction of ocular motion, chemosis, proptosis, a dusky red or necrotic nasal turbinate on the affected side, and a sharply demarcated area of necrosis on the hard palate (strictly respecting the midline) may be present. Invasion of the globe or ophthalmic artery may lead to blindness and that of the orbit to cavernous sinus thrombosis. Pulmonary mucormycosis manifests as progressive, severe necrotizing pneumonia.

DIAGNOSIS The diagnosis is typically made histologically. The agents of mucormycosis appear as broad, rarely septate hyphae 6–50 μm in diameter. Culture should be attempted, but the yield is low.

R̲x̲ TREATMENT
Regulation of diabetes and reduction of immunosuppression facilitate the treatment of mucormycosis. Craniofacial lesions are treated with extensive surgical debridement and 10–12 weeks of IV amphotericin B at maximal doses. Cure may be achieved in 50% of cases.

MISCELLANEOUS MYCOSES

Fusariosis

Fusarium spp. can cause localized or hematogenously disseminated infection, the latter almost exclusively affecting pts with hematologic malignancy and neutropenia. In disseminated infection, an abrupt onset of fever is followed in two-thirds of cases by the appearance of distinctive skin lesions that resemble ecthyma gangrenosum. Blood cultures have been positive in 59% of pts. Amphotericin B should be given, but recovery depends on reduction in the severity of neutropenia.

Malassezia Infection

Malassezia furfur is a component of the normal skin flora but can cause tinea (pityriasis) versicolor or catheter-related sepsis.

The latter infection occurs predominantly in pts receiving IV lipid and is cured by catheter removal.

Pseudallescheriasis

Pseudallescheria boydii (also called *Petriellidium boydii*) is a mold frequently found in soil. Infection may follow inhalation or direct inoculation. The clinical and histologic manifestations of pseudallescheriasis resemble those of aspergillosis, which is much more common. In the U.S., *P. boydii* is the foremost cause of mycetoma, a chronic suppurative infection of subcutaneous tissue. The diagnosis is based on the demonstration of hyphae in tissues. Cultural confirmation is required to distinguish *P. boydii* from *Aspergillus* spp. Therapy with IV miconazole, itraconazole, or ketoconazole is recommended; the response is typically poor.

Sporotrichosis

Sporotrichosis results from the inoculation of *Sporothrix schenckii* into subcutaneous tissue via minor trauma. Nursery workers, florists, and gardeners acquire the illness from roses, peat moss, and other plants. Lymphangitic sporotrichosis, by far the most common form, is characterized by the appearance of a nearly painless red papule at the site of inoculation. Over the next several weeks, similar lesions form along proximal lymphatic channels. Spread beyond an extremity is rare. Diagnosis is made by culture of a skin biopsy sample or of draining pus. A saturated solution of potassium iodide, given in increasing divided daily doses up to 4.5–9 mL/d for adults, may be curative. Therapy should be continued for a month after the resolution of all lesions. Itraconazole (100–200 mg/d) is an effective alternative. For extracutaneous disease, a prolonged course of amphotericin B may be curative.

For a more detailed discussion, see Bennett JE: Diagnosis and Treatment of Fungal Infections, Chap. 202, p. 1148; Histoplasmosis, Chap. 203, p. 1150; Coccidioidomycosis, Chap. 204, p. 1151; Blastomycosis, Chap. 205, p. 1152; Cryptococcosis, Chap. 206, p. 1153; Candidiasis, Chap. 207, p. 1154; Aspergillosis, Chap. 208, p. 1156; Mucormycosis, Chap. 209, p. 1158; and Miscellaneous Mycoses and *Prototheca* Infections, Chap. 210, p. 1158, in HPIM-14.

PNEUMOCYSTIS CARINII INFECTION

Etiology

Pneumocystis carinii is a eukaryotic organism that causes disease in immunocompromised hosts, particularly those with HIV infection. Research on the basic biology of the organism has been hampered by the lack of a reliable in vitro cultivation system. Its taxonomy has been controversial, although recent studies favor its classification as a fungus.

Epidemiology

P. carinii has a worldwide distribution. It is transmitted by airborne inhalation; person-to-person transmission has been suggested in some instances. *P. carinii* pneumonia (PCP) occurs in premature malnourished infants, children with primary immunodeficiency diseases, pts receiving immunosuppressive therapy (especially glucocorticoids) for cancer and organ transplantation, and pts with AIDS. In AIDS, the incidence of PCP rises dramatically when the CD4 + cell count falls below 200/μl.

Clinical Manifestations

P. carinii Pneumonia Pts with PCP have dyspnea, fever, and nonproductive cough. In AIDS pts, the symptoms may be more subtle with insidious onset, and pts are often ill for several weeks. In non-AIDS pts, symptoms commonly begin after the glucocorticoid dose has been tapered. Physical findings include tachypnea, tachycardia, and cyanosis, but few abnormalities are evident on auscultation of the lungs. CXR classically demonstrates bilateral diffuse infiltrates, but many other patterns have been associated with PCP, including nodular densities, cavitary lesions, upper lobe infiltrates (particularly in pts receiving aerosolized pentamidine prophylaxis), and pneumothorax. Early in the course, the CXR may be normal. Evaluation of arterial blood gas reveals hypoxia and an increase in alveolar-arterial oxygen gradient. Gallium scan demonstrates increased uptake in the lungs.

Extrapulmonary Infection Infection usually remains confined to the lungs, but extrapulmonary infection has been described with a frequency ranging from <1% to 3%. Extrapulmonary *P. carinii* infection is especially common among AIDS pts receiving aerosolized pentamidine prophylaxis. The organs most frequently involved include lymph nodes, liver, spleen, and bone marrow. Other sites include the GI and GU tracts, pancreas, adrenal and thyroid glands, heart, eyes, ears, and skin.

Clinical manifestations vary greatly, and the lesions may be found incidentally on biopsy or in imaging studies or may cause disease related to the organ(s) involved.

Diagnosis

As the clinical presentation may vary, the level of suspicion of infection must be high in populations most at risk. The diagnosis is made by demonstration of the organism with stains, including methenamine silver, toluidine blue, and cresyl echt violet. The immunofluorescence and immunoperoxidase staining procedures, based on commercially available monoclonal antibodies, are sensitive and are used in many laboratories. The mainstay of diagnosis is the staining of specimens obtained by fiberoptic bronchoscopy with bronchoalveolar lavage (BAL). In AIDS pts, in whom the burden of organisms is high, induced sputum may yield a diagnosis. While this technique is simple and noninvasive, its success has varied at different institutions. Transbronchial and open lung biopsy now are reserved for situations in which BAL is not diagnostic.

℞ TREATMENT

Trimethoprim-sulfamethoxazole (TMP-SMZ) is the drug of choice for all forms of pneumocystosis. It is administered PO or IV at a TMP dosage of 15–20 (mg/kg)/d in three or four divided doses. Because this agent is poorly tolerated by pts with HIV infection, resulting in fever, rash, neutropenia, thrombocytopenia, hepatitis, or hyperkalemia in more than half of these pts, alternative regimens are often required. Pentamidine isethionate—4 (mg/kg)/d given as a single slow IV infusion—is about as effective as TMP-SMZ but exerts some toxic effects in most recipients, including hypotension, dysglycemia, azotemia, and cardiac arrhythmias. Other alternatives include TMP plus dapsone, clindamycin plus primaquine, atovaquone, and trimetrexate. Because respiratory decompensation frequently follows initiation of treatment in AIDS pts with moderate to severe PCP, glucocorticoids (e.g., prednisone, 40 mg PO bid tapered to 20 mg PO qd over 3 weeks) are given adjunctively to pts with $P_{A_{O_2}}$ values ≤ 70 mmHg or an alveolar-arterial oxygen gradient ≥ 35 mmHg and have been shown to improve survival. The use of glucocorticoids has not been studied in PCP unrelated to HIV infection. The duration of therapy is 14 d for non-AIDS pts and 21 d for AIDS pts.

Prevention

Pts with AIDS should receive prophylactic therapy for life after an episode of PCP (secondary prophylaxis). Primary prophylaxis is given to AIDS pts with CD4 + cell counts <200/μL, unexplained fever for ≥2 weeks, or a history of oropharyngeal candidiasis. The prophylactic regimen of choice is TMP-SMZ (one double-strength tablet qd). Alternative regimens, necessitated by the high rate of adverse reactions to TMP-SMZ in HIV infection, include TMP-SMZ at reduced dose or frequency; dapsone alone; dapsone, pyrimethamine, and leucovorin; or aerosolized pentamidine in a Respirgard II nebulizer. Indications for prophylaxis of PCP in immunocompromised pts without HIV infection are less clear, but prophylaxis should be given to all such pts after recovery from PCP.

Outpatient/Home Care Considerations

Pts with mild PCP who can tolerate oral therapy may be managed as outpatients. Hospitalized pts may be discharged to complete therapy at home when they are able to breathe room air and tolerate oral therapy.

For a more detailed discussion, see Walzer PD: *Pneumocystis carinii* Infection, Chap. 211, p. 1161, in HPIM-14.

102

PROTOZOAL INFECTIONS

AMEBIASIS

EPIDEMIOLOGY Amebiasis is the third leading cause of death from parasitic disease worldwide. The areas of highest incidence include most developing countries in the tropics, particularly Mexico, Central and South America, India, tropical Asia, and Africa. The main groups at risk in developed countries are travelers, recent immigrants, homosexual men, and residents of institutions. *Entamoeba histolytica*, the intestinal protozoan that causes amebiasis, is acquired by ingestion of viable cysts from fecally contaminated water, food, or hands. Food-borne exposure is most common. Less common modes of transmission include oral and anal sexual practices; rare cases are transmitted by direct rectal inoculation through colonic irrigating devices.

PATHOGENESIS After ingestion, cysts release trophozoites (the only form that invades tissue) into the lumen of the small intestine. While cysts can persist in a moist environment for several weeks, trophozoites are killed rapidly by exposure to air. In most pts trophozoites are harmless commensals, but in some they invade the bowel mucosa, causing symptomatic colitis. In yet other pts, trophozoites invade the bloodstream, causing distant abscesses of the liver, lungs, or brain. Numerous virulence factors have been linked to the ability of amebas to invade through interglandular epithelium, including extracellular proteinase.

CLINICAL MANIFESTATIONS *Intestinal Amebiasis* The most common type of amebic infection is asymptomatic cyst passage. Symptomatic amebic colitis develops 2–6 weeks after ingestion of infectious cysts. Lower abdominal pain and mild diarrhea develop gradually and are followed by malaise, weight loss, and diffuse lower-abdominal or back pain. Cecal involvement may mimic appendicitis. In full-blown dysentery, pts may daily pass 10–12 stools consisting of blood and mucus but little fecal material. Virtually all pts have heme-positive stools; fewer than 40% are febrile. Rarely (most often in children), a more fulminant form occurs, with high fevers, severe abdominal pain, and profuse diarrhea. Pts may develop toxic megacolon. Pts receiving glucocorticoids are at risk for more severe amebiasis. Uncommonly, pts develop a more chronic form of amebiasis, which can be confused with inflammatory bowel disease. *Amebomas* are inflammatory mass lesions due to chronic intestinal amebiasis.

Amebic Liver Abscess Extraintestinal infection frequently involves the liver. Most pts develop symptoms within 5 months. The majority of these pts are febrile and have RUQ pain, which may be dull or pleuritic and may radiate to the shoulder. Point tenderness of the liver and right pleural effusion are common; jaundice is rare. Fewer than one-third of pts have accompanying diarrhea. In some pts, especially those who are older, the illness can have a subacute course with weight loss and hepatomegaly. Only about one-third of pts with chronic presentations are febrile. Amebic liver abscess must be considered in the differential diagnosis of fever of unknown origin, as 10–15% of pts present with fever only. Complications of amebic liver abscesses include pleuropulmonary involvement in 20–30% of pts with sterile effusions, contiguous spread from the liver, and frank rupture into the pleural space, the peritoneum, or the pericardium. Rupture of an amebic abscess, which may occur during medical therapy, usually requires drainage.

Other Extraintestinal Sites   Besides the liver, extraintestinal sites of amebiasis include the GU tract (with painful genital ulcers) and the cerebrum (in fewer than 0.1% of pts).

DIAGNOSIS   The cornerstone of the diagnosis of amebic colitis is the demonstration of trophozoites or cysts of *E. histolytica* on wet mount, iodine-stained concentrates of stool, or trichrome stains of stool or concentrates. A combination of these procedures is positive in 75–95% of cases. At least three fresh stool specimens should be examined. Experience in distinguishing *E. histolytica* from *Entamoeba hartmanni*, *Entamoeba coli*, and *Endolimax nana* is important as these parasites do not cause clinical disease and do not need to be treated. Commercially available serologic tests are positive in more than 90% of cases of invasive disease, including colitis. A positive test suggests active infection, since serologies usually revert to negative in 6–12 months. Liver scans, ultrasound, CT, and MRI are all useful for the detection of liver abscess. Barium enemas and sigmoidoscopy with biopsy are potentially dangerous in acute amebic colitis because of a risk of perforation.

℞ TREATMENT

Asymptomatic cyst carriers should be treated with a luminal amebicide that is poorly absorbed. Three luminal drugs are available in the U.S.—iodoquinol (650 mg PO tid for 20 d), diloxanide furoate (obtainable only through the CDC; 500 mg PO tid for 10 d), and paromomycin (500 mg PO tid for 10 d). Pts with colitis or liver abscess should receive a tissue amebicide and a luminal agent. Metronidazole (750 mg PO or IV tid for 5–10 d) is used for the treatment of amebic colitis or liver abscess. Except in the case of rupture, amebic liver abscesses rarely require drainage.

MALARIA

ETIOLOGY   Four species of the genus *Plasmodium* infect humans: *P. vivax*, *P. ovale*, *P. malariae*, and *P. falciparum*. This last species is responsible for most deaths due to malaria.

EPIDEMIOLOGY   Malaria is the most important parasitic disease of humans, causing 1–3 million deaths annually. The disease is found throughout the tropical regions of the world. *P. falciparum* predominates in sub-Saharan Africa, New Guinea, and Haiti. *P. vivax* is more common in Central America and the Indian subcontinent, but *P. falciparum* has been found with increasing frequency in India over the past decade. *P. falciparum* and *P. vivax* are equally prevalent in South America, eastern Asia, and Oceania. *P. malariae* is less common but is found in most areas (especially West and Central Africa). *P. ovale* is uncommon outside of Africa. Malaria is transmitted by the bite of the female anopheline mosquito.

PATHOGENESIS   Human infection begins with the transfer of sporozoites from the mosquito's salivary glands to the bloodstream during a blood meal. After a period of asexual reproduction in liver cells, the swollen cells rupture, releasing merozoites into the bloodstream and initiating the symptomatic phase of infection. In *P. vivax* and *P. ovale* infection, some intrahepatic forms remain dormant for months and can cause relapses after treatment. Merozoites attach to specific erythrocyte surface receptors and then invade the cell. In *P. vivax* infection, this receptor is related to the Duffy group antigen, whose absence in most West Africans renders them resistant to this form of malaria. After invasion, the parasite grows progressively, consumes and degrades intracellular proteins (principally hemoglobin), and alters the cell membrane.

Host defense also plays a role in malaria. In the nonimmune individual, infection triggers nonspecific host defense mechanisms such as splenic filtration. When parasitized erythrocytes that have evaded splenic filtration rupture, the material released activates macrophages, which release proinflammatory cytokines that cause fever and exert other pathologic effects. The distribution of malaria before the introduction of mosquito control programs paralleled the distribution of sickle cell disease, thalassemia, and G6PD deficiency. These diseases may confer protection against death due to falciparum malaria, as has been demonstrated with the sickle cell trait. With repeated exposure to malaria, a specific immune response develops and limits the degree of parasitemia. Over time, pts are rendered immune to disease but remain susceptible to infection.

CLINICAL MANIFESTATIONS   The first symptoms are nonspecific and include malaise, headache, fatigue, abdominal discomfort, and muscle aches, followed by fever and chills. Nausea, vomiting, and orthostatic hypotension are common. The classic malaria paroxysms, in which fever spikes, chills, and rigors occur at regular intervals, suggest infection with *P. vivax* or *P. ovale*. Most often, the fever is irregular at first. In uncomplicated malaria, mild anemia and a palpable spleen may be the only clinical abnormalities identified. The complications of falciparum malaria include cerebral malaria (obtundation, delirium, or gradual or sudden onset of coma, with seizures common as well), hypoglycemia, lactic acidosis, noncardiogenic pulmonary edema, renal impairment (seen mainly in adults and resembling acute tubular necrosis), hematologic abnormalities (anemia, coagulation defects, DIC in pts with cerebral malaria, and so-called blackwater fever, in which massive hemolysis causes hemoglobinemia, black urine, and renal failure), and aspiration pneumonia. In children, *P. malariae* infection may cause nephrotic syndrome.

DIAGNOSIS   The diagnosis of malaria rests on the demonstration of the asexual form of the parasite in thick or thin smears of peripheral blood. Giemsa is the preferred staining method. The level of parasitemia, which can be determined from either type of smear, is expressed as the number of parasitized erythrocytes per 1000 cells; this figure is then used to derive the number of infected erythrocytes per microliter of blood. A thick smear concentrates the parasites but should be interpreted with care as artifacts are common. Smears should be examined on successive days before a diagnosis of malaria is excluded. It is important to diagnose probable or possible *P. falciparum* infection. Features on smear suggestive of falciparum malaria include double-chromatin dots, multiply infected erythrocytes of normal size, banana-shaped gametocytes, and a parasitemia level of >5%. *P. vivax* infection is characterized by the presence of Schüffner's dots in enlarged erythrocytes; *P. ovale* infection is typified by Schüffner's dots in minimally enlarged erythrocytes that are slightly oval in shape and may have fringed edges. A simple, sensitive, and specific diagnostic test that detects *P. falciparum* histidine-rich protein 2 in fingerprick blood samples has recently been introduced.

℞ TREATMENT

Table 102-1 summarizes malaria therapy. Severe falciparum malaria constitutes a medical emergency. In addition to antimalarial agents, the pt should be given phenobarbital (a single dose of 5–20 mg/kg) to prevent seizures. In comatose pts, the blood glucose level should be measured every 4–6 h; those with levels below 40 mg/dL should receive IV dextrose. Exchange transfusion is indicated for vital organ dysfunction and a parasitemia level of >15% and should be considered for pts with parasitemia levels of 5–15%. Glucocorticoids, urea, heparin, and dextran are of no value.

PREVENTION   Table 102-2 summarizes malaria prophylaxis.

LEISHMANIASIS

EPIDEMIOLOGY   Leishmaniasis is spread by female phlebotomine sandflies. Rodents, small mammals, and canines are

Table 102-1

Recommended Therapeutic Doses of Antimalarial Drugs

Drug	Uncomplicated Malaria (Oral)
Chloroquine	10 mg of base/kg followed by 10 mg/kg at 24 h and 5 mg/kg at 48 h *or* by 5 mg/kg at 12, 24, and 36 h (total dose, 25 mg/kg); for *P.vivax* or *P. ovale,* primaquine (0.25 mg of base/kg/d for 14 d†) added for radical cure
Sulfadoxine/ pyrimethamine	20/1 mg/kg, single oral dose (3 tablets for adults)
Mefloquine	For semi-immunes, 15 mg of base/kg as a single dose; in areas with mefloquine resistance or for nonimmunes, 15 mg/kg followed 8–12 h later by second dose of 10 mg/kg
Quinine	10 mg of salt/kg q8h for 7 d combined with tetracycline‡ (4 mg/kg qid) or doxycycline (3 mg/kg once daily) for 7 d
Quinidine gluconate	—
Artesunate	In combination with 25 mg of mefloquine/kg, 10–12 mg/kg given in divided doses over 3–5 d (e.g., 4 mg/kg for 3 d or 4 mg/kg followed by 1.5 mg/kg/d for 4 d); if used alone, same dose divided over 7 d (usually 4 mg/kg initially followed by 2 mg/kg on days 2 and 3 followed by 1 mg/kg on days 4–7)
Artemether	Same regimen as for artesunate

*Oral treatment should be substituted for parenteral therapy as soon as pt can take tablets by mouth.

†In Oceania and Southeast Asia, the dose should be 0.33–0.5 mg of base/kg. This regimen should not be used in pts with severe variants of G6PD deficiency.

‡Neither tetracycline nor doxycycline should be given to pregnant women or to children <8 years old.

§Alternatively, infusion of 7 mg of salt/kg over 30 min can be followed by 10 mg of salt/kg over 4 h.

Severe Malaria* (Parenteral)

10 mg of base/kg by constant-rate infusion over 8 h followed by
  15 mg/kg over 24 h *or* by 3.5 mg of base/kg by IM or SC injection
  every 6 h (total dose, 25 mg/kg)

—

—

20 mg of salt/kg by IV infusion over 4 h§ followed by 10 mg/kg
  over 2–8 h every 8 h

10 mg of base/kg by constant-rate infusion over 1–2 h followed
  by 0.02 mg/kg per min, with ECG monitoring¶
2.4 mg/kg IV or IM stat followed by 1.2 mg/kg at 12 and 24 h
  and then daily

3.2 mg/kg IM stat followed by 1.6 mg/kg/d

¶Some authorities recommend a lower dose of IV quinidine: 6.2 mg of base/kg
over 1–2 h followed by 0.0125 mg/kg per min.

NOTE: In severe malaria, quinine or quinidine should be used if there is any doubt
about the infecting strain's sensitivity to chloroquine.

SOURCE: White NJ, Breman JG: HPIM-14, p. 1187.

Table 102-2

Prophylaxis for Malaria

Purpose	Regimen for Adults
Suppression in areas without chloroquine resistance	Chloroquine 300 mg of base (500 mg of salt) PO once weekly (from 1 week before exposure through 4 weeks afterward)
Suppression in areas with chloroquine resistance	Mefloquine* 228 mg of base (250 mg of salt) weekly (from 1 week before exposure through 4 weeks afterward)
	Alternatives:
	Doxycycline† 100 mg PO qd for 1–2 d before, during, and for 4 weeks after exposure
	or
	Chloroquine 300 mg/week as above plus proguanil‡ 200 mg qd for 1–2 d before, during, and for 4 weeks after exposure; pts should also carry three 25/500-mg sulfadoxine/pyrimethamine tablets for self-treatment of a febrile illness when medical care is not immediately available

*Mefloquine should not be used by pregnant women or by pts with a history of psychiatric or seizure disorders. It should be used with caution in pts with cardiac conduction abnormalities or pts taking beta-blocker medications.

†Doxycycline should not be given to pregnant women.

‡Not available in the U.S.

SOURCE: Modified from White NJ, Breman JG: HPIM-14, p. 1185.

the common reservoir hosts of *Leishmania* spp.; humans are incidental hosts.

CLINICAL MANIFESTATIONS *Visceral Leishmaniasis (Kala-Azar)* Visceral leishmaniasis is most often caused by *Leishmania donovani*. Visceral infection may remain subclinical or become symptomatic, with an acute, subacute, or chronic course. The usual incubation period ranges from weeks to months. In some settings, inapparent infections far outnumber clinically apparent ones; malnutrition is a risk factor for the development of disease. The term *kala-azar* refers to the classic image of the profoundly cachectic, febrile pt who is heavily parasitized and has life-threatening disease. Splenomegaly is typically more impressive than hepatomegaly and can be massive. Peripheral lymphadenopathy may also be detected. With advanced disease, pancytopenia, hypergammaglobulinemia, and hypoalbuminemia may develop.

Visceral leishmaniasis is becoming an important opportunistic infection in HIV pts from *Leishmania*-endemic areas. Such cases may represent newly acquired or reactivated infections. In these hosts, even relatively avirulent leishmanial strains may disseminate to the viscera. The CD4 cell count is usually below 200/μL when disease becomes clinically evident.

Cutaneous Leishmaniasis Cutaneous leishmaniasis has traditionally been classified as New World (American) or Old World. The former occurs from southern Texas to northern Argentina and is usually caused by the *L. mexicana* complex or the *Viannia* group. The latter is caused by *L. tropica, L. major, L. aethiopica, L. infantum,* and *L. donovani.* The incubation period ranges from weeks to months. The lesion usually begins as a single papule at the site of a sandfly bite and evolves to a nodular and then an ulcerative form, with a central depression surrounded by a raised indurated border. Multiple primary lesions, satellite lesions, regional lymphadenopathy, sporotrichoid subcutaneous nodules, lesional pain or pruritus, and secondary bacterial infection are variably present. Spontaneous resolution of the lesions may require weeks, months, or years; reactivation may occur. *Diffuse cutaneous leishmaniasis* develops in the context of *Leishmania*-specific anergy and manifests as chronic nonulcerative skin lesions. *Leishmaniasis recidivans*, a hyperergic variant with scarce parasites, manifests as a chronic solitary lesion on the cheek that expands slowly despite central healing.

DIAGNOSIS   The diagnosis of leishmaniasis requires demonstration of the organism by smear, slide, or culture of aspirates or biopsy specimens (e.g., spleen, liver, bone marrow, or lymph node for visceral disease). Antibody testing is most helpful diagnostically (>90% sensitive) in visceral leishmaniasis when cutaneous lesions are absent. The sensitivity of antibody testing is only about 50% in pts with visceral disease who are coinfected with HIV. *Leishmania*-specific cell-mediated immunity is undetectable in visceral leishmaniasis. For cutaneous disease, Giemsa-stained thin smears (e.g., of skin scrapings) and leishmanin skin-test reactivity are of value.

Rx TREATMENT

Visceral disease is treated with a pentavalent antimonial (Sb^v)—i.e., 20 mg/kg IV or IM qd for 28 d. Factors such as primary drug resistance or concurrent HIV infection of the host may mandate more prolonged therapy or use of an alternative or adjunctive agent. For drug-resistant cases in normal hosts, amphotericin B (0.5–1 mg/kg IV qd or qod, up to a total dose of 7–20 mg/kg) or pentamidine (2–4 mg/kg IV or IM qd or qod for at least 15 doses) are alternatives. The choice of whether and how to treat cutaneous disease should be based on the location, evolution, and chronicity of the infection. For optimal efficacy, Sb^v is given (20 mg/kg IV or IM qd for 20 d). Ketoconazole (adult dose, 600 mg/d PO for 28 d) and itraconazole (adult dose, 200 mg bid for 28 d) are modestly active against certain species and strains. Local or topical therapy should be considered only for infections that do not have the potential to disseminate.

TRYPANOSOMIASIS

Chagas' Disease

EPIDEMIOLOGY   Chagas' disease (American trypanosomiasis) is a zoonosis caused by *Trypanosoma cruzi*, a parasite found only in the Americas. The disease is transmitted to humans primarily by infected reduviid bugs, which are spottily distributed from the southern U.S. to southern Argentina. Infection can also be transmitted by transfusion of infected blood as well as vertically from mother to fetus. Human *T. cruzi* infection is a health problem primarily among the rural poor of Central and South America.

CLINICAL MANIFESTATIONS   The first signs of acute Chagas' disease begin about a week after infection. An indurated area of erythema and swelling (the *chagoma*), accompanied by lymphadenopathy, may appear. *Romaña's sign* (unilateral painless palpebral and periocular edema) occurs when the conjunctiva is the portal of entry. Local signs are followed by fever, anorexia, and edema of the face and lower extremities. Severe myocarditis is a rare but potentially fatal complication. Acute symptoms resolve spontaneously, after which pts enter the asymptomatic or indeterminate phase of chronic *T. cruzi* infection. Symptomatic, chronic Chagas' disease develops years or even decades later, with manifestations attributable principally to cardiac and/or GI involvement. Cardiomyopathy, rhythm disturbances, or thromboemboli may occur. RBBB is the most common ECG abnormality. GI manifestations include mesoesophagus (causing dysphagia, odynophagia, chest pain, and regurgitation) and megacolon (leading to abdominal pain, chronic constipation, obstruction, perforation, septicemia, and even death).

DIAGNOSIS   The diagnosis of acute Chagas' disease requires the detection of parasites, which may be found by examination of fresh blood or buffy coat or of thick or thin blood smears. Mouse inoculation and culture of blood in special media can be attempted. Xenodiagnosis is a last resort. Chronic disease is diagnosed by serology. CF, immunofluorescence, and ELISA are all available, but their utility is limited by false-positive results.

℞ TREATMENT

Nifurtimox, the only drug active against *T. cruzi* that is available in the U.S., reduces the duration and severity of acute disease. It is only moderately effective in eradicating parasites. Treatment should be started as early as possible at a daily dose of 8–10 mg/kg for adults, 12.5–15 mg/kg for adolescents, and 15–20 mg/kg for children 1–10 years of age. Treatment is given orally in four divided doses each day for 90–120 d. There is no satisfactory therapy for chronic infection. Nifurtimox may be obtained from the CDC (tel. no. 770-639-3670).

Sleeping Sickness

EPIDEMIOLOGY   Sleeping sickness (African trypanosomiasis) is caused by parasites of the *Trypanosoma brucei* complex and is transmitted to humans by tsetse flies. About 20,000 new cases are reported annually, a figure that surely understates the true incidence.

CLINICAL MANIFESTATIONS   A painful chancre may appear at the site of inoculation. The disease is divided into stages. Stage I, during which hematogenous and lymphatic dissemination occurs, is characterized by fever, lymphadenopathy, pruritus, and circinate rash. Stage II (CNS invasion) is characterized by the insidious development of neurologic manifestations, such as daytime somnolence, halting speech, extrapyramidal signs, and ataxia, and by progressive CSF abnormalities. Neurologic impairment eventually ends in coma and death. East African trypanosomiasis (caused by *T. brucei rhodesiense*) follows a more acute course than West African trypanosomiasis (caused by *T. brucei gambiense*).

DIAGNOSIS   Definitive diagnosis requires detection of the parasite, which may be achieved in a number of ways, depending on the chronicity of the infection. A CSF examination is mandatory in all pts suspected of having African trypanosomiasis. Serology is variably sensitive and specific and is most useful for epidemiologic surveys.

TREATMENT

Drugs for the treatment of this infection are available through the CDC. The choice of regimens is based on the stage of disease and the parasite subspecies.

TOXOPLASMOSIS

EPIDEMIOLOGY   Cats are the definitive host for *Toxoplasma gondii*, which is transmitted to humans by ingestion of contaminated oocysts from the soil or of bradyzoites in undercooked meat. In the U.S., mutton and pork are far more likely to be contaminated than is beef. The seroprevalence of antibody to *T. gondii* varies by geographic location and population age. Transplacental transmission occurs overall in about one-third of cases in which the mother acquires infection during pregnancy. The risk of transmission and the potential consequences for the fetus vary according to the time in pregnancy at which maternal infection occurs. Only about 15% of women infected in the first trimester transmit infection, but neonatal disease is most severe in these cases; 65% of women infected in the third trimester transmit infection, but the infant is usually asymptomatic at birth.

CLINICAL MANIFESTATIONS   *Immunocompetent Patients*   Acute infection is usually asymptomatic and may go unrecognized in 80–90% of children and adults who acquire infection postnatally. Acute toxoplasmosis is characterized by lymphadenopathy, which, while most often cervical, is generalized in 20–30% of symptomatic pts. Headache, malaise, fatigue, and fever develop in 20–40% of pts with lymphadenopathy. Symptoms usually resolve within several weeks. Lymphadenopathy may persist for months.

Ocular Infection   *T. gondii* causes 35% of cases of chorioretinitis in the U.S. and Europe. Most such infections are acquired congenitally.

Immunocompromised Patients   Pts who have AIDS or who are receiving chemotherapy for a lymphoproliferative disorder are at greatest risk for acute infection. More than 95%

of toxoplasmosis cases in AIDS pts represent reactivated latent infection. Encephalitis occurs in most of these cases, typically when CD4 cell counts are <100/μL. Manifestations referable to CNS disease occur in more than 50% of immunocompromised hosts with acute toxoplasmosis. Symptoms and signs include altered mental status (75%), fever (10–72%), seizures (33%), headaches (56%), and focal neurologic abnormalities (60%) and are attributable to encephalopathy, meningoencephalitis, and/or mass lesions.

DIAGNOSIS While *T. gondii* can be cultured in the peritoneal cavities of mice or identified in histologic specimens, serologic testing is the routine diagnostic method. The Sabin-Feldman dye test, the indirect fluorescent antibody test, and the ELISA all satisfactorily measure circulating IgG antibody, which can appear as early as 2–3 weeks after infection and persists for life. Simultaneous testing for IgM antibody is necessary to determine the timing of infection; the methods used are double-sandwich IgM-ELISA and IgM-immunosorbent assay. The former is more sensitive for detecting fetal and neonatal infections. In AIDS pts, a positive IgG serology and compatible neuroradiographic findings are sufficient for a presumptive diagnosis. On CT or MRI, pts with *Toxoplasma* encephalitis have focal or multifocal lesions; these lesions are usually ring-enhancing on CT. If presumptive therapy for toxoplasmosis fails to result in early radiologic improvement, a brain biopsy should be considered; lymphoma, in particular, may have an identical radiographic appearance. The persistence of IgG antibody or a positive IgM titer after the first week of life is suggestive of congenitally acquired infection. However, up to 25% of infected newborns may be seronegative and have normal routine physical exams. Thus, specific end-organ assessment (eye, brain) may be necessary to establish the diagnosis.

℞ **TREATMENT**

Immunocompetent pts with acute toxoplasmosis generally do not require therapy. For immunocompromised pts, the preferred regimen is pyrimethamine (a 200-mg PO loading dose followed by 50–75 mg/d) plus sulfadiazine (4–6 g/d PO, divided qid), along with leucovorin (10–15 mg/d). If hypersensitivity or toxicity develops, pyrimethamine (75 mg/d) plus clindamycin (450 mg tid) is an alternative regimen. Glucocorticoids are often used to treat intracerebral edema. After 4–6 weeks (or when radiographic improvement becomes evident), the pt may be switched to chronic suppressive therapy with pyrimethamine (25–50 mg/d) plus sulfadiazine (2–

4 g/d); pyrimethamine alone (50–75 mg/d) may be sufficient. Pts with ocular infection can be treated for 1 month. Congenitally infected neonates are treated with daily pyrimethamine (0.5–1 mg/kg) and sulfadiazine (100 mg/kg) for 1 year. Therapy with spiramycin (100 mg/kg qd) plus prednisone (1 mg/kg qd) is also efficacious. A variety of other regimens are available for pts in whom long-term therapy is limited by toxicity. Dapsone may be substituted for sulfadiazine. For pts with AIDS and *Toxoplasma* encephalitis, pyrimethamine (25–75 mg/d) plus clindamycin (300–1200 mg IV qid) is effective, as is pyrimethamine plus clarithromycin. Atovaquone (750 mg tid or qid) is a third-line agent. For prophylaxis in AIDS pts with CD4 counts below 100/μL, TMP-SMZ alone or the combination of pyrimethamine, dapsone, and leucovorin may be used.

PROTOZOAL INTESTINAL INFECTIONS

Giardiasis

EPIDEMIOLOGY Giardiasis is one of the most common parasitic infections worldwide and is the most common cause of waterborne epidemics of gastroenteritis in the U.S. Infection follows ingestion of the cyst form of *Giardia lamblia*. Person-to-person transmission may take place (e.g., among children in day-care centers, among residents of institutions where fecal hygiene is poor, and between homosexuals). Food-borne transmission has also been documented.

CLINICAL MANIFESTATIONS Manifestations may range from asymptomatic infection to fulminant diarrhea and malabsorption. The usual incubation period is 1–3 weeks; symptoms may develop suddenly or gradually. Early symptoms include diarrhea, abdominal pain, bloating, belching, flatus, nausea, and vomiting. Diarrhea is common, but upper intestinal manifestations may predominate. The duration of acute symptoms is usually >1 week; diarrhea may abate earlier. In chronic giardiasis, diarrhea may not be prominent, but increased flatus, loose stools, sulfurous burping, and (in some cases) weight loss occur. Fever is uncommon, as is the presence of blood or mucus in the stool.

DIAGNOSIS Giardiasis is diagnosed by the identification of cysts in the feces or of trophozoites in the feces or small intestine. Repeat examinations of stool or examination of aspirated duodenal fluid or of tissue from a small-intestinal biopsy may be required. A sensitive and specific alternative is to test for parasitic antigen in stool.

℞ **TREATMENT**
Metronidazole (250 mg PO tid for 5 d) is curative in more
than 80% of cases. Furazolidone (100 mg PO qid for 7–10
d) is somewhat less effective but more palatable to children.
Pts in whom initial treatment fails can be retreated with a
longer course. Those who remain infected should be evaluated
for reinfection through close personal contacts or environmental sources and for hypogammaglobulinemia. In particularly
refractory cases, prolonged treatment with metronidazole (750
mg PO tid for 21 d) has been successful. Paromomycin can
be used in pregnant pts with symptomatic giardiasis.

Cryptosporidiosis

EPIDEMIOLOGY Cryptosporidiosis is acquired by ingestion of oocysts. Water is the primary source in outbreaks; the
oocysts are resistant to killing by routine chlorination. Crypt-
osporidial infection may cause symptomatic diarrhea in immunocompetent hosts, but pts with immunodeficiencies (especially
AIDS) are at greatest risk.

CLINICAL MANIFESTATIONS The diarrhea of cryptosporidiosis characteristically is watery, nonbloody, and profuse. Abdominal pain, nausea, anorexia, fever, and weight loss
may occur. In immunocompetent hosts, diarrhea resolves in 1–
2 weeks. In immunocompromised hosts, especially AIDS pts,
diarrhea may be chronic and profuse and may cause significant
fluid and electrolyte losses. Stool volumes may reach 25 L/d.

DIAGNOSIS The diagnosis is made by the demonstration of
oocysts in stool. Concentration methods as well as modified
acid-fast or immunofluorescent staining enhance detection. Intestinal biopsy may also be useful.

℞ **TREATMENT**
There is no effective therapy for this infection, although paromomycin (500–750 mg qid) may be partially effective for
some HIV-infected pts. Supportive treatment is used, including fluid and electrolyte replacement and the administration of antidiarrheal agents.

Isosporiasis

CLINICAL MANIFESTATIONS Acute infection with
Isospora belli begins abruptly with fever, abdominal pain, and
watery nonbloody diarrhea and may last for weeks or months.
In AIDS and other immunocompromised pts, the infection may
not be self-limited but rather may resemble cryptosporidiosis,

with chronic profuse watery diarrhea. Eosinophilia, not found in other enteric protozoan infections, may develop.

DIAGNOSIS The diagnosis is made by the demonstration in stool of large oocysts revealed by modified acid-fast staining. Repeated stool examinations, sampling of duodenal contents by aspiration or a string test, or even small-bowel biopsy may be required.

℞ TREATMENT

I. belli does respond to treatment. TMP-SMZ (160/800 mg PO qid for 10 d, then bid for 3 weeks) has proved effective. Pyrimethamine (50–75 mg/d PO) may be used in pts with sulfonamide intolerance. Relapses can occur in AIDS pts, necessitating maintenance therapy with TMP-SMZ (160/800 mg) three times a week or with sulfadoxine (500 mg) plus pyrimethamine (25 mg) once a week.

Cyclosporiasis

CLINICAL MANIFESTATIONS *Cyclospora cayetanensis* is globally distributed. Waterborne transmission is one means of its acquisition by humans. Infection may be asymptomatic or may manifest as diarrhea, a flulike illness, flatulence, and burping. The illness may be self-limited, may wax and wane, or may persist for >1 month.

DIAGNOSIS The diagnosis can be made by detection of spherical 8- to 10-μm oocysts in the stool. The oocysts are refractile, are variably acid-fast, and fluoresce under UV light.

℞ TREATMENT

Cyclosporiasis is effectively treated with TMP-SMZ (160/800 mg PO bid for 7 d). HIV-infected pts may require suppressive maintenance therapy.

Microsporidiosis

ETIOLOGY AND CLINICAL MANIFESTATIONS Microsporidia are obligate intracellular spore-forming protozoa that have recently been recognized as agents of human disease, especially among people infected with HIV. Six genera are recognized. *Enterocytozoon bieneusi* and *Encephalitozoon intestinalis* cause chronic diarrhea and wasting in AIDS pts; these organisms are found in 10–40% of pts with chronic diarrhea. Disseminated disease due to *E. intestinalis* may also occur, with fever, diarrhea, sinusitis, cholangitis, and bronchiolitis.

DIAGNOSIS The diagnosis of tissue infection may require electron microscopy, although intracellular spores (0.5–2 μm × 1–4 μm) may be seen in tissue sections stained with hematoxylin and eosin, Giemsa, or Gram's stain.

℞ **TREATMENT**

Definitive therapies for microsporidial infections remain to be established.

For a more detailed discussion, see Reed SL: Amebiasis and Infection with Free-Living Amebas, Chap. 215, p. 1176; White NJ, Breman JG: Malaria and Other Diseases Caused by Red Blood Cell Parasites, Chap. 216, p. 1180; Herwaldt BL: Leishmaniasis, Chap. 217, p. 1189; Kirchhoff LV: Trypanosomiasis, Chap. 218, p. 1193; Kasper LH: *Toxoplasma* Infection, Chap. 219, p. 1197; and Nash TE, Weller PF: Protozoal Intestinal Infections and Trichomoniasis, Chap. 220, p. 1202, in HPIM-14.

103

HELMINTHIC INFECTIONS

TRICHINOSIS

EPIDEMIOLOGY *Trichinella* spp. infect carnivorous and omnivorous animals worldwide. Both humans and animals acquire the infection by ingesting meat containing encysted *Trichinella* larvae. Swine are the most common human vector. From 50 to 100 human cases are reported in the U.S. each year. Most mild cases probably remain undiagnosed.

PATHOGENESIS AND CLINICAL MANIFESTATIONS Light infections are usually asymptomatic. With heavy infection, clinical symptoms parallel the stages of the parasite's life cycle: Enteric invasion during the first week may cause diarrhea or constipation, abdominal pain, nausea, and vomiting. Larval migration during the second week is associated with fever, hypereosinophilia, periorbital and facial edema, and splinter hemorrhages. Maculopapular rash, myocarditis, pneumonitis, or encephalitis may develop. Encystment of larvae in muscle beginning in the second to third week is associated with myalgia, muscle edema, and weakness. The most commonly involved muscle groups are the extraocular muscles, the biceps, and the muscles of the jaw, neck, lower back, and diaphragm.

DIAGNOSIS The diagnosis is made histologically by the finding of larvae in a fresh specimen of muscle, which should be compressed between glass slides and examined microscopically. At least 1 g of involved muscle should be biopsied. The yield is highest near tendinous insertions. A rise in the titer of parasite-specific antibody may also be diagnostic but usually does not occur until after the third week of infection.

℞ **TREATMENT**

No agents are currently available for the treatment of *Trichinella* larvae in muscle. Thiabendazole (25 mg/kg PO bid for 5–7 d) and mebendazole (400 mg PO tid) are active against the early, enteric stage of the infection. For cases with severe myositis or myocarditis, prednisone (1 mg/kg PO qd for 5 d) is beneficial.

PREVENTION Larvae encysted in pork may be killed by cooking the meat until it is no longer pink or by freezing it at −15°C for 3 weeks. *T. nativa*, the species prevalent among arctic carnivores, is relatively tolerant of freezing.

VISCERAL AND OCULAR LARVA MIGRANS

PATHOGENESIS AND EPIDEMIOLOGY Visceral larva migrans (toxocariasis) is a syndrome caused by nematodes parasitic for nonhuman species. Human infection is a dead end for the parasite. The nematode larvae do not develop into adult worms. Instead, their migration through host tissues elicits an eosinophilic inflammatory response. Humans acquire toxocariasis mainly by eating soil contaminated with puppy feces containing infective *Toxocara canis* eggs. Seropositivity rates may exceed 20% among U.S. kindergarten children.

CLINICAL MANIFESTATIONS Most light infections are asymptomatic; eosinophilia may be the lone clue. Characteristic manifestations of heavier infection include fever, malaise, anorexia, weight loss, cough, wheezing, rash, and hepatosplenomegaly. Extraordinary eosinophilia is often present; eosinophils may constitute 90% of the WBCs. Half of pts with symptomatic pneumonitis have transient pulmonary infiltrates. Ocular disease occurs when larvae invade the eye. A granulomatous mass develops around the larvae and may be mistaken for retinoblastoma. The spectrum of ocular involvement also includes endophthalmitis, uveitis, and chorioretinitis.

DIAGNOSIS The clinical diagnosis of toxocariasis is confirmed by an ELISA positive for toxocaral antibodies. Since *Toxocara* larvae do not develop into adult worms in humans, eggs are not found in the stool.

Rx TREATMENT

Available anthelmintic drugs have not been shown conclusively to alter the course of larva migrans. In pts with severe disease, glucocorticoids may be used to reduce inflammatory complications. For ocular disease, treatment is unsatisfactory; the roles of glucocorticoids and anthelmintics are controversial.

CUTANEOUS LARVA MIGRANS

Cutaneous larva migrans ("creeping eruption") is a serpiginous skin eruption caused by burrowing larvae of animal hookworms, most commonly *Ancylostoma braziliense*.

PATHOGENESIS AND CLINICAL MANIFESTATIONS Larvae hatch from eggs passed in canine or feline feces and mature in the soil, after which they can penetrate human skin to initiate infection. Erythematous, pruritic lesions form along the tortuous tracks of their migration; the larvae may advance several centimeters per day.

DIAGNOSIS The diagnosis is readily made on clinical grounds. A skin biopsy rarely yields diagnostic material.

Rx TREATMENT

Without treatment, larvae die out after several weeks. Symptoms are alleviated by treatment with thiabendazole (25 mg/kg PO bid or a 10% suspension applied topically for 2–5 d), ivermectin (a single dose of 150–200 µg/kg), or albendazole (200 mg bid for 2 d).

ASCARIASIS

Ascaris lumbricoides (roundworm) is the largest intestinal nematode parasite of humans, reaching up to 40 cm in length.

EPIDEMIOLOGY *Ascaris* is widely distributed in tropical and subtropical regions and in other humid areas, such as the rural southeastern U.S. An estimated 1 billion people are infected worldwide.

PATHOGENESIS   Infective eggs present in soil are ingested. Larvae hatch in the intestine, traverse the mucosa to gain access to the bloodstream, and are transported to the lung, where they break into the alveoli, ascend the bronchial tree, are swallowed, and return to the small intestine. There they become adult worms. Mature females produce many thousands of eggs each day.

CLINICAL MANIFESTATIONS   Clinical disease arises from pulmonary hypersensitivity or from intestinal events. Fever, cough, and eosinophilia may develop during the stage of pulmonary migration. Eosinophilic pneumonitis (Loeffler's syndrome) may be evident on CXR. Light intestinal infection is usually asymptomatic. A heavy intestinal burden of adult worms may cause obstruction and malabsorption. A lone worm migrating to aberrant sites (e.g., the biliary tree) may also cause disease.

DIAGNOSIS   The characteristic eggs may be seen on microscopic examination of stool. Adult worms may be passed.

R̲ₓ TREATMENT
Mebendazole and albendazole are effective, but their use is contraindicated in pregnancy or for heavy infection. Pyrantel pamoate and piperazine citrate are safe in pregnancy.

STRONGYLOIDIASIS

Strongyloides stercoralis is distinguished by a capacity, unusual among helminths, to replicate in humans. This capacity permits ongoing cycles of autoinfection from endogenously produced larvae. Strongyloidiasis can thus persist for decades; at times of host immunocompromise, the larvae may disseminate widely, with catastrophic results (autoinfection syndrome).

EPIDEMIOLOGY   *S. stercoralis* is spottily distributed in tropical areas and other hot, humid regions. It is endemic in parts of the southern U.S. This nematode is also found among residents of mental institutions, where hygiene is poor, and among persons who have lived in endemic areas abroad.

PATHOGENESIS   Filariform larvae in fecally contaminated soil penetrate human skin, travel via the bloodstream to the lung, penetrate into the alveoli, ascend the airway, are swallowed, reach the small bowel, and there mature into adult worms. In autoinfection, larvae invade through the colonic wall or perianal skin.

CLINICAL MANIFESTATIONS In uncomplicated strongyloidiasis, pts may be asymptomatic or have mild cutaneous and/or abdominal symptoms, including recurrent urticaria (especially involving the wrists and/or buttocks), "larva currens" (a pathognomonic response to subcutaneous migrating larvae, which may advance up to 10 cm/h), nausea, diarrhea, GI bleeding, and epigastric pain aggravated by eating. Eosinophilia is common and may fluctuate with time. Pulmonary symptoms are rare. In autoinfection syndrome, larvae may invade the GI tract, lungs, CNS, liver, kidneys, and peritoneum and may facilitate the development of gram-negative sepsis, pneumonia, or meningitis.

DIAGNOSIS In uncomplicated strongyloidiasis, the finding of rhabditiform larvae in stool or intestinal aspirates is diagnostic. A sensitive ELISA for *Strongyloides* antigens is available. For suspected disseminated strongyloidiasis, filariform larvae should be sought in stool, sputum, and other sites of potential dissemination.

℞ TREATMENT

For uncomplicated infection, thiabendazole (25 mg/kg PO bid) should be administered for 2 d. For disseminated infection, treatment should be extended for at least 5–7 d.

LYMPHATIC FILARIASIS

PATHOGENESIS AND EPIDEMIOLOGY The agents of lymphatic filariasis (*Wuchereria bancrofti* throughout the tropics and subtropics, *Brugia malayi* in India and the Far East, and *Brugia timori* in Indonesia) are transmitted by mosquitoes. In excess of 80 million people are affected. The adult filariae reside in lymphatics and lymph node sinuses. The presence of the worms and the host's inflammatory response to them lead to lymphatic compromise. Death of the worms enhances inflammation and fibrosis, ultimately causing lymphatic obstruction and lymphedema.

CLINICAL MANIFESTATIONS Common manifestations include asymptomatic microfilaremia, hydrocele, acute lymphangitis/lymphadenitis (which may be associated with "filarial fever"), and lymphatic obstruction.

DIAGNOSIS A definitive diagnosis is made only by detection of the parasite, which can be difficult. By virtue of their location in lymphatics, the adults are inaccessible. Microfilariae should be sought in blood and hydrocele fluid. The timing of blood sampling is critical and should be based on the periodicity of the microfilariae suspected to be involved. Interpretation of serologic findings is complicated by cross-reactivity of filarial antigens with antigens of other helminths and by the sensitization of some uninfected residents of endemic areas to filarial antigens through exposure to infected mosquitoes. PCR-based assays have been developed.

℞ TREATMENT

Therapy with diethylcarbamazine (DEC, 6 mg/kg daily in either single or divided doses for 2–3 weeks) clears microfilariae. Single-dose ivermectin may be equally efficacious. To minimize acute reactions to antigens released by dying filariae, gradual upward titration of the DEC dose or premedication with glucocorticoids may be useful.

ONCHOCERCIASIS

EPIDEMIOLOGY   Onchocerciasis ("river blindness") is caused by the filarial nematode *Onchocerca volvulus*. Some 13 million people are infected in equatorial Africa and Latin America. Onchocerciasis is the second leading infectious cause of blindness worldwide.

PATHOGENESIS   Infective larvae are deposited on human skin by the bites of infected blackflies. The larvae develop into adults, which reside in subcutaneous nodules. After an interval ranging from months to ~3 years, microfilariae begin to be released, migrate out of the nodule and throughout the tissues, and concentrate in the dermis. Onchocerciasis affects primarily the skin, eyes, and lymph nodes. The damage is elicited by the microfilariae, not by the adult worms.

CLINICAL MANIFESTATIONS   Pruritus and generalized papular rash are common; the pruritus can be incapacitating. Subcutaneous onchocercomata contain adult worms. Lesions may develop in any part of the eye. Ocular lesions include sclerosing keratitis (the leading cause of onchocercal blindness in Africa), anterior uveitis, iridocyclitis, and chorioretinal atrophy. Secondary glaucoma or optic atrophy may occur.

DIAGNOSIS   Definitive diagnosis depends on detection of an adult worm in an excised nodule or of microfilariae in a skin snip. For identification of the latter form, snips should be incubated for 2–4 h in saline on a glass slide and examined by low-power microscopy.

℞ TREATMENT

The main goals of therapy are to prevent the development of irreversible lesions and to ease symptoms. Nodules on the head must be excised to avoid ocular infection. Ivermectin is administered orally in a single dose of 150 µg/kg, either annually or semiannually. Contraindications to treatment include pregnancy, breast-feeding, CNS disorders that compromise the blood-brain barrier, and an age of <5 years. Ivermectin does not kill adult worms. Suramin, which does, is toxic and therefore is recommended only if total cure is necessary.

SCHISTOSOMIASIS

EPIDEMIOLOGY　*Schistosoma mansoni* is found in parts of South America, some Caribbean islands, Africa, and the Middle East; *S. japonicum*, in the Far East; *S. haematobium*, in Africa and the Middle East; and *S. mekongi*, along the Mekong River in Indochina. Worldwide, some 200 million people may be infected with schistosomes. Only a small minority of them develop significant disease.

PATHOGENESIS　Cercariae, released from freshwater snails, penetrate unbroken human skin. As they mature into schistosomes, they reach the portal vein, where males and females pair. They then migrate to the venules of the bladder and ureters (*S. haematobium*) or mesentery (*S. mansoni, S. japonicum, S. mekongi*) and begin to deposit eggs. Some mature ova are extruded into the intestinal or urinary lumina, from which they may reach water and perpetuate the life cycle. The persistence of other ova in tissues leads to a granulomatous host response and fibrosis. Factors governing disease manifestations include the intensity and duration of infection, the location of egg deposition, and the genetic characteristics of the host.

CLINICAL MANIFESTATIONS　Acute schistosomiasis, or Katayama fever, occurs in visitors to endemic areas and lasts up to 3 months. It is frequently mistaken for typhoid fever. Years of heavy infection with *S. mansoni*, *S. japonicum*, or *S. mekongi* can lead to periportal (Symmers') hepatic fibrosis, presinusoidal portal hypertension, splenomegaly, and esophageal varices. *S. haematobium* prefers the veins of the urinary tract. It may cause hematuria and dysuria at all stages of infection and may produce ureteral and vesicular fibrosis and calcification in the chronic stage. Cor pulmonale and immune-complex glomerulonephritis may occur with any of these four schistosome species.

Table 103-1

Treatment of Schistosomiasis

Species	Drug	Total Dose* (mg/kg of Body Weight)
S. haematobium	Praziquantel	40
	Metrifonate†	22.5–30
S. mansoni		
Americas and Caribbean	Oxamniquine	15
	Praziquantel	40
Africa and Middle East	Oxamniquine	60
	Praziquantel	40
S. japonicum or *S. mekongi*	Praziquantel	60

*All recommended drugs are given orally.
†Available from the Parasitic Diseases Division, Center for Infectious Diseases, Centers for Disease Control and Prevention, Atlanta, GA 30333.
SOURCE: Nash TE: HPIM-14, p. 1220.

DIAGNOSIS The diagnosis is established by the identification in urine (*S. haematobium*), feces, or tissues of the characteristic oval eggs with single spinous processes.

℞ TREATMENT
See Table 103-1.

TAENIASIS AND DIPHYLLOBOTHRIASIS

PATHOGENESIS Cysticercal larvae are ingested in undercooked beef (*Taenia saginata*), pork (*Taenia solium*), or fish (*Diphyllobothrium latum*) and develop into mature tapeworms within the definitive human host. For *T. solium*, humans can also be the intermediate host: ingestion of *T. solium* eggs, their embryonation, and dissemination of the larvae lead to cysticercosis.

CLINICAL MANIFESTATIONS Adult tapeworm infections may be asymptomatic or may cause mild abdominal discomfort, nausea, change in appetite, and/or weight loss. Proglottids may be visible in stool. *D. latum* infections are associated with vitamin B_{12} deficiency. CNS cysticercosis can cause seizures, hydrocephalus, and signs of elevated intracranial pressure.

Regimen

Single dose or two doses of 20 mg/kg
Single dose of 7.5 to 10 mg/kg given every other week $\times$ 3

Single dose with food
Single dose or two doses of 20 mg/kg 4 h apart with food
15 mg/kg twice a day for 2 days with food
Single dose or two doses of 20 mg/kg 4 h apart with food
20 mg/kg every 4 h with food

DIAGNOSIS　With adult tapeworm infection, eggs or proglottids (worm segments) are detectable in stool. Cysticercosis is diagnosed definitively by the finding of cysticerci in involved tissue and presumptively by the finding of characteristic neuroradiographic lesions and compatible serology in a pt with an appropriate epidemiologic background.

R_x TREATMENT

For infection with adult worms, a single dose of praziquantel (5–10 mg/kg) is highly effective. Vitamin B_{12} should be given parenterally if the pt is B_{12} deficient. Treatment of the symptoms of neurocysticercosis consists of praziquantel (50 mg/kg qd in 3 doses for 15 d) or albendazole (15 mg/kg qd in 3 doses for 8–28 d); hospitalization and concomitant glucocorticoid therapy are advisable. Ocular, spinal, or cerebral ventricular lesions may require excision.

ECHINOCOCCOSIS

PATHOGENESIS AND EPIDEMIOLOGY　Infection occurs through human ingestion of eggs of the dog tapeworms. Embryos penetrate the intestinal mucosa, enter the portal circulation, and disseminate to various organs, especially the liver and lungs. Brood capsules and daughter cysts develop within hydatid cysts. New larvae, called *scolices*, develop within the brood capsules. *Echinococcus granulosus* occurs in livestock-raising regions outside North America. *E. multilocularis* predominates in arctic and subarctic zones. *E. vogeli* is found only in Central and South America. *E. multilocularis* vesicles are locally invasive.

CLINICAL MANIFESTATIONS Enlargement of cysts may progress for 5–20 years before the development of symptoms, which are typically related to compressive or mass effects. Hepatic echinococcosis may present as abdominal pain, a palpable RUQ mass, or biliary obstruction. Cyst rupture may produce fever, pruritus, urticaria, or anaphylaxis and leads to multifocal dissemination. *E. multilocularis* infection mimics hepatic malignancy, with liver destruction, extension into vital structures, and (in occasional cases) metastasis.

DIAGNOSIS The CT finding of daughter cysts within the larger cyst is pathognomonic for *E. granulosus* infection. MRI, ultrasound, and—for pulmonary disease—plain films may be diagnostically helpful. Serology is negative in up to 50% of pts. Aspiration poses a risk of rupture and dissemination but, with CT guidance, has been used successfully in some centers.

℞ **TREATMENT**
When feasible, surgery is the definitive method of treatment. The exact role of chemotherapy is undefined. As medical therapy, albendazole (400 mg PO bid for 12 weeks) is most efficacious against hepatic and pulmonary cysts. Multiple courses of treatment may be necessary.

For a more detailed discussion, see Liu LX, Weller PF: Trichinosis and Infections with Other Tissue Nematodes, Chap. 221, p. 1206; Liu LX, Weller PF: Intestinal Nematodes, Chap. 222, p. 1208; Nutman TB, Weller PF: Filariasis and Related Infections (Loiasis, Onchocerciasis, and Dracunculiasis), Chap. 223, p. 1212; Nash TE: Schistosomiasis and Other Trematode Infections, Chap. 224, p. 1217; and Nutman TB, Weller PF: Cestodes, Chap. 225, p. 1224, in HPIM-14.

104

PHYSICAL EXAMINATION OF THE HEART

General examination of a pt with suspected heart disease should include vital signs (respiratory rate, pulse, blood pressure), skin color, clubbing, edema, evidence of decreased perfusion (cool and sweaty skin), and hypertensive changes in optic fundi. Important findings on cardiovascular examination include:

CAROTID ARTERY PULSE (Fig. 104-1)

1. *Pulsus parvus:* Weak upstroke due to decreased stroke volume (hypovolemia, LV failure, aortic or mitral stenosis).
2. *Pulsus tardus:* Delayed upstroke (aortic stenosis).
3. *Bounding pulse:* Hyperkinetic circulation, aortic regurgitation, patent ductus arteriosus, marked vasodilatation.
4. *Pulsus bisferiens:* Double systolic pulsation in aortic regurgitation, hypertrophic cardiomyopathy.
5. *Pulsus alternans:* Regular alteration in pulse pressure amplitude (severe LV dysfunction).
6. *Pulsus paradoxus:* Exaggerated inspiratory fall (>10 mmHg) in systolic bp (pericardial tamponade, obstructive lung disease).

JUGULAR VENOUS PULSATION (JVP) (Fig. 104-2)

Jugular venous distention develops in right-sided heart failure,

A. Hypokinetic Pulse   B. Parvus et Tardus Pulse   C. Hyperkinetic Pulse

D. Bisferiens Pulse   E. Dicrotic Pulse + Alternans

FIGURE 104-1   Carotid artery pulse patterns.

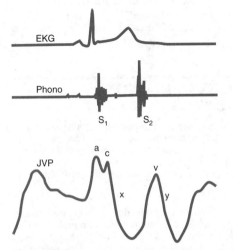

FIGURE 104-2 Normal jugular venous pressure recording.

constrictive pericarditis, pericardial tamponade, obstruction of superior vena cava. JVP normally *falls* with inspiration but may *rise* (Kussmaul's sign) in constrictive pericarditis. Abnormalities in examination include:

1. *Large "a" wave:* Tricuspid stenosis (TS), pulmonic stenosis, AV dissociation (right atrium contracts against closed tricuspid valve).
2. *Large "v" wave:* Tricuspid regurgitation, atrial septal defect.
3. *Steep "y" descent:* Constrictive pericarditis.
4. *Slow "y" descent:* Tricuspid stenosis.

PRECORDIAL PALPATION Cardiac apical impulse is normally localized in the fifth intercostal space, midclavicular line (Fig. 104-3). Abnormalities include:

1. *Forceful apical thrust:* Left ventricular hypertrophy.
2. *Lateral and downward displacement of apex impulse:* Left ventricular dilatation.
3. *Prominent presystolic impulse:* Hypertension, aortic stenosis, hypertrophic cardiomyopathy.
4. *Double systolic apical impulse:* Hypertrophic cardiomyopathy.
5. *Sustained "lift" at lower left sternal border:* Right ventricular hypertrophy.

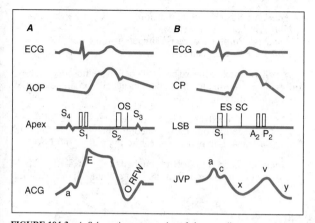

FIGURE 104-3 *A.* Schematic representation of electrocardiogram, aortic pressure pulse (AOP), phonocardiogram recorded at the apex, and apex cardiogram (ACG). On the phonocardiogram, S_1, S_2, S_3, and S_4 represent the first through fourth heart sounds; OS represents the opening snap of the mitral valve, which occurs coincident with the O point of the apex cardiogram. S_3 occurs coincident with the termination of the rapid-filling wave (RFW) of the ACG, while S_4 occurs coincident with the *a* wave of the ACG. *B.* Simultaneous recording of electrocardiogram, indirect carotid pulse (CP), phonocardiogram along the left sternal border (LSB), and indirect jugular venous pulse (JVP). ES, ejection sound; SC, systolic click.

6. *Dyskinetic (outward bulge) impulse:* Ventricular aneurysm, large dyskinetic area post MI, cardiomyopathy.

AUSCULTATION

HEART SOUNDS (Fig. 104-3) S_1 *Loud:* Mitral stenosis, short PR interval, hyperkinetic heart, thin chest wall. *Soft:* Long PR interval, heart failure, mitral regurgitation, thick chest wall, pulmonary emphysema.

S_2 Normally A_2 precedes P_2 and splitting increases with inspiration; abnormalities include:

- *Widened* splitting: Right bundle branch block, pulmonic stenosis, mitral regurgitation.
- *Fixed* splitting (no respiratory change in splitting): Atrial septal defect.
- *Narrow* splitting: Pulmonary hypertension.
- *Paradoxical* splitting (splitting *narrows* with inspiration): Aortic stenosis, left bundle branch block, CHF.

- *Loud* A$_2$: Systemic hypertension.
- *Soft* A$_2$: Aortic stenosis (AS).
- *Loud* P$_2$: Pulmonary arterial hypertension.
- *Soft* P$_2$: Pulmonic stenosis (PS).

S$_3$ Low-pitched, heard best with bell of stethoscope at apex, following S$_2$; normal in children; after age 30–35, indicates LV failure or volume overload.

S$_4$ Low-pitched, heard best with bell at apex, preceding S$_1$; reflects atrial contraction into a noncompliant ventricle; found in AS, hypertension, hypertrophic cardiomyopathy, and CAD.

Opening Snap (OS) High-pitched; follows S$_2$ (by 0.06–0.12s), heard at lower left sternal border and apex in mitral

Table 104-1

Heart Murmurs

SYSTOLIC MURMURS

Ejection-type	Aortic outflow tract
	Aortic valve stenosis
	Hypertrophic obstructive cardiomyopathy
	Aortic flow murmur
	Pulmonary outflow tract
	Pulmonic valve stenosis
	Pulmonic flow murmur
Holosystolic	Mitral regurgitation
	Tricuspid regurgitation
	Ventricular septal defect
Late-systolic	Mitral or tricuspid valve prolapse

DIASTOLIC MURMURS

Early diastolic	Aortic valve regurgitation
	Pulmonic valve regurgitation
Mid-to-late diastolic	Mitral or tricuspid stenosis
	Flow murmur across mitral or tricuspid valves
Continuous	Patent ductus arteriosus
	Coronary AV fistula
	Ruptured sinus of Valsalva aneurysm

stenosis (MS); the more severe the MS, the shorter the OS–S_2 interval.

Ejection Clicks High-pitched sounds following S_1; observed in dilatation of aortic root or pulmonary artery, congenital AS (loudest at apex) or PS (upper left sternal border); the latter decreases with inspiration.

Midsystolic Clicks At lower left sternal border and apex, often followed by late systolic murmur in mitral valve prolapse.

HEART MURMURS (Table 104-1, Fig. 104-4)

Systolic Murmurs May be "crescendo-decrescendo" ejection type, pansystolic, or late systolic; right-sided murmurs (e.g., tricuspid regurgitation) typically increase with inspiration. A number of simple maneuvers produce characteristic changes depending on cause of murmur (Table 104-2).

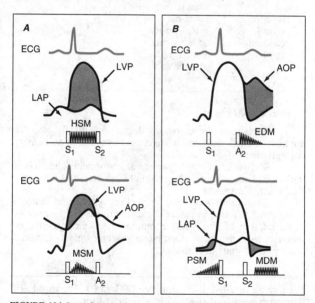

FIGURE 104-4 *A.* Schematic representation of ECG, aortic pressure (AOP), left ventricular pressure (LVP), and left atrial pressure (LAP). The hatched areas indicated a transvalvular pressure difference during systole. HSM, holosystolic murmur; MSM, midsystolic murmur. *B.* Graphic representation of ECG, aortic pressure (AOP), left ventricular pressure (LVP) and left atrial pressure (LAP) with hatched areas indicating transvalvular diastolic pressure difference. EDM, early diastolic murmur; PSM, presystolic murmur; MDM, middiastolic murmur.

Table 104-2

Heart Murmurs and Responsible Lesions

Lesion	Type of murmur	Maneuver			
		Valsalva	Hand Grip	Squat	Stand
Aortic stenosis	Crescendo-decrescendo	↓	↓	↑	↓
Mitral regurgitation	Holosystolic	↓	↑	↑	↓
Ventricular septal defect	Holosystolic	↓	↑	↑	↓
Mitral valve prolapse	Late systolic (follows click)	↑	↓	↓	↑
Hypertrophic obstructive cardiomyopathy	Harsh, diamond-shaped at left sternal border; holosystolic at apex	↑	↓	↓	↑

Diastolic Murmurs

1. *Early diastolic murmurs:* Begin immediately after S_2, are high-pitched, and usually are caused by aortic or pulmonary regurgitation.

2. *Mid-to-late diastolic murmurs:* Low-pitched, heard best with bell of stethoscope; observed in MS or TS; less commonly due to atrial myxoma.

3. *Continuous murmurs:* Present in systole and diastole (envelops S_2); found in patent ductus arteriosus and sometimes in coarctation of aorta; less common causes are systemic or coronary AV fistula, aortopulmonary septal defect, ruptured aneurysm of sinus of Valsalva.

For a more detailed discussion, see O'Gara PT, Braunwald E: Approach to the Patient with a Heart Murmur, Chap. 34, p. 198; and O'Rourke RA, Braunwald E: Physical Examination of the Cardiovascular System, Chap. 227, p. 1231, in HPIM-14.

105

ELECTROCARDIOGRAPHY AND ECHOCARDIOGRAPHY

STANDARD APPROACH TO THE ECG

Normally, standardization is 1.0 mV per 10 mm, and paper speed is 25 mm/s (each horizontal small box = 0.04 s).

HEART RATE   Beats/min = 300 divided by the number of *large* boxes (each 5 mm apart) between consecutive QRS complexes. For faster heart rates, divide 1500 by number of *small* boxes (1 mm apart) between each QRS.

RHYTHM   *Sinus rhythm* is present if every P wave is followed by a QRS, PR interval ≥0.12 s, every QRS is preceded by a P wave, and the P wave is upright in leads I, II, and III. Arrhythmias are discussed in Chap. 107.

MEAN AXIS   If QRS is primarily positive in limb leads I and II, then axis is *normal*. Otherwise, find limb lead in which QRS is most isoelectric (R = S). The mean axis is perpendicular to that lead (Fig. 105-1). If the QRS complex is *positive* in that perpendicular lead, then mean axis is in the direction of that lead; if *negative*, then mean axis points directly away from that lead.

Left-axis deviation (≤30°) occurs in diffuse left ventricular disease, inferior MI; also in left anterior hemiblock (small r, deep S in leads II, III, aVF).

Right-axis deviation (>90°) occurs in right ventricular hypertrophy (R > S in V_1) and left posterior hemiblock (small Q and tall R in leads II, III, and aVF). Mild right-axis deviation is seen in thin, healthy individuals (up to 110°).

INTERVALS   (Normal values in parentheses)

PR   (0.12–0.20 s)

- *Short:* (1) preexcitation syndrome (look for slurred QRS upstroke due to "delta" wave), (2) nodal rhythm (inverted P in aVF).
- *Long:* first-degree AV block (Chap. 107).

QRS   (0.06–0.10 s)

- *Widened:* (1) ventricular premature beats, (2) bundle branch blocks: *right* (RsR′ in V_1, deep S in V_6) and *left* (RR′ in V_6) (see Fig. 105-2), (3) toxic levels of certain drugs (e.g., quinidine), (4) severe hypokalemia.

QT   (≤0.43 s; <50% of RR interval)

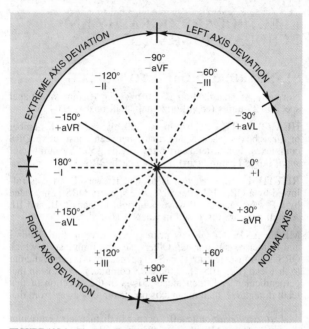

FIGURE 105-1 Electrocardiographic lead systems: The hexaxial frontal plane reference system to estimate electrical axis. Determine leads in which QRS deflections are maximum and minimum. For example, a maximum positive QRS in I which is isoelectric in aVF is oriented to 0°. Normal axis ranges from −30° to +90°. An axis > +90° is right axis deviation and < −30° is left axis deviation.

- *Prolonged:* congenital, hypokalemia, hypocalcemia, drugs (quinidine, procainamide, tricyclics).

HYPERTROPHY

- *Right atrium:* P wave ≥2.5 mm in lead II.
- *Left atrium:* P biphasic (positive, then negative) in V_1, with terminal negative force wider than 0.04 s.
- *Right ventricle:* R > S in V_1 and R in V_1 > 5 mm; deep S in V_6; right-axis deviation.
- *Left ventricle:* S in V_1 plus R in V_5 or V_6 ≥35 mm or R in aVL > 11 mm.

INFARCTION (Figs. 105-3 and 105-4)
Q-wave MI: Pathologic Q waves (≥0.04 s and ≥25% of total QRS height) in leads shown in Table 105-1; acute *non-Q-wave MI* shows ST-T changes in these leads without Q wave

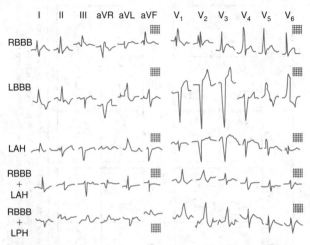

FIGURE 105-2 Intraventricular conduction abnormalities. Illustrated are right bundle branch block (RBBB); left bundle branch block (LBBB); left anterior hemiblock (LAH); right bundle branch block with left anterior hemiblock (RBBB + LAH); and right bundle branch block with left posterior hemiblock (RBBB + LPH). (*Reproduced from Myerburg RJ: HPIM-12.*)

development. A number of conditions (other than acute MI) can cause Q waves (Table 105-2).

ST-T WAVES

- *ST elevation:* Acute MI, coronary spasm, pericarditis (concave upward), LV aneurysm.
- *ST depression:* Digitalis effect, strain (due to ventricular hypertrophy), ischemia, or nontransmural MI.
- *Tall peaked T:* Hyperkalemia; acute MI ("hyperacute T").
- *Inverted T:* Non-Q-wave MI, ventricular "strain" pattern, drug effect (e.g., digitalis), hypokalemia, hypocalcemia, increased intracranial pressure (e.g., subarachnoid bleed).

INDICATIONS FOR ECHOCARDIOGRAPHY
(Fig. 105-5)

VALVULAR STENOSIS Both native and artificial valvular stenosis can be evaluated, and severity can be determined by Doppler [peak gradient = $4 \times$ (peak velocity)^2].

VALVULAR REGURGITATION Structural lesions (e.g., flail leaflet, vegetation) resulting in regurgitation may be identi-

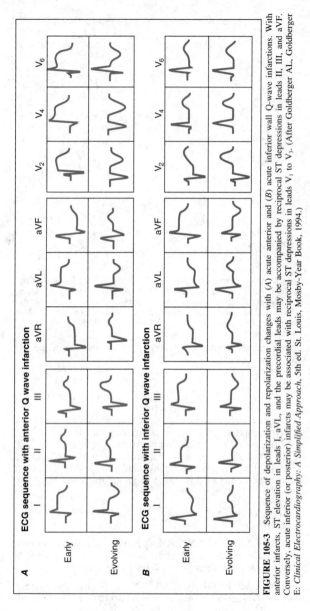

FIGURE 105-3 Sequence of depolarization and repolarization changes with (A) acute anterior and (B) acute inferior wall Q-wave infarctions. With anterior infarcts, ST elevation in leads I, aVL, and the precordial leads may be accompanied by reciprocal ST depressions in leads II, III, and aVF. Conversely, acute inferior (or posterior) infarcts may be associated with reciprocal ST depressions in leads V_1 to V_3. (After Goldberger AL, Goldberger E: *Clinical Electrocardiography: A Simplified Approach*, 5th ed. St. Louis, Mosby-Year Book, 1994.)

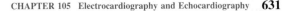

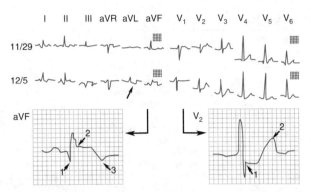

FIGURE 105-4 Acute inferior wall myocardial infarction. The ECG of 11/29 shows minor nonspecific ST-segment and T-wave changes. On 12/5 an acute myocardial infarction occurred. There are pathologic Q waves (1), ST-segment elevation (2), and terminal T-wave inversion (3) in leads II, III, and aVF indicating the location of the infarct on the inferior wall. Reciprocal changes in aVL (small arrow). Increasing R-wave voltage with ST depression and increased voltage of the T wave in V_2 is characteristic of true posterior wall extension of the inferior infarction. (*Reproduced from Myerburg RJ: HPIM-12.*)

fied. Echo can demonstrate whether ventricular function is normal; Doppler (Fig. 105-6) can identify and estimate severity of regurgitation through each valve.

VENTRICULAR PERFORMANCE   Global and regional wall motion abnormalities of both ventricles can be assessed; ventricular hypertrophy/infiltration may be visualized; evidence of pulmonary hypertension may be obtained.

Table 105-1

Leads with Abnormal Q Waves in MI

Leads with Abnormal Q Waves	Site of Infarction
V_1–V_2	Anteroseptal
V_3–V_4	Apical
I, aVL, V_5–V_6	Anterolateral
II, III, aVF	Inferior
V_1–V_2 (tall R, *not* deep Q)	True posterior

Table 105-2

Differential Diagnosis of Q Waves (with Selected Examples)

Physiologic or positional factors
1. Normal variant "septal" q waves
2. Normal variant Q waves in V_1 to V_2, aVL, III, and aVF
3. Left pneumothorax or dextrocardia

Myocardial injury or infiltration
1. Acute processes: myocardial ischemia or infarction, myocarditis, hyperkalemia
2. Chronic processes: myocardial infarction, idiopathic cardiomyopathy, myocarditis, amyloid, tumor, sarcoid, scleroderma

Ventricular hypertrophy/enlargement
1. Left ventricular (poor R-wave progression)*
2. Right ventricular (reversed R-wave progression)
3. Hypertrophic cardiomyopathy

Conduction abnormalities
1. Left bundle branch block
2. Wolff-Parkinson-White patterns

---

* Small or absent R waves in the right to midprecordial leads.
SOURCE: After Goldberger AL: *Myocardial Infarction: Electrocardiographic Differential Diagnosis*, 4th ed. St. Louis, Mosby-Year Book 1991.

CARDIAC SOURCE OF EMBOLISM   May visualize atrial or ventricular thrombus, intracardiac tumors, and valvular vegetations. Yield of identifying cardiac source of embolism is *low* in absence of cardiac history or physical findings. Transesophageal echocardiography is more sensitive than standard transthoracic study for this purpose.

ENDOCARDITIS   Vegetation visualized in more than half of pts (transesophageal echo has much higher sensitivity), but management is generally based on clinical findings, not echo. Complications of endocarditis (e.g., valvular regurgitation) may be evaluated.

CONGENITAL HEART DISEASE   Echo, Doppler, and contrast echo (rapid IV injection of saline) are noninvasive procedures of choice in identifying congenital lesions.

AORTIC ROOT   Aneurysm and dissection of the aorta may be evaluated and complications (aortic regurgitation, tamponade) assessed (Chap. 116).

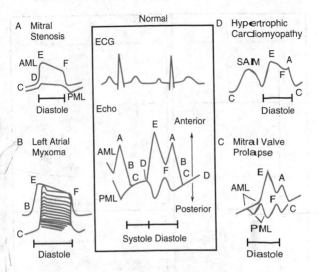

FIGURE 105-5 A schematic presentation of the normal M-mode echocardiographic (Echo) recording of anterior (AML) and posterior mitral leaflet (PML) motion is shown in the center with the simultaneous ECG. Abnormal mitral echocardiograms which occur in (*A*) mitral stenosis, (*B*) left atrial myxoma, (*C*) mitral valve prolapse, and (*D*) obstructive hypertrophic cardiomyopathy are also depicted. In the ECHO, the A point represents the end of anterior movement resulting from left atrial contraction, the CD segment represents the closed position of both mitral leaflets during ventricular systole, and point E ends the anterior movement as the leaflet opens. The slope EF results from posterior motion of the AML during rapid ventricular filling. In obstructive hypertrophic cardiomyopathy, SAM represents systolic anterior movement. (*Reproduced from Wynne J, O'Rourke RA, Braunwald E: HPIM-10, p. 1333.*)

HYPERTROPHIC CARDIOMYOPATHY, MITRAL VALVE PROLAPSE, PERICARDIAC EFFUSION Echo is the diagnostic technique of choice for identifying these conditions.

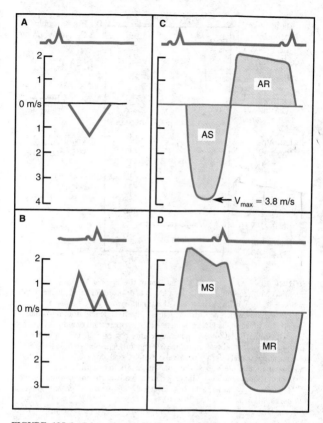

FIGURE 105-6 Schematic presentation of normal Doppler flow across the aortic (*A*) and mitral valves (*B*). Abnormal continuous wave Doppler profiles are depicted in *C*. Aortic stenosis (AS) [peak transaortic gradient $= 4 \times V_{max}^2 = 4 \times (3.8)^2 = 58$ mmHg] and regurgitation (AR). *D.* Mitral stenosis (MS) and regurgitation (MR).

For a more detailed discussion, see Goldberger AL: Electrocardiography, Chap. 228, p. 1237, in HPIM-14.

106

PREOPERATIVE EVALUATION OF CARDIOVASCULAR DISEASE

Goal is to determine if cardiovascular disease is present, assess its severity and stability, and intervene if necessary to minimize surgical risk. Greatest cardiovascular risk occurs with aortic (or other major vascular), intrathoracic, or intraperitoneal procedures or emergent operations in patients of advanced age (see Table 106-1).

HISTORY   Assess for history of MI, angina, CHF, valvular disease, hypertension, symptomatic arrhythmia. Note pertinent concomitant illnesses (e.g., cerebrovascular disease, diabetes mellitus, pulmonary or renal disease, anemia). Review pt's functional capacity in daily life (e.g., ability to perform housework, climb stairs, exercise).

PHYSICAL EXAMINATION   Evaluate for uncontrolled hypertension, signs of CHF (jugular venous distention, rales, S_3), previously unknown heart murmurs, carotid bruits. Inspect for pallor, cyanosis, poor nutritional state.

LABORATORY   Examine *ECG* for evidence of previous MI (Q waves) or arrhythmias. Inspect *CXR* for signs of CHF (e.g.,

Table 106-1

Cardiac Risk of Noncardiac Procedures

Risk	Procedure
High (>5%)	Aortic (or other major vascular) operations
	Emergent operation in patient of advanced age
Intermediate (<5%)	Intrathoracic or intraperitoneal procedures
	Carotid endarterectomy
	Orthopedic operations
	Prostate surgery
Low (<1%)	Endoscopy
	Cataract surgery
	Breast procedures
	Superficial skin operations

SOURCE: Modified from Eagle KA et al. *Circulation*, 93:1278, 1996, with permission.

cardiomegaly, vascular redistribution, Kerley B lines). Additional testing is dictated by specific underlying cardiovascular disease and nature of the planned operation. see Fig. 106-1 for clinical predictors of increased perioperative risk of MI, CHF, or death and approaches to preoperative evaluation.

SPECIFIC CARDIAC CONDITIONS

CORONARY ARTERY DISEASE Consider postponing purely elective operations for 6 months following an MI. Pts with stable CAD can be evaluated per algorithm in Fig. 106-1. Surgical risk is generally acceptable in pts with class I–II symptoms (e.g., able to climb one flight carrying grocery bags) and in those with low-risk results from noninvasive testing (see Table 114-1 for recommended forms of stress testing). For those with high-risk results (Chap. 114) or very limited functional capacity, consider coronary angiography. Perioperative beta-blocker therapy reduces incidence of coronary events and should be included in medical regimen if no contraindications (see Chap. 114).

HEART FAILURE This is a major predictor of perioperative risk. Regimen of ACE inhibitor and diuretics should be optimized preoperatively to minimize risk of either pulmonary congestion or intravascular volume depletion postoperatively.

ARRHYTHMIAS These are often markers for underlying CHF, CAD, drug toxicities (e.g., digitalis), or metabolic abnormalities (e.g., hypokalemia, hypomagnesemia), which should be identified and corrected. Indications for antiarrhythmic therapy or pacemakers are same as in nonsurgical situations (see Chap. 107). Notably, asymptomatic ventricular premature beats generally do not require suppressive therapy preoperatively.

VALVULAR DISEASES Those portending greatest surgical risk are advanced aortic or mitral stenosis (see Chap. 110), which should be repaired, if severe or symptomatic, prior to elective surgery. Ensure adequate ventricular rate control in mitral stenosis with atrial fibrillation (using beta blocker, digoxin, verapamil, or diltiazem). Endocarditis prophylaxis is indicated for operations associated with transient bacteremias (see Chap. 72).

HYPERTENSION This carries a risk of labile bp or hypertensive episodes perioperatively. Control elevated pressure preoperatively (Chap. 115), especially using beta blocker if possible which should be continued perioperatively. If pheochromocytoma is a possibility, surgery should be delayed for evaluation because of high anesthetic risk.

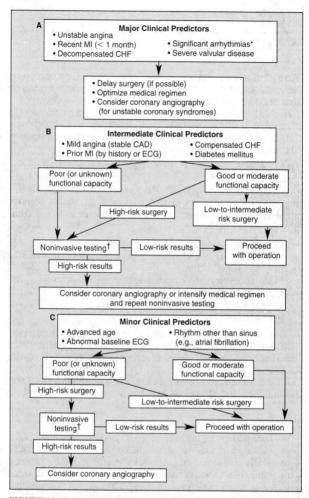

FIGURE 106-1 Approach to preoperative cardiac evaluation. *Significant arrhythmias include: (1) High-grade AV block, (2) symptomatic ventricular arrhythmias, and (3) supraventricular arrhythmias with uncontrolled ventricular rate. †Exercise testing is preferred (treadmill, bicycle, arm ergometry). Perform with echo or nuclear scintigraphy if baseline ST-T waves preclude ECG interpretation. If unable to exercise, consider pharmacologic (e.g., dobutamine or dipyridamole) test with echo or nuclear imaging, or ambulatory ECG monitoring, if baseline ST-T waves normal. (Modified from Eagle KA et al. *Circulation* 93:1278, 1996, with permission.)

107

ARRHYTHMIAS

Arrhythmias may appear in the presence or absence of structural heart disease; they are more serious in the former. Conditions that provoke arrhythmias include (1) myocardial ischemia, (2) CHF, (3) hypoxemia, (4) hypercapnia, (5) hypotension, (6) electrolyte disturbances (especially involving K, Ca, and Mg), (7) drug toxicity (digoxin, antiarrhythmic agents that prolong QT interval), (8) caffeine, (9) ethanol.

DIAGNOSIS Examine ECG for evidence of ischemic changes (Chap. 105), prolonged QT interval, and characteristics of Wolff-Parkinson-White (WPW) syndrome (see below). See Fig. 107-1 for diagnosis of tachyarrhythmias; always identify atrial activity and relationship between P waves and QRS complexes. To aid the diagnosis:

- Obtain long rhythm strip of leads II, aVF, or V_1. Double the ECG voltage and increase paper speed to 50 mm/s to help identify P waves.
- Place accessory ECG leads (right-sided chest, esophageal, right-atrial) to help identify P waves. Record ECG during carotid sinus massage (Table 107-1) for 5 s. *Note:* Do not massage both carotids simultaneously.

Tachyarrhythmias with wide QRS complex beats may represent ventricular tachycardia or supraventricular tachycardia with aberrant conduction. Factors favoring *ventricular tachycardia* include (1) AV dissociation, (2) QRS >0.14 s, (3) LAD, (4) no response to carotid sinus massage, (5) morphology of QRS is similar to that of previous ventricular premature beats.

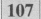 **TREATMENT**

    Tachyarrhythmias (Tables 107-1 and 107-2) Precipitating causes (listed above) should be corrected. If pt is hemodynamically compromised (angina, hypotension, CHF), proceed to immediate cardioversion. *Note:* Do not cardiovert sinus tachycardia; exercise caution if digitalis toxicity is suspected. Initiate drugs as indicated in the tables; follow drug levels and ECG intervals (esp. QRS and QT). Reduce dosage for pts with hepatic or renal dysfunction as indicated in Table 107-2. Drug efficacy is confirmed by ECG (or Holter) monitoring, stress testing, and in special circumstances, invasive electrophysiologic study.

    Antiarrhythmic agents all have potential toxic side effects, including *provocation* of ventricular arrhythmias, esp. in pts with LV dysfunction or history of sustained ventricular ar-

Atrial Rate / Ventric Rate — Rhythm & Rate Disturbances

A. Ectopic atrial contraction

– | N II

B. Sinus tachycardia

100+ / 100+ 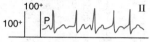 II

C. Paroxysmal supraventricular tachycardia

160 | 160 II

D. Paroxysmal atrial tachycardia with block (2:1)

160 | 80 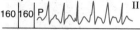 II

E. Atrial flutter (2:1 block)

300 | 150 II

F. Atrial fibrillation

500+ | Variable II

G. Ectopic ventricular contractions

– | N II

H. Ventricular tachycardia

70 | 150 V-1

I. Ventricular fibrillation

– | – II

Atrial Rate / Ventric Rate — Conduction Disturbances

J. First degree heart block

70 | 70

K. Second degree heart block

80 | 40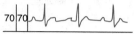

L. Third degree heart block (complete H. B.)

80 | 40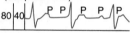

M. Wenckebach

80 | 50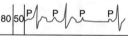

N. Wolff-Parkinson-White with delta waves

70 | 70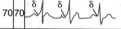

O. Wolff-Parkinson-White without delta waves

70 | 70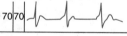

P. Right bundle branch block

70 | 70 V_1 V_6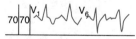

Q. Left bundle branch block

70 | 70 V_1 V_6

FIGURE 107-1   Tachyarrhythmias. (Reproduced by Sobel BE, Braunwald E: HPIM-9, p. 1052.)

Table 107-1

Clinical and Electrocardiographic Features of Common Arrhythmias

Rhythm	Example (Fig. 107-1)	Atrial Rate	Features	Carotid Sinus Massage	Precipitating Conditions	Initial Treatment
NARROW QRS COMPLEX						
Atrial premature beats	A	—	P wave abnormal; QRS width normal	—	Can be normal; or due to anxiety, CHF, hypoxia, caffeine, abnormal electrolytes (K^+, Ca^{2+}, Mg^{2+})	Remove precipitating cause; if symptomatic: beta blocker
Sinus tachycardia	B	100–160	Normal P wave	Rate gradually slows	Fever, dehydration, pain, CHF, hyperthyroidism, COPD	Remove precipitating cause; if symptomatic: beta blocker
Paroxysmal SVT	C	140–250	P wave "peaked" or inverted in leads II, III, aVF	Abruptly converts to sinus rhythm (or no effect)	Healthy individuals; preexcitation syndromes (see text)	Vagal maneuvers; if unsuccessful: adenosine, verapamil, beta blocker, cardioversion (150 J)
Paroxysmal atrial tachycardia with block	D	130–250	Upright "peaked" P; 2:1, 3:1, 4:1 block	No effect on atrial rate; block may ↑	Digitalis toxicity	Hold digoxin, correct [K^+]; phenytoin (250 mg IV over 5 min)

640

		Rate	ECG	Carotid sinus massage	Associations	Treatment
Atrial flutter	E	250–350	"Sawtooth" flutter waves; 2:1, 4:1 block	↑ Block; ventricular rate ↓	Mitral valve disease, hypertension, pulmonary embolism, pericarditis, postcardiac surgery, hyperthyroidism, obstructive lung disease, EtOH, idiopathic	1. Slow the ventricular rate: beta blocker, verapamil, or digoxin 2. Convert to NSR (after anticoagulation if chronic) with group I (A or C)* agent or amiodarone; may require electrical cardioversion (flutter: 50 J; fib: 100–200 J). Atrial flutter may respond to rapid atrial pacing
Atrial fibrillation	F	>350	No discrete P; irregularly spaced QRS	Ventricular rate ↓		
Multifocal atrial tachycardia		100–220	More than 3 different P wave shapes with varying PR intervals	No effect	Severe respiratory insufficiency	Treat underlying lung disease; verapamil may be used to slow ventricular rate

(continued)

Table 107-1 (Continued)

Clinical and Electrocardiographic Features of Common Arrhythmias

Rhythm	Example (Fig. 107-1)	Atrial Rate	Features	Carotid Sinus Massage	Precipitating Conditions	Initial Treatment
WIDE QRS COMPLEX						
Ventricular premature beats	G		Fully compensatory pause between normal beats	No effect	Coronary artery disease, myocardial infarction, CHF, hypoxia, hypokalemia, digitalis toxicity, prolonged QT interval (congenital or drugs: quinidine and other antiarrhythmics, tricyclics, phenothiazines)	May not require therapy;‡ use beta blocker or same drugs as ventricular tachycardia. If unstable: electrical conversion (100 J); otherwise: Acute (IV): lidocaine, procainamide, bretylium; chronic (PO) prevention: group IA, IB, IC, III drugs*
Ventricular tachycardia	H		QRS rate 100–250; slightly irregular rate	No effect		
Ventricular fibrillation	I		Erratic electrical activity only	No effect	Prolonged QT interval (congenital or drugs;	Immediate defibrillation (200–400 J)

642

Torsades de pointes	Ventricular tachycardia with sinusoidal oscillations of QRS height	No effect		IV magnesium; overdrive pacing; lidocaine; isoproterenol (unless CAD present); bretylium. Drugs that prolong QT interval (e.g., quinidine) are contraindicated.
Supraventricular tachycardias with aberrant ventricular conduction	P wave typical of the supraventricular rhythm; wide QRS complex due to conduction through partially refractory pathways		Etiologies of the respective supraventricular rhythms listed above; atrial fibrillation with rapid, wide QRS may be due to preexcitation (WPW)	Same as treatment of respective supraventricular rhythm; if ventricular rate rapid (>200), treat as WPW (see text)

* Antiarrhythmic drug groups listed in Table 107-2.
‡ Indications for treating VPCs listed in Chap. 113.

† Decrease digoxin dose when starting quinidine.
NOTE: J, joules.

Table 107-2

Antiarrhythmic Drugs

Drug	Loading Dose	Maintenance Dose	Side Effects	Excretion
Group IA				
Quinidine sulfate	IV: 500–1000 mg	PO: 200–400 mg q6h	Diarrhea, tinnitus, QT prolongation, hypotension, anemia, thrombocytopenia	Hepatic
Quinidine gluconate		PO: 324–628 mg q8h		Hepatic
Procainamide	IV: 500–1000 mg	IV: 2–5 mg/min	Nausea, lupus-like syndrome, agranulocytosis, QT prolongation	Renal and hepatic
		PO: 500–1000 mg q4h		
Sustained-release:		PO: 1000–2500 mg q12h		
Disopyramide		PO: 100–300 mg q6–8h	Myocardial depression, AV block, QT prolongation, anticholinergic effects	Renal and hepatic
Sustained-release:		PO: 200–400 mg q12h		
Group IB				
Lidocaine	IV: 1 mg/kg bolus followed by 0.5 mg/kg bolus q8–10 min to total 3 mg/kg	IV: 1–4 mg/min	Confusion, seizures, respiratory arrest	Hepatic
Tocainide		PO: 400–600 mg q8h	Nausea, confusion, tremors, lupus-like reaction	Hepatic and renal

Drug	IV Dose	Oral Dose	Side Effects	Clearance
Mexiletine		PO: 100–300 mg q6–8h	Nausea, tremor, gait disturbance	Hepatic
Group IC				
Flecainide		PO: 50–200 mg q12h	Nausea, exacerbation of ventricular arrhythmia, prolongation of PR and QRS intervals	Hepatic and renal
Propafenone		PO: 150–300 mg q8h		Hepatic and renal
Group II				
Propranolol	IV: 0.5–1 mg/min to 0.15–0.2 mg/kg	PO: 10–200 mg q6h	CHF, bradycardia, AV block, bronchospasm	Hepatic
Group III				
Amiodarone	IV: 75–150 mg over 20–30 min; IV: 0.5 mg/min	PO: 800–1400 mg qd × 1–2 weeks; PO: 200–600 mg qd	Thyroid abnormalities, pulmonary fibrosis, hepatitis, corneal microdeposits, bluish skin, QT prolongation	—
Bretylium	IV: 5–10 mg/kg	IV: 0.5–2.0 mg/min	Hypertension, orthostatic hypotension, nausea, parotid pain	Renal
Sotalol		PO: 80–160 mg q12h	Fatigue, bradycardia, exacerbation of ventricular arrhythmia	Renal
Group IV				
Verapamil	IV: 2.5–10 mg	PO: 120–480 mg qd	AV block, CHF, hypotension, constipation	Hepatic

(continued)

Table 107-2 (Continued)

Antiarrhythmic Drugs

Drug	Loading Dose	Maintenance Dose	Side Effects	Excretion
Diltiazem	IV: 0.25 mg/kg over 2 min; can repeat with 0.35 mg/kg after 15 min	IV: 5–15 mg/h PO: 120–360 mg/d	—	—
Other				
Digoxin	IV, PO: 0.75–1.5 mg over 24 h	IV, PO: 0.125–0.25 mg qd	Nausea, AV block, ventricular and supraventricular arrhythmias	Renal
Adenosine	IV: 6-mg bolus; if no effect then 12-mg bolus	—	Transient hypotension or atrial standstill	—

rhythmias. Drug-induced QT prolongation and associated torsades de pointes ventricular tachycardia (see Table 107-1) is most common with group IA agents; the drug should be discontinued if the QTc interval (QT divided by square root of RR interval) increases by more than 25%. Antiarrhythmic drugs should be avoided in pts with asymptomatic ventricular arrhythmias after MI, since mortality risk increases.

Chronic Atrial Fibrillation   Evaluate potential underlying cause (e.g., thyrotoxicosis, mitral stenosis, excessive ethanol consumption, pulmonary embolism). Pts with risk factors for stroke (e.g., valvular heart disease, hypertension, CAD, CHF, age >75) should receive warfarin anticoagulation (INR 2.0–3.0; use caution to keep INR < 3.0 in pts >age 75). Substitute aspirin 325 mg/d for pts without these risk factors or if contraindication to warfarin exists. Control ventricular rate (60–80 bpm at rest, <100 bpm with mild exercise) with beta blocker, digoxin, or calcium channel blocker (verapamil, diltiazem). Consider cardioversion (after ≥3 weeks therapeutic anticoagulation), especially if symptomatic despite rate control: use group IA, IC, or III (amiodarone, sotalol) agent (usually initiate with inpatient monitoring), followed, within a few days, by electrical cardioversion (usually 100–200 J). Anticoagulation should be continued for an additional 3 weeks after successful cardioversion.

PREEXCITATION SYNDROME (WPW)   Conduction occurs through an accessory pathway between atria and ventricles. Baseline ECG typically shows a short PR interval and slurred upstroke of the QRS ("delta" wave) (Fig. 107-1*N*). Associated tachyarrhythmias are of two types:

- *Narrow QRS complex tachycardia* (antegrade conduction through AV node): usually paroxysmal supraventricular tachycardia. Treat cautiously with IV verapamil, digoxin, or propranolol (see Table 107-2).
- *Wide QRS complex tachycardia* (antegrade conduction through accessory pathway): often associated with AF with a very *rapid* (>250/min) ventricular rate (which may degenerate into VF). If hemodynamically compromised, immediate cardioversion is indicated; otherwise, treat with IV lidocaine or procainamide, *not* digoxin or verapamil.

AV BLOCK

FIRST DEGREE (See Fig. 107-1*J*)   Prolonged, constant PR interval (>0.20 s). May be normal or secondary to increased vagal tone or digitalis; no treatment required.

SECOND DEGREE *Mobitz I (Wenckebach)* (See Fig. 107-1*M*) Narrow QRS, progressive increase in PR interval until a ventricular beat is dropped, then sequence is repeated. Seen with drug intoxication (digitalis, beta blockers), increased vagal tone, inferior MI. Usually transient, no therapy required; if symptomatic, use atropine (0.6 mg IV, repeated × 3–4) or temporary pacemaker.

Mobitz II (See Fig. 107-1*K*) Fixed PR interval with occasional dropped beats, in 2:1, 3:1, or 4:1 pattern; the QRS complex is usually wide. Seen with MI or degenerative conduction system disease; a dangerous rhythm—may progress suddenly to complete AV block; pacemaker is indicated.

THIRD DEGREE (COMPLETE AV BLOCK) (See Fig. 107-1*L*) Atrial activity is not transmitted to ventricles; atria and ventricles contract independently. Seen with MI, digitalis toxicity, or degenerative conduction system disease. Permanent pacemaker is indicated, except when associated transiently with inferior MI or in asymptomatic congenital heart block.

For a more detailed discussion, see Josephson ME et al: The Bradyarrhythmias, Chap. 230, p. 1253; and The Tachyarrhythmias, Chap. 231, p. 1261, in HPIM-14.

108

CONGESTIVE HEART FAILURE AND COR PULMONALE

HEART FAILURE

DEFINITION Heart failure is a condition in which the heart is unable to pump sufficient blood for metabolizing tissues or can do so only from an abnormally elevated filling pressure. It is important to identify the *underlying* nature of the cardiac disease and the factors that precipitate acute CHF.

UNDERLYING CARDIAC DISEASE Includes states that depress ventricular function (coronary artery disease, hypertension, dilated cardiomyopathy, valvular disease, congenital heart disease) and states that restrict ventricular filling (mitral stenosis, restrictive cardiomyopathy, pericardial disease).

ACUTE PRECIPITATING FACTORS Include (1) increased Na intake, (2) noncompliance with anti-CHF medications, (3) acute MI (may be silent), (4) exacerbation of hypertension, (5) acute arrhythmias, (6) infections and/or fever, (7) pulmonary embolism, (8) anemia, (9) thyrotoxicosis, (10) pregnancy, and (11) acute myocarditis or infective endocarditis.

SYMPTOMS Due to inadequate perfusion of peripheral tissues (fatigue, dyspnea) and elevated intracardiac filling pressures (orthopnea, paroxysmal nocturnal dyspnea, peripheral edema).

PHYSICAL EXAMINATION Jugular venous distention, S_3, pulmonary congestion (rales, dullness over pleural effusion, peripheral edema, hepatomegaly, and ascites).

LABORATORY CXR can reveal cardiomegaly, pulmonary vascular redistribution, Kerley B lines, pleural effusions. Left ventricular contraction can be assessed by *echocardiography* or *radionuclide ventriculography*. In addition, echo can identify underlying valvular, pericardial, or congenital heart disease, as well as regional wall motion abnormalities typical of coronary artery disease.

CONDITIONS THAT MIMIC CHF *Pulmonary Disease* Chronic bronchitis, emphysema, and asthma (see Chaps. 119 and 121); look for sputum production and abnormalities on CXR and pulmonary function tests.

Other Causes of Peripheral Edema Liver disease, varicose veins, and cyclic edema, none of which results in jugular

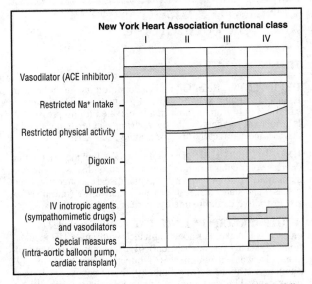

FIGURE 108-1   Overview of the treatment of heart failure. (From RA Kelly and TW Smith in *Heart Failure: Cardiac Function and Dysfunction.* in WS Colucci (ed). *Atlas of Heart Diseases*, vol 4, F. Braunwald (series ed), Philadelphia, Current Medicine, 1995.)

venous distention. Edema due to renal dysfunction is often accompanied by elevated serum creatinine and abnormal urinalysis (see Chap. 17).

R TREATMENT

Aimed at symptomatic relief, removal of precipitating factors, and control of underlying cardiac disease. Overview of treatment shown in Fig. 108-1; notably, ACE inhibitor should be begun early, even in pts with asymptomatic LV dysfunction. Once symptoms develop:

1.   *Decrease cardiac workload:* Reduce physical activity, including periods of bed rest. Prevent deep venous thrombosis with heparin 5000 U SC bid.

2.   *Control excess fluid retention:* (a) *Dietary sodium restriction* (eliminate salty foods, e.g., potato chips, canned soups, bacon, salt added at table); more stringent requirements (<2 g NaCl/d) in advanced CHF. If dilutional hyponatremia

present, restrict fluid intake (<1000 mL/d). (b) *Diuretics* (see Table 17-1): *Loop diuretics* (e.g., furosemide 20–120 mg/d PO or IV) are most potent and unlike thiazides remain effective when GFR <25 mL/min. Combine loop diuretic with thiazide or metolazone for augmented effect. Potassium-sparing diuretics are useful adjunct to reduce potassium loss. They should *not* be added in pts receiving ACE inhibitors, to avoid *hyper*kalemia.

During diuresis, obtain daily weights aiming for loss of 1–1.5 kg/d.

3. *Vasodilators* (Table 108-1): Recommended as standard CHF therapy. Venous dilators (e.g., nitrates) reduce pulmonary congestion; arterial dilators (e.g., hydralazine) augment forward stroke volume, particularly if systemic vascular resistance (SVR) is markedly elevated or mitral or aortic regurgitation is present. ACE inhibitors are mixed (arterial and venous) dilators and are particularly effective and well tolerated. They, and to a lesser extent the combination of hydralazine plus nitrates, have been shown to prolong life in pts with symptomatic CHF. ACE inhibitors also have been shown to delay the onset of CHF in pts with asymptomatic LV dysfunction and to lower mortality when begun soon after acute MI. Vasodilators may result in significant hypotension in pts who are volume depleted, so start at lowest dosage (e.g., captopril 6.25 mg PO tid); pt should remain supine for 2–4 h after the initial doses. Direct-acting vasodilator (e.g., hydralazine) may be added to ACE inhibitor therapy, if needed.

In sicker, hospitalized pts, IV vasodilator therapy (see Table 108-1) is monitored by placement of a pulmonary artery catheter and indwelling arterial line. Nitroprusside is a potent mixed vasodilator for pts with markedly elevated SVR. It is metabolized to thiocyanate, then excreted via the kidneys. To avoid thiocyanate toxicity (seizures, altered mental status, nausea), follow thiocyanate levels in pts with renal failure or if administered for more than 2 d.

4. *Digoxin* is useful in heart failure due to (a) marked systolic dysfunction (LV dilatation, low ejection fraction, S_3) and (b) heart failure associated with atrial fibrillation and rapid ventricular rate. Unlike ACE inhibitors, digoxin does not prolong survival in heart failure pts. Not indicated in CHF due to pericardial disease, restrictive cardiomyopathy, or mitral stenosis (unless atrial fibrillation is present). Digoxin is contraindicated in hypertrophic cardiomyopathy and in pts with AV conduction blocks.

Digoxin loading dose is administered over 24 h (0.5 mg PO/IV, followed by 0.25 mg q6h to achieve total of 1.0–1.5

Table 108-1

Vasodilators for Treatment of CHF

Drug and Site of Action*	Dose	Adverse Effects
IV AGENTS		
Nitroprusside, V = A	0.5–10 (μg/kg)/min	Thiocyanate toxicity (blurred vision, tinnitus, delirium) can occur during prolonged therapy or in renal failure
Nitroglycerin, V > A	10 μg/min–10 (μg/kg)/min	May cause hypotension if LV filling pressure is low
ORAL AGENTS		
ACE inhibitors, V = A		Angioedema, cough, hyperkalemia, leukopenia. Reduce diuretic dosage to prevent azotemia
Captopril	6.25–50 mg tid	
Enalapril	2.5–10 mg bid	
Lisinopril	5–40 mg tid	
Hydralazine†, A	50–200 mg tid	May cause drug-induced lupus or angina due to reflex tachycardia
Nitrates†, V (e.g., isosorbide dinitrate)	10–40 mg tid	Drug tolerance may develop with more frequent administration

* V, venous; A, arterial.
† Hydralazine and nitrates are often used together to achieve combined venous and arterial effect.

mg). Subsequent dose (0.125–0.25 mg qd) depends on age, weight, and renal function and is guided by measurement of serum digoxin level. The addition of quinidine increases serum digoxin level; therefore, digoxin dosage should be halved. Verapamil, amiodarone, and spironolactone also increase serum digoxin level but to a lesser extent.

Digitalis toxicity may be precipitated by hypokalemia, hypoxemia, hypercalcemia, hypomagnesemia, hypothyroidism, or myocardial ischemia. Early signs of toxicity include anorexia, nausea, and lethargy. *Cardiac toxicity* includes ventricular extrasystoles and ventricular tachycardia and fibrillation; atrial tachycardia with block; sinus arrest and sinoatrial block; all degrees of AV block. *Chronic* digitalis intoxication may cause cachexia, gynecomastia, "yellow" vision, or confusion. At first sign of digitalis toxicity, discontinue the drug; maintain serum K concentration between 4.0 and 5.0 mmol/L. Bradyarrhythmias and AV block may respond to atropine (0.6 mg IV); otherwise, a temporary pacemaker may be required. Digitalis-induced ventricular arrhythmias are treated with lidocaine or phenytoin (Chap. 107). Antidigoxin antibodies are available for massive overdose.

5. *Beta-adrenoreceptor blockers* are generally avoided in CHF. However, some pts with moderate (classes II and III) symptoms *may* benefit from gradually augmented doses of, e.g., carvedilol, metoprolol, or bucindolol. Start with low dose (e.g., carvedilol starting with 3.125 mg bid) and increase over 8 weeks to 25–50 mg bid.

6. *IV sympathomimetic amines* (see Table 113-2) are administered to hospitalized pts for refractory symptoms or acute exacerbation of CHF. They are contraindicated in hypertrophic cardiomyopathy. *Dobutamine* [2.5–10 (μg/kg)/min], the preferred agent, augments cardiac output without significant peripheral vasoconstriction or tachycardia. *Dopamine* at low dosage [1–5 (μg/kg)/min] facilitates diuresis; at higher dosage (5–10 μg/kg/min) positive inotropic effects predominate; peripheral vasoconstriction is greatest at dosage greater than 10 μg/kg/min. *Amrinone* [5–10 (μg/kg)/min after a 0.75 mg/kg bolus] is a nonsympathetic positive inotrope and vasodilator. Vasodilators and inotropic agents may be used together for additive effect.

Patients with severe refractory CHF with less than 6 months expected survival, who meet stringent criteria, may be candidates for cardiac transplantation.

COR PULMONALE

Right ventricular enlargement resulting from *primary* lung disease; leads to RV hypertrophy and eventually to RV failure. Etiologies include the following:

- *Pulmonary parenchymal or airway disease.* Chronic obstructive lung disease (COPD), interstitial lung diseases, bronchiectasis, cystic fibrosis (Chaps. 121 and 124).
- *Pulmonary vascular disease.* Recurrent pulmonary emboli, primary pulmonary hypertension (PHT), vasculitis, sickle cell anemia.

- *Inadequate mechanical ventilation.* Kyphoscoliosis, neuro-muscular disorders, marked obesity, sleep apnea.

SYMPTOMS Depend on underlying disorder but include dyspnea, cough, fatigue, and sputum production (in parenchymal diseases).

PHYSICAL EXAMINATION Tachypnea, cyanosis, clubbing are common. RV impulse along left sternal border, loud P_2, right-sided S_4. If RV failure develops, elevated jugular venous pressure, hepatomegaly with ascites, pedal edema.

LABORATORY *ECG* RV hypertrophy and RA enlargement (Chap. 105); tachyarrhythmias are common.

CXR RV and pulmonary artery enlargement; if PHT present, tapering of the pulmonary artery branches. Pulmonary function tests and arterial blood gases characterize intrinsic pulmonary disease.

Echocardiogram RV hypertrophy; LV function typically normal. If imaging is difficult because of air in distended lungs, RV volume and wall thickness can be evaluated by MRI. If pulmonary emboli suspected, obtain radionuclide lung scan.

℞ **TREATMENT**

Aimed at underlying pulmonary disease and may include bronchodilators, antibiotics, and oxygen administration. If RV failure is present, treat as CHF, instituting low-sodium diet and diuretics; digoxin must be administered cautiously (toxicity increased due to hypoxemia, hypercapnia, acidosis). Loop diuretics must also be used with care to prevent significant metabolic alkalosis that blunts respiratory drive. Supraventricular tachyarrhythmias are common and treated with digoxin, quinidine, or verapamil (*not* beta blockers). Chronic anticoagulation with warfarin is indicated when pulmonary hypertension is accompanied by RV failure.

For a more detailed discussion, see Braunwald E: Heart Failure, Chap. 233, p. 1287; and Cor Pulmonale, Chap. 238, p. 1324, in HPIM-14.

109

CONGENITAL HEART DISEASE IN THE ADULT

ATRIAL SEPTAL DEFECT (ASD)

HISTORY   Usually asymptomatic until third or fourth decades, when exertional dyspnea, fatigue, and palpitations may develop. Symptoms often associated with pulmonary hypertension (see below).

PHYSICAL EXAMINATION   Parasternal RV lift, wide fixed splitting of S_2, systolic flow murmur along sternal border, diastolic flow rumble across tricuspid valve, prominent jugular venous v wave.

ECG   Incomplete RBBB. LAD common with ostium primum (lower septal) defect.

CXR   Increased pulmonary vascular markings, prominence of RV and main pulmonary artery (LA enlargement *not* usually present).

ECHOCARDIOGRAM   RA and RV enlargement; Doppler shows abnormal turbulent transatrial flow. Echo contrast (agitated saline) injection into peripheral vein may visualize transatrial shunt.

RADIONUCLIDE ANGIOGRAM   Noninvasively estimates ratio of pulmonary flow to systemic flow (PF:SF).

℞ TREATMENT

In the absence of contraindications an ASD with PF:SF >1.5:1.0 should be surgically repaired. Surgery is contraindicated with significant pulmonary hypertension and PF:SF <1.2:1.0. Medical management includes antiarrhythmic therapy for associated atrial fibrillation or supraventricular tachycardia (Chap. 107) and standard therapy for symptoms of CHF (Chap. 108).

VENTRICULAR SEPTAL DEFECT (VSD)

Congenital VSDs may close spontaneously during childhood. Symptoms relate to size of the defect and pulmonary vascular resistance.

HISTORY   CHF in infancy. Adults may be asymptomatic or develop fatigue and reduced exercise tolerance.

PHYSICAL EXAMINATION Systolic thrill and holosystolic murmur at lower left sternal border, loud P_2, S_3; flow murmur across mitral valve.

ECG Normal with small defects. Large shunts result in LA and LV enlargement.

CXR Enlargement of main pulmonary artery, LA, and LV, with increased pulmonary vascular markings.

ECHOCARDIOGRAM LA and LV enlargement; defect may be visualized; Doppler shows high-velocity flow in RV outflow tract, near the defect.

℞ TREATMENT

Fatigue and mild dyspnea are treated with digitalis, mild diuretics, and afterload reduction (Chap. 108). Surgical closure is indicated if PF:SF>1.5:1. Antibiotic prophylaxis for endocarditis is important.

PATENT DUCTUS ARTERIOSUS (PDA)

Abnormal communication between the descending aorta and pulmonary artery; associated with birth at high altitudes and maternal rubella.

HISTORY Asymptomatic or dyspnea on exertion and fatigue.

PHYSICAL EXAMINATION Hyperactive LV impulse; loud systolic-diastolic "machinery" murmur at upper left sternal border. If pulmonary hypertension develops, diastolic component of the murmur may disappear.

ECG LV hypertrophy is common; RV hypertrophy with pulmonary hypertension.

CXR Increased pulmonary vascular markings; enlarged main pulmonary artery, ascending aorta, LV; occasional calcification of ductus.

ECHOCARDIOGRAPHY Hyperdynamic, enlarged LV; the PDA can often be visualized on two-dimensional echo; Doppler demonstrates abnormal flow contained within it.

℞ TREATMENT

In absence of pulmonary hypertension, PDA should be ligated to prevent infective endocarditis, LV dysfunction, and pulmonary hypertension. Transcatheter closure may be possible in selected pts.

PROGRESSION TO PULMONARY HYPERTENSION (PHT)

Pts with significant, uncorrected ASD, VSD, or PDA may develop progressive, irreversible PHT with shunting of desaturated blood into the arterial circulation (right-to-left shunting). Fatigue, light-headedness, and chest pain due to RV ischemia are common, accompanied by cyanosis, clubbing of digits, loud P_2, murmur of pulmonary valve regurgitation, and signs of RV failure. ECG and echocardiogram show RV hypertrophy. Surgical correction of congenital defects contraindicated with severe PHT and right-to-left shunting.

PULMONIC STENOSIS (PS)

A transpulmonary valve gradient <50 mmHg rarely causes symptoms, and progression tends not to occur. Higher gradients result in dyspnea, fatigue, light-headedness, chest pain (RV ischemia).

PHYSICAL EXAMINATION   Shows jugular venous distention with prominent *a* wave, RV parasternal impulse, wide splitting of S_2 with soft P_2, ejection click followed by "diamond-shaped" systolic murmur at upper left sternal border, S_4.

ECG   RA and RV enlargement in advanced PS.

CXR   Often shows poststenotic dilatation of the pulmonary artery and RV enlargement.

ECHOCARDIOGRAPHY   RV hypertrophy and "doming" of the pulmonic valve. Doppler accurately measures transvalvular gradient.

℞ TREATMENT

Prophylaxis for infective endocarditis is mandatory. Moderate or severe stenosis (gradient >50 mmHg) requires surgical (or balloon) valvuloplasty.

COARCTATION OF THE AORTA

Aortic constriction just distal to the origin of the left subclavian artery is a surgically correctable form of hypertension (Chap. 115). Usually asymptomatic, but it may cause headache, fatigue, or claudication of lower extremities.

PHYSICAL EXAMINATION   Hypertension in upper extremities; delayed femoral pulses with decreased pressure in lower extremities. Pulsatile collateral arteries can be palpated in the intercostal spaces. Systolic (and sometimes diastolic) murmur is best heard over the mid-upper back.

ECG   LV hypertrophy.

CXR   Notching of the ribs due to collateral arteries; "figure 3" appearance of distal aortic arch.

℞ TREATMENT

Surgical correction, although hypertension may persist. Antibiotic prophylaxis against endocarditis is required even after correction. Recoarctation after surgical repair may be amenable to percutaneous balloon dilatation.

For a more detailed discussion, see Friedman WF, Child JS: Congenital Heart Disease in the Adult, Chap. 235, p. 1300, in HPIM-14.

110

VALVULAR HEART DISEASE

MITRAL STENOSIS (MS)

ETIOLOGY   Most commonly rheumatic, although history of acute rheumatic fever is now uncommon; congenital MS is an uncommon cause, observed primarily in infants.

HISTORY   Symptoms most commonly begin in the fourth decade, but MS often causes severe disability by age 20 in economically deprived areas. Principal symptoms are dyspnea and pulmonary edema precipitated by exertion, excitement, fever, anemia, paroxysmal tachycardia, pregnancy, sexual intercourse, etc.

PHYSICAL EXAMINATION   Peripheral and facial cyanosis in severe MS. Right ventricular lift; palpable S_1; opening snap (OS) follows A_2 by 0.06 to 0.12 s; OS–A_2 interval inversely proportional to severity of obstruction. Diastolic rumbling murmur with presystolic accentuation in sinus rhythm. Duration of murmur correlates with severity of obstruction.

COMPLICATIONS   Hemoptysis, pulmonary embolism, pulmonary infection, systemic embolization; endocarditis is *uncommon* in pure MS.

LABORATORY   *ECG*   Typically shows atrial fibrillation (AF) or left atrial (LA) enlargement when sinus rhythm is present. Right-axis deviation and RV hypertrophy in the presence of pulmonary hypertension.

CXR   Shows LA and RV enlargement and Kerley B lines.

Echocardiogram   Most useful noninvasive test; shows inadequate separation, calcification and thickening of valve leaflets, and LA enlargement. Doppler echocardiogram allows estimation of transvalvular gradient and mitral valve area (Chap. 105).

[Rx] **TREATMENT**   (See Fig. 110-1)
Pts should receive prophylaxis for rheumatic fever (penicillin) and infective endocarditis (Chap. 72). In the presence of dyspnea, medical therapy for heart failure; digitalis; beta blockers; or verapamil; to slow ventricular rate in AF, diuretics, and sodium restriction. Anticoagulants for pts with AF and/or history of systemic and pulmonic emboli. Open mitral valvuloplasty in the presence of symptoms and mitral orifice ≤ approximately 1.2 cm². In selected pts, without mitral regurgitation, percutaneous balloon valvuloplasty is frequently a successful alternative to surgery.

MITRAL REGURGITATION (MR)

ETIOLOGY   Rheumatic heart disease in approximately 50%. Other causes: mitral valve prolapse, ischemic heart disease with papillary muscle dysfunction, LV dilatation of any cause, mitral annular calcification, hypertrophic cardiomyopathy, infective endocarditis, congenital.

CLINICAL MANIFESTATIONS   Fatigue, weakness, and exertional dyspnea. Physical examination: sharp upstroke of arterial pulse, LV lift, S_1 diminished: wide splitting of S_2; S_3; loud holosystolic murmur and often a brief early-mid-diastolic murmur.

ECHOCARDIOGRAM   Enlarged LA, hyperdynamic LV; Doppler echocardiogram helpful in diagnosing and assessing severity of MR.

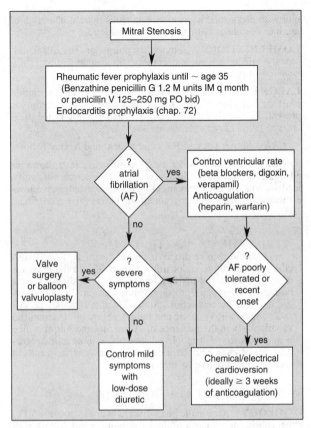

FIGURE 110-1 Management of mitral stenosis.

℞ **TREATMENT** (See Fig. 110-2)

As for heart failure (see Chap. 108), including diuretics and digoxin. Afterload reduction (ACE inhibitors, hydralazine, or IV nitroprusside) decreases the degree of regurgitation, increases forward cardiac output, and improves symptomatology. Endocarditis prophylaxis is indicated, as is anticoagulation in the presence of atrial fibrillation. Surgical treatment,

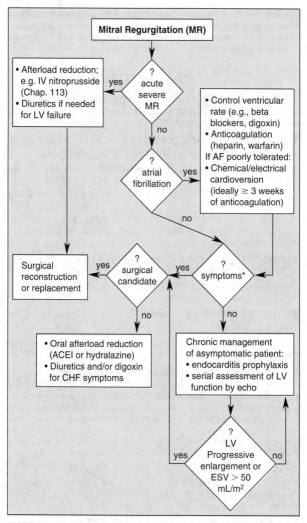

FIGURE 110-2   Management of advanced mitral regurgitation. *Including class II symptoms of LV end-systolic volue (ESV) elevated; ACEI, angiotensin converting-enzyme inhibitors.

either valve repair or replacement, is indicated in the presence of symptoms and impairment of LV function. Operation should be carried out *before* development of severe chronic heart failure.

MITRAL VALVE PROLAPSE (MVP)

ETIOLOGY   Most commonly idiopathic; ?familial; may accompany rheumatic fever, ischemic heart disease, atrial septal defect, the Marfan syndrome.

PATHOLOGY   Redundant mitral valve tissue with myxedematous degeneration and elongated chordae tendineae.

CLINICAL MANIFESTATIONS   More common in females. Most pts are asymptomatic and remain so. Most common symptoms are atypical chest pain and a variety of supraventricular and ventricular arrhythmias. Most important complication is severe MR resulting in LV failure. Rarely, systemic emboli from platelet-fibrin deposits on valve. Sudden death is a *very rare* complication.

PHYSICAL EXAMINATION   Mid or late systolic click(s) followed by late systolic murmur; exaggeration by Valsalva maneuver, reduced by squatting and isometric exercise (Chap. 104).

ECHOCARDIOGRAM   Shows posterior displacement of posterior (occasionally anterior) mitral leaflet late in systole.

℞ TREATMENT

Asymptomatic pts should be reassured, but if systolic murmur is present and/or typical echocardiographic findings with MR, prophylaxis for infective endocarditis is indicated. Valve repair or replacement for pts with severe mitral regurgitation; anticoagulants for pts with history of embolization.

AORTIC STENOSIS (AS)

ETIOLOGY   Often congenital; rheumatic AS is usually associated with rheumatic mitral valve disease. Idiopathic, calcific AS is a degenerative disorder common in the elderly and usually mild.

SYMPTOMS   Dyspnea, angina, and syncope are cardinal symptoms; they occur late, after years of obstruction.

PHYSICAL EXAMINATION   Weak and delayed arterial pulses with carotid thrill. Double apical impulse; A_2 soft or absent; S_4 common. Diamond-shaped systolic murmur $\geq$grade 3/6, often with systolic thrill.

LABORATORY *ECG and CXR* Often show LV hypertrophy, but not useful for predicting gradient.

Echocardiogram Shows thickening of LV wall, calcification and thickening of aortic valve cusps. Dilatation and reduced contraction of LV indicate poor prognosis. Doppler useful for estimating gradient and calculating valve area.

℞ TREATMENT

Avoid strenuous activity in severe AS, even in asymptomatic phase. Treat heart failure in standard fashion (see Chap. 108), but *avoid afterload reduction*. Valve replacement is indicated in adults with symptoms resulting from AS and hemodynamic evidence of severe obstruction. Operation should be carried out *before* frank failure has developed.

AORTIC REGURGITATION (AR)

ETIOLOGY Rheumatic in 70%; also may be due to infective endocarditis, syphilis, aortic dissection, or aortic dilatation due to cystic medial necrosis; three-fourths of pts are males.

CLINICAL MANIFESTATIONS Exertional dyspnea and awareness of heart beat, angina pectoris, and signs of LV failure. Wide pulse pressure, waterhammer pulse, capillary pulsations (Quincke's sign), A_2 soft or absent, S_3 common. Blowing, decrescendo diastolic murmur along left sternal border (along right sternal border with aortic dilatation). May be accompanied by systolic murmur of augmented blood flow.

LABORATORY *ECG and CXR* LV enlargement.

Echocardiogram Increased excursion of posterior LV wall, LA enlargement, LV enlargement, high-frequency diastolic fluttering of mitral valve. Doppler studies useful in detection and quantification of AR.

℞ TREATMENT

Standard therapy for LV failure (see Chap. 108). Surgical valve replacement should be carried out in pts with severe AR when symptoms develop or in asymptomatic pts with LV dysfunction (LV ejection fraction <50%, LV end-systolic volume >55 mL/m², or end-systolic diameter >55 mm) by echocardiography.

TRICUSPID STENOSIS (TS)

ETIOLOGY Usually rheumatic; most common in females; almost invariably associated with MS.

CLINICAL MANIFESTATIONS Hepatomegaly, ascites, edema, jaundice, jugular venous distention with slow y descent (Chap. 104). Diastolic rumbling murmur along left sternal border increased by inspiration with loud presystolic component. Right atrial and superior vena caval enlargement on x-ray.

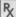 **TREATMENT**
In severe TS, surgical relief is indicated and usually requires valve replacement.

TRICUSPID REGURGITATION (TR)

ETIOLOGY Usually functional and secondary to marked RV dilatation of any cause and often associated with pulmonary hypertension.

CLINICAL MANIFESTATIONS Severe RV failure, with edema, hepatomegaly, and prominent v waves in jugular venous pulse with rapid y descent (Chap. 104). Systolic murmur along sternal edge is increased by inspiration.

TREATMENT
Intensive diuretic therapy. In severe cases (in absence of severe pulmonary hypertension), surgical treatment consists of tricuspid annuloplasty or valve replacement.

For a more detailed discussion, see Braunwald E: Valvular Heart Disease, Chap. 237, p. 1311, in HPIM-14.

111

CARDIOMYOPATHIES AND MYOCARDITIS

DILATED CARDIOMYOPATHY (CMP)

Symmetrically dilated left ventricle (LV), with poor systolic contractile function; right ventricle (RV) commonly involved.

ETIOLOGY Previous myocarditis or "idiopathic" most common; also toxins (ethanol, doxorubicin), connective tissue disorders, muscular dystrophies, "peripartum." Severe coronary disease/infarctions or chronic aortic/mitral regurgitation may behave similarly.

SYMPTOMS Congestive heart failure (Chap. 108); tachyarrhythmias and peripheral emboli from LV mural thrombus occur.

PHYSICAL EXAMINATION Jugular venous distention (JVD), rales, diffuse and dyskinetic LV apex, S_3, hepatomegaly, peripheral edema; murmurs of mitral and tricuspid regurgitation are common.

LABORATORY *ECG* Left bundle branch block and ST-T-wave abnormalities common.

CXR Cardiomegaly, pulmonary vascular redistribution, pulmonary effusions common.

Echocardiogram LV and RV enlargement with globally impaired contraction. *Regional* wall motion abnormalities suggest coronary artery disease rather than primary cardiomyopathy.

℞ TREATMENT

Standard therapy of CHF (Chap. 108); vasodilator therapy with ACE inhibitor or hydralazine-nitrate combination shown to improve longevity. Chronic anticoagulation with warfarin, recommended for very low ejection fraction ($<25\%$), if no contraindications. Antiarrhythmic drugs (Chap. 107) indicated for symptomatic or sustained arrhythmias (guided by invasive electrophysiologic study) but may cause proarrhythmic side effects; implanted internal defibrillator is often a better alternative. Possible trial of immunosuppressive drugs, if active myocarditis present on RV biopsy (controversial as long-term efficacy has not been demonstrated). In selected pts, consider cardiac transplantation.

RESTRICTIVE CARDIOMYOPATHY

Increased myocardial "stiffness" impairs ventricular relaxation; diastolic ventricular pressures are elevated. Etiologies include infiltrative disease (amyloid, sarcoid, hemochromatosis, eosinophilic disorders), myocardial fibrosis, and fibroelastosis.

SYMPTOMS Are of CHF, although right-sided heart failure often predominates with peripheral edema and ascites.

PHYSICAL EXAMINATION Signs of right-sided heart failure: JVD, hepatomegaly, peripheral edema, murmur of tricuspid regurgitation. Left-sided signs also may be present.

LABORATORY *ECG* Low limb lead voltage, sinus tachycardia, ST-T-wave abnormalities.

CXR Mild LV enlargement.

Echocardiogram Bilateral atrial enlargement; increased ventricular thickness ("speckled pattern") in infiltrative disease, especially amyloidosis. Systolic function is usually normal, but may be mildly reduced.

Cardiac Catheterization Increased LV and RV diastolic pressures with "dip and plateau" pattern; RV biopsy useful in detecting infiltrative disease (rectal biopsy useful in diagnosis of amyloidosis).

Note: Must distinguish restrictive cardiomyopathy from constrictive pericarditis, which is surgically correctable (see Table 111-1).

℞ TREATMENT

Salt restriction and diuretics ameliorate pulmonary and systemic congestion; digitalis is not indicated unless systolic function impaired or atrial arrhythmias present. *Note:* Increased sensitivity to digitalis in amyloidosis. Anticoagulation often indicated, particularly in pts with eosinophilic endomyocarditis. For specific therapy of hemochromatosis and sarcoidosis, see Chaps. 320 and 342, respectively, in HPIM-14.

HYPERTROPHIC OBSTRUCTIVE CARDIOMYOPATHY (HOCM)

Marked LV hypertrophy; often asymmetric, without underlying cause. Systolic function is normal; increased LV stiffness results in elevated diastolic filling pressures.

SYMPTOMS Secondary to elevated diastolic pressure, dynamic LV outflow obstruction, and arrhythmias; dyspnea on exertion, angina, and presyncope; sudden death may occur.

Table 111-1

Constrictive Pericarditis vs. Restrictive Cardiomyopathy

	Constrictive Pericarditis	Restrictive Cardiomyopathy
Prominent palpable cardiac apex	No	Often present
Cardiac size	Normal	May be enlarged
S_3, S_4	Absent (pericardial knock possible)	Often present
Calcification of pericardium on x-ray	Frequent	Absent
Systolic function	Normal	May be depressed
"Dip and plateau"	Yes	Yes
LV vs. RV diastolic pressure	Equal	LV usually higher
RV biopsy	Normal	Abnormal: may show infiltrative disease

PHYSICAL EXAMINATION   Brisk carotid upstroke with pulsus bisferiens; S_4, harsh systolic murmur along left sternal border, blowing murmur of mitral regurgitation at apex; murmur changes with Valsalva and other maneuvers (see Chap. 104).

LABORATORY   *ECG*   LV hypertrophy with prominent "septal" Q waves in leads I, aVL, V_{5-6}. Periods of atrial fibrillation or ventricular tachycardia are often detected by Holter monitor.

Echocardiogram   LV hypertrophy, often with asymmetric septal hypertrophy (ASH) and $\geq 1.3 \times$ thickness of LV posterior wall; LV contractile function excellent with small endsystolic volume. If LV outflow tract obstruction is present, systolic anterior motion (SAM) of mitral valve and midsystolic partial closure of aortic valve are present. Doppler shows early systolic accelerated blood flow through LV outflow tract. Carotid pulse tracing shows "spike and dome" configuration.

Table 111-2

Characteristics of the Cardiomyopathies

Dilated	Restrictive	Hypertrophic
VENTRICULAR CHARACTERISTICS		
LV (and usually RV) chamber dilatation	Impaired relaxation (reduced compliance); often due to ventricular infiltration	Marked hypertrophy, often asymmetric with septal thickness > LV free wall
PHYSICAL EXAMINATION		
Dyskinetic LV apex with biventricular CHF: rales, S₃, JVD, peripheral edema; may have murmurs of mitral and tricuspid regurgitation	Predominant right-sided CHF: JVD, hepatomegaly, peripheral edema	Brisk carotid upstroke; prominent S₄, harsh systolic murmur at left sternal border plus apical murmur of mitral regurgitation
CHEST X-RAY		
Four-chamber cardiac enlargement; pulmonary vascular redistribution	Mild cardiac enlargement	Mild cardiac enlargement
ECHOCARDIOGRAM		
Ventricular dilatation and global contractile impairment	Systolic function usually normal or mildly decreased; increased ventricular wall thickness in infiltrative disease; marked biatrial enlargement typical	Left ventricular hypertrophy, often asymmetric (septal thickness ≥1.3 × LV free wall); systolic anterior motion of mitral valve; mitral regurgitation and outflow gradient by Doppler

℞ TREATMENT

Strenuous exercise should be avoided. Beta blockers, vera-pamil, or disopyramide used individually to reduce symptoms. Digoxin, other inotropes, diuretics, and vasodilators are *contraindicated*. Endocarditis antibiotic prophylaxis (Chap. 72) is necessary when outflow obstruction or mitral regurgitation is present. Antiarrhythmic agents, especially amiodarone, may suppress atrial and ventricular arrhythmias. Consider implantable automatic defibrillator for pts with high-risk ventricular arrhythmias. Surgical myectomy may be useful in pts refractory to medical therapy.

Table 111-2 summarizes distinguishing features of the cardiomyopathies.

MYOCARDITIS

Inflammation of the myocardium most commonly due to acute viral infection; may progress to chronic dilated cardiomyopathy. Myocarditis may develop in pts with HIV infection or Lyme disease.

HISTORY   Fever, fatigue, palpitations; if LV dysfunction is present, then symptoms of CHF are present. Viral myocarditis may be preceded by URI.

PHYSICAL EXAMINATION   Fever, tachycardia, soft S_1; S_3 common.

LABORATORY   CK-MB isoenzyme may be elevated in absence of MI. Convalescent antiviral antibody titers may rise.

ECG   Transient ST-T-wave abnormalities.

CXR   Cardiomegaly.

Echocardiogram   Depressed LV function; pericardial effusion present if accompanying pericarditis present.

℞ TREATMENT

Rest; treat as CHF (Chap. 108); immunosuppressive therapy (steroids and azathioprine) may be considered if RV biopsy shows active inflammation, but long-term efficacy not demonstrated.

For a more detailed discussion, see Wynne J, Braunwald E: The Cardiomyopathies and Myocarditides, Chap. 239, p. 1328, in HPIM-14.

PERICARDIAL DISEASE

ACUTE PERICARDITIS

CAUSES   See Table 112-1

HISTORY   Chest pain, which may be intense, mimicking acute MI, but characteristically sharp, pleuritic, and positional (relieved by leaning forward); fever and palpitations are common.

PHYSICAL EXAMINATION   Rapid or irregular pulse, coarse pericardial friction rub, which may vary in intensity and is loudest with pt sitting forward.

LABORATORY   *ECG*   (See Table 112-2) Diffuse ST elevation (concave upward) usually present in all leads except aVR and V_1; PR-segment depression may be present; *days* later (unlike acute MI), ST returns to baseline and T-wave inversion develops. Atrial premature beats and atrial fibrillation may appear. Differentiate from ECG of early repolarization variant (ERV) (ST-T ratio <0.25 in ERV, but >0.25 in pericarditis).

CXR   Increased size of cardiac silhouette if large (>250 mL) pericardial effusion present, with "water bottle" configuration.

Echocardiogram   Most sensitive test for detection of pericardial effusion, which commonly accompanies acute pericarditis (Fig. 112-1).

Table 112-1

Most Common Causes of Pericarditis

Idiopathic
Infections (particularly viral)
Acute myocardial infarction
Metastatic neoplasm
Radiation therapy for tumor (up to 20 years earlier)
Chronic renal failure
Connective-tissue disease (rheumatoid arthritis, SLE)
Drug reaction (e.g., procainamide, hydralazine)
"Autoimmune" following heart surgery or myocardial infarction (several weeks/months later)

Table 112-2

ECG in Acute Pericarditis vs. Acute (Q-wave) MI

ST-Segment Elevation	ECG Lead Involvement	Evolution of ST and T Waves	PR-Segment Depression
PERICARDITIS			
Concave upward	All leads involved except aVR and V$_1$	ST remains elevated for several days; after ST returns to baseline, T waves invert	Yes, in majority
ACUTE MI			
Convex upward	ST elevation over infarcted region only; reciprocal ST depression in opposite leads	T waves invert within hours, while ST still elevated; followed by Q wave development	No

℞ TREATMENT

Aspirin 650–975 mg qid or NSAIDs (e.g., indomethacin 25–75 mg qid); for *severe*, *refractory* pain, prednisone 40–60 mg/d is used and tapered over several weeks or months. Intractable, prolonged pain or frequently recurrent episodes may require pericardiectomy. Anticoagulants are relatively contraindicated in acute pericarditis because of risk of pericardial hemorrhage.

CARDIAC TAMPONADE

Life-threatening emergency resulting from accumulation of pericardial fluid under pressure; impaired filling of cardiac chambers and decreased cardiac output.

ETIOLOGY   Previous pericarditis (most commonly metastatic tumor, uremia, acute MI, viral or idiopathic pericarditis),

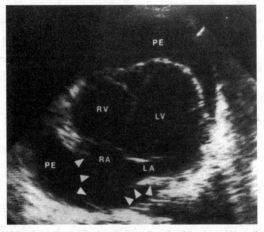

FIGURE 112-1 Two-dimensional echocardiogram of a patient with a malignant pericardial effusion and cardiac tamponade. There is a large pericardial effusion (PE) adjacent to the borders of the right ventricle (RV), right atrium (RA), and left ventricle (LV). The effusion is sufficiently large that fluid is also present behind the left atrium (LA). Diastolic compression (white arrowheads) of both the right and left atria is present. [From Lorell B: Pericardial diseases in *Heart Disease,* 5th ed, E. Braunwald (ed). Philadelphia, Saunders, 1997, with permission].

cardiac trauma, or myocardial perforation during catheter or pacemaker placement.

HISTORY   Hypotension may develop suddenly; subacute symptoms include dyspnea, weakness, confusion.

PHYSICAL EXAMINATION   Tachycardia, hypotension, pulsus paradoxus (inspiratory fall in systolic blood pressure >10 mmHg), jugular venous distention with preserved x descent, but loss of y descent; heart sounds distant. If tamponade develops subacutely, peripheral edema, hepatomegaly, and ascites are frequently present.

LABORATORY   *ECG*   Low limb lead voltage; large effusions may cause electrical alternans (alternating size of QRS complex due to swinging of heart).

CXR   Enlarged cardiac silhouette if large (>250 mL) effusion present.

Echocardiogram Swinging motion of heart within large effusion; prominent respiratory alteration of RV dimension with RA and RV collapse during diastole.

Cardiac Catheterization Confirms diagnosis; shows equalization of diastolic pressures in all four chambers; pericardial = RA pressure.

R̲x̲ TREATMENT

Immediate pericardiocentesis and IV volume expansion.

CONSTRICTIVE PERICARDITIS

Rigid pericardium leads to impaired cardiac filling, elevation of systemic and pulmonary venous pressures, and decreased cardiac output. Results from healing and scar formation in some pts with previous pericarditis. Viral, tuberculosis, previous cardiac surgery, uremia, neoplastic pericarditis are most common causes.

HISTORY Gradual onset of dyspnea, fatigue, pedal edema, abdominal swelling; symptoms of LV failure uncommon.

PHYSICAL EXAMINATION Tachycardia, jugular venous distention (prominent *y* descent) which increases further on inspiration (Kussmaul's sign); hepatomegaly, ascites, peripheral edema are common; sharp diastolic sound, "pericardial knock" following S_2 sometimes present.

LABORATORY *ECG* Low limb lead voltage; atrial arrhythmias are common.

CXR Rim of pericardial calcification in 50% of pts.

Echocardiogram Thickened pericardium, normal ventricular contraction.

CT or MRI More precise than echocardiogram in demonstrating thickened pericardium.

Cardiac Catheterization Equalization of diastolic pressures in all chambers; ventricular pressure tracings show "dip and plateau" appearance (to distinguish from restrictive cardiomyopathy; see Table 111-1). Pts with constrictive pericarditis should be investigated for tuberculosis (Chap. 89).

R̲x̲ TREATMENT

Surgical stripping of the pericardium. Progressive improvement ensues over several months.

_____ *Approach to the Patient* _____

with Asymptomatic Pericardial Effusion of Unknown Cause

If careful history and physical exam do not suggest etiology, the following may lead to diagnosis:

- Skin test and cultures for tuberculosis (Chap. 89)
- Serum albumin and urine protein measurement (nephrotic syndrome)
- Serum creatinine and BUN (renal failure)
- Thyroid function tests (myxedema)
- ANA (SLE and other collagen-vascular disease)
- Search for a primary tumor (especially lung and breast)

For a more detailed discussion, see Braunwald E: Pericardial Disease, Chap. 240, p. 1334, in HPIM-14.

113

ACUTE MYOCARDIAL INFARCTION

Early recognition and immediate treatment of acute MI are essential; diagnosis is based on characteristic history, ECG, and evolution of cardiac enzymes.

SYMPTOMS   Chest pain similar to angina (Chap. 2) but more intense and persistent (>30 min); not fully relieved by rest or nitroglycerin, often accompanied by nausea, sweating, apprehension. However, 25% of MIs are clinically silent.

PHYSICAL EXAMINATION   Pallor, diaphoresis, tachycardia, S_4, dyskinetic cardiac impulse may be present. If CHF exists: rales, S_3. Jugular venous distention is common in right ventricular infarction.

ECG   *Q-wave MI*   ST elevation, followed by T-wave inversion, then Q-wave development (Chap. 105) over several hours.

Non-Q-wave MI   ST depression followed by persistent ST-T-wave changes *without* Q-wave development. Comparison with old ECG helpful.

CARDIAC ENZYMES   Time course is important for diagnosis; creatine phosphokinase (CK) level should be checked every 8 h for first day: CK rises within 4–8 h, peaks at 24 h, returns to normal by 48–72 h. CK-MB isoenzyme is more specific for MI but may also be elevated with myocarditis or after electrical cardioversion. Total CK (but not CK-MB) rises (two- to three-fold) after IM injection, vigorous exercise, or other skeletal muscle trauma. A ratio of CK-MB mass: CK activity ≥2.5 suggests acute MI. CK-MB peaks earlier (about 8 h) following acute reperfusion therapy (see below). Cardiac-specific troponin T and troponin I are highly specific for myocardial injury and remain elevated for 1–2 weeks. LDH peaks at days 3–4 and remains elevated as long as 14 d; LDH_1 isoenzyme is more specific for MI than total LDH.

NONINVASIVE IMAGING TECHNIQUES   Useful when diagnosis of MI is not clear. *Echocardiography* detects infarct-associated regional wall motion abnormalities (but cannot distinguish acute MI from a previous myocardial scar). Echo is also useful in detecting RV infarction, LV aneurysm, and LV thrombus. *Myocardial perfusion imaging* (thallium 201 or technetium 99m-sestamibi) is sensitive for regions of decreased perfusion but is not specific for acute MI.

℞ TREATMENT

Initial Therapy

Goal is to relieve pain, minimize extent of infarcted tissue, and prevent/treat arrhythmias and mechanical complications. Early thrombolytic therapy with streptokinase, reteplase (rPA), or tissue plasminogen activator (tPA) can reduce infarct size and mortality and limit LV dysfunction. In appropriate candidates (Figs. 113-1 and 113-2), thrombolysis should be initiated as quickly as possible (ideally within 30 min) in the emergency room or coronary care unit (CCU); pts treated within 3 h of initial symptoms benefit the most. Complications include bleeding, reperfusion arrhythmias, and, in the case of streptokinase, allergic reactions. Anticoagulation [aspirin (initially 160–325 mg chewed at time of admission, then 160–325 mg PO qd) and heparin] is begun concurrently with the thrombolytic agent (see Fig. 113-1). Subsequent coronary arteriography is reserved for pts with recurrent angina or positive exercise test prior to discharge. In pts with contraindi-

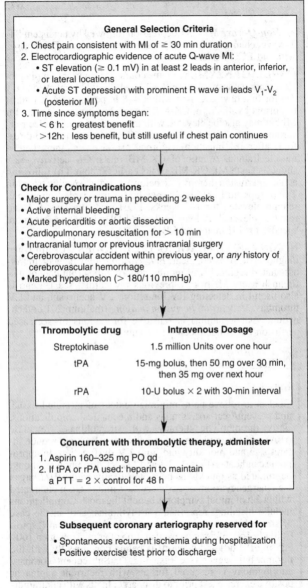

FIGURE 113-1 Approach to thrombolytic therapy of pts with acute MI.

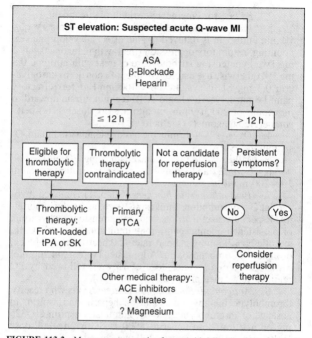

FIGURE 113-2 Management strategies for pts with MI. All pts suspected of having a Q-wave MI (i.e., ST-segment elevation on ECG) should receive aspirin (ASA), beta blockers (in the absense of contraindications), and heparin. Heparin is probably not required in pts receiving steptokinase (SK). Pts treated within 12 h eligible for thrombolytic therapy should receive it expeditiously or be considered for primary PTCA. Immediate, primary PTCA is also to be considered when lytic therapy is contraindicated. Pts treated after 12 h should receive initial medical therapy noted above and, on an individual basis, may be candidates for ACE inhibitors (particularly if LV function is impaired).

cations to thrombolytic therapy (see Fig. 113-1), primary percutaneous transluminal coronary angioplasty (PTCA) can be undertaken to restore coronary flow. Primary PTCA may be preferred over thrombolytic therapy in cardiogenic shock, in pts of advanced age (>70), and in some highly experienced centers, especially if delay can be minimized.

Additional Standard Treatment

(whether or not thrombolytic therapy is administered):

1. Hospitalize in CCU with continuous ECG monitoring.

2.   *IV line* for emergency arrhythmia treatment.

3.   *Pain control:* (a) Morphine sulfate 2–4 mg IV q5–10 min until pain is relieved or side effects develop [nausea, vomiting, respiratory depression (treat with naloxone 0.4–1.2 mg IV), hypotension (if bradycardic, treat with atropine 0.5 mg IV; otherwise use careful volume infusion)]; (b) nitroglycerin 0.3 mg SL if systolic bp >100 mmHg; for refractory pain: IV nitroglycerin (begin at 10 μg/min, titrate upward to maximum of 200 μg/min, monitoring bp closely); (c) beta-adrenergic antagonists (see below).

4.   *Oxygen* 2–4 L/min by nasal cannula (maintain O_2 saturation >90%).

5.   Mild *sedation* (e.g., diazepam 5 mg PO qid).

6.   *Soft diet* and stool softeners (e.g., docusate sodium 100–200 mg/d).

7.   *Beta-adrenergic blockers* (Chap. 115) reduce myocardial O_2 consumption, limit infarct size, and reduce mortality. Especially useful in pts with hypertension, tachycardia, or persistent ischemic pain; contraindications include CHF, systolic bp <95 mmHg, heart rate <50 beats/min, AV block, or history of bronchospasm. Administer IV (e.g., metoprolol 5 mg q5–10 min to total dose of 15 mg), followed by PO regimen (e.g., metoprolol 25–100 mg bid).

8.   *Anticoagulation/antiplatelet agents:* Pts who receive thrombolytic therapy are begun on heparin and aspirin. In absence of thrombolytic therapy, administer aspirin 80–325 mg qd and low-dose heparin (5000 U SC q12h). Full-dose IV heparin (PTT 2 × control) followed by oral anticoagulants is recommended for pts with severe CHF, presence of ventricular thrombus by echocardiogram, or large dyskinetic region in anterior MI. Oral anticoagulants are continued for 3 to 6 months, then replaced by aspirin.

9.   *ACE inhibitors* reduce mortality in pts following acute MI and should be prescribed early in hospitalization for pts who are hemodynamically stable—e.g., captopril (6.25 mg PO test dose) advanced to 50 mg PO tid. ACE inhibitors should be continued indefinitely in pts with CHF or those with asymptomatic LV dysfunction [ejection fraction (EF) ≤40%].

10.   *Serum magnesium* level should be measured and repleted if necessary to reduce risk of arrhythmias.

COMPLICATIONS

VENTRICULAR ARRHYTHMIAS   Isolated ventricular premature beats (VPBs) occur frequently. Precipitating factors should be corrected (hypoxemia, acidosis, hypokalemia, hypercalcemia, hypomagnesemia, CHF, arrhythmogenic drugs). Routine beta-blocker administration (see above) diminishes ventricular ectopy. Other in-hospital antiarrhythmic therapy should be reserved for pts with sustained ventricular arrhythmias.

Management of acute MI pts with ST depression and/or T-wave inversion is outlined in Fig. 113-3.

VENTRICULAR TACHYCARDIA If hemodynamically unstable, perform immediate electrical countershock (unsynchronized discharge of 200–300 J). If hemodynamically tolerated, use IV lidocaine [bolus of 1.0–1.5 mg/kg, infusion of 20–50 (μg/kg)/min; use lower infusion rate ($\approx$1 mg/min) in pts of advanced age or those with CHF or liver disease], IV procainamide (bolus of 15 mg/kg over 20–30 min; infusion of 1–4 mg/min) or IV amiodarone (bolus of 75–150 mg over 10–15 min; infusion of 1.0 mg/min for 6 h, then 0.5 mg/min).

VENTRICULAR FIBRILLATION VF requires immediate defibrillation (200–400 J). If unsuccessful, initiate CPR and standard resuscitative measures (Chap. 27). Ventricular arrhythmias that appear several days or weeks following MI often reflect pump failure and may warrant invasive electrophysiologic study.

ACCELERATED IDIOVENTRICULAR RHYTHM Wide QRS complex, regular rhythm, rate 60–100 beats/min is common and usually benign; if it causes hypotension, treat with atropine 0.6 mg IV.

SUPRAVENTRICULAR ARRHYTHMIAS *Sinus tachycardia* may result from CHF, hypoxemia, pain, fever, pericarditis, hypovolemia, administered drugs. If no cause is identified, may treat with beta blocker (see Table 115-2). For persistent sinus tachycardia (>120), use Swan-Ganz catheter to differentiate CHF from decreased intravascular volume. Other *supraventricular arrhythmias* (paroxysmal supraventricular tachycardia, atrial flutter, and fibrillation) are often secondary to CHF, in which digoxin (Chap. 108) is treatment of choice. In absence of CHF, may also use verapamil or propranolol (Chap. 107). If hemodynamically unstable, proceed with electrical cardioversion.

BRADYARRHYTHMIAS AND AV BLOCK (See Chap. 107) In *inferior MI*, usually represent heightened vagal tone or discrete AV nodal ischemia. If hemodynamically compromised (CHF, hypotension, emergence of ventricular arrhythmias), treat with atropine 0.5 mg IV q5min (up to 2 mg). If no response, use temporary external or transvenous pacemaker. Isoproterenol should be avoided. In *anterior MI*, AV conduction defects usu-

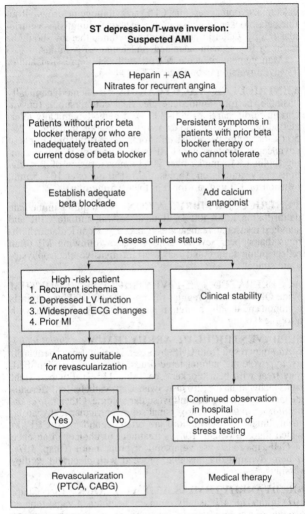

FIGURE 113-3 Management of pts with acute MI and ST depression and/or T-wave inversion.

Table 113-1

Indications for Swan-Ganz Catheter in Acute Myocardial Infarction

1. Moderate to severe CHF
2. Hypotension not corrected by volume infusion
3. Unexplained sinus tachycardia or tachypnea
4. Suspected acute mitral regurgitation or ventricular septal rupture
5. To manage IV vasodilator therapy

---

ally reflect extensive tissue necrosis. Consider temporary external or transvenous pacemaker for (1) complete heart block, (2) Mobitz type II block (Chap. 107), (3) new bifascicular block (LBBB, RBBB + left anterior hemiblock, RBBB + left posterior hemiblock), (4) any bradyarrhythmia associated with hypotension or CHF.

CONGESTIVE HEART FAILURE   CHF may result from systolic "pump" dysfunction, increased LV diastolic "stiffness," and/or acute mechanical complications.

Symptoms   Dyspnea, orthopnea, tachycardia.

Examination   Jugular venous distention, S_3 and S_4 gallop, pulmonary rales; systolic murmur if acute mitral regurgitation or ventricular septal defect (VSD) have developed.

℞ **TREATMENT**   (See Chaps. 29 and 108)
Initial therapy includes diuretics (begin with furosemide 10–20 mg IV), inhaled O_2, and vasodilators, particularly nitrates [PO, topical, or IV (Chap. 108) unless pt is hypotensive (systolic bp <100 mmHg)]; digitalis is usually of little benefit in acute MI unless supraventricular arrhythmias are present. Diuretic, vasodilator, and inotropic therapy (Table 113-2) best guided by invasive hemodynamic monitoring (Swan-Ganz pulmonary artery catheter, arterial line) particularly in pts with accompanying hypotension (see Tables 113-1 and 113-3 and Fig. 113-2). In acute MI, optimal pulmonary capillary wedge pressure (PCW) is 15–20 mmHg; in the absence of hypotension, PCW >20 mmHg is treated with diuretic plus vasodilator therapy [IV nitroglycerin (begin at 10 μg/min) or

Table 113-2

Intravenous Vasodilators and Inotropic Drugs Used
in Acute MI

Drug	Usual Dosage Range	Comment
Nitroglycerin	10 μg/min–10 (μg/kg)/min	May improve coronary blood flow to ischemic myocardium
Nitroprusside	0.5–10 (μg/kg)/min	More potent vasodilator, but improves coronary blood flow less than nitroglycerin With therapy >24 h or in renal failure, watch for thiocyanate toxicity (blurred vision, tinnitus, delirium)
Dobutamine	2–20 (μg/kg)/min	Results in ↑ cardiac output, ↓ PCW, but does not raise bp
Dopamine	2–10 (μg/kg)/min (sometimes higher)	More appropriate than dobutamine if hypotensive Hemodynamic effect depends on dose: (μg/kg/min) <5 ↑ renal blood flow 2.5–10 positive inotrope >10 vasoconstriction
Amrinone	0.75 mg/kg bolus, then 5–15 (μg/kg)/min	Positive inotrope and vasodilator Can combine with dopamine or dobutamine May result in thrombocytopenia
Milrinone	50 mg/kg bolus, then 0.375–0.75 (μg/kg)/min	Ventricular arrhythmias may result

Table 113-3

Hemodynamic Complications in Acute MI

Condition	Cardiac Index, (L/min)/m²	PCW, mmHg	Systolic bp, mmHg	Treatment
Uncomplicated	>2.5	≤18	>100	—
Hypovolemia	<2.5	<15	<100	Successive boluses of normal saline. In setting of inferior wall MI, consider RV infarction (esp. if RA pressure >10)
Volume overload	>2.5	>20	>100	Diuretic (e.g., furosemide 10–20 mg IV) Nitroglycerin: topical paste of IV (Table 113-2)
LV failure	<2.5	>20	>100	Diuretic (e.g., furosemide 10–20 mg IV) IV nitroglycerin (or if hypertensive, use IV nitroprusside)
Severe LV failure	<2.5	>20	<100	If bp ≥90: IV dobutamine ± IV nitroglycerin or sodium nitroprusside. If bp <90: IV dopamine. If accompanied by pulmonary edema: attempt diuresis with IV furosemide; may be limited by hypotension. If new systolic murmur present, consider acute VSD or mitral regurgitation
Cardiogenic shock	<1.8	>20	<90 with oliguria and confusion	IV dopamine Intraaortic balloon pump Coronary angioplasty may be life-saving

NOTE: PCW, pulmonary artery wedge pressure; RV, right ventricle; LV, left ventricle.

683

nitroprusside (begin at 0.5 μg/kg per min)] and titrated to optimize bp, PCW, and systemic vascular resistance (SVR).

$$SVR = \frac{(\text{mean arterial pressure}) - (\text{mean RA pressure}) \times 80}{\text{cardiac output}}$$

Normal SVR = 900–1350 dyn · s/cm^5. If PCW >20 mmHg and pt is hypotensive (Table 113-3 and Fig. 113-4), evaluate for VSD or acute mitral regurgitation, add dobutamine [begin at 1–2 (μg/kg)/min], titrate upward to maximum of 10 (μg/kg)/min; beware of drug-induced tachycardia or ventricular ectopy.

If CHF improves on parenteral vasodilator therapy, oral therapy follows with ACE inhibitor (e.g., captopril, enalapril, or lisinopril—Chap. 115) or the combination of nitrates plus hydralazine (Chap. 108).

CARDIOGENIC SHOCK   Severe LV failure with hypotension (bp <80 mmHg) *and* elevated PCW (>20 mmHg), accompanied by oliguria (<20 mL/h), peripheral vasoconstriction, dulled sensorium, and metabolic acidosis.

R$_X$ **TREATMENT**   (See Chap. 28, Fig. 113–4)
Swan-Ganz catheter and intraarterial bp monitoring are essential; aim for mean PCW of 18–20 mmHg with adjustment of volume (diuretics or infusion) as needed. Intraaortic balloon counterpulsation may be necessary to maintain bp and reduce PCW. Administer high concentration of O$_2$ by mask; if pulmonary edema coexists, intubation and mechanical ventilation should be considered. Acute mechanical complications (see below) should be sought and promptly treated.

If cardiogenic shock develops within 4 h of first MI symptoms, acute reperfusion by PTCA may markedly improve LV function.

Hypotension also may result from *RV MI*, which should be suspected in the setting of inferior or posterior MI, if jugular venous distention and elevation of right-heart pressures predominate (rales are typically absent and PCW may be normal); right-sided ECG leads typically show ST elevation, and echocardiography may confirm diagnosis. *Treatment* consists of volume infusion, gauged by PCW and arterial pressure. Noncardiac causes of hypotension should be considered: hypovolemia, acute arrhythmia, or sepsis.

ACUTE MECHANICAL COMPLICATIONS   Ventricular septal rupture and acute mitral regurgitation due to papillary muscle ischemia/infarct develop during the first week following MI and are characterized by sudden onset of CHF and new

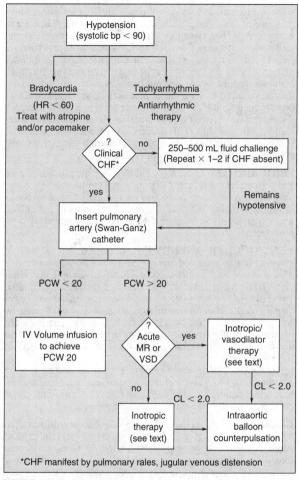

FIGURE 113-4   Approach to hypotension in pts with acute myocardial infarction; PCW, pulmonary capillary wedge pressure.

systolic murmur. Echocardiography with Doppler can confirm presence of these complications. PCW tracings may show large v waves in either condition, but an oxygen "step-up" as the catheter is advanced from RA to RV suggests septal rupture. Acute medical therapy of these conditions includes vasodilator therapy (IV nitroprusside: begin at 10 μg/min and titrate to maintain systolic bp $\simeq$ 100 mmHg); intraaortic balloon pump may be required to maintain cardiac output. Surgical correction is postponed for 4–6 weeks after acute MI if pt is stable; surgery should not be deferred if pt is unstable. Acute ventricular free-wall rupture presents with sudden loss of bp, pulse, and consciousness, while ECG shows an intact rhythm; emergent surgical repair is crucial, and mortality is high.

PERICARDITIS Characterized by *pleuritic, positional* pain and pericardial rub (Chap. 112); atrial arrhythmias are common; must be distinguished from recurrent angina. Often responds to aspirin 650 mg PO qid. Anticoagulants should be withheld when pericarditis is suspected to avoid development of tamponade.

VENTRICULAR ANEURYSM Localized "bulge" of LV chamber due to infarcted myocardium. *True aneurysms* consist of scar tissue and do not rupture. However, complications include CHF, ventricular arrhythmias, and thrombus formation. Typically, ECG shows persistent ST-segment elevation, longer than 2 weeks after initial infarct; aneurysm is confirmed by echocardiography and by left ventriculography. The presence of thrombus within the aneurysm, or a large aneurysmal segment due to anterior MI, warrants oral anticoagulation with warfarin for 3–6 months.

In contrast, *pseudoaneurysm* is a form of cardiac rupture contained by a local area of pericardium and organized thrombus; direct communication with the LV cavity is present; surgical repair usually necessary to prevent rupture.

RECURRENT ANGINA Usually associated with transient ST-T-wave changes; signals high incidence of reinfarction; when it occurs in early post-MI period (2 weeks), proceed directly to coronary arteriography in most pts, to identify those who would benefit from PTCA or coronary artery bypass surgery.

DRESSLER'S SYNDROME Syndrome of fever, pleuritic chest pain, pericardial effusion which may develop 2–6 weeks following acute MI; pain and ECG characteristic of pericarditis (Chap. 112); usually responds to aspirin or NSAIDs. Reserve glucocorticoid therapy (prednisone 1 mg/kg PO qd) for those with severe, refractory pain.

SECONDARY PREVENTION

Submaximal exercise testing should be performed prior to or soon after discharge. A positive test (Chap. 114) in certain subgroups (angina at a low workload, a large region of provocable ischemia, or provocable ischemia with a reduced LV ejection fraction) suggests need for cardiac catheterization to evaluate myocardium at risk of recurrent infarction. *Beta blockers* (e.g., timolol 10 mg bid, metoprolol 25–100 mg bid) should be prescribed routinely for at least 2 years following acute MI (see Table 115-1), unless contraindications present (asthma, CHF, bradycardia, "brittle" diabetes). Aspirin (80–325 mg/d) is administered to reduce incidence of subsequent infarction, unless contraindicated (e.g., active peptic ulcer, allergy). If the LVEF ≤40%, an ACE inhibitor (e.g., captopril 6.25 mg PO tid, advanced to target dose of 50 mg PO tid) should be used indefinitely.

Modification of cardiac risk factors must be encouraged: discontinue smoking; control hypertension, diabetes, and serum lipids (target LDL ≤100 mg/dL) (Chap. 169); and pursue graduated exercise.

For a more detailed discussion, see Antman EM, Braunwald E: Acute Myocardial Infarction, Chap. 243, p. 1352, in HPIM-14.

114

CHRONIC CORONARY ARTERY DISEASE

Angina pectoris, the most common clinical manifestation of CAD, results from an imbalance between myocardial O_2 supply and demand, most commonly resulting from atherosclerotic coronary artery obstruction. Other major conditions that upset this balance and result in angina include aortic valve disease (Chap. 110), hypertrophic cardiomyopathy (Chap. 111), and coronary artery spasm (see below).

SYMPTOMS Angina is typically associated with exertion or emotional upset; relieved quickly by rest or nitroglycerin (see Chap. 2). Major risk factors are cigarette smoking, hypertension, hypercholesterolemia ($\uparrow$LDL fraction; $\downarrow$HDL), diabetes, and family history of CAD below age 55.

PHYSICAL EXAMINATION Often normal; arterial bruits or retinal vascular abnormalities suggest generalized atherosclerosis; S_4 is common. During acute anginal episode, other signs may appear: loud S_3 or S_4, diaphoresis, rales, and a transient murmur of mitral regurgitation due to papillary muscle ischemia.

LABORATORY *ECG* May be normal between anginal episodes or show old infarction (Chap. 105). During angina, ST- and T-wave abnormalities typically appear (ST-segment depression reflects subendocardial ischemia; ST-segment elevation may reflect acute infarction or transient coronary artery spasm). Ventricular arrhythmias frequently accompany acute ischemia.

Stress Testing Enhances diagnosis of CAD (see Fig. 114-1). Exercise is performed on treadmill or bicycle until target heart rate is achieved or pt becomes symptomatic (chest pain, light-headedness, hypotension, marked dyspnea, ventricular tachycardia) or develops diagnostic ST-segment changes. Useful information includes duration of exercise achieved; peak heart rate and bp; depth, morphology, and persistence of ST-segment depression; and whether and at which level of exercise pain, hypotension, or ventricular arrhythmias develop. *Thallium 201* (or technetium 99 sestamibi) imaging increases sensitivity and specificity and is particularly useful if baseline ECG abnormalities prevent interpretation of test (e.g., LBBB). *Note:* Exercise testing should not be performed in pts with acute MI, unstable angina, or severe aortic stenosis. If the pt is unable to exercise, intravenous dipyridamole (or adenosine) testing can be performed in conjunction with thallium or sestamibi imaging or a dobutamine echocardiographic study can be obtained (see Table 114-1).

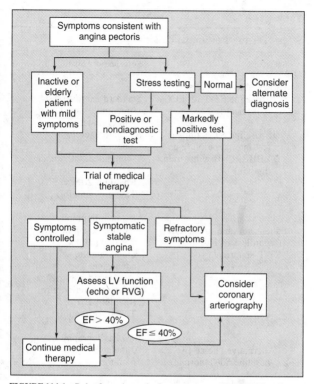

FIGURE 114-1 Role of exercise testing in management of CAD. RVG, radionuclide ventriculogram; EF, left ventricular ejection fraction. (Modified from Lilly LS, in J Noble ed. *Textbook of Primary Care Medicine*, St. Louis, Mosby, 1996, p. 224.)

Some pts do not experience chest pain during ischemic episodes with exertion ("silent ischemia") but are identified by transient ST-T-wave abnormalities during stress testing or Holter monitoring (see below).

Coronary Arteriography The definitive test for assessing severity of CAD; major indications are (1) angina refractory to medical therapy, (2) markedly positive exercise test (≥2-mm ST-segment depression or hypotension with exercise) suggestive of left main or three-vessel disease, (3) recurrent angina or positive exercise test after MI, (4) to assess for coronary

Table 114-1

Stress Testing Recommendations

Subgroup	Recommended Study
Patient able to exercise	
If baseline ST-T on ECG is isoelectric	Standard exercise test (treadmill, bicycle, or arm ergometry)
If baseline ST-T impairs test interpretation (e.g., LBBB, LVH with strain, digoxin)	Standard exercise test (above) combined with *either* Perfusion scintigraphy (thallium 201 or Tc99m-sestamibi) *or* Echocardiography
Patient *not* able to exercise (regardless of baseline ST-T abnormality)	Pharmacologic stress test (IV dobutamine, dipyridamole, or adenosine) combined with *either* Perfusion scintigraphy (thallium 201 or Tc99m-sestamibi) *or* Echocardiography
Alternative choice (if baseline ST-T normal)	Ambulatory ECG monitor

artery spasm, and (5) to evaluate pts with perplexing chest pain in whom noninvasive tests are not diagnostic.

℞ TREATMENT

General

- Identify and treat risk factors: mandatory cessation of smoking; treatment of diabetes, hypertension, and lipid disorders (Chap. 169).
- Correct exacerbating factors contributing to angina: marked obesity, CHF, anemia, hyperthyroidism.
- Reassurance and pt education.

Table 114-2

Examples of Commonly Used Nitrates

	Usual Dose	Recommended Dosing Frequency
SHORT-ACTING AGENTS		
Sublingual TNG	0.3–0.6 mg	As needed
Aerosol TNG	0.4 mg (1 inhalation)	As needed
Sublingual ISDN	2.5–10 mg	As needed
LONG-ACTING AGENTS		
ISDN		
Oral	5–30 mg	tid
Sustained-action	40 mg	bid (once in A.M., then 7 h later)
TNG ointment (2%)	0.5–2	qid (with one 7–10-nitrate-free interval)
TNG skin patches	0.1–0.6 mg/h	Apply in morning, remove at bedtime
ISMO		
Oral	20–40 mg	bid (once in A.M., then 7 h later)
Sustained-action	30–240 mg	qd

NOTE: TNG, nitroglycerin; ISDN, isosorbide dinitrate; ISMO, isosorbide mononitrate.

Drug Therapy

Sublingual nitroglycerin (TNG 0.3–0.6 mg); may be repeated at 5-min intervals; warn pts of possible headache or light-headedness; teach prophylactic use of TNG prior to activity that regularly evokes angina. If chest pain persists for more than 10 min despite 2–3 TNG, pt should report promptly to nearest medical facility for evaluation of possible unstable angina or acute MI.

Long-Term Angina Suppression

Three classes of drugs are used, frequently in combination:
Long-Acting Nitrates May be administered by many routes (Table 114-2); start at the lowest dose and frequency

to limit tolerance and side effects of headache, light-headedness, tachycardia.

Beta Blockers (See Table 115-2) All have antianginal properties; β_1-selective agents are less likely to exacerbate airway or peripheral vascular disease. Dosage should be titrated to resting heart rate of 50–60 beats/min. *Contraindications* to beta blockers include CHF, AV block, bronchospasm, "brittle" diabetes. Side effects include fatigue, bronchospasm, depressed LV function, impotence, depression, and masking of hypoglycemia in diabetics.

Calcium Antagonists (See Table 115-4) Useful for stable and unstable angina, as well as coronary vasospasm. Combination with other antianginal agents is beneficial, but verapamil should be administered very cautiously or not at all to pts on beta blockers or disopyramide (additive effects on LV dysfunction). Use sustained-release, not short-acting, calcium antagonists; the latter may increase coronary mortality.

Aspirin 80–325 mg/d reduces the incidence of MI in chronic stable angina, following MI, and in asymptomatic men. It is recommended in pts with CAD in the absence of contraindications (GI bleeding or allergy).

Mechanical Revascularization

Percutaneous Coronary Revascularization Performed on anatomically suitable stenoses of native vessels and bypass grafts; pts should generally be sufficiently symptomatic to warrant consideration of bypass surgery. With angioplasty (PTCA) initial relief of angina occurs in 85–90% of pts; however, stenosis recurs in 30–45% within 6 months (more commonly in pts with initial unstable angina, incomplete dilation, diabetes, or stenoses containing thrombi). If restenosis occurs, PTCA can be repeated with success and risks like original procedure. Potential complications include dissection or thrombosis of the vessel and uncontrolled ischemia or CHF. Complications are most likely to occur in pts with CHF, long eccentric stenoses, calcified plaque, female gender, and dilation of an artery that perfuses a large segment of myocardium with inadquate collaterals. Placement of an intracoronary stent in suitable pts reduces the restenosis rate to 20–30% at 6 months. PTCA also has been successful in some pts with recent *total* coronary occlusion (<3 months).

Coronary Artery Bypass Surgery (CABG) For angina refractory to medical therapy or when the latter is not tolerated (and when lesions are not amenable to PTCA) or if severe CAD is present (left main, three-vessel disease with impaired LV function). CABG is preferred over PTCA in diabetics with CAD in ≥2 vessels because of better survival.

The relative advantages of PTCA and CABG are summarized in Table 114-3.

UNSTABLE ANGINA

Includes (1) new onset (<2 months) of severe angina, (2) angina at rest or with minimal activity, (3) recent increases in frequency and intensity of chronic angina, (4) recurrent angina within several days of acute MI without reelevation of cardiac enzymes.

℞ TREATMENT

- Admit to continuous ECG-monitored floor.
- Identify and treat exacerbating factors (hypertension, arrhythmias, CHF, acute infection).
- Anticoagulation: IV heparin (aim for PTT 2× control) × 3–5 d; plus aspirin 325 mg/d.
- Rule out MI by ECG and cardiac enzymes.
- Maximize therapy with oral nitrates, beta blockers (to reduce heart rate to 50–70 beats per minute). Reserve use of calcium antagonists for those with refractory pain.
- For refractory pain: IV TNG (begin at 10 μg/min); titrate dosage to alleviate pain, but maintain systolic bp ≥100 mmHg.
- Refractory unstable angina warrants coronary arteriography and possible PTCA or CABG. If symptoms are controlled on medical therapy, a predischarge exercise test should be performed to assess need for coronary arteriography.

CORONARY VASOSPASM

Intermittent focal spasm of a coronary artery; often associated with atherosclerotic lesion near site of spasm. Chest discomfort is similar to angina but more severe and occurs typically at rest, with transient ST-segment elevation. Acute infarction or malignant arrhythmias may develop during spasm-induced ischemia. Evaluation includes observation of ECG (or ambulatory Holter monitor) for transient ST elevation; diagnosis confirmed at coronary angiography using provocative (e.g., IV acetylcholine) testing. *Treatment* consists of long-acting nitrates and calcium antagonists. Prognosis is better in pts with anatomically normal coronary arteries than those with fixed coronary stenoses.

Table 114-3

Comparison of Revscularization Procedures in
Multivessel Disease

Procedure	Advantages	Disadvantages
Precutaneous coronary revascularization (angioplasty and/or stenting)	Less invasive Shorter hospital stay Lower initial cost Easily repeated Effective in relieving symptoms	Restenosis High incidence of incomplete revascularization Relative inefficiency in patients with severe left ventricular dysfunction Uncertain long-term outcome (>10 years) Limited to specific anatomic subsets Poor outcome in diabetics with 2 plus coronary disease
Coronary artery bypass grafting	Effective in relieving symptoms Improved survival in certain subsets, including diabetics Ability to achieve complete revascularization Wider applicability	Cost Increased risk of a repeat procedure due to late graft closure Morbidity

SOURCE: Modified from DP Faxon, in GA Beller (ed), *Chronic Ischemic Heart Disease*, in E Braunwald (series ed), *Atlas of Heart Diseases*, Philadelphia, Current Medicine, 1994.

SILENT ISCHEMIA

Myocardial ischemia that develops without anginal symptoms; detected by Holter monitoring or exercise electrocardiography; occurs mainly in pts who also have *symptomatic* ischemia but is sometimes demonstrated in totally asymptomatic individuals. *Management* is guided by exercise electrocardiography, often with radionuclide scintigraphy, to assess severity of myocardial ischemia. Pts with evidence of severe silent ischemia are candidates for coronary arteriography. It has *not* been demonstrated that pts with silent ischemia without marked abnormalities on exercise testing require chronic anti-ischemic therapy. However, aspirin and lipid-lowering therapy (if LDL > 130 mg/dL) are recommended.

For a more detailed discussion, see Selwyn AP, Braunwald E: Ischemic Heart Disease, Chap. 244, p. 1365; and Baim DS, Grossman W: Coronary Angioplasty and Other Therapeutic Applications of Cardiac Catheterization, Chap. 245, p. 1375, in HPIM-14.

115

HYPERTENSION

DEFINITION   Chronic elevation in bp >140/90; etiology unknown in 90–95% of pts ("essential hypertension"). Always consider a secondary correctable form of hypertension, especially in pts under age 30 or those who become hypertensive after 55. Isolated systolic hypertension (systolic > 160, diastolic <90) most common in elderly pts, due to reduced vascular compliance.

SECONDARY HYPERTENSION

RENAL ARTERY STENOSIS   Due either to atherosclerosis (older men) or fibromuscular dysplasia (young women). Presents with sudden onset of hypertension, refractory to usual antihypertensive therapy. Abdominal bruit often audible; mild hypokalemia due to activation of the renin-angiotensin-aldosterone system may be present.

RENAL PARENCHYMAL DISEASE   Elevated serum creatinine and/or abnormal urinalysis, containing protein, cells, or casts.

COARCTATION OF AORTA   Presents in children or young adults; constriction is usually present in aorta at origin of left subclavian artery. Exam shows diminished, delayed femoral pulsations; late systolic murmur loudest over the midback. CXR shows indentation of the aorta at the level of the coarctation and rib notching (due to development of collateral arterial flow).

PHEOCHROMOCYTOMA   A catecholamine-secreting tumor, typically of the adrenal medulla, that presents as paroxysmal or sustained hypertension in young to middle-aged pts. Sudden episodes of headache, palpitations, and profuse diaphoresis are common. Associated findings include chronic weight loss, orthostatic *hypotension*, and impaired glucose tolerance. Pheochromocytomas may be localized to the bladder wall and may present with micturition-associated symptoms of catecholamine excess. Diagnosis is suggested by elevated urinary catecholamine metabolites in a 24-h urine collection (see below); the tumor is then localized by CT scan or angiography.

HYPERALDOSTERONISM   Due to aldosterone-secreting adenoma or bilateral adrenal hyperplasia. Should be suspected when hypokalemia is present in a hypertensive pt off diuretics (see Chap. 163).

OTHER CAUSES Oral contraceptive usage, Cushing's and adrenogenital syndromes (Chap. 163), thyroid disease (Chap. 162), hyperparathyroidism (Chap. 167), and acromegaly (Chap. 160).

_____ *Approach to the Patient* _____

History

Most pts are asymptomatic. Severe hypertension may lead to headache, epistaxis, or blurred vision.
   Clues to Specific Forms of Secondary Hypertension Use of birth control pills or glucocorticoids, paroxysms of headache, sweating, or tachycardia (pheochromocytoma); history of renal disease or abdominal traumas (renal hypertension).

Physical Examination

Measure bp with appropriate-sized cuff (large cuff for large arm). Measure bp in both arms as well as a leg (to evaluate for coarctation). Signs of hypertension include retinal arteriolar changes (narrowing/nicking); left ventricular lift, loud A_2, S_4. Clues to secondary forms of hypertension include cushingoid appearance, thyromegaly, abdominal bruit (renal artery stenosis), delayed femoral pulses (coarctation of aorta).

Laboratory Workup (See Table 115-1)

   Screening Tests for Secondary Hypertension Should be carried out on all pts with documented hypertension: (1) serum creatinine, BUN, and urinalysis (renal parenchymal disease), (2) serum K measured off diuretics (hypokalemia prompts workup for hyperaldosteronism or renal artery stenosis), (3) CXR (rib notching or indentation of distal aortic arch in coarctation of the aorta), (4) ECG (LV hypertrophy suggests chronicity of hypertension), (5) other useful screening blood tests include CBC, glucose, cholesterol, triglycerides, calcium, uric acid.
   Further Workup Indicated for specific diagnoses if screening tests are abnormal or bp is refractory to antihypertensive therapy: (1) renal artery stenosis: captopril renogram, renal duplex ultrasound, digital subtraction angiography, renal arteriography, and measurement of renal vein renin; (2) Cushing's syndrome: dexamethasone suppression test (Chap. 163); (3) pheochromocytoma: 24-h urine collection for catecholamines, metanephrines, and vanillylmandelic acid; (4) primary hyperaldosteronism: depressed plasma renin activity and hypersecretion

Table 115-1

Classification of Hypertensive and Arteriosclerotic Retinopathy

| Degree | Hypertension | | | | | Arteriolosclerosis | |
| | Arterioles | | | | | | |
	General Narrowing AV ratio*	Focal Spasm†	Hemor-rhages	Exudates	Papil-ledema	Arteriolar Light Reflex	AV Crossing Defects‡
Normal	3:4	1:1	0	0	0	Fine yellow line, red blood column	None
Grade I	1:2	1:1	0	0	0	Broadened yellow line, red blood column	Mild depression of vein

	*	†					
Grade II	1:3	2:3	0	0	0	Broad yellow line, "copper wire," blood column not visible	Depression or humping of vein
Grade III	1:4	1:3	+	+	0	Broad white line, "silver wire," blood column not visible	Right-angle deviation, tapering, and disappearance of vein under arteriole; distal dilation of vein
Grade IV	Fine, fibrous cords	Obliteration of distal flow	+	+	+	Fibrous cords, blood column not visible	Same as grade III

* Ratio of arteriolar to venous diameters.
† Ratio of diameters of region of spasm to proximal arteriole.
‡ Arteriolar length and tortuosity increase with severity.

Table 115-2

Beta Blockers

	Usual Dose, (PO)
NONSELECTIVE AGENTS	
Carteolol*	2.5–10 mg qd
Labetolol†	100–600 mg bid
Nadolol	20–120 mg qd
Penbutolol*	20 mg qd
Pindolol*	5–30 mg bid
Propranolol,	20–60 mg qid
sustained-action	80–160 mg qd
Timolol	5–15 mg bid
BETA$_1$-SELECTIVE AGENTS	
Acebutolol*	200–600 mg bid
Atenolol	25–100 mg qd
Betaxolol	10–20 mg qd
Metoprolol	25–150 mg bid
sustained-action	50–100 mg qd

* Also has beta-agonist activity.
† Also has alpha$_1$ blocking properties.
Side effects: Bradycardia (less common in those with beta-agonist activity), GI discomfort, CHF, bronchospasm (less common with beta$_1$-selective agents), exacerbation of diabetes or impaired response to insulin-induced hypoglycemia, impotence.

of aldosterone, both of which fail to change with volume expansion; (5) renal parenchymal disease (see Chaps. 128–137).

℞ TREATMENT

DRUG THERAPY OF ESSENTIAL HYPERTENSION

Goal is to control hypertension with minimal side effects using a single drug if possible (Fig. 115-1). First-line agents include ACE inhibitors, calcium antagonists, beta blockers, diuretics, and alpha-adrenergic receptor blockers.

Beta Blockers (Table 115-2) Particularly effective in young pts with "hyperkinetic" circulation. Begin with low

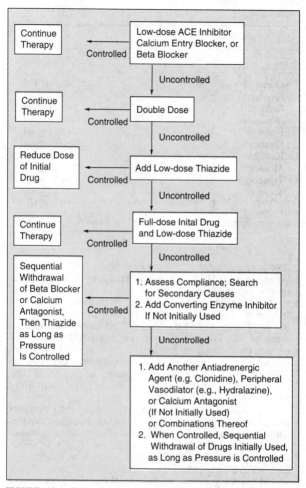

FIGURE 115-1 Schematic approach to the treatment of the pt with hypertension in whom a specific form of therapy is unavailable or unknown.

Table 115-3

ACE Inhibitors

	Dose (PO)
Captopril	12.5–75 mg bid
Enalapril	2.5–40 mg qd
Lisinopril	5–40 mg qd
Benazapril	10–40 mg qd
Fosinopril	10–40 mg qd
Quinapril	10–80 mg qd
Ramipril	2.5–20 mg qd
Moexipril	7.5–30 mg qd
Trandolapril	2–4 mg qd

NOTE: Dosage of ACE inhibitors (except fosinopril) should be reduced in pts with renal failure.

Side effects: Hypotension, angiodema, cough, rash, azotemia, hyperkalemia.

dosage (e.g., atenolol 25 mg qd). Relative contraindications: bronchospasm, CHF, AV block, bradycardia, and "brittle" insulin-dependent diabetes.

ACE Inhibitors (Table 115-3) Well tolerated with low frequency of side effects. May be used as monotherapy or in combination with beta blockers, calcium antagonists, or diuretics. Side effects are uncommon and include rash, angioedema, proteinuria, or leukopenia, particularly in pts with elevated serum creatinine. A nonproductive cough may develop in the course of therapy, requiring an alternative regimen. Note that renal function may deteriorate as a result of ACE inhibitors in pts with bilateral renal artery stenosis.

Potassium supplements and potassium-sparing diuretics should not be combined with ACE inhibitors, unless hypokalemia is documented. If pt is intravascularly volume depleted, hold diuretics for 2–3 d prior to initiation of ACE inhibitor, which should then be administered at very low dosage (e.g., captopril 6.25 mg bid).

For pts who do not tolerate ACE inhibitors because of cough or angioedema, consider angiotensin receptor antagonists (e.g. Losartan) instead.

Calcium Antagonists (Table 115-4) Direct arteriolar vasodilators; all have negative inotropic effects (particularly verapamil) and should be used cautiously if LV dysfunction is present. Verapamil, and to a lesser extent diltiazem, can result in bradycardia and AV block so combination with beta blockers is generally avoided. Use sustained release formulations, as short-acting dihydropyridine calcium channel blockers may increase incidence of coronary events.

Diuretics (see Table 17-1) Thiazides preferred over loop diuretics because of longer duration of action; however, the latter are more potent when GFR < 25 mL/min. Major side effects include hypokalemia, hyperglycemia, and hyperuricemia, which can be minimized by using low dosage (e.g., hydrochlorothiazide 12.5–50 mg qd). Diuretics are particularly effective in elderly and black pts. Prevention of hypokalemia is especially important in pts on digitalis glycosides.

Alpha-1 Receptor Blockers These drugs (e.g. Prazosin, 1–10 mg bid or Terazosin, 1–20 mg qd) are usually well tolerated, but may cause postural hypotension; dosage should be advanced slowly. These agents also improve symptoms of benign prostatic hypertrophy, thus are of particular benefit in hypertensive men with this condition.

If bp proves refractory to drug therapy, work up for secondary forms of hypertension, especially renal artery stenosis and pheochromocytoma (see HPIM-14, p. 1387 for detailed list of antihypertensives).

SPECIAL CIRCUMSTANCES

Pregnancy Safest antihypertensives include methyldopa (250–1000 mg PO bid-tid), hydralazine (10–150 mg PO bid-tid), and beta blockers. Calcium channel blockers also appear to be safe in pregnancy.

Renal Failure Standard thiazide diuretics may not be effective. Consider metolazone, furosemide, or bumetanide, alone or in combination.

Malignant Hypertension Diastolic bp > 120 mmHg is a medical emergency. Immediate therapy is mandatory if there is evidence of cardiac decompensation (CHF, angina), encephalopathy (headache, seizures, visual disturbances), or deteriorating renal function. Drugs to treat hypertensive crisis are listed in Table 115-5. Replace with PO antihypertensive as pt becomes asymptomatic and diastolic bp improves.

Table 115-4

Calcium Channel Antagonists

	Usual Dose (PO)	Adverse Effects
Verapamil SR formulation	40–120 mg tid-qid 120–480 mg qd-bid	Hypotension, bradycardia AV block, heart failure, constipation, ↑ digoxin level

Diltiazem
  SR formulation
  CD formulation
	30–90 mg tid-qid
	60–180 mg bid
	180–300 mg qd
		Hypotension, peripheral edema, bradycardia, AV block, heart failure

Dihydropyridines Nifedipine	10–30 mg tid-qid	Tachycardia, hypotension, peripheral edema, headache, flushing
Nicardipine* SR formulation	20–40 mg tid 30–60 mg bid	
Isradipine*	2.5–10 mg bid	
Felodipine*	5–10 mg qd	
Amlodipine*	2.5–10 mg qd	

* Least negatively inotropic agents.

Table 115-5

Treatment of Malignant Hypertension and Hypertensive Crisis

	Dosage	Adverse Effects
Nitroprusside*	IV: 0.5–8.0 (μg/kg)/min	Hypotension; after 24 h watch for thiocyanate toxicity (tinnitus, blurred vision, altered mental state)
Nitroglycerin*	IV: 5–100 μg/min	Hypotension, headache
Labetolol	IV: 20-80 mg q10min (maximum of 300 mg) or 20 mg IV bolus, then 1–2 mg/min infusion	Hypotension, bradycardia, AV block, bronchospasm
Enalaprilat	IV: 1.25 mg q6h	Angioedema, hyperkalemia
Hydralazine	IV: 5–10 mg IV q10-15min (maximum of 50 mg)	Reflex tachycardia, avoid in pts with CAD or suspected aortic dissection
Diazoxide	IV: 50 mg q5-10min (maximum of 600 mg)	Na^+ retention†, hyperglycemia
Trimethaphan	IV: 0.5–5 mg/min	Tachycardia, abdominal pain, urinary retention

* Intraarterial bp monitoring recommended to avoid rapid fluctuations in bp.
† Administer furosemide 20-80 mg IV concurrently to prevent Na^+ retention.

For a more detailed discussion, see Williams GH: Approach to the Patient with Hypertension, Chap 35, p. 202, Hypertensive Vascular Disease, Chap. 246, p. 1380, in HPIM-14.

116

DISEASES OF THE AORTA

AORTIC ANEURYSM

Abnormal widening of the abdominal or thoracic aorta; in ascending aorta most commonly secondary to cystic medial necrosis or atherosclerosis; aneurysms of descending thoracic and abdominal aorta are primarily atherosclerotic.

HISTORY May be clinically silent, but thoracic aortic aneurysms often result in deep, diffuse chest pain, dysphagia, hoarseness, hemoptysis, dry cough; abdominal aneurysms result in abdominal pain or thromboemboli to the lower extremities.

PHYSICAL EXAMINATION Abdominal aneurysms are often palpable, most commonly in periumbilical area. Pts with ascending thoracic aneurysms may show features of Marfan's syndrome (see HPIM-14, Chap. 348).

LABORATORY *CXR* Enlarged aortic silhouette (thoracic aneurysm); confirm abdominal aneurysm by *abdominal plain film* (rim of calcification), *ultrasound*, *CT scan*, or *MRI*. Contrast aortography is often performed preoperatively. If clinically suspected, obtain serologic test for syphilis, especially if ascending thoracic aneurysm shows thin shell of calcification.

℞ **TREATMENT**

Control of hypertension (Chap. 115) is essential. Surgical resection of aortic aneurysms >6 cm in diameter, for persistent pain despite bp control, or for evidence of rapid expansion. In pts with Marfan's syndrome, thoracic aortic aneurysms >5 cm usually warrant repair.

AORTIC DISSECTION (Fig. 116-1)

Potentially life-threatening condition in which disruption of aortic intima allows dissection of blood into vessel wall; may involve ascending aorta (type II), descending aorta (type III) or both (type I). Alternative classification: Type A—dissection involves ascending aorta; type B—limited to descending aorta. Involvement of the ascending aorta is most lethal form.

ETIOLOGY Ascending aortic dissection associated with hypertension, cystic medial necrosis, Marfan's syndrome (see HPIM-14, Chap. 348); descending dissections commonly associated with atherosclerosis or hypertension. Incidence is increased in pts with coarctation of aorta, bicuspid aortic valve,

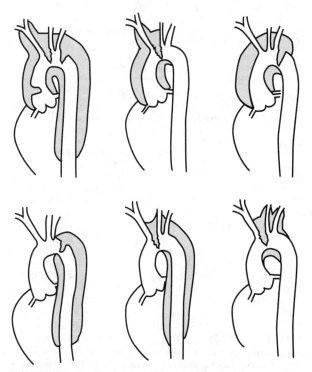

FIGURE 116-1 Classification of aortic dissections. Stanford classification: Top panels illustrate type A dissections that involve the ascending aorta independent of site of tear and distal extension; type B dissections (bottom panels) involve transverse and/or descending aorta without involvement of the ascending aorta. DeBakey classification: Type I dissection involves ascending to descending aorta (top left); type II dissection is limited to ascending or transverse aorta, without descending aorta (top center + top right); type III dissection involves descending aorta only (bottom left). (From DC Miller, in RM Doroghazi, EE Slater, eds., *Aortic Dissection.* New York, McGraw-Hill, 1983, with permission.)

and rarely in third trimester of pregnancy in otherwise normal women.

SYMPTOMS Sudden onset of severe anterior or posterior chest pain, with "ripping" quality; maximal pain may travel if dissection propagates. Additional symptoms relate to obstruction of aortic branches (stroke, MI), dyspnea (acute aortic regurgitation), or symptoms of low cardiac output due to cardiac tamponade (dissection into pericardial sac).

Table 116-1

Treatment of Aortic Dissection

Drug	Dose
PREFERRED REGIMEN	
Sodium nitroprusside	20–400 µg/min IV
plus a beta blocker:	
Propranolol *or*	0.5 mg IV; then 1 mg q 5 min, to total of 0.15 mg/kg
Esmolol	500 µg/kg IV over 1 min; then 50-200 µg/kg/min
Or (if beta blocker contraindicated):	
Reserpine	1–2 mg IM q4-6h
ALTERNATIVE REGIMENS	
Trimethaphan camsylate *or*	2 mg/min IV; then titrate to bp
Labetolol	1–2 mg/min IV

PHYSICAL EXAMINATION   Sinus tachycardia common; if cardiac tamponade develops, hypotension, pulsus paradoxus, and pericardial rub appear. Asymmetry of carotid or brachial pulses, aortic regurgitation, and neurologic abnormalities associated with interruption of carotid artery flow are common findings.

LABORATORY *CXR*   Widening of mediastinum; dissection can be confirmed by *CT scan*, *MRI*, or *ultrasound* (esp. transesophageal echocardiography). Aortography recommended if results of these imaging techniques are not definitive.

R̲x̲ **TREATMENT**
Reduce cardiac contractility and treat hypertension to maintain systolic bp between 100 and 120 mmHg using IV agents (Table 116-1), e.g., sodium nitroprusside accompanied by a beta blocker (aiming for heart rate of 60 beats per min), followed by oral therapy. Direct vasodilators (hydralazine, diazoxide) are contraindicated because they may increase shear stress. Ascending aortic dissection (type A) requires

surgical repair emergently or, if pt can be stabilized with medications, semielectively. Descending aortic dissections are stabilized medically (maintain systolic bp between 110 and 120 mmHg) with oral antihypertensive agents (esp. beta blockers); immediate surgical repair is not necessary unless continued pain or extension of dissection is observed (serial MRI or CT scans).

OTHER ABNORMALITIES OF THE AORTA

ATHEROSCLEROSIS OF ABDOMINAL AORTA   Particularly common in presence of diabetes mellitus or cigarette smoking. Symptoms include intermittent claudication of the buttocks and thighs and impotence (Leriche syndrome); femoral and other distal pulses are absent. Diagnosis is established by noninvasive leg pressure measurements and Doppler velocity analysis, and confirmed by aortography. Aortic-femoral bypass surgery is required for symptomatic treatment.

TAKAYASU'S ("PULSELESS") DISEASE   Arteritis of aorta and major branches in young women. Anorexia, weight loss, fever, and night sweats occur. Localized symptoms relate to occlusion of aortic branches (cerebral ischemia, claudication, and loss of pulses in arms). ESR is increased; diagnosis confirmed by aortography. Glucocorticoid and immunosuppressive therapy may be beneficial, but mortality is high.

For a more detailed discussion, see Dzau VJ, Creager MA: Diseases of the Aorta, Chap. 247, p. 1394, in HPIM-14.

PERIPHERAL VASCULAR DISEASE

Occlusive or inflammatory disease that develops within the peripheral arteries, veins, or lymphatics.

ARTERIOSCLEROSIS OF PERIPHERAL ARTERIES

HISTORY *Intermittent claudication* is muscular cramping with exercise; quickly relieved by rest. Pain in buttocks and thighs suggests aortoiliac disease; calf muscle pain implies femoral or popliteal artery disease. More advanced arteriosclerotic obstruction results in pain at rest; painful ulcers of the feet (painless in diabetics) may result.

PHYSICAL EXAMINATION Decreased peripheral pulses, blanching of affected limb with elevation, dependent rubor (redness). Ischemic ulcers or gangrene of toes may be present.

LABORATORY Doppler ultrasound of peripheral pulses before and during exercise localizes stenoses; contrast arteriography performed only if reconstructive surgery or angioplasty is considered.

℞ TREATMENT
Most pts can be managed medically with daily exercise program, careful foot care (esp. in diabetics), treatment of hypercholesterolemia, and local debridement of ulcerations. Abstinence from cigarettes is mandatory. Pts with severe claudication, rest pain, or gangrene are candidates for arterial reconstructive surgery; percutaneous transluminal angioplasty can be performed in selected pts.

OTHER CONDITIONS THAT IMPAIR PERIPHERAL ARTERIAL FLOW *Arterial Embolism* Due to thrombus or vegetation within the heart or aorta or paradoxically from a venous thrombus through a right-to-left intracardiac shunt.

History Sudden pain or numbness in an extremity in absence of previous history of claudication.

Physical Exam Absent pulse, pallor, and decreased temperature of limb distal to the occlusion. Lesion is identified by angiography and requires immediate anticoagulation and surgical embolectomy.

℞ **TREATMENT**

Thrombolytic therapy (e.g., Streptokinase, urokinase) may be effective for thrombus within atherosclerotic vessel or arterial bypass graft.

Vasospastic Disorders Manifest by Raynaud's phenomenon in which cold exposure results in triphasic color response: blanching of the fingers, followed by cyanosis, then redness. Usually a benign disorder. However, suspect an underlying disease (e.g., scleroderma) if tissue necrosis occurs, if disease is unilateral, or if it develops after age 50.

℞ **TREATMENT**

Keep extremities warm; calcium channel blockers (nifedipine 30–90 mg PO qd or alpha-adrenergic antagonists (e.g., prazocin 1–5 mg tid) may be effective.

Thromboangiitis Obliterans (Buerger's Disease) Occurs in young men who are heavy smokers and involves both upper and lower extremities; nonatheromatous inflammatory reaction develops in veins and small arteries leading to superficial thrombophlebitis and arterial obstruction with ulceration or gangrene of digits. Abstinence from tobacco is essential.

VENOUS DISEASE

SUPERFICIAL THROMBOPHLEBITIS Benign disorder characterized by erythema, tenderness, and edema along involved vein. Conservative therapy includes local heat, elevation, and anti-inflammatory drugs such as aspirin. More serious conditions such as cellulitis or lymphangitis may mimic this, but these are associated with fever, chills, lymphadenopathy, and red superficial streaks along inflamed lymphatic channels.

DEEP VENOUS THROMBOSIS (DVT) More serious condition that may lead to pulmonary embolism (Chap. 123). Particularly common in pts on prolonged bed rest, those with chronic debilitating disease, and those with malignancies (Table 117-1).

History Pain or tenderness in calf or thigh, usually unilateral; may be asymptomatic, with pulmonary embolism as primary presentation.

Physical Exam Often normal; local swelling or tenderness to deep palpation may be present over affected vein.

Laboratory Most helpful noninvasive testing is ultrasound imaging of the deep veins. Doppler studies or impedance ple-

Table 117-1

Conditions Associated with an Increased Risk for Development of Venous Thrombosis

Surgery
Orthopedic, thoracic, abdominal, and genitourinary procedures
Neoplasms
Pancreas, lung, ovary, testes, urinary tract, breast, stomach
Trauma
Fractures of spine, pelvis, femur, tibia
Immobilization
Acute myocardial infarction, congestive heart failure, stroke, postoperative convalescence
Pregnancy
Estrogen use (for replacement or contraception)
Hypercoagulable states
Resistance to activated protein C; deficiencies of antithrombin III, protein C, or protein S; circulating lupus anticoagulant; myeloproliferative disease; dysfibrinogenemia; disseminated intravascular coagulation
Venulitis
Thromboangiitis obliterans, Behçet's disease, homocysteinuria
Previous deep vein thrombosis

thysmography also may be useful. These noninvasive studies are most sensitive for proximal (upper leg) DVT, less sensitive for calf DVT. Invasive venography is used when diagnosis not clear. MRI is useful for diagnosis of DVT within the pelvic veins or in the superior or inferior vena cavae.

℞ TREATMENT

Systemic anticoagulation with heparin (5000- to 10,000-U bolus, followed by continuous IV infusion to maintain a PTT at $2\times$ normal) for 5–7 d, followed by warfarin PO (overlap with heparin for 3–4 d and continue for at least 3 months if proximal deep veins involved). Adjust warfarin dose to maintain prothrombin time at INR 2.0–3.0.

DVT can be prevented by early ambulation following surgery or with low-dose heparin during prolonged bed rest (5000 U SC bid-tid), supplemented by pneumatic compression boots. Following knee or hip surgery, warfarin (INR 2.0–3.0) is an effective regimen. Low-molecular-weight heparins are also effective in preventing DVT after general or orthopedic surgery.

LYMPHEDEMA

Chronic, painless edema, usually of the lower extremities; may be primary (inherited) or secondary to lymphatic damage or obstruction (e.g., recurrent lymphangitis, tumor, filariasis).

PHYSICAL EXAMINATION Marked pitting edema in early stages; limb becomes indurated with *non*pitting edema chronically. Differentiate from chronic *venous* insufficiency, which displays hyperpigmentation, stasis dermatitis, and superficial venous varicosities.

LABORATORY Abdominal and pelvic ultrasound or CT to identify obstructing lesions. Lymphangiography or lymphoscintigraphy (rarely done) to confirm diagnosis. If *unilateral* edema, differentiate from DVT by noninvasive venous studies (above).

℞ TREATMENT
(1) Meticulous foot hygiene to prevent infection, (2) leg elevation, (3) compression stockings and/or pneumatic compression boots. Diuretics should be *avoided* to prevent intravascular volume depletion.

For a more detailed discussion, see Creager MA, Dzau VJ: Vascular Diseases of the Extremities, Chap. 248, p. 1398, in HPIM-14.

118

RESPIRATORY FUNCTION AND DIAGNOSIS

DISTURBANCES OF RESPIRATORY FUNCTION

The respiratory system includes not only the lungs but also the CNS, chest wall (diaphragm, abdomen, intercostal muscles), and pulmonary circulation. Prime function of the system is to exchange gas between inspired air and venous blood.

DISTURBANCES IN VENTILATORY FUNCTION (Figs. 118-1 and 118-2) Ventilation is the process whereby lungs deliver fresh air to alveoli. Measurements of ventilatory function consist of quantification of air in the lungs [total lung capacity (TLC), residual volume (RV)] and the rate at which air can be expelled from the lungs [forced vital capacity (FVC), forced expiratory volume in 1 s (FEV$_1$)] during a forced exhalation from TLC. Expiratory flow rates may be plotted against lung volumes yielding a flow-volume curve (see HPIM-14, Fig. 250-4, p. 1412).

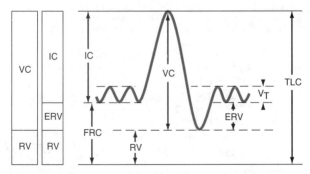

FIGURE 118-1 Lung volumes, shown by block diagrams (*left*) and by a spirographic tracing (*right*). TLC, total lung capacity; VC, vital capacity; RV, residual volume; IC, inspiratory capacity; ERV, expiratory reserve volume; FRC, functional residual capacity; V$_T$, tidal volume. (From Weinberger SE, Drazen JM: HPIM-14.)

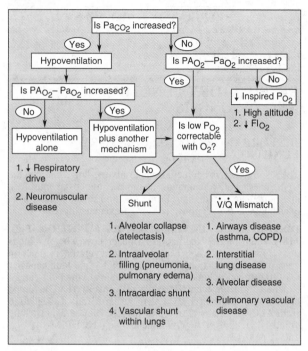

FIGURE 118-2 Flow diagram outlining the diagnostic approach to the pt with hypoxemia (Pa_{O_2} <80 mmHg). $PA_{O_2} - Pa_{O_2}$ is usually <15 mmHg for subjects ≤30 years old, and increases ~3 mmHg per decade after age 30.

Two major patterns of abnormal ventilatory function are restrictive and obstructive patterns (Tables 118-1 and 118-2). In obstructive pattern:

- Hallmark is decrease in expiratory flow rate, i.e., FEV_1.
- Ratio FEV_1/FVC is reduced.
- TLC is normal or increased.
- RV is elevated due to trapping of air during expiration.

In restrictive disease:

- Hallmark is decrease in TLC.
- May be caused by pulmonary parenchymal disease or extra-parenchymal (neuromuscular such as myasthenia gravis or chest wall such as kyphoscoliosis).
- Pulmonary parenchymal disease usually occurs with a re-

Table 118-1

Common Respiratory Diseases by Diagnostic Categories

OBSTRUCTIVE

Asthma	Bronchiectasis
Chronic obstructive lung disease (chronic bronchitis, emphysema)	Cystic fibrosis Bronchiolitis

RESTRICTIVE—PARENCHYMAL

Sarcoidosis	Pneumoconiosis
Idiopathic pulmonary fibrosis	Drug- or radiation-induced interstitial lung disease

RESTRICTIVE—EXTRAPARENCHYMAL

Neuromuscular	Muscular dystrophies*
Diaphragmatic weakness/paralysis	Cervical spine injury*
	Chest wall
Myasthenia gravis*	Kyphoscoliosis
Guillain-Barré syndrome*	Obesity
	Ankylosing spondylitis*

*Can have inspiratory and expiratory limitation (see text).

Table 118-2

Alterations in Ventilatory Function

	TLC	RV	VC	FEV₁/FVC
Obstructive	N to ↑	↑	↓	↓
Restrictive				
Pulmonary parenchymal	↓	↓	↓	N to ↑
Extraparenchymal— inspiratory	↓	N to ↓	↓	N
Extraparenchymal— inspiratory + expiratory	↓	↑	↓	Variable

NOTE: N, normal.
SOURCE: Adapted from Weinberger SE, Drazen JM: HPIM-14, p. 1412.

duced RV but extraparenchymal disease (with expiratory dysfunction) occurs with an increased RV.

DISTURBANCES IN PULMONARY CIRCULATION
Pulmonary vasculature transmits the RV output, approximately 5 L/min at a low-pressure. Perfusion of lung greatest in dependent portion. Assessment requires measuring pulmonary vascular pressures and cardiac output to derive pulmonary vascular resistance. Pulmonary vascular resistance rises with hypoxia, intraluminal thrombi, scarring, or loss of alveolar beds.

All diseases of the respiratory system causing hypoxia are capable of causing pulmonary hypertension. However, pts with hypoxemia due to chronic obstructive lung disease, interstitial lung disease, chest wall disease, and obesity-hypoventilation–sleep apnea are particularly likely to develop pulmonary hypertension.

DISTURBANCES IN GAS EXCHANGE
Primary functions of the respiratory system are to remove CO_2 and provide O_2. Normal tidal volume is about 500 mL, and normal frequency is 15 breaths per minute for a total ventilation of 7.5 L/min. Because of dead space, alveolar ventilation is 5 L/min.

Partial pressure of CO_2 in arterial blood (Pa_{CO_2}) is directly proportional to amount of CO_2 produced each minute ($\dot{V}_{CO_2}$) and inversely proportional to alveolar ventilation ($\dot{V}A$).

$$Pa_{CO_2} = 0.863 \times \dot{V}_{CO_2}/\dot{V}A$$

Gas exchange is critically dependent on proper matching of ventilation and perfusion.

Assessment of gas exchange requires measurement of arterial blood gases. The actual content of O_2 in blood is determined by both P_{O_2} and hemoglobin.

Arterial P_{O_2} can be used to measure alveolar-arterial O_2 difference (A-a gradient). Increased A-a gradient (normal <15 mmHg, rising by 3 mmHg each decade after age 30) indicates impaired gas exchange.

In order to calculate A-a gradient, the alveolar P_{O_2} (PA_{O_2}) must be calculated:

$$PA_{O_2} = FI_{O_2} \times (PB - P_{H_2O}) - Pa_{CO_2}/R$$

where FI_{O_2} = fractional concentration of inspired O_2 (0.21 breathing room air), PB = barometric pressure (760 mmHg at sea level), P_{H_2O} = water vapor pressure (47 mmHg when air is saturated at 37°C), and R = respiratory quotient (the ratio of CO_2 production to O_2 consumption, usually assumed to be 0.8).

Adequacy of CO_2 removal is reflected in the partial pressure of CO_2 in arterial blood.

Because measurement of arterial blood gases necessitates arterial puncture, noninvasive techniques may be useful, particularly to determine trends in gas exchange over time. The pulse oximeter measures oxygen saturation Sa_{O_2} rather than Pa_{O_2}. While widely used, clinicians must be aware that (1) the relationship between Sa_{O_2} and Pa_{O_2} is curvilinear, flattening above a Pa_{O_2} of 60 mmHg, (2) poor peripheral perfusion may interfere with the oximeter's function, and (3) the oximeter provides no information about P_{CO_2}.

Ability of gas to diffuse across the alveolar-capillary membrane is assessed by the diffusing capacity of the lung (DL_{CO}). Carried out with low concentration of carbon monoxide during a single 10-s breath-holding period or during 1 min of steady breathing. Value depends on alveolar-capillary surface area, pulmonary capillary blood volume, degree of ventilation-perfusion ($\dot{V}/\dot{Q}$) mismatching, and thickness of alveolar-capillary membrane.

MECHANISMS OF ABNORMAL FUNCTION Four basic mechanisms of hypoxemia are (1) $\downarrow$ inspired P_{O_2}, (2) hypoventilation, (3) shunt, and (4) $\dot{V}/\dot{Q}$ mismatch. Diffusion block contributes to hypoxemia only under selected circumstances. Approach to the hypoxemic pt is shown in Fig. 118-2.

The essential mechanism underlying all cases of hypercapnia is inadequate alveolar ventilation. Potential contributing factors include (1) increased CO_2 production, (2) decreased ventilatory drive, (3) malfunction of the respiratory pump or increased airways resistance, and (4) inefficiency of gas exchange (increased dead space or $\dot{V}/\dot{Q}$ mismatch) necessitating a compensatory increase in overall minute ventilation.

DIAGNOSTIC PROCEDURES

NONINVASIVE PROCEDURES *Radiography* No CXR pattern is sufficiently specific to *establish* a diagnosis; instead, the CXR serves to *detect* disease, assess magnitude, and guide further diagnostic investigation. Fluoroscopy provides a dynamic image of the chest and is particularly helpful in localizing lesions poorly visible on the CXR. Both fluoroscopy and standard tomography have largely been supplanted by thoracic CT, which is now routine in evaluation of pts with pulmonary nodules and masses. CT is especially helpful in the assessment of pleural lesions. Contrast enhancement also makes thoracic CT useful in differentiating tissue masses from vascular structures. High-resolution CT has largely replaced bronchography in the evaluation of surgical bronchiectasis. MRI is generally less useful than CT but is preferred in evaluation of abnormalities at the lung apex, adjacent to the spine, and at the thoracoabdominal junction.

Skin Tests Specific skin test antigens are available for tuberculosis, histoplasmosis, coccidioidomycosis, blastomycosis, trichinosis, toxoplasmosis, and aspergillosis. A positive delayed reaction (type IV) to a tuberculin test indicates only prior infection, not active disease. Immediate (type I) and late (type III) dermal hypersensitivity to *Aspergillus* antigen supports diagnosis of allergic bronchopulmonary aspergillosis in pts with a compatible clinical illness.

Sputum Exam Sputum is distinguished from saliva by presence of bronchial epithelial cells and alveolar macrophages. Sputum exam should include gross inspection for blood, color, and odor, as well as microscopic inspection of carefully stained smears. Culture of expectorated sputum may be misleading owing to contamination with oropharyngeal flora. Sputum samples induced by inhalation of nebulized, warm, hypertonic saline can be stained using immunofluorescent techniques for the presence of *Pneumocystis carinii*.

Pulmonary Function Tests May indicate abnormalities of airway function, alterations of lung volume, and disturbances of gas exchange. Specific patterns of pulmonary function may assist in differential diagnosis. PFTs also may provide objective measures of therapeutic response, e.g., to bronchodilators.

Pulmonary Scintigraphy Scans of pulmonary ventilation and perfusion aid in the diagnosis of pulmonary embolism. Quantitative ventilation-perfusion scans also are used to assess surgical resectability of lung cancer in pts with diminished respiratory function. *Gallium scanning* may be used to identify inflammatory disease of the lungs or mediastinal lymph nodes. Inflammatory activity of the lungs detected with gallium may be associated with diffuse interstitial infections. Gallium uptake by the lungs also may occur in *P. carinii* pneumonia (PCP).

INVASIVE PROCEDURES ***Bronchoscopy*** Permits visualization of airways, identification of endobronchial abnormalities, and collection of diagnostic specimens by lavage, brushing, or biopsy. The fiberoptic bronchoscope permits exam of smaller, more peripheral airways than the rigid bronchoscope, but the latter permits greater control of the airways and provides more effective suctioning. These features make rigid bronchoscopy particularly useful in pts with central obstructing tumors, foreign bodies, or massive hemoptysis. The fiberoptic bronchoscope increases the diagnostic potential of bronchoscopy, permitting biopsy of peripheral nodules and diffuse infiltrative diseases as well as aspiration and lavage of airways and airspaces. Fiberoptic biopsy is particularly useful in diagnosing diffuse infectious processes, lymphangitic spread of cancer, and granulomatous diseases.

Video-Assisted Thoracic Surgery Now commonly used for diagnosis of pleural lesions as well as peripheral parenchymal infiltrates and nodules. Has largely replaced "open biopsy"; may be used therapeutically.

Percutaneous Needle Aspiration of the Lung Usually performed under CT guidance to obtain cytologic or microbiologic specimens from local pulmonary lesions.

Bronchoalveolar Lavage (BAL) An adjunct to fiberoptic bronchoscopy permitting collection of cells and liquid from distal air spaces. Useful in diagnosis of PCP, other infections, and some interstitial diseases.

Thoracentesis and Pleural Biopsy Thoracentesis should be performed as an early step in the evaluation of any pleural effusion of uncertain etiology. Analysis of pleural fluid helps differentiate transudate from exudate (Chap. 125). (Exudate: pleural fluid LDH >200 IU, pleural fluid/serum protein >0.5, pleural fluid/serum LDH >0.6.) Pleural fluid pH <7.2 suggests that an exudate associated with an infection is an empyema and will almost certainly require drainage. WBC count and differential; glucose, P_{CO_2}, amylase, Gram stain, culture, and cytologic exam should be performed on all specimens. Rheumatoid factor and complement may also be useful. Closed pleural biopsy can also be done when a pleural effusion is present; particularly useful when tuberculosis is suspected.

Pulmonary Angiography The definitive test for pulmonary embolism; also may reveal AV malformations.

Mediastinoscopy Diagnostic procedure of choice in pts with disease involving mediastinal lymph nodes. However, lymph nodes in left superior mediastinum must be approached via *mediastinotomy*.

For a more detailed discussion, see Weinberger SE, Drazen JM: Disturbances of Respiratory Function, Chap. 250, p. 1410; and Weinberger SE, Drazen JM: Diagnostic Procedures in Respiratory Diseases, Chap. 251, p. 1417; in HPIM-14.

119

ASTHMA AND HYPERSENSITIVITY PNEUMONITIS

ASTHMA

DEFINITION Increased responsiveness of lower airways to multiple stimuli; episodic, and with reversible obstruction; may range in severity from mild without limitation of pt's activity to severe and life-threatening. Obstruction persisting for days or weeks is known as *status asthmaticus*.

EPIDEMIOLOGY AND ETIOLOGY Some 4–5% of adults and up to 10% of children are estimated to experience episodes of asthma. Basic abnormality is airway hyperresponsiveness to both specific and nonspecific stimuli. All pts demonstrate enhanced bronchoconstriction in response to inhalation of methacholine or histamine (nonspecific bronchoconstrictor agents). Some pts may be classified as having *allergic asthma;* these experience worsening of symptoms on exposure to pollens or other allergens. They characteristically give personal and/or family history of other allergic diseases, such as rhinitis, urticaria, and eczema. Skin tests to allergens are positive; serum IgE may be ↑. Bronchoprovocation studies may demonstrate positive responses to inhalation of specific allergens.

A significant number of asthmatic pts have negative allergic histories and do not react to skin or bronchoprovocation testing with specific allergens. Many of these develop bronchospasm after a URI. These pts are said to have *idiosyncratic asthma*.

Some pts experience worsening of symptoms on *exercise* or exposure to *cold air* or *occupational* stimuli. Many note increased wheezing following *viral URI* or in response to *emotional stress*.

PATHOGENESIS Common denominator underlying the asthmatic diathesis is nonspecific hyperirritability of the tracheobronchial tree. The etiology of airway hyperresponsiveness in asthma is unknown, but airway inflammation is believed to play a fundamental role. Airway reactivity may fluctuate, and fluctuations correlate with clinical symptoms. Airway reactivity may be increased by a number of factors: allergenic, pharmacologic, environmental, occupational, infectious, exercise-related, and emotional. Among the more common are airborne allergens, aspirin, beta-adrenergic blocking agents (e.g., propranolol, timolol), sulfites in food, air pollution (ozone, nitrogen dioxide), and respiratory infections.

_____ *Approach to the Patient* _____

History Symptoms: wheezing, dyspnea, cough, fever, sputum production, other allergic disorders. Possible precipitating factors (allergens, infection, etc.); asthma attacks often occur at night. Response to medications. Course of previous attacks (e.g., need for hospitalization, steroid treatment).

Physical Exam General: tachypnea, tachycardia, use of accessory respiratory muscles, cyanosis, pulsus paradoxus (accessory muscle use and pulsus paradoxus correlate with severity of obstruction). Lungs: adequacy of aeration, symmetry of breath sounds, wheezing, prolongation of expiratory phase, hyperinflation. Heart: evidence for CHF. ENT/skin: evidence of allergic nasal, sinus, or skin disease.

Laboratory While PFT findings are not diagnostic, they are very helpful in judging severity of airway obstruction and in following response to therapy in both chronic and acute situations. Forced vital capacity (FVC), FEV_1, maximum mid- and peak expiratory flow rate (MMEFR, PEFR), FEV_1/FVC are decreased; RV and TLC increased during episodes of obstruction; $D_{L_{CO}}$ usually normal or slightly increased. Reduction of FEV_1 to <25% predicted or <0.75 L after administration of a bronchodilator indicates severe disease. CBC may show eosinophilia. IgE may show mild elevations; marked elevations may suggest evidence of allergic bronchopulmonary aspergillosis (ABPA). Sputum examination: eosinophilia, Curschmann's spirals (casts of small airways), Charcot-Leyden crystals; presence of large numbers of neutrophils suggests bronchial infection. Arterial blood gases: uniformly show hypoxemia during attacks; usually hypocarbia and respiratory alkalosis present; normal or elevated P_{CO_2} worrisome as may suggest severe respiratory muscle fatigue and airways obstruction. CXR not always necessary: may show hyperinflation, patchy infiltrates due to atelectasis behind plugged airways; important when complicating infection is a consideration.

DIFFERENTIAL DIAGNOSIS "All that wheezes is not asthma": CHF; chronic bronchitis/emphysema; upper airway obstruction due to foreign body, tumor, laryngeal edema; carcinoid tumors (usually associated with stridor, not wheezing); recurrent pulmonary emboli; eosinophilic pneumonia; vocal cord dysfunction; systemic vasculitis with pulmonary involvement.

℞ **TREATMENT**

Five major categories of pharmacologic therapy after removal, if possible, of inciting agent:

1. *Beta-adrenergic agonists:* Inhaled route provides most rapid effect and best therapeutic index; resorcinols (metaproterenol, terbutaline, fenoterol), saligenins (albuterol), and catecholamines (isoproterenol, isoetharine) may be given by nebulizer or metered-dose inhaler. Epinephrine, another catecholamine, 0.3 mL of 1:1000 solution SC (for use in acute situations in absence of cardiac history). In general, resorcinols and saligenins are preferred as first-line agents due to high selectivity for the respiratory tract and absence of significant cardiac effects. Salmeterol, a very long acting congener of albuterol (9–12 mL), is not recommended for acute attacks. IV administration of beta-adrenergic agents for severe asthma is not considered justified due to the risk of toxicity.

2. *Methylxanthines:* Theophylline and various salts; adjust dose to maintain blood level between 5 and 15 μg/mL; may be given PO or IV (as aminophylline). Theophylline clearance varies widely and is reduced with age, hepatic dysfunction, cardiac decompensation, cor pulmonale, febrile illness. Many drugs also alter theophylline clearance (decrease half-life: cigarettes, phenobarbitol, phenytoin; increase half-life: erythromycin, allopurinol, cimetidine, propranolol). In children and young-adult smokers, a loading dose of 6 mg/kg is given, followed by an infusion of 1.0 (mg/kg)/h for 12 h, after which the infusion is reduced to 0.8 (mg/kg)/h. In other pts not on theophylline, the loading dose remains the same, but the infusion rate is reduced to 0.1–0.5 (mg/kg)/h. In pts already taking theophylline, the loading dose is withheld or reduced. Theophylline compounds have lost favor in asthma therapy due to narrow toxic-therapeutic margin.

3. *Glucocorticoids:* Prednisone 40-60 mg PO daily, followed by tapering schedule of 50% reduction every 3–5 d; hydrocortisone 4 mg/kg IV loading dose followed by 3 mg/kg q6h; methylprednisolone 50–100 mg IV q6h. Evidence is accumulating that very large doses of glucocorticoids have no advantage over more conventional doses. Steroids in acute asthma require 6 h or more to have an effect. Inhaled glucocorticoid preparations are important adjuncts to chronic therapy; not useful in acute attacks. Effects of inhaled steroids are dose-dependent. Inhaled steroids are now recommended, in many guidelines, as a mainstay of outpatient management and should be started in any pt not easily controlled with inhaled adrenergic agents.

4. *Cromolyn sodium and Nedocromil sodium:* Not bronchodilators; useful in chronic therapy for prevention, not useful during acute attacks; administered as metered-dose inhaler or nebulized powder, 2 puffs daily. A trial of 4–6 weeks is often necessary to determine effectiveness.

5. *Anticholinergics:* Aerosolized atropine and related compounds, such as ipratropium, a nonabsorbable quaternary ammonium. May enhance the bronchodilation achieved by sympathomimetics but is slow acting (60–90 min to peak bronchodilation). Ipratropium may be given by metered-dose inhaler, 2 puffs up to every 6 h. Expectorants and mucolytic agents add little to the management of acute or chronic asthma.

Framework for Management

Emergencies Aerosolized beta$_2$ agonists are the primary therapy of acute episodes of asthma. Give every 20 min for 3 doses, then every 2 h until attack subsides. Aminophylline may speed resolution after first hour in 5–10% of pts. Paradoxical pulse, accessory muscle use, and marked hyperinflation indicate severe disease and mandate arterial blood gas measurement and monitoring of PEFR or FEV$_1$. PEFR $\leq 20\%$ predicted on presentation with failure to double after 60 min of treatment suggests addition of steroid therapy. Failure of PEFR to improve to $\geq 70\%$ of baseline with emergency treatment suggests need for hospitalization, with final decision made on individual factors (symptoms, past history, etc.). PEFR $\leq 40\%$ after emergency treatment mandates admission.

Chronic Treatment First-line therapy again consists of beta$_2$ agonists. Persistence of symptoms should prompt addition of an anti-inflammatory agent (glucocorticoids or a mast cell–stabilizing agent). Medication adjustments should be based on objective measurement of lung function (PEFR, FEV$_1$) and pts should monitor PEFR regularly.

HYPERSENSITIVITY PNEUMONITIS

DEFINITION Hypersensitivity pneumonitis (HP) or extrinsic allergic alveolitis is an immunologically mediated inflammation of lung parenchyma involving alveolar walls and terminal airways secondary to repeated inhalation of a variety of organic dusts by a susceptible host.

ETIOLOGY A number of inhaled substances have been implicated (see Table 253-1, p. 1427, in HPIM-14). These substances are usually organic antigens, particularly thermophilic actinomycetes, but may include inorganic compounds such as isocyanates.

CLINICAL MANIFESTATIONS Symptoms may be acute, subacute, or chronic depending on the frequency and intensity of exposure to the causative agent; in acute form, cough, fever, chills, dyspnea appear 6–8 h after exposure to antigen; in subacute and chronic forms, temporal relationship to antigenic exposure may be lost and insidiously increasing dyspnea may be predominant symptom.

DIAGNOSIS *History* Occupational history and history of possible exposures and relationship to symptoms are very important.

Physical Exam Nonspecific; may reveal rales in lung fields, cyanosis in advanced cases.

Laboratory Serum precipitins to offending antigen may be present but are not specific; eosinophilia is not a feature. CXR: nonspecific changes in interstitial structures; pleural changes or hilar adenopathy rare. PFTs and ABGs: restrictive pattern possibly associated with airway obstruction; diffusing capacity decreased; hypoxemia at rest or with exercise. Bronchoalveolar lavage may show increased lymphocytes of suppressor-cytotoxic phenotype. Lung biopsy may be necessary in some pts who do not have sufficient other criteria; transbronchial biopsy may suffice, but open lung biopsy is frequently necessary.

DIFFERENTIAL DIAGNOSIS Other interstitial lung diseases, including sarcoidosis, idiopathic pulmonary fibrosis, lung disease associated with collagen-vascular diseases, drug-induced lung disease; eosinophilic pneumonia; allergic bronchopulmonary aspergillosis; silo-fillers' disease; "pulmonary mycotoxicosis" or "atypical" farmer's lung; infection.

℞ TREATMENT

Avoidance of offending antigen is essential. Chronic form may be partially irreversible at the time of diagnosis. Prednisone 1 (mg/kg)/d for 7–14 d, followed by tapering schedule over 2–6 weeks to lowest possible dose. Pts with acute form usually recover without glucocorticoids.

For a more detailed discussion, see McFadden ER Jr: Asthma, Chap. 252, p. 1419; and Hunninghake GW, Richerson HB: Hypersensitivity Pneumonitis and Eosinophilic Pneumonias, Chap. 253, p. 1426, in HPIM-14.

ENVIRONMENTAL LUNG DISEASES

Approach to the Patient

Ask about workplace and work history in detail: Specific contaminants? Availability and use of protective devices? Ventilation? Do coworkers have similar complaints? Ask about every job; short-term exposures may be significant. CXR is very valuable but may over- or underestimate functional impact of pneumoconioses. PFTs may both quantify impairment and suggest the nature of exposure.

An individual's dose of an environmental agent is influenced by intensity as well as by physiologic factors (ventilation rate and depth).

OCCUPATIONAL EXPOSURES AND PULMONARY DISEASE

INORGANIC DUSTS *Asbestosis* Exposures may occur in mining, milling, and manufacture of asbestos products; construction trades (pipefitting, boilermaking); and manufacture of safety garments, filler for plastic material, and friction materials (brake and clutch linings). Major health effects of asbestos include pulmonary fibrosis (asbestosis) and cancers of the respiratory tract, pleura, and peritoneum.

Asbestosis is a diffuse interstitial fibrosing disease of the lung that is directly related to intensity and duration of exposure, usually requiring ≥10 years of moderate to severe exposure. PFTs show a restrictive pattern. CXR reveals irregular or linear opacities, greatest in lower lung fields. High-resolution CT may show distinct changes of subpleural curvilinear lines 5–10 cm in length. *Pleural plaques* indicate past exposure. Excess frequency of *lung cancer* occurs 15 to 20 years after first asbestos exposure. Smoking substantially increases risk of lung cancer after asbestos exposure but does not alter risk of *mesotheliomas,* which peaks 30 to 35 years after (an often brief) initial exposure.

Silicosis Exposure to free silica (crystalline quartz) occurs in mining, stone cutting, abrasive industries, blasting, quarrying, farming. Short-term, high-intensity exposures (as brief as 10 months) may produce acute silicosis—rapidly fatal pulmonary fibrosis with radiographic picture of profuse miliary infiltration or consolidation. Longer-term, less-intense exposures are associated with upper lobe fibrosis and hilar adenopathy ≥15 years after exposure. Fibrosis is nodular and may lead to pulmonary restriction and airflow obstruction. Pts with silicosis are at higher than normal risk for tuberculosis, and pts with chronic silicosis and a positive PPD warrant antituberculous treatment.

Coal Worker's Pneumoconiosis (CWP) Symptoms of simple CWP are additive to the effects of cigarette smoking on chronic bronchitis and obstructive lung disease. X-ray signs of simple CWP are small, irregular opacities (reticular pattern) that may progress to small, rounded opacities (nodular pattern). Complicated CWP is indicated by roentgenographic appearance of nodules >1 cm in diameter in upper lung fields; DL_{CO} is reduced.

Berylliosis Beryllium exposure may produce acute pneumonitis or chronic interstitial pneumonitis. Histology is indistinguishable from sarcoidosis.

ORGANIC DUSTS *Cotton Dust (Byssinosis)* Exposures occur in production of yarns for cotton, linen, and rope making. (Flax, hemp, and jute produce a similar syndrome.) Chest tightness occurs typically on first day of work week. In 10–25% of workers, disease may be progressive with chest tightness persisting throughout the work week. After 10 years, recurrent symptoms are associated with airflow obstruction. Therapy includes bronchodilators, antihistamines, and elimination of exposure.

Grain Dust Farmers and grain elevator operators are at risk. Symptoms are those of cigarette smokers—cough, mucus production, wheezing, and airflow obstruction.

Farmer's Lung Persons exposed to moldy hay with spores of thermophilic actinomycetes may develop a hypersensitivity pneumonitis. Acute farmer's lung causes fever, chills, malaise, cough, and dyspnea 4–8 h after exposure. Chronic low-intensity exposure causes interstitial fibrosis.

TOXIC CHEMICALS Many toxic chemicals can affect the lung in the form of vapor and gases.

Smoke inhalation Kills more fire victims than does thermal injury. Severe cases may develop pulmonary edema. CO poisoning causing O_2 desaturation may be fatal. Early endoscopy may distinguish thermal upper airway injury from diffuse lower airway damage due to toxic constituents of inhaled smoke.

Agents used in the manufacture of synthetic materials may produce sensitization to isocyanates, aromatic amines, and aldehydes. Repeated exposure causes some workers to develop productive cough, asthma, or low-grade fever and malaise.

Fluorocarbons, transmitted from a worker's hands to cigarettes, may be volatilized. The inhaled agent causes fever, chills, malaise, and sometimes wheezing. Occurring in plastics workers, the syndrome is termed *polymer fume fever.*

℞ TREATMENT

Treatment of environmental lung diseases almost invariably involves avoidance of toxic substance. Inorganic dust inhalation produces fibrosis without inflammation, unresponsive to pharmacologic treatment. Acute organic dust exposures may respond to glucocorticoids.

GENERAL ENVIRONMENTAL EXPOSURES

Air Pollution   Difficult to relate specific health effects to any single pollutant. Symptoms and diseases of air pollution are also the noncogenic conditions associated with cigarette smoking (respiratory infections, airway irritation).

Passive Cigarette Smoking   Increased respiratory illness and reduced lung function have been found in children of smoking parents. Lung cancer risk is elevated in adults exposed to passive smoke.

Radon   Risk factor for lung cancer, exacerbated by cigarette smoke.

PRINCIPLES OF MANAGEMENT

With many environmental agents, lung disease occurs years after exposure. If exposure continues, inciting agent must be eliminated, usually by removing pt from workplace. Pulmonary fibrosis (e.g., asbestosis, CWP) is not responsive to glucocorticoids. Therapy of occupational asthma follows usual guidelines (see Chap. 119). Lung cancer screening has not yet proven effective, even in high-risk occupations.

For a more detailed discussion, see Speizer FE: Environmental Lung Diseases, Chap. 254, p. 1429, in HPIM-14.

121

CHRONIC BRONCHITIS, EMPHYSEMA, AND ACUTE RESPIRATORY FAILURE

Definitions

Chronic Bronchitis   Excessive tracheobronchial mucus secretion sufficient to cause cough with expectoration for at least 3 months of the year for 2 consecutive years.

Simple Chronic Bronchitis   Characterized by mucoid sputum production.

Chronic Mucopurulent Bronchitis   Characterized by recurrent purulent sputum in the absence of localized suppurative disease (e.g., bronchiectasis).

Chronic Asthmatic Bronchitis   Cough and mucus hypersecretion associated with dyspnea and wheezing with acute respiratory infections or exposure to inhaled irritants.

Emphysema   Distention of air spaces distal to the terminal bronchioles with destruction of alveolar septa.

Chronic Obstructive Lung Disease (COLD)   Condition with chronic expiratory airflow obstruction due primarily to emphysema, often exacerbated by airways inflammation and bronchospasm. In absence of bronchiectasis, amount of sputum production does not relate to functional impairment. Obstruction is assessed by the expiratory FVC maneuver. Severity of obstruction may fluctuate in COLD, but some degree of obstruction is always present.

Pathology

Chronic bronchitis is associated with hyperplasia and hypertrophy of submucosal mucous glands. There is goblet cell hyperplasia, mucosal edema and inflammation, and increased smooth muscle in small airways. Emphysema may be panacinar (affecting both central and peripheral portions of the acinus) or centriacinar (primary involvement of respiratory bronchioles and alveolar ducts and little involvement of peripheral acini). Panacinar and centriacinar emphysema may exist in the same lung, and both produce similar physiologic changes, primarily increased wasted ventilation.

Pathogenesis

1. *Cigarette smoking:* Responsible for most cases of chronic bronchitis and emphysema; also causes obstruction of small airways in young, asymptomatic persons. Inflammation

caused by smoking accelerates normal loss of elastic tissue in lung. Nonsmokers who remain in the presence of cigarette smokers (passive smokers) are significantly exposed to tobacco products. Children of smoking parents may experience more frequent and severe respiratory infections and have a higher prevalence of respiratory symptoms. However, a causal connection between passive smoking and chronic obstructive lung diseases has not been established.

2. *Occupational exposures:* Dust or gases such as cotton dust and toluene diisocyanate accelerate decline of pulmonary function in COLD.

3. *Acute infections:* May contribute to exacerbations of COLD and lead to chronic obstruction.

4. *Familial aggregation of emphysema:* Occurs with deficiency of alpha$_1$-antitrypsin, a protease inhibitor.

5. *Air pollution:* Although exacerbations of chronic bronchitis and mortality rates from emphysema and bronchitis are associated with air pollution, the role of pollutants in the pathogenesis of COLD is unclear.

Clinical Manifestations

COLD is a progressive disorder even when contributing factors are eliminated and aggressive therapy is instituted. Progression is inevitable since loss of lung elastic tissue is a normal part of aging. Although loss of elastic tissue (emphysema) underlies COLD in all cases, two distinct clinical syndromes exist (Table 121-1). Early development of hypercarbia and secondary manifestations of hypoxia in "Blue Bloater" may reflect genetic or acquired blunting of chemosensitivity (ventilatory response to hypoxia and hypercarbia).

"Pink Puffer" Scant sputum production but prominent exertional dyspnea; asthenic body build, tachypnea, prolonged expiration, hyperresonant chest, diminished breath sounds. Gas exchange is impaired with mildly reduced arterial P_{O_2} and low or normal P_{CO_2}. PFTs show reduced maximal flow rates and diffusing capacity and evidence of gas trapping. Cor pulmonale and hypercapneic respiratory failure occur late in the course.

"Blue Bloater" Chronic cough and mucus production; dyspnea is less prominent. Pts are often cyanotic and overweight; auscultation reveals coarse rhonchi and wheezes. RV heave, RV S_3, and edema are present. Arterial blood gases are severely deranged: both arterial P_{O_2} and P_{CO_2} (in mmHg) may be in high 40s to low 50s. Maximal expiratory flow rates are reduced, residual volume is moderately elevated, and diffusing

Table 121-1

Chronic Obstructive Lung Disease: Salient Features of the Two Types

	Pink Puffer	Blue Bloater
Age at time of diagnosis, yrs	60±	50±
Dyspnea	Severe	Mild
Cough	After dyspnea starts	Before dyspnea starts
Sputum	Scanty, mucoid	Copious, purulent
Bronchial infections	Less frequent	More frequent
Respiratory insufficiency episodes	Often terminal	Repeated
Chest film	"Hyperinflation" ± bullous changes, small heart	Increased bronchovascular markings at bases, large heart
Chronic Pa_{CO_2}	35–40 mmHg	50–60 mmHg
Chronic Pa_{O_2}	65–75 mmHg	45–60 mmHg
Hematocrit	35–45%	50–55%
Pulmonary hypertension:		
Rest	None to mild	Moderate to severe
Exercise	Moderate	Worsens
Cor pulmonale	Rare, except terminally	Common
Elastic recoil	Severely decreased	Normal
Resistance	Normal to slight increase	High
Diffusing capacity	Decreased	Normal to slight decrease

SOURCE: From Honig EG, Ingram RH Jr: HPIM-14, p. 1454.

capacity normal or slightly decreased. Episodes of respiratory failure are frequent, but recovery usually occurs with therapy.

℞ TREATMENT

Because emphysema is untreatable, therapeutic efforts are directed at prevention and management of reversible airways obstruction.

Assessment   In addition to Hx and physical exam, pts should receive a CXR as well as PFTs (spirometry, lung volumes, $D_{L_{CO}}$, arterial blood gases). Effects of inhaled bronchodilator should be assessed after acute administration. However, failure to see an acute response does not rule out improvement with sustained treatment. PFTs should be repeated regularly with and between exacerbations.

Prevention   COLD is progressive; however, the decline is accelerated by smoking, and all pts should be urged to quit. Eliminate aerosol sprays and occupational factors that may accelerate disease. Administer yearly influenza vaccinations.

Infections   Increases in sputum purulence, volume, and viscosity suggest infection. Nonbacterial infections precipitate most exacerbations, but antibiotics lower intensity and duration of symptoms, and a broad-spectrum antibiotic should be administered for 7–10 d with evidence of a change in sputum quality.

Bronchodilators   Sympathomimetics and anticholinergics may alleviate symptoms by reducing bronchial tone. Selective beta$_2$-stimulating drugs (albuterol and metaproterenol, 2 puffs q4–6h, metered-dose inhaler) are associated with fewest side effects. Ipratropium, an anticholinergic agent, is also available in metered-dose inhaler (2 puffs q6–8h) and is considered by many to be the bronchodialator of first choice for pts with COLD. Glucocorticoids should be employed when other measures are insufficient and only with objective documentation of improvement. Oral prednisone should be started at 30 mg/d, with serial PFTs to assess response. The dose should be tapered to the lowest effective level and should be stopped if there is no objective improvement. Long-term oral glucocorticoid therapy should be used rarely. The role of inhaled glucocorticoids remains undefined.

Other   Bronchopulmonary drainage is important in pts with mucus hypersecretion. Continuous O_2 should be given when severe hypoxia is present (P_{O_2} < 55 mmHg) and/or there is evidence of cor pulmonale. Exercise programs do not improve lung function but may increase task-specific exercise tolerance. If body weight is less than 85% of ideal, nutritional supplements may reduce fatigability and breathlessness. Supplementation should not replace an evaluation of weight loss, however. In some pts with disabling dyspnea, lung volume reduction surgery may provide symptomatic relief. A multicenter, cooperative study is underway to define appropriate candidates and indications. In selected pts with refractory symptoms, lung transplantation can substantially improve symptoms and function. As for volume-reduction surgery, indications for transplantation are in evolution.

ACUTE RESPIRATORY FAILURE

Diagnosis Made on the basis of arterial blood gas from baseline (P_{O_2} drop $\geq 10-15$ mmHg and/or increase in P_{CO_2} associated with pH ≤ 7.30).

Precipitating Factors Infection, cardiac decompensation, exacerbation of bronchospasm, pneumothorax, pulmonary thromboembolism, and sedative administration all may precipitate respiratory failure.

℞ TREATMENT

1. Maintain oxygenation with low-flow O_2 therapy (1–2L/min by nasal prongs or 24% by Venturi mask) to achieve a P_{O_2} in the mid-50s. If O_2 results in a large increase in arterial P_{CO_2} with acidosis, mechanical ventilation may be required; do not stop O_2 administration abruptly.
2. Treat infection (antibiotics), administer diuretics for CHF, remove secretions (postural drainage), reverse bronchoconstriction (aminophylline, inhaled sympathomimetics at intervals of 1–2 h, oral or IV glucocorticoids equivalent to 30 mg prednisone each day).
3. Noninvasive positive-pressure ventilation (by mask) may help avoid intubation.

Complications Arrhythmias, heart failure, pulmonary thromboembolism, GI hemorrhage.

For a more detailed discussion, see Honig EG, Ingram RH Jr: Chronic Bronchitis, Emphysema, and Airway Obstruction, Chap. 258, p. 1451, in HPIM-14.

122

UPPER AND LOWER RESPIRATORY TRACT INFECTIONS

HEAD AND NECK INFECTIONS

NOSE AND FACE (See also Chap. 76) Furunculosis (boils) should be treated promptly with local heat and oral antistaphylococcal antibiotics to avoid spread to the cavernous sinuses. Impetigo and erysipelas are caused by group A β-hemolytic streptococci and rarely by *Staphylococcus aureus*. Erysipelas, a well-demarcated cellulitis that is raised in a plateau, requires IV antibiotics active against these pathogens (e.g., oxacillin, 2 g q4h) in adults. Mucormycosis, a life-threatening infection in pts with neutropenia or diabetic ketoacidosis, presents as black crusts overlying necrotic tissue within the nasal cavity; surgical debridement and IV antifungal therapy are indicated.

PARANASAL SINUSES *Etiology* Acute sinusitis can be caused by *Streptococcus pneumoniae,* other streptococci, *Haemophilus influenzae* (not type b), *Moraxella,* and—in the ICU—*S. aureus* and gram-negative organisms. Viruses are isolated in one-fifth of cases. Pathogens of chronic sinusitis can also include anaerobes.

Pathogenesis Obstruction of ostia in the anterior ethmoid and middle meatal complex by retained secretions, mucosal edema (often caused by an antecedent viral respiratory infection), or polyps promotes sinusitis. Barotrauma and ciliary transport defects also can predispose to infection. Nasal cannulation beyond 48 h is the chief risk factor for nosocomial sinusitis.

Clinical Manifestations A consistent clinical feature of bacterial sinusitis is the unusually prolonged persistence of cold symptoms. Facial pain or pressure (often positional), nasal congestion, and purulent nasal or postnasal drainage are frequent manifestations of bacterial sinusitis. Fever develops in about half of pts with acute maxillary sinusitis. Chronic sinusitis features congestion and discharge but rarely fever. Serious complications include orbital cellulitis, frontal subperiosteal abscess (Pott's puffy tumor), and intracranial processes such as epidural abscess, subdural empyema, meningitis, cerebral abscess, and septic dural vein (including cavernous sinus) thrombophlebitis.

Diagnosis Nasal cultures are nondiagnostic. Radiographs are unnecessary for a new, clinically evident case of sinusitis. CT scanning allows assessment of orbital, sphenoid, and bony involvement but may also show reversible acute changes in pts with a common cold. MRI should be limited to the evaluation of fungal infection and tumor; MR angiography (MRA) is used to evaluate vascular complications.

℞ TREATMENT

Ostial patency and bacterial eradication are the goals of therapy. Humidification, hydration, and use of vasoconstricting drugs (but not antihistamines) are indicated. Amoxicillin or trimethoprim-sulfamethoxazole (TMP-SMZ) may be effective for first-time cases; more expensive alternative agents include amoxicillin/clavulanate (40 mg/kg daily, divided tid; up to 500 mg per dose) or a second-generation cephalosporin (e.g., cefuroxime axetil, 250 mg bid for pts >2 years old and 125 mg for pts <2 years old). Treatment should be administered for 1–2 weeks. Where gram-negative pathogens are common, therapy for nosocomial sinusitis should be guided by culture data.

Outpatient and Home Care Considerations Most persons with bacterial sinusitis may be treated as outpatients with oral antibiotics. Severe disease (i.e., with systemic toxicity) should be treated with IV antibiotics. Adjunctive surgery to widen ostia and drain thick secretions may be necessary in severe cases or when disease fails to respond to initial IV therapy.

EAR *Etiology* Viral URI, which can cause edema of the eustachian tube mucosa, often precedes or accompanies episodes of acute otitis media. *S. pneumoniae, H. influenzae* (usually nontypable), and *Moraxella catarrhalis* are the pathogens most commonly isolated from the middle ear. Chronic otitis most often yields *Pseudomonas aeruginosa, S. aureus,* and aerobic gram-negative rods. Anaerobes, often mixed with aerobes, are implicated in half of cases of chronic otitis media. Otitis externa, or swimmer's ear, may be due to *Staphylococcus, Streptococcus,* and *Pseudomonas* spp. *P. aeruginosa* causes invasive ("malignant") otitis externa in diabetic pts.

Pathogenesis Untreated acute or recurrent otitis media leads to chronic otitis with otorrhea. Tympanic membrane perforation and cholesteatoma are associated with chronic infection. Mastoid air cells are connected with the middle ear cavity and thus are involved in otitis media. Alkalinization of the external canal leads to bacterial overgrowth and otitis externa.

Clinical Manifestations Acute otitis media can cause pain, hearing loss, fever, leukocytosis, and a red, bulging, or perforated eardrum. Serous otitis media, a leading cause of hearing loss in children, features a dull retracted membrane with fluid.

Mastoiditis can cause inferolateral displacement of the pinna and a red fluctuant mass behind it. Chronic otitis with otorrhea is a chronically draining ear. In necrotizing otitis externa, there is severe pain and swelling of the external auditory canal.

Diagnosis Direct viewing of the tympanic membrane is required. CT scanning confirms mastoiditis and bony necrosis from malignant otitis externa.

℞ TREATMENT

Treatment is empiric. The agents used include amoxicillin, amoxicillin/clavulanate, TMP-SMZ, and cefuroxime axetil, each given for 10 d for acute otitis media at the same doses used for sinusitis. Drainage is indicated for unresolved or recurrent infection. Surgical therapy, along with a prolonged course of topical antibiotic drops, has been the mainstay of treatment for chronic otitis media. Debridement, antibacterial ear drops, IV antipseudomonal antibiotics, and control of coexisting diabetes are indicated for malignant otitis externa.

Outpatient and Home Care Considerations Most persons with acute otitis media may be treated as outpatients with oral antibiotics. Severe disease (i.e., with systemic toxicity) should be treated with IV antibiotics, and the ear should be drained for both therapeutic and diagnostic purposes.

MOUTH AND PHARYNX *Etiology* Oral anaerobes cause gingivitis. Herpesviruses infect the lip, buccal mucosa, tongue, and pharyngeal wall. Group A coxsackievirus causes herpangina. Yeast, usually a *Candida* species, causes thrush. Group A β-hemolytic streptococci cause exudative pharyngitis, as can *Neisseria gonorrhoeae, Corynebacterium diphtheriae, Mycoplasma pneumoniae, Chlamydia pneumoniae,* EBV, herpes simplex virus, and adenovirus. Respiratory syncytial, parainfluenza, and influenza viruses cause nonexudative pharyngitis.

Clinical Manifestations Acute pharyngitis features sore throat with erythema, exudate, and edema. Associated peritonsillar abscess causes fever, pain, dysphagia and odynophagia, tonsillar asymmetry, and "hot-potato" voice.

Diagnosis For exudative pharyngitis, the rapid strep test is specific for group A *Streptococcus.* However, since this test is not sufficiently sensitive, a throat swab should be inoculated for culture if the rapid test is negative. Herpes simplex is confirmed by culture or immunofluorescence staining. *Neisseria* must be isolated on selective medium. *Candida* is identified in oral lesions with use of a KOH preparation.

℞ TREATMENT

Penicillin or erythromycin (500 mg qid for 10 d) treats streptococcal pharyngitis and helps prevent rheumatic fever but not poststreptococcal glomerulonephritis. Peritonsillar abscess requires incision and drainage. Oral nystatin or clotrimazole—or, in severe cases, systemic antifungal therapy—controls thrush.

LARYNX *Etiology* Acute epiglottitis due to *H. influenzae* type b in children is a life-threatening condition that may cause complete airway obstruction. Croup (laryngotracheobronchitis) is attributable to parainfluenza virus, other respiratory viruses, and *M. pneumoniae.*

Pathogenesis Rapidly developing cellulitis of the epiglottis and surrounding tissues can obstruct the airway. Most pts with *Haemophilus* infection are bacteremic. Croup features circumferential inflammation of the larynx.

Clinical Manifestations Epiglottitis causes fever, hoarseness, odynophagia, and airway obstruction. Pts usually lean forward, drooling. Croup features a brassy "seal's bark" cough, with or without stridor, in children below age 3.

Diagnosis An edematous, cherry red epiglottis and a "thumb sign" on lateral neck film indicate epiglottitis. Direct fiberoptic examination requires a secured airway. Subglottic narrowing on lateral neck film indicates croup.

℞ TREATMENT

Epiglottitis must be managed in the ICU with airway observation or intubation, oxygen as needed, and administration of cefuroxime or a third-generation cephalosporin for 7–10 d. If the pt has unvaccinated household contacts <4 years old, they and all other members of the household should receive prophylaxis with rifampin (20 mg/kg daily, up to 600 mg) to eliminate carriage. Pts with severe croup must be hospitalized for close observation, humidification, and oxygen as indicated.

DEEP NECK SPACES *Etiology* Group A streptococci, *Peptostreptococcus, Prevotella, Porphyromonas,* and *Fusobacterium* are the common isolates from infections of the deep neck spaces.

Pathogenesis Infections originate in dental abscesses, sites of oral infections and sinusitis, and retropharyngeal lymph nodes and track into the lateral pharyngeal, submandibular, or retropharyngeal spaces. Airway obstruction, septic thrombophlebitis, or mediastinitis can develop.

Clinical Manifestations In lateral pharyngeal space infection, fever, leukocytosis, deep neck pain, medial pharyngeal wall displacement, and trismus may develop. Associated septic thrombosis of the internal jugular vein causes rigors, fever spikes, and mandibular angle tenderness. Carotid artery rupture occurs rarely. Ludwig's angina—infection of the submandibular or sublingual space—presents as pain, fever, drooling, inflammation of the mouth floor, and posterior and superior tongue displacement. Infection of the retropharyngeal space can produce dysphagia, "hot-potato" voice, cervical rigidity, dyspnea, or stridor. Mediastinitis, airway obstruction, or rupture into the airway and aspiration pneumonia can occur.

Diagnosis CT scanning and, for vascular involvement, MRA define the site of infection.

℞ TREATMENT

Treatment consists of ampicillin/sulbactam (3.1 g qid) or clindamycin/ceftriaxone, with surgical drainage mandatory in either case.

PNEUMONIA

ETIOLOGY Pneumonia is an infection of the pulmonary parenchyma caused by various bacterial species, mycoplasmas, chlamydiae, rickettsiae, viruses, fungi, and parasites. Compromised hosts are particularly vulnerable to pulmonary infections caused by a variety of pathogens.

EPIDEMIOLOGY Factors such as travel history, exposure to pets, exposure to other people who are ill, occupation, age, presence or absence of teeth, season of the year, geographic location, smoking status, and HIV status all influence the types of pathogens to consider in the etiology of pneumonia.

PATHOGENESIS The most common mechanism for acquiring pneumonia is aspiration of organisms from the oropharynx. The usual organisms are aerobic gram-positive cocci and anaerobes that colonize the oropharynx. Normally, 50% of adults aspirate during sleep. Aspiration increases with impaired consciousness—e.g., in alcoholics and drug users; in pts with stroke or seizure, other neurologic or swallowing disorders, or nasogastric or endotracheal tubes; and during or after anesthesia. Aerobic gram-negative bacilli colonize the oropharynx or stomach more frequently in hospitalized or institutionalized pts than in other individuals. Other routes of transmission for pneumonia include inhalation of infected particles (diameter <5 μm), hematogenous spread, contiguous spread from another infected site, and direct inoculation from open trauma to the chest.

CLINICAL MANIFESTATIONS The "typical" pneumonia syndrome is characterized by the sudden onset of fever, cough productive of purulent sputum, and pleuritic chest pain; signs of pulmonary consolidation; and a lobar infiltrate on CXR. This syndrome is most commonly caused by *S. pneumoniae* and other bacterial pathogens. The "atypical" pneumonia syndrome is characterized by a more gradual onset, a dry cough, a prominence of extrapulmonary symptoms (e.g., headache, malaise, myalgias, sore throat, GI distress), and minimal signs on physical exam (other than rales) despite an abnormal, often patchy or diffuse pattern on CXR. Atypical pneumonia is classically caused by *M. pneumoniae* but may also be due to *Legionella pneumophila, Chlamydia pneumoniae,* oral anaerobes, *Pneumocystis carinii,* and *S. pneumoniae.*

Other, rarer pathogens causing atypical pneumonia include *Chlamydia psittaci, Coxiella burnetii, Francisella tularensis, Histoplasma capsulatum,* and *Coccidioides immitis.* While recent data suggest that the distinction between typical and atypical pneumonia syndromes may be less reliable than was once thought, the differences are of some diagnostic value.

DIAGNOSIS *Radiography* Findings on CXR range from lobar consolidation with air bronchograms to diffuse patchy interstitial infiltrates. Other findings include multiple nodules suspicious for septic emboli, cavitation, pleural effusion, and hilar adenopathy.

Sputum Examination Whenever possible, sputum should be obtained and evaluated grossly for purulence and blood and by Gram's stain. The presence of >25 PMNs and <25 epithelial cells per high-power field suggests that the specimen is adequate. The finding of mixed flora on Gram's stain suggests anaerobic infection. The presence of a single, predominant type of organism suggests the etiology of the pneumonia. Sputum may also be examined directly for acid-fast organisms and by special stain or immunofluorescence for *Legionella* or *Pneumocystis.* Sputum culture may also yield the causative agent but is usually less sensitive than Gram's stain.

Blood Cultures Since sputum examination and culture do not always reveal a pathogen, blood for cultures should be obtained before therapy begins.

Other Diagnostic Maneuvers Sputum induction (with ultrasonic nebulization of 3% saline), bronchoscopy with bronchoalveolar lavage or protected brush specimens, transtracheal aspiration, thoracentesis, percutaneous lung puncture, open lung biopsy, acute and convalescent serology, and chest CT are all useful in selected cases.

℞ TREATMENT

See Table 122-1 for clinical syndromes, likely organisms, and antibiotic choices. See Table 122-2 for doses of antibiotics used for inpatient treatment of pneumonia.

Outpatient and Home Care Considerations Some persons with pneumonia may be treated as outpatients with oral antibiotics. Criteria for hospitalization of pts with pneumonia are listed in Table 122-3.

LUNG ABSCESS

CLINICAL MANIFESTATIONS Lung abscess is usually a complication of the aspiration of oral anaerobes. In most pts it is a subacute disease with an indolent presentation. The pt usually has a cough that may or may not be productive of large quantities of purulent, foul-smelling sputum and often has fevers, night sweats, and weight loss. Pleuritic chest pain and blood-streaked sputum also may be seen.

DIAGNOSIS CXR usually shows a cavitary lesion with an air-fluid level, often in dependent, poorly ventilated portions of the lung. The sputum is not necessarily foul-smelling but usually contains a mixed flora revealed by Gram's stain.

℞ TREATMENT

The treatment of choice is clindamycin (600 mg q8h IV, then 300–450 mg PO); ampicillin (2 g IV q6h) or amoxicillin (500 mg PO tid) with metronidazole (500 mg PO q6h); ampicillin/sulbactam; or amoxicillin/clavulanate. Antibiotics rarely need to be directed at each organism isolated if the abscess is aspirated. Treatment should be continued until CXR findings have resolved, which may require months.

Table 122-1

Treatment of Pneumonia

Syndrome	Common Organisms	Antibiotic(s)
Community-acquired		
Lobar	*S. pneumoniae, H. influenzae, M. catarrhalis*	Penicillin*, erythromycin, SGC, TGC, ampicillin/sulbactam†
Atypical	*M. pneumoniae, Legionella* spp., *C. pneumoniae*	Erythromycin, clarithromycin
Aspiration (mixed flora)	Anaerobes	Clindamycin, ampicillin/sulbactam, amoxicillin + metronidazole
Hospital-acquired	*S. aureus*	Nafcillin, vancomycin
	Enteric gram-negative bacilli or *P. aeruginosa*	Ceftazidime ± antipseudomonal aminoglycoside, ticarcillin/clavulanate ± aminoglycoside, imipenem, ciprofloxacin
	Mixed flora	Ceftazidime + clindamycin (or metronidazole) ± aminoglycoside, imipenem ± aminoglycoside, ticarcillin/clavulanate or piperacillin/tazobactam ± aminoglycoside
Postinfluenza	*S. pneumoniae, S. aureus*	Nafcillin, vancomycin

*For susceptible strains of *S. pneumoniae.* When resistance is suspected, use TGC; in life-threatening cases, add vancomycin.

†Ampicillin/sulbactam does not cover penicillin-resistant *S. pneumoniae.*

ABBREVIATIONS: SGC, second-generation cephalosporin; TGC, third-generation cephalosporin.

742

Table 122-2

Dosage of Antimicrobial Agents for the Treatment of Pneumonia in Hospitalized Patients*

Drug	Dosage
Ampicillin/sulbactam	3 g IV q6h
Aztreonam	2 g IV q8h
Cefazolin	1–2 g IV q8h
Cefotaxime, ceftizoxime	1–2 g q8–12h
Ceftazidime	2 g IV q8h
Ceftriaxone	1–2 g IV q12–24h
Cefuroxime	750 mg IV q8h
Ciprofloxacin	400 mg IV or 750 mg PO q12h
Clindamycin	600–900 mg IV q8h
Erythromycin	0.5–1.0 g IV q6h
Gentamicin (or tobramycin)	5 mg/kg/d in 3 equally divided doses IV q8h
Imipenem	500 mg IV q6h
Metronidazole	500 mg IV or PO q6h
Nafcillin	2 g IV q4h
Penicillin G	1–3 million units IV q4–6h
Ticarcillin/clavulanate	3.1 g IV q4h
Vancomycin	1 g IV q12h

*Dosage must be modified for pts with renal failure.

SOURCE: Levison ME: HPIM-14, p. 1443.

Table 122-3

Criteria for Hospitalization of Patients with Pneumonia

1. Elderly pt (>65 years of age)
2. Significant comorbidity (e.g., kidney, heart, or lung disease; diabetes mellitus; neoplasm; immunosuppression)
3. Leukopenia (<5000 white blood cells/μL) not attributable to a known condition
4. *Staphylococcus aureus,* gram-negative bacilli, or anaerobes as the suspected cause of pneumonia
5. Suppurative complications (e.g., empyema, arthritis, meningitis, endocarditis)
6. Failure of outpatient management
7. Inability to take oral medication
8. Tachypnea (>30/min); tachycardia (>140/min); hypotension (<90 mmHg systolic); hypoxemia (arterial P_{O_2}, <60 mmHg); acute alteration of mental status

SOURCE: Levison ME: HPIM-14, p. 1441.

For a more detailed discussion, see Durand M, Joseph M, Baker AS: Infections of the Upper Respiratory Tract, Chap. 30, p. 179; and Levison ME: Pneumonia, Including Necrotizing Pulmonary Infections (Lung Abscess), Chap. 255, p. 1437, in HPIM-14.

123

PULMONARY THROMBOEMBOLISM AND PRIMARY PULMONARY HYPERTENSION

PULMONARY EMBOLISM (PE) (See Fig. 123-1)

NATURAL HISTORY Immediate result is obstruction of pulmonary blood flow to the distal lung. Respiratory consequences include (1) wasted ventilation (lung ventilated but not

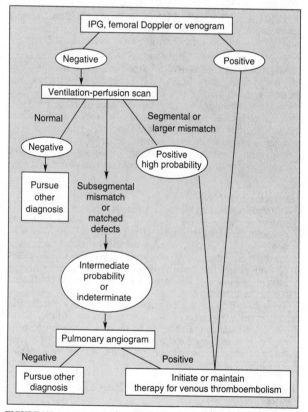

FIGURE 123-1 Flowchart used in diagnosis of pulmonary embolism (PE). IPG, impedance plethysmogram. (Reproduced from Moser KM: HPIM-13.)

perfused), (2) atelectasis that occurs 2–24 h following PE, and (3) widened alveolar-arterial P_{O_2} gradient, usually with arterial hypoxemia. Hemodynamic consequences may include (1) pulmonary hypertension, (2) acute RV failure, and (3) decline in cardiac output. These occur only when significant fraction of pulmonary vasculature is obstructed. Infarction of lung tissue is uncommon, occurring only with underlying cardiac or pulmonary disease.

SYMPTOMS Sudden onset of dyspnea most common; chest pain, hemoptysis accompany infarction; syncope may indicate massive embolism.

PHYSICAL EXAMINATION Tachypnea and tachycardia common; RV gallop; loud P_2 and prominent jugular *a* waves suggest RV failure; temperature >39°C uncommon. Hypotension suggests massive PE.

LABORATORY FINDINGS Routine studies contribute little to diagnosis; normal CXR does not exclude PE, but normal perfusion scintiscan is not seen with a clinically significant embolism. Detection of venous thrombosis with impedance plethysmography, femoral ultrasound, or venography should prompt therapy for venous thromboembolism in a pt with a suspicion of embolism. A segmental or larger perfusion defect with normal ventilation ("mismatch") is highly suggestive of PE; pulmonary angiography remains a definitive test.

℞ **TREATMENT**   (See Fig. 123-2)
IV heparin [18(U/kg)/h] by continuous infusion is therapy for most pts after an initial bolus of 80 U/kg; usual goal is to maintain activated PTT 1.5–2.0 × control; heparin is continued 7 to 10 d for deep venous thrombosis (DVT) and 10 d for thromboembolism. Most pts receive minimum of 3 months of oral coumadin therapy after PE. Thrombolytic therapy hastens resolution of venous thrombi and is probably indicated for pts with massive embolism and systemic hypotension. Surgical therapy is rarely employed for DVT or acute PE. IVC interruption (clip or filter) is used in pts with recurrent PE despite anticoagulants and in those who cannot tolerate anticoagulants. Surgical extraction of old emboli may be helpful in pts with chronic pulmonary hypertension due to repeated PE without spontaneous resolution.

PRIMARY PULMONARY HYPERTENSION (PPH)

HISTORY Uncommon condition. Typical pt is female aged 20–40. At presentation, symptoms are usually of recent onset,

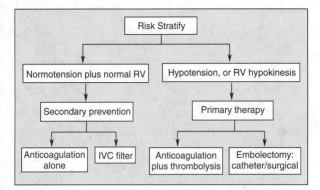

FIGURE 123-2 Acute PTE management: Risk stratification. RV, right ventricular; IVC, inferior vena cava. (From Goldhaber SZ: HPIM-14.)

and natural history is ordinarily less than 5 years. Early symptoms are nonspecific—hyperventilation, chest discomfort, anxiety, weakness, fatigue. Later, dyspnea develops and precordial pain on exertion occurs in 25–50%. Effort syncope occurs very late and signifies ominous prognosis.

PHYSICAL EXAMINATION Prominent *a* wave in jugular venous pulse, right ventricular heave, narrowly split S_2 with accentuated P_2. Terminal course is characterized by signs of right-sided heart failure. *CXR:* RV and central pulmonary arterial prominence. Pulmonary arteries taper sharply. *ECG:* RV enlargement, right axis deviation, and RV hypertrophy. *Echocardiogram:* RA and RV enlargement and tricuspid regurgitation. See Fig. 123-3.

DIFFERENTIAL DIAGNOSIS Other disorders of heart, lungs, and pulmonary vasculature must be excluded. Lung function studies will identify chronic pulmonary disease causing pulmonary hypertension and cor pulmonale. Interstitial diseases (PFTs, CT scan) and hypoxic pulmonary hypertension (ABGs, Sa_{O_2}) should be excluded. Perfusion lung scan should be performed to exclude chronic PE. Pulmonary arteriogram and even open lung biopsy may be required to distinguish PE from PPH. Rarely, pulmonary hypertension is due to parasitic disease (schistosomiasis, filariasis). Cardiac disorders to be excluded include pulmonary artery and pulmonic valve stenosis. Pulmonary artery and ventricular and atrial shunts with pulmonary vascular disease (Eisenmenger reaction) should be sought. Silent mitral stenosis should be excluded by echocardiography.

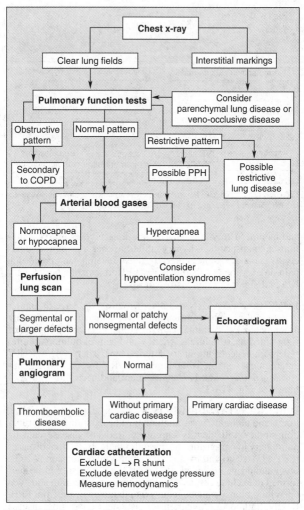

FIGURE 123-3   An algorithm for the workup of a pt with unexplained pulmonary hypertension. (Adapted with permission from Rich S: HPIM-14.)

℞ TREATMENT

Course is usually one of progressive deterioration despite treatment; therapy is palliative, but treatment has improved in recent years. Main focus of therapy is vasodilator drugs. Must lower pulmonary artery pressure and pulmonary vascular resistance while preserving systemic pressure. High doses of calcium channel antagonists (e.g., nifedipine, 120–240 mg/d, or diltiazem, 540–900 mg/d) may reduce pulmonary pressure and resistance, but fewer than half of pts with primary pulmonary hypertension respond. Recent evidence suggests prostacyclin is effective in selected pts. Some experts recommend anticoagulation for all pts. Pts who fail medical therapy may be considered for transplantation.

For a more detailed discussion, see Rich S: Primary Pulmonary Hypertension, Chap. 260, p. 1466; and Goldhaber SZ: Pulmonary Thromboembolism, Chap. 261, p. 1469, in HPIM-14.

INTERSTITIAL LUNG DISEASE (ILD)

Chronic, nonmalignant, noninfectious diseases of the lower respiratory tract characterized by inflammation and derangement of the alveolar walls; >180 separate diseases of known and unknown cause. Each group can be divided into subgroups according to the presence or absence of histologic evidence of granulomas in interstitial or vascular areas (Table 124-1).

DIAGNOSTIC EVALUATION   Rarely, clinical syndrome can be related to causative agent, but histologic exam is usually necessary. With exception of sarcoidosis, which can often be diagnosed by transbronchial biopsy, most infiltrative diseases require open lung biopsy for diagnosis. Gallium scans and bronchoalveolar lavage do not yield a specific diagnosis but help to document the extent and character of inflammation.

INDIVIDUAL ILDs

IDIOPATHIC PULMONARY FIBROSIS   *History*   Average age of 50 at presentation, but range is infancy to old age. Sometimes familial. First manifestations are dyspnea, effort intolerance, and dry cough. Detailed work history essential. Dyspnea and coughing often accompanied by constitutional symptoms (fatigue, anorexia, weight loss). One-third of pts date symptoms to aftermath of viral respiratory infection.

Physical Exam   Late inspiratory crackles at posterior lung bases. Signs of pulmonary hypertension and clubbing occur late in course.

Laboratory Findings   ESR may be elevated. Hypoxemia is common, but polycythemia is rare. Circulating immune-complex titers and serum immunoglobulin levels may be elevated.

Imaging Studies   CXR usually reveals diffuse reticulonodular markings, prominent in lower lung zones. About 14% of biopsy-proven cases have normal CXR. High-resolution CT may show abnormalities when CXR normal.

PFTs   Typically restrictive pattern (see Fig. 118-1) with reduced total lung capacity. $D_{L_{CO}}$ often decreased; mild hypoxemia, which worsens with exercise.

Bronchoalveolar Lavage   Cells recovered (alveolar macrophages, lymphocytes, neutrophils, eosinophils) may reflect the type of alveolar inflammation in specific disorders.

Table 124-1

Major Categories of Alveolar and Interstitial Inflammatory Lung Diseases (ILDs)

Known Cause	Unknown cause

LUNG RESPONSE: ALVEOLITIS, INTERSTITIAL INFLAMMATION, AND FIBROSIS

Asbestos	Idiopathic pulmonary fibrosis
Fumes, gases	Collagen vascular diseases
Drugs (antibiotics) and chemotherapy drugs	Pulmonary hemorrhage syndromes:
Radiation	Goodpasture's syndrome, idiopathic pulmonary hemosiderosis
Aspiration pneumonia	Pulmonary alveolar proteinosis
Residual of adult respiratory distress syndrome	Lymphocytic infiltrative disorders
	Eosinophilic pneumonias
	Lymphangioleiomyomatosis
	Amyloidosis
	Graft vs. host disease (bone marrow transplantation)

LUNG RESPONSE: AS ABOVE BUT WITH GRANULOMA

Hypersensitivity pneumonitis (organic dusts)	Sarcoidosis
Inorganic dusts: beryllium silica	Langerhans cell granulomatosis (eosinophilic granuloma)
	Granulomatous vasculitides: Wegener's granulomatosis, allergic granulomatosis of Churg-Strauss, lymphomatoid granulomatosis
	Bronchocentric granulomatosis

SOURCE: From Reynolds HY: HPIM-14, p. 1461.

ILD ASSOCIATED WITH COLLAGEN-VASCULAR DISORDERS Usually follows development of collagen-vascular disorder; typically mild but occasionally fatal.

RHEUMATOID ARTHRITIS (RA) 50% of pts with RA have abnormal lung function, 25% have abnormal CXR. Rarely causes symptoms.

PROGRESSIVE SYSTEMIC SCLEROSIS Fibrosis with little inflammation; poor prognosis. Must be distinguished from pulmonary vascular disease.

SLE Uncommon complication. When it occurs, it is most often an acute, inflammatory patchy process.

LANGERHANS CELL GRANULOMATOSIS (EOSINOPHILIC GRANULOMA OR HYSTIOCYTOSIS X) Disorder of the dendritic cell system, related to Letterer-Siwe and Hand-Schüller-Christian diseases. Develops between 20 and 40 years of age; 90% are present or former smokers. Complicated frequently by pneumothoraces. No therapy available.

CHRONIC EOSINOPHILIC PNEUMONIA Affects females more than males. Often have history of chronic asthma. Symptoms include weight loss, fever, chills, fatigue, dyspnea. CXR shows "photonegative pulmonary edema" pattern with central sparing. Very responsive to glucocorticoids.

IDIOPATHIC PULMONARY HEMOSIDEROSIS Characterized by recurrent pulmonary hemorrhage; may be life-threatening. Not associated with renal disease.

GOODPASTURE'S SYNDROME Relapsing pulmonary hemorrhage, anemia, and renal failure. Adult males most commonly affected. Circulating anti-basement membrane antibodies.

INHERITED DISORDERS ILD may be associated with tuberous sclerosis, neurofibromatosis, Gaucher's disease, Hermansky-Pudlak syndrome, and Niemann-Pick disease.

℞ TREATMENT

Most important is removal of causative agent. With exception of pneumoconioses, which are generally not treated except for discontinuation of further exposure and some other specific disorders, therapy is directed toward suppressing the inflammatory process, usually with glucocorticoids. After diagnosis, pts given oral prednisone, 1 (mg/kg)/d, for 8–12 weeks. Response is assessed by symptoms and PFTs. For idiopathic pulmonary fibrosis and some other disorders, if pt fails to respond to prednisone, consider immunosuppressive therapy with cyclophosphamide, 1.0 (mg/kg)/d, added to prednisone, 0.25 (mg/kg)/d. Smoking cessation, supplemental oxygen (when P_{O_2} <55 mmHg), and therapy for right-sided heart failure and bronchospasm may all improve symptoms.

For a more detailed discussion, see Reynolds HY: Interstitial Lung Diseases, Chap. 259, p. 1460, in HPIM-14.

DISEASES OF THE PLEURA, MEDIASTINUM, AND DIAPHRAGM

PLEURAL DISEASE

PLEURITIS Inflammation of pleura may occur with pneumonia, tuberculosis, pulmonary infarction, and neoplasm. Pleuritic pain without physical and x-ray findings suggests epidemic pleurodynia (viral inflammation of intercostal muscles); hemoptysis and parenchymal involvement on CXR suggest infection or infarction. Pleural effusion without parenchymal disease suggests postprimary tuberculosis, subdiaphragmatic abscess, mesothelioma, connective tissue disease, or primary bacterial infection of pleural space.

PLEURAL EFFUSION May or may not be associated with pleuritis. In general, effusions due to pleural disease resemble plasma (exudates); effusions with normal pleura are ultrafiltrates of plasma (transudates). Exudates have at least one of the following criteria: high total fluid/serum protein ratio (>0.5), pleural fluid LDH greater than two-thirds of the normal upper limit, or pleural/serum LDH activity ratio >0.6. Leading causes of transudative pleural effusions in the U.S. are left ventricular failure, pulmonary embolism, and cirrhosis. Leading causes of exudative effusions are bacterial pneumonia, malignancy, viral infection, and pulmonary embolism. With empyema, pH <7.2, WBCs ↑ (>1000/mL), and glucose ↓. If neoplasm or tuberculo-

Table 125-1

Evaluation of Pleural Fluid

	Transudate	Exudate
Typical appearance	Clear	Clear, cloudy, or bloody
Protein		
Absolute value	<3.0 g/dL	>3.0 g/dL*
Pleural fluid/ serum ratio	<0.5	>0.5
Lactic dehydrogenase		
Absolute value	<200 IU/L	>200 IU/L
Pleural fluid/ serum ratio	<0.6	>0.6
Glucose	>60 mg/dL (usually same as in blood)	Variable; often <60 mg/dL
Leukocytes	<1000/mL	>1000/mL
Polymorphonuclear	<50%	Usually >50% in acute inflammation
Erythrocytes	<5000/mL†	Variable
Pleural biopsy indicated?	No	Parapneumonic/ other acute inflammation
	Yes	Chronic/subacute or undiagnosed effusion

*Less in hypoproteinemic states.

†Assuming atraumatic tap.

sis is considered, closed pleural biopsy or thoracoscopic biopsy should be performed (see Table 125-1, Fig. 125-1). Despite full evaluation, no cause for effusion will be found in 25% of pts.

POSTPRIMARY TUBERCULOSIS EFFUSIONS Fluid is exudative with predominant lymphocytosis; bacilli are rarely seen on smear, and fluid culture is positive in fewer than 20%; tuberculin test may be nonreactive early in illness; closed biopsy required for diagnosis.

NEOPLASTIC EFFUSIONS Most often lung cancer, breast cancer, or lymphoma. Fluid is exudative; fluid cytology and

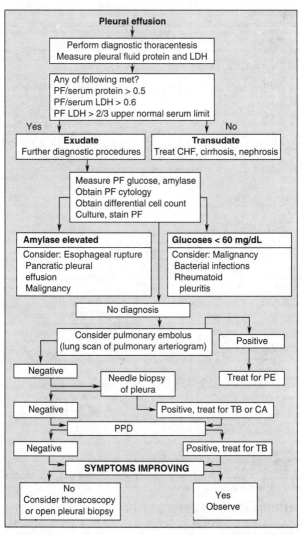

FIGURE 125-1 Approach to the diagnosis of pleural effusions. The special tests are summarized in Table 125–2. PF, pleural fluid; PE, pulmonary embolism. (From Light RW: HPIM-14.)

Table 125-2

Special Tests for Pleural Effusions

	Transudate	Exudate
RBC	<10,000/mL	>100,000/mL suggests neoplasm, infarction, trauma; >10,000 to <100,000/mL is indeterminate
WBC	<100/mL	Usually >1000/mL
Differential WBC	Usually >50% lymphocytes or mononuclear cells	>50% lymphocytes (tuberculosis, neoplasm) >50% polymorphonuclear (acute inflammation)
pH	>7.3	>7.3 (inflammatory)
Glucose	Same as blood (±)	Low (infection) Extremely low (rheumatoid arthritis, occasionally neoplasm)
Amylase		>500 units/mL (pancreatitis; occasionally neoplasm, infection)
Specific proteins		Low C3, C4 components of complement (SLE, rheumatoid arthritis) Rheumatoid factor Antinuclear factor

SOURCE: From Ingram RH Jr, HPIM-11, p. 1125.

pleural biopsy will confirm diagnosis in 60%; pleural sclerosis with bleomycin or minocycline may be required for management (see Table 125-2).

RHEUMATOID ARTHRITIS (RA) Exudative effusions may precede articular symptoms; very low glucose and pH; usually males.

PANCREATITIS Typically left-sided; up to 15% of pts with pancreatitis; high pleural fluid amylase is suggestive but also may occur with effusions due to neoplasms, infection, and esophageal rupture.

EOSINOPHILIC EFFUSION   Defined as more than 10% eosinophils; nonspecific finding may occur with viral, bacterial, traumatic, and pancreatic effusions and may follow prior thoracentesis.

HEMOTHORAX   Most commonly follows blunt or penetrating trauma. Pts with bleeding disorders may develop hemothorax following trauma or invasive procedures on pleura. Adequate drainage mandatory to avoid fibrothorax and "trapped" lung.

PARAPNEUMONIC EFFUSION/EMPYEMA   An effusion associated with contiguous infection. The term *complicated parapneumonic effusion* refers to effusions that require tube thoracostomy for their resolution. Empyema is pus in the pleural space with positive Gram's stain. Tube thoracostomy of parapneumonic effusions is indicated if any of the following applies: (1) gross pus is present, (2) organisms are visible on Gram's stain of pleural fluid, (3) pleural fluid glucose is <50 mg/dL, or (4) pleural fluid pH is below 7.00 and 0.15 units less than arterial pH. If closed drainage does not result in marked symptomatic improvement in several days, open drainage is indicated, usually accomplished through a videoscope.

PNEUMOTHORAX (PNTX)   Spontaneous PNTX most commonly occurs between 20 and 40 years of age; causes sudden, sharp chest pain and dyspnea. Treatment depends on size—if small, observation is sufficient; if large, closed drainage with chest tube is necessary. 50% suffer recurrence, and application of irritants either by surgery or through chest tube may be required so that surfaces become adherent (pleurodesis). Complications include hemothorax, cardiovascular compromise secondary to tension PNTX, and bronchopleural fistula. Many interstitial and obstructive lung diseases may predispose to PNTX.

MEDIASTINAL DISEASE

MEDIASTINITIS   Usually infectious. Routes of infection include esophageal perforation or tracheal disruption (trauma, instrumentation, eroding carcinoma). Radiographic hallmarks include mediastinal widening, air in mediastinum, pneumo- or hydropneumothorax. Therapy usually involves surgical drainage and antibiotics.

TUMORS AND CYSTS   Most common mediastinal masses in adults are metastatic carcinomas and lymphomas. Sarcoido-

Table 125-3

Nature of Masses in Various Locations in Mediastinum

Superior	Anterior and Middle	Posterior
Lymphoma	Lymphoma	Neurogenic tumors
Thymoma	Metastatic carcinoma	Lymphoma
Retrosternal thyroid	Teratodermoid	Hernia (Bochdalek)
Metastatic carcinoma	Bronchogenic cyst	Aortic aneurysm
Parathyroid tumors	Aortic aneurysm	
Zenker's diverticulum	Pericardial cyst	
Aortic aneurysm		

sis, infectious mononucleosis, and AIDS may produce mediastinal lymphadenopathy. Neurogenic tumors, teratodermoids, thymomas, and bronchogenic cysts account for two-thirds of remaining mediastinal masses. Specific locations for specific etiologies (see Table 125-3). Evaluation includes CXR, CT, and when diagnosis remains in doubt, mediastinoscopy and biopsy.

NEUROGENIC TUMORS Most common primary mediastinal neoplasms; majority are benign; vague chest pain and cough.

TERATODERMOIDS Anterior mediastinum; 10–20% undergo malignant transformation.

THYMOMAS 10% primary mediastinal neoplasms; one-quarter are malignant; myasthenia gravis occurs in half.

SUPERIOR VENA CAVA SYNDROME Dilation of veins of upper thorax and neck, plethora, facial and conjunctival edema, headache, visual disturbances, and reduced state of consciousness; most often due to malignant disease—75% bronchogenic carcinoma, most others lymphoma.

DISORDERS OF DIAPHRAGM

DIAPHRAGMATIC PARALYSIS *Unilateral Paralysis*
Usually caused by phrenic nerve injury due to trauma or mediastinal tumor, but nearly half are unexplained; usually asymptomatic; suggested by CXR, confirmed by fluoroscopy.

Bilateral Paralysis May be due to high cervical cord injury, motor neuron disease, poliomyelitis, polyneuropathies, bilateral phrenic involvement by mediastinal lesions, after cardiac surgery, dyspnea; paradoxical abdominal motion should be sought in supine pts.

For a more detailed discussion, see Light, RW: Disorders of the Pleura, Mediastinum, and Diaphragm, Chap. 262, p. 1472, in HPIM-14.

126

DISORDERS OF VENTILATION, INCLUDING SLEEP APNEA

ALVEOLAR HYPOVENTILATION Exists when arterial P_{CO_2} increases above the normal 37–43 mmHg. In most clinically important chronic hypoventilation syndromes, Pa_{CO_2} is 50–80 mmHg.

CAUSE Alveolar hypoventilation always is (1) a defect in the metabolic respiratory control system, (2) a defect in the respiratory neuromuscular system, or (3) a defect in the ventilatory apparatus (Table 126-1).

Disorders associated with impaired respiratory drive, defects in respiratory neuromuscular system, and upper airway obstruction produce an increase in Pa_{CO_2}, despite normal lungs, because of a decrease in overall minute ventilation.

Disorders of chest wall, lower airways, and lungs produce an increase in Pa_{CO_2}, despite a normal or increased minute ventilation.

Increased Pa_{CO_2} leads to respiratory acidosis, compensatory increase in HCO_3^-, and decrease in Pa_{O_2}.

Hypoxemia may induce secondary polycythemia, pulmonary hypertension, right heart failure. Gas exchange worsens during sleep, resulting in morning headache, impaired sleep quality, fatigue, daytime somnolence, mental confusion (Fig. 126-1).

Table 126-1

Chronic Hypoventilation Syndromes

Mechanism	Site of Defect	Disorder
Impaired respiratory drive	Peripheral and central chemoreceptors	Carotid body dysfunction, trauma
		Prolonged hypoxia
		Metabolic alkalosis
	Brainstem respiratory neurons	Bulbar poliomyelitis, encephalitis
		Brainstem infarction, hemorrhage, trauma
		Brainstem demyelination, degeneration
		Chronic drug administration
		Primary alveolar hypoventilation syndrome
Defective respiratory neuromuscular system	Spinal cord and peripheral nerves	High cervical trauma
		Poliomyelitis
		Motor neuron disease
		Peripheral neuropathy
	Respiratory muscles	Myasthenia gravis
		Muscular dystrophy
		Chronic myopathy
Impaired ventilatory apparatus	Chest wall	Kyphoscoliosis
		Fibrothorax
		Thoracoplasty
		Ankylosing spondylitis
		Obesity-hypoventilation
	Airways and lungs	Laryngeal and tracheal stenosis
		Obstructive sleep apnea
		Cystic fibrosis
		Chronic obstructive pulmonary disease

SOURCE: Phillipson EA: HPIM-14, p. 1476.

HYPOVENTILATION SYNDROMES

PRIMARY ALVEOLAR Cause unknown; rare; thought to arise from defect in metabolic respiratory control system; key diagnostic finding is chronic respiratory acidosis without respi-

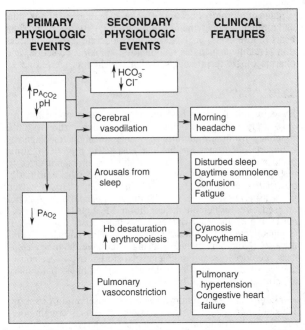

PRIMARY PHYSIOLOGIC EVENTS	SECONDARY PHYSIOLOGIC EVENTS	CLINICAL FEATURES

FIGURE 126-1 Physiologic and clinical features of alveolar hypoventilation. $P_{A_{CO_2}}$, alveolar P_{CO_2}. (After Phillipson EA: HPIM-14.)

ratory muscle weakness or impaired ventilatory mechanics. Some pts respond to respiratory stimulants and supplemental O_2.

RESPIRATORY NEUROMUSCULAR Several primary neuromuscular disorders produce chronic hypoventilation (see Table 126-1). Hypoventilation usually develops gradually, but acute, superimposed respiratory loads (e.g., viral bronchitis with airways obstruction) may precipitate respiratory failure. Diaphragm weakness is a common feature, with orthopnea and paradoxical abdominal movement in supine posture. Testing reveals low maximum voluntary ventilation and reduced maximal inspiratory and expiratory pressures. Therapy involves treatment of underlying condition. Many pts benefit from mechanical ventilatory assistance at night (often through nasal mask) or the entire day (typically through tracheostomy).

OBESITY-HYPOVENTILATION Massive obesity imposes a mechanical load on the respiratory system. Small percentage of morbidly obese pts develop hypercapnia, hypoxemia, and ultimately polycythemia, pulmonary hypertension, and right heart failure. Most pts have mild to moderate airflow obstruction. Treatment includes weight loss, smoking cessation, and pharmacologic respiratory stimulants such as progesterone.

SLEEP APNEA

By convention, apnea is defined as cessation of airflow for >10 s. Hypopneas are defined as reduction in airflow (<50% baseline). Minimum number of events per night for diagnosis is uncertain, but most pts have at least 10-15/h of sleep. Some pts have *central apnea* with transient loss of neural drive to respiratory muscles during sleep. Vast majority have primarily *obstructive apnea* with occlusion in the upper airway. Sleep plays a permissive role in collapse of upper airway. Alcohol and sedatives exacerbate the condition. Most pts have structural narrowing of upper airway. Most pts have obstruction at nasal or palatal level. Mandibular deformities (retrognathia) also predispose. Symptoms include snoring, excessive daytime sleepiness, memory loss, and impotence. Nocturnal hypoxia, a consequence of apnea, may contribute to arrhythmias, pulmonary hypertension, and right heart failure.

Diagnosis   This requires overnight observation of the pt. The definitive test for obstructive sleep apnea is overnight polysomnography, including sleep staging and respiratory monitoring.

[Rx] **TREATMENT**   (See Table 126-2)
Therapy is directed at increasing upper airway size, increasing upper airway tone, and minimizing upper airway collapsing pressures. Weight loss often reduces disease severity. Majority of pts with severe sleep apnea require nasal continuous positive airway pressure (nasal C-PAP). Mandibular positioning device (dental) may treat pts with mild or moderate disease. Surgery (uvulopalatopharyngoplasty) is usually reserved for pts who fail other therapies.

HYPERVENTILATION

Increased ventilation, causing Pa_{CO_2} <37 mmHg. Causes include lesions of the CNS, metabolic acidosis, anxiety, drugs (e.g., salicylates), hypoxemia, hypoglycemia, hepatic coma, and sepsis. Hyperventilation also may occur with some types of lung disease, particularly interstitial disease and pulmonary edema.

Table 126-2

Management of Obstructive Sleep Apnea (OSA)

Mechanism	Mild to Moderate OSA	Moderate to Severe OSA
↑ Upper airway muscle tone	Avoidance of alcohol, sedatives	Tricyclics
↑ Upper airway lumen size	Weight reduction Avoidance of supine posture Oral prosthesis	Uvulopalato-pharyngoplasty
↓ Upper airway subatmospheric pressure Bypass occlusion	Improved nasal patency	Nasal continuous positive airway pressure Tracheostomy

SOURCE: Phillipson EA: HPIM-14, p. 1482.

For a more detailed discussion, see Phillipson EA: Disorders of Ventilation, Chap. 263, p. 1476, and Sleep Apnea, Chap. 264, p. 1480, in HPIM-14.

127

PULMONARY INSUFFICIENCY AND ACUTE RESPIRATORY DISTRESS SYNDROME (ARDS)

ARDS is a descriptive term applied to many acute, diffuse infiltrative lung lesions of diverse etiologies (see Table 127-1) with severe arterial hypoxemia.

Clinical Characteristics and Pathophysiology

Earliest sign is often tachypnea followed by dyspnea. Arterial blood gas shows reduction of P_{O_2} and P_{CO_2} with widened alveolar-arterial O_2 difference. Physical exam and CXR may be normal initially. With progression, pt becomes cyanotic, dyspneic, and increasingly tachypneic. Crackles become audible diffusely, and CXR shows diffuse, bilateral, interstitial and alveolar infiltrates.

ARDS increases lung water without increasing hydrostatic forces. Toxic gases (chlorine, NO_2, smoke) and gastric acid

Table 127-1

Conditions That May Lead to the Acute Respiratory Distress Syndrome

1. Diffuse pulmonary infections (e.g., viral, bacterial, fungal, *Pneumocystis*)
2. Aspiration (e.g., gastric contents with Mendelson's syndrome, water with near drowning)
3. Inhalation of toxins and irritants (e.g., chlorine gas, NO_2, smoke, ozone, high concentrations of oxygen)
4. Narcotic overdose pulmonary edema (e.g., heroin, methadone, morphine, dextropropoxyphene)
5. Nonnarcotic drug effects (e.g., nitrofurantoin)
6. Immunologic response to host antigens (e.g., Goodpasture's syndrome, systemic lupus erythematosus)
7. Effects of nonthoracic trauma with hypotension
8. In association with systemic reactions to processes initiated outside the lung (e.g., gram-negative septicemia, hemorrhagic pancreatitis, amniotic fluid embolism, fat embolism)
9. Postcardiopulmonary bypass ("pump lung," "postperfusion lung")

SOURCE: Honig EG, Ingram RH Jr: HPIM-14, p. 1484.

aspiration damage the alveolar-capillary membrane directly, whereas sepsis increases alveolar-capillary permeability by producing activation and aggregation of formed blood elements. Though radiologically diffuse, regional lung dysfunction is nonhomogeneous with severe ventilation-perfusion imbalance and actual shunting of blood through collapsed alveoli.

℞ TREATMENT

Early in illness, supplemental O_2 may be sufficient to correct hypoxemia, but with progression mechanical ventilatory support is necessary. Goal of therapy is to provide adequate tissue O_2 delivery—determined by arterial oxygen saturation (Sa_{O_2}), hemoglobin (Hb), cardiac output, and blood flow distribution. Reasonable objective is to achieve 90% saturation (Pa_{O_2} 8 kPa or 60 mmHg) with the lowest inspired O_2 concentration practical to avoid O_2 toxicity (FI_{O_2} <0.6). Hb should be ≥100 g/L (≥10 g/dL). Cardiac output is supported as necessary with IV fluids and inotropic agents. Pulmonary artery catheter insertion may be necessary for accurate assessment of ventricular filling pressures, hemodynamics, and O_2 transport. Because airspace disease is nonhomogeneous, large-volume breaths are administered preferentially to normal areas of lung, causing alveolar overdistention and furthering lung injury ("volutrauma"). Avoidance of overdistention is accomplished by using pressure-cycled mechanical ventilation with maximal distending pressure of 35 cmH2O. Positive end-expiratory pressure (PEEP, 15 cmH2O) is used to prevent alveolar collapse. Pressure limitation frequently results in hypoventilation and hypercarbia. Inadequate oxygenation is corrected with: (1) prone positioning, which improves gas exchange; and (2) prolonged inspiratory times (inverse ratio ventilation), which increases mean lung volumes. Experimental techniques such as inhaled nitric oxide may also be used to improve ventilation-perfusion matching.

Complications

1. *LV failure* is a common, easily missed complication, particularly in pts receiving mechanical ventilation.
2. *Secondary bacterial infection* may be obscured by the diffuse roentgenographic changes.
3. *Bronchial obstruction* may be caused by endotracheal or tracheostomy tubes.
4. *Pneumothorax and pneumomediastinum* may cause abrupt deterioration in pts receiving mechanical ventilation.

Prognosis

Overall mortality rate is 50% and varies with the intrinsic mortality of the underlying condition, but preliminary studies suggest new ventilator strategies may reduce mortality. If ARDS occurs as a result of extrapulmonic sepsis, multiple organ failure often supervenes.

For a more detailed discussion, see Honig EG, Ingram RH Jr: Acute Respiratory Distress Syndrome, Chap. 265, p. 1483, in HPIM-14.

128

APPROACH TO PATIENT WITH RENAL DISEASE

The approach to renal disease begins with recognition of particular syndromes on the basis of findings such as presence or absence of azotemia, proteinuria, hypertension, edema, abnormal UA, electrolyte disorders, abnormal urine volumes, or infection (Table 128-1).

Acute Renal Failure (See Chap. 129)

Clinical syndrome is characterized by a rapid, severe decrease in GFR (rise in serum creatinine and BUN), usually with reduced urine output. Extracellular fluid expansion leads to edema, hypertension, and CHF. Hyperkalemia, hyponatremia, and acidosis are common. Etiologies include ischemia, nephrotoxic injury due to drugs or endogenous pigments, sepsis, severe renovascular disease, or conditions related to pregnancy. Prerenal and postrenal failure are potentially reversible causes.

RAPIDLY PROGRESSIVE GLOMERULONEPHRITIS Loss of renal function occurs over weeks to months. Pts are initially nonoliguric and may have recent flulike symptoms; later, oliguric renal failure with uremic symptoms supervenes. Pulmonary manifestations range from asymptomatic infiltrates to life-threatening hemoptysis. UA shows hematuria, proteinuria, and RBC casts.

ACUTE GLOMERULONEPHRITIS (See Chap. 132) An acute illness with sudden onset of hematuria, edema, hypertension, oliguria, and elevated BUN and creatinine. Mild pulmonary congestion may be present. An antecedent or concurrent infection or multisystem disease may be causative, or glomerular disease may exist alone. Hematuria, proteinuria, and pyuria are usually present, and RBC casts confirm the diagnosis. Serum complement may be decreased.

Chronic Renal Failure (See Chap. 130)

Progressive permanent loss of renal function over months to years does not cause symptoms of uremia until GFR is reduced to about 25% of normal. Hypertension may occur early. Later,

Table 128-1

Initial Clinical and Laboratory Data Base for Defining Major Syndromes in Nephrology

Syndromes	Important Clues to Diagnosis	Common Findings
Acute or rapidly progressive renal failure	Anuria Oliguria Documented recent decline in GFR	Hypertension, hematuria Proteinuria, pyuria Casts, edema
Acute nephritis	Hematuria, RBC casts Azotemia, oliguria Edema, hypertension	Proteinuria Pyuria Circulatory congestion
Chronic renal failure	Azotemia for >3 months Prolonged symptoms or signs of uremia Symptoms or signs of renal osteodystrophy Kidneys reduced in size bilaterally Broad casts in urinary sediment	Hematuria, proteinuria Casts, oliguria Polyuria, nocturia Edema, hypertension Electrolyte disorders
Nephrotic syndrome	Protienuria >3.5 g per 1.73 m^2 per 24 h Hypoalbuminemia Hyperlipidemia Lipiduria	Casts Edema
Asymptomatic urinary abnormalities	Hematuria Proteinuria (below nephrotic range) Sterile pyuria, casts	
Urinary tract infection	Bacteriuria >10^5 colonies per milliliter Other infectious agent documented in urine Pyuria, leukocyte casts Frequency, urgency Bladder tenderness, flank tenderness	Hematuria Mild azotemia Mild proteinuria Fever

(*continued*)

Table 128-1 (*Continued*)

Initial Clinical and Laboratory Data Base for Defining Major Syndromes in Nephrology

Syndromes	Important Clues to Diagnosis	Common Findings
Renal tubule defects	Electrolyte disorders	Hematuria
	Polyuria, nocturia	"Tubular" proteinuria
	Symptoms or signs of renal osteodystrophy	Enuresis
	Large kidneys	
	Renal transport defects	
Hypertension	Systolic/diastolic hypertension	Proteinuria
		Casts
		Azotemia
Nephrolithiasis	Previous history of stone passage or removal	Hematuria
	Previous history of stone seen by x-ray	Pyuria
	Renal colic	Frequency, urgency
Urinary tract obstruction	Azotemia, oliguria, anuria	Hematuria
	Polyuria, nocturia, urinary retention	Pyuria
	Slowing of urinary stream	Enuresis, dysuria
	Large prostrate, large kidneys	
	Flank tenderness, full bladder after voiding	

SOURCE: Modified from Coe FL, Brenner BM: HPIM-14.

manifestations include anorexia, nausea, vomiting, insomnia, weight loss, weakness, paresthesia, bleeding, serositis, anemia, acidosis, and hyperkalemia. Causes include diabetes mellitus, hypertension, urinary tract obstruction, interstitial nephritis. Indications of chronicity include long-standing azotemia, anemia, hyperphosphatemia, hypocalcemia, shrunken kidneys, renal osteodystrophy by x-ray, or findings on renal biopsy.

Nephrotic Syndrome (See Chap. 132)

Defined as heavy albuminuria (>3.5 g/d in the adult) with or without edema, hypoalbuminemia, hyperlipidemia, and varying degrees of renal insufficiency. Can be idiopathic or due to drugs, infections, neoplasms, multisystem or hereditary diseases. Complications include severe edema, thromboembolic events, infection, and protein malnutrition.

Asymptomatic Urinary Abnormalities

Hematuria may be due to neoplasms, stones, or infection at any level of the urinary tract, sickle cell disease, or analgesic abuse. Renal parenchymal causes are suggested by RBC casts, proteinuria, or dysmorphic RBCs in urine. Pattern of gross hematuria may be helpful in localizing site. Hematuria with low-grade proteinuria may be due to benign recurrent hematuria or IgA nephropathy. Modest *proteinuria* may be an isolated finding due to fever, exertion, CHF, or upright posture. Renal causes include diabetes mellitus, amyloidosis, or other mild glomerular disease. *Pyuria* can be caused by UTI, interstitial nephritis, SLE, or renal transplant rejection. "Sterile" pyuria is associated with UTI treated with antibiotics, glucocorticoid therapy, acute febrile episodes, cyclophosphamide therapy, pregnancy, renal transplant rejection, genitourinary trauma, prostatitis, cystourethritis, tuberculosis and other mycobacterial infections, fungal infection, *Haemophilus influenzae,* anaerobic infection, fastidious bacteria, and bacterial L forms.

Urinary Tract Infection (See Chap. 134)

Generally defined as greater than 10^5 bacteria/mL of urine. Levels between 10^2 and 10^5/mL may indicate infection but are usually due to poor sample collection, especially if mixed flora are present. Adults at risk are sexually active women or anyone with urinary tract obstruction, reflux, catheterization, or neurogenic bladder. Prostatitis, urethritis, and vaginitis may be distinguished by quantitative urine culture. Flank pain, nausea, vomiting, fever, and chills indicate kidney infection. UTI is a common cause of sepsis.

Renal Tubular Defects (See Chap. 133)

Generally inherited, they include anatomic defects (polycystic kidneys, medullary cystic disease, medullary sponge kidney) detected in the evaluation of hematuria, flank pain, infection, or renal failure of unknown cause and disorders of tubular transport that cause glucosuria, aminoaciduria, stones, or rickets. Fanconi syndrome is a generalized tubular defect that can be hereditary or due to drugs, heavy metals, multiple myeloma, amyloidosis, or renal transplantation. Nephrogenic diabetes insipidus (polyuria, polydypsia, hypernatremia, hypernatremic dehydration) and renal tubular acidosis are additional causes.

Hypertension (See Chap. 115)

Blood pressure $\geq 140/90$ mmHg may affect 20% of the U.S. adult population and when inadequately controlled is an important cause of cerebrovascular accident, MI, CHF, and renal failure. Hypertension is usually asymptomatic until cardiac, renal, or neurologic symptoms appear. Most is idiopathic and occurs between ages 25 and 45.

Nephrolithiasis (See Chap. 136)

Causes colicky pain, UTI, hematuria, dysuria, or unexplained pyuria. Stones may be found on routine x-ray. Most are radiopaque Ca stones, associated with a high level of urinary Ca excretion. Staghorn calculi are large, branching radiopaque stones within the renal pelvis due to recurrent infection. Uric acid stones are radiolucent. UA may reveal hematuria, pyuria, or pathologic crystals.

Urinary Tract Obstruction (See Chap. 137)

Causes variable symptoms depending on whether it is acute or chronic, unilateral or bilateral, complete or partial, and on underlying etiology. It is an important reversible cause of unexplained renal failure. Upper tract obstruction may be silent or produce flank pain, hematuria, and renal infection. Bladder symptoms may be present in lower tract obstruction. Functional consequences include polyuria, anuria, nocturia, acidosis, hyperkalemia, and hypertension. A flank or suprapubic mass may be found on physical exam.

For a more detailed discussion, see Coe FL, Brenner BM: Approach to the Patient with Diseases of the Kidneys and Urinary Tract, Chap. 268, p. 1495, in HPIM-14.

129

ACUTE RENAL FAILURE

Definition

Acute renal failure (ARF), defined as a measurable increase in the serum creatinine (Cr) concentration (usually relative increase of 50% or absolute increase of 0.5 to 1.0 mg/dL) occurs in approximately 5% of hospitalized pts. It is associated with a substantial increase in in-hospital mortality and morbidity. ARF can be anticipated in some clinical circumstances (e.g., before radiocontrast exposure or major surgery), and there are no specific pharmacologic therapies proven helpful at preventing or reversing the condition. Maintaining optimal renal perfusion and intravascular volume appears to be important in most clinical circumstances.

Differential Diagnosis

The separation into three broad categories (prerenal, intrinsic renal, and postrenal failure) is of great clinical utility (Table 129-1). *Prerenal failure* is most common among hospitalized pts. It may result from true volume depletion (e.g., diarrhea, vomiting, GI or other hemorrhage) or "effective circulatory volume depletion," i.e., reduced renal perfusion in the setting of adequate or excess blood volume. Reduced renal perfusion may be seen in CHF (due to reduced cardiac output and/or potent vasodilator therapy), hepatic cirrhosis (due most likely to arteriovenous shunting), nephrotic syndrome and other states of severe hypoproteinemia (total serum protein <5 g/dL), and renovascular disease (because of fixed stenosis at the level of the main renal artery or large branch vessels). Several drugs can reduce renal perfusion, most notably NSAIDs. ACE-inhibitors may reduce GFR but do *not* tend to reduce renal perfusion.

Causes of *intrinsic* renal failure depend on the clinical setting. Among hospitalized pts, especially on surgical services or in intensive care units, acute tubular necrosis (ATN) is the most common diagnosis. Allergic interstitial nephritis, usually due to antibiotics (e.g., penicillins, cephalosporins, sulfa drugs, quinolones, and rifampin) may also be responsible. These conditions are relatively uncommon in the outpatient setting. There, intrinsic disease due to glomerulonephritis or pyelonephritis predominates.

Postrenal failure is due to urinary tract obstruction, which is also more common among ambulatory rather than hospitalized pts. More common in men than women, it is most often caused by ureteral or urethral blockade. Occasionally, stones or renal papillae may cause more proximal obstruction.

Table 129-1

Common Causes of Acute Renal Failure

PRERENAL

Volume depletion
  Blood loss
  GI fluid loss (e.g., vomiting, diarrhea)
  Overzealous diuretic use
Volume overload with reduced renal perfusion
  Congestive heart failure
    Low-output with systolic dysfunction
    "High-output" (e.g., anemia, thyrotoxicosis)
  Hepatic cirrhosis
  Severe hypoproteinemia
Renovascular disease
Drugs
  NSAIDs, cyclosporine, amphotericin B
Other
  Hypercalcemia, "third spacing" (e.g., pancreatitis, sys-
    temic inflammatory response), hepatorenal syndrome

INTRINSIC

Acute tubular necrosis (ATN)
  Hypotension or shock, prolonged prerenal azotemia, post-
    operative sepsis syndrome, rhabdomyolysis, hemolysis,
    drugs
    Radiocontrast, aminoglycosides, cisplatin
Other tubulointerstitial disease
  Allergic interstitial nephritis
  Pyelonephritis (bilateral, or unilateral in single functional
    kidney)
  Heavy metal poisoning
Atheroembolic disease
Glomerulonephritis
  "Rapidly progressive"
    Wegener's granulomatosis
    Anti-GBM disease (Goodpasture's syndrome)
    PAN and other pauci-immune GN
  Immune complex–mediated
    Subacute bacterial endocarditis, SLE, cryoglobulinemia
      (with or without hepatitis C infection), postinfectious
      GN
  Other
    IgA nephropathy (Henoch-Schönlein purpura), HUS/
      TTP, preeclampsia

(continued)

Table 129-1 (Continued)

Common Causes of Acute Renal Failure

POSTRENAL (URINARY TRACT OBSTRUCTION)

Bladder neck obstruction, bladder calculi
Prostatic hypertrophy
Ureteral obstruction due to compression
    Pelvic or abdominal malignancy, retroperitoneal fibrosis
Nephrolithiasis
Papillary necrosis with obstruction

NOTE: GBM, glomerular basement membrane; PAN, polyarteritis nodosa.

Characteristic Findings and Diagnostic Workup

All pts with ARF manifest some degree of azotemia (increased BUN and Cr). Other clinical features depend on the etiology of renal disease. Pts with prerenal azotemia due to volume depletion usually demonstrate orthostatic hypotension, tachycardia, low JVP, and dry mucous membranes. Pts with prerenal azotemia and CHF may show jugular venous distention, an S_3 gallop, and peripheral and pulmonary edema. Therefore, the physical exam is critical in the workup of pts with prerenal ARF. In general, the BUN/Cr ratio tends to be high (>20:1), more so with volume depletion and CHF than with cirrhosis. The uric acid may also be disproportionately elevated in noncirrhotic prerenal states (due to increased proximal tubular absorption overall). Urine chemistries tend to show low urine Na (<10–20 mmol/L, <<10 with hepatorenal syndrome) and a fractional excretion of sodium (FENa) << 1% (Table 129-2). The UA typically shows hyaline and a few granular casts, without cells or cellular casts. Renal ultrasonography is usually normal.

Pts with *intrinsic renal disease* present with varying complaints. Glomerulonephritis (GN) is often accompanied by hypertension and mild to moderate edema (associated with Na retention and proteinuria, and sometimes with hematuria). The urine chemistries may be indistinguishable from those in pts with prerenal failure; in fact, some pts with GN have renal hypoperfusion (due to glomerular inflammation and ischemia) with resultant hyperreninemia leading to hypertension. The urine sediment is most helpful in these cases. RBC, WBC, and cellular casts are characteristic of GN; RBC casts are rarely seen in other conditions (i.e., high specificity). In the setting of inflammatory nephritis (GN or interstitial nephritis, see below),

Table 129-2

Urine Diagnostic Indices in Differentiation of Prerenal versus Intrinsic Renal Azotemia

Diagnostic Index	Typical Findings	
	Prerenal Azotemia	Intrinsic Renal Azotemia
Fractional excretion of sodium (%)* $$\frac{U_{Na} \times P_{Cr}}{P_{Na} \times U_{Cr}} \times 100$$	<1	>1
Urine sodium concentration (mmol/L)	<10	>20
Urine creatinine to plasma creatinine ratio	>40	>20
Urine urea nitrogen to plasma urea nitrogen ratio	>8	<3
Urine specific gravity	>1.018	<1.015
Urine osmolality (mosmol/kg H_2O)	>500	<300
Plasma BUN/creatinine ratio	>20	<10–15
Renal failure index* $$\frac{U_{Na}}{U_{Cr}/P_{cr}}$$	<1	>1
Urinary sediment	Hyaline casts	Muddy brown granular casts

*Most sensitive indices.

NOTE: U_{Na}, urine sodium concentration; P_{Cr}, plasma creatinine concentration; P_{Na}, plasma sodium concentration; U_{Cr}, urine creatinine concentration.

there may be increased renal echogenicity on ultrasonography, so-called "medical renal disease." Unlike pts with GN, pts with interstitial diseases are less likely to have hypertension or proteinuria. Hematuria and pyuria may present on UA; the classic sediment finding in allergic interstitial nephritis is a predominance (>10%) of urinary eosinophils with Wright's or Hansel's stain. WBC casts may also be seen, particularly in cases of pyelonephritis.

Pts with postrenal ARF due to urinary tract obstruction are usually less severely ill than pts with prerenal or intrinsic renal disease, and their presentation may be delayed until azotemia is markedly advanced (BUN > 150, Cr > 12–15 mg/dL). An associated impairment of urinary concentrating ability often "protects" the pt from complications of volume overload. Urinary electrolytes typically show a FENa >1%, and microscopic examination of the urinary sediment is usually bland. Ultrasonography is the key diagnostic tool. More than 90% of pts with postrenal ARF show obstruction of the urinary collection system on ultrasound (e.g., dilated ureter, calyces); false negatives include hyperacute obstruction and encasement of the ureter and/or kidney by tumor, functionally obstructing urinary outflow without structural dilatation.

Rx **TREATMENT**

This should focus on providing etiology-specific supportive care. For example, pts with prerenal failure due to GI fluid loss may experience relatively rapid correction of their ARF after the administration of IV fluid to expand volume. The same treatment in prerenal pts with CHF would be counterproductive; in this case, treatment of the underlying disease with vasodilators and/or inotropic agents would more likely be of benefit.

There are relatively few intrinsic renal causes of ARF for which there is safe and effective therapy. ARF associated with vasculitis may respond to high-dose glucocorticoids and cytotoxic agents (e.g., cyclophosphamide); plasmapheresis and plasma exchange may be useful in other selected circumstances [e.g., Goodpasture's syndrome and hemolytic-uremic syndrome/thrombotic thrombocytopenic purpura (HUS/TTP), respectively]. Antibiotic therapy may be sufficient for the treatment of ARF associated with pyelonephritis or endocarditis. There are conflicting data regarding the utility of glucocorticoids in allergic interstitial nephritis. Many practitioners advocate their use with clinical evidence of progressive renal insufficiency despite discontinuation of the offending drug, or with biopsy evidence of potentially reversible, severe disease.

The treatment of urinary tract obstruction often involves consultation with a urologist. Interventions as simple as Foley catheter placement to as complicated as multiple ureteral stents and/or nephrostomy tubes may be required.

Dialysis for ARF and Recovery of Renal Function Most cases of community- and hospital-acquired ARF resolve with conservative supportive measures, time, and patience. If nonprerenal ARF continues to progress, dialysis must be considered. Traditional indications include: volume overload refractory to diuretic agents; hyperkalemia; encephalopathy not otherwise explained; pericarditis, pleuritis, or other inflammatory serositis; and severe metabolic acidosis, compromising respiratory or circulatory function. The inability to provide requisite fluids for antibiotics, inotropes and other drugs, and/or nutrition should also be considered an indication for dialysis.

Dialytic options for ARF include (1) intermittent hemodialysis (IHD), (2) peritoneal dialysis (PD), and (3) continuous renal replacement therapy (CRRT, i.e., continuous arteriovenous or venovenous hemodiafiltration). Most pts are treated with IHD. The use of a noncellulosic membrane for IHD may limit renal injury in selected pt groups. At many centers, CRRT is prescribed only in pts intolerant of IHD, usually because of hypotension; other centers use it as the modality of choice for pts in intensive care units.

For a more detailed discussion, see Brady HR, Brenner BM: Acute Renal Failure, Chap. 270, p. 1504, in HPIM-14.

130

CHRONIC RENAL FAILURE (CRF) AND UREMIA

Epidemiology

The prevalence of CRF, defined as a long-standing, irreversible impairment of renal function is thought to be substantially greater than the number of pts with end-stage renal disease (ESRD), now > 300,000 in the U.S. There is a spectrum of disease related to decrements in renal function; clinical and therapeutic issues differ greatly depending on whether the GFR reduction is moderate (e.g., 20–60 mL/min) or severe (<20 mL/min). Dialysis is usually required to control symptoms of uremia with GFR <5–10 mL/min. Common causes of CRF are outlined in Table 130-1.

Differential Diagnosis

The first step in the differential diagnosis of CRF is establishing its chronicity, i.e., disproving a major acute component. The

Table 130-1

Common Causes of Chronic Renal Failure

Diabetic nephropathy
Hypertensive nephrosclerosis*
Glomerulonephritis
Renovascular disease (ischemic nephropathy)
Polycystic kidney disease
Reflux nephropathy and other congenital renal diseases
Interstitial nephritis, including analgesic nephropathy
HIV-associated nephropathy
Transplant allograft failure ("chronic rejection")

* Often diagnosis of exclusion; very few pts undergo renal biopsy; may be occult renal disease with hypertension.

most common means of determining disease chronicity is the renal ultrasound, which is used to measure kidney size. In general, kidneys that have shrunk (<10–11.5 cm, depending on body size) are more likely affected by chronic disease. While reasonably specific (few false positives), reduced kidney size is only a moderately sensitive marker for CRF; i.e., there are several relatively common conditions in which kidney disease may be chronic, without any reduction in renal size.

Diabetic nephropathy, HIV-associated nephropathy, and infiltrative diseases such as multiple myeloma may be associated with relatively large kidneys despite chronicity. Renal biopsy is a more reliable means of proving chronicity; a predominance of glomerulosclerosis or interstitial fibrosis argues strongly for chronic disease. Hyperphosphatemia and other metabolic derangements are not reliable indicators in distinguishing acute from chronic disease.

Once chronicity has been established, clues from the physical exam, laboratory panel, and urine sediment evaluation can be used to determine etiology. A detailed Hx will identify important comorbid conditions, such as diabetes, HIV seropositivity, or peripheral vascular disease. The family Hx is paramount in the workup of autosomal dominant polycystic kidney disease or hereditary nephritis (Alport's syndrome). An occupational Hx may reveal exposure to environmental toxins or culprit drugs (including over-the-counter agents, such as analgesics).

Physical exam may demonstrate abdominal masses (i.e., polycystic kidneys), diminished pulses (i.e., atherosclerotic peripheral vascular disease), or an abdominal bruit (i.e., renovascular disease). The Hx and exam may also yield important data garding severity of disease. The presence of foreshortened fingers (due to resorption of the distal phalangeal tufts) and/or subcutaneous nodules may be seen with advanced renal failure and secondary hyperparathyroidism. Excoriations (uremic pruritus), pallor (anemia), muscle wasting, and a nitrogenous fetor are all signs of advanced chronic renal disease, as are pericarditis, pleuritis, and asterixis, complications of particular concern that usually prompt the initiation of dialysis.

LABORATORY FINDINGS Serum and urine laboratory findings typically provide additional information useful in determining the etiology and severity of CRF. Heavy proteinuria (>3.5 g/d), hypoalbuminemia, hypercholesterolemia, and edema suggest nephrotic syndrome (see Chap. 132), pointing toward diabetic nephropathy, membranous nephropathy, focal segmental glomerulosclerosis, minimal change disease, amyloid, and HIV-associated nephropathy as principal causes. Proteinuria may decrease slightly with decreasing GFR but rarely to normal levels. Hyperkalemia and metabolic acidosis may complicate all forms of CRF eventually but are more prominent in pts with interstitial renal diseases.

The Uremic Syndrome

The culprit toxin(s) responsible for the uremic syndrome remain elusive. The serum creatinine (Cr) is the most common laboratory surrogate of renal function. The creatinine clearance (Cr_{Cl}) is calculated as the urine concentration divided by serum concentration multiplied by the urine flow rate; it approximates the GFR and is a more reliable indicator of renal function than the serum Cr alone. Uremic symptoms tend to develop with serum Cr > 6–8 mg/dL, or Cr_{Cl} < 10 mL/min.

Symptoms include anorexia, weight loss, dyspnea, fatigue, pruritus, sleep and taste disturbance, and confusion and other forms of encephalopathy. Key findings on physical exam include hypertension, jugular venous distention, pericardial and/or pleural friction rub, muscle wasting, asterixis, excoriations and ecchymoses. Laboratory abnormalities may include: hyperkalemia, hyperphosphatemia, metabolic acidosis, hypocalcemia, hyperuricemia, anemia, and hypoalbuminemia. Most of these abnormalities resolve with renal dialysis or transplantation (Chap. 131).

℞ TREATMENT

Hypertension complicates most forms of CRF and warrants aggressive treatment to reduce the risk of stroke and potentially to slow the progression of renal disease (see below). Volume overload contributes to hypertension in many cases, and potent diuretic agents are frequently required. Anemia can be reversed with recombinant human erythropoetin (rHuEPO); 2000–4000 units subcutaneously once or twice weekly can normalize Hb concentrations in most pts.

Hyperphosphatemia can be controlled with judicious restriction of dietary potassium and the use of postprandial phosphate binders, usually calcium-based salts (calcium carbonate or acetate). Hyperkalemia should be controlled with dietary potassium restriction. Sodium polystyrene sulfonate (Kayexalate) can be used in refractory cases, although dialysis should be considered if the potassium >6 mmol/L on repeated occasions. If these conditions cannot be conservatively controlled, dialysis should be instituted (Chap. 131). It is also advisable to begin dialysis if severe anorexia, weight loss, or hypoalbuminemia develop, as it has been definitively shown that outcomes for dialysis pts with malnutrition are particularly poor.

Slowing Progression of Renal Disease   Prospective clinical trials have explored the roles of blood pressure control and dietary protein restriction on the rate of progression of renal failure. Control of hypertension is of some benefit, although ACE inhibitors appear to exert unique beneficial effects, most likely due to their effects on intrarenal hemodynamics. These effects are most pronounced in pts with diabetic nephropathy and in those without diabetes but with significant proteinuria (>1 g/d). Dietary protein restriction may offer an additional benefit, particularly in these same subgroups.

For a more detailed discussion, see Lazarus JM, Brenner BM: Chronic Renal Failure, Chap. 271, p. 1513, in HPIM-14.

131

DIALYSIS AND TRANSPLANTATION

DIALYSIS

OVERVIEW   Initiation of dialysis usually depends on a combination of the pt's symptoms, comorbid conditions, and laboratory parameters. Unless a living donor is identified, transplantation is deferred by necessity, due to the scarcity of cadaveric donor organs (median waiting time 2–4 years at most transplant centers). Dialytic options include (in order of prevalence in U.S.): in-center hemodialysis, continuous ambulatory peritoneal dialysis, nocturnal cycled peritoneal dialysis, and home-hemodialysis. Roughly 75% of U.S. pts are started on hemodialysis.

HEMODIALYSIS   This requires direct access to the circulation, either via a native arteriovenous fistula, usually at the wrist (a "Brescia-Cimino" fistula); an arteriovenous graft, usually made of polytetrafluoroethylene; or a stiff, large-bore intravenous catheter. Blood is pumped through hollow fibers of an artificial kidney (the "dialyzer") and bathed with a solution of favorable chemical composition (isotonic, free of urea and other nitrogenous compounds, and generally low in potassium). Most pts undergo dialysis thrice weekly, usually for 3–4 h. The efficiency of dialysis is largely dependent on the duration of dialysis, the blood flow rate, dialysate flow rate, and surface area of the dialyzer. More intense dialysis is associated with reduced morbidity and mortality.

Complications of hemodialysis are outlined in Table 131-1. Many of these relate to the process of hemodialysis as an intense, intermittent therapy. In contrast to the native kidney or to perito-

Table 131-1

Complications of Hemodialysis

Hypotension
Accelerated vascular disease
Rapid loss of residual renal function
Access thrombosis
Access or catheter sepsis
Dialysis-related amyloidosis
Protein-calorie malnutrition
Hemorrhage
Dyspnea/hypoxemia*
Leukopenia*

*Particularly with first use of conventional modified cellulosic dialyzer.

Table 131-2

Complications of Peritoneal Dialysis

Peritonitis
Hyperglycemia
Hypertriglyceridemia
Obesity
Hypoproteinemia
Dialysis-related amyloidosis
Insufficient clearance due to vascular disease or other
   factors
Uremia secondary to loss of residual renal function

neal dialysis (PD), both major dialytic functions (i.e., clearance of solutes and fluid removal, or "ultrafiltration") are accomplished over relatively short time periods. The rapid flux of fluid can cause hypotension, even without a pt reaching "dry weight." This entity is common in diabetic pts whose neuropathy prevents the compensatory responses (vasoconstriction and tachycardia) to intravascular volume depletion. Occasionally, confusion or other CNS symptoms will occur. The dialysis "disequilibrium syndrome" refers to the development of headache, confusion, and rarely seizures, in association with rapid solute removal early in the pt's dialysis history, before adaptation to the procedure.

PERITONEAL DIALYSIS (PD) This does not require direct access to the circulation; rather, it obligates placement of a peritoneal ("Tenckoff") catheter that allows infusion of a dialysate solution into the abdominal cavity, which allows transfer of solutes (i.e., urea, potassium, other uremic molecules) across the peritoneal membrane, which serves as the "artificial kidney." This solution is similar to that used for hemodialysis, except that it must be sterile, and uses lactate, rather than bicarbonate, to provide base equivalents. PD is far less efficient at cleansing the bloodstream than hemodialysis and therefore requires a much longer duration of therapy. Pts generally have the choice of performing their own "exchanges" (2–3 L of dialysate, 4–5 times during daytime hours) or using an automated device at night. Compared with hemodialysis, PD offers the major advantages of (1) independence and flexibility, and (2) a more gentle hemodynamic profile.

Complications are outlined in Table 131-2. Peritonitis is the most important complication. In addition to the ill effects of the systemic inflammatory response, protein loss is magnified severalfold during the peritonitis episode. If severe or prolonged, an episode of peritonitis may prompt removal of the Tenckoff catheter or even discontinuation of the modality (i.e., switch to hemodialysis). Gram-positive organisms (especially *Staphylococcus aureus* and other *Staph* spp.) predominate; *Pseudomonas* or fungal (usually *Candida*) infections tend to be more resistant to medical therapy. Antibiotic administration may be intravenous or intraperitoneal in severe cases.

RENAL TRANSPLANTATION

With the advent of more potent and well-tolerated immunosuppressive regimens and further improvements in short-term graft survival, renal transplantation remains the treatment of choice for most pts with end-stage renal disease. Results are best with living-related transplantation, in part because of optimized tissue matching and in part because waiting time can be eliminated. Many centers have recently begun to perform living-unrelated donor (e.g., spousal) transplants. Graft survival in these cases has been superior to that observed with cadaveric transplants, although less favorable than living-related transplants. Factors that influence graft survival are outlined in Table 131-3. Contraindications to renal transplantation are outlined in Table 131-4.

REJECTION Immunologic rejection is the major hazard to the short-term success of renal transplantation. Rejection may be (1) hyperacute (immediate graft dysfunction due to presensitization) or (2) acute (sudden change in renal function occurring within weeks to months). Rejection is characterized by a rise in serum Cr, hypertension, fever, reduced urine output, and occasionally graft tenderness. A percutaneous renal transplant biopsy confirms the diagnosis. Treatment usually consists of a "pulse" of methylprednisolone (500–1000 mg/d for 3 days). In refractory or particularly severe cases, 7–10 days of a monoclonal antibody directed at human T lymphocytes (OKT3) may be given.

IMMUNOSUPPRESSION Maintenance immunosuppressive therapy usually consists of a two- or three-drug regimen, with each drug targeted at a different stage in the immune response. Cyclosporine is the cornerstone of immunosuppressive therapy. The most potent of orally available agents, its routine use has markedly improved short-term graft survival. Side effects of cyclosporine include hypertension, hyperkalemia, resting tremor, hirsutism, gingival hypertrophy, hyperlipidemia, hyperuricemia, and a slowly progressive loss of renal function with characteristic histopathologic patterns (also seen in exposed recipients of heart and liver transplants).

Table 131-3

Some Factors that Influence Graft Survival in Renal Transplantation

HLA mismatch	Decreases graft survival
Presensitization (preformed antibodies)	Decreases graft survival
Pretransplant blood transfusion	Increases graft survival (however, may lead to presensitization)
Very young or older donor age	Decreases graft survival
Female donor sex	Decreases graft survival
African-American donor race (compared with Caucasian)	Decreases graft survival
Older recipient age	Increases graft survival
African-American recipient race (compared with Caucasian)	Decreases graft survival
Prolonged cold ischemia time	Decreases graft survival
Large recipient body size	Decreases graft survival

Prednisone is frequently used in conjunction with cyclosporine, at least for the first several years following successful graft function. Side effects of prednisone include hypertension, glucose intolerance, Cushingoid features, osteoporosis, hyperlipidemia, acne, and depression and other mood disturbances.

Until recently, azathioprine was the most commonly used "third drug" in combination with cyclosporine and prednisone, although mycophenolate mofetil has become more popular in the past 1–2 years. Azathioprine is generally well tolerated; side effects include leukopenia (and occasionally anemia and thrombocytopenia), liver dysfunction, alopecia, and squamous cell carcinoma of the skin. The drug-drug interaction between azathioprine and allopurinol may complicate treatment of gout (a frequent complication of cyclosporine therapy). Mycophenolate mofetil has a similar mode of action and side-effect profile compared with azathioprine but appears to be more effective at preventing or reversing rejection.

Tacrolimus (FK-506) is similar in efficacy and side-effect profile to cyclosporine although it has been used more widely in liver than kidney transplantation. It is occasionally employed

Table 131-4

Contraindications to Renal Transplantation

ABSOLUTE CONTRAINDICATIONS

Active glomerulonephritis
Active bacterial or other infection
Active or very recent malignancy
HIV infection
Hepatitis B surface antigenemia
Severe degrees of comorbidity (e.g., advanced atherosclerotic vascular disease)

RELATIVE CONTRAINDICATIONS

Age greater than 70 years
Severe psychiatric disease
Moderately severe degrees of comorbidity
Hepatitis C infection with chronic hepatitis or cirrhosis
Noncompliance with dialysis or other medical therapy
Primary renal diseases
    Primary focal sclerosis with prior recurrence in transplant
    Multiple myeloma
    Amyloid
    Oxalosis

in pts with subacute or chronic rejection poorly controlled with cyclosporine. Other immunosuppressive agents are undergoing active clinical investigation.

OTHER COMPLICATIONS Infection and neoplasia are important complications of renal transplantation. Infection is common in the heavily immunosuppressed host (e.g., cadaveric transplant recipient with multiple episodes of rejection requiring steroid or other treatment). The culprit organism depends in part on characteristics of the donor and recipient and timing following transplantation. In the first month, bacterial organisms predominate. After 1 month, there is a significant risk of systemic infection with CMV, particularly in recipients without prior exposure whose donor was CMV positive. Prophylactic use of ganciclovir or high-titer CMV immune globulin can reduce the risk of disease. Later on, there is a substantial risk of fungal and related infections, especially in pts who are unable to taper prednisone to <20–30 mg per day. Daily low-dose trimethoprim-sulfamethoxazole is effective at reducing the risk of *Pneumocystis carinii* infection.

EBV-associated lymphoproliferative disease is the most important neoplastic complication of renal transplantation, especially in pts who receive polyclonal (antilymphocyte globulin, used at some centers for induction of immunosuppression) or monoclonal antibody therapy. Non-Hodgkin's lymphoma and squamous cell carcinoma of the skin are also more common in this population.

For a more detailed discussion, see Carpenter CB, Lazarus JM: Dialysis and Transplantation: Chap. 272, p. 1520, in HPIM-14.

132

GLOMERULAR DISEASES

ACUTE GLOMERULONEPHRITIS (AGN)

Characterized by development, over days, of azotemia, hypertension, edema, hematuria, proteinuria, and sometimes oliguria. Salt and water retention are due to reduced GFR and may result in circulatory congestion. RBC casts on UA confirm Dx. Proteinuria usually <3 g/d. Most forms of AGN are mediated by humoral immune mechanisms. Clinical course depends on underlying lesion (see Table 132-1).

ACUTE POSTSTREPTOCOCCAL GN The prototype and most common cause in childhood. Nephritis develops 1–3 weeks after pharyngeal or cutaneous infection with "nephritogenic" strains of group A beta-hemolytic streptococci. Dx depends on a positive pharyngeal or skin culture, rising antibody titers, and hypocomplementemia. Renal biopsy reveals diffuse proliferative GN. Treatment consists of correction of fluid and electrolyte imbalance. In most cases the disease is self-limited, although the prognosis is less favorable and urinary abnormalities are more likely to persist in adults.

POSTINFECTIOUS GN May follow other bacterial, viral, and parasitic infections. Examples are bacterial endocarditis,

Table 132-1

Causes of Acute Glomerulonephritis

I. Infectious diseases
   A. Poststreptococcal glomerulonephritis*
   B. Nonstreptococcal postinfectious glomerulonephritis
      1. Bacterial: infective endocarditis,* "shunt nephritis," sepsis,* pneumococcal pneumonia, typhoid fever, secondary syphilis, meningococcemia
      2. Viral: hepatitis B, infectious mononucleosis, mumps, measles, varicella, vaccinia, echovirus, and coxsackievirus
      3. Parasitic: malaria, toxoplasmosis
II. Multisystem diseases: SLE,* vasculitis,* Henoch-Schönlein purpura,* Goodpasture's syndrome
III. Primary glomerular diseases: mesangiocapillary glomerulonephritis, Berger's disease (IgA nephropathy),* "pure" mesangial proliferative glomerulonephritis
IV. Miscellaneous: Guillain-Barré syndrome, irradiation of Wilm's tumor, self-administered diphtheria-pertussis-tetanus vaccine, serum sickness

*Most common causes.

SOURCE: Glassock RJ, Brenner BM: HPIM-13.

sepsis, hepatitis B, and pneumococcal pneumonia. Features are milder than with poststreptococcal GN. Control of primary infection usually produces resolution of GN.

SLE (LUPUS)   Renal involvement is due to deposition of circulating immune complexes. Clinical features include arthralgias, skin rash, serositis, hair loss, and CNS disease. Nephrotic syndrome with renal insufficiency is common. Renal biopsy reveals mesangial, focal, or diffuse GN and membranous nephropathy. Diffuse GN, the most common finding, is characterized by an active sediment, severe proteinuria, and progressive renal insufficiency and may have an ominous prognosis. Pts have a positive ANA, anti-dsDNA, and ↓ complement. Treatment includes glucocorticoids and cytotoxic agents. Oral or IV monthly cyclophosphamide is most commonly employed. Azathioprine may be of benefit in some pts.

GOODPASTURE'S SYNDROME   Characterized by lung hemorrhage, GN, and circulating antibody to basement membrane, usually in young men. Hemoptysis may precede nephritis. Rapidly progressive renal failure is typical. Circulating anti-glomerular basement membrane (GBM) antibody and linear immunofluorescence on renal biopsy establish Dx. Linear IgG is also present on lung biopsy. Plasma exchange may produce remission. Severe lung hemorrhage is treated with IV glucocorticoids. Disease isolated to the kidney ("anti-GBM disease") may also occur.

HENOCH-SCHÖNLEIN PURPURA A generalized vasculitis causing GN, purpura, arthralgias, and abdominal pain; occurs mainly in children. Renal involvement is manifested by hematuria and proteinuria. Serum IgA is increased in half of pts. Renal biopsy is useful for prognosis. Treatment is symptomatic.

VASCULITIS *Polyarteritis nodosa* causes hypertension, arthralgias, neuropathy, and renal failure. Similar features plus palpable purpura and asthma are common in *hypersensitivity angiitis. Wegener's granulomatosis* involves upper respiratory tract and kidney and responds to cyclophosphamide.

RAPIDLY PROGRESSIVE GLOMERULONEPHRITIS

Characterized by gradual onset of hematuria, proteinuria, and renal failure, which progresses over a period of weeks to months. Crescentic GN is usually found on renal biopsy. The causes are outlined in Table 132-2. Prognosis for preservation of renal function is poor. Fifty percent of pts require dialysis within 6 months of diagnosis. Combinations of glucocorticoids in pulsed doses, cytotoxic agents (azathioprine, cyclophosphamide), and intensive plasma exchange may be useful, although no prospective clinical trial data are available.

NEPHROTIC SYNDROME (NS)

Characterized by albuminuria (>3.5 g/d) and hypoalbuminemia (<30 g/L) and accompanied by edema, hyperlipidemia, and lipiduria. Complications include renal vein thrombosis and other thromboembolic events, infection, vitamin D deficiency, protein malnutrition, and drug toxicities due to decreased protein binding.

In adults, a minority of cases are secondary to diabetes mellitus, SLE, amyloidosis, drugs, neoplasia, or other disorders (see Table 132-3). By exclusion, the remainder are idiopathic. Renal biopsy is required to make the diagnosis and determine therapy in idiopathic NS.

MINIMAL CHANGE DISEASE Causes about 15% of idiopathic NS in adults. Blood pressure is normal; GFR is normal or slightly reduced; urinary sediment is benign or may show

Table 132-2

Causes of Rapidly Progressive Glomerulonephritis

I. Infectious diseases
   A. Poststreptococcal glomerulonephritis*
   B. Infective endocarditis*
   C. Occult visceral sepsis
   D. Hepatitis B infection (with vasculitis and/or cryoglobulinemia)
   E. HIV infection (?)

II. Multisystem diseases
   A. Systemic lupus erythematosus*
   B. Henoch-Schönlein purpura*
   C. Systemic necrotizing vasculitis (including Wegener's granulomatosis)*
   D. Goodpasture's syndrome*
   E. Essential mixed (IgG/IgM) cryoglobulinemia
   F. Malignancy
   G. Relapsing polychondritis
   H. Rheumatoid arthritis (with vasculitis)

III. Drugs
   A. Penicillamine*
   B. Hydralazine
   C. Allopurinol (with vasculitis)
   D. Rifampin

IV. Idiopathic or primary glomerular disease
   A. Idiopathic crescentic glomerulonephritis*
      1. Type I—with linear deposits of Ig (anti-GBM antibody–mediated)
      2. Type II—with granular deposits of Ig (immune complex–mediated)
      3. Type III—with few or no immune deposits of Ig ("pauci-immune")
      4. Antineutrophil cytoplasmic antibody–induced, ? forme fruste of vasculitis
   B. Superimposed on another primary glomerular disease
      1. Mesangiocapillary (membranoproliferative glomerulonephritis)* (especially type II)
      2. Membranous glomerulonephritis*
      Berger's disease (IgA nephropathy)*

* Most common causes.

SOURCE: Glassock RJ, Brenner BM: HPIM-13.

Table 132-3

Causes of Nephrotic Syndrome (NS)

Systemic Causes (25%)	Glomerular Disease (75%)
Diabetes mellitus, SLE, amyloidosis	Membranous (40%)
Drugs: gold, penicillamine, probenecid, street heroin, captopril, NSAIDs	Minimal change disease (15%)
	Focal glomerulosclerosis (15%)
Infections: bacterial endocarditis, hepatitis B, shunt infections, syphilis, malaria	Membranoproliferative GN (7%)
	Mesangioproliferative GN (5%)
Malignancy: Hodgkin's and other lymphomas, leukemia, carcinoma of breast, GI tract	

SOURCE: Modified from Glassock RJ, Brenner BM: HPIM-13.

few RBCs. Protein selectivity is variable in adults. Recent URI, allergies, or immunizations are present in some cases. ARF may rarely occur, particularly among elderly persons. Renal biopsy shows only foot process fusion on electron microscopy. Remission of proteinuria with glucocorticoids carries a good prognosis; cytotoxic therapy may be required for relapse. Progression to renal failure is uncommon. Focal sclerosis has been suspected in some cases refractory to steroid therapy.

MEMBRANOUS GN   Characterized by subepithelial IgG deposits; accounts for 45% of adult NS. Pts present with edema and nephrotic proteinuria. Blood pressure, GFR, and urine sediment are usually normal at initial presentation. Hypertension, mild renal insufficiency, and abnormal urine sediment develop later. Renal vein thrombosis is common. Underlying diseases such as SLE, hepatitis B, and solid tumors and exposure to such drugs as captopril or penicillamine should be sought. Some pts progress to end-stage renal disease (ESRD); men and persons with very heavy proteinuria are at highest risk—glucocorticods are frequently prescribed but are rarely effective. Cytotoxic agents (chlorambucil or cyclophosphamide) may promote complete or partial remission in some pts.

FOCAL GLOMERULOSCLEROSIS   Involves fibrosis of portions of some (primarily juxtamedullary) glomeruli and is found in 15% of pts with NS. Hypertension, reduced GFR, and hematuria are typical. African-Americans are disproportionately affected.   Some cases may be a late stage of minimal change disease or be due to heroin abuse, vesicoureteral reflux, or AIDS. Fewer than half undergo remission with glucocorticoids; half progress to renal failure in 10 years. Focal glomerulosclerosis may recur in a renal transplant. Presence of azotemia or hypertension reflects poor prognosis.

MEMBRANOPROLIFERATIVE GLOMERULONE-PHRITIS (MPGN) Mesangial expansion and proliferation extend into the capillary loop. Two ultrastructural variants exist. In MPGN I, subendothelial electron-dense deposits are present, C3 is deposited in a granular pattern indicative of immune-complex pathogenesis, and IgG and the early components of complement may or may not be present. In MPGN II, the lamina densa of the GBM is transformed into an electron-dense character, as is the basement membrane in Bowman's capsule and tubules. C3 is found irregularly in the GBM. Small amounts of Ig (usually IgM) are present, but early components of complement are absent. Serum complement levels are decreased. MPGN affects young adults. Blood pressure and GFR are abnormal, and the urine sediment is active. Some have acute nephritis or hematuria. Similar lesions occur in SLE and hemolytic-uremic syndrome. Infection with hepatitis C virus has been linked to MPGN. Treatment with interferon α has resulted in remission of renal disease in some cases. Glucocorticoids, cytotoxic agents, antiplatelet agents, and plasmapheresis have been used with limited success. MPGN may recur in allografts.

DIABETIC NEPHROPATHY Common cause of NS. Pathologic changes include diffuse and/or nodular glomerulosclerosis, nephrosclerosis, chronic pyelonephritis, and papillary necrosis. *Clinical features* include proteinuria, hypertension, azotemia, and bacteriuria. Although prior duration of diabetes mellitus (DM) is variable, proteinuria may develop 10–15 years after onset, progress to NS, and then lead to renal failure over 3–5 years. Other complications of DM are common; retinopathy is nearly universal. Treatment with ACE inhibitors delays the onset of nephropathy and should be instituted in all pts tolerant to that class of drug. Aggressive management of hypertension and restriction of dietary protein may slow decline of renal function.

Evaluation of NS is shown in Table 132-4.

ASYMPTOMATIC URINARY ABNORMALITIES

Proteinuria in the nonnephrotic range and/or hematuria unaccompanied by edema, reduced GFR, or hypertension can be due to multiple causes (see Table 132-5).

Table 132-4

Evaluation of Nephrotic Syndrome

24-h urine for protein; creatinine clearance
Serum albumin, cholesterol, complement
Urine protein electrophoresis
Rule out SLE, diabetes mellitus
Review drug exposure
Renal biopsy
Consider malignancy (in elderly pt with membranous GN or minimal change disease)
Consider renal vein thrombosis (if membranous GN or symptoms of pulmonary embolism are present)

BERGER'S DISEASE, IgA NEPHROPATHY The most common cause of recurrent hematuria of glomerular origin; is most frequent in young men. Episodes of macroscropic hematuria are present with flulike symptoms, without skin rash, abdominal pain, or arthritis. Renal biopsy shows diffuse mesangial deposition of IgA, often with lesser amounts of IgG, nearly always by C3 and properdin but not by C1q or C4. Prognosis is variable; 50% develop ESRD within 25 years; men with heavy proteinuria are at highest risk. Glucocorticoids and other immunosuppressive agents have not proved successful. A recent trial of fish oil supplementation suggested a modest therapeutic benefit.

CHRONIC GLOMERULONEPHRITIS Characterized by persistent urinary abnormalities, slow progressive impairment of renal function, symmetrically contracted kidneys, moderate to heavy proteinuria, abnormal urinary sediment (especially RBC casts), and x-ray evidence of normal pyelocalyceal systems. The time to progression to ESRD is variable, hastened by uncontrolled hypertension and infections.

GLOMERULOPATHIES ASSOCIATED WITH MULTISYSTEM DISEASE (See Table 132-6)

Table 132-5

Glomerular Causes of Asymptomatic Urinary Abnormalities

I. Hematuria with or without proteinuria
  A. Primary glomerular diseases
    1. Berger's disease (IgA nephropathy)*
    2. Mesangiocapillary glomerulonephritis
    3. Other primary glomerular hematurias accompanied by "pure" mesangial proliferation, focal and segmental proliferative glomerulonephritis, or other lesions
    4. "Thin basement membrane" disease (? forme fruste of Alport's syndrome)
  B. Associated with multisystem or hereditary diseases
    1. Alport's syndrome and other "benign" familial hematurias*
    2. Fabry's disease
    3. Sickle cell disease
  C. Associated with infections
    1. Resolving poststreptococcal glomerulonephritis*
    2. Other postinfectious glomerulonephritides*
II. Isolated nonnephrotic proteinuria
  A. Primary glomerular diseases
    1. "Orthostatic" proteinuria*
    2. Focal and segmental glomerulosclerosis*
    3. Membranous glomerulonephritis*
  B. Associated with multisystem or heredofamilial diseases
    1. Diabetes mellitus*
    2. Amyloidosis*
    3. Nail-patella syndrome

*Most common.

SOURCE: Glassock RJ, Brenner BM: HPIM-13.

For a more detailed discussion, see Brady HR, O'Meara YM, Brenner BM: The Major Glomerulopathies, Chap. 274, p. 1536; and O'Meara YM, Brady HR, Brenner BM: Glomerulopathies Associated with Multisystem Diseases, Chap. 275, p. 1545, HPIM-14.

Table 132-6

Serologic Findings in Selected Multisystem Diseases Causing Glomerular Disease

Disease	C3	Ig	FANA	Anti-dsDNA	Anti-GBM	Cryo-Ig	CIC	ANCA
SLE	↓↓	↑IgG	+++	++	−	++	+++	±
Goodpasture's syndrome	−	−	−	−	+++	−	±	−
Henoch-Schönlein purpura	↑↓	↑IgA	−	−	−	+	++	−
Polyarteritis	↓↑	↑IgG	+	±	−	+	+++	++
Wegener's granulomatosis	→	↑IgA, IgE	−	−	−	±	+++	+++
Cryoglobulinemia	→	±↑IgG, IgA, IgD, IgE	−	−	−	+++	+++	−
Multiple myeloma	−	↑IgG	−	−	−	+	−	−
Waldenström's macroglobulinemia	−	↑IgM	−	−	−	−	−	−
Amyloidosis	−	± Ig	−	−	−	−	−	−

NOTE: C3, C3 component; Ig, immunoglobulin levels; FANA, fluorescent antinuclear antibody assay; anti-dsDNA, antibody to double-stranded (native) DNA; anti-GBM, antibody to glomerular basement membrane antigens; cryo-Ig, cryoimmunoglobulin; CIC, circulating immune complexes; ANCA, antineutrophil cytoplasmic antibody; −, normal; +, occasionally slightly abnormal; ++, often abnormal; +++, severely abnormal.

SOURCE: Glassock RJ, Brenner BM: HPIM-13.

133

RENAL TUBULAR DISEASE

Tubulointerstitial diseases constitute a diverse group of acute and chronic, hereditary and acquired disorders involving renal tubules and supporting structures (Table 133-1). Functionally, they may result in nephrogenic diabetes insipidus (DI) with polyuria, nocturia, non-anion-gap metabolic acidosis, salt-wasting, and hypo- or hyperkalemia. Azotemia is common, owing to associated glomerular fibrosis and/or ischemia. Compared with glomerulopathies, proteinuria and hematuria are less dramatic, and hypertension is less common. Functional consequences of tubular dysfunction are outlined in Table 133-2.

Acute (Allergic) Interstitial Nephritis (AIN)

Drugs are a leading cause of this type of renal failure, usually identified by a gradual rise in the serum creatinine at least several days after the institution of therapy, occasionally accompanied by fever, eosinophilia, rash, and arthralgias. In addition to azotemia, there may be evidence of tubular dysfunction (e.g., hyperkalemia, metabolic acidosis). Drugs that commonly cause AIN include: semisynthetic (i.e., methicillin, oxacillin, or nafcillin) and other penicillins, cephalosporins, sulfonamides, quinolones, rifampin, allopurinol, and cimetidine; NSAIDs may cause AIN with or without nephrotic syndrome. Urinalysis shows hematuria, pyuria, and eosinophiluria on Hansel's or Wright's stain.

Renal dysfunction usually improves after withdrawal of the offending drug, but complete recovery may be delayed and incomplete. In uncontrolled studies, glucocorticoids have been shown to promote earlier recovery of renal function. Other than kidney biopsy, no specific diagnostic tests are available. Acute pyelonephritis may also cause AIN, although it is rarely associated with renal failure, unless bilateral (or present in a single functioning kidney) or complicated by urinary tract obstruction, sepsis syndrome, or volume depletion.

Chronic Interstitial Nephritis (IN)

Analgesic nephropathy is an important cause of chronic renal failure (CRF) that results from the cumulative (in quantity and duration) effects of combination analgesic agents, usually phenacetin and aspirin. It is a more common cause of end-stage renal disease in Australia/New Zealand than elsewhere owing to the larger per capita ingestion of analgesic agents in that region of the world. Transitional cell carcinoma may develop. *Analgesic nephropathy* should be suspected in pts with a history of chronic headache or back pain with CRF that is otherwise

Table 133-1

Principal Causes of Tubulointerstitial Disease of the Kidney

TOXINS

Endogenous toxins
  Analgesic nephropathy*
  Lead nephropathy
  Miscellaneous nephrotoxins (e.g., antibiotics, cyclo-
    sporine, radiographic contrast media, heavy metals)*†
Metabolic toxins
  Acute uric acid nephropathy
  Gouty nephropathy*
  Hypercalcemic nephropathy
  Hypokalemic nephropathy
  Miscellaneous metabolic toxins (e.g., hyperoxaluria,
    cystinosis, Fabry's disease)

NEOPLASIA

Lymphoma
Leukemia
Multiple myeloma

IMMUNE DISORDERS

Hypersensitivity nephropathy*†
Sjögren's syndrome
Amyloidosis
Transplant rejection
HIV-associated nephropathy

(continued)

unexplained. Manifestations include papillary necrosis, calculi, sterile pyuria, and azotemia. Metabolic causes of chronic IN include: hypercalcemia (with nephrocalcinosis), oxalosis (primary or secondary, e.g., with intestinal malabsorption, leading to nephrocalcinosis), hypokalemia, and hyperuricemia or hyperuricosuria. Chronic IN can occur in association with several systemic diseases, including sarcoidosis, Sjögren's syndrome, tuberculosis, and following radiation or chemotherapy exposure (e.g., ifosfamide, cisplatin).

Table 133-1 (*Continued*)

Principal Causes of Tubulointerstitial Disease of the Kidney

VASCULAR DISORDERS

> Arteriolar nephrosclerosis*
> Atheroembolic disease
> Sickle cell nephropathy
> Acute tubular necrosis*†
> Medullary cystic disease
> Medullary sponge kidney
> Polycystic kidney disease

HEREDITARY RENAL DISEASES

> Hereditary nephritis (Alport's syndrome)

INFECTIOUS INJURY

> Acute pyelonephritis*†
> Chronic pyelonephritis

MISCELLANEOUS DISORDERS

> Chronic urinary tract obstruction*
> Vesicoureteral reflux*
> Radiation nephritis

*Common.

†Typically acute.

Polycystic Kidney Disease

Autosomal dominant polycystic kidney disease (ADPKD) is the most important hereditary renal disease (except perhaps for "essential" hypertension!). It is characterized clinically by episodic flank pain, hematuria (often gross), hypertension, and/or urinary infection in the third or fourth decade. The kidneys are often palpable and occasionally of very large size. Hepatic cysts and intracranial Berry aneurysms may also be present.

The expression of ADPKD is variable. Some persons discover the disease incidentally in late adult life, having had mild to moderate hypertension earlier. More often, azotemia is progressive and unfortunately does not appear to respond favorably to ACE inhibition or to the restriction of dietary protein intake. The diagnosis is usually made by ultrasonogra-

Table 133-2

Transport Dysfunctions of Tubulointerstitial Disease

Defect	Cause(s)
Reduced GFR*	Obliteration of microvasculature and obstruction of tubules
Fanconi syndrome	Damage to proximal tubular reabsorption of glucose, amino acids, phosphate, and bicarbonate
Hyperchloremic acidosis*	1. Reduced ammonia production 2. Inability to acidify the collecting duct fluid (distal renal tubular acidosis) 3. Proximal bicarbonate wasting
Tubular or small-molecular-weight proteinuria*	Failure of proximal tubule protein reabsorption
Polyuria, isothenuria*	Damage to medullary tubules and vasculature
Hyperkalemia*	Potassium secretory defects including aldosterone resistance
Salt wasting	Distal tubular damage with impaired sodium reabsorption

* Common

phy. Renal cysts are common (50% of persons >50 years have at least one cyst), and multiple renal cysts do not necessarily indicate the presence of ADPKD.

Renal Tubular Acidosis (RTA)

This describes a number of pathophysiologically distinct entities of tubular function whose common feature is the presence of a non-anion-gap metabolic acidosis. Diarrhea and RTA together constitute the vast majority of cases of non-anion-gap metabolic acidosis.

Distal (Type 1) RTA   Pts are unable to acidify the urine despite acidosis; it may be inherited (autosomal dominant) or acquired due to autoimmune and inflammatory diseases (e.g., Sjögren's syndrome, sarcoidosis), urinary tract obstruction, or amphotericin B therapy. Type I RTA may be associated with hypokalemia, hypercalciuria, and osteomalacia.

Proximal (Type II) RTA There is a defect in bicarbonate reabsorption, usually associated with glycosuria, aminoaciduria, phosphaturia, and uricosuria (indicating proximal tubular dysfunction); it may be inherited or acquired due to myeloma, renal transplantation, or drugs (e.g., ifosfamide, L-lysine). Treatment requires large doses of bicarbonate, which aggravates hypokalemia.

Type IV RTA Due to a defect in ammonium excretion, acidosis is accompanied by hyperkalemia and usually with low renin and aldosterone levels (and minimal response to exogenous mineralocorticoid). It is associated with diabetes, other forms of glomerulosclerosis, and many forms of advanced CRF (especially with tubulointerstitial component).

$\boxed{\text{R}_{\text{X}}}$ TREATMENT

Tubulointerstitial diseases associated with exogenous toxins (e.g., analgesic nephropathy, lead and other heavy metal nephropathy) should be treated by withdrawal of the offending toxin. Primary oxalosis may require liver (or combined liver-kidney) transplantation, but secondary oxalosis can be improved with a low-oxalate diet, generous fluid intake, and supplemental calcium salts with meals to bind intestinal oxalate and prevent hyperoxalemia/hyperoxaluria. Hypercalcemia due to multiple causes (e.g., primary hyperparathyroidism, vitamin D excess, thiazide therapy, milk-alkali syndrome) can usually be corrected once recognized. Pts with pyelonephritis due to reflux or recurrent UTI with ADPKD may benefit from suppressive antibiotic therapy. The treatment of RTA depends on type but focuses on correction of the acidosis and prevention of nephrolithiasis (type I), vitamin D deficiency and other metabolic complications (type II), and severe hyperkalemia (type IV).

For a more detailed discussion, see Brenner BM, Levy E, Hostetter TH: Tubulointerstitial Diseases of the Kidney, Chap. 276, p. 1553, in HPIM-14.

134

URINARY TRACT INFECTIONS

URETHRITIS, CYSTITIS, AND PYELONEPHRITIS

ETIOLOGY *Escherichia coli* causes ~80% of uncomplicated UTIs (those unassociated with catheters, urologic abnormalities, or calculi); *Proteus, Klebsiella,* and *Enterobacter* account for lesser percentages of cases. *Staphylococcus saprophyticus* causes 10–15% of acute symptomatic UTIs in young women. Pathogens in recurrent or catheter-associated infection, in infections following urologic manipulation, and in the setting of genitourinary (GU) obstruction or calculi include *E. coli, Proteus, Klebsiella, Enterobacter, Pseudomonas,* and *Serratia* as well as enterococci and *Staphylococcus aureus.* Isolation of *S. aureus* from the urine should always arouse suspicion of staphylococcal bacteremia and secondary infection of the kidney. Agents causing acute urinary symptoms and pyuria in the absence of demonstrable bacteriuria include *Chlamydia trachomatis, Neisseria gonorrhoeae,* and herpes simplex virus. *Candida* and other fungal species commonly colonize the urine of catheterized or diabetic pts.

PATHOGENESIS In the vast majority of UTIs, bacteria gain access to the bladder via the urethra. Ascent of bacteria from the bladder may follow and may lead to upper tract disease. Risk factors for UTIs include female gender, sexual activity, pregnancy, GU obstruction, neurogenic bladder dysfunction, and vesicoureteral reflux. Hematogenous pyelonephritis occurs most often in debilitated pts. Staphylococcemia or candidemia may lead to metastatic renal parenchymal infection.

EPIDEMIOLOGY UTIs may be categorized as catheter-associated (nosocomial) or non-catheter-associated (community-acquired). Acute infections are very common; the vast majority of symptomatic cases involve young women, for whom sexual activity augments the risk of infection. UTIs are rare among men under the age of 50. The development of asymptomatic bacteriuria parallels that of symptomatic infection: it, too, is rare among men under age 50 but common among women between ages 20 and 50 and very common among the elderly of either sex. Bacteriuria develops in at least 10–15% of hospitalized pts with indwelling urethral catheters; the risk of infection is about 3–5% per day of catheterization.

CLINICAL MANIFESTATIONS Bacteriuria can be asymptomatic. Dysuria, frequency, urgency, and suprapubic pain signal cystitis. One-third of pts with such symptoms and significant bacteriuria have concomitant, clinically silent upper tract disease. On the other hand, ~30% of women with acute dysuria do not have significant bacteriuria; some of them have urethritis due to a sexually transmitted pathogen (e.g., *N. gonorrhoeae, C. trachomatis,* or herpesvirus). Manifestations of acute pyelonephritis may include fever, shaking chills, nausea, vomiting, and diarrhea as well as flank pain and dysuria.

DIAGNOSIS Women with symptoms characteristic of acute uncomplicated cystitis may reasonably be treated empirically, either on the basis of Hx and physical findings alone or after confirmatory microscopy or leukocyte esterase determination. Urine should be cultured, however, when the diagnosis of cystitis is uncertain, when upper tract infection is suspected, or when any complicating factors are present. A colony count of $\geq 10^5$/mL in a voided midstream specimen generally indicates infection. In symptomatic women with pyuria, counts of only 10^2–10^4/mL of *E. coli, Klebsiella, Proteus,* or *S. saprophyticus* may also indicate infection, as does bacteriuria to any degree in a suprapubic aspirate or the presence of $\geq 10^2$ bacteria/mL in urine obtained by catheterization. Microscopy of urine from symptomatic pts can be of great value: the finding of bacteria on a gram-stained, unspun specimen indicates a colony count of at least 10^5/mL. The finding of bacteriuria with leukocyte casts suggests pyelonephritis. Asymptomatic bacteriuria should be documented twice before treatment is instituted. All males with UTI and any pt with obstructive disease and non-catheter-associated infection should be evaluated urologically.

℞ TREATMENT

Treat acute uncomplicated cystitis in nonpregnant women whose posttreatment follow-up can be ensured with single doses of trimethoprim-sulfamethoxazole (TMP-SMZ; 4 single-strength tablets) or a quinolone. Use a 3-d course of TMP-SMZ (1 double-strength tablet bid) or a quinolone in uncomplicated cases of longer standing or when follow-up is less reliable. Give a 7- to 14-d course to females with complicated cystitis and to all males with cystitis. Acute cystitis in pregnancy can be managed with 3–7 d of amoxicillin, nitrofurantoin, or a cephalosporin. For women with acute urethritis, choose treatment according to the suspected pathogen—e.g., doxycycline (100 mg PO bid × 7 d) for *C. trachomatis.* For acute uncomplicated pyelonephritis, a 14-d course of a fluoroquinolone, an aminoglycoside, or a third-generation cephalosporin is usually adequate. TMP-SMZ is also acceptable in areas where resistance to this agent among *E. coli* strains causing pyelonephritis remains low. Mildly symptomatic pts can be treated orally from the outset; all others should receive IV therapy until their condition improves. Complicated UTIs require broad-spectrum therapy (e.g., ceftriaxone, 1 g IV q12h) until specific sensitivity data become available. Confirmed asymptomatic bacteriuria calls for 7 d of treatment with an oral agent to which the isolate is sensitive. Recurrent symptomatic bacteriuria warrants prophylaxis daily or thrice weekly with agents such as nitrofurantoin (50 mg) or TMP-SMZ (80/400 mg).

PROSTATITIS

ETIOLOGY In non-catheter-associated cases, acute bacterial prostatitis is usually due to common gram-negative urinary tract pathogens (*E. coli* or *Klebsiella*). In catheter-associated cases, nosocomially acquired gram-negative rods or enterococci may also be involved. *E. coli, Klebsiella, Proteus,* or other uropathogenic organisms may also cause chronic prostatitis. Evidence for causative roles of *Ureaplasma urealyticum* and *C. trachomatis* in chronic prostatitis is inconclusive.

CLINICAL MANIFESTATIONS Acute bacterial prostatitis is characterized by fever, chills, dysuria, and extreme prostatic tenderness. It may occur spontaneously (generally in young men) or in association with an indwelling urethral catheter. Chronic bacterial prostatitis is often asymptomatic, and the prostate usually feels normal on palpation; perineal or lower back pain or obstructive symptoms develop in some cases. A pattern of relapsing cystitis in a middle-aged man suggests the diagnosis and is due to intermittent spread of the prostatic infection.

DIAGNOSIS Cultures of urine usually yield the bacterial pathogen. Vigorous prostatic massage should be avoided. Gram's staining of urine may be particularly useful in guiding empiric therapy for catheter-associated cases.

℞ **TREATMENT**
For acute prostatitis in which gram-negative pathogens are detected in the urine, initially use IV TMP-SMZ (160/800 mg bid), a cephalosporin, a fluoroquinolone, or an aminoglycoside; for cases in which gram-positive cocci are detected, use nafcillin (1–2 g q4h) or a cephalosporin. For catheter-associated acute prostatitis, use a fluoroquinolone, a third-generation cephalosporin, or an aminoglycoside until the etiologic agent has been isolated and tested for sensitivity. For treatment of chronic prostatitis, fluoroquinolones (e.g., ci-

profloxacin, 500 mg bid) have been more successful than other agents but must be given for at least 12 weeks to be effective.

For a more detailed discussion, see Stamm WE: Urinary Tract Infections and Pyelonephritis, Chap. 131, p. 817, in HPIM-14.

| 135 |

RENOVASCULAR DISEASE

Ischemic injury to the kidney depends on the rate, site, severity, and duration of vascular compromise. Manifestations range from painful infarction to acute renal failure (ARF), impaired GFR, hematuria, or tubular dysfunction. Renal ischemia of any etiology may cause renin-mediated hypertension.

Acute Occlusion of a Renal Artery

Can be due to thrombosis or embolism (from valvular disease, endocarditis, mural thrombi, or atrial arrhythmias).

Thrombosis of Renal Arteries   This is an important cause of deterioration of renal function, esp. in the elderly. Large renal infarcts cause pain, vomiting, nausea, hypertension, fever, proteinuria, hematuria, and elevated LDH and AST. In unilateral lesion, renal functional loss depends on contralateral function. IVP or radionuclide scan shows unilateral hypofunction; ultrasound is normal. Renal arteriography establishes diagnosis. With occlusions of large arteries, surgery may be the initial therapy; anticoagulation should be used for occlusions of small arteries.

Renal Atheroembolism   Usually arises when aortic angiography or surgery causes cholesterol embolization of small renal vessels. Renal insufficiency may develop suddenly or gradually. Associated findings are GI or retinal ischemia with cholesterol emboli visible on fundoscopic examination, neurologic deficits, livedo reticularis, toe gangrene, and hypertension. Skin or renal biopsy may be necessary for diagnosis. Heparin is contraindicated.

Renal Vein Thrombosis

This occurs in a variety of settings, including pregnancy, oral contraceptive use, trauma, nephrotic syndrome, dehydration (in infants), extrinsic compression of the renal vein (lymph nodes, aortic aneurysm, tumor), and invasion of the renal vein by renal cell carcinoma. Definitive Dx is established by selective renal renography. Streptokinase may be effective.

Renal Artery Stenosis

Main cause of renovascular hypertension; due to (1) atherosclerosis (two-thirds of cases; usually men aged >60 years, advanced retinopathy) or (2) fibromuscular dysplasia (a third of cases; usually white women aged <45 years, brief history of hypertension). Renal hypoperfusion activates renin-angiotensin-aldosterone axis. Suggestive clinical features include onset of hypertension <30 or >50 years of age, bruits, hypokalemic alkalosis, acute onset of hypertension or malignant hypertension, and hypertension resistant to medical therapy. Malignant hypertension (Chap. 115) also may be caused by renal vascular occlusion. Nitroprusside or calcium antagonists are generally effective in lowering bp.

The gold standard in diagnosis of renal artery stenosis is arteriography. Digital subtraction angiography is often useful to minimize IV contrast dye load. The least invasive and most reliable preliminary test in pts with normal renal function is the captopril renogram when combined with (1) postcaptopril plasma renin activity measurement of ≥ 12 (μg/L)/h, (2) an absolute increase of plasma renin activity of ≥ 10 (μg/L)/h, and (3) increase in plasma renin of $\geq 150\%$ or $\geq 400\%$ if baseline plasma renin activity is ≤ 3 (μg/L)/h. Measurement of renal vein renin may be necessary to demonstrate functional significance of a lesion.

Surgical revascularization achieves best results in fibromuscular disease. Those with localized atherosclerosis, esp. ostial lesions, also do well, but mortality is higher; surgery in pts with diffuse or bilateral lesions is best reserved for urgent cases who have failed medical management.

Angioplasty is most successful with fibromuscular disease and nonoccluded, nonostial atherosclerotic lesions; has a low complication rate and cost. In many pts (the elderly, those with impaired renal function, or those with high surgical risk), pharmacotherapy is employed. Converting-enzyme inhibitors are ideal drugs except in pts with bilateral stenosis or disease in solitary kidney.

Ischemic Nephropathy

In addition to the association between renal artery stenosis and hypertension, there is an important (and less well recognized) association between renal artery stenosis and progressive chronic renal failure. Because most pts do not undergo either kidney biopsy or angiography prior to the initiation of dialysis, it is difficult to estimate the incidence of renovascular disease as a primary cause of end-stage renal disease (some have suggested up to 15–20%, even greater among elderly).

The presence of widespread atherosclerotic vascular disease, asymmetric kidney size and function, and hypertension suggest renovascular disease; episodic "flash" pulmonary edema, renal insufficiency, and ARF in response to a trial of ACE inhibitors suggests that the disease may be severe and bilateral.

Revascularization with the goal of preservation of renal function is sometimes entertained. Angioplasty is less often successful than for fibromuscular dysplasia, although stenting may offer the potential for better "noninvasive" results. Whether with surgical or angiographic intervention, it appears that kidneys <8 cm in size are unlikely to recover substantial renal function. The use of aspirin and lipid-lowering agents is advisable in pts with evidence of renovascular disease, regardless of revascularization options.

Scleroderma

May cause sudden oliguric renal failure and severe hypertension due to small vessel occlusion in previously stable pts. Aggressive control of bp with converting-enzyme inhibitors and dialysis improves survival and may restore renal function.

Arteriolar Nephrosclerosis

Persistent hypertension causes arteriosclerosis of the renal arterioles and loss of renal function (nephrosclerosis). Benign nephrosclerosis is associated with loss of cortical kidney mass and thickened afferent arterioles and mild to moderate impairment of renal function. Malignant nephrosclerosis is characterized by accelerated rise in bp and the clinical features of malignant hypertension, including renal failure (see Chap. 115). Aggressive control of the bp usually can halt or reverse the deterioration of renal function, and some pts have a return of renal function to near normal.

Hemolytic-Uremic Syndrome

Characterized by ARF, microangiopathic hemolytic anemia, and thrombocytopenia; increasingly recognized in adults; may be preceded by a prodrome of bloody diarrhea and abdominal pain. Fibrin deposition leads to small vessel occlusion. Lack of fever or CNS involvement helps to distinguish it from thrombotic thrombocytopenic purpura. Treatment is symptomatic; prognosis for recovery of renal function is poor.

Toxemias of Pregnancy

Preeclampsia is characterized by hypertension, proteinuria, edema, consumptive coagulopathy, sodium retention, and hyperreflexia; *eclampsia* is the further development of seizures. Glomerular swelling causes renal insufficiency. Coagulation abnormalities and ARF may occur. Treatment consists of bed rest, sedation, control of neurologic manifestations with magnesium sulfate, control of hypertension with vasodilators, and delivery of the infant.

Vasculitis

Renal complications are frequent and severe in polyarteritis nodosa, hypersensitivity angiitis, Wegener's granulomatosis, and other forms of vasculitis (see Chap. 151). Therapy is directed toward the underlying disease.

Sickle Cell Nephropathy

The hypertonic and relatively hypoxic renal medulla coupled with slow blood flow in the vasa recta favors sickling. Papillary necrosis, cortical infarcts, functional tubule abnormalities (nephrogenic diabetes insipidus), glomerulopathy, nephrotic syndrome, and, rarely, end-stage renal disease may be complications.

For a more detailed discussion, see Badr KF, Brenner BM: Vascular Injury to the Kidney, Chap. 277, p. 1558, in HPIM-14.

136

NEPHROLITHIASIS

Renal calculi are common, affecting approximately 1% of the population, and recurrent in more than half of pts. Stone formation begins when urine becomes supersaturated with insoluble components due to (1) low volume, (2) excessive excretion of selected compounds, or (3) other factors (e.g., urinary pH) that diminish solubility. Approximately 75% of stones are Ca-based (the majority are Ca oxalate; also Ca phosphate and other mixed stones), 15% struvite (magnesium-ammonium-phosphate), 5% uric acid, and 1% cystine, depending on the metabolic disturbance(s) from which they arise.

Signs and Symptoms

Stones in the renal pelvis may be asymptomatic or cause hematuria alone; with passage, obstruction may occur at any site along the collecting system. Obstruction related to the passing of a stone leads to severe pain, often radiating to the groin, sometimes accompanied by intense visceral symptoms (i.e., nausea, vomiting, diaphoresis, light-headedness), hematuria, pyuria, UTI, and, rarely, hydronephrosis. Staghorn calculi are associated with recurrent UTI with urea-splitting organisms (*Proteus, Klebsiella, Providencia, Morganella,* and others).

Stone Composition

Most stones are composed of Ca oxalate. These may be associated with hypercalciuria or hyperoxaluria. Hypercalciuria can be seen in association with a very high Na diet (or exogenous saline administration), furosemide or other loop diuretic therapy, distal (type I) renal tubular acidosis, sarcoidosis, Cushing's syndrome, conditions associated with hypercalcemia (e.g., primary hyperparathyroidism, vitamin D excess, milk-alkali syndrome), or may be idiopathic.

Hyperoxaluria may be seen with intestinal (especially ileal) malabsorption syndromes (e.g., inflammatory bowel disease, pancreatitis), due to the binding of intestinal Ca by fatty acids within the bowel lumen to form soaps, allowing free oxalate to be absorbed (and then excreted via the urinary tract). Ca oxalate stones may also form due to (1) a deficiency of urinary citrate, an inhibitor of stone formation that is underexcreted with metabolic acidosis; and (2) hyperuricosuria (see below). Ca phosphate stones are much less common and tend to occur in the setting of an abnormally high urinary pH (7–8), usually in association with a complete or partial distal (type I) RTA.

Struvite stones form in the collecting system when infection with urea-splitting organisms is present. Struvite is the most

Table 136-1

Workup for an Outpatient with a Renal Stone

1. Dietary and fluid intake history
2. Careful medical history and physical examination, focusing on systemic diseases
3. Abdominal flat plate examination
4. Serum chemistries: BUN, creatinine (Cr), uric acid, calcium, phosphate, chloride, bicarbonate
5. Timed urine collections (at least one day during week, one day on weekend): Cr, Na, K, urea nitrogen, uric acid, calcium, phosphate, oxalate, citrate, magnesium

common component of staghorn calculi and obstruction. Risk factors include previous UTI, nonstruvite stone disease, urinary catheters, neurogenic bladder (e.g., with diabetes or multiple sclerosis), and instrumentation.

Uric acid stones develop when the urine is saturated with uric acid in the presence of dehydration and an acid urine pH. Pts with myeloproliferative disorders (esp. after treatment with chemotherapy), gout, acute and chronic renal failure, and following cyclosporine therapy often develop hyperuricemia and hyperuricosuria and are at risk for stones if the urine volume diminishes. Hyperuricosuria without hyperuricemia may be seen in association with certain drugs (e.g., probenecid, high-dose salicylates).

Cystine stones are the result of a rare inherited defect of renal and intestinal transport resulting in overexcretion of cystine. Stones begin in childhood and are a rare cause of staghorn calculi; they occasionally lead to end-stage renal disease. Stones are more likely to form in acidic urinary pH.

Workup

Although some have advocated a complete workup after a first stone episode, others would defer that evaluation until there has been evidence of recurrence or if there is no obvious cause (e.g., low fluid intake during the summer months with obvious dehydration). Table 136-1 outlines a reasonable workup for an outpatient with an uncomplicated kidney stone.

℞ TREATMENT

Treatment of renal calculi is often empiric, based on odds (Ca oxalate most common stones) or clinical Hx. Sometimes a stone is recovered and can be analyzed for content. Stone analysis is advisable, especially for pts with more complex

Table 136-2

Specific Therapies for Nephrolithiasis

Stone Type	Dietary Modifications	Other
Calcium oxalate	Increase fluid intake Moderate sodium intake Moderate oxalate intake Moderate protein intake Moderate fat intake	Citrate supplementation (calcium or potassium salts > sodium) Cholestyramine or other therapy for fat malabsorption Thiazides if hypercalciuric Allopurinol if hyperuricosuric
Calcium phosphate	Increase fluid intake Moderate sodium intake	Thiazides if hypercalciuric
Struvite	Increase fluid intake; same as calcium oxalate if evidence of calcium oxalate nidus for struvite	Mandelamine and vitamin C or daily suppressive antibiotic therapy (e.g., trimethoprim-sulfamethoxazole)
Uric acid	Increase fluid intake Moderate dietary protein intake	Allopurinol
Cystine	Increase fluid intake	Alkali therapy Penicillamine

NOTE: Sodium excretion correlates with calcium excretion.

presentations or recurrent disease. An increase in fluid intake to at least 2.5–3 L/day is advisable, regardless of the type of stone. Conservative recommendations for pts with Ca oxalate stones (i.e., low salt, low fat, moderate protein diet) are thought to be healthful in general and therefore probably worth a try in pts whose condition is otherwise uncomplicated. Table 136-2 outlines stone-specific therapies for pts with complex or recurrent nephrolithiasis.

For a more detailed discussion, see Asplin JR, Coe FL, Favus MJ: Nephrolithiasis, Chap. 279, p. 1569, in HPIM-14.

137

URINARY TRACT OBSTRUCTION

Urinary tract obstruction (UTO), a potentially reversible cause of renal failure (RF), should be considered in all cases of acute or abrupt worsening of chronic RF. Consequences depend on duration and severity and whether the obstruction is unilateral or bilateral. UTO may occur at any level from collecting tubule to urethra. It is preponderant in women (pelvic tumors), elderly men (prostatic disease), diabetic pts (papillary necrosis), pts with neurologic diseases (spinal cord injury or multiple sclerosis, with neurogenic bladder), or in individuals with retroperitoneal lymphadenopathy or fibrosis, vesicoureteral reflux, nephrolithiasis, or other causes of functional urinary retention (e.g., anticholinergic drugs).

Clinical Manifestations

Pain can occur in some settings (obstruction due to stones) but is not common. In men, there is frequently a history of prostatism. Physical exam may reveal an enlarged bladder by percussion over the lower abdominal wall. Other findings depend on the clinical scenario. Prostatic hypertrophy can be determined by digital rectal examination. A bimanual examination in women may show a pelvic or rectal mass. The workup of pts with RF suspected of having UTO is shown in Fig. 137-1. Laboratory studies may show marked elevations of BUN and creatinine; if the obstruction has been of sufficient duration, there may be evidence of tubulointerstitial disease (e.g., hyperkalemia, non-anion-gap metabolic acidosis, mild hypernatremia). Urinalysis is most often benign or with a small number of cells; heavy proteinuria is rare. An opaque (all but uric acid) stone may be visualized on abdominal radiography.

Ultrasonography can be used to assess the degree of hydronephrosis and the integrity of the renal parenchyma; CT or intravenous urography may be required to localize the level of obstruction. Calyceal dilation is commonly seen; it may be absent with hyperacute obstruction, upper tract encasement by tumor or retroperitoneal fibrosis, or indwelling staghorn calculi. Kidney size may indicate the duration of obstruction. It should be noted that unilateral obstruction may be prolonged and severe (ultimately leading to loss of renal function in the obstructed kidney), with no hint of abnormality on physical exam and laboratory survey.

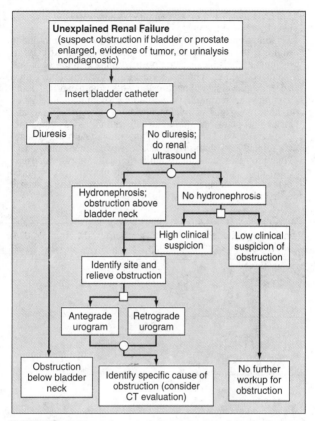

FIGURE 137-1 Diagnostic approach for urinary tract obstruction in unexplained renal failure. Circles represent diagnostic procedures, and squares indicate clinical decisions based on available data. CT, computed tomography.

℞ TREATMENT

Management of acute RF associated with UTO is dictated by (1) the level of obstruction (upper vs. lower tract), and (2) the acuity of the obstruction and its clinical consequences, including renal dysfunction and infection. Benign causes of UTO, including bladder outlet obstruction and nephrolithiasis, should be ruled out as conservative management, including

Foley catheter placement and IV fluids, respectively, will usually relieve the obstruction in most cases.

Among more seriously ill pts, ureteral obstruction due to tumor is the most common and concerning cause of UTO. If technically feasible, ureteral obstruction due to tumor is best managed by cystoscopic placement of a ureteral stent. Otherwise, the placement of nephrostomy tubes with external drainage may be required. IV antibiotics should also be given if there are signs of pyelonephritis or urosepsis. Fluid and electrolyte status should be carefully monitored after obstruction is relieved. There may be a physiologic natriuresis/diuresis related to volume overload. However, there may be an "inappropriate" natriuresis/diuresis related to (1) elevated urea nitrogen, leading to an osmotic diuresis; and (2) acquired nephrogenic diabetes insipidus. Hypernatremia, sometimes to a severe degree, may develop.

For a more detailed discussion, see Seifter JL, Brenner BM: Urinary Tract Obstruction, Chap. 280, p. 1574, in HPIM-14.

ESOPHAGEAL DISEASES

DYSPHAGIA

OROPHARYNGEAL   Difficulty initiating swallowing; food sticks at level of suprasternal notch; nasopharyngeal regurgitation; aspiration. Not to be confused with globus sensation, the feeling of a constant lump in the throat.

Solids Only   Carcinoma, aberrant vessel, congenital web (Plummer-Vinson syndrome), cervical osteophyte.

Solids and Liquids   Cricopharyngeal bar (e.g., hypertensive or hypotensive upper esophageal sphincter), Zenker's diverticulum, myasthenia gravis, steroid myopathy, hyperthyroidism, hypothyroidism, myotonic dystrophy, amyotrophic lateral sclerosis, multiple sclerosis, parkinsonism, stroke, and bulbar and pseudobulbar palsy.

ESOPHAGEAL   Food sticks in mid or lower sternal area (dysphagia is often referred to suprasternal notch); odynophagia (pain on swallowing); regurgitation; aspiration.

Solids Only Initially   If intermittent: lower esophageal (Schatzki) ring. If progressive: peptic stricture (with heartburn), carcinoma (no heartburn), lye stricture.

Solids and Liquids   If intermittent: diffuse esophageal spasm (with chest pain). If progressive: scleroderma (with heartburn), achalasia (no heartburn).

NONCARDIAC CHEST PAIN

Accounts for up to 30% of pts presenting with angina pectoris—coronary arteries are normal angiographically. History and physical examination often cannot distinguish cardiac from noncardiac chest pain. Exclude cardiac disease first.

CAUSES   Gastroesophageal reflux disease, esophageal motility disorder, peptic ulcer disease, gallstones, psychiatric disease (anxiety, panic attacks, depression). Also consider microvascular angina, mitral valve prolapse. Associated with irritable bowel syndrome.

EVALUATION Consider a trial of antireflux therapy (e.g., omeprazole); if no response, 24-h ambulatory luminal pH testing; if negative, esophageal manometry may be considered (see below). Trial of imipramine 50 mg PO qhs may be worthwhile. Psychiatric evaluation in selected cases.

ESOPHAGEAL MOTOR DISORDERS

Patients with esophageal motility disturbances may have a spectrum of manometric findings ranging from nonspecific abnormalities to defined clinical entities.

ACHALASIA (1) Hypertensive lower esophageal sphincter (LES); (2) incomplete relaxation of LES; (3) loss of peristalsis in smooth-muscle portion of esophageal body.

Causes Primary (idiopathic) or secondary due to Chagas' disease, lymphoma, carcinoma, chronic idiopathic intestinal pseudoobstruction, ischemia, neurotropic viruses, drugs, toxins, radiation, postvagotomy.

Diagnosis CXR: absence of gastric air bubble. Barium swallow: dilated esophagus with distal beaklike narrowing and air-fluid level. Endoscopy: exclude tumor; particularly with onset over age 50. Manometry: normal or elevated LES pressure, decreased LES relaxation, absent peristalsis.

℞ TREATMENT
Pneumatic (forceful) balloon dilatation—effective in 85%, risk of perforation (3–5%), bleeding; injection of botulinum toxin into LES at endoscopy—effective and safe but symptoms often recur within 12 months; myotomy of LES (Heller procedure)—effective, risk of reflux esophagitis (10–30%); can be done laparoscopically in many patients. Trial of calcium antagonists (e.g., nifedipine 10–20 mg or isosorbide dinitrate 5–10 mg SL ac) in pts at high risk for dilatation or surgery.

SPASTIC DISORDERS *Diffuse Esophageal Spasm* Multiple spontaneous and swallow-induced contractions of the esophageal body that are of simultaneous onset, long duration, and repetitive occurrence.

Causes Primary (idiopathic) or secondary due to reflux esophagitis, emotional stress, diabetes, alcoholism, neuropathy, radiation, ischemia, collagen-vascular disease.

Variants Nutcracker esophagus: high-amplitude (≥ 180 mmHg) peristaltic contractions; particularly associated with chest pain or dysphagia, but correlation between symptoms and manometric findings is inconsistent. Condition may resolve over time or evolve into diffuse spasm. Associated with increased frequency of depression, anxiety, and somatization.

Diagnosis Barium swallow: corkscrew esophagus, pseudodiverticula, in diffuse spasm. Manometry: spasm—contractions in esophageal body that are of simultaneous onset, high amplitude, long duration, and repetitive occurrence; in nutcracker esophagus, contractions are peristaltic and of high amplitude; possible provocation with edrophonium, ergonovine, bethanecol, etc. (first exclude coronary artery disease).

℞ **TREATMENT**

Trials of anticholinergics (usually of limited value), nitrates (isosorbide dinitrate 5–10 mg SL or 10–30 mg PO ac), Ca antagonists (e.g., diltiazem 60–90 mg PO tid); balloon dilatation may be attempted in some cases refractory to medical therapy; longitudinal myotomy of esophageal circular muscle in severe, resistant cases. Consider drug therapy for depression and psychological intervention.

SCLERODERMA (1) Aperistalsis due to atrophy of esophageal smooth muscle $\pm$ fibrosis; (2) incompetent LES leading to reflux esophagitis, stricture. Treat as for reflux (see below).

GASTROESOPHAGEAL REFLUX

PATHOPHYSIOLOGY

FACTORS THAT PROMOTE GASTROESOPHAGEAL REFLUX (1) Increased gastric volume (after meal, gastric stasis, acid hypersecretion); (2) contents near gastroesophageal junction (bending, recumbency); (3) increased gastric pressure (obesity, tight clothes, pregnancy, ascites); (4) loss of LES–gastric pressure gradient: LES pressure decreased by smoking, anticholinergics, Ca antagonists, pregnancy, progesterone, scleroderma. Hiatal hernia promotes reflux and impairs clearance of acid from esophagus. In most cases, the primary mechanism of reflux relates to frequent transient LES relaxations; less often basal LES pressure is decreased.

Heartburn Occurrence may depend on amount refluxed and frequency; $\downarrow$ esophageal clearance by gravity and peristalsis; $\downarrow$ neutralization by salivary secretion.

Esophagitis   Results when refluxed acid (or bile) overwhelms esophageal mucosal defenses. Aspirin and NSAIDs appear to be cofactors.

CLINICAL FEATURES   Heartburn, regurgitation, nausea, dysphagia due to stricture, aspiration; complications: esophageal ulcer, bleeding, Barrett's esophagus (replacement of squamous with columnar epithelium, premalignant), adenocarcinoma.

DIAGNOSIS   History often suffices; further testing in atypical or refractory cases.

* Barium swallow: detects strictures, ulcers; frequent false-negatives for reflux or esophagitis.
* Endoscopy and mucosal biopsy: detects esophagitis and Barrett's esophagus; may be normal in gastroesophageal reflux.
* Bernstein test: reproduction of symptoms with 0.1 N HCl but not normal saline infused by tube into esophagus; less sensitive than 24-h esophageal luminal pH recording.
* ^{99m}Tc sulfur colloid scintiscan: to document and quantitate reflux; unreliable. 24-h ambulatory esophageal luminal pH recording: most sensitive test for reflux.

Rx **TREATMENT**

General   Weight reduction; sleeping with head elevated or on wedge; avoidance of smoking, large meals, caffeine, alcohol, chocolate, fatty foods, citrus juices, NSAIDs.

Medical Therapy   Antacids, H_2-receptor blockers, sucralfate, or omeprazole (initial doses as for peptic ulcer; Chap. 139); higher than "standard" doses of H_2-receptor blockers may be required (e.g., cimetidine 800 mg PO bid, ranitidine 300 mg PO bid, famotidine 40 mg or higher doses PO bid) or consider adding an agent to increase LES pressure and enhance gastric emptying—cisapride 10–20 mg PO ac or metoclopramide 10–20 mg PO ac + hs (latter has more side effects: tremor, spasms, parkinsonism, elevated prolactin). Long-term therapy usually necessary. Omeprazole 20–40 mg PO qAM or 20 mg PO bid, or lansoprazole 30–60 PO qAM or 30 mg PO bid (substituted benzimidazoles and H^+, K^+-ATPase inhibitors) are most effective agents, even in severe esophagitis or cases resistant to H_2-receptor blockers; long-term use is often necessary (first eradicate *Helicobacter pylori*, if present, to reduce risk of atrophic gastritis). Dilate strictures. Surgical therapy (Belsey repair, Nissen fundoplication, Hill repair) in severe and refractory cases; laparoscopic fundoplication appears promising. Surveillance endoscopy and biopsies for dysplasia q1–2 years in patients with Barrett's esophagus.

OTHER FORMS OF ESOPHAGITIS

HERPES ESOPHAGITIS Caused by herpesvirus I or II, varicella-zoster, or cytomegalovirus. In immunocompromised persons (e.g., those with AIDS), may present with odynophagia, dysphagia, fever, bleeding; diagnosis by endoscopy with biopsy, brush cytology, culture.

℞ TREATMENT

May be self-limited in immunocompetent person; viscous lidocaine for pain; in prolonged cases and in immunocompromised hosts, herpes and varicella esophagitis are treated with acyclovir 5–10 mg/kg IV q8h for 10–14 d, then 200–400 mg PO 5 times daily; CMV is treated with ganciclovir 5 mg/kg IV q12h until healing, which may take weeks to months. In nonresponders, an alternative is foscarnet 60 mg/kg IV q12h for 21 d.

CANDIDA ESOPHAGITIS In immunocompromised hosts (e.g., AIDS), malignancy, diabetes, hypoparathyroidism, hemoglobinopathy, SLE, corrosive esophageal injury; may present with odynophagia, dysphagia, oral thrush (in 50%); diagnosis, endoscopy (yellow-white plaques or nodules on friable, red mucosa) with brushings (KOH stain), biopsy, culture. In patients with AIDS and suggestive symptoms, empiric therapy can be tried first.

℞ TREATMENT

Oral nystatin (100,000 U/mL) 5 mL q6h or clotrimazole 10-mg tablet sucked q6h. In immunocompromised host, fluconazole 100–200 mg PO daily for 1–3 weeks is treatment of choice; alternative is itraconazole 200 mg PO bid or ketoconazole 200–400 mg PO daily; long-term maintenance therapy often required; poorly responsive pts may respond to fluconazole 400 mg PO qd or can be treated with amphotericin 10–15 mg IV q6h for a total dose of 300–500 mg.

PILL-RELATED ESOPHAGITIS Doxycycline, tetracycline, aspirin, NSAIDs, KCl, quinidine, ferrous sulfate, clindamycin, alprenolol, alendronate. Predisposing factors: recumbency after swallowing pills with small sips of water; anatomic factors (e.g., enlarged left atrium or ectatic aorta impinging on esophagus).

R̽ TREATMENT

Withdraw offending drug; antacids; dilate any resulting stricture.

OTHER CAUSES OF ESOPHAGITIS IN AIDS Mycobacterial infections, *Cryptosporidium*, *Pneumocystis carinii*, idiopathic esophageal nonspecific or giant ulcers (possible cytopathic effect of HIV, may respond to systemic glucocorticoids).

ESOPHAGEAL CANCER (See Chap. 60)

For a more detailed discussion, see Goyal RK: Dysphagia, Chap. 40, p. 228, and Diseases of the Esophagus, Chap. 283, p. 1588, in HPIM-14.

139

PEPTIC ULCER AND RELATED DISORDERS

PEPTIC ULCER DISEASE

Most commonly in duodenal bulb (duodenal ulcer—DU) and stomach (gastric ulcer—GU). May also occur in esophagus, pyloric channel, duodenal loop, jejunum, Meckel's diverticulum. Results when "aggressive" factors (gastric acid, pepsin) overwhelm "defensive" factors involved in mucosal resistance (gastric mucus, bicarbonate, microcirculation, prostaglandins, mucosal "barrier"), effects of *Helicobacter pylori*.

CAUSES AND RISK FACTORS *General* Major role for *H. pylori*, spiral urease-producing organism that colonizes gastric antral mucosa in up to 100% of persons with DU and 80% with GU. Also found in normals (increasing prevalence with age) and those of low socioeconomic status. Invariably associated with histologic evidence of active chronic gastritis, which over years can lead to atrophic gastritis and gastric cancer.

Other major cause of ulcers is NSAIDs (those not due to *H. pylori*). Fewer than 1% are due to gastrinoma (Zollinger-Ellison syndrome). Other risk factors and associations: hereditary (? increased parietal cell number), smoking, hypercalcemia, mastocytosis, blood group O (antigens may bind *H. pylori*). Unproven: stress, coffee, alcohol.

DU   Mild gastric acid hypersecretion resulting from (1) increased release of gastrin, presumably due to (a) stimulation of antral G cells by cytokines released by inflammatory cells and (b) diminished production of somatostatin by D cells, both resulting from *H. pylori* infection; and (2) an exaggerated acid response to gastrin due to an increased parietal cell mass resulting from gastrin stimulation. These abnormalities reverse rapidly with eradication of *H. pylori*. However, a mildly elevated maximum gastric acid output in response to exogenous gastrin persists in some patients long after eradication of *H. pylori*, suggesting that gastric acid hypersecretion may be, in part, genetically determined. *H. pylori* may also result in elevated serum pepsinogen levels. Mucosal defense in duodenum is compromised by toxic effects of *H. pylori* infection on patches of gastric metaplasia that result from gastric acid hypersecretion or rapid gastric emptying. Other risk factors include glucocorticoids, NSAIDs, chronic renal failure, renal transplantation, cirrhosis, chronic lung disease.

GU   *H. pylori* is also principal cause. Gastric acid secretory rates usually normal or reduced, possibly reflecting earlier age of infection by *H. pylori* than in DU patients. Gastritis due to reflux of duodenal contents (including bile) may play a role. Chronic salicylate or NSAID use may account for 15–30% of GUs and increase risk of associated bleeding, perforation.

CLINICAL FEATURES   *DU*   Burning epigastric pain 90 min to 3 h after meals, often nocturnal, relieved by food.

GU   Burning epigastric pain made worse by or unrelated to food; anorexia, food aversion, weight loss (in 40%). Great individual variation. Similar symptoms may occur in persons without demonstrated peptic ulcers ("nonulcer dyspepsia"); less responsive to standard therapy.

COMPLICATIONS   Bleeding, obstruction, penetration causing acute pancreatitis, perforation, intractability.

DIAGNOSIS   *DU*   Upper endoscopy or upper GI barium radiography.

GU   Upper endoscopy preferable to exclude possibility that ulcer is malignant (brush cytology, ≥6 pinch biopsies of ulcer margin). Radiographic features suggesting malignancy: ulcer within a mass, folds that do not radiate from ulcer margin, a large ulcer (>2.5–3 cm).

DETECTION OF *H. PYLORI* Detection of antibodies in serum (inexpensive, preferred when endoscopy is not required); rapid urease test of antral biopsy (when endoscopy is required). Urea breath test generally used to confirm eradication of *H. pylori*, if necessary.

℞ TREATMENT

Medical

Objectives: pain relief, healing, prevention of complications, prevention of recurrences. For GU, exclude malignancy (follow endoscopically to healing). Dietary restriction unnecessary with contemporary drugs; discontinue NSAIDs; smoking may prevent healing and should be stopped. Eradication of *H. pylori* markedly reduces rate of ulcer relapse and is indicated for all DUs and GUs associated with *H. pylori* (see Table 139-1). Acid suppression is generally included in regimen. Standard drugs (H_2-receptor blockers, sucralfate, antacids) heal 80–90% of DUs and 60% of GUs in 6 weeks; healing is more rapid with omeprazole (see Table 139-1).

Surgery

For complications (persistent or recurrent bleeding, obstruction, perforation) or, uncommonly, intractability (first screen for surreptitious NSAID use and gastrinoma). For DU, see Table 139-2. For GU, perform subtotal gastrectomy.

Complications of Surgery (1) Obstructed afferent loop (Billroth II), (2) bile reflux gastritis, (3) dumping syndrome (rapid gastric emptying with abdominal distress + postprandial vasomotor symptoms), (4) postvagotomy diarrhea, (5) bezoar, (6) anemia (iron, B_{12}, folate malabsorption), (7) malabsorption (poor mixing of gastric contents, pancreatic juices, bile; bacterial overgrowth), (8) osteomalacia and osteoporosis (vitamin D and Ca malabsorption), (9) gastric remnant carcinoma.

_____ *Approach to Dyspeptic Patient* _____

Optimal approach uncertain. Serologic testing for *H. pylori* and treating, if present, may be cost-effective. Other options include trial of acid suppressive therapy, endoscopy only in treatment failures, or initial endoscopy in all cases.

GASTROPATHIES

EROSIVE GASTROPATHIES   Hemorrhagic gastritis, multiple gastric erosions. Caused by aspirin and other NSAIDs (lower risk with newer agents, e.g., nabumetone and etodolac, which do not inhibit gastric mucosal prostaglandins) or severe stress (burns, sepsis, trauma, surgery, shock, or respiratory, renal, or liver failure). May be asymptomatic or associated with epigastric discomfort, nausea, hematemesis, or melena. Diagnosis by upper endoscopy.

℞ TREATMENT

Removal of offending agent and maintenance of O_2 and blood volume as required. For prevention of stress ulcers in critically ill pts, hourly oral administration of liquid antacids (e.g., Maalox 30 mL), IV H_2-receptor antagonist (e.g., cimetidine 300 mg bolus + 37.5–50 mg/h IV), or both is recommended to maintain gastric pH $\geq$ 4. Alternatively, sucralfate slurry 1 g PO q6h can be given; does not raise gastric pH and may thus avoid increased risk of aspiration pneumonia associated with liquid antacids. As above (Table 139-1), misoprostol 200 (µg PO qid or profound acid suppression (e.g., famotidine 40 mg PO bid) can be used with NSAIDs to prevent NSAID-induced ulcers.

NONEROSIVE GASTRITIS   *Fundal Gland (Type A) Gastritis*   Three patterns: superficial gastritis, atrophic gastritis, gastric atrophy. Generally asymptomatic, common in elderly; atrophic types may be associated with achlorhydria, pernicious anemia, and increased risk of gastric cancer (value of screening endoscopy uncertain).

   Superficial (Type B) Gastritis   Usually antral and caused by *H. pylori* (see above). Often asymptomatic but may be associated with dyspepsia. May also lead to atrophic gastritis, gastric atrophy, gastric lymphoid follicles, and low-grade gastric B cell lymphomas. Infection early in life or in setting of malnutrition or low gastric acid output is associated with gastritis of entire stomach (including body) and increased risk of gastric cancer. Eradication of *H. pylori* (see Table 139-1) is associated with resolution of gastritis, but clinical benefit and cost-effectiveness are uncertain in absence of documented ulcer.

SPECIFIC TYPES OF GASTROPATHY OR GASTRITIS   Alcoholic gastropathy (submucosal hemorrhages), Ménétrier's disease (hypertrophic gastropathy), eosinophilic gastritis, granulomatous gastritis, Crohn's disease, sarcoidosis, infections (tu-

Table 139-1

Drugs Used in the Treatment of Peptic Ulcer

Drug and Mechanism	Dose	Side Effects
"Triple therapy": eradication of *H. pylori*	Bismuth subsalicylate 2 tabs qid, amoxicillin 500 mg qid or tetracycline 500 mg tid, plus metronidazole 250 mg tid. Treat for 2 weeks (combine with H$_2$ receptor antagonist or proton pump inhibitor)	Cumbersome; diarrhea, pseudomembranous colitis
"Dual therapy": eradication of *H. pylori* (plus proton pump inhibition)	Omeprazole 40 mg/d in the morning plus clarithromycin 500 mg tid. Treat for 2 weeks.	As for omeprazole and triple therapy, but frequency of side effects lower and cost greater
"New triple therapy": eradication of *H. pylori* (plus proton pump inhibition)	Omeprazole 20 mg bid plus either clarithromycin 250 mg bid and metronidazole 500 mg bid *or* clarithromycin 500 mg bid and amoxicillin 1 g bid. Treat for one week.	Frequency of side effects lower than for standard triple therapy but cost greater
Ranitidine bismuth citrate plus antibiotic: eradication of *H. pylori*	Ranitidine bismuth citrate 400 mg bid for 4 weeks plus clarithromycin 500 mg tid for first 2 weeks	Taste disturbance and diarrhea most common

Drug	Dose	Adverse Effects
Cimetidine: H$_2$ receptor blockade	300 mg qid or 400 mg bid or 800 mg at bedtime	Uncommon: antiandrogen (high doses), ↑ creatinine, ↓ hepatic drug metabolism, ↑ serum aminotransferase levels, rare blood dyscrasias
Ranitidine: H$_2$ receptor blockade	150 mg bid or 300 mg at bedtime	As for cimetidine but antiandrogen and drug metabolism effects are less frequent; rare cases of hepatitis
Famotidine: H$_2$ receptor blockade	40 mg at bedtime	As for ranitidine
Nizatidine: H$_2$ receptor blockade	300 mg at bedtime	Probably as for ranitidine
Misoprostol: raises prostaglandin levels (enhances mucosal defense, reduces gastric acid secretion)	200 mg qid for prevention of NSAID-induced ulcers	Diarrhea, uterine contraction (do not use in women of childbearing age)
Sucralfate: coats ulcers, binds pepsin	1 g 1 h before meals and at bedtime or 2 g bid	Constipation, binding to coadministered drugs
Omeprazole: inhibits H$^+$, K$^+$-ATPase (proton pump) in gastric parietal cell	20 mg/d in the morning	↓ Hepatic drug metabolism; prolonged use in high doses in rats causes gastric carcinoids
Lansoprazole: proton pump inhibitor	30 mg/d in the morning	As for omeprazole
Antacids: acid neutralization	140 mmol 1 h and 3 h after eating and at bedtime (e.g., 30 mL Maalox); lower doses (15 mL after eating and at bedtime) appear to be as effective	Diarrhea (Mg), constipation (Al), osteomalacia, milk-alkali syndrome (elevated serum, CA, P, BUN, creatinine, HCO$_3$; due to CaCO$_3$)

Table 139-2

Surgical Treatment of Duodenal Ulcer

Operation	Recurrence Rate	Complication Rate
Vagotomy + antrectomy (Billroth I or II)*	1%	Highest
Vagotomy and pyloroplasty	10%	Intermediate
Parietal cell (proximal gastric, superselective) vagotomy	≥10%	Lowest

* Billroth I, gastroduodenostomy; Billroth II, gastrojejunostomy.

berculosis, syphilis, fungi, viruses, parasites), pseudolymphoma, radiation, corrosive gastritis.

ZOLLINGER-ELLISON (Z-E) SYNDROME (GASTRINOMA)

Consider when ulcer disease is severe, refractory to therapy, associated with ulcers in atypical locations, or associated with diarrhea. Tumors usually pancreatic or in duodenum (submucosal, often small), may be multiple, slowly growing; >60% malignant; 25% associated with MEN 1, i.e., multiple endocrine neoplasia type 1 (gastrinoma, hyperparathyroidism, pituitary neoplasm), often duodenal, small, multicentric, less likely to metastasize to liver than pancreatic gastrinomas but often metastasize to local lymph nodes.

DIAGNOSIS *Suggestive* Basal acid output >15 mmol/h; basal/maximal acid output >60%; endoscopy or upper GI radiograph: large mucosal folds.

Confirmatory Serum gastrin >1000 ng/L or rise in gastrin of 200 ng/L following IV secretin and, if necessary, rise of 400 ng/L following IV calcium (see Table 139-3).

DIFFERENTIAL DIAGNOSIS *Increased Gastric Acid Secretion* Z-E syndrome, antral G cell hyperplasia or hyperfunction (? due to *H. pylori*), postgastrectomy retained antrum, renal failure, massive small bowel resection, chronic gastric outlet obstruction.

Normal or Decreased Gastric Acid Secretion Pernicious anemia, chronic gastritis, gastric cancer, vagotomy, pheochromocytoma.

Table 139-3

Differential Diagnostic Tests

Condition	Fasting Gastrin	Gastrin Response to	
		IV Secretin	Food
DU	N* (≤150 ng/L)	NC†	Slight ↑
Z-E	↑ ↑ ↑	↑ ↑ ↑	NC
Antral G (gastrin) cell hyperplasia	↑	↑, NC	↑↑↑

* N, normal.
† NC, no change.

℞ TREATMENT

Omeprazole, beginning at 60 mg PO qAM and increasing until maximal gastric acid output is <10 mmol/h before next dose, is drug of choice during evaluation and in pts who are not surgical candidates; dose can often be reduced over time. Traditionally, tumor localization has been attempted with ultrasound, IV bolus-enhanced CT, MRI (best for hepatic metastases), selective angiography, and, in selected cases, venous sampling for gastrin after selective arterial injection of secretin. Recently, radiolabeled octreotide scanning has emerged as the most sensitive test for detecting primary tumors and metastases; may be supplemented by endoscopic ultrasonography. Exploratory laparotomy with resection of primary tumor and solitary metastases when possible. In pts with MEN 1, tumor is often multifocal and unresectable; treat hyperparathyroidism first (hypergastrinemia may improve). For unresectable tumors, parietal cell vagotomy may enhance control of ulcer disease by drugs. Chemotherapy for metastatic tumor to control symptoms (e.g., streptozocin and 5-fluorouracil); 40% partial response rate.

For a more detailed discussion, see Friedman LS, Peterson WL: Peptic Ulcer and Related Disorders, Chap. 284, pp. 1596, in HPIM-14.

INFLAMMATORY BOWEL DISEASES

Chronic inflammatory disorders of unknown etiology involving the GI tract. Peak occurrence between ages 15 and 35, but onset may occur at any age. Pathogenesis of IBD involves activation of immune cells by unknown inciting agent (?microorganism, dietary component, bacterial or self-antigen) leading to release of cytokines and inflammatory mediators. Genetic component suggested by increased risk in first-degree relatives of pts with IBD and concurrence of type of IBD, location of Crohn's disease, and clinical course. Reported associations include HLA-DR2 in Japanese patients with ulcerative colitis and a Crohn's disease–related gene on chromosome 16. Other potential pathogenic factors include serum antineutrophil cytoplasmic antibodies (ANCA) in 70% of pts with ulcerative colitis and granulomatous angiitis (vasculitis) in Crohn's disease. Acute flares may be precipitated by infections, NSAIDs, stress. Onset of ulcerative colitis often follows cessation of smoking.

ULCERATIVE COLITIS (UC)

PATHOLOGY Colonic *mucosal* inflammation; rectum almost always involved, with inflammation extending continuously (no skip areas) proximally for a variable extent; histologic features include epithelial damage, inflammation, crypt abscesses, loss of goblet cells.

CLINICAL MANIFESTATIONS Bloody diarrhea, mucus, fever, abdominal pain, tenesmus, weight loss; spectrum of severity (majority of cases are mild, limited to rectosigmoid). In severe cases dehydration, anemia, hypokalemia, hypoalbuminemia.

COMPLICATIONS Toxic megacolon, colonic perforation; cancer risk related to extent and duration of colitis; often preceded by or coincident with dysplasia (neoplastic changes in individual epithelial cells), which may be detected on surveillance colonoscopic biopsies.

DIAGNOSIS Sigmoidoscopy/colonoscopy: mucosal erythema, granularity, friability, exudate, hemorrhage, ulcers, inflammatory polyps (pseudopolyps). Barium enema: loss of haustrations, mucosal irregularity, ulcerations.

CROHN'S DISEASE (CD)

PATHOLOGY Any part of GI tract, usually terminal ileum and/or colon; *transmural* inflammation, bowel wall thickening, linear ulcerations, and submucosal thickening leading to cobble-stone pattern; discontinuous (skip areas); histologic features include transmural inflammation, granulomas (often absent), fissures, fistulas.

CLINICAL MANIFESTATIONS Fever, abdominal pain, diarrhea (often without blood), fatigue, weight loss, growth retardation in children; acute ileitis mimicking appendicitis; anorectal fissures, fistulas, abscesses. Clinical course falls into three broad patterns: (1) inflammatory, (2) stricturing, and (3) fistulizing.

COMPLICATIONS Intestinal obstruction (edema vs. fibrosis); rarely toxic megacolon or perforation; intestinal fistulas to bowel, bladder, vagina, skin, soft tissue, often with abscess formation; bile salt malabsorption leading to cholesterol gallstones and/or oxalate kidney stones; intestinal malignancy; amyloidosis.

DIAGNOSIS Sigmoidoscopy/colonoscopy, barium enema, upper GI and small-bowel series: nodularity, rigidity, ulcers that may be deep or longitudinal, cobblestoning, skip areas, strictures, fistulas. CT may show thickened, matted bowel loops or an abscess.

DIFFERENTIAL DIAGNOSIS

INFECTIOUS ENTEROCOLITIS *Shigella*, *Salmonella*, *Campylobacter*, *Yersinia* (acute ileitis), *Plesiomonas shigelloides*, *Aeromonas hydrophilia*, *E. coli* serotype O157:H7, *Gonorrhea*, *Lymphogranuloma venereum*, *Clostridium difficile* (pseudomembranous colitis), tuberculosis, amebiasis, cytomegalovirus, AIDS.

OTHERS Ischemic bowel disease, diverticulitis, radiation enterocolitis, bile salt–induced diarrhea (ileal resection), drug-induced colitis (e.g., NSAIDs), bleeding colonic lesion (e.g., neoplasm), irritable bowel syndrome (no bleeding), microscopic (lymphocytic) or collagenous colitis (chronic watery diarrhea)—normal colonoscopy, but biopsies show superficial colonic epithelial inflammation and, in collagenous colitis, a thick subepithelial layer of collagen; response to aminosalicylates and glucocorticoids variable.

EXTRAINTESTINAL MANIFESTATIONS (UC AND CD)

1. *Joint:* Peripheral arthritis—parallels activity of bowel disease; ankylosing spondylitis and sacroiliitis (associated with HLA-B27)—activity independent of bowel disease.

2. *Skin:* Erythema nodosum, aphthous ulcers, pyoderma gangrenosum, cutaneous Crohn's disease.
3. *Eye:* Episcleritis, iritis, uveitis.
4. *Liver:* Fatty liver, "pericholangitis" (intrahepatic sclerosing cholangitis), primary sclerosing cholangitis, cholangiocarcinoma, chronic hepatitis.
5. *Others*: Autoimmune hemolytic anemia, phlebitis, pulmonary embolus (hypercoaguable state).

℞ TREATMENT

Supportive Antidiarrheal agents (diphenoxylate and atropine, loperamide) in mild disease; IV hydration and blood transfusions in severe disease; parenteral nutrition or defined enteral formulas—effective as primary therapy in CD, although high relapse rate when oral feeding is resumed; should not replace drug therapy; important role in preoperative preparation of malnourished pt; emotional support.

Sulfasalazine and Aminosalicylates Active component of sulfasalazine is 5-aminosalicylic acid (5-ASA) linked to sulfapyridine carrier; useful in colonic disease of mild to moderate severity (1–1.5 g PO qid); efficacy in maintaining remission demonstrated only for UC (500 mg PO qid). Toxicity (generally due to sulfapyridine component): dose-related—nausea, headache, rarely hemolytic anemia—may resolve when drug dose is lowered; idiosyncratic—fever, rash, neutropenia, pancreatitis, hepatitis, etc.; miscellaneous—oligospermia. Newer aminosalicylates are as effective as sulfasalazine but with fewer side effects. Enemas containing 4 g of 5-ASA (mesalamine) may be used in distal UC, 1 nightly retained qhs until remission, then q2hs or q3hs. Suppositories containing 500 mg of 5-ASA may be used in proctitis. Oral formulations of 5-ASA are described in Table 140-1.

Glucocorticoids Useful in severe disease and ileal or ileocolonic CD. Prednisone 40–60 mg PO qd, then taper; IV hydrocortisone 100 mg tid or equivalent in hospitalized pts; IV ACTH drip (120 U qd) may be preferable in first attacks of UC. Nightly hydrocortisone retention enemas in proctosigmoiditis. Numerous side effects make long-term use problematic.

Immunosuppressive Agents Azathioprine, 6-mercaptopurine 50 mg PO qd up to 2.0 or 1.5 mg/kg qd, respectively. Useful as steroid-sparing agents and in intractable or fistulous CD (may require 2- to 6-month trial before efficacy seen). Toxicity—immunosuppression, pancreatitis, ? carcinogenicity. Avoid in pregnancy.

Metronidazole Appears effective in colonic CD (500 mg

Table 140-1

The Aminosalicylates

Drug (Brand Name)	Formulation	Initial Dose	Maintenance Dose	Comments
Sulfasalazine (Azulfidine)	5-ASA linked to sulfapyridine, split by bacteria in colon	500 mg PO bid; increase over 1 week to 1–1.5 g qid	500 mg PO qid	Numerous side effects (see text)
Olsalazine (Dipentum)	5-ASA linked to 5-ASA, split in colon	500–1000 mg PO bid	500 mg PO bid	Causes diarrhea in 20% of cases, may improve with dose reduction, administration with meals
Mesalamine (Asacol)	5-ASA coated with acrylic resin, released in alkaline pH (terminal ileum, colon)	400–800 mg PO tid, can increase to 1600 mg tid	400–800 mg PO tid	May help in terminal ileitis as well as colitis
Mesalamine (Pentasa)	5-ASA microspheres coated with ethyl cellulose, slowly released throughout small bowel and colon	1 g PO qid	500 mg– 1 g PO qid	Effective in small bowel CD and UC

PO bid) and refractory perineal CD (10–20 mg/kg PO qd). Toxicity—peripheral neuropathy, metallic taste, ? carcinogenicity. Avoid in pregnancy. Other antibiotics (e.g., ciprofloxacin 500 mg PO bid) may be of value in terminal ileal and perianal CD, and broad-spectrum IV antibiotics are indicated for fulminant colitis and abscesses.

   Others   Cyclosporine (potential value in a dose of 4 (mg/kg)/d IV for 7–14 d in severe UC and possibly intractable Crohn's fistulas); experimental—methotrexate, chloroquine, fish oil, nicotine, others.

Surgery

UC: Colectomy (curative) for intractability, toxic megacolon (if no improvement with aggressive medical therapy in 24–48 h), cancer, dysplasia. Ileal pouch–anal anastomosis is operation of choice in UC but contraindicated in CD and in elderly. CD: Resection for fixed obstruction (or stricturoplasty), abscesses, persistent symptomatic fistulas, intractability.

For a more detailed discussion, see Glickman RM: Inflammatory Bowel Disease: Ulcerative Colitis and Crohn's Disease, Chap. 286, p. 1633, in HPIM-14.

141

COLONIC AND ANORECTAL DISEASES

IRRITABLE BOWEL SYNDROME (IBS)

Characterized by altered bowel habits, abdominal pain, and absence of detectable organic pathology. Most common GI disease in clinical practice. Three types of clinical presentations: (1) spastic colon (chronic abdominal pain and constipation), (2) alternating constipation and diarrhea, or (3) chronic, painless diarrhea.

PATHOPHYSIOLOGY   Probably heterogeneous group of disorders. Reported abnormalities include altered colonic motility at rest and in response to stress, cholinergic drugs, cholecystokinin; altered small-intestinal motility; enhanced visceral sensation (lower pain threshold in response to gut distention); and abnormal extrinsic innervation of the gut. Patients presenting with IBS to a physician have an increased frequency of psychological disturbances—depression, hysteria, obsessive-compulsive disorder. Specific food intolerances and malabsorption of bile acids by the terminal ileum may account for a few cases.

CLINICAL MANIFESTATIONS   Onset often before age 30; females/males = 2:1. Abdominal pain and irregular bowel habits. Additional symptoms often include abdominal distention, relief of abdominal pain with bowel movement, increased frequency of stools with pain, loose stools with pain, mucus in stools, and sense of incomplete evacuation. Associated findings include pasty stools, ribbony or pencil-thin stools, heartburn, bloating, back pain, weakness, faintness, palpitations, urinary frequency.

DIAGNOSIS   Often by history; consider sigmoidoscopy and barium radiographs to exclude inflammatory bowel disease or malignancy; consider excluding giardiasis, intestinal lactase deficiency, hyperthyroidism.

℞ TREATMENT

Reassurance and supportive physician-patient relationship, avoidance of stress or precipitating factors, dietary bulk (fiber, psyllium extract, e.g., Metamucil 1 tbsp daily or bid); for diarrhea, trials of loperamide (2 PO qA.M. then 1 PO after each loose stool to a maximum of 8/d, then titrate), diphenoxylate (Lomotil)(up to 2 PO qid), or cholestyramine (up to 1 packet mixed in water PO qid); for pain, anticholinergics (e.g., dicyclomine HCl 10–40 mg PO qid) or hyoscyamine as Levsin 1–2 PO q4h prn. Amitryptiline 25–50 mg PO qhs or other antidepressants in low doses may relieve pain. Leuprolide acetate (gonadotrophin-releasing hormone analogue), psychotherapy, hypnotherapy of possible benefit in severe refractory cases.

DIVERTICULAR DISEASE

Herniations or saclike protrusions of the mucosa through the muscularis at points of nutrient artery penetration; possibly due to increased intraluminal pressure, low-fiber diet; most common in sigmoid colon.

Clinical Presentations and Treatment

1. *Asymptomatic* (detected by barium enema or colonoscopy).
2. *Pain*: Recurrent left lower quadrant pain relieved by defecation; alternating constipation and diarrhea. Diagnosis by barium enema.
3. *Diverticulitis*: Pain, fever, altered bowel habits, tender colon, leukocytosis. Best confirmed and staged by CT after opacification of bowel. (In patients who recover with medical therapy, perform elective barium enema or colonoscopy in 4–6 weeks to exclude cancer.) Complications: pericolic abscess, perforation, fistula (to bladder, vagina, skin, soft tissue), liver abscess, stricture. Frequently require surgery or, for abscesses, percutaneous drainage.
4. *Hemorrhage*: Usually in absence of diverticulitis, often from ascending colon and self-limited. If persistent, manage with mesenteric arteriography and intraarterial infusion of vasopressin, or surgery.

℞ **TREATMENT**
   Pain   High-fiber diet, psyllium extract (e.g., Metamucil 1 tbsp PO qd or bid), anticholinergics (e.g., dicyclomine HCl 10-40 mg PO qid).
   Diverticulitis   NPO, IV fluids, antibiotics (e.g., cefoxitin 2 g IV q6h or imipenem 500 mg IV q6–8h); for ambulatory patients, ampicillin or tetracycline 500 mg PO qid (clear liquid diet); surgical resection in refractory or frequently recurrent cases, young persons (<age 50), immunosuppressed pts, or when there is inability to exclude cancer.

INTESTINAL PSEUDOOBSTRUCTION

Recurrent attacks of nausea, vomiting, and abdominal pain and distention mimicking mechanical obstruction; may be complicated by steatorrhea due to bacterial overgrowth.

CAUSES   *Primary*: Familial visceral neuropathy, familial visceral myopathy, idiopathic. *Secondary*: Scleroderma, amyloidosis, diabetes, celiac disease, parkinsonism, muscular dystrophy, drugs, electrolyte imbalance, postsurgical.

℞ TREATMENT

For acute attacks: intestinal decompression with long tube. Oral antibiotics for bacterial overgrowth (e.g., metronidazole 250 mg PO tid, tetracycline 500 mg PO qid, or ciprofloxacin 500 mg bid 1 week out of each month, usually in an alternating rotation of at least two antibiotics). Avoid surgery. In refractory cases, consider long-term parenteral hyperalimentation.

VASCULAR DISORDERS (SMALL AND LARGE INTESTINE)

MECHANISMS OF MESENTERIC ISCHEMIA   (1) Occlusive: embolus (atrial fibrillation, valvular heart disease); arterial thrombus (atherosclerosis); venous thrombosis (trauma, neoplasm, infection, cirrhosis, oral contraceptives, antithrombin-III deficiency, protein S or C deficiency, lupus anticoagulant, factor V Leiden mutation, idiopathic); vasculitis (SLE, polyarteritis, rheumatoid arthritis, Henoch-Schönlein purpura); (2) nonocclusive: hypotension, heart failure, arrhythmia, digitalis (vasoconstrictor).

ACUTE MESENTERIC ISCHEMIA   Periumbilical pain out of proportion to tenderness; nausea, vomiting, distention, GI bleeding, altered bowel habits. Abdominal x-ray shows bowel distention, air-fluid levels, thumbprinting (submucosal edema) but may be normal early in course. Peritoneal signs indicate infarcted bowel requiring surgical resection. Early celiac and mesenteric arteriography is recommended in all cases following hemodynamic resuscitation (avoid vasopressors, digitalis). Intraarterial vasodilators (e.g., papaverine) can be administered to reverse vasoconstriction. Laparotomy indicated to restore intestinal blood flow obstructed by embolus or thrombosis or to resect necrotic bowel. Postoperative anticoagulation indicated in mesenteric venous thrombosis, controversial in arterial occlusion.

CHRONIC MESENTERIC INSUFFICIENCY   "Abdominal angina": dull, crampy periumbilical pain 15–30 min after a meal and lasting for several hours; weight loss; occasionally diarrhea. Evaluate with mesenteric arteriography for possible bypass graft surgery.

ISCHEMIC COLITIS Usually due to nonocclusive disease in pt with atherosclerosis. Severe lower abdominal pain, rectal bleeding, hypotension. Abdominal x-ray shows colonic dilatation, thumbprinting. Sigmoidoscopy shows submucosal hemorrhage, friability, ulcerations; rectum often spared. Conservative management (NPO, IV fluids); surgical resection for infarction or postischemic stricture.

COLONIC ANGIODYSPLASIA

In persons over age 60, vascular ectasias, usually in right colon, account for up to 40% of cases of chronic or recurrent lower GI bleeding. May be associated with aortic stenosis. Diagnosis by arteriography (clusters of small vessels, early and prolonged opacification of draining vein) or colonoscopy (flat, bright red, fernlike lesions). For bleeding, treat by colonoscopic electro- or laser coagulation, band ligation, arteriographic embolization, or, if necessary, right hemicolectomy.

COLONIC POLYPS AND COLON CANCER
(See Chap. 60)

ANORECTAL DISEASES

HEMORRHOIDS Due to increased hydrostatic pressure in hemorrhoidal venous plexus (associated with straining at stool, pregnancy). May be external, internal, thrombosed, acute (prolapsed or strangulated), or bleeding. Treat pain with bulk laxative and stool softeners (psyllium extract, dioctyl sodium sulfosuccinate 100–200 mg/d), sitz baths 1–4/d, witch hazel compresses, analgesics as needed. Bleeding may require rubber band ligation or injection sclerotherapy. Operative hemorrhoidectomy in severe or refractory cases.

ANAL FISSURES Medical therapy as for hemorrhoids. Internal anal sphincterotomy in refractory cases.

PRURITUS ANI Often of unclear cause; may be due to poor hygiene, fungal or parasitic infection. Treat with thorough cleansing after bowel movement, topical glucocorticoid, antifungal agent if indicated.

ANAL CONDYLOMAS (Genital Warts) Wart-like papillomas due to sexually transmitted papillomavirus. Treat with cautious application of liquid nitrogen or podophyllotoxin or with intralesional alpha interferon. Tend to recur.

For a more detailed discussion, see Isselbacher KJ, Epstein A: Diverticular, Vascular, and Other Disorders of the Intestine and Peritoneum, Chap. 288, p. 1648, in HPIM-14.

142

CHOLELITHIASIS, CHOLECYSTITIS, AND CHOLANGITIS

CHOLELITHIASIS

There are three major types of gallstones: cholesterol, pigment, and mixed stones. Mixed and cholesterol gallstones contain more than 70% cholesterol monohydrate. Pigment stones have less than 10% cholesterol and are composed primarily of calcium bilirubinate. In the U.S., 80% of stones are cholesterol or mixed, 20% pigment.

EPIDEMIOLOGY   One million new cases of cholelithiasis per year in the U.S. Increased incidence in American Indians and with obesity, diabetes, ileal disease, pregnancy, estrogen or oral contraceptive use, type IV hyperlipidemia, and cirrhosis. Females/males = 4:1.

SYMPTOMS AND SIGNS   Many gallstones are "silent," i.e., present in asymptomatic pts. Symptoms occur when stones produce inflammation or obstruction of the cystic or common bile ducts. Major symptoms: (1) biliary colic, which is usually constant; RUQ or epigastric pain that occurs 30–90 min after meals, lasts for several hours, and occasionally radiates to the right scapula or back; (2) nausea, vomiting. Physical exam may be normal or show epigastric or RUQ tenderness.

LABORATORY   Occasionally, mild and transient elevations in bilirubin [<85 μmol/L (<5 mg/dL)] accompany biliary colic.

IMAGING   Only 10% of gallstones are radioopaque. Ultrasonography is best diagnostic test. The oral cholecystogram requires a functioning gallbladder and serum bilirubin <51 μmol/L (<3 mg/dL) (see Table 142-1).

DIFFERENTIAL DIAGNOSIS   Includes peptic ulcer disease, gastroesophageal reflux, irritable bowel syndrome, and hepatitis.

℞ TREATMENT

Since risk of developing complications requiring surgery is small in asymptomatic pts, elective cholecystectomy should be reserved for: (1) symptomatic pts (i.e., biliary colic despite low-fat diet); (2) persons with previous complications of cholelithiasis (see below); and, (3) asymptomatic pts with an increased risk of complications (calcified or nonfunctioning gallbladder, cholesterolosis, adenomyomatosis). Patients with gallstones >2 cm or with an anomalous gallbladder containing stones should also be considered for surgery. Laparoscopic cholecystectomy is minimally invasive and is the procedure of choice for most patients undergoing elective cholecystectomy. Oral dissolution agents (chenodeoxycholic acid, ursodeoxycholic acid) partially or completely dissolve radiolucent stones in 50% of selected pts but are ineffective in dissolving large, radioopaque, or pigment stones and those within a poorly opacified gallbladder following oral cholecystography. Recurrence is likely if the medication is stopped. Extracorporeal shockwave lithotripsy followed by medical litholytic therapy is effective in selected pts with solitary radiolucent gallstones. Direct dissolution of gallstones using solvents such as methyl-*tert*-butyl ether instilled through a percutaneously placed biliary catheter should be considered experimental.

COMPLICATIONS   See "Acute Cholecystitis" below.

ACUTE CHOLECYSTITIS

Acute inflammation of the gallbladder usually caused by cystic duct obstruction by an impacted stone.

ETIOLOGY   90% calculous; 10% acalculous; latter caused by prolonged acute illness, fasting, hyperalimentation leading to gallbladder stasis, vasculitis, carcinoma of gallbladder or common bile duct, some gallbladder infections (*Leptospira*, *Streptococcus*, etc.).

SYMPTOMS AND SIGNS   (1) RUQ or epigastric pain; (2) nausea, vomiting, anorexia; and (3) fever. Examination typically reveals RUQ tenderness; palpable RUQ mass found in 20% of

Table 142-1

Radiologic and Imaging Modalities for Biliary Tract Disease

Plain films of abdomen	Rarely useful for diagnosis of gallstones
	Can exclude other causes of abdominal pain (intestinal obstruction, perforated ulcer)
Ultrasound	High sensitivity/specificity for detecting gallstones
	Dilated ducts suggest ductal obstruction
	Intramural gas, pericholecystic fluid suggest gallbladder inflammation or infection
	Cannot definitively exclude choledocholithiasis
Scintigraphy (HIDA)	High sensitivity/specificity for acute cholecystitis
Oral cholecystogram	Seldom used for diagnosis of gallstone disease
	Can help select pts for nonsurgical therapy
CT scan	Useful if suspicion of cancer is high
Endoscopic retrograde cholangiopancreatography	Delineates lower limit of common bile duct (CBD) obstruction
	Therapeutic intervention possible
Percutaneous transhepatic cholangiography	Delineates upper limit of CBD obstruction
MR cholangiography	Promising noninvasive technique to evaluate the ductal system

pts. Murphy's sign is present when deep inspiration or cough during palpation of the RUQ produces increased pain or inspiratory arrest.

LABORATORY   Mild leukocytosis; serum bilirubin, alkaline phosphatase, and SGOT may be mildly elevated.

IMAGING Ultrasonography is useful for demonstrating gallstones and occasionally a phlegmonous mass surrounding the gallbladder. Radionuclide scans (HIDA, DISIDA, etc.) may identify cystic duct obstruction.

DIFFERENTIAL DIAGNOSIS Includes acute pancreatitis, appendicitis, pyelonephritis, peptic ulcer disease, hepatitis, and hepatic abscess.

℞ TREATMENT

Bowel rest, nasogastric suction, IV fluids and electrolytes, analgesia (meperidine or pentazocine), and antibiotics (ampicillin, cephalosporins, or aminoglycosides) are the mainstays of treatment. Diabetic, septic, or debilitated pts should receive combination antibiotic therapy. Acute symptoms will resolve in 75% of patients. Surgery is definitive and should be performed as soon as feasible (within 24–48 h of admission). Delayed surgery is reserved for pts with high risk of emergent surgery and where the diagnosis is in doubt.

COMPLICATIONS Empyema, hydrops, gangrene, perforation, fistulization, gallstone ileus, porcelain gallbladder.

CHRONIC CHOLECYSTITIS

ETIOLOGY Chronic cholecystitis usually caused by gallstones.

SYMPTOMS AND SIGNS Often nonspecific; include dyspepsia, fatty food intolerance, and abdominal pain.

LABORATORY Tests are usually normal.

IMAGING Ultrasonography preferred; usually shows gallstones within a contracted gallbladder (see Table 142-1).

DIFFERENTIAL DIAGNOSIS Peptic ulcer disease, esophagitis, irritable bowel syndrome.

℞ TREATMENT

Surgery indicated if pt is symptomatic.

CHOLEDOCHOLITHIASIS/CHOLANGITIS

SYMPTOMS AND SIGNS Choledocholithiasis may present as an incidental finding, biliary colic, obstructive jaundice, cholangitis, or pancreatitis. Cholangitis usually presents as fever, RUQ pain, and jaundice (Charcot's triad).

LABORATORY Elevations in serum bilirubin, alkaline phosphatase, and aminotransferases. Leukocytosis usually accompanies cholangitis. Amylase is elevated in 15% of cases.

IMAGING Ultrasonography may reveal dilated bile ducts but is not sensitive for detecting common duct stones. Endoscopic retrograde cholangiopancreatography or transhepatic cholangiography will confirm the diagnosis (see Table 142-1).

DIFFERENTIAL DIAGNOSIS Acute cholecystitis, renal colic, perforated viscus, pancreatitis.

℞ TREATMENT

Cholecystectomy with choledocholithotomy and T-tube drainage of the bile ducts is the treatment of choice for most pts with choledocholithiasis. If retained calculi are evident on a follow-up T-tube cholangiogram, percutaneous basket extraction should be performed. In elderly or poor-surgical-risk pts, endoscopic papillotomy with stone extraction is possible. Cholangitis treated like acute cholecystitis; bowel rest, hydration, and analgesia are the mainstays; stones should be removed surgically or endoscopically.

COMPLICATIONS Cholangitis, obstructive jaundice, gallstone-induced pancreatitis, and secondary biliary cirrhosis.

PRIMARY SCLEROSING CHOLANGITIS (PSC)

PSC is a sclerosing inflammatory process involving the biliary tree.

ETIOLOGY Males outnumber females and most patients are 25–45 years old. Associations: ulcerative colitis (60% of cases of PSC), AIDS, rarely Crohn's disease and retroperitoneal fibrosis.

SYMPTOMS AND SIGNS Pruritus, RUQ pain, jaundice, fever, weight loss, and malaise. May progress to cirrhosis with portal hypertension.

LABORATORY Evidence of cholestasis (elevated bilirubin and alkaline phosphatase) common.

RADIOLOGY/ENDOSCOPY Transhepatic or endoscopic cholangiograms reveal stenosis and dilation of the intra- and extrahepatic bile ducts.

DIFFERENTIAL DIAGNOSIS Cholangiocarcinoma, Caroli's disease (cystic dilation of bile ducts), *Fasciola hepatica* infection, echinococcosis, and ascariasis.

R_X TREATMENT

No satisfactory therapy. Cholangitis should be treated as outlined above. Cholestyramine may control pruritus. Supplemental vitamin D and calcium may retard bone loss. Urodeoxycholic acid, methotrexate, and cyclosporine appear promising as therapies. Surgical relief of biliary obstruction may be appropriate but has a high complication rate. The efficacy of colectomy for pts with ulcerative colitis is uncertain. Liver transplantation should be considered in pts with endstage cirrhosis.

For a more detailed discussion, see Greenberger NJ, Isselbacher KJ: Diseases of the Gallbladder and Bile Ducts, Chap. 302, p. 1725, in HPIM-14.

143

PANCREATITIS

ACUTE PANCREATITIS

The differentiation between acute and chronic pancreatitis is based on clinical criteria. In acute pancreatitis, there is restoration of normal pancreatic function; in the chronic form, there is permanent loss of function and pain may predominate. There are two pathologic types of acute pancreatitis: edematous and necrotizing.

ETIOLOGY Most common causes in the U.S. are alcohol and cholelithiasis. Others include abdominal trauma; postoperative or postendoscopic retrograde cholangiopancreatography (ERCP); metabolic (e.g., hypertriglyceridemia, hypercalcemia, renal failure); hereditary pancreatitis; infection (e.g., mumps, viral hepatitis, coxsackievirus, ascariasis, *Mycoplasma*); opportunistic infections (CMV, *Cryptococcus*, *Candida*, TB); medications (e.g., azathioprine, sulfonamides, thiazides, furosemide, estrogens, tetracycline, valproic acid, pentamidine); vasculitis (e.g., lupus, necrotizing angiitis, thrombotic thrombocytopenic purpura); penetrating peptic ulcer; obstruction of the ampulla of Vater (e.g., regional enteritis); pancreas divisum.

SYMPTOMS AND SIGNS   Can vary from mild abdominal pain to shock. *Common symptoms*: (1) steady, boring midepigastric pain radiating to the back that is frequently increased in the supine position; (2) nausea, vomiting. *Physical exam*: (1) low-grade fever, tachycardia, hypotension; (2) erythematous skin nodules due to subcutaneous fat necrosis; (3) basilar rales, pleural effusion (often on the left); (4) abdominal tenderness and rigidity, diminished bowel sounds, palpable upper abdominal mass; (5) Cullen's sign: blue discoloration in the periumbilical area due to hemoperitoneum; (6) Turner's sign: blue-red-purple or green-brown discoloration of the flanks due to tissue catabolism of hemoglobin.

LABORATORY

1.   *Serum amylase*: Large elevations ($>3 \times$ normal) virtually assure the diagnosis if salivary gland disease and intestinal perforation/infarction are excluded. However, normal serum amylase does not exclude the diagnosis of acute pancreatitis, and the degree of elevation does not predict severity of pancreatitis. Amylase levels typically return to normal in 48–72 h.

2.   *Urinary amylase-creatinine clearance ratio* may be helpful in distinguishing between pancreatitis and other causes of hyperamylasemia (e.g., macroamylasemia) but is invalid in the presence of renal failure. Simultaneous serum and urine amylase values are used. $C_{am}/C_{Cr} = (am_{urine} \times Cr_{serum}) / (am_{serum} \times Cr_{urine})$. Normal value is less than 4%.

3.   *Serum lipase* level is more specific for pancreatic disease and remains elevated for 7–14 d.

4.   *Other tests*: *Hypocalcemia* occurs in approximately 25% of pts. *Leukocytosis* (15,000–20,000/µL) occurs frequently. *Hypertriglyceridemia* occurs in 15% of cases and can cause a spuriously normal serum amylase level. Hyperglycemia is common. *Serum bilirubin*, *alkaline phosphatase*, and *aspartate aminotransferase* can be transiently elevated. *Hypoalbuminemia* and marked elevations of serum lactic dehydrogenase (LDH) are associated with an increased mortality rate. *Hypoxemia* is present in 25% of pts. Arterial pH <7.32 may spuriously elevate serum amylase. The ECG may demonstrate ST-segment and T-wave abnormalities.

Imaging

1.   *Abdominal radiographs* are abnormal in 50% of pts but are not specific for pancreatitis. Common findings include total

or partial ileus ("sentinel loop") and spasm of transverse colon. Useful for excluding diagnoses such as intestinal perforation.

2. *Ultrasound* often fails to visualize the pancreas because of overlying intestinal gas but may detect gallstones or edema or enlargement of the pancreas.

3. *CT* can confirm diagnosis of pancreatitis (edematous pancreas) and is useful for predicting and identifying late complications.

DIFFERENTIAL DIAGNOSIS Intestinal perforation (especially peptic ulcer), cholecystitis, acute intestinal obstruction, mesenteric ischemia, renal colic, myocardial ischemia, aortic dissection, connective tissue disorders, pneumonia, and diabetic ketoacidosis.

℞ TREATMENT

Most (90%) cases subside over a period of 3–7 d. Conventional measures: (1) analgesics, such as meperidine; (2) IV fluids and colloids; (3) no oral alimentation; (4) treatment of hypocalcemia, if symptomatic; (5) antibiotics only if there is established infection. Not effective: cimetidine (or related agents), nasogastric suction, glucagon, peritoneal lavage, and anticholinergic medications. Pts with mild pain, minimal vomiting, and adequate hydration can be treated as outpatients if careful monitoring and follow-up are feasible. Precipitating factors (alcohol, medications) must be eliminated. Elderly pts and those with tachycardia, fever, hypoglycemia, or hypocalcemia should be hospitalized, even though symptoms are mild. In mild or moderate pancreatitis, a clear liquid diet can usually be started after 3–6 d. Fulminant pancreatitis usually requires aggressive fluid support and meticulous management of cardiovascular collapse, respiratory insufficiency, and pancreatic infection. Laparotomy with removal of necrotic material and adequate drainage should be considered if pt continues to deteriorate despite conventional therapy. Pts with severe gallstone-induced pancreatitis often benefit from early (<3 d) papillotomy.

COMPLICATIONS Increased mortality with respiratory failure, shock, massive colloid requirements, hypocalcemia, or hemorrhagic peritoneal fluid. *Early*: Shock, GI bleeding, common duct obstruction, ileus, splenic infarction or rupture, DIC, subcutaneous fat necrosis, ARDS, pleural effusion, hematuria, acute renal failure, sudden blindness. *Late*: (1) *Pancreatic phlegmon* (a solid mass of swollen, inflamed pancreas) should be suspected if abdominal pain, fever, and hyperamylasemia persist for more than 5 d. Phlegmons may become secondarily infected resulting in abscess formation (see below). (2) *Pancreatic pseudocysts* develop over 1–4 weeks in 15% of pts. Abdominal pain is the usual complaint, and a tender upper abdominal mass may be present. Can be detected by abdominal ultrasound or CT. In pts who are stable and uncomplicated, treatment is supportive; if there is no resolution within 6 weeks, consider CT-guided needle aspiration/drainage, surgical drainage, or resection. In pts with an expanding pseudocyst or complicated by hemorrhage, rupture, or abscess, surgery should be performed. (3) *Pancreatic abscess* (signaled by fever, leukocytosis, ileus, and rapid deterioration in a pt recovering from pancreatitis) is most often due to *E. coli*. The diagnosis of pancreatic infection can be established by CT-guided needle aspiration of phlegmons and pseudocysts. Treatment consists of antibiotic therapy and surgical drainage. (4) *Pancreatic ascites and pleural effusions* are usually due to disruption of the main pancreatic duct. Treatment involves nasogastric suction and parenteral alimentation for 2–3 weeks. If medical management fails, pancreatography followed by surgery should be performed.

CHRONIC PANCREATITIS   Chronic pancreatitis may occur as recurrent episodes of acute inflammation superimposed upon a damaged pancreas or as chronic damage with pain and malabsorption. The causes of relapsing pancreatitis are similar to acute pancreatitis.

ETIOLOGY   Chronic alcoholism most frequent in U.S.; also hypertriglyceridemia, hypercalcemia, hereditary pancreatitis, hemochromatosis, and cystic fibrosis. In 25% of adults, etiology is unknown.

SYMPTOMS AND SIGNS   *Pain* is cardinal symptom. Weight loss, steatorrhea, and other signs and symptoms of malabsorption common. Physical exam often unremarkable.

LABORATORY   No specific laboratory test for chronic pancreatitis. Serum amylase and lipase levels are often normal. Serum bilirubin and alkaline phosphatase may be elevated. Steatorrhea (fecal fat concentration ≥9.5%) late in the course. The bentiromide test, a simple, effective test of pancreatic exocrine function may be helpful. D-Xylose urinary excretion test is usually normal. Impaired glucose tolerance is present in over 50% of pts. Secretin stimulation test is a relatively sensitive test for pancreatic exocrine deficiency.

IMAGING   *Plain films of the abdomen* reveal pancreatic calcifications in 30–60%. *Ultrasound* and *CT scans* may show pseudocysts or dilation of the pancreatic duct. *ERCP* often reveals irregular dilation of the main pancreatic duct and pruning of the branches.

DIFFERENTIAL DIAGNOSIS Important to distinguish from pancreatic carcinoma; may require radiographically guided biopsy.

℞ TREATMENT

Aimed at controlling pain and malabsorption. Intermittent attacks treated like acute pancreatitis. Alcohol and large, fatty meals must be avoided. Narcotics for severe pain, but subsequent addiction is common. Pts unable to maintain adequate hydration should be hospitalized, while those with milder symptoms can be managed on an ambulatory basis. Surgery may control pain if there is a ductal stricture. Subtotal pancreatectomy may also control pain but at the cost of exocrine insufficiency and diabetes. Malabsorption is managed with a low-fat diet and pancreatic enzyme replacement (8 conventional tablets or 3 enteric-coated tablets with meals). Because pancreatic enzymes are inactivated by acid, agents that reduce acid production (e.g., omeprazole or sodium bicarbonate) may improve their efficacy (but should not be given with enteric-coated preparations). Insulin may be necessary to control serum glucose.

COMPLICATIONS Vitamin B_{12} malabsorption in 40% of alcohol-induced and all cystic fibrosis cases. Impaired glucose tolerance. Nondiabetic retinopathy due to vitamin A and/or zinc deficiency. GI bleeding, icterus, effusions, subcutaneous fat necrosis, and bone pain occasionally occur. Increased risk for pancreatic carcinoma. Narcotic addiction common.

For a more detailed discussion, see Greenberger NJ, Toskes, PP, Isselbacher KJ: Acute and Chronic Pancreatitis, Chap. 304, p. 1741, in HPIM-14.

144

ACUTE HEPATITIS

VIRAL HEPATITIS

Clinically characterized by malaise, nausea, vomiting, diarrhea, and low-grade fever followed by dark urine, jaundice, and tender hepatomegaly; may be subclinical and detected on basis of elevated aspartate and alanine aminotransferase (AST and ALT) levels. Hepatitis B may be associated with immune-complex phenomena, including arthritis, serum-sickness–like illness, glomerulonephritis, and polyarteritis nodosa. Hepatitis-like illnesses may be caused not only by hepatotropic viruses (A, B, C, D, E), but also by other viruses (Epstein-Barr, CMV, coxsackievirus, etc.), alcohol, drugs, hypotension and ischemia, and biliary tract disease. (See Table 144-1.)

HEPATITIS A (HAV) 27-nm picornavirus (hepatovirus) with single-stranded RNA genome. Clinical course: See Fig. 144-1.

Outcome Recovery within 6–12 months, occasionally after one or two apparent clinical and serologic relapses; in some cases, pronounced cholestasis suggesting biliary obstruction may occur; rare fatalities (fulminant hepatitis), no chronic carrier state.

Diagnosis IgM anti-HAV in acute or early convalescent serum sample.

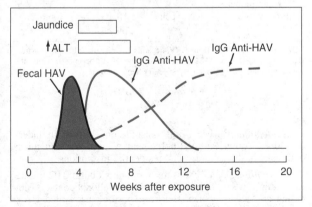

FIGURE 144-1 Scheme of typical clinical and laboratory features of HAV. (Reproduced from Dienstag JL, Isselbacher KJ, HPIM-14).

Table 144-1

The Hepatitis Viruses

	HAV	HBV	HCV
Viral Properties			
Size nm	27	42	~55
Nucleic acid	RNA	DNA	RNA
Genome length, kb	7.5	3.2	9.4
Classification	Picorna-virus	Hepadna-virus	Flavivirus-like
Incubation, days	15–45	30–180	15–160
Transmission			
Fecal-oral	+ + +	—	—
Percutaneous	Rare	+ + +	+ + +
Sexual	?	+ +	Uncommon
Perinatal	—	+ + +	Uncommon
Clinical Features			
Severity	Usually mild	Moderate	Mild
Chronic infection	No	1–2%; up to 90% in neonates	80–90%
Carrier state	No	Yes	Yes
Fulminant hepatitis	0.1%	1%	Rare
Hepatocellular carcinoma	No	Yes	Yes
Prophylaxis	IG; vaccine	HBIG; vaccine	None

NOTE: HAV, hepatitis A virus; HBV, hepatitis B virus; HCV, hepatitis C virus; HDV, hepatitis D virus; HEV, hepatitis E virus; HGV, hepatitis G virus; IG, imune globulin; + +, sometimes; + + +, often; ?, possibly.

Epidemiology   Fecal-oral transmission; endemic in under-developed countries; food-borne and waterborne epidemics; outbreaks in day-care centers, residential institutions.

Prevention   After exposure: immune globulin 0.02 mL/kg IM within 2 weeks to household and institutional contacts (not casual contacts at work). Before exposure: inactivated HAV vaccine 0.5–1 mL IM (dose depends on formulation); half dose

HDV	HEV	HGV
~36	~32	?
RNA	RNA	RNA
1.7	7.5	9.4
—	Calicivirus-like or alpha-virus-like	Flavivirus
21–140	14–63	?
—	+ + +	?
+ + +	—	+ +
+ +	—	?
+	—	?
May be severe	Usually mild	Mild
Common	No	Yes
Yes	No	Yes
Up to 20% in superinfection	10–20% in pregnant women	?
?	No	?
None (HBV vaccine for susceptibles)	None	None

to children; repeat at 6–12 months; target travelers, military recruits, animal handlers, day-care personnel.

HEPATITIS B (HBV) 42-nm hepadnavirus with outer surface coat (HBsAg), inner nucleocapsid core (HBcAg), DNA polymerase, and partially double-stranded DNA genome of 3200 nucleotides. Circulating form of HBcAg is HBeAg, a marker of viral replication and infectivity. Multiple serotypes and genetic heterogeneity. Course: see Fig. 144-2.

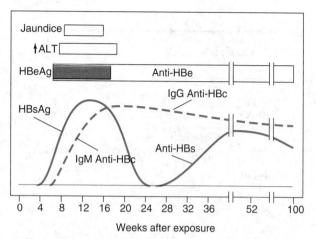

Weeks after exposure

FIGURE 144-2 Scheme of typical clinical and laboratory features of HBV. (Reproduced from Dienstag JL, Isselbacher KJ, HPIM-14.)

Outcome Recovery >90%, fulminant hepatitis (<1%), chronic hepatitis or carrier state (only 1–2% of immunocompetent adults; higher in neonates, elderly, immunocompromised), cirrhosis and hepatocellular carcinoma (especially following chronic infection beginning in infancy or early childhood) (Chap. 146).

Diagnosis HBsAg in serum (acute or chronic infection); IgM anti-HBc (early anti-HBc indicative of acute or recent infection). Most sensitive test is detection of HBV DNA in serum; not generally required for routine diagnosis.

Epidemiology Percutaneous (needlestick), sexual, or perinatal transmission. Endemic in sub-Saharan Africa and Southeast Asia, where up to 20% of population acquire infection, usually early in life.

Prevention After exposure: hepatitis B immune globulin (HBIG) 0.06 mL/kg IM immediately after needlestick, within 14 days of sexual exposure, or at birth (HBsAg+ mother) in combination with vaccine series. Before exposure: recombinant hepatitis B vaccine 10–20 μg IM (dose depends on formulation); half dose to children, 40-μg dose to immunocompromised adults; at 0, 1, and 6 months; deltoid, not gluteal injection. Has been targeted to high-risk groups (e.g., health workers, gay men, IV drug users, hemodialysis pts, hemophiliacs, household and sexual contacts of HBsAg carriers, all neonates in endemic

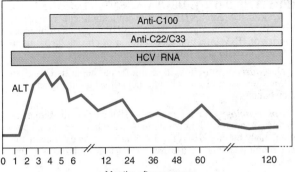

FIGURE 144-3 Serologic course of acute hepatitis type C progressing to chronicity. HCV RNA is detectable before the ALT elevation. Antibody to C22 and anti-C33 appears during acute hepatitis C, whereas antibody to C100 appears 1 to 3 months later. (Reproduced from Dienstag JL, Isselbacher KJ, HPIM-14.)

areas, or high-risk neonates in lower-risk areas). Universal vaccination of all children is now recommended in U.S.

HEPATITIS C (HCV) Caused by flavi-like virus with RNA genome of over 9000 nucleotides (similar to yellow fever virus, dengue virus); some genetic heterogeneity. Incubation period 7–8 weeks. Course often clinically mild and marked by fluctuating elevations of serum aminotransferase levels; >50% likelihood of chronicity, leading to cirrhosis in over 20%.

Diagnosis Anti-HCV in serum. Current second- and third-generation enzyme immunoassay detects antibody to epitopes designated C200, C33c, C22-3; may appear after acute illness but generally present by 3–5 months after exposure. Most sensitive test is detection of HCV RNA in serum; not generally required (Fig. 144-3).

Epidemiology Percutaneous transmission accounts for over 90% of transfusion-associated hepatitis cases. Intravenous drug use accounts for over 50% of reported cases. Little evidence for frequent sexual or perinatal transmission.

Prevention Exclusion of paid blood donors, testing of donated blood for anti-HCV. Anti-HCV detected by enzyme immunoassay in blood donors with normal ALT is often falsely positive (30%); result should be confirmed with recombinant immunoblot assay (RIBA), which correlates with presence of HCV RNA in serum.

HEPATITIS D (HDV, DELTA AGENT) Defective 37-nm RNA virus that requires HBV for its replication; either *coinfects* with HBV or *superinfects* a chronic HBV carrier. Enhances severity of HBV infection (acceleration of chronic hepatitis to cirrhosis, occasionally fulminant acute hepatitis).

Diagnosis Anti-HDV in serum (acute hepatitis D—often in low titer, is transient; chronic hepatitis D—in higher titer, is sustained).

Epidemiology Endemic among HBV carriers in Mediterranean basin, areas of South America, etc. Otherwise spread percutaneously among HBsAg + IV drug users or by transfusion in hemophiliacs and to a lesser extent among HBsAg + gay men.

Prevention Hepatitis B vaccine (noncarriers only).

HEPATITIS E (HEV) Caused by 29 to 32-nm agent thought to be related to caliciviruses. Responsible for waterborne epidemics of hepatitis in India, parts of Asia and Africa, and Mexico. Self-limited illness with high (10–20%) mortality rate in pregnant women.

HEPATITIS G (HGV) Recently identified flavivirus with RNA genome of over 9000 nucleotides (distantly related to HCV). Though common (detected in 1.7% of U.S. blood donors) and associated with viremia lasting for years, HGV does not appear to cause significant liver disease.

R̲x̲ TREATMENT

Activity as tolerated, high-calorie diet (often tolerated best in morning), IV hydration for severe vomiting, cholestyramine up to 4 g PO qid for severe pruritus, avoid hepatically metabolized drugs; no role for glucocorticoids. Liver transplantation for fulminant hepatic failure and grades III–IV encephalopathy.

TOXIC AND DRUG-INDUCED HEPATITIS

DOSE-DEPENDENT (DIRECT HEPATOTOXINS) Onset is within 48 h, predictable, necrosis around terminal hepatic venule—e.g., carbon tetrachloride, benzene derivatives, mushroom poisoning, acetaminophen, or microvesicular steatosis (e.g., tetracyclines, valproic acid).

IDIOSYNCRATIC Variable dose and time of onset, small number of exposed persons affected, may be associated with fever, rash, arthralgias, eosinophilia. In many cases, mechanism may actually involve toxic metabolite, possibly determined on genetic basis—e.g., isoniazid, halothane, phenytoin, methyldopa, carbamazepine, diclofenac, oxacillin, sulfonamides.

℞ TREATMENT

Supportive as for viral hepatitis; withdraw suspected agent. Liver transplantation if necessary.

ACUTE HEPATIC FAILURE

Massive hepatic necrosis with impaired consciousness occurring within 8 weeks of the onset of illness.

CAUSES Infections (viral, including HAV, HBV, HCV (rarely), HDV, HEV, bacterial, rickettsial, parasitic), drugs and toxins, ischemia (shock), Budd-Chiari syndrome, idiopathic chronic active hepatitis, acute Wilson's disease, microvesicular fat syndromes (Reye's syndrome, acute fatty liver of pregnancy).

CLINICAL MANIFESTATIONS Neuropsychiatric changes—delirium, personality change, stupor, coma; cerebral edema—suggested by profuse sweating, hemodynamic instability, tachyarrhythmias, tachypnea, fever, papilledema, decerebrate rigidity (though all may be absent); deep jaundice, coagulopathy, bleeding, renal failure, acid-base disturbance, hypoglycemia, acute pancreatitis, cardiorespiratory failure, infections (bacterial, fungal).

ADVERSE PROGNOSTIC INDICATORS Age <10 or >40, certain causes (e.g., halothane, hepatitis C), duration of jaundice >7 d before onset of encephalopathy, serum bilirubin >300 μmol/L (>18 mg/dL), coma (survival <20%), rapid reduction in liver size, respiratory failure, marked prolongations of PT, factor V level <20%. In acetaminophen overdose, adverse prognosis is suggested by blood pH <7.30, serum creatinine >266 μmol/L (>3 mg/dL), markedly prolonged PT.

℞ TREATMENT

Endotracheal intubation often required. Monitor serum glucose—IV D10 or D20 as necessary. Prevent gastrointestinal bleeding with H_2-receptor antagonists and antacids (maintain gastric pH ≥3.5). In many centers intracranial pressure is monitored—more sensitive than CT in detecting cerebral edema. Value of dexamethasone for cerebral edema unclear; IV mannitol may be beneficial. Liver transplantation should be considered in pts with grades III–IV encephalopathy and other adverse prognostic indicators.

For a more detailed discussion, see Dienstag JL, Isselbacher KJ: Acute Viral Hepatitis, Chap. 295, p. 1677, in HPIM-14.

145

CHRONIC HEPATITIS

A group of disorders characterized by a chronic inflammatory reaction in the liver for at least 6 months.

OVERVIEW

ETIOLOGY Hepatitis B virus (HBV), hepatitis C virus (HCV), hepatitis D virus (HDV, delta agent), drugs (methyldopa, nitrofurantoin, isoniazid, dantrolene), autoimmune hepatitis, Wilson's disease, hemochromatosis, alpha$_1$ antitrypsin deficiency.

HISTOLOGIC CLASSIFICATION (Table 145-1)

PRESENTATION Wide clinical spectrum ranging from asymptomatic serum aminotransferase elevations to apparently acute, even fulminant, hepatitis. Common symptoms include fatigue, malaise, anorexia, low-grade fever; jaundice is frequent in severe disease. Some pts may present with complications of cirrhosis; ascites, variceal bleeding, encephalopathy, coagulopathy, and hypersplenism. In chronic hepatitis B or C and autoimmune hepatitis, extrahepatic features may predominate.

CHRONIC HEPATITIS B

Follows up to 1–2% of cases of acute hepatitis B in immunocompetent hosts; more frequent in immunocompromised hosts. Spectrum of disease: asymptomatic antigenemia, chronic hepatitis, cirrhosis, hepatocellular cancer; *early phase* often associated with continued symptoms of hepatitis, elevated aminotrans-

Table 145-1

Histologic Classification of Chronic Hepatitis

| | Inflammatory Activity | | Degree of Fibrosis | |
| | Portal | Hepatic | | |
Grade	Tracts	Lobule	Stage	Fibrosis
0	None or minimal	None	1	No fibrosis or limited to within expanded portal tracts
1	Portal inflammation	Inflammation, no necrosis	2	Periportal fibrosis or portal-to-portal septa with intact architecture
2	Mild limiting plate necrosis	Focal necrosis	3	Septal fibrosis with architectural distortion
3	Moderate limiting plate necrosis	Severe focal cell damage	4	Cirrhosis
4	Severe limiting plate necrosis	Bridging necrosis		

ferase levels, presence in serum of HBeAg and HBV DNA, and presence in liver of replicative form of HBV; *later phase* in some pts may be associated with clinical and biochemical improvement, disappearance of HBeAg and HBV DNA and appearance of anti-HBe in serum, and integration of HBV DNA into host hepatocyte genome. In Mediterranean area, a frequent variant is characterized by a severe and rapidly progressive course and HBV DNA with anti-HBe in serum, due to a mutation in the pre-C region of the HBV genome that prevents HBeAg synthesis (may appear during course of chronic wild-type HBV infection as a result of immune pressure and may also account for some cases of fulminant hepatitis B). Chronic hepatitis B ultimately leads to cirrhosis in 25–40% of cases (particularly in pts with HDV superinfection or the pre-C mutation) and hepatocellular carcinoma in many of these pts (particularly when chronic infection is acquired early in life).

EXTRAHEPATIC MANIFESTATIONS (IMMUNE-COMPLEX-MEDIATED) Rash, urticaria, arthritis, polyarteritis, polyneuropathy, glomerulonephritis.

℞ TREATMENT

Standard approach is interferon-α 5 million units qd or 10 million units three times per week × 4 months for serum HBeAg/HBV-DNA-positive pts with symptoms, elevated aminotransferase levels, and biopsy evidence of chronic hepatitis. Results in HBeAg anti-HBe seroconversion with clinical, biochemical, and histologic improvement in up to 40% of cases. Best predictor of response is serum HBV DNA level <200 ng/L. Poor responders: pts positive for anti-HDV or HIV, adult carriers infected in childhood, immunocompromised pts, persons infected with HBeAg-negative "pre-core" mutant. Common side effects: flulike reactions, bone marrow depression, precipitation of autoimmune diseases including thyroid disease, CNS symptoms, anorexia, sleep disturbance. In pts with lower aminotransferase levels (<100 U/L), efficacy of interferon may be enhanced by a priming prednisone course, 60 mg PO qd, tapering over 6 weeks, but this approach may result in fatal flare of hepatitis B and is not recommended. Avoid interferon in pts with decompensated cirrhosis (e.g., ascites, jaundice, coagulopathy, encephalopathy). The nucleoside analogues lamivudine and famciclovir appear promising.

CHRONIC HEPATITIS C

Follows at least 70% of cases of transfusion-associated and sporadic hepatitis C. Clinically mild, often waxing and waning aminotransferase elevations; mild chronic hepatitis on liver biopsy. Associated with essential mixed cryoglobulinemia, porphyria cutanea tarda, membranoproliferative glomerulonephritis, and lymphocytic sialadenitis. Diagnosis confirmed by detecting anti-HCV in serum. May lead to cirrhosis in 20% or more of cases after 20 years.

℞ TREATMENT

Therapy with interferon-α 3 million units 3 times per week for 12–18 months should be considered in pts with aminotransferase elevations, biopsy evidence of moderate or severe chronic hepatitis, HCV RNA in serum; 50% achieve clinical and biochemical remission or improvement; however, at least

50% of pts relapse within 12 months of treatment and may require retreatment. Higher doses do not improve sustained response rate and cause more side effects. Sustained response is associated with loss of HCV RNA from serum. Poorer response rates are associated with cirrhosis, high serum HCV RNA levels, and HCV genotypes 1a and 1b, which are prevalent in U.S. Benefit in pts with normal or nearly normal serum aminotransferase levels or decompensated cirrhosis is doubtful. Benefit of adding ribavirin, a nucleoside analogue, is under study.

AUTOIMMUNE HEPATITIS

CLASSIFICATION *Type I*: classic autoimmune hepatitis, anti-smooth muscle and/or antinuclear antibodies. *Type II*: associated with anti-liver/kidney microsomal antibodies (anti-LKM), which are directed against cytochrome P4502D6 (seen primarily in southern Europe).

CLINICAL MANIFESTATIONS Classic autoimmune hepatitis (type I): 80% women, third to fifth decades. Abrupt onset (acute hepatitis) in a third. Insidious onset in two-thirds: progressive jaundice, anorexia, hepatomegaly, abdominal pain, epistaxis, fever, fatigue, amenorrhea. Leads to cirrhosis; >50% 5-year mortality if untreated.

EXTRAHEPATIC MANIFESTATIONS Rash, arthralgias, keratoconjunctivitis sicca, thyroiditis, hemolytic anemia, nephritis.

SEROLOGIC ABNORMALITIES Hypergammaglobulinemia, smooth-muscle antibody (40–80%), ANA (20–50%), antimitochondrial antibody (10–20%), false-positive anti-HCV enzyme immunoassay but usually not recombinant immunoblot assay (RIBA). Type II: anti-LKM antibody.

℞ **TREATMENT**
Indicated for symptomatic disease with biopsy evidence of severe chronic hepatitis (bridging necrosis), marked aminotransferase elevations (5- to 10-fold), and hypergammaglobulinemia. Prednisone or prednisolone 30 mg PO qd tapered to 10–15 mg qd over several weeks; often azathioprine 50 mg PO qd is also administered to permit lower glucocorticoid doses and avoid steroid side effects. Monitor LFTs monthly. Symptoms may improve rapidly, but biochemical improvement may take weeks or months and subsequent histologic improvement (to lesion of mild chronic hepatitis or normal biopsy) up to 18–24 months. Withdrawal of glucocorticoids

can be attempted following clinical, biochemical, and histologic remission; relapse occurs in 50–90% of cases (retreat). For frequent relapses, consider maintenance therapy with low-dose glucocorticoids or azathioprine 2(mg/kg)/d.

For a more detailed discussion, see Dienstag JL, Isselbacher KJ: Chronic Hepatitis, Chap. 297, p. 1696, in HPIM-14.

146

CIRRHOSIS AND ALCOHOLIC LIVER DISEASE

CIRRHOSIS

Chronic disease of the liver characterized by fibrosis, disorganization of the lobular and vascular architecture, and regenerating nodules of hepatocytes.

CAUSES Alcohol, viral hepatitis (B, C, D), primary or secondary biliary cirrhosis, hemochromatosis, Wilson's disease, alpha$_1$ antitrypsin deficiency, autoimmune hepatitis, Budd-Chiari syndrome, chronic CHF (cardiac cirrhosis), drugs and toxins, schistosomiasis, cryptogenic.

CLINICAL MANIFESTATIONS May be absent.

Symptoms Anorexia, nausea, vomiting, diarrhea, fatigue, weakness, fever, jaundice, amenorrhea, impotence, infertility.

Signs Spider telangiectases, palmar erythema, parotid and lacrimal gland enlargement, nail changes (Muehrcke lines, Terry's nails), clubbing, Dupuytren's contracture, gynecomastia, testicular atrophy, hepatosplenomegaly, ascites, gastrointestinal bleeding (e.g., varices), hepatic encephalopathy.

Laboratory findings Anemia (microcytic due to blood loss, macrocytic due to folate deficiency), pancytopenia (hypersplenism), prolonged PT, rarely overt DIC; hyponatremia, hypokalemic alkalosis, glucose disturbances, hypoalbuminemia, hypoxemia (hepatopulmonary syndrome).

Other associations Gastritis; duodenal ulcer; gallstones. Altered drug metabolism because of decreased drug clearance, metabolism (e.g, by cytochrome P450), and elimination; hypoalbuminemia; and portosystemic shunting.

DIAGNOSTIC STUDIES Depend on clinical setting. Serum: HBsAg, anti-HBc, anti-HBs, anti-HCV, anti-HDV, Fe, total iron-binding capacity, ferritin, antimitochondrial antibody (AMA), smooth-muscle antibody (SMA), anti-KLM antibody, ANA, ceruloplasmin, alpha$_1$ antitrypsin (and pi typing); abdominal ultrasound with doppler study, CT or MRI (may show cirrhotic liver, splenomegaly, collaterals, venous thrombosis), portal venography, and wedged hepatic vein pressure measurement. Definitive diagnosis often depends on liver biopsy (percutaneous, transjugular, or open).

ALCOHOLIC LIVER DISEASE

Three forms: fatty liver, alcoholic hepatitis, cirrhosis; may coexist. History of excessive alcohol use often denied. Severe forms (hepatitis, cirrhosis) associated with ingestion of 80–160 g/d for >5–10 years; women more susceptible than men because of lower levels of gastric alcohol dehydrogenase; polymorphisms of alcohol dehydrogenase and acetaldehyde dehydrogenase genes may also affect susceptibility. Hepatitis B and C may be cofactors in the development of liver disease. Malnutrition may contribute to development of cirrhosis.

FATTY LIVER May follow even brief periods of ethanol use. Often presents as asymptomatic hepatomegaly and mild elevations in biochemical liver tests. Reverses on withdrawal of ethanol; does not lead to cirrhosis.

ALCOHOLIC HEPATITIS Clinical presentation ranges from asymptomatic to severe liver failure with jaundice, ascites, GI bleeding, and encephalopathy. Typically anorexia, nausea, vomiting, fever, jaundice, tender hepatomegaly. Occasional cholestatic picture mimicking biliary obstruction. Aspartate aminotransferase (AST) usually less than 300 U and more than twofold higher than alanine aminotransferase (ALT). Bilirubin may be >170 μmol/L (>10 mg/dL). WBC may be as high as 20,000/μL. Diagnosis defined by liver biopsy findings: hepatocyte swelling, alcoholic hyaline (Mallory bodies), infiltration of PMNs, necrosis of hepatocytes, pericentral venular fibrosis.

Other metabolic consequences of alcoholism Increased NADH/NAD ratio leads to lacticacidemia, ketoacidosis, hyperuricemia, hypoglycemia. Hypomagnesemia, hypophosphatemia. Also mitochondrial dysfunction, induction of microsomal enzymes resulting in altered drug metabolism, lipid peroxidation leading to membrane damage, hypermetabolic state; many features of alcoholic hepatitis are attributable to toxic effects of acetaldehyde and cytokines (IL-1, IL-6, and TNF, released because of impaired detoxification of endotoxin).

Adverse prognostic factors *Short-term*: PT >5 s above control despite vitamin K, bilirubin >170 μmol/L (>10 mg/dL), encephalopathy, hypoalbuminemia, azotemia. Mortality is >35% if (pt's PT in 1 s) − (control PT in 1 s) x 4.6 + serum bilirubin (mg/dL) =>32.
Long-term: severe hepatic necrosis and fibrosis, portal hypertension, continued alcohol consumption.

R⃝ TREATMENT

Abstinence is essential; 8500–12,500 kJ (2000–3000 kcal) diet with 1 g/kg protein (less if encephalopathy). Daily multivitamin, thiamine 100 mg, folic acid 1 mg. Correct potassium, magnesium, and phosphate deficiencies. Transfusions of packed red cells, plasma as necessary. Monitor glucose (hypoglycemia in severe liver disease). Prednisone 40 mg or prednisolone 32 mg PO qd × 1 month may be beneficial in severe alcoholic hepatitis with encephalopathy (in absence of GI bleeding, renal failure, infection). Colchicine 0.6 mg PO bid may slow progression of alcoholic liver disease. *Experimental*: amino acid infusions, propylthiouracil, insulin and glucagon, anabolic steroids. Liver transplantation in carefully selected pts who have been abstinent >6 months.

PRIMARY BILIARY CIRRHOSIS

Progressive nonsuppurative destructive intrahepatic cholangitis. Affects middle-aged women. Presents as asymptomatic elevation in alkaline phosphatase (better prognosis) or with pruritus, progressive jaundice, consequences of impaired bile excretion, and ultimately cirrhosis and liver failure.

CLINICAL MANIFESTATIONS Pruritus, jaundice, xanthelasma, xanthomata, osteoporosis, steatorrhea, skin pigmentation, hepatosplenomegaly, portal hypertension; elevations in serum alkaline phosphatase, bilirubin, cholesterol, and IgM levels.

ASSOCIATED DISEASES Sjögren's syndrome, collagen-vascular diseases, thyroiditis, glomerulonephritis, pernicious anemia, renal tubular acidosis.

DIAGNOSIS AMA in >90-95% (directed against the E₂ component of pyruvate dehydrogenase and other 2-oxo-acid dehydrogenase mitochondrial enzymes). Liver biopsy: stage 1—destruction of interlobular bile ducts, granulomas; stage 2—ductular proliferation; stage 3—fibrosis; stage 4—cirrhosis.

PROGNOSIS Correlates with age, serum bilirubin, serum albumin, prothrombin time, edema.

℞ TREATMENT

Cholestyramine 4 g PO with meals for pruritus; in refractory cases consider rifampin, phototherapy with UVB light, naloxone infusion, plasmapheresis. Vitamin K 10 mg IM qd × 3 (then once a month) for elevated PT due to intestinal bile-salt deficiency. Vitamin D 100,000 U IM q 4 weeks plus oral calcium 1 g qd for osteoporosis (often unresponsive). Vitamin A 25,000–50,000 U PO qd or 100,000 U IM q 4 weeks and zinc 220 mg PO qd may help night blindness. Vitamin E 10 mg IM or PO qd. Substituting dietary fat with medium-chain triglycerides (MCTs) may reduce steatorrhea. Glucocorticoids, D-penicillamine, azathioprine, chlorambucil, cyclosporine of no value. Most widely used agent is ursodeoxycholic acid 12–15 (mg/kg)/d PO in 2 divided doses—improves symptoms and LFTs and slows progression, delaying need for liver transplantation. Colchicine less effective, and methotrexate requires more study. Liver transplantation for end-stage disease.

LIVER TRANSPLANTATION

Consider for chronic, irreversible, progressive liver disease or fulminant hepatic failure when no alternative therapy is available. (Also indicated to correct certain congenital enzyme deficiencies and inborn errors of metabolism.)

CONTRAINDICATIONS *Absolute* Extrahepatobiliary sepsis or malignancy, severe cardiopulmonary disease, AIDS.

Relative Age >70, HIV, extensive previous abdominal surgery, portal and superior mesenteric vein thrombosis, active alcoholism or drug abuse, lack of pt understanding.

INDICATIONS Guidelines: expected death in 2 years; preferably in anticipation of major complication (variceal bleeding, irreversible encephalopathy, severe malnutrition and incapacitating weakness, hepatorenal syndrome); refractory ascites, progressive bone disease, severe pruritus, recurrent bacterial cholangitis, intractable coagulopathy; hepatopulmonary syndrome (intrapulmonary vascular dilatations with increased alveolar-arterial gradient), once considered a contraindication, may reverse with transplantation; bilirubin >170–340 μmol/L (>10–20 mg/dL), albumin <20 g/L (<2 g/dL), worsening coagulopathy; poor quality of life. In fulminant hepatic failure consider for grade III–IV coma (before cerebral edema develops).

SELECTION OF DONOR   Matched for ABO blood group compatibility and liver size (reduced-size grafts may be used, esp. in children). Should be negative for HIV, HBV, and HCV.

IMMUNOSUPPRESSION   Various combinations of tacrolimus or cyclosporine and glucocorticoids, azathioprine, or OKT3 (monoclonal antithymocyte globulin).

MEDICAL COMPLICATIONS AFTER TRANSPLANTATION   Liver graft dysfunction (primary nonfunction, acute or chronic rejection, ischemia, hepatic artery thrombosis, biliary obstruction or leak, recurrent hepatitis B or C); infections (bacterial, viral, fungal, opportunistic); renal dysfunction; neuropsychiatric disorders.

SUCCESS RATE   70–80% long-term survival; less for certain conditions (e.g., chronic hepatitis B, hepatocellular carcinoma).

For a more detailed discussion, see Podolsky DK, Isselbacher KJ: Cirrhosis and Alcoholic Liver Disease, Chap. 298, p. 1704; Dienstag JL: Liver Transplantation, Chap. 301, p. 1721, in HPIM-14.

147

PORTAL HYPERTENSION

An increase in portal vein pressure due to anatomic or functional obstruction to blood flow in the portal venous system.

Normal portal vein pressure is 7–10 mmHg. Indicators of portal hypertension are (1) intraoperative portal vein pressure of >30 cm saline, (2) intrasplenic pressure of >17 mmHg, (3) wedged hepatic vein pressure of >4 mmHg above IVC pressure.

CLASSIFICATION (Table 147-1)

CONSEQUENCES (1) Increased collateral circulation between high-pressure portal venous system and low-pressure systemic venous system: lower esophagus/upper stomach (varices, portal hypertensive gastropathy), rectum (varices, portal hypertensive colopathy), anterior abdominal wall (caput Medusae; flow away from umbilicus), parietal peritoneum, splenorenal; (2) increased lymphatic flow; (3) increased plasma volume; (4) ascites; (5) splenomegaly, possible hypersplenism; (6) portosystemic shunting (including hepatic encephalopathy).

ESOPHAGOGASTRIC VARICES

Bleeding is major life-threatening complication; risk correlates with variceal size above minimal portal venous pressure >12

Table 147-1

Pathophysiologic Classification of Portal Hypertension

Site of obstruction	Pressure		Examples
	Portal	Corrected wedged hepatic vein*	
Presinusoidal	↑	Normal	Splenic AV fistula, portal or splenic vein thrombosis, schistosomiasis
Sinusoidal	↑	↑	Cirrhosis, hepatitis
Postsinusoidal	↑	↑ (May be unmeasureable due to hepatic vein occlusion)	Budd-Chiari syndrome, venoocclusive disease

* Wedged hepatic vein minus inferior vena cava pressure.

Table 147-2

Classification of Cirrhosis According to Child and Turcotte

	Class		
	A	B	C
Serum bilirubin, μmol/L (mg/dL)	<34 (<2)	34–51 (2–3)	>51 (>3)
Serum albumin, g/L (g/dL)	>35 (>3.5)	30–35 (3.0–3.5)	<30 (<3.0)
Ascites	None	Easily controlled	Poorly controlled
Encephalopathy	None	Mild	Advanced
Nutrition	Excellent	Good	Poor
Prognosis	Good	Fair	Poor

mmHg and presence on varices of "red wales." Mortality correlates with severity of underlying liver disease (hepatic reserve), e.g., Child-Turcotte classification (Table 147-2).

DIAGNOSIS   *Esophagogastroscopy*: procedure of choice for acute bleeding. *Upper GI series*: tortuous, beaded filling defects in lower esophagus. *Celiac and mesenteric arteriography*: when massive bleeding prevents endoscopy and to evaluate portal vein patency (portal vein also may be studied by ultrasound with Dopplers and MRI).

℞ **TREATMENT**
See Chap. 13 for general measures to treat GI bleeding.
   Control of acute bleeding   Choice of approach depends on clinical setting and availability.

   1.   Endoscopic band ligation or sclerotherapy—procedure of choice (not always suitable for gastric varices); band ligation is now preferred because of lower complication rate and possibly greater efficacy—application of bands around "pseudopolyp" of varix created by endoscopic suction; sclerotherapy involves direct injection of sclerosant into varix; >90% success rate in controlling acute bleeding; complications (less frequent with band ligation than sclerotherapy)—esophageal ulceration and stricture, fever, chest pain, mediastinitis, pleural effusions, aspiration.

2. Intravenous vasopressin up to 0.4–0.9 U/min until bleeding is controlled for 12–24 h (50–60% success rate, but no effect on mortality), then discontinue or taper (0.1 U/min q6–12h); add nitroglycerin up to 0.6 mg SL q 30 min, 40–400 μg/min IV, or by transdermal patch 10 mg/24 h to prevent coronary and renal vasoconstriction. Maintain systolic bp >90 mmHg. Octreotide 50–250 μg bolus + 50–250 μg/h IV infusion as effective as vasopressin with no serious complications.

3. Blakemore-Sengstaken balloon tamponade: can be inflated for up to 24–48 h; complications—obstruction of pharynx, asphyxiation, esophageal ulceration. Generally reserved for massive bleeding, failure of vasopressin and/or endoscopic therapy.

4. Transjugular intrahepatic portosystemic shunt (TIPS)—radiologic portacaval shunt, reserve for failure of other approaches; risk of hepatic encephalopathy (20–30%), shunt stenosis or occlusion (30–60%), infection.

Prevention of Recurrent Bleeding

1. Repeated endoscopic band ligation or sclerotherapy (e.g., q2–4 weeks) until obliteration of varices. Decreases but does not eliminate risk of recurrent bleeding; effect on overall survival uncertain but compares favorably to shunt surgery.

2. Propranolol or nadolol–nonselective beta blockers that act as portal venous antihypertensives; most effective in well-compensated cirrhotics; generally given in doses that reduce heart rate by 25%.

3. Splenectomy (for splenic vein thrombosis).

4. TIPS—regarded as useful "bridge" to liver transplantation in pt awaiting a donor liver who has failed on pharmacologic therapy.

5. Portosystemic shunt surgery: portacaval (total decompression) or distal splenorenal (Warren) (selective; contraindicated in ascites; ? lower incidence of hepatic encephalopathy). Alternative procedure—devascularization of lower esophagus and upper stomach (Sugiura). Surgery is now generally reserved for pts with compensated cirrhosis (Child's class A) who fail nonsurgical therapy (e.g., band ligation). Liver transplantation should be considered in appropriate candidates. (A previous portosystemic shunt does not preclude subsequent liver transplantation, though best to avoid portacaval shunts in transplant candidates.)

Prevention of Initial Bleed

Recommended for pts at high risk of variceal bleeding—large varices, "red wales." Beta blockers appear to be more effective than sclerotherapy; role of band ligation uncertain.

PROGNOSIS (AND SURGICAL RISK) Correlated with Child and Turcotte classification (see Table 147-2).

HEPATIC ENCEPHALOPATHY

A state of disordered CNS function associated with severe acute or chronic liver disease; may be acute and reversible or chronic and progressive.

CLINICAL FEATURES *Grade 1*: day-night reversal of sleep cycle, somnolence, mild confusion, personality change, asterixis (flapping tremor), abnormal psychometric testing. *Grade 2*: drowsiness, inappropriate behavior. *Grade 3*: stupor, marked confusion, inarticulate speech. *Grade 4*: coma, occasionally extrapyramidal signs, muscle twitching, hyperventilation. Fetor hepaticus (odor of breath and urine caused by mercaptans). Characteristic EEG abnormalities.

PATHOPHYSIOLOGY Failure of liver to detoxify agents noxious to CNS, i.e., ammonia, mercaptans, fatty acids, γ-aminobutyric acid (GABA), due to decreased hepatic function and portosystemic shunting. Ammonia may deplete brain of glutamate, an excitatory neurotransmitter, to form glutamine. False neurotransmitters also may enter CNS due to increased aromatic and decreased branched-chain amino acid levels in blood. Endogenous benzodiazepine agonists may play a role. Blood ammonia most readily measured marker, although may not always correlate with clinical status.

PRECIPITANTS GI bleeding (100 mL = 14–20 g protein), azotemia, constipation, high-protein meal, hypokalemic alkalosis, CNS depressant drugs (e.g., benzodiazepines and barbiturates), hypoxia, hypercarbia, sepsis.

℞ **TREATMENT**

Remove precipitants; reduce blood ammonia by decreasing protein intake (20–30 g/d initially, then 60–80 g/d, vegetable sources); enemas/cathartics to clear gut. Lactulose (converts NH_3 to unabsorbed NH_4^+, produces diarrhea, alters bowel flora) 30–50 mL PO qh until diarrhea, then 15–30 mL tid-qid prn 2–3 loose stools/d. In coma, give as enema (300 mL in 700 mL H_2O). Lactilol, a second-generation disaccharide that is less sweet than lactulose and can be dispensed as a powder, is not yet available in U.S. In refractory cases, add neomycin 1 g PO bid, metronidazole 250 mg PO tid, or vancomycin 1 g PO bid. *Unproven*: IV branched-chain amino acids, levodopa, bromocriptine, keto-analogues of essential amino acids. Flumazenil, a GABA-benzodiazepine receptor antagonist, is effective in some pts but is short-acting and requires continuous IV infusion. Liver transplantation when otherwise indicated.

For a more detailed discussion, see Podolsky DK, Isselbacher KJ: Cirrhosis and Alcoholic Liver Disease, Chap. 298, p. 1704 in HPIM-14.

148

DISEASES OF IMMEDIATE TYPE HYPERSENSITIVITY

DEFINITION These diseases result from IgE-dependent release of mediators from sensitized basophils and mast cells on contact with appropriate antigen (allergen). Associated disorders include anaphylaxis, allergic rhinitis, urticaria, asthma, and eczematous (atopic) dermatitis. *Atopic allergy* implies a familial tendency to the development of these disorders singly or in combination.

PATHOPHYSIOLOGY IgE binds to surface of mast cells and basophils through a high-affinity receptor. Cross-linking of this IgE by antigen causes cellular activation with the subsequent release of preformed and newly synthesized mediators. These include histamine, prostaglandins, leukotrienes (including C4, D4, and E4, collectively known as *slow-reacting substance of anaphylaxis* SRS-A), acid hydrolases, neutral proteases, proteoglycans, and cytokines (see Fig. 310-2, p. 1862, HPIM-14). The mediators have been implicated in many pathophysiologic events associated with immediate type hypersensitivity, such as vasodilatation, increased vasopermeability, smooth-muscle contraction, and chemotactic attraction of neutrophils and other inflammatory cells. The clinical manifestations of each allergic reaction depend largely on the anatomic site(s) and time course of mediator release.

URTICARIA AND ANGIOEDEMA

DEFINITION May occur together or separately. *Urticaria* involves superficial dermis and presents as circumscribed wheals with raised serpiginous borders and blanched centers; wheals may coalesce. *Angioedema* involves deeper layers of skin and may include subcutaneous tissue. These disorders may be classified as (1) IgE-dependent, including atopic, secondary to specific allergens, and physical stimuli, especially cold; (2) complement-mediated (including hereditary angioedema and hives related to serum sickness or vasculitis); (3) nonimmunologic due to direct mast cell–releasing agents or drugs that influence mediator release; and (4) idiopathic.

PATHOPHYSIOLOGY Characterized by massive edema formation in the dermis (and subcutaneous tissue in angioedema). Presumably the edema is due to increased vasopermeability caused by mediator release from mast cells or other cell populations.

DIAGNOSIS History, with special attention to possible offending exposures and/or ingestion as well as the duration of lesions. Vasculitic urticaria typically persists longer than 72 h, whereas conventional urticaria often has a duration of less than 48 h.

- Skin testing to food and/or inhalant antigens.
- Physical provocation, e.g., challenge with vibratory or cold stimuli
- Laboratory examination: complement levels, ESR (neither an elevated ESR nor hypocomplementemia is observed in IgE-mediated urticaria or angioedema); C1-esterase inhibitor levels if history suggests hereditary angioedema; cryoglobulins, hepatitis B antigen, and antibody studies; autoantibody screen.
- Skin biopsy may be necessary.

DIFFERENTIAL DIAGNOSIS Atopic dermatitis, cutaneous mastocytosis (urticaria pigmentosa), systemic mastocytosis.

PREVENTION Identification and avoidance of offending agent(s), if possible.

℞ TREATMENT

- H_1 and H_2 antihistamines may be helpful; e.g., ranitidine 150 mg PO bid; diphenhydramine 25–50 mg PO qid; hydroxyzine 25–50 mg PO qid.
- Cyproheptadine 4 mg PO tid may be helpful.
- Sympathomimetic agents occasionally are useful.
- Topical glucocorticoids are of no value in the management of urticaria and/or angioedema. Because of their long-term toxicity, systemic glucocorticoids should not be used in the treatment of idiopathic, allergen-induced, or physical urticaria.

ALLERGIC RHINITIS

DEFINITION An inflammatory condition of the nose characterized by sneezing, rhinorrhea, and obstruction of nasal passages; may be associated with conjunctival and pharyngeal itching, lacrimation, and sinusitis. Seasonal allergic rhinitis is commonly caused by exposure to pollens, especially from grasses, trees, weeds, and molds. Perennial allergic rhinitis is frequently due to contact with house dust (containing dust mite antigens) and animal danders.

PATHOPHYSIOLOGY Impingement of pollens and other allergens on nasal mucosa of sensitized individuals results in IgE-dependent triggering of mast cells with subsequent release of mediators that cause development of mucosal hyperemia, swelling, and fluid transudation. Inflammation of nasal mucosal surface probably allows penetration of allergens deeper into tissue, where they contact perivenular mast cells. Obstruction of sinus ostia may result in development of secondary sinusitis, with or without bacterial infection.

DIAGNOSIS Accurate history of symptoms correlated with time of pollenation of plants in a given locale; special attention must be paid to other potentially sensitizing antigens such as pets.

- Physical examination: nasal mucosa may be boggy or erythematous; nasal polyps may be present; sinuses may demonstrate decreased transillumination; conjunctivae may be inflamed or edematous; manifestations of other allergic conditions (e.g., asthma, eczema) may be present.
- Skin tests to inhalant and/or food antigens.
- Nasal smear may reveal large numbers of eosinophils; presence of neutrophils may suggest infection.
- Total and specific serum IgE (as assessed by immunoassay) may be elevated.

DIFFERENTIAL DIAGNOSIS Vasomotor rhinitis, URI, irritant exposure, pregnancy with nasal mucosal edema, rhinitis medicamentosa, nonallergic rhinitis with eosinophilia, rhinitis due to use of beta-adrenergic agents.

PREVENTION Identification and avoidance of offending antigen(s).

 TREATMENT

- Antihistamines, e.g., sustained-release chlorpheniramine 12 mg PO bid, terfenedine 60 mg PO bid, astemizole 10 mg PO qd, loratidine 10 mg PO qd. Note: life-threatening cardiac arrhythmias have occurred due to inhibition of the metabolism of terfenadine or astemizole by concomitantly administered macrolide antibiotics (such as erythromycin and clarithromycin) or broad-spectrum antifungal agents such as ketoconazole or itraconazole. The use of either terfenadine or astemizole is contraindicated in combination with these drugs and in individuals with concomitant medical illnesses that impair hepatic function or predispose to cardiac arrhythmias.

- Oral sympathomimetics, e.g., pseudoephedrine 30–60 mg PO qid; may aggravate hypertension; combination antihistamine/decongestant preparations may balance side effects and provide improved patient convenience.
- Topical vasoconstrictors—should be used sparingly due to rebound congestion and chronic rhinitis associated with prolonged use
- Topical nasal steroids, e.g., beclomethasone 2 sprays in each nostril bid–tid.
- Topical nasal cromolyn sodium 1–2 sprays in each nostril qid.
- Hyposensitization therapy if more conservative therapy is unsuccessful.

SYSTEMIC MASTOCYTOSIS

DEFINITION A systemic disorder characterized by mast cell hyperplasia; generally recognized in bone marrow, skin, GI mucosa, liver, and spleen. Classified as: (1) indolent, (2) associated with concomitant hematologic disorder, (3) aggressive, and (4) mastocytic leukemia.

PATHOPHYSIOLOGY AND CLINICAL MANIFESTATIONS The clinical manifestations of systemic mastocytosis are due to tissue occupancy by the mast cell mass, the tissue response to that mass (fibrosis), and the release of bioactive substances acting both locally (urticaria pigmentosa, crampy abdominal pain, gastritis, peptic ulcer) and at distal sites (headache, pruritus, flushing, vascular collapse). Clinical manifestations may be aggravated by alcohol, use of narcotics (e.g., codeine), ingestion of NSAIDs.

DIAGNOSIS May be made by measurement of urinary or blood levels of mast cell products including histamine, histamine metabolites, prostaglandin D_2 (PGD_2) metabolites, or mast cell tryptase, and tissue or bone marrow biopsy demonstrating increased mast cell density. Other studies including bone scan, skeletal survey, GI contrast studies may be helpful. Other flushing disorders (e.g., carcinoid syndrome, pheochromocytoma) should be excluded.

Rx TREATMENT

- H_1 and H_2 antihistamines.
- Proton pump inhibitor for gastric hypersecretion.
- Oral cromolyn sodium for diarrhea and abdominal pain.
- NSAIDs (in nonsensitive pts) may help by blocking PGD_2 production.
- Systemic glucocorticoids may help but frequently are associated with complications.

For a more detailed discussion, see Austen KF: Disease of Immediate Type Hypersensitivity, Chap. 310, p. 1860, in HPIM-14.

149

PRIMARY IMMUNODEFICIENCY DISEASES

DEFINITION   Disorders involving the cell-mediated (T cell) or antibody-mediated (B cell) pathways of the immune system; some disorders may manifest abnormalities of both pathways. Pts are prone to development of recurrent infections and, in certain disorders, lymphoproliferative neoplasms. *Primary disorders* may be congenital or acquired; some are familial in nature. *Secondary disorders* are not caused by intrinsic abnormalities of immune cells but may be due to infection (such as in AIDS; see HPIM-14, Chap. 308), treatment with cytotoxic drugs, radiation therapy, or lymphoreticular malignancies. Pts with disorders of antibody formation are chiefly prone to infection with encapsulated bacterial pathogens (e.g., streptococci, *Haemophilus*, meningococcus), and *Giardia*. Individuals with T cell defects are generally susceptible to infections with viruses, fungi, and protozoa.

CLASSIFICATION

Severe Combined Immunodeficiency (SCID)

Congenital (autosomal recessive or X-linked); affected infants rarely survive beyond 1 year. Dysfunction of both cellular and humoral immunity:

- *Swiss-type*: Autosomal recessive; severe lymphopenia involving B and T cells.
- *Adenosine deaminase (ADA) deficiency*: Autosomal recessive; has been treated with gene therapy.
- *X-linked SCID*: Characterized by an absence of peripheral T cells and natural killer cells. B lymphocytes are present in normal numbers but are functionally defective. These pts have a mutation in the gene that encodes the γ chain common to the interleukin (IL)-2, -4, -9, -15 receptors, thus disrupting the action of these important lymphokines. The same phenotype seen in X-linked SCID can be inherited as an autosomal recessive disease due to mutations in the JAK3 protein kinase gene. This enzyme associates with the common γ chain of the receptors for IL-2, -4, -9, and -15 and is a key element in the signal transduction pathways used by these receptors.

Rx TREATMENT
Bone marrow transplantation is useful in some SCID pts.

T Cell Immunodeficiency

- *DiGeorge's syndrome*: Maldevelopment of organs derived embryologically from third and fourth pharyngeal pouches (including thymus); associated with congenital cardiac defects, parathyroid hypoplasia with hypocalcemic tetany, abnormal facies, thymic aplasia; serum Ig levels may be normal but specific antibody responses are impaired.
- *T cell receptor (TCR) complex deficiency*: Immunodeficiencies due to inherited mutations of the CD3γ and CD3ε components of the TCR complex have been identifed. CD3γ mutations result in a selective defect in CD8 T cells, whereas CD3ε mutations lead to a preferential reduction in CD4 T cells.
- *MHC class II deficiency*: Antigen-presenting cells from pts with this rare disorder fail to express the class II molecules DP, DQ, and DR on their surface, which results in limited development of CD4 + T cells in the thymus and defective interaction of CD4 T cells and antigen-presenting cells in the periphery. Affected pts experience recurrent bronchopul-

monary infections, chronic diarrhea, and severe viral infections.

* *Inherited deficiency of purine nucleoside phosphorylase*: Functions in same salvage pathway as ADA; cellular dysfunction may be related to intracellular accumulation of purine metabolites.

* *Ataxia-telangiectasia*: Autosomal recessive; cerebellar ataxia, oculocutaneous telangiectasia, immunodeficiency; not all pts have immunodeficiency; lymphomas common; IgG subclasses may be abnormal.

℞ TREATMENT

Treatment for T cell disorders is complex and largely investigational.

Immunoglobulin Deficiency Syndromes

* *X-linked agammaglobulinemia*: Due to a mutation in the Bruton's tyrosine kinase (Btk) gene. Marked deficiency of circulating B lymphocytes; all Ig classes low; recurrent sinopulmonary infections and chronic echovirus encephalitis, including vaccine-aquired poliomyelitis infection, are common complications.

* *Transient hypogammaglobulinemia of infancy*: This occurs between 3 and 6 months of age as maternally derived IgG levels decline.

* *Isolated IgA deficiency*: Most common immunodeficiency; the majority of affected individuals do not have increased infections; antibodies against IgA may lead to anaphylaxis during transfusion of blood or plasma; may be associated with deficiencies of IgG subclasses; often familial.

* *IgG subclass deficiencies*: Total serum IgG may be normal, yet some individuals may be prone to recurrent sinopulmonary infections due to selective deficiencies of certain IgG subclasses.

* *Common variable immunodeficiency*: Heterogeneous group of syndromes characterized by panhypogammaglobulinemia, deficiency of IgG and IgA, or selective IgG deficiency and recurrent sinopulmonary infections; associated conditions include chronic giardiasis, intestinal malabsorption, atrophic gastritis with pernicious anemia, lymphoreticular neoplasms, arthritis, and autoimmune diseases.

* *X-linked immunodeficiency with increased IgM*: In most pts this syndrome results from genetic mutation in the gene encoding CD40 ligand, a transmembrane protein expressed by activated T cells and necessary for normal T and B cell

Table 149-1

INITIAL SCREENING ASSAYS

Complete blood count with differential smear
Serum immunoglobulin levels: IgM, IgG, IgA, IgD, IgE

OTHER READILY AVAILABLE ASSAYS

Quantification of blood mononuclear cell populations by immunofluorescence assays employing monoclonal antibody markers†
  T cells: CD3, CD4, CD8, TCRαβ, TCRγδ
  B cells: CD19, CD20, CD21, Ig(μ, δ, γ, α, κ, λ), Ig-associated molecules (α, β)
  NK cells: CD16
  Monocytes: CD15
  Activation markers: HLA-DR, CD25, CD80 (B cells)
T cell functional evaluation
  1. Delayed hypersensitivity skin tests (PPD, *Candida* histoplasmin, tetanus toxoid)
  2. Proliferative response to mitogens (anti-CD3 antibody, phytohemagglutinin, concanavalin A) and allogeneic cells (mixed lymphocyte response)
  3. Cytokine production
B cell functional evaluation
  1. Natural or commonly acquired antibodies: isohemagglutinins; antibodies to common viruses (influenza, rubella, rubeola) and bacterial toxins (diphtheria, tetanus)
  2. Response to immunization with protein (tetanus toxoid) and carbohydrate (pneumococcal vaccine, *H. influenzae B* vaccine) antigens
  3. Quantitative IgG subclass determinations
Complement
  1. CH_{50} assays (classic and alternative pathways)
  2. C3, C4, and other components
Phagocyte function
  1. Reduction of nitroblue tetrazolium
  2. Chemotaxis assays
  3. Bactericidal activity

---

* Together with a history and physical examination, these tests will identify more than 95 percent of pts with primary imunodeficiencies.

† The menu of monoclonal antibody markers may be expanded or contracted to focus on particular clinical questions.

cooperation, germinal center formation, and immunoglobulin isotype switching. Pts exhibit increased serum IgM with low or absent IgG and IgA and recurrent sinopulmonary infections; pts also exhibit T lymphocyte abnormalities with increased susceptibility to infection with opportunistic pathogens (*Pneumocystis carinii*). Associated conditions include neutropenia, autoimmune diseases, and lymphoreticular neoplasms.

- Isolated deficiency of IgM.

℞ **TREATMENT**

Intravenous immunoglobulin administration (only for pts who have recurrent bacterial infections and are deficient in IgG):

- starting dose 200–400 mg/kg given every 3–4 weeks.
- Adjust dose to keep trough IgG level ≥400 mg/dL.
- Usually done in outpatient setting.
- Decision to treat based on severity of clinical symptoms and response to antigenic challenge

MISCELLANEOUS IMMUNODEFICIENCY SYNDROMES

- Mucocutaneous candidiasis.
- X-linked lymphoproliferative syndrome.
- Immunodeficiency with thymoma.
- Wiskott-Aldrich syndrome.
- Hyper-IgE syndrome.
- Metabolic abnormalities associated with immunodeficiency

For a more detailed discussion, see Cooper MD, Lawton AR III: Primary Immune Deficiency Diseases, Chapter 307 in HPIM-14.

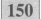

150

SLE, RA, AND OTHER CONNECTIVE TISSUE DISEASES

CONNECTIVE TISSUE DISEASE

DEFINITION Heterogeneous disorders that share certain common features, including inflammation of skin, joints, and other structures rich in connective tissue, as well as altered patterns of immunoregulation, including production of autoantibodies and abnormalities of cell-mediated immunity. While certain distinct clinical entities may be defined, manifestations may vary considerably from one pt to the next, and overlap of clinical features between and among specific diseases is common.

SYSTEMIC LUPUS ERYTHEMATOSUS (SLE)

DEFINITION AND PATHOGENESIS Disease of unknown etiology in which tissues and cells are damaged by deposition of pathogenic autoantibodies and immune complexes. Genetic, environmental, and sex hormonal factors are likely of pathogenic importance. T and B cell hyperactivity, production of autoantibodies with specificity for nuclear antigenic determinants, and abnormalities of T cell function occur.

CLINICAL MANIFESTATIONS 90% of cases are women, usually of child-bearing age; more common in blacks than whites. Course of disease is often one of periods of exacerbation and relative quiescence. May involve virtually any organ system and have a wide range of disease severity. Common features include:

- *Constitutional*—fatigue, fever, malaise, weight loss
- *Cutaneous*—rashes (especially malar "butterfly" rash), photosensitivity, vasculitis, alopecia, oral ulcers
- *Arthritis*—inflammatory, symmetric, nonerosive
- *Hematologic*—anemia (may be hemolytic), neutropenia, thrombocytopenia, lymphadenopathy, splenomegaly, venous or arterial thrombosis
- *Cardiopulmonary*—pleuritis, pericarditis, myocarditis, endocarditis
- *Nephritis*
- *GI*—peritonitis, vasculitis
- *Neurologic*—organic brain syndromes, seizures, psychosis, cerebritis

Drug-Induced Lupus A clinical and immunologic picture similar to spontaneous SLE may be induced by drugs; in particular: procainamide, hydralazine, isoniazid, chlorpromazine, methyldopa. Features are predominantly constitutional, joint, and pleuropericardial; CNS and renal disease are rare. All pts have antinuclear antibodies (ANA); antihistone antibodies may be present, but antibodies to dsDNA and hypocomplementemia are uncommon. Most pts improve following withdrawal of offending drug.

EVALUATION

- Hx and physical exam
- Presence of ANA is a cardinal feature, but a (+) ANA is not specific for SLE. Laboratory assessment should include: CBC, ESR, ANA and subtypes (antibodies to dsDNA, ssDNA, Sm, Ro, La, histone), complement levels (C3, C4, CH50), serum immunoglobulins, VDRL, PT, PTT, anticardiolipin antibody, lupus anticoagulant, UA.
- Appropriate radiographic studies
- ECG
- Consideration of renal biopsy if evidence of glomerulonephritis

DIAGNOSIS Made in the presence of four or more published criteria (see Table 312-3, p. 1876, in HPIM-14).

℞ TREATMENT

Choice of therapy is based on type and severity of disease manifestations (Fig. 150-1). Goals are to control acute, severe flares and to develop maintenance strategies where symptoms are suppressed to an acceptable level. The toxicity of therapy must always be considered. Useful agents include:

- *NSAIDs* (e.g., ibuprofen 400–800 mg tid–qid).
- *Antimalarials* (hydroxychloroquine 400 mg/d)—may improve constitutional, cutaneous, articular manifestations. Ophthalmologic evaluation required before and during Rx to rule out ocular toxicity.
- *Systemic glucocorticoids*—may be necessary for life-threatening or severely disabling manifestations.
- *Cytotoxic agents*—beneficial in active glomerulonephritis; may be required for severe disease not successfully controlled by acceptable doses of steroids.

  1. Cyclophosphamide—most effective and most toxic; administered as IV pulse 10–15 mg/kg every 4 weeks. Daily oral dosing 1.5–2.5 (mg/kg)/d can also be used but has a greater risk of urinary bladder toxicity.
  2. Azathioprine 2–3 (mg/kg)/d—indicated in pts who cannot take cyclophosphamide.

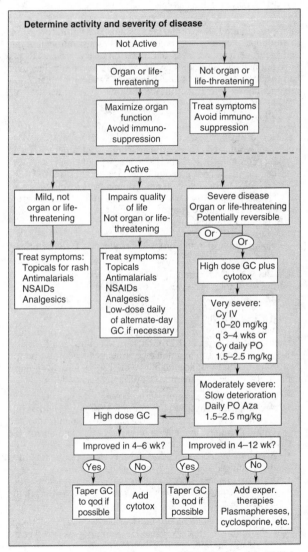

FIGURE 150-1 Algorithm for the treatment of SLE. GC, glucocorticoids; high-dose GC, methylprednisolone 1000 mg, IV, qd × 3, then 1 to 2 mg/kg prednisone per day orally, or 1 to 2 mg/kg prednisone per day orally; cytotox, cytotoxic drugs such as cyclophosphamide (Cy) and azathioprine (Aza); qod, alternate day therapy.

- Anticoagulation may be indicated in pts with thrombotic complications.

RHEUMATOID ARTHRITIS (RA)

DEFINITION AND PATHOGENESIS   A chronic multisystem disease of unknown etiology characterized by persistent inflammatory synovitis, usually involving peripheral joints in a symmetric fashion. Although cartilaginous destruction, bony erosions, and joint deformity are hallmarks, the course of RA can be variable. An association with HLA-DR4 has been noted; both genetic and environmental factors may play a role in initiating disease. The propagation of RA is an immunologically mediated event in which joint injury occurs from synovial hyperplasia, lymphocytic infiltration of synovium, and local production of cytokines and chemokines by activated lymphocytes, macrophages, and fibroblasts.

CLINICAL MANIFESTATIONS   RA occurs in ~0.8% of the population; women affected 3 times more often than men; prevalence increases with age, onset most frequent in 4th and 5th decades.
   Articular manifestations—typically a symmetric polyarthritis of peripheral joints with pain, tenderness, and swelling of affected joints; morning stiffness is common; PIP and MCP joints frequently involved; joint deformities may develop after persistent inflammation.
   Extraarticular manifestations:

- Cutaneous—rheumatoid nodules, vasculitis
- Pulmonary—nodules, interstitial disease, BOOP, pleural disease, Caplan's syndrome [sero(+) RA associated with pneumoconiosis]
- Ocular—keratoconjunctivitis sicca, episcleritis, scleritis
- Hematologic—anemia, Felty's syndrome (splenomegaly and neutropenia)
- Cardiac—pericarditis, myocarditis
- Neurologic—myelopathies secondary to cervical spine disease, entrapment, vasculitis.

EVALUATION

- Hx and physical exam with careful examination of all joints.
- Rheumatoid factor is present in 85% of pts; its presence correlates with severe disease, nodules, extraarticular features.
- Other laboratories: CBC, ESR.
- Synovial fluid analysis—useful to rule out crystalline disease, infection.

- Radiographs—juxtaarticular osteopenia, joint space narrowing, marginal erosions. CXR should be obtained.

DIAGNOSIS Not difficult in pts with typical established disease. May be confusing early. New criteria are more sensitive and specific (see Table 313-2, p. 1885, in HPIM-14).

Differential Diagnosis Gout, SLE, psoriatic arthritis, infectious arthritis, osteoarthritis, sarcoid.

R̲x̲ TREATMENT

Goals: lessen pain, improve/maintain function, prevent long-term joint damage, control of systemic involvement. Increasing trend to treat RA more aggressively earlier in disease course (Fig. 150-2).

- Pt education on disease, joint protection
- Physical and occupational therapy—strengthen periarticular muscles, consider assistive devices.
- Aspirin or NSAIDs.
- Intrarticular glucocorticoids.
- Systemic glucocorticoids.
- Disease-modifying drugs—e.g., methotrexate; oral or IM gold salts; hydroxychloroquine; sulfasalazine; D-penicillamine; azathioprine; cyclosporin. Each agent has individual toxicities—pt education and monitoring required.
- Surgery—may be considered for severe functional impairment due to deformity.

SYSTEMIC SCLEROSIS (SCLERODERMA, SSc)

DEFINITION AND PATHOGENESIS Multisystem disorder characterized by inflammatory, vascular, and fibrotic changes of skin and various internal organ systems (chiefly GI tract, lungs, heart, and kidney). Pathogenesis unclear; involves immunologic mechanisms leading to vascular endothelial damage and activation of fibroblasts.

CLINICAL MANIFESTATIONS

- Cutaneous—edema followed by fibrosis of the skin (chiefly extremities, face, trunk); telangiectasis; calcinosis; Raynaud's phenomenon
- Arthralgias and/or arthritis
- GI—esophageal hypomotility; intestinal hypofunction
- Pulmonary—fibrosis, pulmonary hypertension
- Cardiac—pericarditis, cardiomyopathy, conduction abnormalities

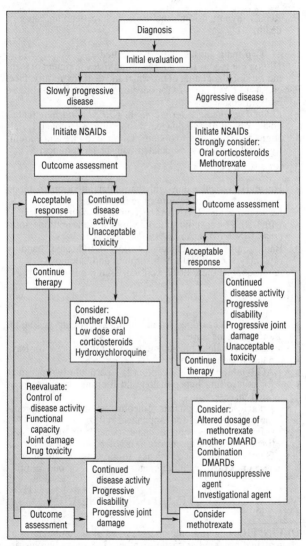

FIGURE 150-2   Algorithm for the medical management of rheumatoid arthritis. (Courtesy of the University of Texas Southwestern Medical Center, Office of Continuing Education.)

- Renal—hypertension; renal crisis/failure (leading cause of death).

    Two main subsets can be identified:
    Diffuse cutaneous scleroderma—rapid development of symmetric skin thickening of proximal and distal extremity, face, and trunk. At high risk for development of visceral disease early in course.
- *Limited cutaneous scleroderma* or *CREST syndrome* (calcinosis, *R*aynaud's, *e*sophageal dysmotility, *s*clerodactyly, *t*elangiectasias)—skin involvement limited to face and extremity distal to elbows; associated with better prognosis.

EVALUATION

- Hx and physical exam with particular attention to blood pressure (heralding feature of renal disease).
- Laboratories: ESR, ANA (anticentromere pattern associated with CREST), specific antibodies may include antitopoisomerase I (Scl-70), UA
- Radiographs: CXR, barium swallow if indicated, hand x-rays may show distal tuft resorption and calcinosis.
- Additional studies: ECG, consider skin biopsy.

℞ TREATMENT

- Education regarding warm clothing, smoking cessation, antireflux measures
- Calcium channel blockers (e.g., nifedipine) useful for Raynaud's phenomenon
- ACE inhibitors (e.g., captopril)—particularly important for controlling hypertension and limiting progression of renal disease.
- Antacids, H_2 antagonists, omeprazole, and metoclopramide may be useful for esophageal reflux.
- D-Penicillamine—controversial benefit to reduce skin thickening and prevent organ involvement.
- Glucocorticoids—no efficacy in slowing progression of SSc; indicated for inflammatory myositis or pericarditis.

MIXED CONNECTIVE TISSUE DISEASE (MCTD)

DEFINITION Syndrome characterized by a combination of clinical features similar to those of SLE, SSc, polymyositis, and RA; unusually high titers of circulating antibodies to a nuclear ribonucleoprotein (RNP) are found.

CLINICAL MANIFESTATIONS   Raynaud's phenomenon, polyarthritis, swollen hands or sclerodactyly, esophageal dysfunction, pulmonary fibrosis, inflammatory myopathy. Renal involvement occurs in about 25%. Laboratory abnormalities include high-titer ANAs, very high titers of antibody to RNP, positive rheumatoid factor in 50% of pts.

EVALUATION   Similar to that for SLE and SSc.

TREATMENT
Little published data. Treat based upon manifestations with similar approach to that used if feature occurred in SLE/SSc/polymyositis/RA.

SJÖGREN'S SYNDROME

DEFINITION   An immunologic disorder characterized by progressive lymphocytic destruction of exocrine glands most frequently resulting in symptomatic eye and mouth dryness; can be associated with extraglandular manifestations; predominantly affects middle-age females; may be primary or secondary when it occurs in association with other autoimmune diseases.

CLINICAL MANIFESTATIONS

- *Constitutional*—fatigue
- *Sicca symptoms*—keratoconjunctivitis sicca (KCS) and xerostomia
- *Dryness of other surfaces*—nose, vagina, trachea, skin
- *Extraglandular features*—arthralgia/arthritis, Raynaud's, lymphadenopathy, interstitial pneumonitis, vasculitis (usually cutaneous), nephritis, lymphoma.

EVALUATION

- Hx and physical exam—with special attention to oral, ocular, lymphatic exam and presence of other autoimmune disorders.
- Presence of autoantibodies is a hallmark of disease (ANA, RF, anti-Ro, anti-La)
- Other laboratories—ESR, CBC, renal, liver, and thyroid function tests, SPEP (hypergammaglobulinemia or monoclonal gammopathy common), UA.
- Ocular studies—to diagnose and quantitate KCS; Schirmer's test, Rose bengal staining.
- Oral exam—unstimulated salivary flow, dental exam.
- Labial salivary gland biopsy—demonstrates lymphocytic infiltration and destruction of glandular tissue.

DIAGNOSIS   Criteria often include: KCS, xerostomia, (+) serologic features of autoimmunity. Positive lip biopsy considered necessary in some series—should be performed in setting of objective KCS/xerostomia with negative serologies.

℞ TREATMENT

- Regular follow-up with dentist and ophthalmologist.
- Symptomatic relief of dryness with artificial tears, ophthalmic lubricating ointments, nasal saline sprays, frequent sips of water, sugarless candy, moisturizing skin lotions.
- Bromhexine or pilocarpine—may help sicca manifestations.
- Hydroxychloroquine—may help arthralgias.
- Glucocorticoids—not effective for sicca Sx but may have role in treatment of extraglandular manifestations.

POLYMYOSITIS/DERMATOMYOSITIS

DEFINITION   *Polymyositis* is a condition of presumed autoimmune etiology in which the skeletal muscle is damaged by an inflammatory process dominated by lymphocytic infiltration. The term *dermatomyositis* is used when polymyositis is accompanied by characteristic skin changes.

CLASSIFICATION

- *Group I: Primary idiopathic polymyositis*—female:male 2:1.
- *Group II: Primary idiopathic dermatomyositis*—skin changes may precede or follow muscle changes.
- *Group III: Dermatomyositis (or polymyositis) associated with neoplasia*—malignancy may precede or follow onset of myositis by up to 2 years; commonly associated malignancies: lung, ovary, breast, GI tract, myeloproliferative disorders.
- *Group IV: Childhood dermatomyositis (or polymyositis) associated with vasculitis*—vasculitis may involve skin and visceral organs.
- *Group V: Polymyositis (or dermatomyositis) associated with collagen-vascular disease*—RA, scleroderma, SLE, MCTD most frequently associated.

CLINICAL MANIFESTATIONS

Symptoms

- Proximal muscle weakness—difficulty climbing stairs, combing hair, arising from chair

- Weakness of neck flexors—unable to raise head from pillow
- Muscle pain or tenderness
- Dysphagia—25% at presentation
- Dyspnea—respiratory impairment in 5%

Physical Examination

- Muscle weakness proximal > distal
- Skin lesions: localized or diffuse erythema, maculopapular eruption, scaling eczematoid dermatitis, exfoliative dermatitis, classic lilac-colored (heliotrope) rash on eyelids, nose, cheeks, forehead, trunk, extremities, nailbeds, knuckles (Gottron's papules)
- Subcutaneous calcification—see especially in childhood disease
- Complete evaluation is important to look for features suggestive of neoplasm or other connective tissue diseases.

EVALUATION

- CPK, aldolase, SGOT, SGPT, LDH usually elevated.
- In setting of very high CPK, check urine myoglobin and renal function.
- Autoantibodies—anti-Jo-1 seen in 50% of pts with polymyositis and 15% with dermatomyositis, other antibodies may be seen in association with other connective tissue diseases.
- ECG abnormal in 5-10% cases at presentation.
- EMG—abnormal in 40% of cases; markedly increased insertional activity seen with motor unit action potentials, which show low amplitude, are polyphasic, and have abnormally early recruitment.
- MRI—may identify sites of muscle involvement and guide biopsy location.
- Skeletal muscle pathology—patchy process; inflammatory cells, destruction of muscle fibers with a phagocytic reaction, and perivascular inflammatory cell infiltration.

DIAGNOSIS Diagnosis strongly suggested by presence of muscle weakness, elevation of CK, abnormal EMG. Pts with dermatomyositis who have skin rash may not require muscle biopsy. In polymyositis, biopsy usually needed to make a firm diagnosis and rule out other myopathies.

Differential Diagnosis Inclusion body myositis, metabolic myopathies, infectious myositis, toxic myopathies, neuromuscular disorders, endocrine and electrolyte disorders, myositis associated with sarcoidosis, polymyalgia rheumatica, eosinophilia myalgia syndrome.

℞ TREATMENT

- Prednisone 1–2 (mg/kg)/day, tapered after strength improves and CK declines. Approximately 75% of pts have good clinical response to steroids alone. The onset of steroid-induced myopathy may complicate therapy.
- Cytotoxic agents: should be considered for severe disease, inadequate response to steroids, relapsing disease, steroid-induced complications. Methotrexate 7.5–15 mg/week, azathioprine 2.5–3.5 (mg/kg)/day, cyclophosphamide 1–2 (mg/kg)/day reported to be beneficial but have significant side effects.
- The possibility of malignancy should be kept in mind, especially in elderly pts with dermatomyositis.
- Physical therapy

For a more detailed discussion, see Hahn BH: Systemic Lupus Erythematosus, Chap. 312, p. 1874; Lipsky PE: Rheumatoid Arthritis, Chap. 313, p. 1880; Gilliland BC: Systemic Sclerosis (Scleroderma), Chap. 314, p. 1888; Moutsopoulos HM: Sjögren's Syndrome, Chap. 316, p. 1901; Tandan R: Dermatomyositis and Polymyositis, Chap. 315, p. 1896, in HPIM-14.

151

VASCULITIS

Definition and Pathogenesis

A clinicopathologic process characterized by inflammation of and damage to blood vessels, compromise of vessel lumen, and resulting ischemia. Clinical manifestations depend on size and location of affected vessel. Most vasculitic syndromes appear to be mediated in whole or in part by immune mechanisms. May be primary or sole manifestation of a disease or secondary to another disease process. Unique vasculitic syndromes can be identified that can differ greatly with regards to clinical features, disease severity, histology, and treatment.

Classification

CLASSIC POLYARTERITIS NODOSA (PAN) Medium-sized muscular arteries involved; frequently associated with arteriographic aneurysms; commonly affects renal arteries, liver, GI tract, peripheral nerves, skin, heart; can be associated with hepatitis B.

MICROSCOPIC POLYANGIITIS Small-vessel vasculitis that can affect the glomerulus and lungs; medium-sized vessels may also be affected.

WEGENER'S GRANULOMATOSIS Granulomatous vasculitis of upper and lower respiratory tracts together with glomerulonephritis; upper airway lesions affecting the nose and sinuses can cause purulent or bloody nasal discharge, mucosal ulceration, septal perforation, and cartilaginous destruction (saddlenose deformity). Lung involvement may be asymptomatic or cause cough, hemoptysis, dyspnea; eye involvement may occur; renal involvement accounts for most deaths.

ALLERGIC ANGIITIS AND GRANULOMATOSIS (CHURG-STRAUSS DISEASE) Granulomatous vasculitis of multiple organ systems, particularly the lung; characterized by asthma, peripheral eosinophilia, eosinophilic tissue infiltration; glomerulonephritis can occur.

POLYANGIITIS OVERLAP SYNDROME Primary systemic vasculitis that does not precisely fit into a single diagnostic category.

GIANT CELL (OR TEMPORAL) ARTERITIS Inflammation of medium- and large-sized arteries; primarily involves temporal artery but systemic involvement may occur; symptoms include headache, jaw/tongue claudication, scalp tenderness, fever, musculoskeletal symptoms (polymyalgia rheumatica); sudden blindness from involvement of optic vessels is a dreaded complication.

TAKAYASU'S ARTERITIS Vasculitis of the large arteries with strong predilection for aortic arch and its branches; most common in young women; presents with inflammatory or ischemic symptoms in arms and neck, systemic inflammatory symptoms, aortic regurgitation.

HENOCH-SCHÖNLEIN PURPURA Characterized by involvement of skin, GI tract, kidneys; more common in children; may recur after initial remission.

PREDOMINANTLY CUTANEOUS VASCULITIS (HY-PERSENSITIVITY VASCULITIS) Heterogeneous group of disorders; common feature is small-vessel involvement; skin disease usually predominates.

Exogenous Stimuli Proved or Suspected

- Serum sickness and serum sickness–like reactions
- Drug-induced vasculitis
- Vasculitis associated with infectious diseases

Endogenous Antigens Likely Involved

- Vasculitis associated with neoplasms
- Vasculitis associated with connective tissue disorders
- Vasculitis associated with other underlying diseases
- Vasculitis associated with congenital deficiencies of complement system.

MISCELLANEOUS VASCULITIC SYNDROMES

- Mucocutaneous lymph node syndrome (Kawasaki disease)
- Isolated vasculitis of the central nervous system
- Thromboangiitis obliterans (Buerger's disease)
- Behçet's syndrome
- Cogan's syndrome
- Erythema elevatum diutinum

Evaluation (See Fig. 151-1)

- Thorough Hx and physical exam—special reference to ischemic manifestations and systemic inflammatory signs/symptoms.
- Laboratories—important in assessing organ involvement: CBC with differential, ESR, renal function tests, UA. Should also be obtained to rule out other diseases: ANA, rheumatoid factor, anti-GBM, hepatitis B/C serologies, HIV.
- Antineutrophil cytoplasmic autoantibodies (ANCA)—cytoplasmic pattern associated with Wegener's granulomatosis; presence of ANCA is adjunctive and should not be used in place of biopsy as a means of diagnosis.
- Radiographs—CXR should be performed even in the absence of symptoms.
- Diagnosis—can only be made by arteriogram or biopsy of affected organ(s).

Differential Diagnosis

Guided by organ manifestations. In many instances includes infections and neoplasms, which must be ruled out prior to beginning immunosuppressive therapy.

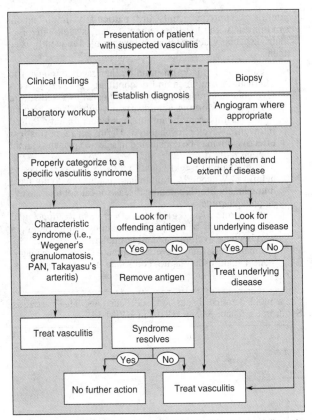

FIGURE 151-1 Algorithm for the approach to a pt with suspected diagnosis of vasculitis.

℞ TREATMENT

Therapy is based on the specific vasculitic syndrome and its manifestations. Immunosuppressive therapy should be avoided in disease that rarely results in irreversible organ system dysfunction or that usually does not respond to such agents (e.g., predominantly cutaneous vasculitis). Glucocorticoids alone may control temporal arteritis and Takayasu's arteritis. Cytotoxic agents are particularly important in syndromes with life-threatening organ system involvement, especially active glomerulonephritis. Frequently used agents:

- Prednisone 1 (mg/kg)/d initially, then tapered; convert to alternate-day regimen and discontinue.
- Cyclophosphamide 2 (mg/kg)/d, adjusted to avoid severe leukopenia. Morning administration with a large amount of fluid is important in minimizing bladder toxicity. Pulsed intravenous cyclophosphamide (1 g/m^2 per month) is less effective but may be considered in selected pts who cannot tolerate daily dosing.
- Methotrexate in weekly doses up to 25 mg/week may be helpful in Wegener's granulomatosis pts who do not have immediately life-threatening disease or cannot tolerate cyclophosphamide.
- Azathioprine 2 (mg/kg)/d. Less effective in treating active disease but may be useful in maintaining remission in pts who become cyclophosphamide intolerant.
- Plasmapheresis may have an adjunctive role in management if manifestations not controlled by above measures.

For a more detailed discussion, see Fauci AS: The Vasculitis Syndromes, Chap. 319, p. 1910, in HPIM-14.

152

SARCOIDOSIS

Definition

A systemic granulomatous disease of unknown etiology. Affected organs are characterized by an accumulation of T lymphocytes and mononuclear phagocytes, noncaseating epithelioid granulomas, and derangements of normal tissue architecture.

Pathophysiology

Mononuclear cells, mostly T helper lymphocytes and mononuclear phagocytes, accumulate in affected organs followed by formation of granulomas. It does not appear that this process injures parenchyma by releasing mediators; rather, organ dysfunction results from the accumulated inflammatory cells distorting the architecture of the affected tissue. Severe damage of parenchyma can lead to irreversible fibrosis.

Clinical Manifestations

In 10–20% of cases, sarcoidosis may first be detected as asymptomatic hilar adenopathy. Sarcoid manifests clinically in organs where it affects function or where it is readily observed. Onset may be acute or insidious.

Acute sarcoid—20–40% of cases. Two acute syndromes: *Lofgren's syndrome*: hilar adenopathy, erythema nodosum, acute arthritis presenting in one or both ankles spreading to involve other joints; *Heerfordt-Waldenström syndrome*: parotid enlargement, fever, anterior uveitis, facial nerve palsy.

Insidious onset—40–70% of cases. Respiratory Sx most common presenting feature with constitutional or extrathoracic Sx less frequent.

Disease manifestations of sarcoid include:

- Constitutional symptoms—fever, weight loss, anorexia, fatigue.
- Lung—most commonly involved organ; 90% with sarcoidosis will have abnormal CXR some time during course. Features include: hilar adenopathy, alveolitis, interstitial pneumonitis; airways may be involved and cause obstruction to airflow; pleural disease and hemoptysis are uncommon.
- Lymph nodes—intrathoracic nodes enlarged in 75–90% of pts.
- Skin—25% will have skin involvement; lesions include erythema nodosum, plaques, maculopapular eruptions, subcutaneous nodules, and lupus pernio (indurated blue-purple shiny lesions on face, fingers, and knees).

- Eye—uveitis in approximately 25%; may progress to blindness.
- Upper respiratory tract—nasal mucosa involved in up to 20%, larynx 5%.
- Bone marrow and spleen—mild anemia and thrombocytopenia may occur.
- Liver—involved on biopsy in 60–90%; rarely important clinically.
- Kidney—parenchymal disease, nephrolithiasis secondary to abnormalities of calcium metabolism.
- Nervous system—cranial/peripheral neuropathy, chronic meningitis, pituitary involvement, space-occupying lesions, seizures.
- Heart— disturbances of rhythm and/or contractility, pericarditis.
- Musculoskeletal—dactylitis, chronic mono- or oligoarthritis of knee, ankle, PIP.
- Other organ systems affected: endocrine/reproductive, exocrine glands, GI.

Evaluation

- Hx and physical exam to rule out exposures and other causes of interstitial lung disease.
- CBC, Ca^{2+}, LFTs, ACE, PPD and control skin tests.
- CXR, ECG, PFTs.
- Biopsy of lung or other affected organ.
- Bronchoalveolar lavage and gallium scan of lungs may help decide when treatment is indicated and may help to follow therapy; however, these are not uniformly accepted.

Diagnosis

Made on basis of clinical, radiographic, and histologic findings. Biopsy of lung or other affected organ is mandatory to establish diagnosis before starting therapy. Transbronchial lung biopsy usually adequate to make diagnosis. No blood findings are diagnostic. Differential includes neoplasms, infections, HIV, other granulomatous processes.

℞ TREATMENT

Many cases remit spontaneously; therefore, deciding when treatment is necessary is difficult and controversial. Significant involvement of the eye, heart, or CNS or progressive lung disease is the main indication for treatment. Glucocorticoids are mainstay of therapy. Usual therapy is prednisone 1 (mg/kg)/d for 4–6 weeks followed by taper over 2–3 months.

Anecdotal reports suggest that cyclosporine may be useful in extrathoracic sarcoid not responding to glucocorticoids.

Outcome

Most pts with acute disease are left with no significant sequelae. Overall, 50% of pts with sarcoid have some permanent organ dysfunction; in 15–20% disease remains active or recurrent; death directly due to disease occurs in 10% of cases. Respiratory tract abnormalities cause most of the morbidity and mortality related to sarcoid.

For a more detailed discussion, see Crystal RG: Sarcoidosis, Chap. 320, p. 1922, in HPIM-14.

153

ANKYLOSING SPONDYLITIS

Definition

Chronic and progressive inflammatory disease of the axial skeleton with sacroiliitis (usually bilateral) as its hallmark. Involvement of limb joints other than hips and shoulders is uncommon. Most frequently presents in young men in second or third decade; strong association with histocompatibility antigen HLA-B27. In Europe, also known as Marie-Strumpell or Bechterew's disease.

Clinical Manifestations

- Back pain and stiffness—not relieved by lying down, often present at night forcing pt to leave bed, worse in the morning, improves with activity, insidious onset, duration >3 months (often called symptoms of "inflammatory" back pain).
- Peripheral joint pain (especially hip).
- Chest pain from involvement of thoracic skeleton and muscular insertions.
- Extra/juxtaarticular pain—due to "enthesitis": inflammation

at insertion of tendons and ligaments into bone; frequently affects greater trochanter, iliac crests, ischial tuberosities, tibial tubercles, heels.
- Extraarticular findings include acute anterior uveitis in about 20% of pts, aortitis, aortic insufficiency, GI inflammation, cardiac conduction defects, amyloidosis, bilateral upper lobe pulmonary fibrosis.
- Constitutional symptoms may occur: fever, fatigue, weight loss.
- Neurologic complications related to spinal fracture/dislocation (can occur with even minor trauma), atlantoaxial subluxation, cauda equina syndrome.

Physical examination:
- Tenderness over involved joints
- Diminished chest expansion
- Diminished anterior flexion of lumbar spine (Schober test)

Evaluation

- ESR and C-reactive protein elevated in majority.
- Mild anemia.
- Rheumatoid factor and ANA negative.
- HLA-B27 may be helpful in pts with inflammatory back Sx but negative x-rays.
- Radiographs: early may be normal. Sacroiliac joints: usually symmetric; bony erosions with "pseudowidening" followed by fibrosis and ankylosis. CT can detect changes earlier than plain x-ray. Spine: squaring of vertebrae; syndesmophytes; ossification of annulus fibrosis and anterior longitudinal ligament causing "bamboo spine." Sites of enthesitis may ossify and be visible on x-ray.

Diagnosis

Modified New York criteria widely used: radiographic evidence of sacroiliitis plus one of: (1) Hx of inflammatory back pain symptoms, (2) lumbar motion limitation, (3) limited chest expansion.

DIFFERENTIAL DIAGNOSIS Spondyloarthropathy associated with reactive arthritis, psoriatic arthritis, enteropathic arthritis (Fig. 153-1). Diffuse idiopathic skeletal hyperostosis.

℞ TREATMENT
- Exercise program to maintain posture and mobility is key to management.

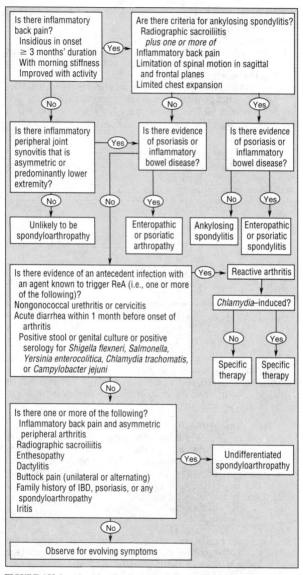

FIGURE 153-1 Algorithm for diagnosis of the spondyloarthropathies.

- NSAIDs (e.g., indomethacin 75 mg slow-release qd or bid) useful in most pts.
- Sulfasalazine 2–3 g/d may be useful.
- No therapeutic role for systemic glucocorticoids or other immunosuppressive has been documented in ankylosing spondylitis.
- Adjunctive therapy includes intraarticular glucocorticoids for persistent enthesitis or peripheral synovitis; ocular glucocorticoids for uveitis; surgery for severely affected or deformed joints.

For a more detailed discussion, see Taurog JD, Lipsky PE: Ankylosing Spondylitis, Reactive Arthritis, and Undifferentiated Spondyloarthropathy, Chap. 317, p. 1904, in HPIM-14.

154

DEGENERATIVE JOINT DISEASE

Definition

Degenerative joint disease or osteoarthritis (OA) is a disorder characterized by progressive deterioration and loss of articular cartilage accompanied by proliferation of new bone and soft tissue in and around involved joint.

- *Primary (idiopathic) OA*: no underlying cause is apparent.
- *Secondary OA:* a predisposing factor is present such as trauma, repetitive stress (occupation, sports), congenital abnormality, metabolic disorder, or other bone/joint disease.
- *Erosive OA*: term often applied to pts who have hand DIP/PIP OA associated with synovitis and radiographic central erosions of the articular surface.

Pathogenesis

Initial changes begin in cartilage, with change in arrangement and size of collagen fibers. Proteases lead to loss of cartilage matrix. Proteoglycan synthesis initially undergoes a compensatory increase but eventually falls off, leading to full-thickness cartilage loss.

Clinical Manifestations

OA is the most common form of joint disease. It can affect almost any joint, but usually occurs in weight-bearing and frequently used joints such as the knee, hip, spine, and hands. The hand joints that are typically affected are the DIP, PIP, or first CMC (thumb base); MCP involvement is rare.

SYMPTOMS

- Use-related pain affecting one or a few joints (rest and nocturnal pain less common).
- Stiffness after rest or in morning may occur but usually brief (<30 min).
- Loss of joint movement or functional limitation.
- Joint instability.
- Joint deformity.
- joint crepitation ("crackling").

PHYSICAL EXAMINATION

- Chronic monarthritis or asymmetric oligo/polyarthritis.
- Firm or "bony" swellings of the joint margins, e.g., Heberden's nodes (hand DIP) or Bouchard's nodes (hand PIP).
- Mild synovitis with a cool effusion can occur but is uncommon.
- Crepitance—audible creaking or crackling of joint on passive or active movement
- Deformity, e.g., OA of knee may involve medial, lateral, or patellofemoral compartments resulting in varus or valgus deformities.
- Restriction of movement, e.g., limitation of internal rotation of hip.
- Objective neurologic abnormalities may be seen with spine involvement (may affect intervertebral disks, apophyseal joints, and paraspinal ligaments).

Evaluation

- Routine lab work usually normal.
- ESR usually normal but may be elevated in pts who have synovitis.
- Rheumatoid factor, ANA studies negative.
- Joint fluid is straw-colored with good viscosity; fluid WBCs <2000/μL; of value in ruling out crystal-induced arthritis or infection.
- Radiographs may be normal at first but as disease progresses

may show joint space narrowing, subchondral bone sclerosis, subchondral cysts, and osteophytes. Erosions are distinct from those of rheumatoid and psoriatic arthritis as they occur subchondrally along the central portion of the joint surface.

Diagnosis

Usually established on basis of pattern of joint involvement, radiographic features, normal laboratory tests, and synovial fluid findings.

DIFFERENTIAL DIAGNOSIS   Osteonecrosis, Charcot joint, rheumatoid arthritis, psoriatic arthritis, crystal-induced arthritides.

 TREATMENT

- Pt education, weight reduction, appropriate use of cane and other supports, isometric exercises to strengthen muscles around affected joints.
- Topical capsaicin cream may help relieve hand or knee pain.
- Acetaminophen, salicylates, or NSAIDs.
- Intraarticular glucocorticoid injections may provide symptomatic relief but should be performed infrequently as cartilage breakdown may be accelerated if performed too often.
- Systemic glucocorticoids have no place in the treatment of OA.
- Surgery may be considered in pts with intractable pain and loss of function who are unresponsive to other measures.

For a more detailed discussion, see Brandt KD: Osteoarthritis, Chap. 322, p. 1935, in HPIM-14.

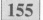

GOUT, PSEUDOGOUT, AND RELATED DISEASES

GOUT

Definition

The term *gout* is applied to a spectrum of manifestations that may occur singly or in combination. Hyperuricemia is the biologic hallmark of gout. When present, plasma and extracellular fluids become supersaturated with uric acid, which, under the right conditions, may crystallize and result in clinical gout.

Pathogenesis

Uric acid is the end product of purine nucleotide degradation; its production is closely linked to pathways of purine metabolism, with the intracellular concentration of 5-phosphoribosyl-1-pyrophosphate (PRPP) being the major determinant of the rate of uric acid biosynthesis. Uric acid is excreted primarily by the kidney through mechanisms of glomerular filtration, tubular secretion and reabsorption. Hyperuricemia may thus arise in a wide range of settings that cause overproduction or reduced excretion of uric acid or a combination of the two (see Table 344-1, p. 2159, HPIM-14).

ACUTE GOUTY ARTHRITIS   Monosodium urate (MSU) crystals present in the joint are phagocytosed by leukocytes; release of inflammatory mediators and lysosomal enzymes leads to recruitment of additional phagocytes into the joint and to synovial inflammation.

Clinical Manifestations

- *Acute inflammatory arthritis.* Usually an exquisitely painful monarthritis but may be polyarticular and accompanied by fever; podagra (attack in the great toe) is the site of first attack in half and may occur eventually in 90%. Attack will generally subside spontaneously after days to weeks. Although some pts may have a single attack, 75% have a second attack within 2 years. Differential diagnosis includes septic arthritis, reactive arthritis, calcium pyrophosphate deposition (CPPD) disease, rheumatoid arthritis.
- *Tenosynovitis.*
- *Chronic tophaceous arthritis. Tophi:* aggregates of MSU crystals surrounded by a giant cell inflammatory reaction. Occurs in the setting of long-standing gout.

- *Extraarticular tophi.* Often occur in olecranon bursa, helix and anthelix of ears, ulnar surface of forearm, Achilles tendon.
- *Urate nephrosis.* Deposition of MSU crystals in interstitium and pyramids. Can cause chronic renal insufficiency.
- *Acute uric acid nephropathy.* Reversible cause of acute renal failure due to precipitation of urate in the tubules; pts receiving cytotoxic treatment for neoplastic disease are at risk.
- *Uric acid nephrolithiasis.* Responsible for 10% of renal stones in United States.

Evaluation

- Synovial fluid analysis—only definitive method of diagnosing gouty arthritis is joint aspiration and demonstration of characteristic needle-shaped negatively birefringent MSU crystals by polarizing microscopy. Gram stain and culture should be performed on all fluid to rule out infection.
- Serum uric acid—normal levels do not rule out gout.
- Urine uric acid—excretion of >800 mg/d on regular diet in the absence of drugs suggests overproduction.
- Screening for risk factors—renal insufficiency, hyperlipidemia, diabetes.
- If overproduction is suspected, measurement of erythrocyte HGPRT and PRPP levels may be indicated.
- Joint x-rays—may demonstrate erosions late in disease.
- If renal stones suggested: abdominal flat plate (stones often radiolucent), possibly IVP.
- Chemical analysis of renal stones.

℞ TREATMENT

Asymptomatic Hyperuricemia   As only about 5% of hyperuricemic pts develop gout, treatment of asymptomatic hyperuricemia is not indicated. Exception is pts about to receive cytotoxic therapy for neoplasms.

Acute Gouty Arthritis   Treatment is given for symptomatic relief only as attack is self-limited and will resolve spontaneously. Toxicity of therapy must be considered in each pt.

- Analgesia.
- NSAIDs—Rx of choice when not contraindicated.
- Colchicine—generally only effective within first 24 h of attack; overdose has potentially life-threatening side effects; use is contraindicated in pts with renal insufficiency, cytopenias, LFTs >2× normal, sepsis. PO—0.6 mg qh until pt improves, has GI side effects, or maximal dose of 5 mg is reached. IV—dangerous and best avoided; if used,

give no more than 2 mg over 24 h and no further drug for 7 days following; IV must never be given in a pt who has received PO colchicine.
- Intraarticular glucocorticoids—septic arthritis must be ruled out prior to injection.
- Systemic glucocorticoids—brief taper may be considered in pts with a polyarticular gouty attack for whom other modalities are contraindicated and where articular or systemic infection has been ruled out.

Uric Acid Lowering Agents Indications for initiating uric acid–lowering therapy include recurrent frequent acute gouty arthritis, polyarticular gouty arthritis, tophaceous gout, renal stones, cytotoxic therapy prophylaxis. Should not start during an attack. Initiation can precipitate an acute flare; consider concomitant PO colchicine 0.6 mg qd until uric acid <5.0 mg/dL, then discontinue.

- Allopurinol. Decreases uric acid synthesis by inhibiting xanthine oxidase. Must be dose-reduced in renal insufficiency. Has significant side effects and drug interactions.
- Uricosuric drugs (probenecid, sulfinpyrazone). Increases uric acid excretion by inhibiting its tubular reabsorption; ineffective in renal insufficiency; should not be used in these settings: age >60, renal stones, tophi, increased urinary uric acid excretion, cytotoxic therapy prophylaxis.

PSEUDOGOUT

Definition and Pathogenesis

CPPD disease is characterized by acute and chronic inflammatory joint disease, usually affecting older individuals. The knee and other large joints most commonly affected. Calcium deposits in articular cartilage (chondrocalcinosis) may be seen radiographically; these are not always associated with symptoms.

CPPD may be hereditary; idiopathic, associated chiefly with aging; or occur secondary to hyperparathyroidism, hemochromatosis, hypophosphatasia, hypomagnesemia, hypothyroidism, gout, ochronosis, joint trauma, severe medical illness, or surgery.

Crystals are not thought to form in synovial fluid but probably are shed from articular cartilage into joint space where they are phagocytosed by neutrophils and incite an inflammatory response.

Clinical Manifestations

Acute "pseudogout"—occurs in approximately 25% of pts with CPPD disease; knee is most frequently involved, but other joints may be affected; involved joint is erythematous, swollen, warm, and painful; most pts have evidence of chondrocalcinosis. A minority will have involvement of multiple joints.

Degenerative CPPD disease—chronic arthropathy with progressive degenerative changes in multiple joints. Common sites include knee, wrist, MCP, hips, and shoulders. These pts may also have intermittent acute attacks.

Diagnosis

- Made by demonstration of calcium pyrophosphate dihydrate crystals (appearing as short blunt rods, rhomboids, and cuboids with weak positive birefringence) in synovial fluid.
- Radiographs may demonstrate chondrocalcinosis and degenerative changes (joint space narrowing, subchondral sclerosis/cysts).
- Secondary causes of CPPD should be considered in pts <50 years old.

DIFFERENTIAL DIAGNOSIS OA, RA, gout, septic arthritis.

℞ TREATMENT

- NSAIDs
- Intraarticular injection of glucocorticoids
- Colchicine is variably effective.

HYDROXYAPATITE ARTHROPATHY

Calcium hydroxyapatite (HA) deposition can cause a calcific bursitis or tendinitis and arthropathy primarily affecting the shoulder and knee. Abnormal HA accumulation can occur idiopathically or secondary to tissue damage, hypercalcemia, hyperparathyroidism, or chronic renal failure. HA is an important factor in *Milwaukee shoulder*, a destructive arthropathy of the elderly that occurs in the shoulders and knees. HA crystals are small; clumps may stain purplish on Wright's stain and bright red with alizarin red S. Definitive identification requires electron microscopy or x-ray diffraction studies. Radiographic appearance resembles CPPD disease. *Treatment*: NSAIDs, repeated aspiration, and rest of affected joint.

CALCIUM OXALATE DEPOSITION DISEASE

CaOx crystals may be deposited in joints in primary oxalosis (rare) or secondary oxalosis (a complication of end-stage renal disease). Clinical syndrome similar to gout and CPPD disease. *Treatment*: marginally effective.

For a more detailed discussion, see Wortmann RL: Gout and Other Disorders of Purine Metabolism, Chap. 344, p. 2158; and Reginato AJ, Hoffman GS: Arthritis due to Deposition of Calcium Crystals, Chap. 323, p. 1941, in HPIM-14.

156

PSORIATIC ARTHRITIS

Definition

Psoriatic arthritis is a chronic inflammatory arthritis that affects 5–42% of people with psoriasis. Some pts, especially those with spondylitis, will carry the HLA-B27 histocompatibility antigen. Onset of psoriasis usually precedes development of joint disease; approximately 15% of pts develop arthritis prior to onset of skin disease.

Patterns of Joint Involvement

- Asymmetric oligoarthritis: most common pattern affecting 16–70% (mean 47%); often involve DIP/PIP of hands and feet, knees, wrists, ankles; "sausage digits" may be present, reflecting tendon sheath inflammation.
- Symmetric polyarthritis (25%) resembles rheumatoid arthritis except rheumatoid factor is negative, absence of rheumatoid nodules.
- Predominantly distal interphalangeal joint involvement (10%): high frequency of association with psoriatic nail changes.
- "Arthritis mutilans" (3–5%): aggressive, destructive form of arthritis with severe joint deformities and bony dissolution.
- Spondylitis and/or sacroiliitis: axial involvement is present

in 20–40% of pts with psoriatic arthritis; may occur in absence of peripheral arthritis.

Evaluation

- Negative tests for rheumatoid factor.
- Hypoproliferative anemia, elevated ESR.
- Hyperuricemia may be present.
- HIV should be suspected in fulminant disease.
- Inflammatory synovial fluid and biopsy without specific findings.
- Radiographic features include erosion at joint margin, bony ankylosis, tuft resorption of terminal phalanges, "pencil-in-cup" deformity (bone proliferation at base of distal phalanx with tapering of proximal phalanx), axial skeleton with asymmetric sacroiliitis, asymmetric nonmarginal syndesmophytes.

Diagnosis

Suggested by: pattern of arthritis and inflammatory nature, absence of rheumatoid factor, radiographic characteristics, presence of skin and nail changes of psoriasis (see Fig. 153-1).

Rx TREATMENT

- Pt education, physical and occupational therapy.
- NSAIDs.
- Intraarticular steroid injections—useful in some settings. Systemic glucocorticoids should rarely be used as may induce rebound flare of skin disease upon tapering.
- Gold salts IM or PO—helpful in some pts, significant side-effect profile.
- Methotrexate (5–25 mg PO weekly)—in advanced cases, especially with severe skin involvement, significant side-effect profile.

For a more detailed discussion, see Schur PH: Psoriatic Arthritis and Arthritis Associated with Gastrointestinal Diseases, Chap. 325, p. 1949, in HPIM-14.

157

REACTIVE ARTHRITIS AND REITER'S SYNDROME

Definition

Reiter's syndrome describes the triad of arthritis, conjunctivitis, and nongonococcal urethritis. This term is largely of historic interest and is now considered to be part of the spectrum of *reactive arthritis,* an acute nonpurulent arthritis complicating an infection elsewhere in the body (usually genitourinary or enteric) that may be accompanied by extraarticular features.

Pathogenesis

Up to 85% of pts possess the HLA-B27 alloantigen. It is thought that in individuals with appropriate genetic background, reactive arthritis may be triggered by an enteric infection with any of several *Shigella, Salmonella, Yersinia,* and *Campylobacter* species; by genitourinary infection with *Chlamydia trachomatis;* and possibly by other agents.

Clinical Manifestations

The sex ratio following enteric infection is 1:1, but genitourinary acquired reactive arthritis is predominantly seen in young males. In a majority of cases Hx will elicit Sx of genitourinary or enteric infection 1–4 weeks prior to onset of other features.

- Constitutional—fatigue, malaise, fever, weight loss.
- Arthritis—usually acute, asymmetric, oligoarticular, involving predominantly lower extremities; sacroiliitis may occur.
- Enthesitis—inflammation at insertion of tendons and ligaments into bone; "sausage digit," plantar fasciitis, and Achilles tendinitis common.
- Ocular features—conjunctivitis, usually minimal; uveitis, keratitis, and optic neuritis rarely present.
- Urethritis—discharge intermittent and may be asymptomatic.
- Other urogenital manifestations—prostatitis, cervicitis, salpingitis.
- Mucocutaneous lesions—painless lesions on glans penis (*circinate balanitis*) and oral mucosa in approximately a third of pts; *keratoderma blenorrhagica*: cutaneous vesicles that become hyperkerotic, most common on soles and palms.
- Uncommon manifestations—pleuropericarditis, aortic regurgitation, neurologic manifestations, secondary amyloidosis.

- Reiter's syndrome is associated with and may be the presenting Sx of HIV.

Evaluation

- Pursuit of *Chlamydia* infection by culture, DFA, or EIA of secretions from throat, urethra, cervix.
- Stool cultures may secure Dx of enteric pathogen.
- Rheumatoid factor and ANA negative.
- Mild anemia, leukocytosis, elevated ESR may be seen.
- HLA-B27 may be helpful in atypical cases.
- HIV screening should be performed in all pts.
- Synovial fluid analysis—often very inflammatory; negative for crystals or infection.
- Radiographs—erosions may be seen with new periosteal bone formation, ossification of entheses, sacroiliitis (often unilateral).

Differential Diagnosis

Includes septic arthritis (gram $+/-$), gonococcal arthritis, crystalline arthritis, psoriatic arthritis (see Fig. 153-1).

℞ TREATMENT

- Prolonged administration of antibiotics may benefit *Chlamydia*-induced disease.
- NSAIDs (e.g., indomethacin 25–50 mg PO tid) benefit most pts.
- Intraarticular glucocorticoids.
- Sulfasalazine up to 3 g/d in divided doses may help some pts with persistent arthritis.
- Cytotoxic therapy, such as azathioprine [1–2 (mg/kg)/d] or methotrexate (7.5–15 mg/week) may be considered for debilitating disease refractory to other modalities; contraindicated in HIV disease.
- Uveitis may require therapy with ocular or systemic glucocorticoids.

Outcome

Prognosis is variable; a third will have recurrent or sustained disease, with 15–25% developing permanent disability.

For a more detailed discussion, see Taurog JD, Lipsky PE: Ankylosing Spondylitis, Reactive Arthritis, and Undifferentiated Spondyloarthropathy, Chap. 317, p. 1904, in HPIM-14.

158

OTHER ARTHRITIDES

ENTEROPATHIC ARTHRITIS

Both peripheral and axial arthritis may be associated with ulcerative colitis or Crohn's disease. The arthritis can occur after or before the onset of intestinal symptoms. Peripheral arthritis is episodic, asymmetric, and most frequently affects knee and ankle. Attacks usually subside within several weeks and characteristically resolve completely without residual joint damage. Enthesitis (inflammation at insertion of tendons and ligaments into bone) can occur with manifestations of "sausage digit," Achilles tendinitis, plantar fasciitis. Axial involvement can manifest as spondylitis and/or sacroiliitis (often symmetric). Laboratory findings are nonspecific; rheumatoid factor absent; radiographs of peripheral joints usually normal; axial involvement is often indistinguishable from ankylosing spondylitis (see Fig. 153-1).

Treatment   Directed at underlying inflammatory bowel disease; NSAIDs may alleviate joint symptoms; sulfasalazine may benefit peripheral arthritis.

INTESTINAL BYPASS ARTHRITIS   Some pts will develop arthritis-dermatitis following intestinal bypass surgery. Possibly related to bacterial overgrowth. Symptoms may be relieved by NSAIDs, suppression of bacterial overgrowth with tetracycline or other antibiotics, or surgical reanastomosis of bypassed segment.

WHIPPLE'S DISEASE   Characterized by arthritis in up to 90% of pts that usually precedes appearance of intestinal symptoms. Usually polyarticular, symmetric, transient but may become chronic. GI and joint manifestations respond to antibiotic therapy.

NEUROPATHIC JOINT DISEASE

Also known as *Charcot's joint*, this is a severe destructive arthropathy that occurs in joints deprived of pain and position sense; may occur in diabetic neuropathy, tabes dorsalis, syringomyelia, amyloidosis, spinal cord or peripheral nerve injury. Usually begins in a single joint but may spread to involve other joints. Joint effusions are usually noninflammatory but can be hemorrhagic. Radiographs can reveal either bone resorption or new bone formation with bone dislocation and fragmentation.

Treatment   Stabilization of joint; surgical fusion may improve function.

RELAPSING POLYCHONDRITIS

An idiopathic disorder characterized by recurrent inflammation of cartilaginous structures. Cardinal manifestations include ear and nose involvement with floppy ear and saddle nose deformities, inflammation and collapse of tracheal and bronchial cartilaginous rings, asymmetric episodic nondeforming polyarthritis. Other features can include scleritis, conjunctivitis, iritis, keratitis, aortic regurgitation, glomerulonephritis and other features of systemic vasculitis. Diagnosis is made clinically and may be confirmed by biopsy of affected cartilage.

Treatment   Glucocorticoids (prednisone 40–60 mg/d with subsequent taper) may suppress acute features and reduce the severity/frequency of recurrences; cytotoxic agents may be considered for unresponsive disease.

HYPERTROPHIC OSTEOARTHROPATHY

Syndrome consisting of periosteal new bone formation, digital clubbing, and arthritis. Most commonly seen in association with lung carcinoma but also occurs with chronic lung or liver disease; congenital heart, lung, or liver disease in children; and idiopathic and familial forms. Symptoms include burning and aching pain most pronounced in distal extremities. Radiographs show periosteal thickening with new bone formation of distal ends of long bones.

Treatment   Identify and treat associated disorder; aspirin, NSAIDs, other analgesics, vagotomy or percutaneous nerve block may help to relieve symptoms.

FIBROMYALGIA

A common disorder characterized by pain, aching, stiffness of trunk and extremities, and presence of a number of specific tender points. More common in women than men. Frequently associated with sleep disorders. Diagnosis is made clinically; evaluation reveals soft tissue tender points but no objective joint abnormalities by exam, laboratory, or radiograph.

Treatment   Benzodiazepines or tricyclics for sleep disorder, local measures (heat, massage, injection of tender points), NSAIDs.

REFLEX SYMPATHETIC DYSTROPHY SYNDROME (RSDS)

A syndrome of pain and tenderness, usually of a hand or foot, associated with vasomotor instability, trophic skin changes, and rapid development of bony demineralization. Frequently, development will follow a precipitating event (local trauma, myocardial infarction, stroke, or peripheral nerve injury). Early recognition and treatment can be effective in preventing disability.

Treatment Options include pain control, application of heat or cold, exercise, sympathetic nerve block, and short courses of high-dose prednisone in conjunction with physical therapy.

POLYMYALGIA RHEUMATICA (PMR)

Clinical syndrome characterized by aching and morning stiffness in the shoulder girdle, hip girdle, or neck for >1 month, elevated ESR, and rapid response to low-dose prednisone (15 mg qd). Rarely occurs before age 50. PMR can occur in association with giant cell (temporal) arteritis, which requires treatment with higher doses of prednisone. Evaluation should include a careful history to elicit Sx suggestive of giant cell arteritis (see Chap. 151), ESR, labs to rule out other processes usually include RF, ANA, CBC, CPK, SPEP, and renal, hepatic, and thyroid function tests.

Treatment Pts rapidly improve on prednisone 10–20 mg qd but may require treatment over months to years.

OSTEONECROSIS (AVASCULAR NECROSIS)

Caused by death of cellular elements of bone, believed to be due to impairment in blood supply. Frequent associations include glucocorticoid treatment, connective tissue disease, trauma, sickle cell disease, embolization, alcohol use. Commonly involved sites include femoral and humeral heads, femoral condyles, proximal tibia. Hip disease is bilateral in >50% of cases. Clinical presentation is usually the abrupt onset of articular pain. Early changes are not visible on plain radiograph and are best seen by MRI, later stages demonstrate bone collapse ("crescent sign"), flattening of articular surface with joint space loss.

Treatment Limited weight bearing of unclear benefit, NSAIDs for Sx. Surgical procedures to enhance blood flow may be considered in early-stage disease but are of controversial efficacy; joint replacement may be necessary in late-stage disease for pain unresponsive to other measures.

PERIARTICULAR DISORDERS

BURSITIS Inflammation of the thin-walled bursal sac surrounding tendons and muscles over bony prominences. The subacromial and greater trochanteric bursae are most commonly involved.

Treatment   Prevention of aggravating conditions, rest, NSAIDs, and local glucocorticoid injections.

TENDINITIS   May involve virtually any tendon but frequently affects tendons of the rotator cuff around shoulder, especially the supraspinatus. Pain is dull and aching but becomes acute and sharp when tendon is squeezed below acromion.

Treatment   NSAIDs, glucocorticoid injection, and physical therapy may be beneficial. The rotator cuff tendons or biceps tendon may rupture acutely, frequently requiring surgical repair.

CALCIFIC TENDINITIS   Results from deposition of calcium salts in tendon, usually supraspinatus. The resulting pain may be sudden and severe.

ADHESIVE CAPSULITIS   ("frozen shoulder") Results from conditions that enforce prolonged immobility of shoulder joint. Shoulder is painful and tender to palpation, and both active and passive range of motion is restricted.

Treatment   Spontaneous improvement may occur; NSAIDs, local injections of glucocorticoids, and physical therapy may be helpful.

For a more detailed discussion, see Schur PH: Psoriatic Arthritis and Arthritis Associated with Gastrointestinal Diseases, Chap. 325, p. 1949; and Gilliland BC: Relapsing Polychondritis and Other Arthritides, Chap. 326, p. 1951, in HPIM-14.

159

AMYLOIDOSIS

Definition

A disease characterized by deposition of the fibrous protein amyloid in one or more sites of the body. Clinical manifestations depend on anatomic distribution and intensity of amyloid protein deposition and range from local deposition with little significance to involvement of virtually any organ system with consequent severe pathophysiologic changes.

Classification

Chemical characterization reveals several varieties of amyloid fibrils associated with different clinical situations (see Table 309-1, p. 1857, in HPIM-14):

- *Light chain amyloidosis* (AL): most common form of systemic amyloidosis seen in clinical practice; occurs in primary idiopathic amyloidosis and amyloid associated with multiple myeloma.
- *Amyloid A amyloidosis* (AA): occurs in secondary amyloidosis as a complication of chronic inflammatory disease and in familial Mediterranean fever (FMF).
- *Heredofamilial amyloidoses*
- $A\beta_2M$: Chronic hemodialysis-related amyloid; identical to beta$_2$ microglobulin.
- *Localized* or *organ-limited amyloidoses*: includes Aβ: found in neuritic plaques and cerebrovascular walls of pts with Alzheimer's disease and Down's syndrome.

Clinical Manifestations

Clinical features are varied and depend entirely on biochemical nature of the fibril protein. Frequent sites of involvement:

- Kidney—seen with AA and AL; proteinuria, nephrosis, azotemia.
- Liver—occurs in AA, AL, and heredofamilial; hepatomegaly.
- Skin—characteristic of AL but can be seen in AA; raised waxy papules.
- Heart—common in AL and heredofamilial; CHF, cardiomegaly, arrhythmias.
- GI—common in all types; GI obstruction or ulceration, hemorrhage, protein loss, diarrhea, macroglossia, disordered esophageal motility.
- Joints—usually AL, frequently with myeloma; periarticular

amyloid deposits, "shoulder pad sign": firm amyloid deposits in soft tissue around the shoulder, symmetric arthritis of shoulders, wrists, knees, hands.

- Nervous system—prominent in heredofamilial; peripheral neuropathy, postural hypotension, dementia. Carpal tunnel syndrome may occur in AL and $A\beta_2M$.
- Respiratory—lower airways can be affected in AL, localized amyloid can cause obstruction along upper airways.
- Hematologic—selective clotting factor deficiency.

Diagnosis

Requires demonstration of amyloid in a biopsy of affected tissue using appropriate stains (e.g., Congo red). Aspiration of abdominal fat pad or biopsy of rectal mucosa may demonstrate amyloid fibrils. Electrophoresis and imunoelectrophoresis of serum and urine may assist in detecting paraproteins.

Prognosis

Outcome is variable and depends on type of amyloidosis and organ involvement. Average survival of AL amyloid is ~12 months; prognosis is poor when associated with myeloma. Renal failure and heart disease are the major causes of death.

℞ TREATMENT

There is no specific therapy for any variety of amyloidosis. If present, an underlying disorder should be treated. Primary amyloidosis may respond to regimens incorporating prednisone and alkylating agents, presumably because of the effects of these agents on synthesis of the AL amyloid protein. Colchicine (1–2 mg/d) may prevent acute attacks in FMF and thus may block amyloid deposition. Renal transplantation may be effective in selected pts.

For a more detailed discussion, see Sipe JD, Cohen AS: Amyloidosis, Chap. 309, p. 1856, in HPIM-14.

160

DISORDERS OF THE ANTERIOR PITUITARY AND HYPOTHALAMUS

The anterior pituitary produces growth hormone (GH), prolactin (PRL), luteinizing hormone (LH), follicle-stimulating hormone (FSH), thyroid-stimulating hormone (TSH), and corticotropin (ACTH). Hormone production is under feedback control by target glands, and hence hormone levels in blood increase when target glands fail. The pituitary is also under control of chemical mediators synthesized in the hypothalamus and transported to the pituitary via the portal vessels of the pituitary stalk. With hypothalamic ablation, the levels of GH, LH, FSH, TSH, and ACTH fall, whereas PRL levels increase, indicating that the major hypothalamic influence on the latter is inhibitory. Disorders of the anterior pituitary can cause mass effects, hypopituitarism, or disorders due to excess or deficiency of individual hormones.

MASS LESIONS OF THE SELLA TURCICA AND SUPRASELLAR REGION

Sellar enlargement can be an incidental finding on skull series or cause headache or visual disturbances (bitemporal hemianopsia). Differential diagnosis includes tumors (pituitary adenomas, craniopharyngiomas, meningiomas, metastatic lesions), granulomas, and empty sella syndrome (nontumorous enlargement resulting from protrusion of arachnoid cavity and CSF into the sella). Anterior pituitary hormone production is usually not impaired in the latter. MRI with gadolinium contrast and CT scan with contrast are the most reliable imaging tools available. Pituitary function must be evaluated in all pts with a pituitary mass.

Pituitary adenomas account for 10–15% of intracranial neoplasms and are classified as microadenomas (<1 cm) or macroadenomas (≥1 cm). The presence of a pituitary adenoma is suspected either with symptoms due to mass effects (sellar enlargement, visual field defects, oculomotor palsies, or increased intracranial pressure) or because of evidence of hormone deficiency or excess. Diagnosis is confirmed with laboratory testing (Table 160-1) and imaging studies. The most common

Table 160-1

Pituitary Hormone Evaluation

Hormone	Excess
Growth hormone	A. Measurement of plasma growth hormone 1 h after glucose PO B. Measurement of IGF-I
Prolactin	A. Measurement of basal serum prolactin, preferably fasting
TSH	A. Measurement of T_4, free T_4 index, T_3, TSH, TSH α
Gonadotropins	A. Measurement of FSH, LH, LH β, testosterone, FSH β, FSH response to TRH

ACTH	A. Measurement of urine free cortisol*
	B. Dexamethasone suppression by one of the following:
	  1. Measurement of 8 A.M. plasma cortisol after administration of 1 mg dexamethasone at midnight
	  2. Measurement of 8 A.M. plasma cortisol or 24-h urine 17-hydroxysteroids or free cortisol after 0.5 mg dexamethasone PO q 6 h for 8 doses
	C. High-dose dexamethasone suppression by one of the following:
	  1. Measurement of plasma cortisol after 8 mg dexamethasone PO at midnight
	  2. Measurement of 8 A.M. plasma cortisol or 24-h urine 17-hydroxysteroids or free cortisol after 2 mg dexamethasone q 6 h for 8 doses
	D. Metyrapone response (same protocol as for deficiency testing)†
	E. Response of plasma ACTH and cortisol to ovine corticotropin releasing hormone (1 µg/kg body wt)

Arginine vasopressin (AVP)	A. Measurement of serum sodium and osmolality, urine osmolality in presence of normal renal, adrenal, thyroid function B. Simultaneous measurement of serum osmolality and ADH levels

*Tests 1 and 2 establish the diagnosis of Cushing's syndrome. Tests 3, 4, and 5 localize the Cushing's disease to the pituitary gland. Often bilateral inferior petrosal sinus catheterization will be necessary.

Deficiency

A. Measurement of plasma growth hormone 30, 60, and 120 min after one of the following:
   1. Regular insulin 0.1 to 0.15 unit/kg IV
   2. Levodopa 10 mg/kg PO
   3. L-Arginine 0.5 mg/kg intravenously over 30 min
B. Measurement of IGF-I

A. Measurement of serum prolactin 10 to 20 min after one of the following:
   1. TRH 200 to 500 µg IV
   2. Chlorpromazine 25 mg IM

A. Measurement of T_4, free T_4, free T_4 index, TSH

A. Measurement of basal LH, FSH in postmenopausal women; no measurements in menstruating, ovulating women
B. Testosterone, FSH, and LH in men

A. Measurement of serum cortisol at 30 and 60 min after regular insulin 0.05 to 0.15 units per kilogram IV
B. Metyrapone response by one of the following:
   1. Measurement of plasma 11-deoxycortisol at 8 A.M. after 30 mg/kg body wt metyrapone at midnight (maximal dose 2 g)†
   2. Measurement of 24-h urinary 17-hydroxycorticoids or plasma 11-deoxycortisol day of and day after 750 mg metyrapone q 4 h for 6 doses†
   3. Measurement of 24-h urinary 17-hydroxycorticoids day of and day after 500 mg metyrapone q 2 h for 12 doses†
C. ACTH stimulation test: Measurement of plasma cortisol and aldosterone at 0, 30, and 60 min after IM or IV administration of 0.25 mg cosyntropin
D. ?Response of plasma ACTH and cortisol to ovine corticotropin-releasing hormone (1 µg/kg body weight)

A. Comparison of urine osmolality and serum osmolality under conditions of increased AVP secretion‡

B. Simultaneous measurement of serum osmolality and AVP levels

---

†Give food with metyrapone.
‡May be achieved by water deprivation or saline administration.
SOURCE: Biller BMK, Daniels GH, HPIM-14, p. 1990.

pituitary tumor is the prolactinoma, but adenomas that appear to be nonsecretory cause mild hyperprolactinemia via compression of the pituitary stalk. Some micro- and macroadenomas can be treated medically (ergot alkaloids for prolactinoma or somatostatin analogues for acromegaly). Surgery is indicated for hormonal hypersecretion not responsive to medical therapy, symptoms of mass effects, or increasing tumor size. For macroadenomas, surgery is effective for visual field abnormalities but may not cure hormone excess when residual tumor remains. Complications of surgery include hypopituitarism, diabetes insipidus, CSF rhinorrhea, visual loss, and oculomotor palsy. Radiation therapy is a useful adjunct for treatment of adenomas.

Craniopharyngiomas arise from remnants of Rathke's pouch and are usually manifested in childhood. Children present with symptoms of increased intracranial pressure due to hydrocephalus (80%); visual abnormalities (60%), including field cuts and vision loss; short stature (7–40%); and delayed sexual development (20%). Adults present with visual complaints (80%), headache (40%), personality change (26%), or hypogonadism (35%). Diabetes insipidus and panhypopituitarism may occur. Skull x-ray abnormalities include calcification, sellar enlargement, and signs of increased intracranial pressure. CT scan and MRI are also useful. Therapy often results in major functional deficits. The currently favored approach is biopsy and partial resection followed by conventional radiation.

Pituitary and suprasellar tumors that extend upward can impair the hypothalamus, which produces regulatory hormones and controls many nonendocrine functions (food intake and feeding behavior, temperature regulation, sleep patterns, short-term memory, thirst, and autonomic nervous system function).

HYPOPITUITARISM

Deficiency of one or more pituitary hormones has many etiologies (see Table 160-2). When diabetes insipidus is present, the primary defect is almost invariably in the hypothalamus or the pituitary stalk, often in conjunction with mild hyperprolactinemia and anterior pituitary hypofunction. Diagnosis is based on multiple hormonal tests (see Table 160-1) and requires replacement of missing hormones. Glucocorticoid is the most important and is commonly given as cortisone acetate (20–37.5 mg/d) or prednisone (5–7.5 mg/d). In emergent situations, hydrocortisone hemisuccinate, 75 mg IM/IV q6h, or methylprednisolone sodium succinate, 15 mg IM/IV q6h, is given.

Table 160-2

Causes of Hypopituitarism

A. Isolated hormone deficiencies
  1. Congenital or acquired deficiencies
B. Tumors
  1. Large pituitary adenomas
  2. Pituitary apoplexy
  3. Hypothalamic tumors, e.g., craniopharyngiomas, germinomas, chordomas, meningiomas, gliomas, and others
  4. Metastatic tumors
C. Inflammatory diseases
  1. Granulomatous disease, e.g., sarcoidosis, tuberculosis, syphilis, granulomatous hypophysitis
  2. Eosinophilic granuloma
  3. Lymphocytic hypophysitis (autoimmune)
D. Vascular diseases
  1. Postpartum necrosis (Sheehan's syndrome)
  2. ?Diabetic peripartum necrosis
  3. Carotid aneurysm
E. Destructive-traumatic events
  1. Surgery
  2. Stalk section
  3. Radiation (conventional—hypothalamus; heavy-particle—pituitary)
  4. Trauma
F. Developmental anomalies
  1. Pituitary aplasia
  2. Basal encephalocoele
G. Infiltration
  1. Hemochromatosis
  2. Amyloidosis
H. "Idiopathic" causes: autoimmune disease

SOURCE: Biller BMK, Daniels GH: HPIM-14, p. 1993.

Thyroid hormone deficiency is replaced with levothyroxine (0.1–0.2 mg/d); glucocorticoid replacement should always precede levothyroxine therapy to avoid precipitation of adrenal crisis. Hypogonadism in women is treated with estrogen-progestogen combinations (see Chap. 166) and in men with testosterone either by injection or dermal patch (see Chap. 165). GH deficiency is usually not treated in adults. See Chap. 161 for treatment of diabetes insipidus.

DISORDERS ASSOCIATED WITH INDIVIDUAL HORMONES

PROLACTIN (PRL)   The secretion of PRL, a hormone essential for lactation, is inhibited by dopamine and stimulated by thyroid hormone–releasing hormone (TRH) (although TSH and PRL are under independent control in most physiologic states). *Prolactin excess* has many causes (Table 160-3) and can cause galactorrhea, oligomenorrhea or amenorrhea, and infertility in women. Hyperprolactinemia occurs in 10–40% of women with amenorrhea, and 30% of women with galactorrhea and amenorrhea have prolactinomas. In men impotence and infertility may occur, whereas gynecomastia and galactorrhea are unusual. Hypogonadism is due to inhibition by PRL of the release of LH-releasing hormone (LHRH) from the hypothalamus and subsequent decreased gonadotropin levels. Serum PRL levels should be measured in all pts with hypogonadism, galactorrhea, or unexplained infertility. A PRL level >300 μg/L is diagnostic of pituitary adenoma. When other causes such as pregnancy, the postpartum state, and drug causes are excluded, modest PRL elevation is usually due to pituitary stalk compression and impairment of delivery of dopamine to the gland, most commonly due to the mass effects of nonsecretory adenomas of the pituitary. Dopamine agonists such as bromocriptine lower PRL levels in virtually all hyperprolactinemic pts. Therapy should begin with 1.25 mg PO qhs, increasing gradually up to a maximum of 25 mg/d or until serum PRL is normal. The usual dose is 2.5 mg PO bid. Maximum dosage is usually 25 mg/d. Surgery may be curative for microadenomas, but recurrence is common. Macroadenomas usually shrink with octreotide, but residual tumor or unresponsive tumors may require surgical debulking or radiation therapy. Surgical resection of macroadenomas is usually incomplete, and life-long ergot alkaloid therapy may be necessary.

Prolactin deficiency is manifested as an inability to lactate, which may be the first clue to panhypopituitarism. After TRH administration, an increase in serum prolactin by <200% of baseline suggests PRL deficiency and makes it necessary to evaluate other pituitary hormones.

GROWTH   HORMONE   (GH,   SOMATOTROPIN)
Growth hormone regulates linear growth by stimulating the formation of insulin-like growth factors (IGF-I). Hypothalamic inhibition of GH release is mediated by somatostatin, and hypothalamic stimulation of release is mediated by growth hormone–releasing hormone (GHRH). Evaluation of GH deficiency and excess is described in Table 160-1. *GH excess* leads to gigantism in children and to acromegaly in adults. Soft tissue and bony

Table 160-3

Causes of Hyperprolactinemia

I. Physiologic states
  A. Pregnancy
  B. Nursing (early)
  C. "Stress"
  D. Sleep
  E. Nipple stimulation
  F. Food ingestion
II. Drugs
  A. Dopamine receptor antagonists
    1. Phenothiazines
    2. Butyrophenones
    3. Thioxanthenes
    4. Metoclopramide
  B. Dopamine-depleting agents
    1. Methyldopa
    2. Reserpine
  C. Estrogens
  D. Opiates
  E. Verapamil
III. Disease states
  A. Pituitary tumors
    1. Prolactinomas
    2. Adenomas secreting GH and prolactin
    3. Adenomas secreting ACTH and prolactin (Nelson's syndrome and Cushing's disease)
    4. Nonfunctioning chromophobe adenomas with pituitary stalk compression
  B. Hypothalamic and pituitary stalk disease
    1. Granulomatous diseases especially sarcoidosis
    2. Craniopharyngiomas and other tumors
    3. Cranial irradiation
    4. Stalk section
    5. Empty sella
    6. Vascular abnormalities including aneurysm
    7. Lymphocytic hypophysitis
    8. Metastatic cancer
  C. Primary hypothyroidism
  D. Chronic renal failure
  E. Cirrhosis
  F. Chest wall trauma (including surgery, *herpes zoster*)
  G. Seizures

SOURCE: Biller BMK, Daniels GH: HPIM-14, p. 1975.

overgrowth is manifested by increased hand, foot, jaw, and cranial size; enlargement of the tongue; wide spacing of teeth; and coarsening of facial features. Thickening of the palms, increased skin tags, acanthosis nigricans, oily skin, and obstructive sleep apnea are common. Neurologic symptoms include headaches, paresthesias (including carpal tunnel syndrome), muscle weakness, and arthralgias. Insulin resistance causes diabetes mellitus in one-sixth of pts. Discrete pituitary adenomas are usually present. Basal or random GH levels cannot be used for screening for the diagnosis. The standard diagnostic test is measurement of GH 60–120 min after 100 g oral glucose. Serum GH <5 μg/L is considered normal (GH <2 μg/L is a more rigorous criterion), while acromegalics pts usually have GH >10 μg/L. Basal or random IGF-I levels correlate with disease activity. MRI or CT scan with contrast can define tumor size. Transsphenoidal surgery results in apparent cure rates between 35 and 75%. Pituitary radiation is also used. Bromocriptine may be useful as an adjunct to other modalities in dosages of 20–60 mg/d. Octreotide, a long-acting somatostatin analogue, in doses of 50–250 μg q6–8h SC, lowers GH levels to normal in two-thirds of acromegalic pts and is particularly useful as an adjunct to surgery and/or radiation.

GH deficiency in children leads to short stature and in adults causes minimal changes (fine wrinkling of facial skin and increased sensitivity to insulin in pts with diabetes mellitus). Diagnosis is made by measuring IGF-I levels or by documenting an inadequate rise after insulin-induced hypoglycemia (Table 160-1). GH replacement therapy is effective in children, but the role of GH replacement in adults is not established. Screening laboratory investigations for evaluation of short stature are described in Table 160-4.

GONADOTROPINS   FSH regulates spermatogenesis and growth of the ovarian follicular granulosa cell, and LH controls testosterone production in Leydig cells and ovarian steroidogenesis. The secretion of both hormones is regulated by pulsatile LHRH secretion by the hypothalamus. In postmenopausal women and in men with primary hypogonadism, FSH and LH levels are elevated in the face of low levels of gonadal steroids. *Gonadotropin excess* can arise in several ways. Gonadotropin [usually human chorionic gonadotropin (hCG)] may be secreted ectopically by nonseminoma germ cell tumors, lung carcinomas, hepatomas, and other tumors. FSH-secreting pituitary adenomas are large tumors that are usually recognized in men with decreased libido, decreased serum testosterone, and normal PRL levels. Thyrotropin-releasing hormone (TRH) challenge in such pts may cause enhanced FSH release. No syndrome of FSH hypersecretion is recognized in women. LH-secreting pituitary adenomas are characterized by increased testosterone, elevated LH, normal or low FSH, and (frequently) partial hypopituitarism. Testicular response to hCG is preserved with gonadotropin-secreting adenomas and may help differentiate these tumors from primary hypogonadism.

Congenital isolated *gonadotropin deficiency* is termed *Kall-*

Table 160-4

Screening Laboratory Investigations in Short Stature

Test or X-Ray	Disorder
↓Serum thyroxine	Hypothyroidism
↓IGF-I	GH deficiency
Bone age	Constitutional delay, hypothyroidism, GH deficiency
Lateral skull film	Craniopharyngioma or other CNS lesion
↓Serum calcium	Pseudohypoparathyroidism
↓Serum phosphate	Vitamin D–resistant rickets
↓Serum bicarbonate	Renal tubular acidosis
↑Blood urea nitrogen	Renal failure
↓Complete blood count	Anemia, nutritional disorder
↑Sedimentation rate	Inflammatory disease of bowel
Chromosomal karyotype	Gonadal dysgenesis or other abnormality

SOURCE: Adapted from Hintz RL: HPIM-14, p. 2001.

mann's syndrome and is often associated with anosmia and midline anatomic defects. Acquired isolated gonadotropin deficiency can occur with hemochromatosis and after head trauma; functional gonadotropin deficiency can occur with stress, severe illness, anorexia nervosa, and rigorous physical training.

THYROTROPIN (TSH) *TSH excess* can cause several disorders. Pituitary (TSH-induced) hyperthyroidism can be caused by TSH-secreting adenomas (the characteristic overproduction of TSH alpha subunit causes a ratio of >1:1 serum alpha:intact TSH level). Octreotide may decrease production of TSH and TSH alpha. Pituitary resistance to thyroid hormone can result in hyperthyroidism secondary to TSH overproduction. Primary failure of the thyroid gland causes compensatory hypertrophy of thyrotrophs, increased TSH levels, modest elevations in PRL, and on occasion pituitary thyrotropinonas.

TSH deficiency usually occurs in association with deficiency of other pituitary hormones but may be isolated. Secondary hypothyroidism is associated with low levels of TSH and serum thyroxine. See Chap. 162 for a discussion of thyroid diseases.

CORTICOTROPIN (ACTH) Corticotropin-releasing hormone is the major regulator of ACTH release, and ACTH in turn controls the release of cortisol from the adrenal cortex. ACTH is highest at 4 A.M. and lowest in late evening. *ACTH excess* of pituitary origin (Cushing's disease) is caused by a microadenoma in 90% of cases. Clinical manifestations of cortisol excess are described in Chap. 163. Once the presence of cortisol excess is established, a high-dose overnight dexamethasone (8 mg at midnight) or a 2-day dexamethasone suppression test (2 mg q6h for 8 doses) results in suppression of urine 17-hydroxycorticosteroids and free cortisol and of plasma cortisol, usually by >50%, in cases of ACTH-secreting adenomas. In some instances the inferior petrosal sinuses must be catheterized to localize the site of ACTH overproduction. Transsphenoidal surgery is successful in about 75% of pts. Ectopic ACTH production by lung cancer or bronchial carcinoids can also cause Cushing's syndrome (see Chap. 163).

ACTH deficiency may be isolated or occur in association with other pituitary hormone deficiencies. Temporary ACTH deficiency is common after prolonged glucocorticoid administration. Patients with ACTH deficiency are not hyperkalemic because aldosterone production is usually normal. For evaluation of ACTH deficiency see Table 160-1.

For a more detailed discussion, see Biller BMK, Daniels GH: Neuroendocrine Regulation and Diseases of the Anterior Pituitary and Hypothalamus, Chap. 328, p. 1972; and Hintz RL: Disorders of Growth, Chap. 329, p. 1999, in HPIM-14.

DISORDERS OF THE POSTERIOR PITUITARY

DIABETES INSIPIDUS (DI)

Arginine vasopressin (AVP; antidiuretic hormone, ADH) functions to concentrate urine and conserve water. In *central DI*, insufficient AVP is released in response to physiologic stimuli. Causes include (1) neoplastic or infiltrative lesions of hypothalamus such as pituitary tumors that extend upward, metastatic tumors, leukemia, germinomas, pinealomas, histiocytosis X, and sarcoidosis; (2) pituitary or hypothalamic surgery; (3) severe head injury, usually associated with skull fracture; (4) ruptured cerebral aneurysms; and (5) idiopathic.

MANIFESTATIONS AND LABORATORY FEATURES The onset of polyuria, excessive thirst, and polydipsia can be sudden, and urine volume may be 16–24 L/d. Urine osmolality (<290 mosmol/kg; specific gravity <1.010) is less than that of serum. Increase in serum osmolality stimulates thirst, and dehydration is unusual while pts have free access to water. When water intake is inadequate (postoperatively, head trauma, or other CNS dysfunction), rising serum sodium level and osmolality can cause weakness, fever, mental disturbances, prostration, and death.

DIFFERENTIAL DIAGNOSIS Central DI must be differentiated from other forms of polyuria (Table 161-1). Comparison of urinary osmolality after dehydration with that after AVP administration (Table 161-2) usually defines the cause of polyuria. Urinary osmolality normally rises by $<9\%$ after injection of vasopressin. In central DI, the increase in urinary osmolality after vasopressin is $>9\%$. In *nephrogenic DI* or *potassium depletion*, little change occurs in urine osmolality with dehydration, and there is no further rise with vasopressin. In *primary polydipsia* plasma and urine osmolality are both low, and there is no response to AVP after water deprivation.

℞ TREATMENT
In the absence of brain tumor or systemic disease, treatment is usually successful. For acute therapy of unconscious pts after head trauma or neurosurgery, aqueous vasopressin should be given subcutaneously in doses of 5–10 U q3–6h. For long-term therapy see Table 161-3. Chlorpropamide may be useful in pts with partial AVP deficiency.

Table 161-1

Major Polyuric Syndromes

I. Primary disorders of water intake or output
   A. Excessive water intake
      1. Psychogenic polydipsia
      2. Hypothalamic disease: histiocytosis X, sarcoidosis
      3. Drug-induced polydipsia
         a. Thioridazine
         b. Chlorpromazine
         c. Anticholinergic drugs (dry mouth)
   B. Inadequate tubular reabsorption of filtered water
      1. Vasopressin deficiency
         a. Central diabetes insipidus
         b. Drug-induced inhibition of AVP release (e.g., narcotic antagonists)
      2. Renal tubular unresponsiveness to AVP
         a. Nephrogenic diabetes insipidus (congenital and familial)
         b. Nephrogenic diabetes insipidus (acquired)
            (1) Several chronic renal diseases, after obstructive uropathy, unilateral renal arterial stenosis, after renal transplantation, after acute tubular necrosis
            (2) Potassium deficiencies, including primary aldosteronism
            (3) Chronic hypercalcemias, including hyperparathyroidism
            (4) Drug-induced: lithium, methoxyflurane anesthesia, demeclocycline
            (5) Various systemic disorders: multiple myeloma, amyloidosis, sickle cell anemia, Sjögren's syndrome
II. Primary disorders of renal reabsorption of solutes (osmotic diuresis)
   A. Glucose: diabetes mellitus
   B. Salts, especially sodium chloride
      1. Various chronic renal diseases, especially chronic pyelonephritis
      2. After various diuretics.

SOURCE: Moses AM, Streeten DHP: HPIM-14, p. 2007.

Table 161-2

Dehydration Test

1. Withhold fluids until urinary osmolality becomes stable [an increase of <30 (mmol/kg)/h for at least 3 h] and plasma osmolality exceeds 288 mmol/kg; body weight usually decreases by 1 kg.
2. Administration of 5 U aqueous vasopressin or 1 μg desmopressin by SC injection or 10 μg desmopressin intranasally.
3. Measure urine and plasma osmolality before and 1 h after the injection.

SYNDROME OF INAPPROPRIATE VASOPRESSIN SECRETION (SIADH)

The hyponatremia of SIADH is due to inability to dilute urine; ingested fluids are retained, and extracellular fluid volume is expanded without edema. It may occur by three mechanisms: (1) AVP is synthesized and autonomously released from tumors (usually oat cell carcinoma of lung); (2) nontumorous tissue acquires capacity to synthesize and release AVP autonomously or to stimulate AVP release by pituitary (as in pulmonary tuberculosis, pneumonias, and other pulmonary diseases); (3) pituitary AVP is released inappropriately due to CNS disorders (inflammation, neoplasm, vascular lesions) or to drugs such as morphine (see Table 161-4).

MANIFESTATIONS AND LABORATORY FEATURES Symptoms of weight gain, weakness, lethargy, and mental confusion can ultimately progress to convulsions and coma. Laboratory findings include low BUN, creatinine, uric acid, and albumin; serum Na < 130 mmol/L and plasma osmolality < 270 mmol/L; urine almost always hypertonic to plasma, and urinary Na usually > 20 mmol/L. SIADH should be suspected in hyponatremic pts with urine that is hypertonic to plasma.

DIFFERENTIAL DIAGNOSIS   (1) Depletional hyponatremias, especially due to adrenal insufficiency, salt-losing nephritis, diarrhea, or diuretic therapy; (2) hyponatremic edematous states (CHF, cirrhosis, nephrosis); (3) pseudohyponatremia from hyperlipidemia or severe hyperglycemia; (4) hypothyroidism; and (5) primary polydipsia in which the urine is invariably dilute. Assessment of response to water loading may be useful in establishing diagnosis.

Table 161-3

Agents Used in Treatment of Diabetes Insipidus

	Dose Form	Usual Dose	Duration of Action, h
CENTRAL DIABETES INSIPIDUS			
Hormone replacement:			
Desmo-pressin	2.5-mL intranasal preparation, 100 µg/mL; 1- or 10-mL ampul, for injection, 4 µg/mL	10–20 µg intranasally or 1–4 µg subcutaneously	12–24
Lypressin	5-mL nasal spray, 50 units/mL	2–4 units intranasally	4–6
Arginine vasopressin	10 or 20 units/ampul	5–10 units subcutaneously	3–6
Other agents:			
Chlorprop-amide	100- and 250-mg tablets	200–500 mg daily	
Clofibrate	500-mg capsules	500 mg four times daily	
Carbama-zepine	200-mg tablets	400–600 mg daily	
NEPHROGENIC DIABETES INSIPIDUS			
Hydrochlo-rothiazide	50-mg tablets	50–100 mg daily	
Chlorthal-idone	50-mg tablets	50 mg daily	

SOURCE: Moses AM, Streeten DHP: HPIM-14, p. 2008.

Table 161-4

Causes of Inappropriate Vasopressin Secretion (SIADH)

Malignant neoplasms with autonomous AVP release
    Small cell carcinoma of lung
    Carcinoma of pancreas
    Lymphoma, lymphocytic lymphoma, Hodgkin's disease
    Carcinoma of duodenum
    Thymoma
Nonmalignant pulmonary diseases
    Tuberculosis
    Lung abscess
    Pneumonia
    Viral pneumonitis
    Empyema
    Chronic obstructive pulmonary disease
CNS disorders
    Skull fracture
    Subdural hematoma
    Subarachnoid hemorrhage
    Cerebral vascular thrombosis
    Cerebral atrophy
    Acute encephalitis
    Tuberculous meningitis
    Purulent meningitis
    Guillain-Barré syndrome
    Lupus erythematosus
    Acute intermittent porphyria
Drugs
    Chlorpropamide
    Vincristine
    Vinblastine
    Cyclophosphamide
    Carbamazepine
    Oxytocin
    General anesthesia
    Narcotics
    Tricyclic antidepressants
Miscellaneous causes
    Hypothyroidism
    Positive pressure respiration

SOURCE: Moses AM, Streeten DHP: HPIM-14, p. 2009.

℞ TREATMENT

In mild SIADH, fluid intake should be restricted to 0.8–1 L/d. In severe SIADH, 200–300 mL 5% sodium chloride solution should be given IV over several hours to raise the serum Na to a level at which symptoms will improve. Demeclocycline interferes with renal action of AVP and may be useful when fluid restriction is impractical, but it has delayed onset of action.

For a more detailed discussion, see Moses AM, Streeten DHP: Disorders of the Neurohypophysis, Chap. 330, p. 2003, in HPIM-14.

162

DISEASES OF THE THYROID

The thyroid secretes thyroxine (T_4) and triiodothyronine (T_3), which influence basal metabolic rate and cardiac and neurologic function. Diseases of the thyroid can cause alterations in hormone secretion, enlargement of the gland, or both.

The hypothalamus releases thyrotropin-releasing hormone (TRH), which stimulates release of thyroid-stimulating hormone (TSH) from the anterior pituitary. TSH is secreted into the circulation and binds to receptors on the thyroid gland, where it controls production and release of T_4 and T_3, which in turn inhibit further TSH release from the pituitary (see Chap. 160).

Some T_3 is secreted by the thyroid, but most is produced by deiodination of T_4 in peripheral tissues. Both T_4 and T_3 are bound to carrier proteins [principally thyroid-binding globulin, (TBG), albumin, and thyroid-binding prealbumin (TBPA)] in the circulation (Table 162-1).

HYPOTHYROIDISM

Deficient thyroid hormone secretion can be due to thyroid failure (primary hypothyroidism) or pituitary or hypothalamic disease (secondary hypothyroidism). Symptoms of lethargy, constipa-

Table 162-1

Altered TBG Concentration

Increased	Decreased
Pregnancy	Androgens
Newborn state	Large doses of
Oral contraceptives and other	glucocorticoids
estrogens	Chronic liver disease
Tamoxifen	Severe systemic
Infections and chronic active	illness
hepatitis	Active acromegaly
Biliary cirrhosis	Nephrosis
Acute intermittent porphyria	Inherited trait
Perphenazine	
Inherited trait	

SOURCE: Wartofsky L: HPIM-14, p. 2014.

tion, cold intolerance, stiffness and cramping of muscles, carpal tunnel syndrome, and menorrhagia may be insidious in onset. Intellectual and motor activity slows, appetite declines, weight increases, hair and skin become dry, and the voice deepens. Obstructive sleep apnea may occur. Cardiomegaly is usually due to pericardial effusion. Relaxation phase of deep tendon reflexes is prolonged. The ultimate picture is a dull, expressionless face, sparse hair, periorbital puffiness, large tongue, and pale, doughy, cool skin that may progress into a hypothermic, stuporous state (myxedema coma). Factors that predispose to myxedema coma include cold exposure, trauma, infection, and administration of narcotics. Respiratory depression may cause rise in arterial P_{CO_2}.

Diagnosis Decreased serum T_4 is common to all varieties of hypothyroidism. Serum TSH is increased in primary and normal or decreased in secondary hypothyroidism. Serum cholesterol, creatinine phosphokinase, and lactic dehydrogenase may be elevated, and bradycardia, low-amplitude QRS complexes, and flattened or inverted T waves may be present on ECG.

℞ TREATMENT

Levothyroxine is the preferred treatment. In adults, the initial daily dose of 25 μg/d is increased by 25–50 μg/d at 2- to 3-week intervals until serum TSH is within normal range (an average dose of 112 μg/d). When secondary hypothyroidism is suspected, thyroxine should not be administered until adrenal insufficiency has been evaluated and, if present, treated (see Chap. 146). Myxedema coma is a life-threatening emergency requiring administration of levothyroxine 200–300 μg IV over 5 min along with dexamethasone 2 mg PO/IV q6h. Levothyroxine 100 μg/d can then be given IV/PO until the pt stabilizes.

THYROTOXICOSIS

Manifestations include nervousness, palpitations, emotional lability, sleepiness, tremors, frequent bowel movements, excessive sweating, heat intolerance, oligomenorrhea, amenorrhea, and weight loss despite a well-maintained or increased appetite. Pts are anxious, restless, and fidgety. Skin is warm, moist, and velvety; palms are erythematous; and fingernails may separate from the nail bed (Plummer's nails). Hair is fine and silky, and a fine tremor may involve fingers and tongue. Eye signs include a stare with widened palpebral fissures, infrequent blinking, and lid lag. Cardiovascular findings include a wide pulse pressure,

Table 162-2

Varieties of Thyrotoxicosis

DISORDERS ASSOCIATED WITH THYROID HYPERFUNCTION*

Excess production of TSH (rare)
Abnormal thyroid stimulator
    Graves' disease
    Trophoblastic tumor (hCG)
Intrinsic thyroid autonomy
    Hyperfunctioning adenoma
    Toxic multinodular goiter

DISORDERS NOT ASSOCIATED WITH THYROID HYPERFUNCTION†

Disorders of hormone storage
    Subacute thyroiditis
    Chronic thyroiditis with transient thyrotoxicosis
Extrathyroid source of hormone
    Thyrotoxicosis factitia
    Ectopic thyroid tissue
        Struma ovarii
        Functioning follicular carcinoma

*Associated with increased RAIU unless body iodine burden is excessive.
†Associated with decreased RAIU.
SOURCE: Wartofsky L: HPIM-14, p. 2023.

especially atrial fibrillation, systolic murmurs, and cardiac enlargement.

Several disorders can produce thyrotoxicosis (see Table 162-2).

GRAVES' DISEASE is due to the presence of a circulating thyroid-stimulating immunoglobulin and is manifested by a diffuse goiter and infiltrative ophthalmopathy (with variable ophthalmoplegia, proptosis, and periorbital swelling) and dermopathy (pretibial myxedema).

Diagnosis This is made on the basis of the clinical findings and the presence of elevated levels of serum T_4 and T_3 and suppressed or undetectable levels of TSH. Although not usually required for diagnosis, radioactive iodine uptake (RAIU) is high.

℞ TREATMENT

Treatment is directed at limiting the amount of hormone the gland can produce. Antithyroid drugs interpose a chemical blockage to hormone synthesis (propylthiouracil 200 mg q8h or methimazole 10–20 mg q12h). Leukopenia is the principal side effect. Propranolol can alleviate adrenergic symptoms (40–120 mg/d in divided doses). Ablation of thyroid function can be effected by surgery or radioiodine. Radioiodine is a simple, effective, and economic therapy; as many as 40–70% of pts eventually become hypothyroid after radioiodine. Pts should be followed every 6 weeks after therapy until the residual thyroid function is known to be normal. Radioactive iodine is contraindicated in pregnancy.

Circulating thyroid hormone levels must be reduced rapidly in severe thyrotoxicosis (thyroid storm). Propylthiouracil (PTU) 1 g, followed by 300 mg q6h, is given along with dexamethasone 2 mg PO/IV q6h. Potassium iodide (SSKI) 4–5 drops q6h for 2 days is initiated 2 h after the first dose of PTU. Tachycardia can be titrated with propranolol 10–20 mg IV/PO q6h. Special care in the use of beta blockers is required in the setting of CHF.

During pregnancy it is important to control symptoms with the lowest effective dose of PTU (often <300 mg/d). When control is not achieved during the middle trimester, subtotal thyroidectomy may be required.

Treatment of ophthalmopathy is frequently unsatisfactory. Corneal drying can be prevented during sleep by taping lids closed and using artificial tears. Progressive exophthalmos with chemosis, ophthalmoplegia, or vision loss is treated with large doses of prednisone (120–140 mg/d); orbital radiation or surgical decompression may be useful.

TOXIC NODULAR GOITER (PLUMMER'S DISEASE)
This ordinarily occurs in pts with preexisting goiter, usually in the elderly, and is not associated with circulating thyroid stimulators or with ophthalmopathy. The thyrotoxicosis is less severe than in Graves' disease, but impact on the cardiovascular system may be severe. The diagnosis is as described above, and radioactive iodine is the treatment of choice.

THYROTOXICOSIS ASSOCIATED WITH SUBACUTE THYROIDITIS This is due to leakage of preformed thyroid hormone from the inflamed gland. Thyroid function eventually returns to normal. Mild cases may be treated with aspirin; prednisone (20–40 mg/d) is reserved for severe cases. Propranolol may control symptom.

THYROBLASTIC TUMORS These occasionally secrete so much hCG (a weak TSH agonist) that the thyroid becomes hyperactive. Rarely, the source of excess thyroid hormone is from outside the thyroid, e.g., thyroid hormone ingestion or metastatic thyroid carcinoma (see Table 162-2).

SICK EUTHYROID SYNDROME

Severe illness, physical trauma, or physiologic stress can alter peripheral binding and metabolism of thyroid hormones and regulation of TSH secretion. The most consistent feature is low serum T_3, whereas total serum T_4 may be decreased, normal, or rarely increased. The findings are due to a combination of impaired conversion of T_4 to T_3 and impaired serum binding of hormones. The importance of this syndrome is that it has to be distinguished from mild hypothyroidism or mild hyperthyroidism. Measurements of total serum T_4 or T_3 in conjunction with assessment of hormone binding are generally the most reliable means of making this distinction. Primary alterations in TBG produce changes in T_3 uptake that are inverse to those in serum T_4 and T_3, and as a result, free levels of the hormone remain normal. By contrast, hyper- and hypothyroidism cause changes in free hormone levels in the same directions as those in total serum thyroxine. When estimates of free hormone are low (e.g., in severely ill pts), euthyroid state can be confirmed by measuring TSH.

THYROIDITIS

SUBACUTE THYROIDITIS Usually follows an URI and can be due to any of several viruses. Stretching of the thyroid capsule causes pain over the thyroid or referred pain to lower jaw, ear, or occiput. Onset may be acute with severe pain accompanied by fever and nodularity of the thyroid. ESR may be elevated, and RAIU may be low. Early, mild thyrotoxicosis is present owing to leakage of T_4 from gland. After glandular hormone is depleted, a hypothyroid phase may ensue. Thyroid function eventually returns to normal.

℞ **TREATMENT**

In mild cases, aspirin controls symptoms. In more severe cases, prednisone is generally effective. Propranolol can be used to control thyrotoxic manifestations. When RAIU returns to normal, therapy can be withdrawn without recurrence of symptoms.

HASHIMOTO'S THYROIDITIS (CHRONIC LYMPHO-CYTIC THYROIDITIS) This chronic thyroid inflammation is autoimmune in origin and may coexist with other autoimmune diseases, including pernicious anemia, Sjögren's syndrome, chronic hepatitis, SLE, rheumatoid arthritis, adrenal insufficiency, and diabetes mellitus. Goiter may be asymmetric, and thyroid failure usually supervenes. Initially, serum TSH concentration rises, serum T_4 then declines, and frank hypothyroidism ensues. High titers of thyroid antimicrosomal antibody are almost always present. Such antibodies may cause simultaneous thyroiditis and hyperthyroidism (so-called Hashitoxicosis). Treatment with replacement doses of levothyroxine is indicated and may cause regression of goiter.

THYROID NEOPLASMS

THYROID ADENOMAS These are classified into three types: papillary, follicular, and Hurthle cell. Follicular adenomas are the most common and most likely to function autonomously or cause hyperthyroidism. Surgery or ^{131}I is curative. Hyperfunctioning nodules are rarely malignant.

THYROID CARCINOMAS Carcinomas of follicular epithelium can be anaplastic, follicular, or papillary. Anaplastic carcinoma is rare, highly malignant, and rapidly fatal. Follicular carcinoma may undergo hematogenous spread and is more common in older age groups. Papillary carcinoma has a bimodal frequency with a peak during the second and third decades and again later in life. Medullary carcinomas of the thyroid arise from parafollicular (C) cells and may occur in association with multiple endocrine neoplasia type 2A.

Diagnosis The workup of the solitary thyroid nodule is shown in Fig. 162-1. Features suggesting carcinoma include recent or rapid growth of a nodule or mass, history of neck irradiation, and fixation to surrounding tissues. Serum thyro-

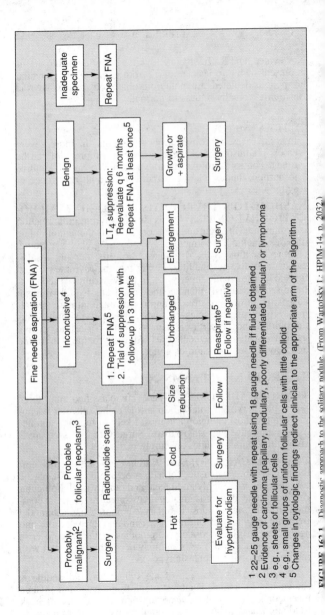

FIGURE 162-1 Diagnostic approach to the solitary nodule. (From Wartofsky L: HPIM-14, p. 2032.)

1 22–25 gauge needle with repeat using 18 gauge needle if fluid is obtained
2 Evidence of carcinoma (papillary, medullary, poorly differentiated, follicular) or lymphoma
3 e.g., sheets of follicular cells
4 e.g., small groups of uniform follicular cells with little colloid
5 Changes in cytologic findings redirect clinician to the appropriate arm of the algorithm

globulin is a tumor marker but is most useful in following the response to therapy in that elevated levels in pts on suppressive therapy signal recurrent or metastatic disease, and a rising level should prompt reevaluation. Calcitonin is a tumor marker for medullary thyroid cancer.

℞ TREATMENT

Near-total thyroidectomy is recommended, with regional lymph node exploration. Levothyroxine therapy is instituted, and approximately 3 weeks after surgery, liothyronine (50–75 μg/d) is substituted since it permits a more rapid increase in TSH secretion when withdrawn 3 weeks later. When the TSH is ≥50 mU/L, a large scanning dose is given of ^{131}I [1850 MBq (50 mCi)], which is often ablative. Suppression therapy with levothyroxine is reinstituted 24–48 h later, and a follow-up whole-body scan is done 1 week later. Ablation may be repeated if more functioning tissue is found. Pts are maintained on levothyroxine therapy and have biannual whole-body scans for the first 3 years and then at 5 years posttherapy. Six weeks before the scan, levothyroxine is changed to liothyronine, which is discontinued 3 weeks later. Once the scan and any additional therapy is complete, levothyroxine is reinstituted 24–48 h later.

NONTOXIC GOITER

Enlargement of thyroid gland (normally 15–25 g) may be generalized or focal and may be associated with normal, increased, or decreased hormone secretion. Most commonly, an etiology cannot be found. In the case of a nontoxic (euthyroid) goiter, clinical manifestations arise solely from the enlargement of the gland. Mechanical sequelae include compression and displacement of trachea or esophagus and obstructive symptoms.

℞ TREATMENT

Treatment is generally aimed at reduction in goiter size or prevention of further growth by suppression of TSH and is achieved by replacing iodine deficiency, removing known goitrogens, or giving graduated doses of levothyroxine to a maximum of 150–200 μg/d. Surgical resection or radioiodine ablation is rarely indicated.

For a more detailed discussion, see Wartofsky L: Diseases of the Thyroid, Chap. 331, p. 2012, in HPIM-14.

163

DISEASES OF THE ADRENAL CORTEX

HYPERFUNCTION OF ADRENAL GLAND

CUSHING'S SYNDROME   This is due to production of excess cortisol (and other hormones) by the adrenal cortex. Some common manifestations (central obesity, hypertension, osteoporosis, muscle weakness, emotional lability, and diabetes mellitus) are nonspecific and may or may not be helpful in diagnosis. More useful findings include easy bruising, typical skin striae, myopathy, fat deposition in the face and interscapular areas (moon facies and buffalo hump), and virilization.

The most common cause of glucocorticoid excess is iatrogenic administration. Excess production of cortisol by the adrenal is usually due to bilateral adrenal hyperplasia secondary to hypersecretion of pituitary ACTH (Cushing's disease) or production of ACTH by nonendocrine tumors (small cell carcinoma of lung, medullary carcinoma of thyroid, or tumors of thymus, pancreas, or ovary). Approximately 25% is due to adenoma or carcinoma of the adrenal.

Levels of plasma cortisol and of urine free cortisol and 17-hydroxycorticosteroid are elevated. Hypokalemia, hypochloremia, and metabolic alkalosis are prominent, particularly with ectopic production of ACTH.

Diagnosis   The Dx of endogenous Cushing's disease requires demonstration of increased cortisol production and of failure to suppress cortisol secretion normally by dexamethasone (see Table 160-2). For initial screening, the overnight dexamethasone test or measurement of 24-h urinary free cortisol is appropriate. Definitive diagnosis is established by demonstrating failure to suppress urinary cortisol to <30 µg/d or plasma cortisol to <5 mg/dL after 0.5 mg dexamethasone q6h for 48 h. Once diagnosis is established, further testing is required to determine etiology (Table 163-1). Low levels of plasma ACTH suggest an adrenal adenoma or carcinoma; high plasma ACTH and adrenal suppression by high-dose dexamethasone suggest an ACTH-producing microadenoma of the pituitary. ACTH-secreting macroadenomas of the pituitary and ectopic sources of ACTH do not suppress with high-dose dexamethasone, and these sources must be differentiated by imaging techniques.

℞ TREATMENT

Therapy of adrenal adenoma or carcinoma requires surgical exploration and excision; stress doses of glucocorticoids must be given pre- and postoperatively. Metastatic and unresectable adrenal carcinomas are treated with mitotane in doses gradually increased to 8–10 g/d in three or four divided doses. Transsphenoidal surgery can be curative for pituitary hypersecretion of ACTH (see Chap. 160). On occasion, debulking of lung carcinoma or resection of carcinoid tumors can cause remission of ectopic Cushing's disease. If the source of ACTH or corticotropin-releasing hormone cannot be resected, bilateral total adrenalectomy or medical management with fluconazole or mitotane may relieve manifestations.

ALDOSTERONISM Aldosteronism is caused by hypersecretion of the adrenal mineralocorticoid aldosterone. *Primary aldosteronism* refers to an adrenal cause and can be due either to an adrenal adenoma or to bilateral adrenal hyperplasia, and the term *secondary aldosteronism* is used when an extraadrenal stimulus is present (Table 163-1). Most pts with primary hyperaldosteronism have headaches and mild diastolic hypertension. Hypokalemia may be severe and is due to loss in the urine; hypernatremia can be due both to Na retention and polyuria secondary to impairment of concentration of urine. Metabolic alkalosis and elevated serum HCO_3 are due to H^+ movement intracellularly and H^+ loss in urine. The ECG may show signs of potassium depletion (U waves, arrhythmias, premature contractions).

Diagnosis The Dx requires (1) diastolic hypertension with unexplained hypokalemia, (2) hyposecretion of renin (as judged

Table 163-1

Causes of Secondary Hyperaldosteronism

Normotensive states
  Pregnancy
  Diuretic therapy
Hypertensive states
  Primary reninism (renin secreting tumors)
  Secondary reninism
    Renal artery stenosis (atherosclerotic, fibromuscular type)
    Arteriolar nephrosclerosis (malignant hypertension)
    Accelerated hypertension
  Diuretic therapy
Bartter's syndrome
Edematous states
  Cirrhosis
  Nephrotic syndrome

by low plasma renin activity levels) that fails to increase appropriately during volume depletion (upright posture, sodium depletion), and (3) hypersecretion of aldosterone that fails to suppress appropriately during volume expansion (salt loading). Abdominal CT/MRI or percutaneous transfemoral bilateral adrenal vein catheterization with simultaneous adrenal venography can localize the adenoma. Secondary hyperaldosteronism (see Table 163-1) is associated with elevated plasma renin activity. Rarely, hypertensive patients with hypokalemic alkalosis have deoxycorticosterone (DOC)-secreting adenomas. Such pts have low renin levels and normal or reduced aldosterone levels.

℞ TREATMENT

Surgery can be curative in pts with adrenal adenoma but is not appropriate for adrenal hyperplasia, which is managed with sodium restriction and spironolactone (25–100 mg/d). Secondary aldosteronism is treated with salt restriction and correction of the underlying cause.

ADRENAL ANDROGEN EXCESS   The syndromes of adrenal androgen excess result from overproduction of dehydroepiandrosterone (DHEA) and androstenedione. Manifestations in women include hirsutism, oligomenorrhea, acne, and virilization. These syndromes can result from hyperplasia, adenoma, or carcinoma. Congenital adrenal hyperplasia is caused by various enzymatic defects in the steroid hormone pathway inherited as an autosomal recessive trait. Deficiency of C-21 hydroxylase (CYP21) is the most common, resulting in virilization of female infants and cortisol deficiency, with or without an associated salt-losing tendency. Other enzyme defects result in a range of phenotypes.

Diagnosis   The diagnosis should be considered in any infant with "failure to thrive," esp. if there is salt-wasting or abnormal genitalia. Late-onset adrenal hyperplasia (partial CYP21 deficiency) is characterized by elevated urinary 17-ketosteroids and plasma DHEA sulfate. Diagnosis can be confirmed by high basal levels of 17-hydroxyprogesterone or elevation of 17-hydroxyprogesterone after ACTH stimulation (1–4 h infusion).

Hirsutism in women is most often idiopathic. The differential diagnosis is found in Table 163-2, and evaluation is described in Table 163-3.

℞ TREATMENT

Therapy of congenital adrenal hyperplasia consists of appropriate doses of glucocorticoids and fludrocortisone. Therapy

Table 163-2

Causes of Hirsutism in Women

Familial
Idiopathic
Ovarian
    Polycystic ovaries; hilus-cell hyperplasia
    Tumor arrhenoblastoma, hilus cell, adrenal rest
Adrenal
    Congenital adrenal hyperplasia
    Noncongenital adrenal hyperplasia (Cushing's)
    Tumor: virilizing carcinoma or adenoma

SOURCE: Williams GH, Dluhy RG: HPIM-14, p. 2050.

of late onset adrenal hyperplasia consists of daily glucocorticoids (dexamethasone 0.25–0.5 mg at night) to suppress ACTH secretion. For adenoma and carcinoma see above.

HYPOFUNCTION OF THE ADRENAL GLAND

ADDISON'S DISEASE   Occurs when >90% of adrenal tissue is destroyed surgically or by tuberculosis, histoplasmosis, coccidioidomycosis, cryptococcosis, or autoimmune mechanisms. Bilateral tumor metastases, amyloidosis, and sarcoidosis are rare causes. Manifestations include fatigue, weakness, anorexia, nausea and vomiting, cutaneous and mucosal pigmentation, hypotension, and occasionally, hypoglycemia. Routine laboratory parameters may be normal, or serum Na, Cl, and HCO_3 can be reduced, while serum K is increased. Extracellular fluid depletion accentuates hypotension.

Diagnosis   Dx requires assessment of adrenal capacity for steroid production. A rapid screening test is to administer 25 U ACTH (cosyntropin) intravenously and measure plasma cortisol levels at baseline, then 30 and 60 min later; an increase of <7 μg/dL above baseline suggests adrenal insufficiency. To differentiate primary from secondary adrenal insufficiency, cosyntropin is infused at a rate of 2 U/h for 24 h. In normal subjects, 17-hydroxysteroid excretion is increased by 25 mg/d, and plasma cortisol levels to >40 μg/dL. In secondary disease, the maximal increase in urinary 17-hydroxysteroid is 3–20 mg/d, and the plasma cortisol ranges from 10–40 μg/dL. Pts with primary disease have even less response.

Table 163-3

Laboratory Evaluation of Hirsutism-Virilizing Syndromes

	Ovarian		Adrenal			Idiopathic
	Polycystic Ovary Syndrome	Ovarian Tumor	Congenital Adrenal Hyperplasia	Adrenal Neoplasm	Cushing's Syndrome	
Urinary 17-ketosteroids, plasma DHEA sulfate	N↑	N	N↑	↑↑↑	N↑	N
Plasma testosterone	N↑	↑↑	N↑	N↑	N↑	N
LH/FSH ratio	N↑	N	N↑	N	N	N
Precursors of cortisol biosynthesis						
Basal	N	N	N↑	N↑	N	N
Following ACTH infusion	N	N	↑↑	N↑	N	N
Cortisol following overnight dexamethasone suppression test	N	N	N	↑	↑	N

NOTE: N, normal; ↑, elevated.

SOURCE: Williams GH, Dluhy RG: HPIM-14, p. 2051.

Ⓡ TREATMENT

In periods of stress the dosage of hydrocortisone should be 100–200 mg/d, and the dose should be tapered for long-term replacement to 15–37.5 mg/d. Fludrocortisone (0.1 mg/d) also may be necessary. In emergencies, a bolus of 100 mg IV hydrocortisone is followed by a continuous infusion of 10 mg/h.

HYPOALDOSTERONISM Isolated aldosterone deficiency accompanied by normal cortisol production occurs with hyporeninism, as an inherited biosynthetic defect, postoperatively following removal of aldosterone-secreting adenomas, during protracted heparin or heparinoid administration, in pretectal disease of the nervous system, and in severe postural hypotension. Most pts present with unexplained hyperkalemia, often exacerbated by salt restriction.

Hyporeninemic hypoaldosteronism is seen most commonly in adults with mild renal failure and diabetes mellitus in association with disproportionate hyperkalemia and metabolic acidosis. Oral fludrocortisone (0.1–0.2 mg daily) restores electrolyte balance if salt intake is adequate. Some pts may require higher doses to correct hyperkalemia.

INCIDENTAL ADRENAL MASSES

Adrenal masses are common findings on abdominal CT or MRI scans. The first step in evaluation is to determine the functional status by measurement of 24-h urinary catecholamines and aldosterone levels and serum postassium and performance of an overnight dexamethasone suppression test. More than 90% of such "incidentalomas" are nonfunctional, and the incidence of adrenal carcinomas is less than 0.01%, the frequency of benign adrenal adenomas. Surgery is appropriate for nonfunctional masses >3 cm in diameter and for all functional masses. When surgery is not performed, scans should be repeated every 3–6 months. For workup of pheochromocytoma, see Chap. 115.

CLINICAL USE OF GLUCOCORTICOIDS

Glucocorticoids are pharmacologic agents for a variety of disorders. Replacement therapy is indicated for pts with Addison's disease (hydrocortisone 15–37.5 mg/d). Steroids are also used in rheumatologic diseases (rheumatoid arthritis, SLE, vasculitis, temporal arteritis), hematologic diseases (hemolytic anemia, leukemia), neurologic (cerebral edema) and pulmonary disorders (sarcoidosis, COPD), and endocrine states (hypercalcemia). As little as 10 mg/d of prednisone for 3 weeks can suppress

Table 163-4

Glucocorticoid Preparations

	Relative Potency		
Generic Name	Glucocorticoid	Mineral-ocorticoid	Dose equivalent
Short-acting			
Hydrocortisone	1.0	1.0	20.0
Cortisone	0.8	0.8	25.0
Intermediate-acting			
Prednisone	4.0	0.8	5.0
Methylprednis-olone	5.0	0.5	4.0
Triamcinolone	5.0	0	4.0
Long-acting			
Dexamethasone	25.0	0	0.75
Betamethasone	25.0	0	0.6

the adrenal axis for up to 1 year. Stress can precipitate adrenal crisis in such pts even months after discontinuation, and these individuals should carry this information in case of emergency. "Stress doses" of glucocorticoids are the equivalent of 80–160 mg/d of hydrocortisone. Long-term glucocorticoid therapy in pharmacologic doses can result in weight gain, hypertension, cushingoid facies, diabetes mellitus, osteoporosis, myopathy, increased intraocular pressure, ischemic bone necrosis, infection, hypercholesterolemia, type IV hyperlipoproteinuria, and other effects. See Table 163-4 for dosage equivalents of glucocorticoids in common use.

For a more detailed discussion, see Williams GH, Dluhy RG: Diseases of the Adrenal Cortex, Chap. 332, p. 2035, in HPIM-14.

164

DIABETES MELLITUS

Manifestations of diabetes mellitus, the most common endocrine disorder, include polyuria, polydipsia, weakness, and weight loss, but some pts present with ketoacidosis or hyperosmolar, nonketotic coma (see Chap. 34) or, rarely, with the long-term complications such as nephropathy or retinopathy. Pts with immune-mediated pancreatic β-cell destruction are typically insulin-dependent (IDDM) and develop ketoacidosis without insulin therapy. Most pts are resistant to the action of insulin and do not secrete enough insulin to prevent hyperglycemia, so called non-insulin-dependent diabetes (NIDDM) and can be treated with diet, oral hypoglycemic agents, or insulin. Secondary forms of diabetes occur with chronic pancreatitis, pheochromocytoma, acromegaly, Cushing's syndrome, and exogenous glucocorticoid administration. Hyperglycemia usually causes polyuria, polydipsia, polyphagia, and weight loss, but the first symptom may be ketoacidosis or hyperosmolar nonketotic coma.

DIAGNOSIS This traditionally requires a fasting plasma glucose of ≥7.8 mmol/L (≥140 mg/dL) on two occasions, although the American Diabetes Association has recommended lowering the diagnostic level to 7 mmol/L (126 mg/dL) on two occasions. Alternatively, following ingestion of 75 g of glucose, the finding of a venous plasma glucose ≥11.1 mmol/L (≥200 mg/dL) after 2 h and on at least one other occasion during the 2-h test is suggestive of the diagnosis.

 TREATMENT

Once diagnosis is established, a diet should be instituted that includes an appropriate number of calories based on ideal body weight, adequate protein, and a carbohydrate intake of about 40–60% of total energy (Chap. 47). Appropriate distribution of food intake is also important. When hyperglycemia in NIDDM cannot be controlled by diet, oral hypoglycemic agents may be administered (see Table 164-1). The usual practice is to prescribe sulfonylureas, increasing the dose to the maximal level as required, and then to add metformin as a second drug when indicated. Troglitazone, which enhances insulin action, is used by some physicians as an additional drug in NIDDM pts who do not have adequate response to insulin or maximal doses of oral agents (although it is not approved by the FDA for the latter purpose).

Insulin is always required for IDDM and for many with

Table 164-1

Oral Hypoglycemic Agents

Agent	Daily Dose, mg	Doses/d	Duration of Action, h
Sulfonylureas			
Acetohexamide	250–1500	1–2	12–18
Chlorpropamide	100–500	1–2	60
Tolazamide	100–1000	1–2	12–14
Tolbutamide	500–3000	2–3	6–12
Glimeripiride	4	1	Up to 24
Glyburide	1.25–20	1–2	Up to 24
Glipizide	2.5–40	1–2	Up to 24
Glibornuride	12.5–100	1–2	Up to 24
Biguanide			
Metformin	1500–2500	1–2	Up to 24
Thiazolidinedione			
Troglitazone	400–600	1	Up to 24

SOURCE: Adapted from Foster DW: HPIM-14, p. 2070.

NIDDM (see Table 164-2). Conventional therapy involves the administration of an intermediate-acting insulin (NPH or lente) once or twice a day with or without small amounts of regular insulin. The standard starting dose is 0.5–1.0 (U/kg)/d before breakfast or a mixture of two-thirds intermediate-acting insulin and one-third of short-acting insulin; an addi-

Table 164-2

Insulin Preparations Available

	Onset of Action, h	Peak Effect, h	Duration of Action, h
Rapid-acting			
Humalog	0.25	1–2	3–4
Regular	0.25–1	2–6	4–12
Semilente	0.25–1	3–6	8–16
Intermediate-acting			
NPH	1.5–4	6–16	12–24
Lente	1–4	6–16	12–28
Long-acting			
Ultralente	3–8	14–24	24–48
Protamine zinc	3–8	14–24	24–48

Table 164-3

Adjusting Insulin Dosage in Conventional Insulin

| Blood Glucose | | Regular Insulin, Units | |
| | | Breakfast | Supper |
mmol/L	mg/dL	(To Be Mixed with Intermediate Dosage)	
2.8–5.5	51–100	8	4
5.6–8.3	101–150	10	5
8.4–11.1	151–200	12	6
11.2–13.9	201 250	14	7
14.0–16.6	251–300	16	8
>16.6	>300	20	10

* Once the pt has most blood sugars in the reasonable range, a prescription can be written for varying the regular insulin dosage as illustrated. The prescription in this case was for a pt in reasonable control on 25 units of NPH plus 10 units of regular before breakfast and 10 units of NPH plus 5 units of regular before supper. Change in metabolic status may require adjustments in both intermediate insulin and the sliding scale of regular insulin.

SOURCE: Foster DW: HPIM-14, p. 2067.

tional injection given before supper contains one-third of the morning dose. The goal for blood glucose control is a glycated hemoglobin level within the normal range. If this goal cannot be achieved, the incidence of long-term complications of diabetes is increased. If pts not controlled on two daily injections are candidates for the rigors of more intensive therapy, they should be referred to a specialty team for a trial of such therapy. Intensive therapy reduces the long-term complications but is associated with more frequent and more severe hypoglycemic episodes. An example of such a regimen is shown in Table 164-3. The treatment of diabetic ketoacidosis and hyperosmolar, nonketotic coma is described in Chap. 34.

LONG-TERM COMPLICATIONS These result in serious morbidity and mortality. Macrovascular complications (atherosclerosis) may cause intermittent claudication, gangrene, coronary artery disease, and stroke. Microvascular complications affect the heart, eyes, kidneys, and nervous system. *Cardiomyopathy* can cause heart failure, despite normal coronary arteries by angiography. *Diabetic retinopathy* can be divided into simple (background) and proliferative forms, a leading cause of blindness. New vessel formation and scarring can cause vitreous hemorrhage, retinal detachment, and blindness. *Renal disease* (*Kimmelstiel-Wilson's disease*) is the most common condition requiring dialysis and renal transplantation in the U.S. The kidneys are initially enlarged. Microalbuminuria then appears with excretion of albumin in the range of 20–200 mg/d. Once macroalbuminuria begins (>200 mg/d), GFR declines about 1 mL/min per month. Azotemia ordinarily begins about 10–12 years after onset of diabetes and may be preceded by nephrotic syndrome. No specific treatment is available, but the rate of progression may be slowed with ACE inhibitors, aggressive control of hypertension, and low-protein diets. Hyporeninemic hypoaldosteronism, associated with renal tubular acidosis, may require alkalinizing solutions (Shohl's) and avoidance of external potassium loads. *Peripheral sensory neuropathy* causes numbness, paresthesias, severe hypesthesias, and pain that may be deep-seated and severe and often worse at night. Absent stretch reflexes and diminished vibratory sensation are early signs. A special problem is foot ulcers, which can almost invariably be prevented with proper foot care. *Autonomic neuropathy* can cause GI manifestations (esophageal dysfunction, delayed gastric emptying, constipation, diarrhea, or malabsorption), orthostatic hypotension, bladder dysfunction including urinary incontinence, myopathy, and (in men) erectile impotence.

For a more detailed discussion, see Foster DW: Diabetes Mellitus, Chap. 334, p. 2060, in HPIM-14.

165

DISORDERS OF THE TESTES AND PROSTATE

THE TESTES

The testes produce sperm and steroid hormones that regulate male sexual function. Inadequate production of sperm can occur as an isolated defect, whereas inadequate formation of testosterone by the Leydig (interstitial) cells usually impairs spermatogenesis secondarily. Classification of abnormalities of testicular function in adults is found in Table 165-1.

ANDROGEN STATUS   This is assessed by documenting the timing and extent of sexual maturation at puberty, rate of beard growth, testicular size, current libido, sexual function, and general strength and energy. If Leydig cell dysfunction occurs prior to onset of puberty, failure of sexual maturation (eunuchoidism) is evidenced by an infantile amount and distribution of body hair, poor development of skeletal muscles, and failure of the epiphyses to close so that the arm span is >5 cm greater than height and the lower body segment is >5 cm longer than the upper body segment (pubis to crown).

At the completion of puberty, plasma testosterone levels reach the adult level of 10–35 nmol/L (3–10 ng/mL) throughout the day, and plasma luteinizing hormone (LH) and follicle-stimulating hormone (FSH) levels are <15 IU/L each. Testicular failure after puberty can be due to either hypothalamic-pituitary defects (*secondary hypogonadism*) or testicular failure (*primary hypogonadism*). Leydig cell failure that occurs after puberty may present as gynecomastia or diminished virilization or libido, and diagnosis requires a high index of suspicion.

Secondary Hypogonadism   This is diagnosed when pooled plasma levels of both testosterone and gonadotropins are low. The most frequent cause is *hypogonadotropic hypogonadism* (*Kallman's syndrome*), which is frequently familial and is characterized by low levels of LH and FSH and, in some, anosmia, midline defects, mental retardation, and cryptorchidism. The disorder is due to impairment of the synthesis and/or release of LH-releasing hormone (LHRH) and consequent impairment of pulsatile release of LH. Untreated pts usually remain indefinitely in the prepubertal state. Administration of gradually increasing doses of testosterone promotes sexual development, but fertility requires gonadotropin therapy. Destruction of the pituitary gland by tumors, infection, trauma, or metastatic disease ordinarily causes hypogonadism as a component of panhypopituitarism. Cushing's syndrome, congenital adrenal hyper-

Table 165-1

Presentation of Adult Abnormalities of Testicular Function

Infertility with Underandrogenization	Infertility with Normal Virilization
HYPOTHALAMIC-PITUITARY ABNORMALITIES	
Panhypopituitarism	
Hypogonadotropic hypogonadism	Isolated FSH deficiency
Cushing's syndrome	Congenital adrenal hyperplasia
Hyperprolactinemia	Hyperprolactinemia
Hemochromatosis	Androgen use
TESTICULAR ABNORMALITIES	
Developmental and structural defects	
Klinefelter's syndrome*	Germinal cell aplasia
XX male	Cryptorchidism
	Varicocele
	Immotile cilia syndrome
Acquired defects	
Viral orchitis*	*Mycoplasma* infection
Trauma	
Radiation	Radiation
Drugs (spironolactone, alcohol, ketoconazole, cyclophosphamide)	Drugs (cyclophosphamide) Environmental toxins
Autoimmunity	Autoimmunity
Granulomatous disease	
Associated with systemic diseases	
Liver disease	Febrile illness
Renal failure	Celiac disease
Sickle cell disease	
Neurologic diseases (myotonic dystrophy and paraplegia)	Neurologic disease (paraplegia)
Androgen resistance	Androgen resistance
ABNORMALITIES OF SPERM TRANSPORT	
	Obstruction of the epididymis or vas deferens (cystic fibrosis, DES exposure, congenital absence)

* The common testicular causes of underandrogenization and infertility in adults—Klinefelter's syndrome and viral orchitis—are associated with small testes.
SOURCE: Griffin JE, Wilson JD: HPIM-14, p. 2092.

plasia, hemochromatosis, and hyperprolactinemia (due to pituitary adenomas or drugs such as phenothiazines) may have suppressed levels of LH and testosterone.

Primary Hypogonadism This is diagnosed when testosterone levels are low and gonadotropin levels are high. *Klinefelter's syndrome* is the most common cause and is due to the presence of one or more extra X chromosomes, usually a 47,XXY karyotype. The testes are small and contain sclerosed tubules; azoospermia is usual. Gynecomastia is common, and variable features include a eunuchoid habitus, mental retardation, and diabetes mellitus. Acquired primary testicular failure usually results from viral orchitis, frequently mumps, but may be due to trauma, radiation damage, or systemic diseases such as amyloidosis, Hodgkin's disease, sickle cell disease, or granulomatous diseases such as leprosy. Testicular failure can occur as part of a generalized disorder of autoimmunity in which multiple primary endocrine deficiencies coexist (polyglandular autoimmune failure). Testicular failure can occur with malnutrition, renal failure, liver disease, and toxins such as lead, alcohol, marijuana, heroin, methadone, and antineoplastic and chemotherapeutic agents. Spironolactone and ketoconazole block the synthesis of testosterone, and spironolactone and cimetidine act as antiandrogens by competing for binding to the androgen receptor.

℞ TREATMENT

Treatment of hypogonadal men with androgens restores normal male secondary sexual characteristics (beard, body hair, external genitalia), male sexual drive, and masculine somatic development (hemoglobin, muscle mass). Parenteral administration of a long-acting testosterone ester (100–200 mg testosterone enanthate at 1- to 3-week intervals) or daily application of transdermal testosterone patches causes a return of testosterone levels to normal.

MALE INFERTILITY This is found in one third of infertile couples (couples who fail to conceive after 1 year of unprotected intercourse). Evaluation of the infertile male should assess androgen status, document the size and consistency of the testes, and determine if a varicocele is present; varicocele may be of etiologic importance in one-third of all male infertility. When the seminiferous tubules are damaged prior to puberty, testes are small (usually <12 mL) and firm, whereas postpubertal damage causes the testes to be soft (the capsule, once enlarged, does not contract to its previous size). Normal ejaculate volume should be >2 mL, with 20–100 million sperm per milliliter,

>60% of which should be mobile. Plasma FSH level may correlate inversely with spermatogenesis.

In addition to secondary impairment of spermatogenesis by androgen deficiency, isolated spermatogenic tubule dysfunction and impaired spermatogenesis can arise from alterations of temperature of testes (*varicocele*), *cryptorchism*, *cystic fibrosis*, or *immotile cilia syndrome*. *Kartagener's syndrome* is a form of the latter disorder with situs inversus.

Defects in the androgen receptor cause resistance to the action of androgen usually associated with defective male phenotypic development, infertility, and underandrogenization. *Disorders of sperm transport* are the cause of infertility in as many as 6% of infertile men with normal virilization. *Ejaculatory obstruction* can be congenital (idiopathic, cystic fibrosis, in utero DES exposure) or acquired (tuberculosis, leprosy, gonorrhea).

IMPOTENCE   This is the failure to achieve erection, ejaculation, or both. Men with sexual dysfunction may complain of loss of libido, inability to initiate or maintain an erection, ejaculatory failure, premature ejaculation, or inability to achieve orgasm. Sexual dysfunction can be psychogenic but usually has an organic component, either secondary to systemic disease, urogenital disorders, or endocrinopathy. Some organic causes of erectile impotence in men can be found in Table 165-2. Evaluation includes a detailed general as well as genital physical exam. Penile abnormalities (Peyronie's disease), testicular size, and gynecomastia should be noted. Peripheral pulses should be palpated, and bruits should be sought. Neurologic exam should assess anal sphincter tone, perineal sensation, and bulbocavernosus reflex. Penile arteriography, electromyography, or pulsed Doppler analyses with high-resolution ultrasound are occasionally performed. Pooled serum testosterone, LH, and prolactin should be measured.

℞ **TREATMENT**

Treatment consists of correction (if possible) of the underlying cause; injection of vasoactive substances such as alprostadil into the corpora cavernosa or urethra or vacuum tumescence devices may be successful, and an orally active phosphodiesterase inhibitor sildenafil is under trial. The insertion of penile prostheses is rarely indicated.

TESTICULAR CANCER   (See Chap. 61)

PROSTATE DISEASE

PROSTATIC HYPERPLASIA   This is an almost universal phenomenon in aging men and is the most common cause of

Table 165-2

Some Organic Causes of Erectile Impotence in Men

I. Endocrine causes
  A. Testicular failure (primary or secondary)
  B. Hyperprolactinemia
II. Drugs
  A. Antiandrogens
    1. Spironolactone
    2. Ketoconazole
    3. H_2 blockers (e.g., cimetidine)
    4. Finasteride
  B. Antihypertensives
    1. Central-acting sympatholytics (e.g., clonidine and methyldopa)
    2. Peripheral acting sympatholytics (e.g., guanadrel)
    3. Beta blockers
    4. Thiazides
  C. Anticholinergics
  D. Antidepressants
    1. Monoamine oxidase inhibitors
    2. Tricyclic antidepressants
  E. Antipsychotics
  F. Central nervous system depressants
    1. Sedatives (e.g., barbiturates)
    2. Antianxiety drugs (e.g., diazepam)
  G. Drugs of habituation or addiction
    1. Alcohol
    2. Methadone
    3. Heroin
    4. Tobacco
III. Penile diseases
  A. Peyronie's disease
  B. Previous priapism
  C. Penile trauma
IV. Neurologic diseases
  A. Anterior temporal lobe lesions
  B. Diseases of the spinal cord
  C. Loss of sensory input
    1. Tabes dorsalis
    2. Disease of dorsal root ganglia
  D. Disease of nervi erigentes
    1. Radical prostatectomy and cystectomy
    2. Rectosigmoid operations
  E. Diabetic autonomic neuropathy and various polyneuropathies

(continued)

Table 165-2 (*Continued*)

Some Organic Causes of Erectile Impotence in Men

V. Vascular disease
   A. Aortic occlusion (Leriche syndrome)
   B. Atherosclerotic occlusion or stenosis of the puden-
      dal and/or cavernosal arteries
   C. Venous leak
   D. Disease of the sinusoidal spaces
   E. Arterial damage from pelvic radiation

SOURCE: McConnell JD, Wilson JD: HPIM-14, p. 287.

outflow obstruction. Symptoms can be minimal if the detrusor muscles of the bladder hypertrophy and compensate for resistance to urine flow. With increasing obstruction, diminution in caliber and force of urinary stream, hesitancy in initiating voiding, postvoiding dribbling, sensation of incomplete emptying, and, on occasion, urinary retention supervene. These obstructive symptoms must be distinguished from irritative symptoms such as dysuria, frequency, and urgency that can result from inflammatory, infectious, or neoplastic causes. As residual urine increases, nocturia, infection, and overflow incontinence may develop.

Prostate size is evaluated during digital rectal examination. Hyperplasia produces a smooth, firm, elastic enlargement, but obstructive symptoms may not correlate with size. Obstruction to outflow is assessed by measurement of urine flow rate and/or residual urine. Urethrocystoscopy may be useful before invasive treatment or to evaluate hematuria.

℞ **TREATMENT**
Watchful waiting may be appropriate when symptoms are minimal because the natural history is neither well understood or predictable. With significant manifestations, treatment should be individualized for severity of symptoms and risks of therapy and may be medical (e.g., 5α-reductase inhibition with finasteride or alpha-adrenergic antagonists such as terazosin) or surgical (usually transurethral prostatectomy).

PROSTATIC CARCINOMA   This is the most common malignancy in men and can be asymptomatic, but most men have extensive disease at diagnosis. Common presenting complaints include dysuria, difficulty in voiding, increased urinary frequency, complete urinary retention, back or hip pain, and hema-

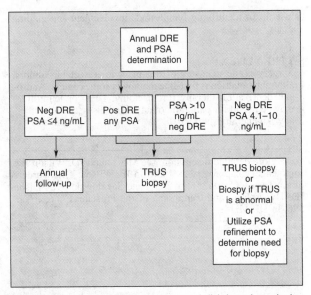

FIGURE 165-1 Schematic for use of the annual digital rectal examination (DRE) and measurement of prostate specific antigen (PSA) as guides for deciding which men should have transrectal prostate biopsy under sonography. There are at least three schools of thought about what to do if the DRE is negative and the PSA is equivocal (4.1–10 ng/dL). (Sagalowsky AI, Wilson JD: HPIM-14, p. 599.)

turia. Serious complications include spinal cord compression, intradural metastasis, venous thromboses, and myelophthisis.

Importance of the rectal exam cannot be overemphasized because the posterior surfaces of the lateral lobes, where carcinoma usually begins, are palpable. Carcinoma is characteristically hard, nodular, and irregular.

Usefulness of prostate specific antigen (PSA) as a screening test is not established due to its insensitivity (35% false negative) and lack of specificity (elevations can occur with hyperplasia, inflammation, or infarction of the prostate). Most urologists feel that prostate biopsy is indicated when a palpable abnormality is detected, when the PSA is >10 ng/dL, or when lower urinary tract symptoms occur in men who have no known cause of obstruction. Biopsy is usually performed transrectally with guidance by ultrasound (TRUS) (see Fig. 165-1). Serum acid phosphatase level is elevated in some localized disease but more commonly with extensive or metastatic disease. Surgical staging is useful for identifying lymph node involvement and guiding therapy.

℞ TREATMENT

Surgery is the mainstay of treatment for resectable tumors, although radiation is first-line therapy in some centers. Androgen deprivation therapy (orchiectomy, DES, or leuprolide) may be useful for palliation of advanced disease. Chemotherapy is generally ineffective.

For a more detailed discussion, see McConnell JD, Wilson JD: Impotence, Chap. 51, p. 286; Griffin JE, Wilson JD: Disorders of the Testes, Chap. 336, p. 2087; and Sagalowsky AI, Wilson JD: Hyperplasia and Carcinoma of the Prostate, Chap. 97, p. 596, in HPIM-14.

166

DISORDERS OF THE OVARY AND FEMALE GENITAL TRACT

MENSTRUAL DISORDERS

ABNORMAL UTERINE BLEEDING During the reproductive years the cycle averages 28 ± 3 days, and the mean duration of flow is 4 ± 2 days. When abnormal uterine bleeding is suspected, other sources such as rectum, bladder, cervix, and vagina must be excluded. In premenarche period, abnormal uterine bleeding may result from trauma, infection, or precocious puberty. Vaginal bleeding following menopause is frequently due to malignancy.

In the absence of pregnancy, abnormal uterine bleeding in women of reproductive age is associated with either ovulatory or anovulatory cycles. Menstrual bleeding with ovulatory cycles is spontaneous, regular in onset, predictable in duration and amount of flow, and often painful. Such abnormal but regular cycles are usually due to anatomic abnormalities of the outflow tract, usually leiomyomas, adenomyosis, endometrial polyps, or uterine synechiae or scarring. Bleeding between cyclic ovulatory menses can be due to cervical or endometrial lesions.

Anovulatory menstrual bleeding (dysfunctional uterine bleeding) is painless, irregular in occurrence, and unpredictable as to amount and duration. Transient disruption of hypothalamic-pituitary-ovarian cycle is a common cause of failure of ovulation in menarchial years. Persistent dysfunctional uterine bleeding in reproductive years is usually due to continuous estrogen effects on the uterus uninterrupted by cyclic progesterone withdrawal, most commonly due to polycystic ovarian disease.

AMENORRHEA   All women of childbearing age with amenorrhea should be assumed to be pregnant until proven otherwise. Even when history and physical exam are not suggestive, pregnancy must be excluded by a suitable screening test.

Primary amenorrhea is defined as failure of menarche by age 16, regardless of the presence or absence of secondary sexual characteristics, whereas *secondary amenorrhea* is failure of menstruation for 6 months in a woman with previous periodic menses. However, the causes of primary and secondary amenorrhea overlap, and it is generally more useful to classify the disorder according to etiology (Fig. 166-1). Initial workup involves careful physical exam, serum prolactin assay, and evaluation of estrogen status.

Anatomic defects of the outflow tract that prevent vaginal bleeding include *absence of vagina, imperforate hymen, transverse vaginal septae,* and *cervical stenosis* and are usually diagnosed by physical exam. When findings are indeterminate, the next diagnostic procedure is to administer medroxyprogesterone acetate 10–20 mg/d PO for 5 d or 100 mg progesterone in oil IM. If estrogen levels are adequate (and outflow tract is intact), menstrual bleeding should occur within 1 week of ending progestogen treatment, and the diagnosis is *chronic anovulation with estrogen present,* usually *polycystic ovarian disease.* If no withdrawal bleeding occurs and the serum prolactin level is normal in the woman with *chronic anovulation with estrogen absent,* plasma gonadotropins should be measured. If gonadotropin levels are increased, the diagnosis is ovarian failure (*gonadal dysgenesis, resistant ovary syndrome,* or *premature ovarian failure*). Chromosomal karyotype should be obtained when gonadal dysgenesis is suspected.

If gonadotropins are normal or decreased, the diagnosis is either hypothalamic-pituitary disease or an anatomic defect of

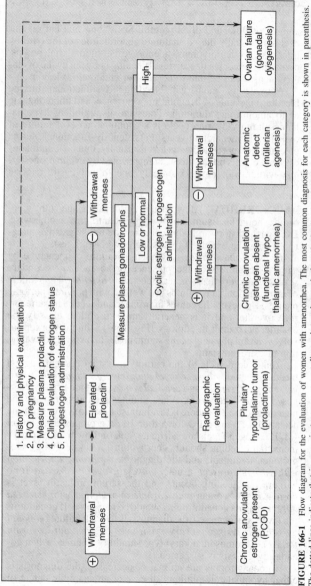

FIGURE 166-1 Flow diagram for the evaluation of women with amenorrhea. The most common diagnosis for each category is shown in parenthesis. The dotted lines indicate that in some instances a correct diagnosis can be reached on the basis of history and physical exam alone. (Reproduced from

outflow tract (see above). When the diagnosis is not clear-cut, it is useful to administer cyclic estrogen plus progestogen (1.25 mg oral conjugated estrogens qd for 3 weeks with 10 mg medroxyprogesterone acetate added for the last 5–7 days of treatment) followed by 10 days of observation. If no bleeding occurs, the diagnosis of *Asherman's syndrome* or other anatomic defects of outflow tract should be confirmed by hysteroscopy or hysterosalpingogram. If withdrawal bleeding occurs following estrogen-progesterone combination, the diagnosis is chronic anovulation with estrogen absent (*hypothalamic amenorrhea*); causes include hypogonadotropic hypogonadism, extreme emotional stress, anorexia nervosa, chronic debilitating disease, pituitary adenomas, craniopharyngiomas, and panhypopituitarism. Radiologic evaluation of pituitary-hypothalamic region may be indicated.

PELVIC PAIN   Pelvic pain may be associated with normal or abnormal menstrual cycles. Severe or incapacitating cramping with ovulatory menses in the absence of demonstrable disorders of the pelvis is termed *primary dysmenorrhea* and is best treated with NSAIDs or oral contraceptive agents. Pelvic pain due to organic causes may be classified as uterine (leiomyomas, adenomyosis, cervical stenosis, infections, cancer), adnexal (salpingo-oophoritis, cysts, neoplasms, torsion, endometriosis), vulvar or vaginal (*Monilia, Trichomonas, Gardnerella,* herpes, condyloma acuminatum, cysts or abscesses of Bartholin's glands), and pregnancy-associated (threatened or incomplete abortion, ectopic pregnancy). Evaluation includes history, pelvic exam, human chorionic gonadotropin measurement, pelvic ultrasound, and laparoscopy or laparotomy in some cases.

Many women experience abdominal discomfort with ovulation (*mittelschmerz*), a dull, aching pain at midcycle that lasts minutes to hours. In addition, ovulatory women may experience somatic symptoms during the few days prior to menses, including edema, breast engorgement, abdominal discomfort, and a symptom of cyclic irritability, depression, and lethargy, a complex known as *premenstrual syndrome.*

MENOPAUSE

During the interval between the reproductive years up to and beyond the last menstrual period, ovarian function is progressively lost, and endocrine, somatic, and psychological changes ensue. Oophorectomy causes more abrupt manifestations. Symptoms are due to vasomotor instability (hot flash), atrophy of urogenital epithelium and skin, decreased size of breasts, and osteoporosis. Nervousness, anxiety, irritability, and depression may occur. Plasma gonadotropins are elevated.

℞ TREATMENT

Estrogen replacement therapy in menopausal women relieves vasomotor instability (hot flashes), prevents atrophy of urogenital epithelium and skin, protects against coronary artery disease, and prevents osteoporosis. The risks of endometrial adenocarcinoma, venous thromboembolism, and hypertension can be minimized by low-dose estrogen administration (0.625 mg/d conjugated estrogen or estraderm skin patches for 25 d/month) with cyclic progestogen (10 mg/d medroxyprogesterone for d 15–25 each month) or continuous low-dose progestogen (2.5 mg/d medroxyprogesterone). Women who have had a hysterectomy do not require progestogen. All women on hormone replacement therapy should have periodic gynecologic examinations.

ORAL CONTRACEPTIVE AGENTS

These are widely used to prevent pregnancy and control dysmenorrhea and anovulatory bleeding. The ideal contraceptive contains the lowest amount of steroid to minimize side effects but sufficient to prevent pregnancy or breakthrough bleeding. Combination oral contraceptive agents contain synthetic estrogen (mestranol or ethinyl estradiol) and synthetic progestogen (norethindrone, norethindrone acetate, norethynodrel, norgestrel, or ethynodiol diacetate). Biphasic or triphasic formulations utilize different agents at different times of the cycle.

Despite overall safety, oral contraceptive users are at risk for deep venous thrombosis, pulmonary embolism, thromboembolic stroke, hypertension, glucose intolerance, and cholelithiasis. Risks are increased with smoking and increasing age, and the drugs should be discontinued in women who experience visual complaints or headaches. Other side effects include minor dyspepsia, breast discomfort, weight gain, pigmentation of the face (chloasma), and psychological effects such as depression and changes in libido. Oral contraceptives are not associated with an increased incidence of cancer of the uterus, cervix, or breast.

Absolute contraindications to the use of oral contraceptives include previous thromboembolic disorders, cerebral vascular or coronary artery disease, known or suspected carcinoma of breasts or other estrogen-dependent neoplasia, undiagnosed genital bleeding, or known or suspected pregnancy. Relative contraindications include hypertension, migraine headaches, diabetes mellitus, uterine leiomyomas, sickle cell anemia, hyperlipidemia, and elective surgery.

For a more detailed discussion, see Carr BR, Bradshaw KD: Disturbances of Menstruation and Other Common Gynecologic Complaints in Women, Chap. 52, p. 289; and Carr BR, Bradshaw KD: Disorders of the Ovary and Female Reproductive Tract, Chap. 337, p. 2097, in HPIM-14.

HYPER- AND HYPOCALCEMIC DISORDERS

HYPERCALCEMIA

Manifestations of hypercalcemia include fatigue, depression, mental confusion, anorexia, nausea, constipation, renal tubule defects, polyuria, and cardiac conduction abnormalities. CNS and GI symptoms can occur at levels of serum calcium >2.9 mmol/L (>11.5 mg/dL), and nephrocalcinosis and impairment of renal function occur when serum calcium is >3.2 mmol/L (>13 mg/dL). The causes of hypercalcemia are listed in Table 167-1. Hyperparathyroidism and malignancy account for 90% of cases.

PARATHYROID-RELATED HYPERCALCEMIA *Primary Hyperparathyroidism* This generalized disorder of bone metabolism is due to increased secretion of parathyroid hormone (PTH) by an adenoma (81%) or carcinoma (4%) in a single gland or by parathyroid gland hyperplasia (15%). Familial hyperparathyroidism may be part of multiple endocrine neoplasia type 1 (MEN 1), which also includes pituitary and pancreatic tumors and hypergastrinemia with peptic ulcer disease (Zollinger-Ellison syndrome), or of MEN 2, in which hyperparathyroidism occurs with pheochromocytoma and medullary carcinoma of the thyroid.

Most pts with hyperparathyroidism are asymptomatic even when the disease involves the kidneys and the skeletal system. Pts frequently have hypercalciuria and polyuria, and Ca can be deposited in the renal parenchyma or form calcium oxalate stones. The characteristic skeletal lesion is osteopenia and occa-

Table 167-1

Classification of Causes of Hypercalcemia

I. Parathyroid-related
   A. Primary hyperparathyroidism
      1. Solitary adenomas
      2. Multiple endocrine neoplasia
   B. Lithium therapy
   C. Familial hypocalciuric hypercalcemia

II. Malignancy-related
   A. Solid tumor with humoral mediation of hypercalcemia (lung, kidney)
   B. Solid tumor with metastases (breast)
   C. Hematologic malignancies (multiple myeloma, lymphoma, leukemia)

III. Vitamin D–related
   A. Vitamin D intoxication
   B. ↑ $1,25(OH)_2D$; sarcoidosis and other granulomatous diseases
   C. Idiopathic hypercalcemia of infancy

IV. Associated with high bone turnover
   A. Hyperthyroidism
   B. Immobilization
   C. Thiazides
   D. Vitamin A intoxication

V. Associated with renal failure
   A. Severe secondary hyperparathyroidism
   B. Aluminum intoxication
   C. Milk-alkali syndrome

SOURCE: Potts JT Jr: HPIM-14, p. 2227.

sionally osteitis fibrosa cystica, in which normal cellular and marrow elements are replaced by fibrous tissue. Resorption of phalangeal tufts, subperiosteal resorption of bone in the digits, and tiny "punched out" lesions in the skull also may be present. Increased bone resorption primarily involves cortical rather than trabecular bone.

Diagnosis is made on clinical grounds and confirmed by demonstration of an inappropriately high PTH level for degree of hypercalcemia. Hypercalcemia may be intermittent or sustained. Serum phosphate is usually low but may be normal. Serum K may be normal or low, and serum Cl is often elevated with a reduced serum bicarbonate (reflecting acidosis and renal phosphate wasting). Hypercalciuria helps to distinguish this disorder from familial hypocalciuric hypercalcemia. ECG may reveal a short QT interval and arrhythmias.

℞ TREATMENT

Treatment of parathyroid adenomas requires the initial management of hypercalcemia if severe and symptomatic. General recommendations that apply to the acute management of hypercalcemia from any cause can be found in Table 167-2. Curative surgical parathyroidectomy should be performed promptly in pts with severe disease. Asymptomatic disease may not require surgery; usual surgical indications include age <50 y, nephrolithiasis, urine Ca >400 mg/d, reduced creatinine clearance, significant reduction in bone mass, or serum Ca >0.25–0.4 mmol/L (1.0–1.6 mg/dL) above the normal range. If neck exploration does not reveal an abnormal gland, ultrasound, CT, radio thallium and technetium studies or intraarterial digital angiography may help localize the abnormal tissue.

Postoperative management requires close monitoring of Ca and phosphorous. Ca supplementation is given for symptomatic hypocalcemia [calcium gluconate or chloride 1 mg/mL in 5% dextrose in water at 0.5–2 (mg/kg)/h or 30–100 mL/h]. Hypomagnesemia should be corrected (deficiency impairs PTH release).

Lithium Lithium causes hypercalcemia in 10% of pts by causing hyperfunction of the parathyroid glands (not adenoma). Elevation of Ca depends on continued administration of lithium, and the drug may be continued if hypercalcemia is asymptomatic. If hypercalcemia and elevated PTH persist with the pt off lithium, parathyroidectomy may be indicated.

Familial hypocalciuric hypercalcemia (FHH) FHH is due to an autosomal dominant mutation of the Ca sensor that results in inappropriate secretion of PTH and enhanced renal Ca resorption (>90% of the filtered load). Most pts are detected on routine screening and are asymptomatic. Hypercalcemia may be detected in affected family members before age 10 (rare in hyperparathyroidism/MEN syndromes). Immunoreactive PTH levels are usually within the normal range. The parathyroid glands are only permissive for the syndrome, and parathyroid resection is not recommended. Medical intervention is also inappropriate.

HYPERCALCEMIA OF MALIGNANCY This common disorder involves 10–15% of lung cancers, is often severe, and can be difficult to manage. Malignancies may cause hypercalcemia by local bone destruction (myeloma, breast carcinoma), by

Table 167-2

Therapies for Severe Hypercalcemia

Treatment	Onset of Action	Duration of Action
MOST USEFUL THERAPIES		
Hydration with saline	Hours	During infusion
Forced diuresis; saline + loop diuretic	Hours	During treatment
Bisphosphonates		
1st generation: etidronate	1–2 days	5–7 days in doses used
2d generation: pamidronate	1–2 days	10–14 days after high dose
Calcitonin	Hours	2–3 days
OTHER THERAPIES		
Gallium nitrate	Day after 5-day administration	7–10 days
Plicamycin	3–4 days	Days
Phosphate		
Oral	24 h	During use
Intravenous	Hours	During use and 24–48 h afterward
Glucocorticoids	Days	Days, weeks
Dialysis	Hours	During use and 24–48 h afterward

Advantages	Disadvantages
Rehydration invariably needed Rapid action	Cardiac decompensation, intensive monitoring electrolyte disturbance hypokalemia, hypomagnesemia
First available bisphosphonate; intermediate onset of action	Hyperphosphatemia; 3-day infusion
High potency; intermediate onset; prolonged duration of action	Fever in 20%; hypophosphatemia hypocalcemia, hypomagnesemia
Rapid onset of action; useful as adjunct in severe hypercalcemia	Often limited calcium lowering, rapid tachyphylaxis
High potency	Length of IV administration; cannot be used with renal failure
Potent antiresorptive	Liver, kidney, and marrow toxicity; bleeding
Low toxicity if P < 4 mg/dL	Limited use except as adjuvant or chronic therapy
Rapid action, highly potent	Ectopic calcification; severe hypocalcemia
Oral therapy, antitumor agent	Active only in certain malignancies; glucocorticoid side effects
Useful in renal failure; onset of effect in hours; can immediately reverse life-threatening hypercalcemia	Complex procedure, reserved for extreme or special circumstances

SOURCE: Potts JT Jr: HPIM-14, p. 2239.

Table 167-3

Differential Diagnosis of Hypercalcemia: Laboratory Criteria

	Blood*			
	Ca	P_i	$1,25(OH)_2D$	iPTH
Primary hyperparathyroidism	↑	↓	↑,↔	↑(↔)
Malignancy-associated hypercalcemia:				
Humoral hypercalcemia	↑↑	↓	↓,↔	↓↔
Local destruction (osteolytic metastases)	↑	↔	↓,↔	↓↔

* Symbols in parentheses refer to values rarely seen in the particular disease.

NOTE: P_i, inorganic phosphate; iPTH, immunoreactive parathyroid hormone.

SOURCE: Potts JT Jr: HPIM-12, p. 1911.

release of parathyroid hormone–related protein (PTHrP) (lung, kidney, squamous cell carcinoma), by activating lymphocytes to release interleukin 1 (IL-1) and tumor necrosis factor (TNF), or by increased synthesis of $1,25(OH)_2$ vitamin D [$1,25(OH)_2D$] (lymphoma) (see Table 167-3).

VITAMIN D–RELATED HYPERCALCEMIA Sarcoidosis and other granulomatous disease (such as tuberculosis and histoplasmosis) cause hypercalcemia by increasing the synthesis of $1,25(OH)_2D$, thus enhancing Ca and phosphorus absorption from the GI tract. Hypercalcemia of this type can be treated by restriction of the intake of Ca and vitamin D, reducing exposure to sunlight, and administration of glucocorticoids. Vitamin D intoxication results from chronic ingestion of large doses of vitamin D (50–100 × normal physiologic requirements, i.e., 50,000–100,000 U/d). Diagnosis can be confirmed by documenting elevated 25(OH)D levels. Treatment is hydration, restriction of vitamin D intake, and in some cases glucocorticoids (100 mg/d hydrocortisone).

HIGH BONE TURNOVER STATES Hyperthyroidism commonly produces a mild elevation of serum Ca with hypercalciuria. Immobilization in adults is rarely associated with hypercalcemia in absence of associated disease. Thiazide diuretics can aggravate hypercalcemia in primary hyperparathyroidism and in high bone turnover states by augmenting PTH responsiveness in target cells of bone and renal tubule. Vitamin A intoxication is a rare cause of hypercalcemia. Therapy is the same as for vitamin D intoxication.

RENAL FAILURE Severe secondary hyperparathyroidism may complicate end-stage renal disease. Patients may have hypocalcemia, hyperphosphatemia, bone pain, ectopic calcification, and pruritus. Concomitant osteomalacia (vitamin D and calcium deficiency), and osteitis fibrosa cystica (excessive PTH action on bone) may be seen. Aluminum intoxication, which can occur with chronic dialysis, results in severe osteomalacia. Potentially fatal hypercalcemia can occur when such pts are treated with vitamin D or calcitriol. Milk-alkali syndrome is characterized by hypercalcemia, alkalosis, and renal failure. Treatment involves dialysis and discontinuing ingestion.

HYPOCALCEMIA

Symptoms include muscle spasms, carpopedal spasm, facial grimacing, laryngeal spasm, seizure, and respiratory arrest. Increased intracranial pressure and papilledema may occur with long-standing hypocalcemia. Other manifestations include irritability, depression, psychosis, intestinal cramps, and chronic malabsorption. Chvostek's and Trousseau's signs are frequently positive, and the QT interval on ECG is prolonged.

Transient hypocalcemia often occurs in critically ill patients with burns, sepsis, and acute renal failure and following transfusion with citrated blood. Hypoalbuminemia can reduce serum Ca below 2.1 mmol/L (8.5 mg/dL), although ionized Ca levels remain normal. Fewer than 10% of hypoalbuminemic, hypocalcemic pts have low levels of ionized Ca, possibly related to alkalosis which increases the binding of Ca to proteins. Medications such as protamine and heparin can suppress Ca levels, and pancreatitis can cause severe hypocalcemia. A classification of hypocalcemia is shown in Table 167-4.

PTH ABSENT *PTH deficiency* may be *hereditary* (isolated PTH deficiency, DiGeorge syndrome), *acquired* (surgery, radiation therapy, hemochromatosis), or part of a polyglandular autoimmune syndrome (adrenal, ovarian, and parathyroid failure; mucocutaneous candidiasis; alopecia; vitiligo; and pernicious anemia). Treatment involves administration of Ca (calcium citrate 950 mg, 2 tablets tid) and vitamin D or calcitriol (0.5 μg/d), adjusted according to serum Ca levels and urinary excretion. Excessive hypercalciuria predisposes to nephrolithiasis, and thiazide diuretics help reduce urinary Ca excretion if a low-sodium diet is followed. Severe hypomagnesemia [<0.4 mmol/L (<1.0 mg/dL)] can cause hypocalcemia due to impaired PTH secretions and reduced peripheral responsiveness. Restoration of to-

Table 167-4

Functional Classification of Hypocalcemia (Excluding Neonatal Conditions)

I. PTH absent
   A. Hereditary hypoparathyroidism
   B. Acquired hypoparathyroidism
   C. Hypomagnesemia
II. PTH ineffective
   A. Chronic renal failure
   B. Active vitamin D lacking
     1. ↓ dietary intake or sunlight
     2. Defective metabolism
       a. Anticonvulsant therapy
       b. Vitamin D–dependent rickets type I
   C. Active vitamin D ineffective
     1. Intestinal malabsorption
     2. Vitamin D–dependent rickets type II
   D. Pseudohypoparathyroidism
III. PTH overwhelmed
   A. Severe, acute hyperphosphatemia
     1. Tumor lysis
     2. Acute renal failure
     3. Rhabdomyolysis
   B. Osteitis fibrosa after parathyroidectomy

SOURCE: Potts JT Jr: HPIM-14, p. 2241.

tal-body magnesium stores leads to rapid reversal of hypocalcemia.

PTH INEFFECTIVE These disorders often involve unavailability of $1,25(OH)_2D$. *Chronic renal failure* results in phosphate retention and impaired $1,25(OH)_2D$ production and action leading to hypocalcemia and secondary hyperparathyroidism. Phosphate binders (aluminum hydroxide), Ca supplements (1–2 g/d), and calcitriol (0.25–1.0 μg/d) are integral to proper management. Vitamin D deficiency occasionally occurs in the elderly. Levels of $25(OH)D$ are low or low normal. Bone biopsy reveals osteomalacia. Treatment is with vitamin D, 1000–2000 U/d, and Ca, 1–1.5 g/d. *Defective vitamin D metabolism* may result from anticonvulsant therapy (phenytoin) and responds to vitamin D, 50,000 U/week, and Ca, 1 g/d. *Vitamin D–dependent rickets type I* is an autosomal recessive disorder due to a defect in conversion of $25(OH)D$ to $1,25(OH)_2D$. Calcitriol in physiologic

Table 167-5

Classification of Pseudohypoparathyroidism (PHP) and Pseudopseudohypoparathyroidism (PPHP)

	PHP-Ia	PHP-Ib	PHP-II	PPHP
Hypocalcemia, hyperphosphatemia	Yes	Yes	Yes	No
Response of urinary cyclic AMP to PTH	↓	↓	Normal	Normal
Serum PTH	↑	↑	↑	Normal
G_s subunit deficiency	Yes	No	No	Yes
Albright's hereditary osteodystrophy	Yes	No	No	Yes
Resistance to hormones in addition to PTH	Yes	No	No	±

SOURCE: Modified from Potts JT Jr.: HPIM-14, p. 2244.

doses is curative. *Vitamin D–dependent rickets type II* is due to defective response to $1,25(OH)_2D$. Plasma levels of $1,25(OH)_2D$ are elevated at least $3 \times$ normal. High doses of vitamin D are required. *Intestinal malabsorption* may result in hypocalcemia, secondary hyperparathyroidism, and severe hypophosphatemia. *Pseudohypoparathyroidism* is due to end-organ unresponsiveness to PTH; a working classification is found in Table 167-5. Treatment is similar to that of hypoparathyroidism except that lower doses of Ca and vitamin D are required.

PTH OVERWHELMED   Occasionally, loss of Ca from extracellular fluid is so severe that PTH cannot compensate (rhabdomyolysis, hypothermia, massive hepatic failure, hematologic malignancies with acute tumor lysis, and acute renal failure). Parathyroidectomy in pts with osteitis fibrosa cystica (now an unusual complication of hyperparathyroidism) can cause hypocalcemia, which is managed with calcitriol and parenteral calcium.

℞ TREATMENT
Symptomatic hypocalcemia of all types may be treated with intravenous calcium chloride or calcium gluconate. Management of chronic hypocalcemia usually requires a vitamin D preparation, commonly calcitriol, and an oral calcium preparation (see Table 167-6).

Table 167-6

Elemental Calcium Content of Various Oral Calcium Preparations

Calcium Preparation	Elemental Calcium Content
Calcium citrate	40 mg/300 mg
Calcium carbonate	400 mg/g
Calcium lactate	80 mg/600 mg
Calcium gluconate	40 mg/500 mg
Calcium carbonate + 5 µg vitamin D_2 (Os-Cal 250)	250 mg/tablet

SOURCE: Potts JT Jr: HPIM-12, p. 1926.

For a more detailed discussion, see Potts JT Jr: Diseases of the Parathyroid Gland and Other Hyper- and Hypocalcemic Disorders, Chap. 354, p. 2227, in HPIM-14.

168

METABOLIC BONE DISEASE

OSTEOPOROSIS

Reduction of bone density to a level that impairs mechanical support can be due to multiple causes. Remodeling of bone (formation and resorption) is continuous, and osteoporosis results either from failure to attain optimal bone mass prior to age 30 or when the rate of bone resorption exceeds the rate of bone formation after peak bone mass is obtained. Vertebrae, wrist, hip, humerus, and tibia are particularly prone to fracture.

In *type I osteoporosis*, disproportionate loss of trabecular bone is associated with fractures of vertebrae and distal forearm in middle-aged, postmenopausal women. Serum parathyroid hormone levels tend to be low or normal. Risk factors include white race, small stature, sedentary life style, and smoking. *Type II osteoporosis* occurs in men and women above age 75 and is associated with fractures of femoral neck, proximal humerus, proximal tibia, and pelvis. Serum parathyroid hormone levels may be high.

Vertebral bodies may collapse anteriorly in lower thoracic and upper lumbar regions after sudden bending, lifting, or jumping movements. Pain is acute and radicular in distribution but usually subsides after days, and pts may be ambulatory in 4–6 weeks. Collapse not associated with pain can cause dorsal kyphosis and exaggerated cervical lordosis (widow's hump).

Blood levels of calcium, phosphorus, and alkaline phosphatase are normal. Mild hypercalciuria may be present. Radiologic studies demonstrate decreased bone mineral density after approximately 30% of bone density is lost; vertebrae become increasingly biconcave, and compression fractures may be visible. More sensitive studies such as single- and dual-photon bone densitometry, quantitative CT, and neutron activation analysis are better for assessing the risk for fracture.

The differential diagnosis is listed in Table 168-1. Other disorders that reduce bone mass include acromegaly, hyperparathyroidism, and malignancies (multiple myeloma, lymphoma, leukemia, carcinomas). Cigarette smoking and glucocorticoids are common factors in loss of bone density.

℞ TREATMENT

Prevention of further loss of bone mass or increase in bone density involves correction of any secondary contributors such as smoking and a variety of more specific therapies. Oral *calcium* (1–1.5 g/d of elemental calcium) is adequate to main-

Table 168-1

Classification of Osteoporosis

Common forms, unassociated with other disease
    Idiopathic osteoporosis (juvenile and adult)
    Type I osteoporosis
    Type II osteoporosis
Disorders in which osteoporosis is a common feature
    Hypogonadism
    Hyperadrenocorticism
    Chronic glucocorticoid administration
    Hyperparathyroidism
    Thyrotoxicosis
    Malabsorption
    Scurvy
    Calcium deficiency
    Immobilization
    Chronic heparin administration
    Systemic mastocytosis
    Adult hypophosphatasia
    Other metabolic bone diseases
Heritable disorders of connective tissue in which osteoporosis is a feature
    Osteogenesis imperfecta
    Homocystinuria due to cystathionine synthase deficiency
    Ehlers-Danlos syndrome
    Marfan's syndrome
Disorders in which the pathogenesis of associated osteoporosis is not understood
    Rheumatoid arthritis
    Malnutrition
    Alcoholism
    Epilepsy
    Primary biliary cirrhosis
    Chronic obstructive pulmonary disease
    Menkes' syndrome

SOURCE: Krane SM, Holick MF: HPIM-14, p. 2249.

tain calcium equilibrium, and regular *exercise* helps to preserve bone mass. *Estrogen* administration to postmenopausal women decreases rate of bone resorption, but bone mass usually does not increase and eventually may decrease. The minimum effective dosage of conjugated estrogen is 0.625 mg/d or the estroderm patch applied twice weekly; progestogen is given with estrogen in a variety of schedules in women with an intact uterus. *Androgen* therapy is equally effective in hypogonadal men with osteoporosis. *Bisphosphonates* that do not inhibit bone mineralization such as alendronate 10 mg/d augment bone density and decrease fractures. *Thiazide diuretics* are useful in high-turnover osteoporosis with hypercalciuria and secondary hyperparathyroidism. *Fluoride* increases new bone formation and reduces fractures in pts at risk but is recommended only for treatment of established vertebral osteoporosis with symptomatic crush fractures because of the increased incidence of hip fracture in some series.

OSTEOMALACIA

Defective mineralization of organic matrix of bone can result from inadequate intake or malabsorption of vitamin D (chronic pancreatic insufficiency, gastrectomy, and steatorrhea of other causes), acquired or inherited disorders of vitamin D metabolism (anticonvulsant therapy or chronic renal failure), chronic acidosis (renal tubular acidosis, acetazolamide ingestion), renal tubular defects that produce hypophosphatemia (Fanconi's syndrome), and chronic administration of aluminum-containing antacids.

CLINICAL MANIFESTATIONS   May be subtle in adults. Skeletal deformities may be overlooked until fractures occur after minimal trauma. Symptoms include diffuse skeletal pain and bony tenderness. Pain in hips may result in an altered gait. Proximal muscle weakness may mimic primary muscle disorders. Decrease in bone density is usually associated with loss of trabeculae and thinning of cortices. Characteristic x-ray finding are radiolucent bands (Looser's zones or pseudofractures) ranging from a few millimeters to several centimeters in length, usually perpendicular to surface of femur, pelvis, scapula, upper fibula, or metatarsals. Changes in serum calcium, phosphorus, 25(OH)D, and 1,25(OH)$_2$D levels vary depending on cause.

℞ TREATMENT

In osteomalacia due to vitamin D deficiency, 2000–4000 IU/d vitamin D$_2$ (cholecalciferol) or D$_3$ (ergocalciferol) is given PO for 6–12 weeks, followed by daily supplements of 200–400 IU. Healing of pseudofractures may be evident within 3–4 weeks. Osteomalacia due to malabsorption requires large doses of vitamin D (up to 100,000 IU/d) and calcium (calcium carbonate 4 g/d). In pts on anticonvulsants, it is usually necessary to continue drugs while administering sufficient vitamin D to bring serum calcium and serum

25(OH)D to the normal range. Dihydrotachysterol (0.2–1.0 mg/d) or calcitriol (0.25 μg/d) is effective in treating hypocalcemia and osteodystrophy of chronic renal failure.

For a more detailed discussion, see Krane SM, Holick MF: Metabolic Bone Disease, Chap. 355, p. 2247, HPIM-14.

169

DISORDERS OF LIPID METABOLISM

LIPID TRANSPORT

EXOGENOUS PATHWAY In the intestinal wall, dietary triglycerides and cholesterol are incorporated into large lipoproteins (chylomicrons), which are transported via lymph to the circulation. Chylomicrons contain apoprotein (apo) CII, which activates lipoprotein lipase in capillaries, thus liberating fatty acids and monoglycerides from the chylomicron. Fatty acids pass through the endothelial cells into adipocytes or muscle. The chylomicron remnants in the circulation are taken up by liver. The net result is to deliver triglycerides to adipose tissue and cholesterol to the liver.

ENDOGENOUS PATHWAY The liver synthesizes triglycerides and secretes them into the circulation together with cholesterol and apo B100 in the form of very low density lipoproteins (VLDL), which carry 5–10 times more triglycerides than cholesterol esters. In the circulation, apos CII and E are added to VLDL. In the capillaries, lipoprotein lipase hydrolyses triglycerides to form VLDL remnants, which either return to the liver for reutilization or are processed to low-density lipoprotein (LDL). LDL is the source of cholesterol for extrahepatic cells, such as adrenal cortex, lymphocytes, muscles, and kidney. LDL binds via the apo B100 component to specific receptors on cell surfaces and then undergoes endocytosis and digestion by lysosomes. The liberated cholesterol is used for membrane synthesis and metabolic requirements. In addition, some oxidized LDL is degraded by a macrophage scavenger system resulting in the formation of cholesterol-laden foam cells. As cell membranes undergo turnover, unesterified cholesterol is released into plasma, where it initially binds to high-density lipoprotein (HDL) and is esterified with fatty acid by lecithin:cholesterol acyltransferase (LCAT). HDL cholesterol esters are transferred to VLDL and eventually to LDL. By this cycle, LDL delivers cholesterol to cells and cholesterol returns from extrahepatic sites via HDL.

HYPERLIPOPROTEINEMIA (See Table 169-1)

Hyperlipoproteinemia in adults is defined as plasma cholesterol >5.2 mmol/L (>200 mg/dL) or triglyceride levels >2.2 mmol/L (>200 mg/dL). An isolated increase in plasma triglycerides indicates that chylomicrons and/or VLDL are increased. An isolated increase of plasma cholesterol indicates elevated LDL. Elevations of both triglycerides and cholesterol are caused by elevations in both VLDL and LDL or in VLDL remnant particles.

FAMILIAL HYPERCHOLESTEROLEMIA This autosomal dominant disorder in the LDL receptor affects 1 in 500 individuals. Heterozygotes with this mutation have a 2- to 3-fold increase in plasma cholesterol and LDL and are prone to accelerated atherosclerosis and premature MI, particularly men. The rare homozygotes have aggressive atherosclerosis that can be manifested in childhood. Xanthomas of tendons and arcus cornea are common. Diagnosis is suggested by finding an isolated increase of plasma cholesterol with normal triglycerides. Every effort should be made to lower plasma cholesterol concentration to normal. *Treatment* is restriction of dietary cholesterol, bile acid–binding resins, and HMG-CoA reductase inhibitors (lovastatin, pravastatin, simvastatin, atorvastatin, or fluvastatin).

FAMILIAL DEFECTIVE APO B This autosomal dominant disorder impairs the synthesis and/or function of the principal binding ligand of the LDL receptor and causes a phenocopy of familial hypercholesterolemia.

POLYGENIC HYPERCHOLESTEROLEMIA Most moderate hypercholesterolemia [<9mmol/L (<350 mg/dL)] arises from an interaction of multiple genetic defects and environmental factors such as diet, age, and exercise. Plasma HDL and triglyceride levels are normal, and xanthomas are not present. *Treatment* includes restriction of dietary cholesterol, HMG-CoA reductase inhibitors, and bile acid–binding resins.

FAMILIAL HYPERTRIGLYCERIDEMIA In this autosomal dominant disorder, increased plasma VLDL causes plasma

Table 169-1

Characteristics of Common Hyperlipidemias

Lipid Phenotype	Plasma Lipid Levels, mmol/L (mg/dL)
ISOLATED HYPERCHOLESTEROLEMIA	
Familial hypercholesterolemia	Heterozygotes: total chol = 7–13 (275–500)
	Homozygotes: total chol > 13 (>500)
Familial defective apo B100	Heterozygotes: total chol = 7–13 (275–500)
Polygenic hypercholesterolemia	Total chol = 6.5–9.0 (250–350)
ISOLATED HYPERTRIGLYCERIDEMIA	
Familial hypertriglyceridemia	TG = 2.8–8.5 (250–750) (plasma may be cloudy)
Familial lipoprotein lipase deficiency	TG > 8.5 (>750) (plasma may be milky)
Familial apo CII deficiency	TG > 8.5 (>750) (plasma may be milky)
HYPERTRIGLYCERIDEMIA AND HYPERCHOLESTEROLEMIA	
Combined hyperlipidemia	TG = 2.8–8.5 (250–750) Total chol = 6.5–13.0 (250–500)
Dysbetalipoproteinemia	TG = 2.8–5.6 (250–500) Total chol = 6.5–13.0 (250–500)

NOTE: Total chol, the sum of free and esterified cholesterol; LDL, low-density lipoprotein; TG, triglycerides; VLDL, very low density lipoproteins; IDL, intermediate-density lipoprotein.

Lipoproteins		
Elevated	Phenotype	Clinical Signs
LDL	IIa	Usually develop xanthomas in adulthood and vascular disease at 30–50 years
LDL	IIa	Usually develop xanthomas and vascular disease in childhood
LDL	IIa	
LDL	IIa	Usually asymptomatic until vascular disease develops; no xanthomas
VLDL	IV	Asymptomatic; may be associated with increased risk of vascular disease
Chylomicrons	I, V	May be asymptomatic; may be associated with pancreatitis, abdominal pain, hepatosplenomegaly
Chylomicrons	I, V	As above
VLDL, LDL	IIb	Usually asymptomatic until vascular disease develops; familial form may also present as isolated high TG or an isolated high LDL cholesterol
VLDL, IDL; LDL normal	III	Usually asymptomatic until vascular disease develops; may have palmar or tuboeruptive xanthomas

SOURCE: From Ginsberg HN, Goldberg IJ: HPIM-14, p. 2142.

triglyceride concentration to range from 2.2–5.6 mmol/L (200–500 mg/dL). Obesity, hyperglycemia, and hyperinsulinemia are characteristic, and diabetes mellitus, ethanol consumption, oral contraceptives, and hypothyroidism may exacerbate the condition. Because atherosclerosis is accelerated, vigorous attempts should be made to control all exacerbating factors, and intake of saturated fat should be minimal. If dietary measures fail, clofibrate or gemfibrozil should be administered.

FAMILIAL LIPOPROTEIN LIPASE DEFICIENCY This rare autosomal recessive disorder results from absence or deficiency in lipoprotein lipase, which in turn retards metabolism of chylomicrons. Accumulation of chylomicrons in plasma causes recurrent bouts of pancreatitis, usually beginning in childhood. Eruptive xanthomas occur on buttocks, trunk, and extremities. Plasma is milky or creamy (lipemic). Symptoms and signs recede when pt is placed on a fat-free diet (<20 g/d). Accelerated atherosclerosis is not a feature.

FAMILIAL APO CII DEFICIENCY This rare autosomal recessive disorder is due to absence of apo CII, an essential cofactor for lipoprotein lipase. As a result, chylomicrons and triglycerides accumulate and cause manifestations similar to those in lipoprotein lipase deficiency. Diagnosis requires demonstration of absence of apo CII by protein electrophoresis. *Treatment* involves the use of fat-free diet.

COMBINED HYPERLIPIDEMIA This inherited disorder can cause different lipoprotein abnormalities in affected individuals, including hypercholesterolemia, hypertriglyceridemia, or both. Atherosclerosis is accelerated. Therapy should be directed at predominant lipid abnormality. All pts should restrict dietary fat and cholesterol and avoid alcohol and oral contraceptives. Elevated triglycerides may respond to clofibrate or gemfibrozil, and a bile acid–binding resin plus HMG-CoA inhibitor may be used when cholesterol is elevated.

DYSBETALIPOPROTEINEMIA This rare disorder is associated with homozygosity for apo E2, but development of disease requires additional environmental and/or genetic factors. Plasma cholesterol and triglycerides are increased due to accumulation of VLDL and chylomicron remnant particles. Severe atherosclerosis involves coronary arteries, internal carotids, and abdominal aorta and causes premature MI, intermittent claudication, and gangrene. Cutaneous xanthomas are distinctive: xanthoma striata palmaris and tuberous or tuberoeruptive xanthomas. Levels of triglyceride and cholesterol are similarly elevated. Diagnosis is established by finding of a broad beta band on lipoprotein electrophoresis. *Treatment* is either clofibrate or gemfibrozil. If present, hypothyroidism and diabetes mellitus must be treated.

SECONDARY HYPERLIPOPROTEINEMIAS Diabetes mellitus, ethanol consumption, oral contraceptives, renal disease, hepatic disease, and hypothyroidism can either cause sec-

Table 169-2

LDL Cholesterol Treatment Guidelines

	Levels of LDL for Beginning Therapy, mmol/L (mg/dL)		
	Diet	Drugs	Goal
No CHD and less than two risk factors	≥4.1(≥160)	≥4.9(≥190)	<4.1(<160)
No CHD but two or more risk factors	≥3.4(≥130)	≥4.1(≥160)	<3.4(<130)
Presence of CHD	>2.6(>100)	>3.4(>130)	<2.6(<100)

SOURCE: From Ginsberg HN, Goldberg IJ: HPIM-14, p. 2146.

ondary hyperlipoproteinemias or worsen prior hyperlipoproteinemic states. In either case, control of aggravating or inciting cause is essential for management.

PREVENTION OF THE COMPLICATIONS OF ATHEROSCLEROSIS

The National Cholesterol Education Program guidelines (Table 169-2) are based on plasma LDL levels and estimations of other risk factors. The goal in pts with the highest risk (secondary prevention after MI and primary treatment of known atherosclerotic heart disease) is to lower LDL cholesterol to <2.6 mmol/L (<100mg/dL). The goal is an LDL cholesterol <3.4 mmol/L (<130 mg/dL) in pts with two or more risk factors for atherosclerotic heart disease [men >age 45, women >age 55 or after menopause, family history of early CHD, hypertension, diabetes mellitus, or HDL cholesterol <0.9 mmol/L (<35 mg/dL)]. Note that one risk factor may be subtracted if HDL cholesterol is >1.8 mmol/L (>70 mg/dL). *Therapy* begins with a low-fat diet (see Chap. 47), but pharmacologic intervention is often required (Table 169-3).

Table 169-3

Hypolipidemic Agents

	Class	
	Bile Acid–Binding Resins	Nicotinic Acid
Dose	Cholestyramine 8–12 g bid or tid Cholestipol 10–15 g bid or tid	Niacin 50–100 mg tid initially then increase to 1.0–2.5 g tid; slow-release niacin 0.5–1.0 g tid
Mode of action	Interrupts enterohepatic circulation of bile acids; ↑ synthesis of new bile acids and LDL receptors	↓ Synthesis of VLDL and LDL
Lipoprotein class affected	↓ LDL cholesterol 20–30% ↑ HDL cholesterol and triglycerides	↓ VLDL cholesterol 25–35% ↓ LDL cholesterol 15–25% HDL may ↑
Side effects	Constipation, gastric discomfort, nausea, hemorrhoidal bleeding	Flushing, tachycardia, atrial arrhythmias, pruritus, dry skin, nausea, diarrhea, hyperuricemia, peptic ulcer disease, glucose intolerance, hepatic dysfunction
Contraindications	Biliary track obstruction, gastric outlet obstruction, hypertriglyceridemia	Peptic ulcer disease, cardiac arrhythmias, liver disease, gout, diabetes mellitus

NOTE: LDL, low-density lipoprotein; HMG-CoA, 3-hydroxy-3-methylglutaryl-coenzyme A; HDL, high-density lipoprotein; VLDL, very low density lipoprotein; LPL, lipoprotein lipase.

SOURCE: From Ginsberg HN, Goldberg IJ: HPIM-14, p. 2146.

Class	
HMG-CoA Reductase Inhibitors	Fibric Acid Derivatives
Lovastatin 10–80 mg/d Pravastatin 10–40 mg/d Simvastatin 5–40 mg/d Fluvastatin 20–40 mg/d Atorvastatin 10–80 mg/d	Gemfibrozil 600 mg bid
↓ Cholesterol synthesis ↑ LDL receptors	↑ LPL and ↑ triglyceride hydrolysis ↓ VLDL synthesis ↑ LDL catabolism
↓ LDL cholesterol 30–40% ↓ VLDL	↓ Triglycerides 20–30% ↑ or ↓ LDL cholesterol ↑ HDL
Abnormal liver function, myositis	↑ Lithogenicity of bile, nausea, abnormal liver functions, myositis
↑ Myositis in patients with renal failure and in patients on gemfibrozil, nicotinic acid, or cyclosporine	Hepatic or biliary disease; ↓ dose in renal insufficiency

For a more detailed discussion, see Ginsberg HN, Goldberg IJ:
Disorders of Lipoprotein Metabolism, Chap. 341, p. 2138, in
HPIM-14.

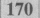

INHERITED METABOLIC DISEASES

HEMOCHROMATOSIS

Hemochromatosis occurs when increased intestinal iron absorption causes Fe deposition, fibrosis, and organ failure of the liver, heart, pancreas, and pituitary. Causes include single-gene mutations (involving a novel class 1–like gene termed *HLA-H*), impaired hematopoiesis (as in sideroblastic anemia and thalassemia), or excessive Fe ingestion. Alcoholic liver disease also may be associated with a moderate increase in hepatic Fe and elevated body Fe stores (Table 170-1).

SYMPTOMS Include weakness, lassitude, weight loss, a bronze pigmentation or darkening of skin, abdominal pain, and loss of libido. Hepatomegaly occurs in 95% of pts, sometimes in the presence of normal LFTs. Other signs include spider angiomas, splenomegaly, arthropathy, ascites, cardiac arrythmias, CHF, loss of body hair, palmar erythema, gynecomastia, and testicular atrophy. The latter is due to pituitary involvement and gonadotropin deficiency and liver failure with estrogen excess. Diabetes mellitus occurs in about 65%, usually in pts with family history of diabetes. Adrenal insufficiency, hypothyroidism, and hypoparathyroidism rarely occur.

Serum Fe, percent transferrin saturation, and serum ferritin levels are increased. Urinary Fe mobilization is elevated after IM deferoxamine. Liver biopsy is the definitive test and should be performed in suspected cases. Once diagnosis is established, family members at risk should be screened with the combined measurements of (1) percent transferrin saturation and (2) serum ferritin measurement. If either test is abnormal, a liver biopsy should be done.

Death in untreated pts results from cardiac failure (30%), cirrhosis (25%), and hepatocellular carcinoma (30%); the latter may develop despite adequate Fe removal.

TREATMENT

Involves removal of excess body Fe, usually by intermittent phlebotomy. Since 1 unit of blood contains about 250 mg Fe, and since 25 g or more of Fe must be removed, phlebotomy is performed weekly for 2–3 years. Less frequent phlebotomy is then used to maintain serum Fe at <27 μmol/L (<150 μg/dL). When given parenterally, chelating agents such as deferoxamine remove 10–20 mg iron per day, a fraction of that mobilized by weekly phlebotomy. Chelation therapy is indicated, however, when phlebotomy is inappropriate.

Table 170-1

Representative Iron Values in Normal Subjects, Patients with Hemochromatosis, and Patients with Alcoholic Liver Disease

Determination	Normal	Symptomatic Hemochromatosis	Homozygotes with Early, Asymptomatic Hemochromatosis	Alcoholic Liver Disease
Plasma iron, μmol/L (μg/dL)	9–27 (50–150)	32–54 (180–300)	Usually elevated	Often elevated
Total iron-binding capacity, μmol/L (μg/dL)	45–66 (250–370)	36–54 (200–300)	36–54 (200–300)	45–66 (250–370)
Transferrin saturation, percent	22–46	50–100	50–100	27–60
Serum ferritin, μg/L	10–200	900–6000	200–500	10–500
Urinary iron,* mg/24 h	0–2	9–23	2.5	Usually <5
Liver iron, μg/g dry wt	300–1400	6000–18,000	2000–4000	300–2000

*After intramuscular administration of 0.5 g deferoxamine.

SOURCE: Powell LW, Isselbacher K: HPIM-14, p. 2150.

PORPHYRIAS

The porphyrias are inherited or acquired disturbances in heme biosynthesis, each of which causes a unique pattern of overproduction, accumulation, and excretion of intermediates of heme synthesis. Manifestations include intermittent nervous system dysfunction and/or sensitivity of skin to sunlight.

INTERMITTENT ACUTE PORPHYRIA   This is an autosomal dominant disorder with variable expressivity. Manifestations include colicky abdominal pain, fever, leukocytosis, vomiting, constipation, port-wine colored urine, and neurologic and psychiatric disturbances. Acute attacks rarely occur before puberty and may last from days to months. Photosensitivity does not occur. Clinical and biochemical manifestations may be precipitated by barbiturates, anticonvulsants, estrogens, oral contraceptives, or alcohol. Diagnosis is established by the Watson-Swartz test. Fresh urine may darken on standing because porphobilinogens polymerize spontaneously to uroporphyrin and porphobilin.

℞ TREATMENT

Treatment involves administration of IV glucose at rates up to 20 g/h or parenteral nutrition if oral feeding is not possible for long periods. Narcotic analgesics may be required during acute attacks for abdominal pain, and phenothiazines are useful for nausea, vomiting, anxiety, and restlessness. If symptoms do not improve in 48 h, hematin (4 mg/kg) should be infused every 12 h for 3–6 days. Treatment between attacks involves adequate nutritional intake, avoidance of drugs known to exacerbate the disease, and prompt treatment of other intercurrent diseases or infections.

PORPHYRIA CUTANEA TARDA   The most common porphyria; characterized by chronic skin lesions and (usually) hepatic disease. It is due to deficiency (inherited or acquired) of uroporphyrinogen decarboxylase. Photosensitivity causes enhanced facial pigmentation, increased fragility of skin, erythema, and vesicular and ulcerative lesions, typically involving face, forehead, and forearms. Liver disease and hepatic siderosis may be related to alcoholism. Diabetes mellitus, SLE, and other autoimmune diseases may coexist. Urine uroporphyrin and coproporphyrin are increased.

℞ TREATMENT

Avoidance of precipitating factors, including abstinence from alcohol, is the first line of therapy and leads to improvement;

decrease in hepatic iron by systematic phlebotomy may ameliorate skin lesions. Chloroquine or hydroxychloroquine may be used in low doses to promote porphyrin excretion in pts unable to undergo or unresponsive to phlebotomy.

CONGENITAL ERYTHROPOIETIC PORPHYRIA A rare autosomal recessive defect that causes chronic photosensitivity, mutilating skin lesions, and hemolytic anemia. Death may occur in childhood. Exposure to sunlight should be avoided.

For a more detailed discussion, see Powell LW, Isselbacher KI: Hemochromatosis, Chap. 342, p. 2149; and Desnik RJ: The Porphyrias, Chap. 343, p. 2152, in HPIM-14.

171

THE NEUROLOGIC EXAMINATION

MENTAL STATUS EXAM

The goal of the mental status exam is to evaluate pt's attention, orientation, memory, insight, judgment, and grasp of general information. Attention is tested by asking the pt to respond every time a specific item recurs in a list. Orientation is evaluated by asking about the pt's name, the day, the date, and the pt's location. Memory can be tested by asking the pt to immediately recall a sequence of numbers and by testing recall of a series of objects after defined times (e.g., 5 and 15 min). More remote memory is evaluated by assessing pt's ability to provide a cogent chronologic history of his or her illness or personal life events. Recall of major historical events or dates or of major current events can be used to assess the pt's knowledge. Evaluation of language function should include assessment of spontaneous speech, naming, repetition, reading, writing, and comprehension. Additional tests such as ability to draw and copy, perform calculations, interpret proverbs or logic problems, identify right vs. left, name and identify body parts, etc. are also important.

CRANIAL NERVE (CN) EXAM

CN I Occlude each nostril sequentially and ask pt to gently sniff a mild test stimulus, such as soap, toothpaste, coffee, or lemon oil, to see if pt can detect and correctly identify the odor.

CN II Check visual acuity with and without correction using a Snellen chart (distance) and Jaeger's test type (near). Map visual fields (VFs) by confrontation testing in each quadrant of visual field for each eye individually. The best method is to sit facing pt (2–3 ft apart), have pt cover one eye gently, and fix uncovered eye on examiner's nose. A small white object (e.g., a cotton-tipped applicator) is then moved slowly from periphery of field toward center until pt appreciates its presence. The pt's VF should be mapped against examiner's for comparison. Formal perimetry and tangent screen exam are essential to identify and delineate small defects. Optic fundi should be examined with an ophthalmoscope, and the color, size, and degree of swelling or elevation of the optic disc recorded. The retinal vessels should be checked for size, regularity, AV nicking at crossing points, hemorrhage, exudates, aneurysms, etc. The retina, including the macula, should be examined for abnormal pigmentation and other lesions.

CNs III, IV, VI Describe size, regularity, and shape of pupils as well as their reaction (direct and consensual) to light and convergence (pt follows an object as it moves closer). Check for lid drooping, lag, or retraction. Ask pt to follow your finger as you move it horizontally to left and right and vertically with each eye first fully adducted then fully abducted. Check for failure to move fully in particular directions and for presence of regular, rhythmic, involuntary oscillations of eyes (nystagmus). Test quick voluntary eye movements (saccades) as well as pursuit (e.g., follow the finger).

CN V Feel the masseter and temporalis muscles as pt bites down and test jaw opening, protrusion, and lateral motion against resistance. Examine sensation over entire face as well as response to touching each cornea lightly with a small wisp of cotton.

CN VII Look for asymmetry of face at rest and with spontaneous as well as emotion-induced (e.g., laughing) movements. Test eyebrow elevation, forehead wrinkling, eye closure, smiling, frowning, check puff, whistle, lip pursing, and chin muscle contraction. Look particularly for differences in strength of lower and upper facial muscles. Taste on the anterior two-thirds of tongue can be affected by lesions of the seventh CN proximal to the chorda tympani. Test taste for sweet (sugar), salt, sour (lemon), and bitter (quinine) using a cotton-tipped applicator moistened in appropriate solution and placed on lateral margin of protruded tongue about halfway back from tip.

CN VIII Check ability to hear tuning fork, finger rub, watch tick, and whispered voice at specified distances with each ear. Check for air vs. mastoid bone conduction (Rinne) and lateralization of a tuning fork placed on center of forehead (Weber). Accurate, quantitative testing of hearing requires formal audiometry. Remember to examine tympanic membranes.

CNs IX, X Check for symmetric elevation of palate-uvula with phonation ("*ahh*"), as well as position of uvula and palatal arch at rest. Sensation in region of tonsils, posterior pharynx, and tongue also may require testing in specific pts. Pharyngeal ("gag") reflex is evaluated by stimulating posterior pharyngeal wall on each side with a blunt object (e.g., tongue blade). Direct examination of vocal cords by laryngoscopy is necessary in some situations.

CN XI Check shoulder shrug (trapezius muscle) and head rotation to each side (sternocleidomastoid muscle) against resistance.

CN XII Examine bulk and power of tongue. Look for atrophy, deviation from midline with protrusion, tremor, and small flickering or twitching movements (fibrillations, fasciculations).

MOTOR EXAM

Power should be systematically tested for major movements at each joint (see Table 171-1). Strength should be recorded using a reproducible scale (e.g., 0 = no movement, 1 = flicker or trace of contraction with no associated movement at a joint, 2 = movement present but cannot be sustained against gravity, 3 = movement against gravity but not against applied resistance, 4 = movement against some degree of resistance, and 5 = full power; values can be supplemented with the addition of + and − signs to provide additional gradations). The speed of movement, the ability to promptly relax contractions, and fatigue with repetition should all be noted. Loss in bulk and size of muscle (atrophy) should be checked for, as well as the presence of irregular involuntary contraction (twitching) of groups of muscle fibers (fasciculations). Involuntary movements should be looked for while pt is at rest, during maintained posture, and with voluntary action. Rhythmic involuntary movements are referred to as tremors, whereas more irregular movements generally fall into the categories of choreoathetosis, ballismus, myoclonus, or tics.

REFLEXES

Important muscle-stretch reflexes to test routinely and the spinal cord segments involved in their reflex arcs include biceps (C5, 6); brachioradialis (C5, 6); triceps (C7, 8); patellar (L3, 4); and Achilles (S1, 2). A common grading scale is 0 = absent, 1 = present but diminished, 2 = normal, 3 = hyperactive, and 4 = hyperactive with clonus (repetitive rhythmic contractions with maintained stretch). The plantar reflex should be tested by using a blunt-ended object such as the point of a key to stroke the outer border of the sole of the foot from the heel toward the base of the great toe. An abnormal response (Babinski sign) is extension (dorsiflexion) of the great toe at the metatarsophalangeal joint. In some cases this may be associated with abduction (fanning) of other toes and variable degrees of flexion at ankle, knee, and hip. (Normal response is plantar flexion of the toes.) Abdominal, anal, and sphincteric reflexes are important in certain situations, as are additional muscle-stretch reflexes.

Table 171-1

Muscles that Move Joints

	Muscle	Nerve	Segmental Innervation
Shoulder	Supraspinatus	Suprascapular n.	C5,6
	Deltoid	Axillary n.	C5,6
Forearm	Biceps	Musculocutaneous n.	C5,6
	Brachioradialis	Radial n.	C5,6
	Triceps	Radial n.	C6,7,8
	Ext. carpi radialis	Radial n.	C5,6
	Ext. carpi ulnaris	P. interosseous n.	C7,8
	Ext. digitorum	P. interosseous n.	C7,8
	Supinator	P. interosseous n.	C6,7
	Flex. carpi radialis	Median n.	C6,7
	Flex. carpi ulnaris	Ulnar n.	C7,8,T1
	Pronator teres	Median n.	C6,7
Wrist	Ext. carpi ulnaris	Ulnar n.	C7,8,T1
	Flex. carpi radialis	Median n.	C6,7
Hand	Lumbricals	Median + ulnar n.	C8,T1
	Interossei	Ulnar n.	C8,T1
	Flex. digitorum	Median + A. interosseous n.	C7,C8,T1
Thumb	Opponens pollicis	Median n.	C8,T1
	Ext. pollicis	P. interosseous n.	C7,8
	Add. pollicis	Median n.	C8,T1
	Abd. pollicis	Ulnar n.	C8,T1
	Flex. pollicis br.	Ulnar n.	C8,T1
Thigh	Iliopsoas	Femoral n.	L1,2,3
	Glutei	Sup. + inf. gluteal n.	L4,L5,S1,S2
	Quadriceps	Femoral n.	L2,3,4
	Adductors	Obturator n.	L2,3,4
	Hamstrings	Sciatic n.	L5,S1,S2
Foot	Gastrocnemius	Tibial n.	S1,S2
	Tibialis ant.	Deep peroneal n.	L4,5
	Peronei	Deep peroneal n.	L5,S1
	Tibialis post.	Tibial n.	L4,5
Toes	Ext. hallucis l.	Deep peroneal n.	L5,S1

Function

Abduction of upper arm
Abduction of upper arm
Flexion of the supinated forearm
Forearm flexion with arm between pronation and supination
Extension of forearm
Extension and abduction of hand at the wrist

Extension and adduction of hand at the wrist

Extension of fingers at the MCP joints
Supination of the extended forearm
Flexion and abduction of hand at the wrist

Flexion and adduction of hand at the wrist

Pronation of the forearm
Extension/adduction at the wrist

Flexion/abduction at the wrist

Extension of fingers at PIP joint with the MCP joint extended and fixed
Abduction/adduction of the fingers
Flexion of the fingers

Touching the base of the 5th finger with thumb

Extension of the thumb
Adduction of the thumb
Abduction of the thumb
Flexion of the thumb

Flexion of the thigh
Abduction, extension, and internal rotation of the leg
Extension of the leg at the knee
Adduction of the leg
Flexion of the leg at the knee
Plantar flexion of the foot
Dorsiflexion of the foot
Eversion of the foot
Inversion of the foot
Dorsiflexion of the great toe

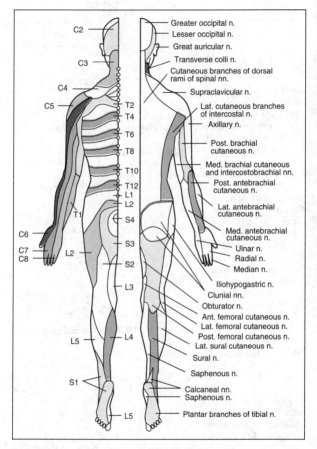

FIGURE 171-1 Posterior view of dermatomes (*left*) and cutaneous areas supplied by individual nerves (*right*). (From HPIM-14, p. 124.)

SENSORY EXAM

For most purposes it is sufficient to test sensation to pinprick, touch, position, and vibration in each of the four extremities (see Figs. 171-1 and -2). Specific problems often require more painstaking evaluation. Pts with cerebral lesions may have ab-

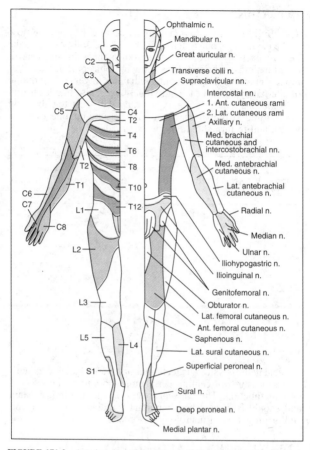

FIGURE 171-2 Anterior view of dermatomes (*left*) and cutaneous areas supplied by individual peripheral nerves (*right*). (From HPIM-14, p. 124.)

normalities in "discriminative sensation" such as the ability to perceive double simultaneous stimuli, to localize stimuli accurately, to identify closely approximated stimuli as separate (two-point discrimination), to identify objects by touch alone (stereognosis), or to judge weights, evaluate texture, or identify letters or numbers written on the skin surface (graphesthesia).

COORDINATION AND GAIT

The ability to move the index finger accurately from the nose to the examiner's outstretched finger and the ability to slide the heel of each foot from the knee down the shin are tests of coordination. Additional tests (drawing objects in the air, following a moving finger, tapping with index finger against thumb or alternately against each individual finger) also may be useful in some pts. The pt's ability to stand with feet together and eyes closed (Romberg test), to walk a straight line (tandem walk), and to turn should all be observed.

For a more detailed discussion, see Martin JB, Hauser SL: Approach to the Patient with Neurologic Disease, Chap. 360, p. 2277, in HPIM-14.

172

DIAGNOSTIC METHODS IN NEUROLOGY

Clinical neurophysiologic techniques provide objective, quantitative measures of central, peripheral, and autonomic nervous system function. They are an extension of the clinical exam and should be used when important for diagnosis, treatment, and/or prognosis of neurologic disorders.

ELECTROENCEPHALOGRAPHY

An EEG records the electrical activity of the brain from multiple electrodes placed on the scalp. It is used primarily in the investigation and management of pts with epilepsy. It is also useful in the evaluation of altered mental status, coma, and brain death. The EEG may show characteristic abnormalities in certain cerebral neurologic disorders. With the advancement of neuroimaging, it has become less important in the localization of structural abnormalities such as brain tumors. Finally, it is used in the evaluation of sleep disorders.

NORMAL EEG RHYTHMS IN ADULTS   In an awake pt lying quietly with eyes closed, an 8–12 Hz alpha rhythm should be present over the posterior head regions and attenuate with eye opening. There may be beta activity (>13 Hz) as well, which is more pronounced with drowsiness and certain drugs. Theta (4–7 Hz) activity is present predominantly over the temporal regions with drowsiness and light sleep. Normal sleep activity includes delta activity (<4 Hz), sleep spindles, and vertex waves.

ABNORMAL EEG RHYTHMS IN ADULTS   The EEG in a pt with epilepsy may show ictal, interictal, or normal activity. An electrographic seizure consists of abnormal, repetitive, rhythmic activity having abrupt onset and termination. Some ictal or interictal patterns are consistent with a certain type of epilepsy. Interictal epileptiform activity in correlation with an appropriate history strongly suggests epilepsy and includes bursts of abnormal discharges containing spikes and sharp waves. Generalized 3-Hz spike-and-wave activity is present in absence seizures. Focal interictal activity makes partial complex seizures more likely. These EEG patterns help to dictate specific treatments and prognosis. A normal EEG does not exclude the diagnosis of epilepsy.

In pts with altered mental status due to an organic cause, there may be generalized or focal slowing of the record. The presence of triphasic waves suggests a metabolic cause. Reactivity of the record correlates with a better prognosis. Loss of reactivity or a burst-suppression pattern is present with severe coma. Electrocerebral silence in the absence of drug overdose or hypothermia implies that useful cognitive recovery will not occur.

Certain cerebral neurologic disorders have characteristic but nonspecific EEG abnormalities. For instance, periodic lateralized epileptiform discharges (PLEDs) can be seen with herpes simplex encephalitis. Generalized periodic complexes in the presence of a dementing disorder are consistent with Creutzfeld-Jakob disease. The EEG does not reliably distinguish between dementia and pseudodementia.

EVOKED POTENTIALS

Evoked potentials (EPs) are averaged time-locked cortical potentials following stimulation of visual, auditory, or somatosensory afferents. Prolongation of the latency of these potentials reflects a lesion in the specific pathway being tested but is nonspecific. They are most often used in the evaluation of possible multiple sclerosis (MS). EPs can demonstrate lesions in multiple areas of white matter and are especially useful if the pt has clinical evidence of only one lesion or vague, ill-defined complaints of questionable organic basis. Other specific uses are discussed below. Precise localization is difficult as the generators of multiple EP components are unknown.

VISUAL EVOKED POTENTIALS (VEPs)   Elicited by monocular stimulation with a reversing checkerboard pattern and recorded from the occipital region of the scalp. A P100 response is recorded at a latency of approximately 100 ms. Latency, amplitude, and symmetry of the response are measured. VEPs are most commonly abnormal with optic neuritis (active or residual) but can be abnormal with other lesions of the optic nerve such as compression or with glaucoma.

BRAINSTEM AUDITORY EVOKED POTENTIALS   Using earphones, clicks presented to one ear produce seven wave forms (I–VII) recorded from the scalp. These are thought to represent successive activation of the auditory nerve (I) and brainstem auditory pathways (cochlear nucleus, II; superior olivary complex, III; lateral lemniscus, IV; inferior colliculus, V; and higher auditory centers, VI, VII). Lesions at or between any of these levels delay or obliterate the waves that follow. It is the most sensitive screening test for acoustic neuroma. Other applications include localization of level of the lesion in coma (usually normal in toxic/metabolic coma or bihemispheric disease and abnormal with brainstem pathology) and hearing evaluation of infants.

SOMATOSENSORY EVOKED POTENTIALS (SEPs)   Generated by delivering multiple small electrical stimuli to large sensory nerve fibers of the limbs to produce afferent volleys recorded at many levels along the somatosensory pathway (proximal peripheral nerve trunks, spinal cord dorsal columns, and primary sensory cortex). The SEP is delayed due to lesions of the proximal sensory nerves or dorsal columns. It can be abnormal in multiple disorders, including MS when there is a lesion in the cord, vitamin B_{12} deficiency, AIDS, cervical stenosis, or Lyme disease. The presence or absence of SEPs may have prognostic significance with coma and spinal cord injury. They can also be used intraoperatively during spine surgery or carotid endarterectomy to indicate possible iatrogenic injury to the cord or parietal cortex, respectively.

COGNITIVE EVOKED POTENTIALS   These are EP components that depend on the mental attention of the subject, also known as event-related or endogenous potentials. Infrequent auditory stimuli presented amongst regularly occurring sounds result in a positive wave (P3 or P300) 300–400 ms after the stimulus. The P3 can be prolonged in dementia but is generally normal in depression or psychiatric illness simulating dementia.

MOTOR EVOKED POTENTIALS   Motor evoked potentials are recorded from the spinal cord or muscle following transcutaneous magnetic stimulation of the motor cortex. Abnormalities have been described in disorders such as MS and motor neuron disease, but the clinical utility of this technique is still being developed.

ELECTROMYOGRAPHY(EMG)/NERVE CONDUCTION STUDIES (NCS)

The EMG/NCS primarily assesses the peripheral nervous system (motor neuron, dorsal root ganglion, peripheral nerve, neuromuscular junction, and muscle). EMG/NCS can be used to localize or exclude a lesion in the peripheral nervous system and to identify characteristics of these lesions that help with diagnosis, treatment, and/or prognosis. For example, neuropathies can be categorized as focal, multifocal, or generalized; sensory or motor; axonal or demyelinating. EMG/NCS is useful to localize and characterize focal neuropathies (location along nerve, axonal or conduction block, complete or partial). The presence and type of spontaneous activity in a myopathy can direct diagnosis and treatment. Some CNS disorders can also be evaluated by EMG (tremor, ataxia, asterixis, myoclonus, and dystonia).

NERVE CONDUCTION STUDIES   NCS involve electrical stimulation of sensory and motor nerves, recording a response over the muscle and distal sensory nerves, respectively. Distal latency, duration, and conduction velocity of the response usually reflect the integrity of myelin. The amplitude reflects the integrity of axons. Late responses include F and H waves, which provide information about the proximal conduction in motor (F waves) or motor and sensory (H waves) nerves. F waves can be particularly important in the early diagnosis of inflammatory neuropathies such as Guillain-Barré syndrome. Blink reflexes evaluate the conduction in branches of the trigeminal and facial nerves.

REPETITIVE STIMULATION   Repetitive stimulation of motor nerves can identify and characterize disorders of the neuromuscular junction. A train of supramaximal stimuli is delivered to a motor nerve, recording over the muscle at rest and after exercise. A decrement of the compound muscle action potential amplitudes is seen in myasthenia gravis and congenital myasthenia. An increment is seen with Lambert-Eaton myasthenic syndrome and botulism.

ELECTROMYOGRAPHY   EMG involves placing a needle in skeletal muscle and recording the electrical activity of the muscle at rest (spontaneous activity) and with activation (motor unit action potentials, or MUAPs). Resting muscle does not show activity except at the motor endplate. Abnormal spontaneous activity, such as fibrillation potentials and positive waves, is seen with denervation and certain types of myopathy. MUAPs are of a characteristic duration and morphology in each muscle. Short-duration MUAPs suggest a myopathic process or disorder of the neuromuscular junction. Long-duration MUAPs are present with axonal neuropathies and motor neuron disease. The pattern of activation (reduced or rapid recruitment) reflects a neurogenic or myopathic process, respectively.

Single Fiber EMG   Single fiber EMG is a sensitive but not specific technique for disorders of the neuromuscular junction. The firing of a pair of muscle fibers from the same motor unit is recorded in the muscle. The variation of the time interval between the two fibers is called *jitter* and disappearance of the second muscle fiber action potential is called *blocking*. An increase in jitter and/or blocking is seen in disorders of the neuromuscular junction.

Quantitative EMG   Various techniques such as macro EMG and motor unit estimates have been developed to quantitate the number and size of motor units in a muscle. These are used in experimental settings.

AUTONOMIC TESTING

Autonomic studies include determination of heart rate variation with respiration, Valsalva ratio, heart rate response to standing/tilting, blood pressure response to sustained hand grip, and a measure of sympathetic skin response. These tests can provide objective evidence of autonomic insufficiency (central or peripheral) and provide a measure of function for small unmyelinated peripheral axons.

LUMBAR PUNCTURE

INDICATIONS   Lumbar puncture is used to obtain pressure measurements and secure a sample of CSF for cellular, chemical, immunologic, and bacteriologic examination in the evaluation of infections of the central nervous system, meningeal cancer, inflammatory neuropathies, acute demyelinating disorders, benign intracranial hypertension, and other unexplained neurologic disorders (see Chap. 197 for normal values). It is also used for adminstration of spinal anesthesia, antibiotics, or antitumor agents and to inject contrast agents for myelography.

CONTRAINDICATIONS Some relative contraindications to lumbar puncture include thrombocytopenia or other disorders of blood coagulation, the presence of local skin or soft tissue infection along the needle tract, and increased intracranial pressure. If increased intracranial pressure is suspected, a head CT or MRI should be performed prior to the study to exclude a mass lesion. CSF should always be obtained with suspected meningitis. A fine-bore (24 gauge) needle should be used. If the pressure is >400 mmHg, the minimal amount of fluid should be removed with administration of mannitol or dexamethasone if needed to prevent herniation.

COMPLICATIONS The most common complication of a lumbar puncture is a positional headache due to persistent leakage of CSF. Treatment is discussed in Chap. 15, in HPIM-14. Seeding of the subarachnoid space with bacteria is rare.

For a more detailed discussion, see Martin JB, Hauser SL: Approach to the Patient with Neurologic Disease, Chap. 360, p. 2277; Aminoff MJ, Electrophysiologic Studies of the Central and Peripheral Nervous Systems, Chap. 361, p. 2282; and Engstrom JW, Martin JB, Chap. 371, p. 2372, in HPIM-14.

173

SEIZURES AND EPILEPSY

Definitions

Seizure: paroxysmal event due to abnormal, excessive, hyper-synchronous discharges from an aggregate of CNS neurons. *Epilepsy:* recurrent seizures due to a chronic, underlying process.

Seizure Classification

Proper seizure classification is vital for diagnostic, therapeutic, and prognostic reasons. *Partial* (or *focal*) *seizures* originate in localized area of cortex; *generalized seizures* involve diffuse regions of the brain in a bilaterally symmetric fashion. *Simple-partial seizures* do not affect consciousness and may have motor, sensory, autonomic, or psychic symptoms. *Complex-partial seizures* include alteration in consciousness coupled with automatisms (e.g., lip smacking, chewing, aimless walking, or other complex motor activities).

Generalized seizures may occur as a primary disorder or result from secondary generalization of a partial seizure. *Tonic-clonic* seizures (grand mal) cause sudden loss of consciousness, loss of postural control, tonic muscular contraction producing teeth-clenching and rigidity in extension (tonic phase), followed by rhythmic muscular jerking (clonic phase). Tongue-biting and incontinence may occur during the seizure. Recovery of consciousness is typically gradual over many minutes to hours. Headache and confusion are common postictal phenomena. In *absence seizures* (*petit mal*) there is sudden, brief impairment of consciousness without loss of postural control. Events rarely last longer than 5–10 s but can recur many times per day. Minor motor symptoms are common, while complex automatisms and clonic activity are not. Other types of generalized seizures include atypical absence, infantile spasms, and tonic, atonic, and myoclonic seizures.

Etiology

Seizure type and age of pt provide important clues to etiology. Important causes of seizures by age group are shown in Table 173-1.

Clinical Evaluation

Careful review of history is essential since diagnosis of seizures and epilepsy is often based solely on clinical grounds. Differential diagnosis commonly includes syncope or psychogenic

Table 173-1

The Causes of Seizures

Neonates (<1 month)	Perinatal hypoxia and ischemia
	Intracranial hemorrhage and trauma
	Acute CNS infection (bacterial and viral meningitis)
	Metabolic disturbances (hypoglycemia, hypocalcemia, hypomagnesemia, pyridoxine deficiency)
	Drug withdrawal
	Developmental disorders (acquired and genetic)
	Genetic disorders
Infants and children (>1 mo and <12 years)	Febrile seizures
	Genetic disorders (metabolic, degenerative, primary epilepsy syndromes)
	CNS infection
	Developmental disorders (acquired and genetic)
	Trauma
	Idiopathic
Adolescents (12–18 years)	Trauma
	Genetic disorders
	Infection
	Brain tumor
	Illicit drug use
	Idiopathic
Young adults (18–35 years)	Trauma
	Alcohol withdrawal
	Illicit drug use
	Brain tumor
	Idiopathic
Older adults (>35 years)	Cerebrovascular disease
	Brain tumor
	Alcohol withdrawal
	Metabolic disorders (uremia, hepatic failure, electrolyte abnormalities, hypoglycemia)
	Alzheimer's disease and other degenerative CNS diseases
	Idiopathic

Table 173-2

Commonly Used Antiepileptic Drugs

Generic Name	Trade Name	Principal Uses	Typical Dosage and Dosing Intervals	Half-Life
Phenytoin (diphenyl-hydantoin)	Dilantin	Tonic-clonic (grand mal) Focal-onset	300–400 mg/d (3–6 mg/kg, adult; 4–8 mg/kg, child) qd-bid	24 h (wide variation, dose-dependent)
Carbama-zepine	Tegretol	Tonic-clonic Focal-onset	600–1800 mg/d (15–35 mg/kg, child) bid-qid	13–17 h
Valproic acid	Depakane Depakote	Tonic-clonic Absence Atypical absence Myoclonic Focal-onset	750–2000 mg/d (20–60 mg/kg) bid-qid	15 h
Phenobar-bital	Luminol	Tonic-clonic Focal-onset	60–180 mg/d (1–4 mg/kg, adult); (3–6 mg/kg, child) qd	90 h (70 h in children)

Therapeutic Range	Adverse Effects		Drug Interactions
	Neurologic	Systemic	
10–20 μg/mL	Ataxia Incoordination Confusion Cerebellar	Gum hyperplasia Lymphadenopathy Hirsutism Osteomalacia Facial coarsening Skin rash	Level increased by isoniazid, sulfonamides Level decreased by carbamazepine, phenobarbital Altered folate metabolism
4–12 μg/mL	Ataxia Dizziness Diplopia Vertigo	Aplastic anemia Leukopenia Gastrointestinal irritation Hepatotoxicity	Level decreased by phenobarbital, phenytoin Level increased by erythromycin, propoxyphene, isoniazid, cimetidine
50–150 μg/mL	Ataxia Sedation Tremor	Hepatotoxicity Thrombocytopenia Gastrointestinal irritation Weight gain Transient alopecia Hyperammonemia	Level decreased by carbamazepine, phenobarbital, phenytoin
10–40 μg/mL	Sedation Ataxia Confusion Dizziness Decreased libido Depression	Skin rash	Level increased by valproic acid, phenytoin Enhances metabolism of other drugs via liver enzyme induction

(*continued*)

Table 173-2 (*Continued*)

Commonly Used Antiepileptic Drugs

Generic Name	Trade Name	Principal Uses	Typical Dosage and Dosing Intervals	Half-Life
Primidone	Mysoline	Tonic-clonic Focal-onset	750–1000 mg/d (10–25 mg/kg) bid-tid	Primidone, 8–15 h Phenobarbital, 90 h
Ethosux-imide	Zarontin	Absence (petit mal)	750–1250 mg/d (20–40 mg/kg) qd-bid	60 h, adult 30 h, child
Gabapentin	Neurontin	Focal-onset	900–2400 mg/d tid-qid	5–9 h
Lamotrigine	Lamictal	Focal-onset Lennox-Gastaut syndrome	150–500 mg/d bid	25 h 14 h (with enzyme-inducers) 59 h (with valproic acid)
Clonazepam	Klonopin	Absence Atypical absence Myoclonic	1–12 mg/d (0.1–0.2 mg/kg) qd-tid	24–48 h
Felbamate	Felbatol	Focal-onset Lennox-Gastaut syndrome	2400–3600 mg/d, (45 mg/kg, child) tid-qid	16–22 h

Therapeutic Range	Adverse Effects		Drug Interactions
	Neurologic	Systemic	
Primidone, 4–12 μg/mL Phenobarbital, 10–40 μg/mL	Same as phenobarbital		
40–100 μg/mL	Ataxia Lethargy Headache	Gastrointestinal irritation Skin rash Bone marrow suppression	
Not established	Sedation Dizziness Ataxia Fatigue	Gastrointestinal irritation	No known significant interactions
Not established	Dizziness Diplopia Sedation Ataxia Headache	Skin rash Stevens-Johnson syndrome	Level decreased by carbamazepine, phenobarbital, phenytoin Level increased by valproic acid
10–70 ng/mL	Ataxia Sedation Lethargy	Anorexia	Level decreased by carbamazepine, phenobarbital
Not established	Insomnia Dizziness Sedation Headache	Aplastic anemia Hepatic failure Weight loss Gastrointestinal irritation	Increases phenytoin, valproic acid, active carbamazepine metabolite

seizures (pseudoseizures). General exam includes search for infection, trauma, toxins, systemic illness, neurocutaneous abnormalities, and vascular disease. Asymmetries in neurologic exam can suggest brain tumor, stroke, trauma, or other focal lesions.

Laboratory Findings

Serum glucose, electrolytes, calcium, magnesium, liver and renal function tests, and CBC are obtained immediately. Toxicology screen is indicated in selected pts, and serum drug levels should be measured in pts taking antiepileptic medication. Pts with a suspected seizure disorder should have a sleep-deprived EEG with activation procedures (hyperventilation, photic stimulation, sleep) to assist in diagnosis and classification of seizures. Almost all pts with a first-time seizure should have an MRI scan to rule out structural abnormalities; CT scanning is reserved for acute situations in which there is a suspicion of infection or mass lesions or when MRI is unavailable. CSF analysis is indicated in patients with suspected infection.

℞ TREATMENT

Acutely, pt should be placed in semiprone position with head to the side to avoid aspiration. Tongue blades or other objects should not be forced between clenched teeth. Oxygen should be given via face mask. Reversible metabolic disorders (e.g., hypoglycemia, hyponatremia, hypocalcemia, drug or alcohol withdrawal) should be promptly corrected. Treatment of status epilepticus is discussed in Chap. 32.

Longer-term therapy includes treatment of underlying conditions, avoidance of precipitating factors, prophylactic therapy with antiepileptic medications or surgery, and addressing various psychological and social issues. Choice of antiepileptic drug therapy (Table 173-2) depends on a variety of factors including seizure type, dosing schedule, and potential side effects. First choice for focal seizures is carbamazepine or phenytoin; for generalized seizures, valproic acid is initial choice, and carbamazepine and phenytoin are alternatives. Therapeutic goal is complete cessation of seizures without side effects using a single drug (monotherapy). If ineffective, medication should be increased to maximal tolerated dose based primarily on clinical response rather than serum levels. If unsuccessful, a second drug should be added, and when control is obtained the first drug can be slowly tapered. Approximately one-third of pts will require polytherapy with two or more drugs. Recently approved drugs used as second-line agents include lamotrigine, gabapentin, and topiramate.

Pts with certain epilepsy syndromes (e.g., temporal lobe epilepsy) are often refractory to medical therapy and will benefit from surgical excision of the seizure focus.

For a more detailed discussion, see Lowenstein DH: Seizures and Epilepsy, Chap. 365, p. 2311, in HPIM-14.

174

CEREBROVASCULAR DISEASES

STROKE

A stroke is the sudden onset of a neurologic deficit from a vascular mechanism. 20% are primary hemorrhages, including subarachnoid and hypertensive lobar and deep cerebral hemorrhages. 80% are related to ischemia; ischemic brain tissue rapidly loses function but can remain viable with potential for recovery for hours. An ischemic deficit that rapidly resolves is termed a *transient ischemic attack* (TIA); 24 h is a useful boundary between TIA and stroke. It is important to differentiate the clinical terms *TIA* and *stroke* from the underlying tissue processes of *ischemia* and *infarction,* as temporal correlation is imperfect. Stroke is the leading cause of adult disability, and much can be done to limit morbidity and mortality through prevention and acute intervention.

PATHOGENESIS   Ischemic stroke is most often due to embolic occlusion of large cerebral vessels. Source of emboli may be the heart, aortic arch, or a more proximate arterial lesion. Primary involvement of intracerebral vessels with atherosclerosis is much less common than in coronary vessels. Small, deep ischemic lesions are most often related to intrinsic small-vessel disease, with hypertension and diabetes as main risk factors. Low-flow strokes are seen with severe proximal stenosis and inadequate collaterals challenged by significant hypotensive episodes. Hemorrhage most frequently results from rupture of aneurysms or small vessels within brain tissue.

CLINICAL PRESENTATION   *Stroke*   Abrupt and dramatic onset of focal neurologic symptoms; temporal pattern can suggest the underlying vascular mechanism. Vascular mechanisms causing TIA are the same as those causing ischemic stroke (Table 174-1). Symptoms reflect the vascular territory involved and provide clues to localization and identification of the vessel and pathology (Table 174-2). Rapid resolution of TIA symptoms suggests resolution of the underlying ischemia, although small areas of tissue infarction are often found when symptoms persist more than 1–2 h. Variability in stroke recovery is influenced by collateral vessels, blood pressure, and specific site and mechanism of vessel occlusion. Reversible ischemia and salvage of tissue at risk have become real concepts with application of thrombolytic and neuroprotective agents.

Intracranial Hemorrhage   Most common types are hypertensive and lobar hemorrhages (50%), ruptured saccular aneurysm, and ruptured arteriovenous malformation (AVM). Vom-

Table 174-1

Causes of Ischemic Stroke

THROMBOSIS

Atherosclerosis
Vasculitis
Collagen vascular diseases: temporal (giant cell) arteritis, polyarteritis nodosa, Wegener's granulomatosis, Takayasu's arteritis, syphilis
Meningitis: tuberculosis, fungi, syphilis, bacteria, herpes zoster
Arterial dissection: carotid, vertebral, intracranial arteries at the base of the brain (spontaneous or traumatic)
Hematologic disorders: polycythemia, thrombocytosis, thrombotic thrombocytopenic purpura, disseminated intravascular coagulation, dysproteinemias, hemoglobinopathies (sickle cell disease)
Miscellaneous: cocaine, amphetamines, moyamoya disease, fibromuscular dysplasia, Binswanger's disease

EMBOLISM

Cardiac source
Atherothrombotic arterial source: bifurcation of common carotid artery, carotid siphon, distal vertebral artery, aortic arch
Unknown source: may be associated with a hypercoagulable state secondary to systemic disease, carcinoma (especially pancreatic), eclampsia, oral contraceptives, lupus, factor C or S deficiency, factor V mutation, etc.

VASOCONSTRICTION

Vasospasm: cerebral vasospasm following subarachnoid hemorrhage
Reversible cerebral vasoconstriction: idiopathic, migraine, eclampsia, trauma

VENOUS

Dehydration, pericranial infection, postpartum and postoperative states, systemic cancer

SOURCE: Easton JD, Hauser SL, Martin JB: HPIM-14, p. 2326.

Table 174-2

Anatomic Localization of Cerebral Lesions in Stroke

Signs and Symptoms	Structures Involved
CEREBRAL HEMISPHERE, LATERAL ASPECT (MIDDLE CEREBRAL A.)	
Hemiparesis	Contralateral parietal and frontal motor cortex
Hemisensory deficit	Contralateral somatosensory cortex
Motor aphasia (Broca's)—hesitant speech with word-finding difficulty and preserved comprehension	Motor speech area, dominant frontal lobe
Central aphasia (Wernicke's)—anomia, poor comprehension, jargon speech	Central, perisylvian speech area, dominant hemisphere
Unilateral neglect, apraxias	Nondominant parietal lobe
Homonymous hemianopsia or quadrantanopsia	Optic radiation in inferior parietal or temporal lobe
Gaze preference with eyes deviated to side of lesion	Center for lateral gaze (frontal lobe)
CEREBRAL HEMISPHERE, MEDIAL ASPECT (ANTERIOR CEREBRAL A.)	
Paralysis of foot and leg with or without paresis of arm	Leg area with or without arm area of contralateral motor cortex
Cortical sensory loss over leg	Foot and leg area of contralateral sensory cortex
Grasp and sucking reflexes	Medial posterior frontal lobe
Urinary incontinence	Sensorimotor area, paracentral lobule
Gait apraxia	Frontal cortices
CEREBRAL HEMISPHERE, INFERIOR ASPECT (POSTERIOR CEREBRAL A.)	
Homonymous hemianopsia	Calcarine occipital cortex
Cortical blindness	Occipital lobes, bilaterally
Memory deficit	Hippocampus, bilaterally or dominant
Dense sensory loss, spontaneous pain dysesthesias, choreoathetosis	Thalamus plus subthalamus

(continued)

Table 174-2 (*Continued*)

Anatomic Localization of Cerebral Lesions in Stroke

Signs and Symptoms	Structures Involved
BRAINSTEM, MIDBRAIN (POSTERIOR CEREBRAL A.)	
Third nerve palsy and contralateral hemiplegia	Third nerve and cerebral peduncle (Weber's syndrome)
Paralysis/paresis of vertical eye movement	Supranuclear fibers to third nerve
Convergence nystagmus, disorientation	Top of midbrain, periaqueductal
BRAINSTEM (PONTOMEDULLARY JUNCTION BASILAR A.)	
Facial paralysis	Seventh nerve, ipsilateral
Paresis of abduction of eye	Sixth nerve, ipsilateral
Paresis of conjugate gaze	"Center" for lateral gaze, ipsilateral
Hemifacial sensory deficit	Tract and nucleus of V, ipsilateral
Horner's syndrome	Descending sympathetic pathways
Diminished pain and thermal sense over half body (with or without face)	Spinothalamic tract, contralateral
Ataxia	Middle cerebellar peduncle and cerebellum
BRAINSTEM, LATERAL MEDULLA (VERTEBRAL A.)	
Vertigo, nystagmus	Vestibular nucleus
Horner's syndrome (miosis, ptosis, decreased sweating)	Descending sympathetic fibers, ipsilateral
Ataxia, falling toward side of lesion	Cerebellar hemisphere or fibers
Impaired pain and thermal sense over half body with or without face	Contralateral spinothalamic tract

iting occurs in most cases, and headache in about one-half. Signs and symptoms not usually confined to a single vascular territory. Hypertensive hemorrhage typically occurs in (1) the putamen, adjacent internal capsule, and central white matter; (2) thalamus; (3) pons; and (4) cerebellum. A neurologic deficit that evolves relentlessly over 5–30 min strongly suggests intra-cerebral bleeding. Ocular signs are important in localization: (1) putaminal—eyes deviated to side opposite paralysis (toward lesion); (2) thalamic—eyes deviated downward, sometimes with unreactive pupils; (3) pontine—reflex lateral eye movements impaired and small (1–2 mm), reactive pupils; (4) cerebellar—eyes deviated to side opposite lesion (early on, in absence of paralysis).

RISK FACTORS Atherosclerosis is a systemic disease af-fecting arteries throughout the body. Multiple factors including hypertension, diabetes, hyperlipidemias, and familial tendencies influence stroke and TIA risk. Cardioembolic risk factors in-clude atrial fibrillation, MI, valvular heart disease, and cardio-myopathy. Prolonged hypertension and diabetes are also specific risk factors for lacunar stroke with small-vessel lipohyalinotic disease. Smoking is a potent risk factor for all vascular mecha-nisms of stroke.

COMPLICATIONS Neurologic deficits can worsen after presentation because of several possible complications. Embolic stroke carries the risk of early recurrence. This can occur from cardiac sources and arterial stenoses and from acute arterial occlusions as distal stump emboli. Large, deep ischemic infarcts can develop hemorrhage into the affected tissue. Large cerebral or cerebellar infarcts can develop edema sufficient to lead to neurologic deterioration. While most intracerebral hemorrhages bleed only briefly, some may continue to expand with resultant mass effect. Seizures are uncommon in acute stroke but develop as a delayed complication in 5–10%.

LABORATORY EVALUATION *CT* Initial CT study without contrast indicated to exclude hemorrhage or other mass lesions. Early signs of ischemic stroke can be recognized within the first few hours of large strokes, but small cortical infarcts can be difficult to assess by CT.

MRI Compared with CT, increased sensitivity for small infarcts of cortex and brainstem.

MR Angiography Special sequences that image blood flow can evaluate patency of intracranial vessels and extracranial carotid and vertebral vessels.

Noninvasive Carotid Tests   Most commonly used are "duplex" studies, combining ultrasound imaging of the vessel with Doppler evaluation of blood flow characteristics.

Cerebral Angiography   "Gold standard" for evaluation of vascular disease. Detects ulcerative lesions, severe stenosis, and mural thrombosis; can also visualize atherosclerotic disease or dissection in carotid siphon or intracranial vessels, demonstrate collateral circulation around the circle of Willis, and show embolic occlusion of cerebral branch vessels. Best method to demonstrate atherothrombotic disease of the basilar artery. It causes substantial morbidity (1–5%) and may precipitate a threatened stroke, thus is used only when noninvasive studies fail to detect an arterial lesion that, if identified, would influence management.

Cardiac Evaluation   Indicated in suspected cardiogenic embolization; ECG, cardiac ultrasound with attention to right-to-left shunts, and 24-h Holter monitoring. In absence of clinical history of heart disease or ECG abnormality, routine cardiac evaluation is unlikely to be useful.

Blood Studies   Routine initial studies include CBC/platelets, electrolytes, ESR, RPR, PT, and PTT. In cases where a hypercoagulable state is suspected, further studies of coagulation are indicated.

℞ TREATMENT

Acute Ischemic Stroke and TIA   Ischemic deficits of <3 h duration, with no hemorrhage by CT criteria, may benefit from thrombolytic therapy with IV recombinant tissue plasminogen activator (rt-PA). This therapy has been shown to improve neurologic outcome, but currently only a small percentage of stroke pts are seen early enough to treat with this agent.

Careful evaluation and treatment are essential to minimize infarction and reduce recurrent stroke risk. Blood pressure should never be lowered precipitously (exacerbates the underlying ischemia), and only in the most extreme situations (systolic blood pressure >220 mmHg) should gradual decreases be undertaken. Intravascular volume should be maintained with isotonic fluids as volume restriction is rarely helpful. Osmotic therapy with mannitol may be necessary to control edema in large infarcts, but isotonic volume must be replaced to avoid hypovolemia. In cerebellar infarction (or hemorrhage), rapid deterioration can occur from brainstem compression and hydrocephalus. These pts require neurosurgical evaluation and careful neurologic monitoring.

Indications for heparin are empirically based; objective clinical data are lacking. IV heparin generally used when atherothrombotic vascular stenosis or occlusion is suspected, particularly in ischemic stroke with progression of symptoms ("stuttering stroke"), unstable TIA (crescendo or recent onset), or posterior circulation involvement. Warfarin may be used long term for atherothrombotic disease when carotid surgery (see below) is not an option or for cardiac sources of embolism (anterior MI, AF, or valvular disease). Antiplatelet agents (aspirin 325 mg/d) may reduce risk of further TIA and stroke in symptomatic pts and provide an alternative to anticoagulation. Surgical endarterectomy benefits many pts with symptomatic severe (>70%) carotid stenosis. Aggressive control of hypertension, hypercholesterolemia, diabetes, and smoking can produce significant risk reduction.

Intracerebral Hemorrhage   Noncontrast head CT will confirm diagnosis. It is important to identify and correct any coagulopathy rapidly. Neurosurgical consultation should be sought for possible urgent evacuation of hematoma, especially in the case of cerebellar hemorrhage. Prophylactic anticonvulsant therapy is usually undertaken in supratentorial hemorrhage, especially when extending to the cortical surface. Treatment for edema and mass effect with mannitol may be necessary, and while steroids may be helpful in some cases, routine use leads to many steroid complications.

SUBARACHNOID HEMORRHAGE

Most common cause of nontraumatic subarachnoid hemorrhage (SAH) is rupture of an intracerebral aneurysm; other etiologies include mycotic aneurysms in subacute bacterial endocarditis, bleeding dyscrasias, and rarely infections or tumors.

CLINICAL PRESENTATION   Sudden, severe headache, often with transient loss of consciousness at onset; vomiting is common. Bleeding may injure adjacent brain tissue and produce focal neurologic deficits. A progressive third nerve palsy with severe headache suggests posterior communicating artery aneurysm.

LABORATORY EVALUATION   *CT*   Noncontrast CT is done first and usually demonstrates the hemorrhage. On occasion, LP is required for diagnosis of suspected SAH if CT is nondiagnostic.

Cerebral Angiography   Necessary to define the anatomy, location, and type of vascular malformation, such as aneurysm or AVM; also assesses vasospasm. Usually done as soon as possible after diagnosis of SAH is made.

ECG   ST-segment changes, prolonged QRS complex, increased QT interval, and prominent or inverted T waves often present; some changes reflect SAH, others indicate associated myocardial ischemic injury.

Blood Studies   Closely follow serum electrolytes and osmolality; hyponatremia frequently develops several days after SAH. Cerebral salt wasting is common, and supplemental sodium used to overcome renal losses.

℞ TREATMENT

Standard management includes bed rest, analgesics, and stool softeners. Anticonvulsants are begun at diagnosis and continued at least until the aneurysm is treated. Risk of early rebleeding is high (20–30% over 2 weeks), thus early treatment (within 1–3 days) is advocated to avoid rerupture and allow aggressive treatment of vasospasm. Neurosurgical clipping of the aneurysm neck is the most common treatment, although newer endovascular techniques are also possible. Severe hydrocephalus may require urgent placement of a ventricular catheter for external CSF drainage. Blood pressure is carefully monitored and regulated to assure adequate cerebral perfusion while avoiding excessive elevations. Symptomatic vasospasm may occur by day 4 and continue through day 14, leading to focal ischemia and possible stroke. Medical treatment, including nimodipine, may minimize the neurologic sequelae of vasospasm. Cerebral perfusion can be improved in vasospasm by increasing mean arterial pressure with vasopressor agents such as neosynephrine or dopamine. Intravascular volume can be expanded with crystalloid to help support maintenance of hypertension. Angioplasty of the cerebral vessels can be effective in cases of severe vasospasm when ischemic symptoms appear despite maximal medical therapy.

For a more detailed discussion, see Easton JD, Hauser SL, Martin JB: Cerebrovascular Diseases, Chap. 366, p. 2325, in HPIM-14.

175

NEOPLASTIC DISEASES OF THE CENTRAL NERVOUS SYSTEM

Clinical Features

Brain tumors present with: (1) progressive focal neurologic deficit, (2) seizure, or (3) a nonfocal neurologic disorder (headache, dementia, personality change, gait disorder). Systemic symptoms suggest metastatic rather than primary brain tumor.

- *Focal neurologic deficit*—due to compression of neurons by tumor or edema
- *Seizures*—caused by stimulation of excitatory, or loss of inhibitory, cortical circuits
- *Nonfocal neurologic disorders*—due to increased intracranial pressure, hydrocephalus, or diffuse tumor spread
- *Headache* associated with brain tumor—caused by focal irritation/displacement of pain-sensitive structures or increased intracranial pressure (papilledema, impaired lateral gaze, increased headache with recumbency
- *Strokelike onset*—may reflect hemorrhage into tumor

Brain tumors may be large at presentation if located in clinically silent region (i.e., prefrontal) or slow-growing; may present with psychiatric disorder if diencephalic, frontal, or temporal lobe location.

Laboratory Evaluation

Primary brain tumors have no systemic features of malignancy, unlike metastases. CSF exam is limited to diagnosis of possible meningitis or meningeal metastases but may cause brain herniation in setting of brain mass. Neuroimaging reveals mass effect (volume of neoplasm and surrounding edema) and contrast enhancement (breakdown of blood-brain barrier permitting leakage of contrast into brain parenchyma). Positron emitting tomography (PET) scanning distinguishes tumor recurrence from delayed brain necrosis following radiation therapy (RT).

℞ TREATMENT

Symptomatic Treatment Glucocorticoids (dexamethasone 12–20 mg/d in divided doses) to reduce edema; prophylaxis with anticonvulsants (phenytoin, carbamazepine, or valproic acid) for tumors involving cortex or hippocampus.

Intracranial Tumors

The only known risk factor is ionizing radiation. Fatal effects of primary brain tumors are caused by local growth. Tissue diagnosis by biopsy essential.

Astrocytomas Most common primary intracranial neoplasm. Prognosis poor if age >65 years, poor baseline functional status, high-grade tumor. Difficult to treat; infiltration along white matter pathways prevents total resection. Imaging studies fail to indicate full tumor extent. Surgery for pathologic diagnosis and to control mass effect. RT prolongs survival and improves quality of life. Systemic chemotherapy with nitrosoureas is only marginally effective, often employed as adjunct to RT for high-grade gliomas. Role of stereotaxic radiosurgery (single dose, highly focused radiation—gamma knife) unclear. Interstitial brachytherapy (stereotaxic implantation of radioactive beads) reserved for tumor recurrence; associated with necrosis of normal brain tissue. For low grade astrocytoma, optimal management is uncertain.

Oligodendrogliomas Supratentorial; mixture of astrocytic and oligodendroglial cells. As oligodendroglial component increases, so does long-term survival; 5-year survival >50%. Total surgical resection often possible; may respond dramatically to chemotherapy.

Ependymomas Derived from ependymal cells; highly cellular. If aggressive histology (cellular atypia, frequent mitotic figures), recurrence is certain. If total excision, 5-year disease-free survival >80%.

Germinomas Tumors of midline brain structures with onset in second decade. Neuroimaging—uniformly enhancing mass; treatment—complete surgical excision; 5-year survival >85%.

Primitive Neuro-Ectodermal Tumors (PNET) 50% in posterior fossa; highly cellular; derived from neural precursor cells. Treatment—surgery, chemotherapy, and RT.

Primary CNS Lymphomas B cell malignancy; most occur in immunosuppressed patients (organ transplantation, AIDS). May present as a single mass lesion (immunocompetent pts) or as multiple mass lesions or meningeal disease (immunosuppressed pts). Prognosis generally poor. In immunocompetent pts RT and combination chemotherapy may increase survival to 18 months or more; AIDS-related cases have survival of 3 months or less.

Meningiomas Extraaxial mass attached to dura; dense and uniform contrast enhancement is diagnostic. Total surgical resection of benign meningiomas is curative. With subtotal resection, local RT reduces recurrence to <10%. Incidental meningiomas may be followed radiologically. Rare aggressive meningiomas—treat with excision and RT.

Tumors Metastatic to Brain Skull metastases rarely invade CNS; may compress adjacent brain or cranial nerves or obstruct intracranial venous sinuses. Common metastases to brain are small cell lung, breast, melanoma, germ cell, and thyroid cancers; rare metastases to brain are prostate and ovarian cancers and Hodgkin's disease. Brain metastases are well demarcated by MRI and enhance with gadolinium; triple-dose contrast is most sensitive for detection; ring enhancement is nonspecific. Differential diagnosis includes brain abscess, radiation necrosis, toxoplasmosis, granulomas, demyelinating lesions, primary brain tumors, CNS lymphomas, stroke, hemorrhage, and trauma. CSF cytology is unnecessary—intraparenchymal metastases rarely shed cells into CSF. One-third of pts with brain metastasis have unknown primary (ultimately small cell lung cancer, melanoma most frequent); primary tumor never identified in 30%. CXR is best screening test for occult cancer; if negative → chest CT. If chest CT negative → CT scan of abdomen and pelvis. Further imaging studies unhelpful if above studies negative. *Treatment* is palliative—glucocorticoids, anticonvulsants, and RT may improve quality of life. Whole brain RT is given, assuming multiple microscopic tumor deposits throughout the brain. A single metastasis may be surgically excised as palliation. Systemic chemotherapy may produce dramatic responses in isolated cases.

Leptomeningeal Metastases Diagnosis by CSF cytology, MRI (nodular meningeal tumor deposits or diffuse meningeal enhancement), or meningeal biopsy. Associated with hydrocephalus due to CSF pathway obstruction; detected by complete neuraxis MRI. Aggressive treatment (intrathecal chemotherapy, focal external beam RT) produces sustained response (~6 months) in 20% of pts.

Spinal Cord Compression from Metastases (See Chap. 188) Expansion of vertebral body metastasis (usually lung, breast, or prostate primary) into epidural space compresses cord. Back pain (>90%) usually precedes development of weakness, sensory level, and incontinence. Early recognition of impending spinal cord compression is essential to avoid devastating sequelae. Diagnosis is by MRI.

Complications of Radiation Therapy Three patterns of radiation injury after RT: acute, early delayed (2–4 months), late delayed (up to 15 years). Clinical course—expanding mass lesion; may resolve spontaneously or with steroids. Progressive radiation necrosis is best treated with surgical resection. Endocrine dysfunction due to hypothalamus or pituitary gland injury may occur.

For a more detailed discussion, see Sagar SM, Israel MA: Tumors of the Nervous System, Chap. 375, p. 2398, in HPIM-14.

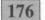

BACTERIAL INFECTIONS OF THE CENTRAL NERVOUS SYSTEM

ACUTE BACTERIAL MENINGITIS

ETIOLOGY The pathogens most frequently involved in bacterial meningitis in immunocompetent adults are *S. pneumoniae* ("pneumococcus") and *N. meningitidis* ("meningococcus"). Predisposing factors for pneumococcal meningitis include distant foci of infection (otitis, sinusitis, pneumonia, endocarditis) and asplenia, sickle cell disease, hypogammaglobulinemia, multiple myeloma, alcoholism, cirrhosis, and recent head trauma with CSF leak. Pts with deficiency of terminal complement components, or properdin, are at increased risk of meningococcal infection, which may also occur in epidemics. Although vaccination has dramatically reduced the incidence of *H. influenzae* meningitis, this organism is still an important cause of meningitis in unvaccinated children (age 3 mos to 18 yrs) and in adults with predisposing risk factors (e.g., otitis, sinusitis, epiglottitis, pneumonia, alcoholism, diabetes, immunocompromise, asplenia). Pts with impaired cell-mediated immunity, neonates, the elderly, diabetics, and alcoholics are at increased risk of infection caused by *L. monocytogenes* and a variety of gram-negative organisms. Pts with recent head trauma, neurosurgery, or ventricular shunts are at increased risk of both gram-negative and staphylococcal infections.

CLINICAL MANIFESTATIONS   85% of adults have headache, fever, and meningismus (stiff neck). Additional signs can include altered consciousness, cranial nerve palsies, seizures, nausea and vomiting, myalgia, sweating, and photophobia. Meningismus and fever may be absent in neonates and elderly pts. Infants may present with listlessness, irritability, feeding problems, or abnormal crying. Rash (erythematous, macular, purpural, petechial) suggests meningococcal infection but may occur with other organisms.

LABORATORY FINDINGS   Lumbar puncture (LP) is critical to the diagnosis of meningitis but should be deferred pending CT or MRI in pts with focal neurologic findings or papilledema. Treatment (see below) must not be delayed in such cases but should be started empirically after obtaining blood cultures. Key CSF findings in bacterial meningitis commonly include a CSF leukocytosis with neutrophilic predominance, an elevated protein, hypoglycorrhachia (decreased glucose), and elevated opening pressure. Mononuclear cells may predominate as infection continues. Cell counts are typically 5–20,000 cells/μL. Counts above 50,000/μL should suggest the possibility of intraventricular rupture of brain abscess. CSF glucose is <40 mg/dL (2.2 mmol/L) in 60% and the CSF-to-serum ratio of glucose concentrations is <0.31 in 70%. Gram stain reveals organisms in 75% of untreated pts, and cultures are positive in 70–80%. Latex agglutination test may be helpful in pts with partially treated meningitis. Blood cultures should always be obtained and are positive in 50% of pts.

[Rx] **TREATMENT**
Recommendations for appropriate antibiotic therapy are in a state of flux. Suggested regimens for empiric therapy are based on the pt's age, immunologic status, presence or absence of recent head trauma or neurosurgery, and CSF Gram stain results. Therapy is then modified based on results of CSF culture. Infants <3 months of age should receive ampicillin plus cefotaxime. Immunocompetent individuals between the ages of 3 mos and 50 yrs can be treated with a third-generation cephalosporin, typically either ceftriaxone or cefotaxime. Adults >50 yrs should also receive ampicillin. Pts with recent head trauma or neurosurgical procedures should be treated with vancomycin plus ceftazidime. Pts with gram-positive cocci seen on CSF Gram stain or cultures positive for *S.*

Table 176-1

Suggested Intravenous Therapy in Acute Bacterial Meningitis

Drug	Adult Dose	Pediatric Dose
Ampicillin	2 g q4h	100 mg/kg q8h
Cefotaxime	2 g q6h	50 mg/kg q6h
Ceftazidime	50–100 mg/kg q8h (6 g/d maximum)	50–100 mg/kg q8h
Ceftriaxone	2 g q12h	50–100 mg/kg q12h
Gentamicin	1.5 mg/kg loading dose then 1–2 mg/kg q8h	
Penicillin G	300,000 (units/kg)/d (24 million units/d maximum)	
Vancomycin	15 mg/kg q6h (2 g/d maximum)	

pneumoniae should be treated with a combination of cefotaxime or ceftriaxone and vancomycin because of the increasing incidence of beta-lactam resistant isolates. Pts with gram-negative cocci on CSF Gram stain or cultures positive for *N. meningitidis* can be treated with penicillin G. Pts with gram-negative bacilli on Gram stain or cultures positive for Enterobacteriaceae should be treated with cefotaxime or ceftriaxone plus gentamicin. In cases with recent head trauma or neurosurgery, because of the increased risk of *Pseudomonas* infection, ceftazidime is the cephalosporin of choice combined with gentamicin. Penicillin G remains the drug of choice for *N. meningitidis* infection, and ceftriaxone or cefotaxime for *H. influenzae* infection. *L. monocytogenes* should be treated with a combination of ampicillin plus gentamicin. Therapy is generally administered for 7–21 days depending on the nature of the infecting organism. Suggested IV doses for adult and pediatric pts are shown in Table 176-1.

Children (>3 mos) should receive adjunctive dexamethasone therapy. Dexamethasone (0.15 mg/kg every 6 h) should be given intravenously, with the initial dexamethasone dose given 20 min before the first antibiotic dose. Treatment should be continued for 4 days. Data concerning the efficacy of dexamethasone treatment in adults is less conclusive than for pediatric use. Dexamethasone may reduce penetration of vancomycin into the CSF.

COMPLICATIONS CNS complications can include increased intracranial pressure, infarction, cerebral sinus or venous thrombosis, seizures, obstructive hydrocephalus, subdural effusion (children), and hearing loss.

BRAIN ABSCESS

A focal suppurative infection involving brain parenchyma.

ETIOLOGY Common etiologic agents include mixed flora, aerobic or microaerophilic streptococci, *S. aureus*, aerobic gram-negative bacilli, and anaerobes. Risk factors include sinusitis, otitis, dental infections, head trauma, neurosurgery, and distant foci of infection.

CLINICAL FEATURES Solitary abscesses involve frontal > temporal > parietal > cerebellar > occipital lobes of the brain, in decreasing order of frequency. Hematogenous spread of infection to brain frequently results in multiple abscesses. Specific clinical features are shown in Table 176-2.

DIAGNOSIS CT and MRI are the most useful diagnostic tools and serve to identify the location and number of abscesses and the presence of associated parameningeal or sinus infection. Typical CT appearance is of a hypodense lesion with a uniformly enhancing ring surrounded by an outer zone of hypodense-appearing edema. Typical features may be absent in early lesions

Table 176-2

Clinical Manifestations of Brain Abscess

Symptoms or Sign	Percent
Headache	50–75
Triad of fever, headache, focal deficit	<50
Fever	40–50
Focal neurologic deficit	~50
Seizures	25–40
Nausea/vomiting	22–50
Nuchal rigidity	~25
Papilledema	~25

NOTE: Other symptoms and signs are dependent on location.

SOURCE: Scheld WM: HPIM-14, p. 2428.

and in pts receiving glucocorticoids. Neoplasms, granulomas, resolving hematomas, and infarcts may resemble abscesses on CT and MRI. LP is contraindicated in pts with suspected or known brain abscess as it rarely adds useful diagnostic information and may precipitate herniation.

Ⓡ TREATMENT

Optimal therapy of encapsulated abscesses includes surgical drainage (aspiration or total excision) and antibiotics. Unencapsulated abscesses ("cerebritis") may respond to antimicrobial therapy alone. Empiric antibiotic therapy should be modified based on the results of abscess cultures. Typical regimens for empiric therapy include cefotaxime (1.5 g IV q4h) plus metronidazole (15 mg/kg loading dose followed by 7.5 mg/kg IV q6h). Nafcillin or oxacillin (2 g IV q4h) should be added in pts with recent head trauma, neurosurgery, or suspected staphylococcal infection. Glucocorticoids should be used only in pts with proven or suspected elevation in intracranial pressure. Prophylactic anticonvulsant therapy is frequently used in pts with abscesess near the cortical surface.

SUBDURAL EMPYEMA

A collection of pus between the dural and arachnoid membranes.

ETIOLOGY   Major pathogens include aerobic and anaerobic streptococci, staphylococci, and aerobic gram-negative bacilli.

PATHOGENESIS   Infection may spread to the subdural space through thrombophlebitis of the valveless cranial emissary veins or by contiguous spread of cranial osteomyelitis. Paranasal sinusitis is a major predisposing factor. Other risk factors include otitis, mastoiditis, cranial trauma, neurosurgery, and distant foci of infection.

CLINICAL MANIFESTATIONS   Empyema can present as a rapidly progressive life-threatening condition. Signs and symptoms reflect the antecedent infection (e.g., sinusitis), meningeal irritation, the presence of a focal CNS lesion, and increased intracranial pressure. These can include fever, headache, nausea and vomiting, declining mental status, focal or generalized seizures, and hemiparesis or hemiplegia.

DIAGNOSIS   CT with contrast enhancement and MRI are the diagnostic procedures of choice. Typical CT appearance is of an area of crescentic hypodensity beneath the cranium, with a fine line of contrast enhancement between the empyema margin and the subjacent cortex. CT and MRI also help delineate associated otitis or sinusitis. LP rarely adds useful information and is contraindicated because of the risk of herniation.

℞ TREATMENT

Subdural empyema is a surgical emergency. Treatment consists of emergent surgical drainage combined with antibiotic treatment. Typical empiric antibiotic regimens include nafcillin or oxacillin (1.5 g IV q4h) plus metronidazole (15 mg/kg IV loading dose followed by 7.5 mg/kg q6h) plus ceftriaxone or cefotaxime. In pts with recent head trauma or neurosurgical procedures, ceftazidime is the broad-spectrum cephalosporin of choice. Treatment should be continued for a minimum of 3–4 weeks, with final duration of therapy determined by the pt's clinical condition and the resolution of infection on neuroimaging studies.

For a more detailed discussion, see Scheld WM: Bacterial Meningitis, Brain Abscess, and Other Suppurative Intracranial Infections, Chap. 377, p. 2419, in HPIM-14.

177

ASEPTIC MENINGITIS, VIRAL ENCEPHALITIS, AND PRION DISEASES

VIRAL MENINGITIS

The syndrome of viral meningitis consists of fever, headache, and meningeal irritation associated with a CSF lymphocytic pleocytosis, slightly elevated protein, and normal glucose. Associated symptoms can include malaise, anorexia, nausea and vomiting, abdominal pain, and diarrhea. The presence of significant impairment in consciousness, seizures, or focal neurologic findings suggests parenchymal involvement and is not typical of uncomplicated viral meningitis.

ETIOLOGY (See Tables 177-1, 177-2) Most cases of viral meningitis are due to enteroviruses, including the majority of culture-negative cases. Other common causes of viral meningitis include herpes simplex virus (HSV) type 2, arboviruses, and HIV. The incidence of enteroviral and arboviral infections is greatly increased during the summer.

DIAGNOSIS CSF polymerase chain reaction (PCR) tests have greatly facilitated diagnosis of viral meningitis and encephalitis. PCR testing is the procedure of choice for rapid, sensitive, and specific identification of viral infections caused by enteroviruses, HSV, EBV, varicella zoster virus (VZV), and CMV. Attempts should also be made to culture virus from CSF and other sites and body fluids including blood, throat swabs, feces, and urine. Serologic studies, including those utilizing paired

Table 177-1

Viruses Causing Aseptic Meningitis*

Common	Less Common	Rare
Enteroviruses	HSV-1	Adenoviruses
Arboviruses	LCMV	CMV
HIV	Mumps	EBV
HSV-2		Influenza A, B; measles; parainfluenza; rubella; VZV

*CMV, cytomegalovirus; EBV, Epstein-Barr virus; HSV, herpes simplex virus; LCMV, lymphocytic choriomeningitis virus; VZV, varicella-zoster virus.

Table 177-2

Seasonal Prevalence of Viruses Commonly Causing Meningitis

Summer–Early Fall	Fall and Winter	Winter and Spring	Nonseasonal
Arboviruses	LCMV	Mumps	HIV
Enteroviruses			HSV

ABBREVIATIONS: See Table 177-1.

CSF and serum specimens, may be helpful for retrospective diagnosis.

℞ TREATMENT

For the majority of cases of viral meningitis, supportive or symptomatic therapy is sufficient and hospitalization is not generally required. Neonates, elderly pts, and immunocompromised pts should be hospitalized, as should pts in whom the diagnosis is uncertain or in whom bacterial or other nonviral causes of meningitis cannot be excluded. The course and severity of meningitis due to HSV, EBV, and VZV may be shortened or ameliorated by antiviral treatment, which can include oral or IV acyclovir or oral valacyclovir or famciclovir, although detailed clinical studies are lacking. Pts with HIV meningitis should be treated with antiretroviral therapy. Additional supportive or symptomatic therapy can include analgesics and antipyretics.

VIRAL ENCEPHALITIS

Viral encephalitis is an infection of the brain parenchyma commonly associated with meningitis ("meningoencephalitis"). Clinical features are those of viral meningitis plus symptoms and signs indicative of brain tissue involvement. These commonly include altered consciousness, seizures, and focal neurologic findings such as aphasia, hemiparesis, involuntary movements, and cranial nerve deficits.

ETIOLOGY (See Table 177-3)   The most common cause of acute sporadic encephalitis is HSV type 1. Arboviruses are responsible for both sporadic and epidemic cases of encephalitis (Table 177-4). Other common viral causes of encephalitis include enteroviruses, mumps, EBV, and VZV.

Table 177-3

Viruses Causing Encephalitis

Common	Less Common	Rare
Arboviruses, enteroviruses, HSV-1, mumps	CMV, EBV, HIV, measles, VZV	Adenoviruses, CTFV, influenza A, LCMV, parainfluenza, rabies, rubella

ABBREVIATIONS: As in Table 177-1; also, CTFV, Colorado tick fever virus.

DIAGNOSIS (See Fig. 177-1) CSF should be examined in all cases of suspected viral encephalitis. The typical CSF profile is similar to that for viral meningitis. The use of CSF PCR tests has dramatically improved the diagnosis of viral encephalitis. CSF PCR allows for rapid and reliable diagnosis of infections due to HSV, EBV, VZV, and enteroviruses. CSF should be sent for culture, although this is often negative. Cultures of blood, throat swab, feces, urine, and skin lesions should also

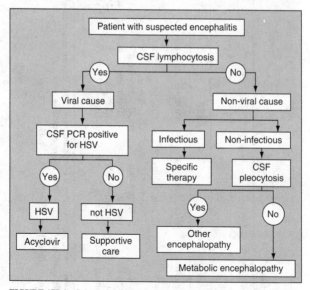

FIGURE 177-1 Scheme for the treatment of patients with suspected encephalitis. HSV, herpes simplex virus. (From Fig. 379-2, HPIM-14, p. 2444.)

Table 177-4

Features of Selected Arbovirus Encephalitides

Feature	Virus				
	WEE	EEE	VEE	SLE	CE
Region	West, midwest	Atlantic and Gulf	South	All	East and north-central
Age	Infants, adults >50 years	Children	Adults	Adults >50 years	Children
Deaths	5–15 percent	50–75 percent	1 percent	2–20 percent	<1 percent
Sequelae	Low to moderate	80 percent	Rare	20 percent	Rare
Vector	Mosquito	Mosquito	Mosquito	Mosquito	Mosquito
Animal host	Birds	Birds	Horses, small mammals	Birds	Rodents

ABBREVIATIONS: CE, California encephalitis virus; EEE, Eastern equine encephalitis virus; SLE, St. Louis encephalitis virus; VEE, Venezuelan equine encephalitis virus; WEE, Western equine encephalitis virus.

SOURCE: From Tyler KL: HPIM-14, p. 2444.

be obtained. Serologic studies, including paired CSF and serum samples, are useful for retrospective diagnosis. MRI is the neuroimaging procedure of choice and will frequently show areas of increased T2 signal. Bitemporal and orbitofrontal areas of increased signal are seen in HSV encephalitis but are not diagnostic. Areas of multifocal increased T2 signal associated with decreased T1 signal and gadolinium enhancement are suggestive of postinfectious immune-mediated demyelination. The EEG may suggest the presence of seizures and may show temporally predominant periodic spikes on a slow, low-amplitude background suggestive of HSV encephalitis.

℞ TREATMENT

All pts with suspected HSV encephalitis should be treated with IV acyclovir (10 mg/kg q8h). Pts with a PCR-confirmed diagnosis of HSV encephalitis should receive a 14-day course of therapy. CSF PCR testing for HSV, performed by an experienced and reliable laboratory, is sufficiently sensitive that with rare exceptions a negative result excludes the diagnosis of HSV encephalitis and allows acyclovir therapy to be discontinued. Acyclovir treatment may also be of benefit to pts with encephalitis due to EBV and VZV, although clinical studies are limited. No specific therapy is currently available for pts with arboviral or enteroviral encephalitis or encephalitis caused by mumps or measles. Pts with encephalitis due to HIV infection should receive appropriate antiretroviral therapy. CMV encephalitis, which occurs almost exclusively in immunocompromised pts, should be treated with ganciclovir, foscarnet, or a combination of the two drugs. Additional treatment should be directed at reducing or controlling fever, elevations in intracranial pressure, and seizures. Appropriate measures should be taken to reduce the risk of aspiration pneumonia, decubitus ulcers, thrombophlebitis, pulmonary emboli, and gastritis.

HERPES ZOSTER (SHINGLES)

CLINICAL FEATURES   Paresthesia or dysesthesia in a dermatomal distribution, followed by a localized cutaneous eruption of clear vesicles on an erythematous base, most commonly involving the lower thoracic (T5-10) dermatomes.

℞ TREATMENT

Oral acyclovir (800 mg 5 times a day), famciclovir (500 mg tid), or valacyclovir (1 g tid) for 7 days if instituted within

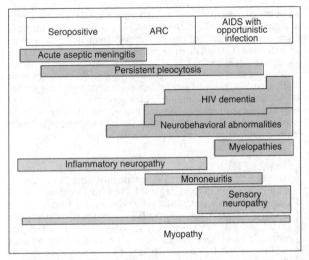

FIGURE 177-2 Relative frequency and timing of major neurologic complications of direct HIV infection. Diseases that affect the CNS are shaded in blue; those that affect the peripheral nervous system are shown with gray shading. Height of the boxes is a relative indicator of the frequency of each type of disease. (From Fig. 379-3, HPIM-14, p. 2446.)

72 h of rash onset will diminish the duration and severity of viral shedding, new lesion formation, and acute pain. A role for antiviral drugs in reducing the incidence of postherpetic neuralgia (PHN), defined as pain persisting for greater than 4–6 weeks after zoster rash, has been suggested but not established. PHN rarely occurs in pts <50 years of age. Treatment can include nonnarcotic analgesics, tricyclic antidepressants, carbamazepine, dilantin, and topical capsaicin ointment. Additional complications of VZV infection can include meningoencephalitis, cerebellitis, myelitis, and granulomatous arteritis.

NEUROLOGIC COMPLICATIONS OF HIV INFECTION

CLINICAL FEATURES Direct neurologic manifestations of HIV infection are myriad. They can involve any part of the nervous system, and can occur at any stage of HIV infection (see Fig. 177-2). Aseptic meningitis may occur at the time of initial infection with HIV. HIV dementia typically occurs late in illness. Pts present with psychomotor slowing, apathy, difficulty with memory and concentration, and gait abnormalities. HIV vacuolar myelopathy also occurs in advanced infection and may mimic the myelopathy of vitamin B_{12} deficiency. Peripheral neuropathies can occur at any stage of illness and may be either axonal or demyelinating, with predominant sensory or sensorimotor involvement.

Secondary neurologic complications of HIV infection result from opportunistic infections and neoplasia and typically occur in immunocompromised pts. Common causes of CNS lesions include toxoplasmosis, progressive multifocal leukoencephalopathy (PML), and primary CNS lymphoma (PCNSL). Infection with CMV can result in retinitis, meningoencephalitis, myelitis, or radiculopathy. VZV infection can produce shingles, disseminated zoster, meningoencephalitis, CNS vasculitis, or myelitis.

R_X TREATMENT

Direct neurologic complications of HIV infection may stabilize or improve with optimization of antiretroviral therapy, including the use of protease inhibitors. The incidence of opportunistic infections appears to be lower in pts in whom antiretroviral therapy results in improvement of immunologic function. Specific therapy is available for treatment of toxoplasmosis, CMV, and VZV. No therapy is currently available for PML. Radiation plus chemotherapy may produce modest increases in survival for selected pts with PCNSL.

PROGRESSIVE MULTIFOCAL LEUKOENCEPHALOPATHY (PML)

CLINICAL FEATURES A progressive multifocal demyelinating disease of the CNS resulting from infection of oligodendrocytes by JC virus. Clinical manifestations reflect the location, extent, and number of lesions and can include mental status impairment, visual field abnormalities, and focal weakness.

DIAGNOSIS MRI typically shows multifocal white matter lesions that do not enhance with contrast and are without mass effect. The CSF cell counts and chemistries are typically normal. Amplification of JC virus DNA from CSF using PCR techniques, in association with the typical clinical and neuroimaging findings, is diagnostic. A negative CSF PCR decreases the likelihood but does not exclude the diagnosis of PML. Definitive diagnosis may require brain biopsy.

℞ TREATMENT

No effective therapy for PML is currently available. Improvement of pts' immune status (e.g., by optimization of antiretroviral therapy in HIV-infected individuals) has been reported to result in stabilization or remission of disease in isolated cases.

TROPICAL SPASTIC PARAPARESIS/ HTLV-ASSOCIATED MYELOPATHY

CLINICAL FEATURES   A slowly progressive spastic paraparesis associated with serologic evidence of infection with human T lymphotropic virus type I (HTLV-I). Clinical findings include spastic leg weakness, hyperactive deep tendon reflexes, and impaired bladder function. Pain and sensory loss may be present but are typically mild.

DIAGNOSIS   CSF may show a lymphocytic pleocytosis, elevated protein, and oligoclonal bands. HTLV-I antibodies are found in serum and CSF. MRI may show areas of demyelination in the spinal cord and cerebrum.

℞ TREATMENT

Myelitis appears to reflect immune-mediated injury to the spinal cord mediated by cytotoxic T lymphocytes rather than direct viral injury. Pts may respond to prednisone or equivalent glucocorticoids.

PRION DISEASES

CLINICAL FEATURES   Prion diseases of the CNS may present as sporadic, rapidly progressive dementia associated with myoclonus (Creutzfeldt-Jakob Disease, CJD), or less commonly as familial forms of rapidly progressive dementia (familial CJD), cerebellar degeneration (Gerstmann-Straussler-Scheinker Disease, GSS), or complex syndromes of insomnia, hallucinations, motor abnormalities, and autonomic and endocrine disturbances (fatal familial insomnia, FFI). Iatrogenic prion diseases can result from use of contaminated corneal or dura grafts, neurosurgical instruments, or cadaveric-derived pituitary hormones. Approximately a dozen cases of an atypical or variant form of CJD characterized by early age of onset and prominent initial neuropsychiatric and behavioral abnormalities followed by ataxia and progressive dementia have been reported from England and France. It has been suggested, but not definitively established, that these cases may be the result of human exposure to food or other products derived from cattle infected with bovine spongiform encephalopathy ("mad cow disease").

DIAGNOSIS CT and MRI are often normal but may show rapidly progressive atrophy or increased T2 signal in the basal ganglia (MRI). CSF cell counts and chemistries are normal. Both CSF and neuroimaging studies may help exclude other diagnoses. It has been reported that the presence in CSF of specific proteins (14-3-3) is suggestive but not diagnostic of CJD. EEG may show periodic sharp wave complexes in CJD, but these are absent or occur only rarely in GSS, FFI, and variant CJD. Definitive diagnosis of sporadic forms of prion disease requires neuropathologic study of brain tissue. Typical findings include neuronal loss, astrogliosis, spongiform changes, absence of inflammatory response, and the presence, in GSS and atypical CJD, of typical plaques containing protease-resistant prion protein. The detection of protease-resistant prion proteins by immunoblotting or immunocytochemistry in appropriately treated brain sections or material establishes the diagnosis. Pts with familial CJD, GSS, or FFI invariably have mutations in the PRNP gene, which encodes the prion protein. Specific polymorphisms in the PRNP gene are also found with increased frequency in pts with sporadic CJD, iatrogenic CJD, and atypical CJD, and may enhance susceptibility to prion diseases.

℞ **TREATMENT**

CNS prion diseases are all inexorably progressive and invariably fatal. No effective treatment is currently available.

For a more detailed discussion see Tyler KL: Aseptic Meningitis, Viral Encephalitis, and Prion Diseases, Chap. 379, p. 2439, in HPIM-14 and HPIM-14 chapters covering specific organisms or infections.

178

MULTIPLE SCLEROSIS (MS)

Characterized by chronic inflammation and selective destruction of CNS myelin; peripheral nervous system is spared. Pathologically, the multifocal scarred lesions of MS are termed *plaques*. Etiology is thought to be autoimmune, with susceptibility determined by genetic and environmental factors. MS affects 350,000 Americans; onset is most often in early to middle adulthood, and women are affected approximately twice as often as men.

Clinical Manifestations

Onset may be dramatic or insidious. Most common are recurrent attacks of focal neurologic dysfunction, typically lasting weeks or months, and followed by variable recovery; some pts initially present with slowly progressive neurologic deterioration. Symptoms often transiently worsen with fatigue, stress, exercise, or heat. The manifestations of MS are protean (Table 178-1) but commonly include weakness and/or sensory symptoms involving a limb, visual difficulties, abnormalities of gait and coordination, urinary urgency or frequency, and abnormal fatigue. Motor involvement can present as a heavy, stiff, weak, or clumsy limb. Localized tingling, "pins and needles," and "dead" sensations are common. Optic neuritis can result in blurring or misting of vision, especially in the central visual field, often with associated retroorbital pain accentuated by eye movement. Involvement of the brainstem may result in diplopia, nystagmus, vertigo, or facial symptoms of pain, numbness, weakness, hemispasm, or

Table 178-1

Initial Symptoms of MS

Symptom	Percent of Cases	Symptom	Percent of Cases
Sensory loss	37	Lhermitte	3
Optic neuritis	36	Pain	3
Weakness	35	Dementia	2
Paresthesia	24	Visual loss	2
Diplopia	15	Facial palsy	1
Ataxia	11	Impotence	1
Vertigo	6	Myokymia	1
Paroxysmal attacks	4	Epilepsy	1
Bladder	4	Falling	1

SOURCE: From Hauser SL, Goodkin DE: HPIM-14, p. 2411.

myokymia (rippling muscular contractions). Ataxia, tremor, and dysarthria may reflect disease of cerebellar pathways. Lhermitte's symptom, a momentary electric-like shock sensation evoked by neck flexion, indicates disease in the cervical spinal cord. Diagnostic criteria for MS are listed in Table 178-2.

Physical Examination

Abnormal signs are usually more widespread than expected from the history and may provide evidence of the multifocal nature of disease process. Check for abnormalities in visual fields, loss of visual acuity, disturbed color perception, optic pallor or papillitis, abnormalities in pupillary reflexes, nystagmus, internuclear ophthalmoplegia (slowness or loss of adduction in one eye with nystagmus in the abducting eye on lateral gaze), facial numbness or weakness, dysarthria, incoordination, ataxia, weakness and spasticity, hyperreflexia, loss of abdominal reflexes, ankle clonus, upgoing toes, sensory abnormalities.

Disease Course

Four general categories of MS exist:

- *Relapsing-remitting MS* is characterized by recurrent attacks of neurologic dysfunction with or without recovery; between attacks, no progression of neurologic impairment is noted.
- *Secondary progressive MS* initially presents with a relapsing-remitting pattern but evolves to be progressive.
- *Primary progressive MS* is characterized by gradual progression of disability from onset.
- *Progressive-relapsing MS* is a rare form that begins with a primary progressive course but superimposed relapses occur.

MS is a chronic illness; 15 years after diagnosis, 20% of pts have no functional limitation, 70% are limited or unable to perform major activities of daily living, and 75% are not employed.

LABORATORY FINDINGS

MRI scans are the most sensitive means of detecting demyelinating lesions; multifocal bright areas on T2-weighted sequences are found in more than 90% of pts. Administration of gadolinium DPTA results in enhancement of active lesions due to disruption of the blood-brain barrier by inflammation. MRI may also help exclude other disorders that can mimic MS. Abnormalities in the CSF may include mild lymphocytic pleocytosis (5–75 cells in 25%), oligoclonal bands (75–90%), elevated IgG (80%), and normal total protein level. Visual, auditory, and somatosensory

Table 178-2

Diagnostic Criteria for MS

1. Examination must reveal objective abnormalities of the CNS.
2. Involvement must reflect predominantly disease of white matter long tracts, usually including (a) pyramidal pathways, (b) cerebellar pathways, (c) medial longitudinal fasciculus, (d) optic nerve, and (e) posterior columns.
3. Examination or history must implicate involvement of two or more areas of the CNS.
   a. MRI may be used to document a second lesion when only one site of abnormality has been demonstrable on examination. A confirmatory MRI must have either four lesions involving the white matter or three lesions if one is periventricular in location. Acceptable lesions must be greater than 3 mm in diameter. For patients older than 50 years, two of the following criteria must also be met: (a) lesion size >5 mm; (b) lesions abut the bodies of the lateral ventricles; or, (c) lesion(s) present in the posterior fossa.
   b. Evoked response testing may be used to document a second lesion not evident on clinical examination.
4. The clinical pattern must consist of (a) two or more separate episodes of worsening involving different sites of the CNS, each lasting at least 24 h and occurring at least 1 month apart, or (b) gradual or step-wise progression over at least 6 months if accompanied by increased CSF IgG synthesis or two or more oligoclonal bands.
5. Age of onset between 15 and 60 years of age.
6. The patient's neurologic condition could not be better attributed to another disease. Laboratory testing that may be advisable in certain cases includes (a) CSF analysis, (b) MRI of the head or spine, (c) serum B_{12} level, (d) human T cell lymphotropic virus type I (HTLV-I) titer, (e) erythrocyte sedimentation rate, (f) rheumatoid factor, antinuclear, anti-DNA antibodies (SLE), (g) serum VDRL, (h) angiotensin-converting enzyme (sarcoidosis), (i) *Borrelia* serology (Lyme disease), (j) very long chain fatty acids (adrenoleukodystrophy), and (k) serum or CSF lactate, muscle biopsy, or mitochondrial DNA analysis (mitochondrial disorders).

(continued)

Table 178-2 (*Continued*)

Diagnostic Criteria for MS

DIAGNOSTIC CATEGORIES

1. *Definite MS:* All six criteria fulfilled.
2. *Probable MS:* All six criteria fulfilled except (a) only one objective abnormality despite two symptomatic episodes or (b) one symptomatic episode despite two or more objective abnormalities.
3. *At risk for MS:* All six criteria fulfilled except one symptomatic episode and one objective abnormality.

SOURCE: From Hauser SL, Goodkin DE: HPIM-14, p. 2413.

evoked response tests may be of value in identifying lesions that are clinically silent. One or more evoked response tests are abnormal in >80% of pts with definite MS. Urodynamic studies often aid in management of bladder symptoms.

℞ **TREATMENT**   (Fig. 178-1 and Table 178-3)
   Prophylaxis Against Relapses   Three treatments are available: Interferon (IFN) β1b (Betaseron), IFNβ1a (Avonex), and copolymer 1 (Copaxone). Each of these therapies reduces annual exacerbation rates by approximately one-third; IFNβ1a most convincingly delays the time to onset of sustained progression. Injection site reactions are common in IFNβ1b and copolymer 1 recipients. Approximately 15% of copolymer 1 recipients experience transient flushing, chest tightness, dyspnea, and palpitations. Approximately 40% of IFNβ1b and 20% of IFNβ1a recipients develop neutralizing antibodies within 12 months of initiating therapy, and these pts appear to lose the benefit of therapy.
   Acute Relapses   Acute relapses that produce functional impairment may be treated with a short course of IV methylprednisolone (MePDN) followed by oral prednisone (PDN). This regimen speeds recovery and may modestly improve the degree of recovery that occurs. Initial attacks of demyelinating disease—typically optic neuritis or myelitis—are treated in a similar fashion, except that all initial attacks—even mild ones—are treated if the MRI scan indicates that multifocal disease is present.
   Chronic Progression   There is a limited role for chronic immunosuppression; these treatments should be administered only with the understanding that they carry risks and that

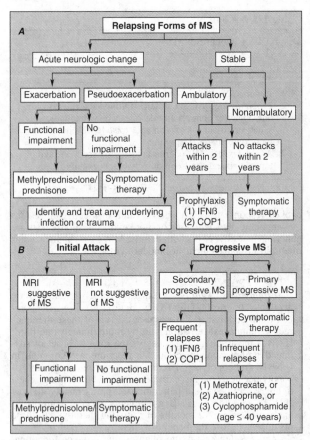

FIGURE 178-1 Therapeutic decision-making for MS. (From Hauser SL, Goodkin DE: HPIM-14.)

efficacy is modest. Monotherapy with either methotrexate or azathioprine is a reasonable initial approach.

Symptomatic Therapy Spasticity may respond to baclofen (15–80 mg/d in divided doses), diazepam (2 mg bid-tid), or tizanidine (2–8 mg tid). Dysesthesia may respond to carbamazepine (100–1200 mg/d in divided doses), phenytoin (300 mg/d), or amitriptyline (50–200 mg/d). Treatment of bladder symptoms is based upon the underlying pathophysiol-

Table 178-3

Disease-Modifying Therapy for MS

1. Prophylaxis against relapses
   a IFNβ1b (Betaseron): 8 million international units (MIU) SC every other day
   b. IFNβ1a (Avonex): 6 MIU IM once weekly
   c. Copolymer 1 (Copaxone): 20 mg SC once daily
2. Acute relapses: methylprednisolone-prednisone
   a. Inpatient administration: methylprednisolone, 250 mg, mixed in 250 mL D_5W and administered over 1–2 h IV q6h for 3 days, followed by oral prednisone (1 mg/kg as single A.M. dose) on days 4–17, 20 mg on day 18, and 10 mg on days 19–21
   b. Outpatient administration: methylprednisolone, 1000 mg slow IV push daily for 3 days, followed by oral prednisone (1 mg/kg as single A.M. dose) on days 4–17, 20 mg on day 18, and 10 mg on days 19–21
3. Chronic Progression
   a. Methotrexate: 7.5–20 mg PO once each week
   b. Azathioprine 2–3 (mg/kg)/d PO

ogy: hyperreflexia is treated with anticholinergics such as oxybutinin (5 mg bid-tid), hyporeflexia with the cholinergic drug bethanecol (10–50 mg tid-qid), and dyssynergia with anticholinergics and intermittent catheterization.

For a more detailed discussion, see Hauser SL, Goodkin DE: Multiple Sclerosis and Other Demyelinating Diseases, Chap. 376, p. 2409, in HPIM-14.

179

ALZHEIMER'S DISEASE AND OTHER DEMENTIAS

DEMENTIA

Dementia is a deterioration in cognitive ability. Memory loss is most common, but other mental faculties may be affected including attention, judgment, comprehension, orientation, learning, calculation, problem solving, mood, and behavior. Agitation or withdrawal, hallucinations, delusions, insomnia, and loss of inhibitions are also common. Dementia is chronic, whereas delirium is an acute condition associated with altered consciousness (agitation with autonomic hyperactivity or lethargy).

DIAGNOSIS The mini-mental status examination is a useful screening test for dementia (Table 179-1). A score of less than 24 points (out of 30) indicates a need for more detailed cognitive and physical assessment.

DIFFERENTIAL DIAGNOSIS Dementia is a syndrome with many causes (Table 179-2); it is essential to exclude treatable etiologies. Pseudodementia (depression) can be difficult to distinguish from dementia, but memory is usually intact on careful testing. Some clinical clues to treatable disorder—gait disturbance, urinary incontinence (normal-pressure hydrocephalus); resting tremor, bradykinesia (Parkinson's disease); neuropathy (vitamin B_{12} deficiency); bradycardia, delayed relaxation of stretch reflexes (hypothyroidism); early-onset seizures (neoplasm); insomnia, anxiety, psychiatric disturbance, seizures (drug intoxication or withdrawal); myoclonus (Creutzfeld-Jakob disease); fever, meningismus (chronic infection); confusion, ophthalmoparesis, ataxia, followed by severe anterograde and retrograde amnesia (Wernicke-Korsakoff syndrome).

EVALUATION An approach to the workup of dementia is outlined in Table 179-3. Brain MRI or CT identifies multiinfarct dementia, brain tumors, subdural hematoma, and normalpressure hydrocephalus. Several laboratory tests (thyroid function, vitamin B_{12}, complete blood count, electrolytes, VDRL) indicated in all pts, with additional tests (e.g., HIV, liver and renal function, LP, toxic screen, angiogram, or brain biopsy) determined by the clinical situation. EEG indicated if seizures or Creutzfeld-Jakob disease suspected.

ALZHEIMER'S DISEASE (AD)

This is the most common cause of dementia; it affects 3–4 million persons in the U.S. and cost >$50 billion dollars/year.

Table 179-1

The Mini-Mental Status Examination

	Points
Orientation	
Name: season/date/day/month/year	5 (1 for each name)
Name: hospital/floor/town/state/ country	5 (1 for each name)
Registration	
Identify three objects by name and ask patient to repeat	3 (1 for each object)
Attention and calculation	
Serial 7s; subtract from 100 (e.g., 93 − 86 − 79 − 72 − 65)	5 (1 for each subtraction)
Recall	
Recall the three objects presented earlier	3 (1 for each object)
Language	
Name pencil and watch	2 (1 for each object)
Repeat "No ifs, ands, or buts",	1
Follow a 3-step command (e.g., "Take this paper, fold it in half, and place it on the table")	3 (1 for each command)
Write "close your eyes" and ask patient to obey written command	1
Ask patient to write a sentence	1
Ask patient to copy a design (e.g., intersecting pentagons)	1
TOTAL	30

SOURCE: Bird TD: HPIM-14, p. 149.

CLINICAL MANIFESTATIONS Pts present with subtle recent memory loss, then develop slowly progressive dementia. Memory loss is often not recognized initially; impaired activities of daily living (keeping track of finances, appointments) draw attention of friends/family. Disorientation, poor judgment, poor concentration, aphasia, apraxia, and alexia occur also. Pts may be frustrated or unaware of deficit. Social graces and superficial conversations are intact until later phases. Death from malnutrition or secondary infection.

PATHOGENESIS Risk factors for AD are old age, positive family history. Pathology: *neuritic plaques* composed of Aβ

Table 179-2

Differential Diagnosis of Dementia

MOST COMMON CAUSES OF DEMENTIA

Alzheimer's disease
Vascular dementia
  Multi-infarct
  Diffuse white matter disease (Binswanger's)

Alcoholism*
Parkinson's disease
Drug/medication intoxication*

LESS COMMON CAUSES OF DEMENTIA

Vitamin deficiencies
  Thiamine (B_1): Wernicke's encephalopathy*
  B_{12} (Pernicious anemia)*
  Nicotinic acid (pellagra)*
Endocrine and other organ failure
  Hypothyroidism*
  Adrenal insufficiency and Cushing's syndrome*
  Hypo- and hyperparathyroidism*
  Renal failure*
  Liver failure*
  Pulmonary failure*
Chronic infections
  HIV
  Neurosyphilis*
  Papovavirus (progressive multifocal leukoencephalopathy)
  Prion (Creutzfeldt-Jakob and Gerstmann-Sträussler-Scheinker disease)
  Tuberculosis, fungal, and protozoal*
  Sarcoidosis*
  Whipple's disease*

Toxic disorders
  Drug, medication, and narcotic poisoning*
  Heavy metal intoxication*
  Dialysis dementia (aluminum)
  Organic toxins
Psychiatric
  Depression (pseudodementia)*
  Schizophrenia*
  Conversion reaction*
Degenerative disorders
  Huntington's disease
  Pick's disease
  Diffuse Lewy body disease
  Progressive supranuclear palsy (Steel-Richardson syndrome)
  Multisystem degeneration (Shy-Drager syndrome)
  Hereditary ataxias (some forms)
  Motor neuron disease [amyotrophic lateral sclerosis (ALS); some forms]
  Frontal lobe dementia
  Cortical basal degeneration
  Multiple sclerosis

(continued)

Table 179-2 (*Continued*)

Differential Diagnosis of Dementia

LESS COMMON CAUSES OF DEMENTIA (*continued*)

Head trauma and diffuse brain damage	Adult Down's syndrome with Alzheimer's
Dementia pugilistica	ALS-Parkinson's-
Chronic subdural hematoma*	Dementia complex of Guam
Postanoxia	Miscellaneous
Postencephalitis	Vasculitis*
Normal-pressure hydrocephalus*	Acute intermittent porphyria*
Neoplastic	Recurrent nonconvulsive seizures*
Primary brain tumor*	Additional conditions in children or adolescents
Metastatic brain tumor*	Hallervorden-Spatz disease
Paraneoplastic limbic encephalitis	Subacute sclerosing panencephalitis
	Metabolic disorders (e.g., Wilson's and Leigh's diseases, leukodystrophies, lipid storage diseases, mitochondrial mutations)

* Potentially treatable dementia.

amyloid and other proteins; *neurofibrillary tangles* composed of abnormally phosphorylated tau protein. An important genetic finding is identification of the *apolipoprotein E* (apo E) gene (chromosome 21) in pathogenesis; the ε4 allele appears to modify age of onset of AD and is associated with sporadic and late-onset familial cases of AD. Apo E testing is not indicated as a predictive test at this time. Rare genetic causes of AD are Down's syndrome (trisomy 21), amyloid precursor protein (APP) gene mutations (chromosome 21), mutations in presenilin I (chromosome 14) and presenilin II (chromosome 1) genes.

℞ TREATMENT

There is no definitive treatment for AD; control of behavioral/ neurologic problems in conjunction with family and caregiv-

Table 179-3

Evaluation of the Demented Patient

Routine Evaluation	Optional Focused Tests
History	HIV
Physical examination	Chest x-ray
Laboratory tests	Lumbar puncture
Thyroid function (TSH)	Liver function
Vitamin B_{12}	Renal function
Complete blood count	Urine toxin screen
Electrolytes	Psychometric testing
VDRL	Apolipoprotein E
CT/MRI	

Occasionally Helpful Tests	
EEG	RBC sedimentation rate
Parathyroid function	Angiogram
Adrenal function	Brain biopsy
Urine heavy metals	

DIAGNOSTIC CATEGORIES

Treatable Causes	Untreatable/Degenerative Dementias
Examples	Examples
Hypothyroidism	Alzheimer's
Thiamine deficiency	Pick's
Vitamin B_{12} deficiency	Huntington's
Normal-pressure hydro-	Diffuse Lewy body
cephalus	disease
Chronic infection	Multi-infarct
Brain tumor	Leukoencephalopathies
Drug intoxication	Parkinson's

Associated Treatable Conditions	Psychiatric Disorders
Depression	Depression
Seizure	Schizophrenia
Insomnia	Conversion reaction
Agitation	
Caregiver "burnout"	
Drug side effects	

ers is essential. Depression is common in early stages and may respond to antidepressants. Mild sedation may help insomnia. Agitation controlled with low-dose haloperidol (0.5–2 mg). Notebooks and posted daily reminders can function as memory aids in early stages. Kitchens, bathrooms, and bedrooms need evaluation for safety. Caregiver burnout is common; nursing home placement may be necessary. Local and national support groups (Alzheimer's Disease and Related Disorders Association) are valuable resources.

Drug therapy is limited. Two centrally acting cholinesterase inhibitors approved for AD; they presumably function via increase in cerebral levels of acetylcholine. Tetrahydroaminoacridine (Tacrine), 80–160 mg/d PO, associated with improved caregiver ratings of pt function and a decreased rate in decline of cognitive test scores. 10–20% of AD pts respond modestly and tolerate side effects (dose-related, nausea, vomiting, and diarrhea). No benefit in late AD; medication is expensive and potentially hepatotoxic. A newer agent, donazepril (Aricept), 5–10 mg/d PO, has the advantages of few side effects and single daily dosage. Estrogen may be helpful in postmenopausal women. Value of vitamin E in prevention is uncertain.

OTHER CAUSES OF DEMENTIA

VASCULAR DEMENTIA This may follow multiple strokelike episodes (multi-infarct dementia) or rarely develop in a slow progressive fashion (diffuse white matter or Binswanger's disease). Unlike AD, focal neurologic signs (e.g., hemiparesis) are usually present at presentation.

NORMAL-PRESSURE HYDROCEPHALUS (NPH) This presents as a gait disorder (ataxic or apractic), dementia, and urinary incontinence; 30–50% of pts respond to ventricular shunting.

HUNTINGTON'S DISEASE This presents as chorea and altered behavior. The disease is autosomal dominant; the abnormal gene has expanded trinucleotide repeat resulting in a protein (huntingtin) with an expanded polyglutamine tract.

For a more detailed discussion, see Bird TD: Memory Loss and Dementia, Chap. 26, p. 142; Bird TD: Alzheimer's Disease and Other Primary Dementias, Chap. 367, p. 2348, in HPIM-14.

PARKINSON'S DISEASE

Clinical Features

Parkinsonism is defined as tremor, rigidity, bradykinesia, and characteristic abnormalities of gait and posture; may occur with many disorders. *Parkinson's disease* (PD) is idiopathic parkinsonism without evidence of more widespread neurologic involvement. Onset between ages 40 and 70 years with insidious progression. Tremor at rest (4–6 Hz); worsens with stress; typically "pill-rolling" tremor of hands. A faster (7–8 Hz) "action tremor" may also occur. Presentation with tremor confined to one limb or one side of body is common. Other findings—rigidity (flexed posture; "cogwheeling" to passive limb movements), bradykinesia (slowness of voluntary movements), fixed expressionless face (facial masking) with reduced blinking, hypophonic voice, drooling, impaired rapid alternating movements, micrographia (small handwriting), reduced arm swing, flexed posture with walking, shuffling gait, difficulty initiating or stopping walking, en-bloc turning (multiple small steps required to turn), retropulsion (tendency to fall backwards). In advanced PD—intellectual deterioration, aspiration pneumonia, and bedsores (due to immobility) common. Normal muscular strength, deep tendon reflexes and sensory exam. Diagnosis based upon history and examination; neuroimaging, EEG, and CSF studies usually normal.

Etiology

Degeneration of pigmented pars compacta neurons of the substantia nigra in the midbrain, which provide dopaminergic input to striatum; accumulation of eosinophilic intraneural inclusion granules (Lewy bodies). Cause of cell death is unknown but may result from generation of free radicals and oxidative stress, perhaps by oxidation of dopamine itself.

Differential Diagnosis

Features of parkinsonism may occur with: depression (paucity of vocal inflection and facial movement); essential tremor (tremor worse with limbs held against gravity; head tremor common; improves with alcohol intake); normal-pressure hydrocephalus (apraxic gait, urinary incontinence, dementia); Wilson's disease (early age of onset, Kayser-Fleischer rings, low serum copper, low ceruloplasmin); Huntington's disease (positive family history, chorea, dementia); drug use (phenothiazines, MPTP); carbon monoxide or manganese poisoning; other degenerations (progressive supranuclear palsy, olivopontocerebellar atrophy, cortical-basal ganglionic degeneration, striatonigral degeneration).

℞ TREATMENT

Exclude other causes of parkinsonism prior to initiating treatment. Goal of treatment is to restore function (i.e., reduce disabling tremor) and not only to lessen clinical signs. Sinemet is the mainstay of treatment in most cases; it is composed of levodopa, the metabolic precurser of dopamine, combined with an extracerebral inhibitor of dopa decarboxylase. A summary of drugs for PD is listed in Table 180-1; an algorithmic approach to management is shown in Fig. 368-1 (HPIM-14, p. 2357). Amantadine is useful for mild symptoms and acts by potentiating release of endogenous dopamine. Tremor responds best to anticholinergic drugs. Sinemet is most helpful for bradykinesia. Late complications: (1) end-dose phenomenon—deterioration shortly before next dose, and (2) on-off phenomenon—abrupt, transient fluctuations without warning or obvious relationship to dosing. On-off may be partially controlled by reducing dosing intervals, restricting dietary protein, and administering levodopa 1 h prior to meals. Response fluctuations to oral levodopa may be reduced by frequent dosing, continuous gastric infusion or parenteral administration. Dopamine agonist drugs (bromocriptine, pergolide) are useful adjuncts to Sinemet. Selegiline, an inhibitor of monoamine oxidase B, may reduce oxidative damage and slow disease progression; its effect, however, is uncertain, and recent safety concerns have been raised. In refractory cases, unilateral pallidotomy may be effective in relieving signs of PD on contralateral side.

Table 180-1

Doses of Drugs Used in Parkinson's Disease

Drug	Trade Name	Dose	Side Effects
Trihexyphe-nidyl	Artane	2–5 mg tid	Dry mouth, blurred vision, confusion
Benztropine	Cogentin	0.5–2 mg tid	Dry mouth, confusion
Carbidopa/levodopa	Sinemet	10/100 to 25/250 mg; increase slowly to tid or qid	Orthostatic hypotension, GI complaints, hallucinations, confusion, chorea, dyskinesias
Amantadine	Symmetrel	100 mg bid	Depression, postural hypotension, psychosis, urinary retention
Bromocriptine	Parlodel	7.5–30 mg daily in divided doses	Postural hypotension, nausea and vomiting, hallucinations, psychosis, dyskinesias
Pergolide	Permax	0.05–3 mg daily in divided doses	Nausea, dizziness, hallucinations, confusion, constipation, postural hypotension, dyskinesias
Selegiline	Eldepryl	5 mg bid	Nausea, dizziness, confusion, hallucinations

For a more detailed discussion, see Aminoff MJ: Parkinson's Disease and Other Extrapyramidal Disorders, Chap. 368, p. 2356, in HPIM-14.

ATAXIC DISORDERS

Clinical Presentation

Various combinations of gait instability, nystagmus, dysarthria (scanning speech), impaired limb coordination, intention tremor (i.e., with movement), hypotonia. *Differential diagnosis:* Vertigo can resemble gait instability of cerebellar disease but produces sensation of head movement in space. Sensory deficits, in particular with neuropathies (Fisher variant of Guillain Barré syndrome), can simulate cerebellar limb ataxia.

_____ *Approach to the Patient* _____

Causes are best grouped by determining whether the ataxia is symmetric or asymmetric and by its time course (Table 181-1). It is also important to distinguish whether ataxia is present in isolation or is part of a multisystem neurologic disorder. Acute symmetric ataxia is usually due to medications (phenytoin), toxins (ethanol, mercury), viral infection, or a postinfectious syndrome (especially varicella). Unilateral ataxia suggests a focal lesion in the ipsilateral cerebellar hemisphere or its connections. Subacute or chronic symmetric ataxia can result from hypothyroidism, vitamin deficiencies [B$_1$ (thiamine), B$_{12}$, E], infections (Lyme disease, tabes dorsalis from syphilis), alcohol, and other toxins. Progressive nonfamilial cerebellar ataxia after age 45 suggests a paraneoplastic syndrome, either subacute cortical cerebellar degeneration (ovarian, breast, small cell lung, Hodgkin's) or opsoclonus-myoclonus (neuroblastoma, breast). An important cause of acute unilateral ataxia is cerebrovascular disease. Cerebellar hemorrhage, or swelling from an ischemic cerebellar infarction, can compress brainstem structures, producing altered consciousness and ipsilateral pontine signs (small pupil, lateral gaze or sixth nerve paresis, facial weakness); limb ataxia may not be prominent. Other focal lesions that produce unilateral or asymmetric ataxia include tumors, multiple sclerosis, progressive multifocal encephalopathy (immunodeficiency states), or congenital malformations.

Inherited Ataxias

May be autosomal dominant, autosomal recessive, or mitochondrial (maternal inheritance); 18 different disorders recognized. Friedreich's ataxia is most common; autosomal recessive; ataxia with areflexia, upgoing toes, vibration and position sense deficits, cardiomyopathy, hammer toes, scoliosis; linked to expanded trinucleotide repeat in intron of "frataxin" gene; a second

Table 181-1

Etiology of Cerebellar Ataxia

Acute (Hours to Days)	Subacute (Days to Weeks)	Chronic (Months to Years)
SYMMETRIC SIGNS		
Alcohol, lithium, diphenylhydantoin, barbiturates (positive history and toxicology screen) Acute viral cerebellitis (CSF supportive of acute viral infection) Postinfection syndrome	Intoxication: mercury, solvents, gasoline, glue; cytotoxic chemotherapeutic drugs Alcoholic-nutritional (vitamin B_1 and B_{12} deficiency) Lyme disease	Paraneoplastic syndrome Hypothyroidism Inherited diseases Tabes dorsalis (tertiary syphilis)
ASYMMETRIC SIGNS		
Vascular: Cerebellar infarction, hemorrhage, or subdural hematoma Infectious: cerebellar abscess (positive mass lesion on MRI/CT, positive history in support of lesion)	Neoplastic: cerebellar glioma or metastatic tumor (positive for neoplasm on MRI/CT) Demyelinating: Multiple sclerosis (history, CSF and MRI are consistent) AIDS-related progressive multifocal leukoencephalopathy (positive HIV test and CD4+ cell count for AIDS)	Stable gliosis secondary to vascular lesion or demyelinating plaque (stable lesion on MRI/CT older than several months) Congenital lesion: Dandy-Walker or Arnold-Chiari malformations (malformation noted on MRI/CT)

SOURCE: Modified from Rosenberg RN: HPIM-14, p. 2363.

genetic form of Friedreich's is associated with vitamin E deficiency. Common dominantly inherited ataxias are spinocerebellar ataxia (SCA) 1 (olivopontocerebellar degeneration; "ataxin-1" gene) and SCA 3 (Machado-Joseph disease); both present with ataxia and brainstem and extrapyramidal signs, and SCA 3 may also have dystonia and amyotrophy; genes for each disorder contain unstable trinucleotide repeats in coding region.

Evaluation

For symmetric ataxias, drug and toxic screens; vitamin B_1, B_{12}, and E levels; thyroid function tests; antibody tests for syphilis and Lyme infection; paraneoplastic autoantibodies (anti-Yo, anti-Ri, anti-Hu); and CSF studies often indicated. Genetic testing is available for many inherited ataxias but should be carried out only with genetic counseling. For unilateral or asymmetric ataxias, MRI or CT scan is the initial test of choice.

℞ TREATMENT

Hypothyroidism, vitamin deficiency, infectious and parainfectious causes of ataxia are treatable. With paraneoplastic ataxias, identification of underlying cancer is important for pt, but as a rule ataxia does not improve following treatment of tumor. Cerebellar hemorrhage and many other mass lesions of the posterior fossa are surgically treated.

For a more detailed discussion, see Rosenberg RN: Ataxic Disorders, Chap. 369, p. 2363, in HPIM-14.

182

MOTOR NEURON DISEASE, INCLUDING ALS

Etiology

Disorders caused by degeneration of motor neurons at all levels of the CNS including anterior horns of the spinal cord, brainstem motor nuclei, and motor cortex. Familial amyotrophic lateral sclerosis (FALS) represents 5–10% of the total and is inherited as an autosomal dominant disorder. Syndromes clinically indistinguishable from classic ALS may result rarely from intoxication with mercury, lead, or aluminum and in hyperparathyroidism, thyrotoxicosis, immunologic or paraneoplastic mechanisms, and hereditary biochemical disorders. Tumors near the foramen magnum, high spinal cord tumors, cervical spondylosis, chronic polyradiculopathies, polymyositis, spinal muscle atrophies, and diabetic, syphilitic, and postpolio amyotrophies can all produce signs and symptoms similar to those seen in ALS and should be carefully considered in differential diagnosis (see Table 182-1).

Clinical History

Onset is usually midlife, with most cases progressing to death in 3–5 years. Common initial symptoms are weakness, muscle wasting, stiffness and cramping, and twitching in muscles of hands and arms. Legs are less severely involved than arms, with complaints of leg stiffness, cramping, and weakness common. Symptoms of brainstem involvement include dysarthria and dysphagia.

Physical Examination

Lower motor neuron disease results in weakness and wasting that often first involves intrinsic hand muscles but later becomes generalized. Fasciculations occur in involved muscles, and fibrillations may be seen in the tongue. Hyperreflexia, spasticity, and upgoing toes in weak, atrophic limbs provide evidence of upper motor neuron disease. Brainstem disease produces wasting of the tongue, difficulty in articulation, phonation, and deglutition, and pseudobulbar palsy (e.g., involuntary laughter, crying). Important additional features that characterize ALS are preservation of intellect, lack of sensory abnormalities, and absence of bowel or bladder dysfunction.

Laboratory Findings

EMG provides objective evidence of muscle denervation, as well as of involvement of muscles innervated by different pe-

Table 182-1

Etiology and Investigation of Motor Neuron Disorders

Diagnostic Categories	Investigations
Structural lesions	MRI scan of head (including
Parasagittal or foramen magnum tumors	foramen magnum), cervical spine
Cervical spondylosis	
Chiari malformation or syrinx	
Spinal cord arteriovenous malformation	
Infections	CSF exam, culture
Bacterial—tetanus, Lyme	Lyme antibody titer
Viral—poliomyelitis, herpes zoster	Antiviral antibody titers
Retroviral myelopathy	HTLV-I titer
Intoxications, physical agents	
Toxins—lead, aluminum, other metals	24-h urine for heavy metals
	Serum and urine for lead, aluminum
Drugs—strychnine, phenytoin	
Electric shock, x-irradiation	
Immunologic mechanisms	Complete blood count
Plasma cell dyscrasias	Sedimentation rate
Autoimmune polyradiculoneuropathy	Immunoprotein electrophoresis
Paraneoplastic	Anti-GM$_1$ antibodies
Paracarcinomatous/ lymphoma	Anti-Hu antibody
	MRI scan, bone marrow biopsy
Metabolic	
Hypoglycemia	Fasting blood sugar (FBS), routine chemistries including calcium
Hyperparathyroidism	Thyroid functions
Hyperthyroidism	
Deficiency of folate, vitamins B$_{12}$, E, and folate	Vitamin B$_{12}$, folate levels
Malabsorption	24-h stool fat, carotene, prothrombin time

(*continued*)

Table 182-1 (*Continued*)

Etiology and Investigation of Motor Neuron Disorders

Diagnostic Categories	Investigations
Hereditary biochemical disorders	
Superoxide dismutase 1 mutation	White blood cell DNA analysis
Androgen receptor defect (Kennedy's disease)	Abnormal CAG insert in androgen receptor gene
Hexosaminidase deficiency	Lysosomal enzyme screen
Infantile α-glucosidase deficiency (Pompe's disease)	
Hyperlipidemia	Lipid electrophoresis
Hyperglycinuria	Urine and serum amino acids
Methylcrotonylglycinuria	CSF amino acids

SOURCE: Brown RH Jr: HPIM-14, p. 2370.

ripheral nerves and nerve roots. Myelography, CT, or MRI may be useful to exclude compressive lesions. CSF is normal. Muscle enzymes (e.g., CK) may be elevated. Serum antibodies to the gangliosides GM_1 and GD_{1b} have been reported in a variable percentage of pts. Pulmonary function studies may aid in management of ventilation. Useful tests to exclude other diseases can include urine and serum screens for heavy metals, thyroid functions, serum immunoelectrophoresis, lysosomal enzyme screens, B_{12} levels, VDRL, CBC, ESR, and serum chemistries. In FALS, one subset have mutations in the gene encoding the cytosolic enzyme superoxide dismutase 1 (SOD1).

Complications

Weakness of ventilatory muscles leads to respiratory insufficiency; dysphagia may result in aspiration pneumonia and compromised energy intake.

℞ TREATMENT

There is no treatment capable of arresting ALS. The drug riluzole produces modest lengthening of survival. It may act by diminishing glutamate release and thereby decreasing excitotoxic neuronal cell death. Several types of secondary motor neuron disorders which resemble ALS are treatable (Table 182-1). All pts should have a careful search for these disorders. A number of motor neuron tropic factors have recently been cloned and biologically characterized. Several are currently undergoing clinical trials for treatment of ALS, but none have yet been found to be of substantial benefit. Supportive care can include home care ventilation and pulmonary support; speech therapy; nonverbal, electronic, or mechanical communication systems for anarthric patients; and dietary management to ensure adequate energy intake. Attention to use of rehabilitative devices (braces, splints, canes, walkers, mechanized wheelchairs) is essential to improve care.

For a more detailed discussion, see Brown RH Jr: Motor Neuron Diseases, Chap. 370, p. 2368, in HPIM-14.

183

APHASIA

Definition

Aphasias are disturbances in the comprehension or production of spoken or written language. Aphasias may be classified based on their clinical manifestations, the anatomic location of the underlying lesion, their etiology, and associated clinical symptoms (see Table 183-1).

Global Aphasia

ETIOLOGY   Occlusion of internal carotid artery (ICA) or middle cerebral artery (MCA) supplying dominant hemisphere (less commonly hemorrhage, trauma, or tumor), resulting in a large lesion of frontal, parietal, and superior temporal lobes.

CLINICAL MANIFESTATIONS   All aspects of speech and language are impaired. Pt cannot read, write, or repeat and has poor auditory comprehension. Speech output is minimal and nonfluent. Usually hemiplegia, hemisensory loss, and homonymous hemianopia are present.

Table 183-1

Clinical Features of Aphasias and Related Conditions

	Comprehension	Repetition of Spoken Language	Naming	Fluency
Wernicke's	Impaired	Impaired	Impaired	Preserved or increased
Broca's	Preserved (except grammar)	Impaired	Impaired	Decreased
Global	Impaired	Impaired	Impaired	Decreased
Conduction	Preserved	Impaired	Impaired	Preserved
Nonfluent (motor) transcortical	Preserved	Preserved	Impaired	Impaired
Fluent (sensory) transcortical	Impaired	Preserved	Impaired	Preserved
Isolation	Impaired	Echolalia	Impaired	No purposeful speech
Anomic	Preserved	Preserved	Impaired	Preserved except for word-finding pauses
Pure word deafness	Impaired only for spoken language	Impaired	Preserved	Preserved
Pure alexia	Impaired only for reading	Preserved	Preserved	Preserved

SOURCE: Mesulam M-M: HPIM-14, p. 136.

1054

Broca's Aphasia (Motor or Nonfluent Aphasia)

ETIOLOGY Core lesion involves dominant inferior frontal convolution (Broca's area), although cortical and subcortical areas along superior sylvian fissure and insula are often involved. Commonly caused by vascular lesions involving the superior division of the MCA, less commonly due to tumor, abscess, metastasis, subdural hematoma, encephalitis.

CLINICAL MANIFESTATIONS Speech output is sparse, slow, effortful, dysmelodic, poorly articulated, and telegraphic. Most pts have severe writing impairment. Comprehension of written and spoken language is relatively preserved. Pt is aware of and visibly frustrated by deficit.

With large lesions, a dense hemiparesis may occur, and the eyes may deviate toward side of lesion. More commonly, lesser degrees of contralateral face and arm weakness are present. Sensory loss is rarely found, and visual fields are intact. Bucco-lingual apraxia is common, the pt having difficulty imitating movements with tongue and lips or performing these movements on command. An apraxia involving the ipsilateral hand may occur due to involvement of fibers in the corpus callosum.

Wernicke's Aphasia (Sensory or Fluent Aphasia)

ETIOLOGY Embolic occlusion of inferior division of dominant MCA (less commonly hemorrhage, tumor, encephalitis, or abscess) involving posterior perisylvian region.

CLINICAL MANIFESTATIONS Although speech sounds grammatical, melodic, and effortless ("fluent"), it is often virtually incomprehensible due to errors in word usage, structure, and tense and the presence of neologisms and paraphasia. Comprehension of written and spoken material is severely impaired, as are reading, writing, and repetition. Pt seems unaware of deficit. Associated clinical symptoms can include parietal lobe sensory deficits and homonymous hemianopia. Motor disturbances are rare.

Conduction Aphasia

Comprehension of speech and writing is largely intact, and speech output is fluent, although paraphasia is common. *Repetition is severely affected.* Most cases are due to lesions involving supramarginal gyrus of dominant parietal lobe, dominant superior temporal lobe, or arcuate fasciculus. Lesions are typically due to an embolus to either the ascending parietal or posterior temporal branch of the dominant MCA. Associated symptoms include contralateral hemisensory loss and hemianopia.

Pure Word Deafness

Almost total lack of auditory comprehension with inability to repeat or write to dictation and relatively preserved spoken language and spontaneous writing. Comprehension of visual or written material is superior to that of auditory information. The lesion(s) are typically in or near the primary auditory cortex (Heschl's gyrus) in the superior temporal gyrus. Causes are infarction, hemorrhage, or tumor.

Pure Word Blindness

Inability to read and often to name colors with preserved speech fluency, language comprehension, repetition, and writing to dictation (alexia without agraphia). Lesion usually involves left occipitostriate cortex and visual association areas as well as fibers in splenium of corpus callosum connecting right and left visual association areas. Most pts have an associated right homonymous hemianopia, hemisensory deficit, and memory disturbance due to vascular lesions involving the left posterior cerebral artery (PCA) territory. Rarely, tumor or hemorrhage may be the cause.

Isolation of Speech Area

Hypotension, ischemia, or hypoxia may result in borderzone infarctions between the anterior cerebral–MCA–PCA territories that spare the sylvian region of the MCA. Pts are severely brain damaged and have parrot-like repetition of spoken words (echolalia) with little or no spontaneous speech or comprehension.

Laboratory Studies in Aphasia

CT scan or MRI usually identify the location and nature of the causative lesion. Angiography helps in accurate definition of specific vascular syndromes.

℞ TREATMENT

Speech therapy may be helpful in treatment of certain types of aphasia.

For a more detailed discussion, see Mesulam M-M: Aphasias and Other Focal Cerebral Disorders, Chap. 25, p. 134, in HPIM-14.

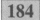

184

CRANIAL NERVE DISORDERS

OLFACTORY NERVE (I)

The sense of smell may be impaired by (1) interference with access of odorant to olfactory neuroepithelium (*transport loss*), e.g., by swollen nasal mucous membrane in URI, allergic rhinitis, or structural changes in naval cavity such as with a deviated septum, nasal polyps, or neoplasm; (2) injury to receptor region (*sensory loss*), e.g., destruction of olfactory neuroepithelium by viral infections, neoplasma, inhalation of toxic chemicals, or radiation to head; and (3) damage to central olfactory pathways (*neural loss*), e.g., by head trauma with or without fractures of cribriform plate, neoplasms of anterior cranial fossa, neurosurgical procedures, neurotoxic drugs, or congenital disorders such as Kallmann's syndrome.

OPTIC NERVE (II)

Visual disturbances may be localized upon examination of globe, retina, or optic disc or may require careful visual field testing to pinpoint. Retinal lesions cause arcuate, central, or centrocecal scotomas. Chiasmal lesions produce bitemporal hemianopias. Homonymous hemianopias arise behind the chiasm and, if complete, are of no further localizing value. When incomplete, an incongruous homonymous hemianopia suggests a lesion in the tract or radiations (tract lesions may have associated optic atrophy and an afferent pupillary defect, whereas pupils in postgeniculate lesions are normal). A congruous (identical) homonymous hemianopia implies a lesion in calcarine cortex.

AQUEOUS HUMOR AND GLAUCOMA Glaucoma is a condition in which elevated intraocular pressure (>22 mmHg) transmitted through aqueous humor damages the optic nerve. It is the leading cause of blindness in the United States.

Open-Angle Glaucoma Rarely causes ocular pain or corneal edema. Visual loss occurs first in the periphery, and visual acuity remains normal until late in the course.

℞ TREATMENT
Topical cholinergic (pilocarpine or carbachol) and beta-blocking (timolol) agents with or without carbonic anhydrase inhibitors (acetazolamide or methazolamide).

Angle-Closure Glaucoma May be precipitated by drugs to dilate the pupil. *Symptoms:* visual loss, pupillary dilation, pain, and when acute, erythema. This is a medical emergency, to be treated with IV mannitol, parenteral acetazolamide, and topical pilocarpine or timolol.

Congenital Glaucoma Rare.

Secondary Glaucoma May be associated with leukemia, sickle cell disease, Waldenström's macroglobulinemia, ankylosing spondylitis, rheumatoid arthritis, sarcoidosis, congenital rubella, onchocerciasis, amyloidosis, osteogenesis imperfecta, neoplastic metastases, neurofibromatosis, Sturge-Weber syndrome, chronic glucocorticoid use, amphetamines, hexamethonium, reserpine, anticholinergics, ocular trauma, and dislocation of the lens (homocystinuria and Marfan's syndrome).

RETINA Causes of retinal disease include *vasculopathies* associated with major medical illnesses (e.g., hypertension, diabetes mellitus); *central retinal artery occlusion* (CRA) (with boxcar segmentation of blood flow in retinal veins, milky white retina, and cherry red spot from preserved vascularity of choroid) due to emboli, temporal arteritis, arteriosclerosis, collagen-vascular disease, hyperviscosity states; *transient monocular blindness* (amaurosis fugax) due to episodic retinal ischemia, usually associated with ipsilateral carotid artery stenosis or embolism of the retinal arteries. Typically, an episode of blindness evolves swiftly (10 to 15 s) and is described as a shade that falls smoothly and painlessly over the field of vision. An altitudinal defect may be described with obliteration of vision from below. Blindness lasts seconds or minutes and then clears slowly and uniformly in reverse sequence. May be distinguished from transient blindness of classic migraine, since the latter often begins with unformed light flashes (photopsia) or zigzag lines (fortification spectra or teichopsia) moving across visual field for several minutes leaving scotomatous/hemianopic defect (although pts may report monocular symptoms). Retinal disease may also ensue from degeneration due to retinitis pigmentosa and associated multisystem diseases and toxic effects of drugs, e.g., phenothiazines or chloroquine.

OPTIC NERVE *Retrobulbar Optic Neuropathy or Optic Neuritis* Characterized by rapid development (hours to days) of impaired vision in one or both eyes, usually due to acute optic nerve demyelination. Most cases occur in childhood, adolescence, or young adulthood. Total blindness is rare. PE: acutely, optic disc and retina are normal or there is papillitis; eye movement or pressure on globe produces pain; affects central more than peripheral vision; and the pupillary light reflex is impaired (swinging flashlight test). CSF is normal or has WBCs (10–20/µL) with or without oligoclonal bands. 50% will develop signs of multiple sclerosis within 15 years. Other causes: postinfectious or disseminated encephalomyelitis, posterior uveitis, vascular lesions of the optic nerve, tumors (optic nerve glioma, neurofibromatosis, meningioma, metastases), and fungal infections.

Anterior Ischemic Optic Neuropathy (AION) Caused by atherosclerotic or inflammatory disease of ophthalmic artery or its branches. Presents as acute painless monocular visual loss with an altitudinal defect. Optic disc is pale and swollen, with splinter peripapillary hemorrhages and normal macula and retina. Evaluation should aggressively rule out temporal arteritis. Occasionally microemboli (e.g., following cardiac surgery) may cause AION.

Toxic or Nutritional Optic Neuropathy Presents as simultaneous impairment of vision in both eyes with central or centrocecal scotomas, developing over days to weeks. Agents: methyl alcohol intoxication, chloramphenicol, ethambutol, isoniazid, streptomycin, sulfonamides, digitalis, ergot, disulfiram, and heavy metal.

Bitemporal Hemianopia Caused by suprasellar extension of a pituitary tumor or saccular aneurysm of circle of Willis, tuberculum sellae meningioma, or rarely, sarcoid, metastases, and Hand-Schüller-Christian disease.

OCULOMOTOR, TROCHLEAR, AND ABDUCENS NERVES (III, IV, VI)

Isolated Third or Sixth Nerve Palsies May be due to diabetes mellitus, neoplasm, increased intracranial pressure (sixth nerve), pontine glioma in children or metastatic nasopharyngeal tumor in adults (sixth nerve), tumor at base of brain (third nerve), ischemic infarction of nerve, aneurysms in the circle of Willis. In compressive third nerve lesions, the pupil is usually dilated, whereas pupils are spared in infarction of the nerve.

Third, Fourth, and Sixth Nerve Lesions May occur at level of their nuclei, along their course from brainstem through subarachnoid space, cavernous sinus, or superior orbital fissure (see Table 184-1).

Table 184-1

Cranial Nerve Syndromes

Site	Cranial Nerves Involved	Usual Cause
Sphenoid fissure (superior orbital)	III, IV, first division V, VI	Invasive tumors of sphenoid bone, aneurysms
Lateral wall of cavernous sinus	III, IV, first division V, VI, often with proptosis	Aneurysms or thrombosis of cavernous sinus, invasive tumors from sinuses and sella turcica, sometimes benign granuloma responsive to steroids
Retrosphenoid space	II, III, IV, V, VI	Large tumors of middle cranial fossa
Apex of petrous bone	V, VI	Petrositis, tumors of petrous bone
Internal auditory meatus	VII, VIII	Tumors of petrous bone (dermoids, etc.), infectious processes, acoustic neuroma
Pontocerebellar angle	V, VII, VIII, and sometimes IX	Acoustic neuroma, meningioma
Jugular foramen	IX, X, XI	Tumors and aneurysms
Posterior latero-condylar space	IX, X, XI, XII	Tumors of parotid gland, carotid body, and metastatic tumor
Posterior retroparotid space	IX, X, XI, XII and Horner syndrome	Tumors of parotid gland, carotid body, lymph nodes; metastatic tumor; tuberculous adenitis

SOURCE: Modified from Martin JB, Beal MF: HPIM-14, p. 2380.

Tolosa-Hunt Syndrome Painful, combined unilateral palsies due to parasellar granuloma.

Pituitary Apoplexy Acute onset of uni- or bilateral ophthalmoplegia and visual field defect with headache and/or drowsiness.

Migrainous Ophthalmoplegia Attacks of ocular palsy in conjunction with typical migraine.

TRIGEMINAL NERVE (V)

Trigeminal Neuralgia (Tic Douloureaux) Frequent, excruciating paroxysms of pain in lips, gums, cheek, or chin (rarely in ophthalmic division of fifth nerve) lasting seconds to minutes. Appears in middle or old age. Pain is often stimulated at trigger points. Sensory deficit cannot be demonstrated. Must be distinguished from other forms of facial pain arising from diseases of jaw, teeth, or sinuses. Tic is rarely caused by herpes zoster or a tumor.

℞ TREATMENT

Carbamazepine (1–1.5 g qd in divided doses) is effective in 75% of cases; follow CBC for rare complications of aplastic anemia. When medications fail, surgical gangliolysis or suboccipital craniectomy for decompression of trigeminal nerve are options.

Trigeminal Neuropathy May be caused by a variety of rare conditions, usually presenting with facial sensory loss or weakness of jaw muscles. These include tumors of middle cranial fossa or trigeminal nerve, metastases to base of skull, or lesions in cavernous sinus (affecting first and second divisions of fifth nerve) or superior orbital fissure (affecting first division of fifth nerve).

FACIAL NERVE (VII)

Lesions of the seventh nerve or nucleus produce hemifacial weakness that includes muscles of forehead and orbicularis oculi; if lesion is in middle ear portion, taste is lost over the anterior two-thirds of tongue and there may be hyperacusis; if lesion is at internal auditory meatus, there may be involvement of auditory and vestibular nerves, whereas pontine lesions usually affect abducens nerve and often corticospinal tract as well. Peripheral nerve lesions with incomplete recovery may result in diffuse continuous contraction of affected facial muscles ± associated movements (synkinesis) of other facial muscle groups and facial spasms.

Bell's Palsy Most common form of idiopathic facial paralysis, found in 23/100,000 annually. Weakness evolves over 12–48 h, sometimes preceded by retroaural pain. Fully 80% recover within several weeks or months.

Rx **TREATMENT**

Involves protection of eye during sleep. Prednisone (60–80 mg qd over 5 d, tapered off over the next 5 d) may be beneficial, but this has not been firmly established.

Ramsay Hunt Syndrome   Caused by herpes zoster infection of geniculate ganglion; distinguished from Bell's palsy by a vesicular eruption in pharynx, external auditory canal, and other parts of the cranial integument.

Acoustic Neuromas   Often compress the seventh nerve.

Pontine Tumors or Infarcts   May cause a lower motor neuron facial weakness.

Bilateral Facial Diplegia   May appear in Guillain-Barré, sarcoidosis, Lyme disease, and leprosy.

Hemifacial Spasm   May appear either as a result of Bell's palsy, with irritative lesions (e.g., acoustic neuroma, basilar artery aneurysm, or aberrant vessel compressing the nerve) or as an idiopathic disorder.

Blepharospasm   Involuntary recurrent spasm of both eyelids occurring in the elderly ± facial spasm. May spontaneously subside.

Rx **TREATMENT**

In severe cases, differential facial nerve section or nerve decompression. Recently, local injection of botulinum toxin into orbicularis occuli has been effective, even with repeated treatment, without morbidity.

VESTIBULAR NERVE (VIII)

Vertigo due to a lesion in the vestibular component of N. VIII is discussed in Chap. 10. Lesions of the auditory nerve cause hearing impairment which can be either *conductive* caused by structural abnormalities in external auditory canal or middle ear due to tumor, infection, trauma, etc., or *sensorineural,* due to damage to hair cells of the organ of Corti secondary to excessive noise, viral infections, ototoxic drugs, temporal bone fractures, meningitis, cochlear otosclerosis, Ménière's disease, or neural damage due largely to cerebellar angle tumors or vascular, demyelinating, or degenerative diseases affecting the central auditory pathways. Brainstem auditory evoked responses (BAERs) are a sensitive and accurate test for distinguishing sensory from neural hearing losses. Audiometry can distinguish conductive from sensorineural hearing losses. Most pts with conductive and asymmetric sensorineural hearing losses should have CT scans of the temporal bone. Sensorineural hearing losses should be evaluated with electronystagmography and caloric testing.

GLOSSOPHARYNGEAL NERVE (IX)

Glossopharyngeal Neuralgia Paroxysmal, intense pain in tonsillar fossa of throat that may be precipitated by swallowing. There is no demonstrable sensory or motor deficit. Other diseases affecting this nerve include herpes zoster or compressive neuropathy when found in conjunction with vagus and accessory nerve palsies due to tumor or aneurysm in region of jugular foramen.

℞ TREATMENT

Carbamazepine or phenytoin is often effective, but surgical division of the ninth nerve near the medulla is sometimes necessary.

VAGUS NERVE (X)

Lesions of vagus nerve cause symptoms of dysphagia and dysphonia. Unilateral lesions produce drooping of soft palate, loss of gag reflex, and "curtain movement" of lateral wall of pharynx with hoarse, nasal voice. Diseases that may involve the vagus include diphtheria (toxin), neoplastic and infectious processes at the meningeal level, tumors and vascular lesions in the medulla, or compression of the recurrent laryngeal nerve by intrathoracic processes.

HYPOGLOSSAL NERVE (XII)

The twelfth cranial nerve supplies the ipsilateral muscles of the tongue. Lesions affecting the motor nucleus may occur in the brainstem (tumor, poliomyelitis, or motor neuron disease), during the course of the nerve in the posterior fossa (platybasia, Paget's disease), or in the hypoglossal canal.

For a more detailed discussion, see Martin JB, Beal MF: Disorders of the Cranial Nerves, Chap. 372, p. 2377, in HPIM-14.

185

METABOLIC ENCEPHALOPATHY

Global disruption of brain function occurs commonly in pts with serious medical illness. Such metabolic encephalopathies usually begin with an alteration in alertness (drowsiness), followed by agitation, confusion, delirium, or psychosis, and progressing to stupor and coma. These states are discussed in Chap. 13.

Evaluation of pt requires careful physical exam for underlying structural brain lesions, CNS infection, and general medical illness. Next, blood should be drawn, glucose and naloxone administered, and electrolytes, toxic screen, CBC, and renal, liver, and thyroid functions measured. A brain CT scan is sometimes necessary to exclude mass lesions, and a CSF exam should be done to exclude meningitis or encephalitis. Common causes of metabolic encephalopathy are listed below with their salient features.

ELECTROLYTE DISORDERS

Hyponatremia is often associated with seizures if the serum Na^+ <120 mmol/L. Too rapid (>12 mmol/L in 24 h) or overcorrection of the serum Na^+ can cause central pontine myelinolysis. Extreme hyperosmolarity due to hypernatremia or hyperglycemia causes tremulousness, convulsions, and coma. Hypokalemia is associated with severe muscle weakness and confusion; hypercalcemia with inattentiveness, somnolence, and depression; hypocalcemia with paresthesia, muscular tetanus, and seizures. Acidosis also produces stupor or coma; D-lactic acidosis produces encephalopathy in pts with jejunoileal shunts.

ENDOCRINE DISORDERS

Confusional states, affective disorders, and psychosis occur in *Cushing's disease* or in pts treated with glucocorticoids. *Hyperthyroidism* can cause restlessness, insomnia, tremor, and agitated delirium. A syndrome of lethargy and depression termed *apathetic hyperthyroidism* occurs in elderly pts. Slowed mentation, depression, dementia, and coma occur in *hypothyroidism* and *Addison's disease.* An inappropriate jocularity and ataxia are sometimes seen in *hypothyroidism,* occasionally with paranoia and psychosis. *Hypoglycemia* causes convulsions and even focal neurologic findings if glucose falls below 1.4–1.7 mmol/L (25–30 mg/dL). Because of its variable clinical presentation and risk of permanent brain injury, hypoglycemia should be considered in all encephalopathies wihtout known cause. Glucose level should be determined and IV dextrose administered. Recurrent hypoglycemia as occurs with islet cell tumor may present as episodic encephalopathy.

MISCELLANEOUS ENCEPHALOPATHIES

HYPERCAPNEIC ENCEPHALOPATHY Frequently accompanied by headache, asterixis, coarse muscular twitching, and sometimes papilledema.

HEPATIC ENCEPHALOPATHY Also causes asterixis, sometimes with fluctuating rigidity; Babinski signs; and seizures. Paroxysms of triphasic slow waves may be found on the EEG. Restriction of dietary protein, oral antibiotics, acidification of colonic contents with lactulose, and treatment of infection constitute standard therapy. Chronic or recurrent hepatic encephalopathy can lead to hepatocerebral degeneration. *Reye's syndrome* is a hepatic encephalopathy seen in children; it is characterized by brain swelling.

ANOXIC-ISCHEMIC ENCEPHALOPATHY Occurs after insults severe enough to cause loss of consciousness; commonly seen after cardiorespiratory failure or arrest, CO poisoning, drowning, and asphyxia. If extreme and sustained, permanent brain injury will result. If brainstem reflexes and spontaneous respirations return promptly, full recovery can occur. Incomplete recovery results in the postanoxic syndromes, i.e., persistent vegetative state, dementia, parkinsonism, cerebellar ataxia, intention myoclonus, Korsakoff's amnesia. Occasionally, delayed cerebral degeneration occurs weeks after an initial recovery from an anoxic insult, especially in CO poisoning.

RENAL DISEASE With uremia, leads to apathy, inattentiveness, and irritability, progressing to delirium and stupor. There is usually myoclonus or seizures. Episodic encephalopathy with seizures, muscle cramps, and headache sometimes complicates rapid dialysis. Dialysis dementia with prominent dysarthria, myoclonus, psychosis, and motor aphasia may be related to aluminum in the dialysate passing into the bloodstream.

HYPERTENSIVE ENCEPHALOPATHY With headache, retinopathy, seizure, and posterior cerebral white matter edema; can complicate pregnancy, renal failure, pheochromocytoma, or primary hypertension. A similar disorder occurs as an adverse reaction to cyclosporine.

NUTRITIONAL ENCEPHALOPATHIES Occur in patients with B_{12}, thiamine, niacin, nicotinic acid, or pyridoxine deficiency. Peripheral neuropathy, spinal cord dysfunction, and mucocutaneous abnormalities are frequent accompaniments. Wernicke's encephalopathy is associated with diplopia, nystagmus, and ataxia. Early treatment with thiamine can prevent a permanent Korsakoff's amnestic state. The encephalopathy of B_{12} deficiency occasionally simulates dementia.

TOXIC ENCEPHALOPATHIES   A recent onset of an encephalopathic condition should lead to blood and urine screening for narcotics, salicylates, hypnotics, antidepressants, phenothiazines, lithium, anticonvulsants, amphetamines, alcohol, arsenic, lead, bismuth, and carbon monoxide.

OTHERS   Illnesses that can present as encephalopathy include bacterial endocarditis, thrombotic thrombocytopenic purpura, multiple fat or air emboli, typhoid fever, AIDS, multiple intracerebral metastases, hepatic porphyria, collagen-vascular disorders, and hyperproliferative hematologic disorders.

For a more detailed dicussion, see Martin JB, Beal MF: Nutritional and Metabolic Diseases of the Nervous System, Chap. 380, p. 2451, in HPIM-14.

186

DISORDERS OF THE AUTONOMIC NERVOUS SYSTEM

The regulation of homeostatic functions is accomplished by the autonomic nervous system (ANS). The ANS regulates physiologic processes critical to survival including blood pressure, blood flow and tissue perfusion; sweating, hunger and satiety; and temperature, thirst, and circadian rhythms. The importance of this regulation is demonstrated by the severity of disability resulting from compromised ANS function.

ANS OVERVIEW

Key features of the ANS are summarized in Table 186-1. Responses to sympathetic (S) or parasympathetic (P) activation often have opposite effects; partial activation of both systems allows for simultaneous integration of multiple body functions. The postganglionic sympathetic input to sweat glands and the adrenal medulla is cholinergic.

Catecholamines exert their effects on two types of receptors, alpha and beta. The alpha$_1$ receptor mediates vasoconstriction. The alpha$_2$ receptor mediates presynaptic inhibition of norepinephrine (NE) release from adrenergic nerves, inhibits acetylcholine (ACh) release from cholinergic nerves, inhibits lipolysis in adipocytes, inhibits insulin secretion, and stimulates platelet aggregation. The beta$_1$ receptor responds to both NE and epinephrine (E) and mediates cardiac stimulation and lipolysis. The beta$_2$ receptor is more responsive to E than NE and mediates vasodilatation and bronchodilation.

Table 186-1

ANS Overview

	Sympathetic NS	Parasympathetic NS
CNS location of preganglionic neurons	C8-L1 cord segments	Brainstem and sacral spinal cord
Neurotransmitter		
Preganglionic	Acetylcholine (ACh)	ACh
Postganglionic	Norepinephrine (NE)	ACh
Mechanism of inactivation	Reuptake	Synaptic cleft metabolism

DISORDERS OF THE ANS

The CNS, peripheral nervous system, or both may be affected; disorders may be generalized, segmental, or focal. Clinical signs and symptoms are often due to interruption of the afferent limb, CNS processing centers, or efferent limb of the reflex arc controlling the autonomic responses. One classification scheme for autonomic disorders is shown in Table 186-2.

The clinical manifestations of autonomic disease are influenced by the organ involved, the normal balance of sympathetic-parasympathetic innervation, the nature of the underlying illness, and the severity and stage of disease progression. Orthostatic hypotension, a postural decrease from the supine to standing position of at least 20 mmHg in systolic or 10 mmHg in diastolic BP sustained for at least 2 min, is often the most disabling feature of autonomic dysfunction. Syncope or near-syncope results when the drop in BP impairs cerebral perfusion and metabolism. Suggestive symptoms that may appear on standing include light-headedness, dimming of vision, nausea, diminished hearing, hyperhidrosis, hypohidrosis, pallor, and weakness.

_____ *Approach to the Patient* _____

The first step in the evaluation of symptomatic orthostasis is the exclusion of treatable causes for postural hypotension. The history should include a review of pt medications (e.g., diuretics) and medical problems (e.g., diabetes). Exaggerated responses to medications may be the first sign of an underlying autonomic disorder. The relationship of symptoms to meals (splanchnic shunting of blood) and awakening in the morning (relative intravascular volume depletion) should be sought. On examination, sustained drops in systolic (>20 mmHg) or diastolic (>10 mmHg) BP after standing for at least 2 min (unassociated with an appropriate increase in pulse rate) are suggestive for an autonomic deficit. Neurologic evaluation should include an examination of mental status (e.g., neurodegenerative disorders), cranial nerves (e.g., impaired downgaze with progressive supranuclear palsy), motor function (e.g., parkinsonian syndromes), and sensory function (e.g., polyneuropathy). Disorders of autonomic function need to be considered in the differential diagnosis of pts with symptoms of impotence, bladder dysfunction (urinary frequency, hesitancy, or incontinence), diarrhea, constipation, or altered sweating (hyperhidrosis or hypohidrosis).

Autonomic Testing

The functional characteristics of the ANS can be assessed by physiologic and pharmacologic tests. The most commonly used

Table 186-2

Classification of ANS Disorders

GENERALIZED ANS DISORDERS

With CNS signs
    Multiple system atrophy
        Shy-Drager syndrome
        Olivopontocerebellar degeneration
        Striatonigral degeneration
    Parkinson's disease
    Huntington's disease
    Hypothalamic disorders
Without CNS signs
    Pure autonomic failure (Bradbury and Eggleston)
    Guillain-Barré syndrome (occasionally accompanied by
      CNS signs)
    Chronic idiopathic anhidrosis
    Postural orthostatic tachycardia syndrome (POTS)
    Raynaud's syndrome
    Familial dysautonomia—Riley-Day syndrome

SEGMENTAL ANS DISORDERS

Diabetes mellitus
Spinal cord and root disorders
Peripheral neuropathy (amyloidosis, porphyria, alcoholism)
Guillain-Barré syndrome
Tabes dorsalis
Lambert-Eaton syndrome
Postprandial hypotension

FOCAL ANS DISORDERS

Reflex sympathetic dystrophy
    Shoulder-hand syndrome
    Causalgia
Horner's syndrome
Reinnervation anomalies
    "Crocodile" tears

physiologic tests assess autonomic aspects of cardiovascular function; they are noninvasive, easy to administer, and provide quantitative information about autonomic function. However, interpretation of physiologic test results requires collection of data under the same circumstances as normal control data. Heart rate variation with deep breathing is a measure of vagal function and is abolished by the administration of atropine. The Valsalva response assesses the afferent limb, central integrity, and efferent limb of the baroreceptor reflex arc. A constant expiratory pressure of 40 mmHg is maintained for 15 s while measuring changes in heart rate and blood pressure. The Valsalva ratio is the maximum heart rate during the maneuver divided by the minimum heart rate following the maneuver. The ratio reflects the integrity of the entire baroreceptor reflex arc and sympathetic efferents to blood vessels (see Chap. 371, HPIM-14). Tilt-table beat-to-beat BP measurements in the supine, 80° tilt, and tilt-back positions can be used to evaluate orthostatic failure in BP control and pts with unexplained syncope.

Other physiologic tests of autonomic function include the quantitative sudomotor axon reflex test (QSART), the thermoregulatory sweat test (TST), and the cold pressor test. The QSART provides a quantitative, regional measure of sweating in response to iontophoresis of ACh. The TST provides a qualitative measure of regional sweating over the entire anterior surface of the body in response to an elevation of body temperature. The cold pressor test is used to assess sympathetic efferent function. For a more complete discussion of autonomic function testing, see Chap. 371, HPIM-14.

SPECIFIC SYNDROMES OF ANS DYSFUNCTION   Diseases of the CNS may cause ANS dysfunction at the level of the hypothalamus, brainstem, or spinal cord (see Table 186-1). Multiple system atrophy (MSA) refers to several overlapping CNS syndromes with a variable combination of symptoms and signs including postural hypotension, impotence, bladder and bowel dysfunction, defective sweating, rigidity, tremor, loss of associative movements, or abnormal eye movements. Pts may present with one symptom or sign (e.g., postural hypotension) and only later develop the full clinical spectrum of MSA. Spinal cord injury may be accompanied by autonomic hyperreflexia affecting bowel, bladder, sexual, temperature regulation, and cardiovascular functions. Dangerous increases or decreases in body temperature may result from the inability to experience the sensory accompaniments of heat or cold exposure below the level of the injury. Markedly increased autonomic discharge (autonomic dysreflexia) can be elicited by bladder pressure or stimulation of the skin or muscles. Bladder distention from palpation, catheter insertion, catheter obstruction, or urinary infection are common and correctable causes of autonomic dysreflexia.

Peripheral neuropathies are the most common cause of

chronic autonomic insufficiency (see Chap. 371, HPIM-14). Autonomic involvement in diabetes may begin at any stage in the disease and often presents with asymptomatic, abnormal vagal function (detectable as reduced heart rate variation with deep breathing). Diabetic enteric neuropathy may result in gastroparesis, nausea and vomiting, malnutrition, and bowel incontinence. Impotence, urinary incontinence, pupillary abnormalities, and postural hypotension may occur as well. Prolongation of the QT interval may occur and enhances the risk of sudden death. The cause of the neuropathy in diabetes is unknown. Autonomic neuropathy occurs in both sporadic and familial forms of amyloidosis. Pts may present with a distal, painful polyneuropathy. Cardiac or renal impairment are the usual causes of death. Alcoholic polyneuropathy results in clinical symptoms of autonomic failure only when the signs of peripheral neuropathy are severe. Blood pressure fluctuation and cardiac arrhythmias can be severe in Guillain-Barré syndrome. The importance of postprandial hypotension among healthy elderly persons and hypertensive pts taking BP medications with meals is drawing increasing attention.

REFLEX SYMPATHETIC DYSTROPHY (RSD) AND CAUSALGIA The role of the ANS in RSD and causalgia is controversial. The lack of an accepted pathogenetic mechanism for these disorders has resulted in a proposed change in nomenclature. Complex regional pain syndrome (CRPS) type I and CRPS type II have been substituted for the terms RSD and causalgia, respectively.

In causalgia, spontaneous pain develops within the territory of an injured nerve and may spread outside, but contiguous to, the distribution of the affected nerve. Allodynia (the perception of a nonpainful stimulus as painful) and hyperpathia (an exaggerated pain response to a mildly painful stimulus) are common. RSD is a regional pain syndrome that develops after trauma. Unlike causalgia, limb symptoms are not confined to the distribution of a single peripheral nerve. Although pain is the primary feature of both causalgia and RSD, there must be vasomotor, sudomotor, or edematous changes to satisfy criteria for diagnosis. Treatment of both disorders is a difficult therapeutic challenge.

℞ **TREATMENT**

In most conditions, management of autonomic failure is limited to alleviating the disability caused by the symptoms. A review of pt medications, relationship of symptoms to meals, pt medical illnesses, and other symptoms of possible autonomic origin is mandatory. Orthostatic hypotension requires treatment only if it causes symptoms. In the early stages, pts can maintain normal function by using simple measures. Alcohol intake and exposure to excessive environmental temperature should be avoided because vaosdilatation can suddenly lower BP. Drugs that affect BP should be used with great caution. Salt intake should be increased to the maximum tolerated. Sleeping in reverse Trendelenburg position (head-up tilt) minimizes supine hypertension. Frequent, small meals are better tolerated by pts with postprandial hypotension. Most eventually require drug therapy for the management of hypotension. Fludrocortisone is the initial drug of choice. Potassium supplements are necessary with chronic administration. Other pharmacologic agents have been used with variable success to elevate BP, but the supine hypertension seen in many pts with autonomic failure often limits pharmacotherapy. Anesthetic management poses unique problems since pts may have abnormal baroreceptor reflexes, sympathetic innervation of peripheral arterioles, abnormal fluid balance, and adrenal medullary insufficiency.

For a more detailed discussion, see Engstrom JW, Martin JB: Disorders of the Autonomic Nervous System, Chap. 371, p. 2372, in HPIM-14.

DISORDERS OF SLEEP AND CIRCADIAN RHYTHMS

Disorders of sleep and wakefulness are among the most common problems seen by clinicians. One-third of adults experience occasional or persistent insomnia. Sleep disruption produced by sleep apnea syndromes, periodic limb movement disorders, and other medical conditions often produces serious impairment of daytime wakefulness and functioning. Recent understanding of the physiology of sleep and wakefulness, the characterization of a number of sleep disorder syndromes, the acceptance of both in-laboratory and ambulatory polysomnography as a clinical tool, and the development of a nosology of sleep disorders (see Table 187-1) have established sleep medicine as a discipline and medical specialty.

Normal Sleep and Wakefulness

Most adults sleep 7–8 h per night in one consolidated period. In some cultures, a shortened nighttime sleep is accompanied by a midafternoon nap. Frequent interruptions of sleep are present in infants and the elderly. Two systems govern the sleep-wake cycle: one that generates sleep and sleep-associated events and the other a circadian pacemaker that times sleep within the 24-h cycle.

Polysomnography is the recording of EEG, EMG, eye movements, oxygen saturation, respiratory effort, air flow, leg movements, body position, and occasionally transesophageal thoracic pressure and infrared videotaping. The initial three parameters define two types of sleep: rapid eye movement (REM) and non-rapid eye movement (NREM) sleep. NREM sleep is further divided into stages 1–4, characterized by increasing arousal thresholds and EEG slowing. REM sleep, also known as "paradoxical sleep," demonstrates a low-voltage, high-frequency EEG resembling the awake EEG but with absent somatic EMG activity and with bursts of rapid eye movements.

The normal nightly sleep architecutre consists of sleep cycles of NREM stages 1–4 within 45 to 60 min, followed by REM sleep. NREM and REM alternate throughout the night with an average period of 90 to 110 min. The architecture of sleep may be altered by endogenous depression, narcolepsy, circadian rhythm disorders, or drug withdrawal; other sleep pathologies, prior sleep history, and normal aging may also distort the sleep patterns.

Table 187-1

International Classification of Sleep Disorders

I. Dyssomnias
    A. Intrinsic sleep disorders
        1. Psychophysiologic insomnia
        2. Idiopathic insomnia
        3. Narcolepsy
        4. Sleep apnea syndromes
        5. Periodic limb movement disorder
        6. Restless legs syndrome
    B. Extrinsic sleep disorders
        1. Inadequate sleep hygiene
        2. Altitude insomnia
        3. Drug- or alcohol-dependent sleep disorders
    C. Circadian rhythm sleep disorders
        1. Time-zone change (jet-lag) syndrome
        2. Shift-work sleep disorder
        3. Delayed sleep phase syndrome
        4. Advanced sleep phase syndrome
II. Parasomnias
    A. Arousal disorders
        1. Confusional arousals
        2. Sleepwalking
        3. Sleep terrors
    B. Sleep-wake transition disorders
        1. Sleep talking
        2. Nocturnal leg cramps
    C. Parasomnias usually associated with REM sleep
        1. Nightmares
        2. Sleep paralysis
        3. Impaired sleep-related penile erections
        4. Sleep-related painful erections
    D. Other parasomnias
        1. Sleep bruxism
        2. Sleep enuresis
III. Sleep disorders associated with medical/psychiatric disorders
    A. Associated with mental disorders
    B. Associated with neurologic disorders
        1. Cerebral degenerative disorders
        2. Parkinsonism
        3. Sleep-related epilepsy
        4. Sleep-related headaches

(continued)

Table 187-1 (*Continued*)

International Classification of Sleep Disorders

    C. Associated with other medical disorders
        1. Nocturnal cardiac ischemia
        2. Chronic obstructive pulmonary disease
        3. Sleep-related asthma
        4. Sleep-related gastroesophageal reflux

SOURCE: Modified from *International Classification of Sleep Disorders,* prepared by the Diagnostic Classification Committee, Thorpy MJ, Chairman, American Sleep Disorders Association, 1990.

Approach to the Patient

A practical classification of sleep disorders describes four types of problems: (1) disorders of initiating and maintaining sleep (insomnia), (2) disorders of excessive daytime sleepiness (fatigue, somnolence), (3) behavioral phenomena occurring during sleep itself (sleepwalking, REM behavioral disorder, periodic leg movements of sleep, etc.), and (4) circadian rhythm disorders associated with jet lag, shift work, and delayed sleep phase syndrome. A careful history of sleep habits supplemented by pt-recorded sleep logs and sleep partner reports is the cornerstone of diagnosis. Objective sleep laboratory recording is necessary to evaluate sleep apnea, narcolepsy, REM behavior disorder, periodic leg movements, and other suspected disorders.

Insomnia

Insomnia is a disorder of initiating or maintaining sleep and/or the perception of poor sleep quality (nonrestorative sleep). The temporal pattern of the insomnia is usually a clue to diagnosis. Sleep-onset insomnia is often psychophysiologic: an anxious preoccupation with the perceived inability to sleep adequately. Sleep maintenance problems are common to chronic medical conditions, sedative/hypnotics overuse, periodic leg movements, altitude insomnia, and some breathing disorders. Early morning awakening is frequently present in depression.

R_x TREATMENT

Insomnia treatment is often challenging but usually effective using several treatment modalities. Cognitive therapy emphasizes understanding the nature of normal sleep, the circadian rhythm, the use of light therapy, and visual imagery to block unwanted thought intrusions. Behavioral modification involves the use of bedtime restriction, set schedules, and careful sleep environment practices. Some pts benefit from the use of low-dose sedating tricyclics, such as 10 mg amitriptylene or the judicious use of benzodiazepine or its congeners. A judicious use would be either short term (1 week) or limited use not to exceed 3 days/week.

Hypersomnias (Disorders of Excessive Daytime Sleepiness)

Inappropriate daytime sleepiness has profound personal, occupational, and societal implications due to cognitive and motor impairments. Differentiation of sleepiness from subjective complaints of fatigue may be difficult. Quantification of daytime sleepiness can be performed in a sleep laboratory using a multiple sleep latency test (MSLT), the repeated daytime measurement of sleep latency under standardized conditions. Common causes include sleep apnea, narcolepsy/cataplexy syndrome, periodic leg movements of sleep, inadequate bed time (common in adolescents and young adults), and medical conditions that disrupt sleep (pain, asthma, nocturnal angina, congestive heart failure, etc.).

Excessive daytime sleepiness may emerge with any condition that causes disruptions of sleep. One example is periodic leg movements of sleep, a disinhibited spinal reflex affecting 1% of the population, producing repetitive stereotyped leg movements that result in subclinical arousals. Treatment with L-dopa, opioids, or clonazepam is often effective. Hypersomnolence can also be present in metabolic, endocrine, and neurologic disorders—uremia, hypothyroidism, hypercalcemia, hypercapnia—and with increased intracranial pressure or hypothalamic disorders.

SLEEP APNEA SYNDROME Respiratory dysfunction during sleep is a common serious cause of excessive daytime sleepiness, often unrecognized by both pts and physicians. Middle-aged men are affected 20 times as frequently as women. Only two-thirds of pts are obese. The pathophysiology is a small, collapsible airway, heralded by snoring and followed by airway obstruction producing repeated arousals and unsustained awakenings. Obstruction is exacerbated by obesity, supine posture, sedatives (especially alcohol), nasal obstruction, and hypothyroidism.

R̲x̲ TREATMENT

This consists of correction of the above factors, positive airway pressure devices, oral appliances, and sometimes surgery (see also Chap. 264, HPIM-14).

NARCOLEPSY/CATAPLEXY Narcolepsy/cataplexy is a disorder of excessive daytime sleepiness and intrusion of REM-related sleep phenomena into wakefulness (cataplexy, hypnagogic hallucinations, and sleep paralysis). Cataplexy, the abrupt loss of muscle tone in arms, legs, or face, is precipitated by emotional stimuli such as laughter or sadness. The excessive daytime sleepiness usually appears in adolescence, and the other phenomena, variably, later in life.

The prevalence is 40/100,000, affecting men and women equally. Nearly all pts are DR2,WQ1-positive, with a strong familial tendency. Well-documented but rare cases occur with brainstem pathology due to trauma, tumors, and multiple sclerosis. Sleep studies such as an MSLT confirm a pathologically short daytime sleep latency and a rapid transition to REM sleep.

R̲x̲ TREATMENT

Treatment for narcolepsy is a combination of stimulants (pemoline, methylphenidate, *d*-amphetamine) and the use of short naps. Tricyclic antidepressants such as imipramine are useful in reducing cataplexy.

Disorders of Circadian Rhythmicity

Insomnia or hypersomnia may occur in disorders of sleep timing rather than sleep generation. Such conditions may be (1) organic—due to a defect in the circadian pacemaker located in the suprachiasmatic nucleus of the hypothalamus, or (2) environmental—due to a disruption of entraining stimuli (light/dark cycle). Common examples of the latter include jet-lag syndrome and shift work. Another sleep cycle disorder, often misdiagnosed as sleep-onset insomnia, is delayed sleep phase syndrome, characterized by late sleep onset and awakening with otherwise normal sleep architecture. These pts almost invariably respond to a rescheduling regimen in which bedtimes are successively delayed by 3 h/day until the desired early bedtime is achieved (chronotherapy). The advanced sleep phase syndrome, frequent in the elderly, moves sleep onset to the early evening hours with early morning awakening. Bright light phototherapy may benefit these pts as well as those with jet lag and shift-work disorders.

For a more detailed discussion, see Czeisler CA, Richardson GS: Disorders of Sleep and Circadian Rhythms, Chap. 27, p. 150, in HPIM-14.

188

SPINAL CORD DISEASES

Diseases of the spinal cord can be devastating, but many are treatable if recognized early (Table 188-1). A working knowledge of relevant spinal cord anatomy is often the key to correct diagnosis (Fig. 188-1).

Table 188-1

Some Treatable Spinal Cord Disorders

Compressive
    Epidural, intradural, or intramedullary neoplasm
    Epidural abscess
    Epidural hemorrhage
    Cervical spondylosis
    Herniated disc
    Posttraumatic compression by fractured or displaced
      vertebra or hemorrhage
Vascular
    Arteriovenous malformation
Inflammatory
    Transverse myelitis
    Multiple sclerosis
Infectious
    Herpes simplex virus type 2 infection
    Parasitic or bacterial infection
Developmental
    Syringomyelia
Metabolic
    Subacute combined degeneration

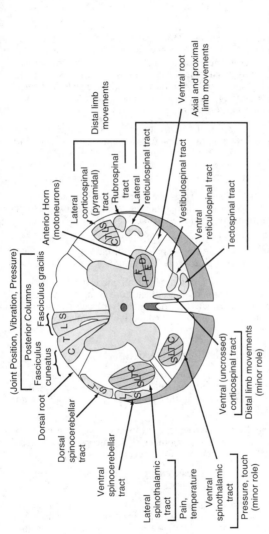

FIGURE 188-1 Transverse section through the spinal cord, composite representation, illustrating the principal ascending (*left*) and descending (*right*) pathways. The lateral and ventral spinothalamic tracts (*dark blue*) ascend contralateral to the side of the body that is innervated. C, cervical; T, thoracic; L, lumbar; S, sacral; D, distal; P, proximal; F, flexors; E, extensors.

Joint Position, Vibration, Pressure)

Posterior Columns

Fasciculus gracilis

Fasciculus cuneatus

Dorsal root

Dorsal spinocerebellar tract

Ventral spinocerebellar tract

Lateral spinothalamic tract

Pain, temperature

Ventral spinothalamic tract

Pressure, touch (minor role)

Ventral (uncrossed) corticospinal tract

Distal limb movements (minor role)

Tectospinal tract

Ventral reticulospinal tract

Vestibulospinal tract

Axial and proximal limb movements

Ventral root

Lateral reticulospinal tract

Rubrospinal tract

Lateral corticospinal (pyramidal) tract

Distal limb movements

Anterior Horn (motoneurons)

Symptoms and Signs

Principal signs are loss of sensation below a horizontal meridian on the trunk ("sensory level"), accompanied by weakness and spasticity.

Sensory Symptoms   Often paresthesia; may begin in one or both feet and ascend. Sensory level to pin sensation or vibration often correlates well with location of transverse lesions. May have isolated pain/temperature sensation loss over the shoulders ("cape" or "syringomyelic" pattern) or loss of sensation to vibration/position on one side of the body and pain/temperature loss on the other.

Motor Impairment   Disruption of corticospinal tracts causes quadriplegia or paraplegia with increased muscle tone, hyperactive deep tendon reflexes, and extensor plantar responses. With acute severe lesions there may be initial flaccidity and areflexia (spinal shock).

Segmental Signs   These are approximate indicators of level of lesion, e.g., band of hyperalgesia/hyperpathia, isolated flaccidity, atrophy, or single lost tendon reflex.

Autonomic Dysfunction   Primarily urinary retention; should raise suspicion of spinal cord disease when associated with back or neck pain, weakness, and/or a sensory level.

Pain   Midline back pain is of localizing value; interscapular pain may be first sign of midthoracic cord compression; radicular pain may mark site of more laterally placed spinal lesion; pain from lower cord (conus medullaris) lesion may be referred to low back.

Specific Signs by Spinal Cord Level

Lesions Near the Foramen Magnum   Weakness of the ipsilateral shoulder and arm, followed by weakness of ipsilateral leg, then contralateral leg, then contralateral arm, with respiratory paralysis.

Cervical Cord   Best localized by noting pattern of motor weakness and areflexia; shoulder (C5), biceps (C6), triceps/finger and wrist extensors (C7), finger flexors (C8).

Thoracic Cord   Localized by identification of a sensory level on the trunk.

Lumbar Cord   Upper lumbar cord lesions paralyze hip flexion and knee extension, whereas lower lumbar lesions affect foot and ankle movements, knee flexion, and thigh extension.

Sacral Cord (Conus Medullaris) Saddle anaesthesia and early bladder/bowel/sexual dysfunction.

Cauda Equina Lesions below spinal cord termination at the L1 vertebral level produce a flaccid, areflexic, asymmetric paraparesis with bladder/bowel dysfunction and sensory loss below L1; pain is common and projected to perineum or thighs.

Intramedullary and Extramedullary Syndromes

Spinal cord disorders may be intramedullary (arising from within the substance of the cord) or extramedullary (compressing the cord or its blood supply). Extramedullary lesions often produce radicular pain, early corticospinal signs, and sacral sensory loss. Intramedullary lesions produce poorly localized burning pain, less prominent corticospinal signs, and often spare perineal/sacral sensation.

Acute and Subacute Spinal Cord Diseases

Commonly due to spinal cord compression (by tumor, infection, spondylosis, or trauma), infarction or hemorrhage, inflammation, or infection. Evaluation consists of MRI scans that provide excellent resolution of the spinal cord and identify most compressive lesions. Plain x-rays or CT of spine may be useful to assess presence of fractures and alignment of vertebral column. CSF analysis useful for infectious and inflammatory processes.

1. *Tumors of spinal cord:* May be metastatic or primary, epidural or intradural; most are epidural metastases from adjacent vertebra. Malignancies commonly responsible: breast, lung, prostate, lymphoma, and plasma cell dyscrasias. Initial symptom is commonly back pain, worse when recumbent, with local tenderness preceding other symptoms by many weeks. Spinal cord compression due to metastases is a medical emergency; *treatment* consists of glucocorticoids (dexamethasone 40 mg daily) to reduce interstitial edema, local radiotherapy initiated as early as possible to the symptomatic lesion, and specific therapy for the underlying tumor type. Intradural tumors are generally benign—meningiomas or neurofibromas; treatment is surgical resection.

2. *Spinal epidural abscess:* Triad of fever, localized spinal pain, and myelopathy (progressive weakness and bladder symptoms); once neurologic signs appear, cord compression rapidly progresses. *Treatment* is emergency decompressive laminectomy with debridement combined with long-term antibiotic therapy.

3. *Spinal epidural hemorrhage and hematomyelia:* Presents as acute transverse myelopathy evolving over minutes or

hours with severe pain. Causes: minor trauma, LP, anticoagulation, hematologic disorder, AV malformation, hemorrhage into tumor—most are idiopathic. *Treatment* is surgical evacuation and correction of any underlying bleeding disorder.

4. *Acute disk protrusion:* Cervical and thoracic disk herniations are less common than lumbar.

5. *Acute trauma with spinal fracture/dislocation:* May not produce myelopathy until mechanical stress further displaces destabilized spinal column.

6. *Inflammatory myelopathies:* Acute transverse myelitis presents as sensory and motor symptoms, often with bladder involvement, evolving over hours to days. May follow infection, vaccination, or be the first sign of multiple sclerosis. Glucocorticoids, consisting of IV methylprednisolone followed by oral prednisone (see Table 178-3), are indicated for moderate to severe symptoms. Rarely, a rapidly ascending necrotic myelopathy may occur as a paraneoplastic syndrome.

7. *Infectious myelopathies:* Herpes zoster is the most common viral agent; schistosomiasis is an important cause worldwide.

8. *Spinal cord infarction:* Anterior spinal artery infarction produces paraplegia or quadriplegia, dissociated sensory loss affecting pain/temperature and sparing vibration/position sensations (supplied by posterior spinal arteries), and loss of sphincter control. Associated conditions: aortic atherosclerosis, dissecting aortic aneurysm, hypotension. *Treatment* is symptomatic.

Chronic Myelopathies

1. *Spondylitic myelopathies:* Presents as neck and shoulder pain, radicular arm pain, and progressive spastic paraparesis with parasthesia and loss of vibration sense; in advanced cases, urinary incontinence may occur. Results from combinations of disk bulging, osteophytic spur formation, partial subluxation, and hypertrophy of the dorsal spinal ligament. *Treatment* is surgical.

2. *Vascular malformations:* An important treatable cause of progressive myelopathy. May occur at any level; diagnosis is made by contrast-enhanced MRI, confirmed by selective spinal angiography. *Treatment* is embolization with occlusion of the major feeding vessels.

3. *Retrovirus-associated myelopathies:* Infection with HTLV-I may produce a slowly progressive spastic paraparesis with variable pain, sensory loss, and bladder disturbance; diagnosis is made by demonstration of specific serum antibody. *Treatment* is symptomatic. A progressive vacuolar myelopathy may also occur in AIDS.

4. *Syringomyelia:* Cavitary expansion of the spinal cord resulting in progressive myelopathy; may be an isolated finding or associated with protrusion of cerebellar tonsils into cervical spinal canal (Chiari type 1) or with incomplete closure of spinal canal (Chiari type 2). Classic presentation is loss of pain/temperature sensation in the neck, shoulders, forearms, or hands with areflexic weakness in the upper limbs and progressive spastic paraparesis; cough headache, facial numbness, or thoracic kyphoscoliosis may occur. Diagnosis is made by MRI; *treatment* is surgical.

5. *Multiple sclerosis:* See Chap. 178

6. *Subacute combined degeneration (vitamin B_{12} deficiency):* Paresthesia in hands and feet, early loss of vibration/position sense, progressive spastic/ataxic weakness, and areflexia due to associated peripheral neuropathy; mental changes ("megaloblastic madness") may be present. Diagnosis is confirmed by a low serum B_{12} level and a positive Schilling test. *Treatment* is vitamin replacement.

7. *Tabes dorsalis:* May present as lancinating pains, gait ataxia, bladder disturbances, and visceral crises. Cardinal signs are areflexia in the legs, impaired vibration/position sense, Romberg's sign, and Argyll Robertson pupils, which fail to constrict to light but react to accomodation.

8. *Familial spastic paraplegia:* Progressive spasticity and weakness in the legs occurring on a familial basis; may be autosomal dominant, recessive, or X-linked.

Complications

Damage to urinary tract due to urinary retention with bladder distention and injury to detrusor muscle; UTI; paroxysmal hypertension or hypotension with volume changes; ileus and gastritis; in high cervical cord lesions, mechanical respiratory failure; severe hypertension and bradycardia in response to noxious stimuli or bladder or bowel distention; pressure sores; venous thrombosis and pulmonary embolism.

For a more detailed discussion, see Hauser SL: Diseases of the Spinal Cord, Chap. 373, p. 2381, in HPIM-14.

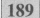

189

PERIPHERAL NEUROPATHIES INCLUDING GUILLAIN-BARRÉ SYNDROME

Peripheral neuropathy (PN) refers to a peripheral nerve disorder of any cause. Nerve involvement may be single (mononeuropathy) or multiple (polyneuropathy); pathology may be axonal or demyelinating. An approach to pts with suspected neuropathy appears in Fig. 189-1.

POLYNEUROPATHY

CLINICAL FEATURES The typical axonal polyneuropathy begins with sensory symptoms (tingling or burning) distally in the toes or feet. Symptoms spread proximally to the ankles, then involve the calves. Ankle reflexes are lost. Once sensory loss reaches the knees, proximal spread extends into the thighs and numbness of fingers appears. This pattern results in a "stocking-glove" distribution of sensory and motor findings. Further progression results in loss of knee reflexes. Light touch may be perceived as uncomfortable (allodynia) or pinprick as excessively painful (hyperpathia). Weakness and atrophy evolve from distal to proximal—initial toe dorsiflexion weakness may progress to bilateral foot drop, intrinsic hand muscle weakness, or (in extreme cases) impairment of muscles needed for ventilation and sphincter function. A family history for neuropathy should be sought, since adult-onset hereditary motor and sensory neuropathy (HMSN II) is not uncommon. In contrast to axonal neuropathy, demyelinating neuropathy does not produce stocking-glove deficits; diffuse loss of reflexes and strength is usual, and nerves are often palpably enlarged.

DIAGNOSTIC EVALUATION Diagnosis is aided by classification into axonal or demyelinating pathology and consideration of the time course of the neuropathy (Table 189-1). EMG is particularly helpful when history and examination do not clarify the diagnosis. EMG can distinguish axonal from demyelinating neuropathy, neuropathy from myopathy, nerve root or plexus disorders from distal nerve involvement, generalized polyneuropathy from mononeuropathy multiplex, and central weakness from peripheral nerve weakness. Sural nerve biopsy is helpful when vasculitis, multifocal demyelination, amyloidosis, leprosy, or sarcoidosis are considerations; biopsy results in lateral foot sensory loss, and rarely a painful neuroma may form at the biopsy site. Screening laboratory studies in a distal, sym-

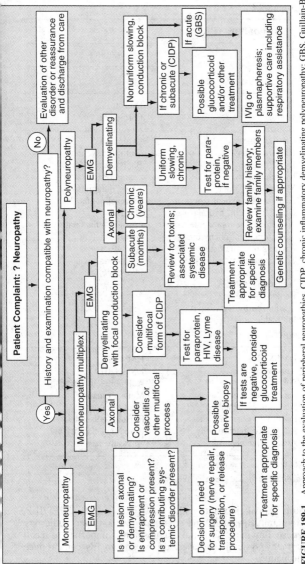

FIGURE 189-1 Approach to the evaluation of peripheral neuropathies. CIDP, chronic inflammatory demyelinating polyneuropathy; GBS, Guillain-Barré syndrome; IVIg, intravenous immune globulin. (From Asbury A: HPIM-14, p. 2458.)

Table 189-1

Polyneuropathies (PN)*

Axonal	Demyelinative
ACQUIRED	
Diabetes	Diabetes
Uremia	Carcinoma
B_{12} deficiency	HIV infection
Critical illness	Lymphoma
HIV infection	Multiple myeloma
Lyme disease	Benign monoclonal
Lymphoma	gammopathy (IgM)
Multiple myeloma	Acute inflammatory
Acute motor axonal neuropathy	demyelinating PN
Drugs: cisplatin, hydralazine,	(AIDP)
isoniazid, metronidazole,	Chronic inflammatory
nitrofurantoin, phenytoin,	demyelinating PN
pyridoxine, vincristine	(CIDP)
Toxins: arsenic, thallium,	Diphtheria toxin
inorganic lead,	Idiopathic
organophosphates	
Benign monoclonal	
gammopathy (IgA, IgG)	
Idiopathic	
HEREDITARY	
HMSN II†	HMSN I
Amyloid	HMSN III
Porphyria	Adrenomyeloneuropathy
Fabry's disease	Metachromatic
Abetalipoproteinemia	leukodystrophy
Friedreich's ataxia	Refsum's disease
Adrenomyeloneuropathy	Hereditary liability to
Ataxia telangiectasia	pressure palsies

*Does not include rare causes.

†Hereditary motor and sensory neuropathy

metric axonal polyneuropathy are Hb A_{1C}, ESR, SPEP/IEP, and vitamin B_{12}, BUN, and creatinine levels. Other studies are suggested by the differential diagnosis; it is important to recall that many systemic diseases, drugs, and toxins can produce neuropathy.

SPECIFIC POLYNEUROPATHIES

1. *Acute inflammatory demyelinating polyneuropathy (AIDP) or Guillain-Barré syndrome* (GBS): an ascending, demyelinating, motor > sensory polyneuropathy accompanied by areflexia, motor paralysis, and elevated CSF total protein without pleocytosis. Over two-thirds are preceded by infection with EBV or other herpesviruses, HIV, other viruses, *Mycoplasma,* or *Campylobacter jejuni* gastroenteritis. Maximum weakness is usually reached in 7–10 d (maximum 4–6 weeks); demyelination by EMG. Most pts are hospitalized; one-third require ventilatory assistance. 85% of pts make a complete or near-complete recovery with supportive care. Plasmapheresis or IV immune globulin (2 g/kg given over 5 d) significantly shorten the course. Glucocorticoids are ineffective. Variants of GBS include Fisher syndrome (ophthalmoparesis, facial diplegia, ataxia, areflexia; associated with antibodies to ganglioside GQ_{1b}) and acute motor axonal neuropathy (more severe course than demyelinating GBS; antibodies to GM_1 in some cases).

2. *Chronic inflammatory demyelinating polyneuropathy (CIDP):* a slowly progressive or relapsing polyneuropathy characterized by diffuse hyporeflexia or areflexia, diffuse weakness, elevated CSF protein without pleocytosis, and demyelination by EMG. Treatment options include glucocorticoids, IV immune globulin, plasmapheresis, or immunosuppressants (azothiaprine, cyclophosphamide, cyclosporine).

3. *Diabetic neuropathy:* typically a distal symmetric, sensorimotor, axonal polyneuropathy, but many variations occur. A mixture of demyelination and axonal loss is frequent. Isolated sixth or third cranial nerve palsies, asymmetric proximal motor neuropathy in the legs, truncal neuropathy, autonomic neuropathy, and an increased frequency of entrapment neuropathy at common sites of nerve compression all occur.

4. *Mononeuropathy multiplex (MM):* defined as involvement of multiple noncontiguous nerves. One-third of adults with MM have an acquired demyelinating disorder that is treatable. The remainder have an axonal disorder; 50% of these have vasculitis—usually due to a connective tissue disorder. In this latter group, immunosuppressive treatment of the underlying disease is indicated.

MONONEUROPATHY

CLINICAL FEATURES Mononeuropathies are usually caused by trauma, compression, or entrapment. Sensory and motor symptoms are in the distribution of a single nerve—most commonly ulnar or median nerves in the arms or peroneal nerve in the leg (Table 189-2). Clinical features favoring conservative

Table 189-2

Common Mononeuropathies—Findings and Treatment

	Median	Ulnar	Common Peroneal
Site	Wrist—carpal tunnel	Elbow—cubital tunnel or condylar groove	Knee—fibular head
Sensory loss	Lateral palm; 1st–3rd finger ± 4th finger	Medial palm; 5th ± 4th finger	Dorsal foot Lateral calf
Motor weakness	Thumb abduction Thumb opposition	Index finger abduction 5th finger abduction	Foot dorsiflexion Foot eversion
Conservative Rx	Wrist splint, NSAIDs	Elbow pad Avoid elbow trauma	Avoid direct compression
Surgical Rx	Transverse carpal ligament section	Cubital tunnel release; ulnar nerve transposition	—

management of median neuropathy at the wrist (carpal tunnel syndrome) or ulnar neuropathy at the elbow include sudden onset, no motor deficit, few or no sensory findings (pain or paresthesia may be present), and no evidence of axonal loss by EMG. Factors favoring surgical decompression include chronic course (lack of response to conservative treatment), motor deficit, and electrodiagnostic evidence of axonal loss. Patterns of weakness, sensory loss, and conservative/surgical treatment options are listed in Table 189-2.

For a more detailed discussion, see Asbury AK: Diseases of the Peripheral Nervous System, Chap. 381, p. 2457, in HPIM-14.

190

MYOPATHIES AND MUSCULAR DYSTROPHIES

MUSCULAR DYSTROPHIES

A disparate group of disorders that are all inherited, progressive degenerations of muscle but vary widely in their clinical and pathologic features and mode of inheritance. The genetics of many of these disorders is now better understood (Table 190-1).

Duchenne Dystrophy

X-linked recessive mutation of the dystrophin gene that affects males almost exclusively. Onset is by age 5; symmetric and relentlessly progressive weakness in hip and shoulder girdle muscles leading to difficulty in climbing, running, jumping, hopping, etc. By age 8–10, most children require leg braces; by age 12, the majority are nonambulatory. Survival beyond age 25 is rare.

Associated Problems Include tendon and muscle contractures (e.g., heel cords), progressive kyphoscoliosis, impaired

Table 190-1

Progressive Muscular Dystrophies

Type	Genetics
Duchenne	X-linked recessive mutation of dystrophin gene
Becker	X-linked recessive mutation of dystrophin gene
Myotonic	Autosomal dominant; expansion of unstable region of DNA at chromosome 19q13.3 (myotonin kinase)
Facioscapulohumeral	Autosomal dominant; frequent mutations at chromosome 4q35
Limb-girdle (includes several disorders)	Autosomal recessive (α-, β-, γ-, and δ-sarcoglycan; and calpain) or autosomal dominant
Oculopharyngeal	Autosomal dominant (French-Canadian or Hispanic background)
Congenital (includes several disorders including Fukuyama and cerebro-ocular-dysplasia types)	Autosomal recessive

SOURCE: Mendell JR, Griggs RC, Ptáček LJ: HPIM-14, p. 2473.

pulmonary function, cardiomyopathy, and intellectual impairment. Muscle weakness is conjoined with palpable enlargement and firmness of some muscles (e.g., calves) resulting initially from hypertrophy and later from replacement of muscle by fat and connective tissue.

Clinical Features	Other Organ System Involvement
Onset before age 5; progressive weakness of girdle muscles; inability to walk after age 12; kyphoscoliosis; respiratory failure in second to third decade	Cardiomyopathy; mental impairment
Onset in early to late childhood; slowly progressive weakness of girdle muscles; retain ability to walk after age 15; respiratory failure after fourth decade	Cardiomyopathy
Onset any decade; slowly progressive weakness of eyelids, face, neck, distal limb muscles; myotonia	Cardiac conduction defects; mental impairment; cataracts; frontal baldness; gonadal atrophy
Onset before age 20; slowly progressive face, shoulder girdle, foot dorsiflexion weakness	Hypertension; deafness
Onset in early childhood to adulthood; slowly progressive weakness of shoulder and hip girdle muscles	Cardiomyopathy
Onset fifth to sixth decade; slowly progressive weakness of extraocular, eyelid, face, and pharyngeal muscles; cricopharyngeal achalasia	
Onset at birth; hypotonia, contractures, and delayed milestones; early respiratory failure in some, static course in others	Cerebral; eye

Laboratory Findings   Include massive elevations (20–100 × normal) of muscle enzymes (CK, aldolase), a myopathic pattern on EMG testing, and evidence of groups of necrotic muscle fibers with regeneration, phagocytosis, and fatty replacement of muscle on biopsy. Diagnosis can be accurately established by determination of dystrophin in muscle tissue by western blot and/or immunochemical staining. Mutations in the dystrophin gene can be identified in approximately two-thirds of pts using a battery of cDNA probes. ECG abnormalities (increased net RS in V_1, deep Q in precordial leads) reflect the presence of cardiomyopathy.

Carrier Detection   Serum CK is elevated in 50% of female carriers. Since the gene and its product (dystrophin) have now been identified, cDNA probes are now available for use in detecting carriers and in prenatal diagnosis.

Complications   Include respiratory failure and infections, aspiration, and acute gastric dilatation. CHF and cardiac arrhythmias may complicate the cardiomyopathy.

℞ TREATMENT

Definitive therapy is not yet available. Prednisone, 0.75 (mg/kg)/d, may significantly alter progression of disease for up to 3 years, but the complications of chronic steroid use often outweigh the benefits. Passive stretching of muscles, tenotomy, bracing, physiotherapy, mechanical assistance devices, and avoidance of prolonged immobility may all be of symptomatic benefit.

Becker Dystrophy (Benign Pseudohypertrophic)

A less severe and rarer dystrophy than Duchenne, with a slower course and later age of onset (5–15) but similar clinical and laboratory features. This disorder also results from defects in the dystrophin gene.

Myotonic Dystrophy

A multisystem disorder in which weakness typically becomes obvious in the second to third decade and initially involves the muscles of the face, neck, and distal extremities. This results in a distinctive facial appearance ("hatchet face") characterized by ptosis, temporal wasting, drooping of the lower lip, and sagging of the jaw. Myotonia manifests as a peculiar inability to relax muscles rapidly following a strong exertion (e.g., after tight hand grip), as well as by sustained contraction of muscles following percussion (e.g., of tongue or thenar eminence).

Associated Problems   Can include frontal baldness, posterior subcapsular cataracts, gonadal atrophy, respiratory and cardiac problems, endocrine abnormalities, intellectual impairment, and hypersomnia. Cardiac complications, including complete heart block, may be life-threatening. Respiratory function should be carefully followed, as chronic hypoxia may lead to cor pulmonale.

Laboratory Studies Show normal or mildly elevated CK, characteristic myotonia and myopathic features on EMG, and a typical pattern of muscle fiber injury on biopsy, including selective type I fiber atrophy.

Genetics Myotonic dystrophy is an autosomal dominant disorder that displays genetic anticipation. Pts have an unstable region of DNA with an increased number of trinucleotide CTG repeats at chromosome location 19q13.3. The protein encoded by the affected gene appears to be a protein kinase. Molecular genetic studies may be useful in early detection and prenatal diagnosis.

℞ TREATMENT

Phenytoin, procainamide, and quinine may help myotonia, but they must be used carefully in pts with heart disease as they may worsen cardiac conduction. Pacemaker insertion may be required for pts with syncope or heart block. Orthoses may control foot drop, stabilize the ankle, and decrease falling.

Facioscapulohumeral Dystrophy

Typically, an autosomal dominant, slowly progressive disorder with onset in the third to fourth decade. Weakness involves facial, shoulder girdle, and proximal arm muscles and can result in atrophy of biceps, triceps, scapular winging, and slope shoulders. Facial weakness results in inability to whistle and loss of facial expressivity. Foot drop and leg weakness may cause falls and progressive difficulty with ambulation.

Laboratory Studies Include normal or slightly elevated CK and mixed myopathic-neuropathic features on EMG and muscle biopsy. Pts have mutations at chromosome 4q35. A genetic probe specific for this site can be used in carrier detection and prenatal diagnosis. Orthoses and other stabilization procedures may be of benefit for selected patients.

LESS COMMON DYSTROPHIES

Limb-Girdle Dystrophy

A constellation of diseases with proximal muscle weakness involving the arms and legs as the core symptom. Age of onset, rate of progression, severity of manifestations, inheritance pattern (autosomal dominant or autosomal recessive) and associated complications (e.g., cardiac, respiratory) vary with the specific subtype of disease. Laboratory findings include elevated CK and myopathic features on EMG and muscle biopsy. At least six distinct autosomal recessive forms have been identified by molecular genetic analysis, four due to mutations in different dystrophin-associated proteins and one due to mutations in the enzyme calpain.

Oculopharyngeal Dystrophy (Progressive External Ophthalmoplegia)

Onset in the fifth to sixth decade of ptosis, limitation of extraocular movements, and facial and cricopharyngeal weakness. Cricopharyngeal muscle weakness results in achalasia, dysphagia, and aspiration. Chronic nature of the eye movement disorder rarely results in diplopia. Most pts are Hispanic or of French-Canadian descent.

METABOLIC MYOPATHIES

These disorders result from abnormalities in utilization by muscle of glucose or fatty acids as sources of energy. Pts present with either an acute syndrome of myalgia, myolysis, and myoglobinuria or chronic progressive muscle weakness. Definitive diagnosis requires biochemical-enzymatic studies of biopsied muscle. However, muscle enzymes, EMG, and muscle biopsy are all typically abnormal and may suggest specific disorders.

Infantile and childhood forms of glycogen storage disorders often have associated disorders of cardiac, hepatic, and endocrine function that overshadow the muscle disease. Childhood and adult forms can mimic muscular dystrophy or polymyositis. In some types the presentation is one of episodic muscle cramps and fatigue provoked by exercise. The ischemic forearm lactate test is helpful as normal postexercise rise in serum lactic acid does not occur. Disorders of fatty acid metabolism present with clinical pictures similar to those described above. In some pts, exercise-induced cramps, myolysis, and myoglobinuria are common; in others, the picture resembles polymyositis or muscular dystrophy. Some pts have benefited from special diets (medium-chain triglyceride-enriched), oral carnitine supplements, or glucocorticoids.

MITOCHONDRIAL MYOPATHIES

More accurately referred to as mitochondrial cytopathies because multiple tissues are usually affected, these disorders result from defects in mitochondrial DNA. The clinical presentations vary enormously: muscle symptoms may include weakness, pain, stiffness, or may even be absent; age of onset ranges from

Table 190-2

Toxic Myopathies

> Focal myopathies: pentazocine, meperidine, heroin
> Generalized myopathies
>> Inflammatory: cimetidine, D-penicillamine, procainamide
>> Muscle weakness and myalgias: zidovudine, chloroquine, clofibrate, colchicine, glucocorticoids, emetine, ε-aminocaproic acid, labetalol, perhexilene, propranolol, vincristine, niacin, cyclosporine
>> Rhabdomyolysis and myoglobinuria: alcohol, heroin, amphetamine, clofibrate, lovastatin, gemfibrozil, ε-aminocaproic acid, phencyclidine, barbiturates, cocaine
>> Malignant hyperthermia: halothane, ethylene, diethyl ether, methoxyflurane, ethyl chloride, trichloroethylene, gallamine, succinylcholine, lidocaine, mepivacaine

SOURCE: Mendell JR, Griggs RC, Ptáček LJ: HPIM-14, 2481.

infancy to adulthood; associated clinical presentations include ataxia, encephalopathy, seizures, strokelike episodes, and recurrent vomiting. The characteristic finding on muscle biopsy is "ragged red fibers," which are muscle fibers with accumulations of abnormal mitochondria. Genetics show a maternal pattern of inheritance because mitochondrial genes are inherited almost exclusively from the oocyte.

MISCELLANEOUS DISORDERS

Myopathies may be associated with endocrine disorders, especially those involving hypo- or hyperfunction of the thyroid, parathyroid, pituitary, and adrenal glands. Drugs (esp. glucocorticoids) and certain toxins (e.g., alcohol) are commonly associated with myopathies (see Table 190-2), as are deficiencies of vitamins D and E. In most cases weakness is symmetric and involves proximal limb girdle muscles. Weakness, myalgia, and cramps are common symptoms. Diagnosis often depends on resolution of signs and symptoms with correction of underlying disorder or removal of offending agent, as muscle enzymes, EMG, and even muscle biopsy may be unremarkable in individual pts.

For a more detailed discussion, see Mendell JR, Griggs RC, Ptáček LJ: Diseases of Muscle, Chap. 383, p. 2473, in HPIM-14.

191

MYASTHENIA GRAVIS (MG)

A neuromuscular disorder resulting in weakness and fatiguability of skeletal muscles, due to autoimmune-mediated decrease in acetylcholine receptors (AChRs) at neuromuscular junctions (NMJs).

Clinical Features

May present at any age. Symptoms fluctuate throughout the day and are provoked by exertion. Characteristic distribution: cranial muscles (lids, extraocular muscles, facial weakness, "nasal" or slurred speech, dysphagia); in 85%, limb muscles (often proximal and asymmetric) become involved. Reflexes and sensation normal. May be limited to extraocular muscles only—particularly in elderly. Complications: aspiration pneumonia (weak bulbar muscles), respiratory failure (weak chest wall muscles), exacerbation of myasthenia due to administration of drugs with neuromuscular junction blocking effects (tetracycline, aminoglycosides, procainamide, propanolol, phenothiazines, lithium).

Pathophysiology

Specific anti-AChR antibodies reduce the number of AChRs at the NMJ. Postsynaptic folds are flattened or "simplified," with resulting inefficient neuromuscular transmission. During repeated or sustained muscle contraction, decrease in amount of Ach released per nerve impulse, combined with decrease in postsynaptic AChRs, results in pathologic fatigue. Thymus is abnormal in 75% of pts (65% hyperplasia, 10% thymoma). Other autoimmune diseases in 10%.

Differential Diagnosis

1. Lambert-Eaton syndrome (autoantibodies to calcium channels in presynaptic motor nerve terminals)—reduced ACh release; associated with malignancy or idiopathic
2. Neurasthenia—weakness/fatigue without underlying organic disorder
3. Penicillamine may cause MG; resolves weeks to months after discontinuing drug
4. Hyperthyroidism
5. Botulism—toxin inhibits presynaptic ACh release
6. Intracranial mass lesion—compression of nerves to extraocular muscles
7. Progressive external ophthalmoplegia—seen in mitochondrial disorders

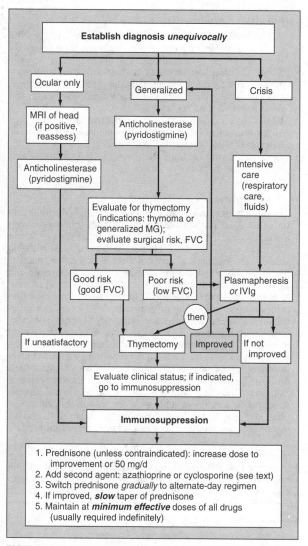

FIGURE 191-1 Algorithm for the management of myasthenia gravis. FVC, forced vital capacity. (From Drachman DM: HPIM-14.)

Laboratory Evaluation

- AChR antibodies—no correlation with disease severity; 80% of all myasthenic pts positive; 50% with ocular findings only are positive; positive antibodies are diagnostic.
- Tensilon (edrophonium) test—a short-acting anticholinesterase—look for rapid and transient improvement of strength; false-positive (placebo response, motor neuron disease) and false-negative tests occur.
- EMG—low frequency (2–4 Hz) repetitive stimulation produces decrement in amplitude of evoked motor responses.
- Chest CT/MRI—search for thymoma.
- Consider thyroid and other studies (e.g., ANA) for associated autoimmune disease.

R̲x̲ **TREATMENT** (see Fig. 191-1)

The anticholinesterase drug pyridostigmine (Mestinon) titrated to assist pt with functional activities (chewing, swallowing, strength during exertion); usual initial dose of 60 mg 3–5 times daily; long-acting tablets help at night. Muscarinic side effects (diarrhea, abdominal cramps, salivation, nausea) blocked with propantheline if required. Plasmapheresis and IV immune globulin [IVIg; 400 (mg/kg)/d × 5 days] provide temporary boost for seriously ill pts; used to improve condition prior to surgery or during myasthenic crisis (severe exacerbation of weakness). Thymectomy improves likelihood of long-term remission in adult (± elderly) pts. Glucocorticoids are a mainstay of treatment; begin prednisone at low dose (15–25 mg/d), increase by 5 mg/d q2–3 days until marked clinical improvement or dose of 50 mg/d is reached. Maintain high dose for 1–3 months, then decrease to alternate-day regimen. Long-term treatment with low-dose prednisone usual. Immunosuppressive drugs (azathioprine, cyclosporine, cyclophosphamide) may spare dose of prednisone required to control symptoms; azathioprine [2–3 (mg/kg)/d] most often used.

For a more detailed discussion, see Drachman DB: Myasthenia Gravis and Other Diseases of the Neuromuscular Junction, Chap. 382, p. 2469, in HPIM-14.

192

APPROACH TO THE PATIENT WITH PSYCHIATRIC SYMPTOMS

Disorders of mood, thinking and behavior may be due to a *primary* psychiatric diagnosis (DSM-IV* Axis I major psychiatric diagnoses) or a personality disorder (DSM-IV Axis II disorders) or may be *secondary* to metabolic abnormalities, drug toxicities, focal cerebral lesions, seizure disorders, or degenerative neurologic disease. Any pt presenting with new onset of psychiatric symptoms must be evaluated for underlying psychoactive substance abuse and/or medical or neurologic illness. Specific psychiatric medications are discussed in Chap. 193.

MAJOR PSYCHIATRIC DISORDERS (AXIS I DIAGNOSES)

Mood Disorders (Major Affective Disorders)

MAJOR DEPRESSION *Clinial Features* Affects 15% of the general population at some point in life. Diagnosis is made when a depressed/irritable mood or a lack of normal interest/pleasure exists for at least 2 weeks, in combination with four or more of the following symptoms: (1) change in appetite plus change in weight; (2) insomnia or hypersomnia; (3) fatigue or loss of energy; (4) motor agitation or retardation; (5) feelings of worthlessness, self-reproach, or guilt; (6) decreased ability to concentrate and make decisions; (7) recurrent thoughts of death or suicide. A small number of pts with major depression will have psychotic symptoms—hallucinations and delusions—with their depressed mood; many present with a "masked depression," unable to describe their psychological distress but with multiple diffuse somatic complaints.

Onset of a first depressive episode is typically in the thirties or forties, although major depression can be found in children and adolescents. Untreated episodes will usually resolve sponta-

*Diagnostic and Statistical Manual, Fourth Edition, American Psychiatric Association

neously in 5–9 months; a small number of pts suffer from chronic, unremitting depression. Half of all pts experiencing a first episode will go on to a recurrent course, with a second episode occurring within 2 years. A family history of mood disorder is common, and tends to predict a recurrent course.

Pts with major depression have abnormal sleep EEGs, abnormal monoamine neurotransmission, and altered function of the hypothalamic-pituitary-adrenal (HPA) axis. These abnormalities disappear with treatment and resolution of the depressive episode. Major depression can be the initial presentation of manic depressive illness.

Suicide   Most suicides occur in pts with a mood disorder, and many pts seek contact with a physician prior to their suicide attempt. Physicians must always inquire about suicide when evaluating a pt with depression. Features that place a pt at high risk for suicidal behavior include: (1) a formulated plan and a method, as well as an intent; (2) concomitant alcohol or other psychoactive substance use; (3) psychotic symptoms; (4) older age; (5) male; (6) Caucasian; (7) social isolation; (8) serious medical illness.

℞ TREATMENT

Patients with suicidal ideation require hospitalization and treatment by a psychiatrist. Most other pts with an uncomplicated unipolar major depression (a major depression that is not part of a cyclical mood disorder) can be successfully treated by a non-psychiatric physician. Vigorous intervention may also decrease the risk of future relapse.

Antidepressant medication is the mainstay of treatment; symptoms are ameliorated after 2–6 weeks at a therapeutic dose. Antidepressants should be continued for 9–12 months, then tapered slowly. Pts must be monitored carefully after termination of treatment since relapse is common. The combination of pharmacotherapy with psychotherapy [usually cognitive-behavioral therapy (CBT)] produces even better and longer-lasting results. Electroconvulsive therapy is reserved for pts with life-threatening depression unresponsive to medication.

BIPOLAR DISORDER (MANIC DEPRESSIVE ILLNESS)
Clinical Features   A cyclical mood disorder in which episodes of major depression are interspersed with episodes of mania or hypomania; 1–2% of the population is affected. Most pts initially present with a manic episode in adolescence or young adulthood, but 20% present with a major depression. Antidepressant therapy is contraindicated in this latter group because

it may provoke a manic episode. Young pts with a first major depressive episode and a family history of bipolar disorder should be referred promptly to a psychiatrist.

With mania, an elevated, expansive mood, irritability, and impulsivity are characteristic. Specific symptoms include: (1) increased motor activity and restlessness; (2) unusual talkativeness; (3) flight of ideas and racing thoughts; (4) inflated self-esteem that can become delusional; (5) decreased need for sleep (often the first feature of an incipient manic episode); (6) decreased appetite; (7) distractability; (8) excessive involvement in risky activities (buying sprees, sexual indiscretions). Pts with full-blown mania can become psychotic.

Untreated, a manic or depressive episode typically lasts for 1–3 months, with cycles of 1–2 episodes per year. Risk for manic episodes increases in the spring and fall. Variants of bipolar disorder include rapid and ultrarapid cycling, or simultaneous mixed manic and depressed episodes. In many pts, especially females, antidepressants trigger rapid cycling and worsen the course of illness. Pts with bipolar disorder are at risk for psychoactive substance use, especially alcohol abuse.

℞ TREATMENT

Bipolar disorder is a serious, chronic illness that requires lifelong monitoring by a psychiatrist. Acutely manic pts often require hospitalization to reduce environmental stimulation and to protect themselves and others from the consequences of their reckless behavior. Mood-stabilizers (lithium, carbamazepine, valproic acid) are highly effective for treatment of acute episodes and for prophylaxis of future episodes. As in unipolar depression, rapid therapeutic intervention may also decrease the risk of future relapse.

Schizophrenia and Other Psychotic Disorders

SCHIZOPHRENIA *Clinical Features* Occurs in 1% of the population worldwide; 30–40% of the homeless are affected. Characterized by a waxing and waning vulnerability to psychosis, i.e., an impaired ability to monitor reality, resulting in altered mood, thinking, language, perceptions, behavior, and interpersonal interactions. Pts usually present between late adolescence and the third decade, often after an insidious premorbid course of subtle psychosocial difficulties. Core psychotic features last 6 months or more and include: (1) delusions, which can be paranoid, jealous, somatic, grandiose, religious, nihilistic, or simply bizarre; (2) hallucinations, often auditory hallucinations of a voice or voices maintaining a running commentary; (3) disorders of language and thinking: incoherence, loosening of associations, tangentiality, illogical thinking; (4) inappropriate affect and bizarre, catatonic, or grossly disorganized behavior.

Many pts stabilize after the first 5 years of illness. 30–40% show a deteriorating course, but at least 25% do well, especially with early intervention. Females tend to have a later age of onset and a more benign course than males. Comorbid substance abuse is common.

℞ TREATMENT

Hospitalization is required for acutely psychotic patients, especially those with violent command hallucinations, who may be dangerous to themselves or others. Traditional antipsychotic medications are effective against hallucinations, agitation, and thought disorder (the so-called positive symptoms) in 60% of pts, but are often less useful for apathy, blunted affect, social isolation, and anhedonia (negative symptoms). The novel antipsychotic medications—clozapine, risperidone, olanzapine, and others—are helpful in a subgroup of pts unresponsive to traditional neuroleptics and have more effect on negative symptoms. Long-acting injectable forms of haloperidol and fluphenazine are ideal for noncompliant pts. Psychosocial intervention, rehabilitation, and family support are also essential.

OTHER PSYCHOTIC DISORDERS These include schizoaffective disorder (where symptoms of chronic psychosis are interspersed with major mood episodes) and delusional disorders (in which a fixed, unshakable delusional belief is held in the absence of the other stigmata of schizophrenia). Pts with somatic delusions can be especially difficult to diagnose; they may become violent towards the physician if they feel misunderstood or thwarted and resist referral to a psychiatrist.

Anxiety Disorders

Characterized by severe, persistent anxiety in the absence of psychosis or a severe change in mood.

PANIC DISORDER Occurs in 1–2% of the population; female:male ratio of 2:1. Onset in second or third decade. Initial presentation is almost always to a nonpsychiatric physician, frequently in the ER, as a possible heart attack or serious respiratory problem. Prompt diagnosis and treatment can greatly reduce morbidity.

Clinical Features Characterized by panic attacks, which are sudden, unexpected, overwhelming paroxysms of terror and apprehension with multiple associated somatic symptoms. Attacks usually last 10–20 min, then slowly resolve spontaneously. Diagnostic criteria for panic disorder require four or more panic attacks within 4 weeks occurring in nonthreatening or nonexertional settings, and attacks must be accompanied by at least four of the following: dyspnea, palpitations, chest pain or discomfort, choking/smothering feelings, dizziness/vertigo/unsteady feelings, feelings of unreality, paresthesia, hot and cold flashes, sweating, faintness, trembling, and fear of dying, going crazy, or doing something uncontrolled during an attack. Panic disorder is often associated with a concomitant major depression.

When the disorder goes unrecognized and untreated, pts start to experience significant morbidity: they become afraid of going out in case they have a panic attack and start to develop anticipatory anxiety, agoraphobia, and other spreading phobias; many turn to self-medication with alcohol or benzodiazepines.

Panic disorder must be differentiated from cardiovascular and respiratory disorders. Conditions that may mimic or worsen panic attacks include hyper- and hypothyroidism, pheochromocytoma, complex partial seizures, hypoglycemia, drug ingestions (amphetamines, cocaine, caffeine, sympathomimetic nasal decongestants), and drug withdrawal (alcohol, barbiturates, opiates, minor tranquilizers).

℞ TREATMENT

Psychotherapy (identifying and aborting panic attacks through relaxation and breathing techniques)—either alone or combined with medication—is highly effective. Tricyclic antidepressants, monoamine oxidase inhibitors, and selective serotonin reuptake inhibitors (SSRIs) all treat the disorder and prevent spontaneous attacks. Clonazepam, alprazolam, or other benzodiazepines may be used in the short-term while waiting for antidepressants to take effect (2–3 weeks).

GENERALIZED ANXIETY DISORDER (GAD)   Characterized by persistent, chronic anxiety but without the specific symptoms of phobic, panic, or obsessive-compulsive disorders; occurs in 2–3% of the population.

Clinical Features   Pts experience persistent motor hyperactivity (shakiness, trembling, restlessness, easy startle), autonomic hyperactivity, apprehensive expectation (anxiety, fear, rumination, anticipation of misfortune, etc.), and vigilance (distractability, poor concentration, insomnia, impatience, and irritability). These symptoms are chronic and pervasive, rather than situational. Secondary depression is common.

℞ **TREATMENT**

Benzodiazepines are the agents of choice when generalized anxiety is severe enough to warrant drug therapy. Many pts, however, become psychologically if not physically dependent on their anxiolytics; a subgroup respond to antidepressants and/or to buspirone, a nonbenzodiazepine anxiolytic. Psychotherapy and relaxation training can be useful.

OBSESSIVE-COMPULSIVE DISORDER (OCD)   A severe disorder present in 4–6% of the population and characterized by recurrent obsessions (persistent intrusive thoughts) and compulsions (repetitive behaviors) that the pt experiences as involuntary, senseless, or repugnant. Pts are often ashamed of their symptoms and only seek help after they have become debilitated.

Clinical Features   Common obsessions include thoughts of violence (such as killing a loved one), obsessive slowness for fear of making a mistake, fears of germs or contamination, and excessive doubt or uncertainty. Examples of compulsions include repeated checking to be assured that something was done properly, hand washing, extreme neatness and ordering behavior, and counting rituals, such as numbering one's steps while walking.

Onset is usually in adolescence, with 65% of cases manifest before age 25. In families of OCD pts, an increased incidence of both OCD and Tourette's syndrome is found. The course of OCD is usually episodic with periods of incomplete remission. Pts with severe disease may become completely housebound. Major depression, substance abuse, and social impairment are common.

℞ **TREATMENT**

Clomipramine and the SSRIs are highly effective. A combination of drug therapy and CBT is most effective for the majority of pts. Referral to a national support organization is also useful.

POSTTRAUMATIC STRESS DISORDER (PTSD)   Occurs in a subgroup of individuals exposed to a severe trauma. Predisposing factors include a prior history of traumatization and/or a diathesis towards anxiety responses. Developmental windows may exist during which full-blown PTSD is more likely to develop (adolescence and early adulthood). Early psychological intervention following a traumatic event may reduce the risk for chronic PTSD.

Clinical Features   Three core sets of symptoms; (1) *reexperiencing,* where the pt unwillingly reexperiences the trauma through recurrent intrusive recollections, recurrent dreams, or by suddenly feeling as if the traumatic event is recurring; (2) *avoidance and numbing,* where the pt experiences reduced responsiveness to, and involvement with, the external world, a sense of a foreshortened future, and avoidance of activities that arouse recollection of the traumatic event; (3) *arousal,* characterized by hypervigilance, hyperalertness, an exaggerated startle response, sleep disturbance, guilt about having survived when others have not or about behavior required for survival, memory impairment or trouble concentrating, and intensification of symptoms by exposure to events that symbolize or resemble the traumatic event.

Patients with PTSD have disturbed HPA function and changes in sleep architecture. Comorbid substance abuse and other mood and anxiety disorders are common. This disorder is extremely debilitating, particularly as it becomes chronic and affects the pt's psychosocial functioning. Most pts require referral to a psychiatrist for ongoing care.

℞ TREATMENT

Medications used with varying success include a combination of an SSRI and trazodone, 50–200 mg qhs for sleep; tricyclic antidepressants; and mood stabilizers. Group psychotherapy (with other trauma survivors), alone or with individual psychotherapy, is useful.

PHOBIC DISORDERS *Clinical Features* Recurring, irrational fears of specific objects, activities, or situations, with subsequent avoidance behavior of the phobic stimulus. Diagnosis is made only when the avoidance behavior is a significant source of distress or interferes with social or occupational functioning.

1. *Agoraphobia:* Fear of being in public places. May occur in absence of panic disorder, but is almost invariably preceded by that condition.

2. *Social phobia:* Persistent irrational fear of, and need to avoid, any situation where there is risk of scrutiny by others, with potential for embarassment or humiliation. Common examples include excessive fear of public speaking and excessive fear of social engagements.

3. *Simple phobias:* Persistent irrational fears and avoidance of specific objects. Common examples include fear of heights (acrophobia), closed spaces (claustrophobia), and animals.

℞ TREATMENT

Agoraphobia is treated as for panic disorder. Propranolol, alprazolam, monoamine oxidase inhibitors, and SSRIs are helpful in treating social phobias. Social and simple phobias respond well to CBT and relaxation techniques and to systematic desensitization and exposure treatment.

PERSONALITY DISORDERS (AXIS II DIAGNOSES)

Defined as an inappropriate, stereotyped, maladaptive use of a certain set of psychological characteristics; affects 5–15% of the general population. The pattern of behavior is enduring and affects the person's relationships and ability to function satisfactorily in life.

Comorbid Axis I diagnosis is common, as is a psychoactive substance use disorder. In medical and surgical settings, pts with personality disorders often become engaged in hostile, manipulative, or unproductive relationships with their physicians. Long-term psychotherapy is beneficial for pts who are motivated to change. Antidepressants and antipsychotic medications can be helpful, particularly for episodes of decompensation.

DSM-IV describes three major categories of personality disorders; patients usually present with a combination of features.

Cluster A Personality Disorders

Affected pts are often characterized as "weird." The *paranoid* personality is suspicious, hypersensitive, guarded, hostile, and can occasionally become threatening or dangerous. The *schizoid* personality is interpersonally isolated, cold, and indifferent, while the *schizotypal* personality is eccentric and superstitious, with magical thinking and unusual beliefs.

Cluster B Personality Disorders

Patients with these disorders are often "wild." The *borderline* personality is impulsive and manipulative, with unpredictable and fluctuating intense moods and unstable relationships, a fear of abandonment, and occasional micropsychotic episodes. The *histrionic* pt is dramatic, engaging, seductive, and attention-seeking. The *narcissistic* pt is self-centered and has an inflated sense of self-importance combined with a tendency to devalue or demean others, while pts with *antisocial* personality disorder use other people to achieve their own ends and engage in exploitative and manipulative behavior with no sense of remorse.

Cluster C Personality Disorders

Patients with these disorders are often "whiny." The *dependent* patient fears separation, tries to engage others to assume responsibility, and often has a help-rejecting style. Patients with *compulsive* personality disorder are meticulous and perfectionistic but also inflexible and indecisive, while those who are *passive-aggressive* request help, appear compliant on the surface, but undo or resist all efforts aimed at change. *Avoidant* pts are anxious about social contact and have difficulty assuming responsibility for their isolation.

For a more detailed discussion, see Reus VI: Mental Disorders, Chap. 385, p. 2485, in HPIM-14.

193

PSYCHIATRIC MEDICATIONS

Four major classes of psychiatric medications are commonly used in adults: (1) antidepressants, (2) anxiolytics, (3) antipsychotics, and (4) mood-stabilizing agents. Nonpsychiatric physicians should become familiar with one or two drugs in each class so that the indications, dose range, efficacy, and potential side effects are well known.

GENERAL PRINCIPLES OF USE

1. Most errors are due to *undermedication* and *impatience*. For a proper medication trial to take place, an effective dose must be taken for an adequate amount of time. For antidepressants, antipsychotics, and mood stabilizers, full effects may take weeks or months to occur.
2. History of a positive response to a medication usually indicates that a response to the same drug will occur again. A family history of a positive response to a specific medication is also useful.
3. Patients who fail to respond to one drug may respond to another in the same class; one should attempt another trial with a drug that has a different mechanism of action or a different chemical structure.

4. Avoid polypharmacy; a pt who is not responding to standard monotherapy probably requires referral to a psychiatrist.
5. Pharmacokinetics may be altered in the elderly, with smaller volumes of distribution, reduced renal and hepatic clearance, longer biologic half-lives, and greater potential for CNS toxicity. The rule with elderly pts is to "start low and go slow."
6. Never stop treatment abruptly; especially true for antidepressants and anxiolytics. In general, medications should be slowly tapered and discontinued over 2–4 weeks.
7. Review possible side effects each time a drug is prescribed; educate pts and family members about side effects and need for patience in awaiting a response.

ANTIDEPRESSANTS

Useful to group according to known actions on CNS monoaminergic systems (Table 193-1). The SSRIs, or selective serotonin reuptake inhibitors, have predominant effects on serotonergic neurotransmission, also reflected in side effect profile. The TCAs, or tricyclic antidepressants, affect noradrenergic and, to a lesser extent, serotonergic neurotransmission but also have anticholinergic and antihistaminic effects. Venlafaxine and mirtazapine have relatively "pure" noradrenergic and serotonergic effects. Bupropion has dopamine reuptake inhibitor properties. Trazodone and nefazodone have mixed effects on serotonin receptors and on other neurotransmitter systems. The MAOIs inhibit monoamine oxidase, the primary enzyme responsible for the degradation of monoamines in the synaptic cleft.

Antidepressants are effective against major depression, particularly when vegetative symptoms and signs are present. In very severe depression with many endogenous features, TCAs or MAOIs are more efficacious than SSRIs. Antidepressants are also useful in treatment of panic disorder, posttraumatic stress disorder, chronic pain syndromes, and generalized anxiety disorder. The SSRIs and the TCA clomipramine successfully treat obsessive-compulsive disorder.

All antidepressants require at least 2 weeks at a therapeutic dose before clinical improvement is observed (probably due to neurotransmitter receptor downregulation and long-term cellular changes related to DNA transcription). All antidepressants have the potential to trigger a manic episode or rapid cycling when given to a pt with bipolar disorder. The MAOIs must not be prescribed concurrently with other antidepressants or with narcotics, as potentially fatal reactions may occur.

ANXIOLYTICS

Antianxiety agents include the benzodiazepines, and the non-benzodiazepine buspirone.

Benzodiazepines bind to stereospecific sites on the gamma-aminobutyric acid receptor and are cross-tolerant with alcohol and with barbiturates. Four clinical properties: (1) sedative, (2) anxiolytic, (3) skeletal muscle relaxant, (4) antiepileptic. Individual drugs differ in terms of potency, onset of action, duration of action (related to half-life and presence of active metabolites), and metabolism (Table 193-2). Benzodiazepines have additive effects with alcohol; like alcohol, they can produce tolerance and physiologic dependence, with serious withdrawal syndromes (tremors, seizures, delirium, and autonomic hyperactivity) if discontinued too quickly, especially for those with short half-lives.

Buspirone is an anxiolytic that is nonsedating, is not cross-tolerant with alcohol, and does not induce tolerance or dependence. It acts via serotonergic pathways, and requires at least 2 weeks at therapeutic doses to achieve full effects.

ANTIPSYCHOTIC MEDICATIONS

These include the typical (or traditional) neuroleptics, which act by blocking dopamine D_2 receptors, and the novel neuroleptics, which act on dopamine, serotonin, and other neuroreceptor systems. Some antipsychotic effect may occur within hours or days of initiating treatment, but full effects usually require 6 weeks to several months of daily, therapeutic dosing.

TYPICAL ANTIPSYCHOTICS   Useful to group into high-, mid-, and low-potency neuroleptics (Table 193-3). High-potency neuroleptics are least sedating, have almost no anticholinergic side effects, and have a strong tendency to induce extrapyramidal side effects (EPSEs) secondary to dopamine receptor blockade. The EPSEs occur within several hours to several weeks of beginning treatment and include acute dystonias, akathisia, and pseudo-parkinsonism. They are treated by judicious dose reduction and by use of anticholinergic and dopamine agonist medications. Low-potency neuroleptics are very sedating, may cause orthostasis, are anticholinergic, and therefore tend not to induce EPSEs. Mid-potency agents are best tolerated by the average pt.

20% of pts treated with typical antipsychotic agents for more than 1 year develop tardive dyskinesia (probably due to dopamine receptor supersensitivity), an abnormal involuntary movement disorder most often observed in the face and distal extremities. Treatment includes gradual withdrawal of the neu-

Table 193-1

Antidepressants

Name	Usual Daily Dose, mg	Side Effects
SSRIs		
Fluoxetine (Prozac)	10–40	Headache; nausea and other GI effects; jitteriness; insomnia; sexual dysfunction; can affect plasma levels of other meds (except sertraline); akathisia rare
Sertraline (Zoloft)	50–200	
Paroxetine (Paxil)	20–40	
Fluvoxamine (Luvox)	50–200	
TCAs		
Amitriptyline (Elavil)	100–300	Anticholinergic (dry mouth, tachycardia, constipation, urinary retention, blurred vision); sweating; tremor; postural hypotension; cardiac conduction delay; sedation; weight gain
Nortriptyline (Pamelor)	50–150	
Imipramine (Tofranil)	100–300	
Desipramine (Norpramin)	100–300	
Doxepin (Sinequan)	100–300	
Clomipramine (Anoframil)	150–300	
Dopamine Reuptake Inhibitor		
Bupropion (Wellbutrin)	225–400	Jitteriness; flushing; seizures in at-risk pts; anorexia; tachycardia; psychosis
Mixed Norepinephrine/ Serotonin Reuptake Inhibitors		
Venlafaxine (Effexor)	75–375	Nausea; dizziness; dry mouth; headaches; increased blood pressure; anxiety and insomnia
Mirtazapine (Remeron)	15–30	Somnolence; weight gain; neutropenia rare

Comments

Once daily dosings, usually in A.M.; fluoxetine has very long half-life; must not be combined with MAOIs

Once daily dosing, usually qhs; blood levels of most TCAs available; can be lethal in O.D. (lethal dose = 2 g); nortriptyline best tolerated, especially by elderly

Tid dosing, but sustained release also available; fewer sexual side effects than SSRIs or TCAs; may be useful for adult ADD

Bid-tid dosing; lower potential for drug-drug interactions than SSRIs; contraindicated with MAOIs.

Once daily dosing

(continued)

Table 193-1 (*Continued*)

Antidepressants

Name	Usual Daily Dose, mg	Side Effects
Mixed-Action Drugs		
Trazodone (Desyrel)	100–600	Sedation; dry mouth; ventricular irritability; postural hypotension; priapism rare
Nefazodone (Serzone)	200–600	Sedation; headache; dry mouth; nausea; constipation
MAOIs		
Phenelzine (Nardil)	30–90	Insomnia; hypotension; anorgasmic; weight gain; hypertensive crisis; tyramine cheese reaction; lethal reactions with SSRIs; serious reactions with narcotics
Tranylcypromine (Parnate)	20–60	

NOTE: ADD, attention deficit disorder; MAOI, monoamine oxidase inhibitor; REM, rapid eye movement; SSRI, selective serotonin reuptake inhibitor; TCA, tricyclic antidepressant.

roleptic, with possible switch to a novel neuroleptic; anticholinergic agents can worsen the disorder.

1–2% of pts exposed to neuroleptics develop neuroleptic malignant syndrome (NMS), a life-threatening complication with a mortality rate as high as 25%; hyperpyrexia, autonomic hyperactivity, muscle rigidity, obtundation, and agitation are characteristic, associated with increased WBC, increased CPK, and myoglobinuria. Treatment involves immediate discontinuation of neuroleptics, supportive care, and use of dantrolene and bromocriptine.

NOVEL ANTIPSYCHOTICS A new class of agents with great promise (Table 193-4); efficacious in treatment-resistant pts, tend not to induce EPSEs or tardive dyskinesia, and appear

Comments

Useful in low doses for sleep because of sedating effects with no anticholinergic side effects

Once daily dosing; no effect on REM sleep unlike other antidepressants

May be more effective in pts with atypical features or treatment-retractory depressions

to have uniquely beneficial properties on negative symptoms and cognitive dysfunction.

MOOD-STABILIZING AGENTS

Three mood-stabilizers in common use: lithium, carbamazepine, and valproic acid (Table 193-4). Useful in acute manic episodes; 1–2 weeks to reach full effect. As prophylaxis, they reduce frequency and severity of both manic and depressed episodes in cyclical mood disorders. Believed to work at various sites of second-messenger signal transduction systems in the CNS. In refractory bipolar disorder, combinations of mood stabilizers are often beneficial.

Table 193-2

Anxiolytics

Name	Equivalent PO dose, mg	Onset of Action
Benzodiazepines:		
Diazepam (Valium)	5	Fast
Flurazepam (Dalmane)	15	Fast
Triazolam (Halcion)	0.25	Intermediate
Lorazepam (Ativan)	1	Intermediate
Alprazolam (Xanax)	0.5	Intermediate
Chlordiazepoxide (Librium)	10	Intermediate
Oxazepam (Serax)	15	Slow
Temazepam (Restoril)	15	Slow
Clonazepam (Klonopin)	0.5	Slow
Non-benzodiazepines		
Buspirone (BuSpar)	7.5	2 weeks

Half-life, h	Comments
20–70	Active metabolites; quite sedating
30–100	Flurazepam is a pro-drug; metabolites are active; quite sedating
1.5–5	No active metabolites; can induce confusion and delirium, especially in elderly
10–20	No active metabolites; direct hepatic glucuronide conjugation; quite sedating
12–15	Active metabolites; not too sedating; may have specific antidepressant and antipanic activity; tolerance and dependence develop easily
5–30	Active metabolites; moderately sedating
5–15	No active metabolites; direct glucuronide conjugation; not too sedating
9–12	No active metabolites; moderately sedating
18–50	No active metabolites; moderately sedating
2–3	Active metabolites; tid dosing—usual daily dose 10–20 mg tid; nonsedating; no additive effects with alcohol; useful for agitation in demented or brain-injured patients

Table 193-3

Antipsychotic Agents

Name	Usual PO Daily Dose, mg	Side Effects
TYPICAL ANTIPSYCHOTICS		
Low-potency		
Chlorpromazine (Thorazine)	100–1000	+ + + Anticholinergic effects; orthostasis;
Thioridazine (Mellaril)	100–800	photosensitivity; cholestasis
Mid-potency		
Trifluoperatine (Stelazine)	2–15	Fewer anticholinergic side effects; fewer
Perphenazine (Trilafon)	4–32	EPSEs than with higher potency agents
High-potency		
Haloperidol (Haldol)	0.5–10	No anticholinergic side effects; EPSEs often prominent
Fluphenazine (Prolixin)	1–10	
Thiothixene (Navane)	2–20	
NOVEL ANTIPSYCHOTICS		
Cloazpine (Clozaril)	200–600	Agranulocytosis (1%); weight gain; seizures; drooling; hyperthermia
Risperidone (Risperdal)	2–8	Orthostasis
Olanzapine (Zyprexa)	10–20	Weight gain
Seroquel (Quietapine)	300–400	Sedation; weight gain; anxiety

NOTE: EPSEs, extrapyramidal side effects.

Sedation	Comments
+ + + + + +	EPSEs usually not prominent; can cause anticholinergic delirium in elderly pts
+ + + +	Well tolerated by most pts
0/+ 0/+ 0/+	Often prescribed in doses that are too high; long-acting injectable forms of haloperidol and fluphenazine available
+ +	Requires weekly WBC
+	Requires slow titration; EPSEs observed with doses >6 mg qd
+ +	Generally well tolerated
+ + +	Bid dosing

For a more detailed discussion, see Reus VI: Mental Disorders, Chap. 385, p. 2485, in HPIM-14.

Table 193-4

Mood-Stabilizing Agents

Name	Usually Daily Dose, mg	Side Effects	Comments
Lithium	600–2400	Tremor, nausea, ataxia, poly-uria–diabetes insipidus, acne, psoriasis, hypo-thyroidism, weight gain, edema, benign leukocytosis	Dose adjusted to serum concentration 0.8–1.2 mEq/L; contra-indicated during pregnancy; diuretics and prostaglandin-synthetase inhibitors can increase lithium to toxic levels; severe toxicity can lead to coma and death
Carbama-zepine (Tegretol)	400–1600	Agranulocytosis and aplastic anemia (rare); dizziness; ataxia; sedation; pruritis; Stevens-Johnson syndrome (rare)	Plasma levels of 8–12 μg/mL needed to treat manic episodes; monitor hepatic, hematologic, and cardiac status; multiple drug interactions, including decrease of blood concentrations of oral contraceptives
Valproic acid	750–1500	Nausea, vomiting, sedation, headache; (tolerance to these side effects usually develops); pancreatitis (rare), hepatitis (rare)	Avoid in hepatic and renal disease; monitor LFTs; plasma levels of 50–100 μg/mL therapeutic

194

ALCOHOLISM

Alcoholism and alcohol abuse are defined by the regular and excessive use of alcohol with concomitant social, occupational, and/or physical problems; alcohol is associated with half of all traffic fatalities and half of all homicides. In alcohol dependence, the regular use of alcohol has resulted in a state of physiologic tolerance and dependence. A pt may never suffer from withdrawal symptoms and still meet criteria for alcohol abuse.

Alcoholism is a multifactorial disorder in which genetic, biologic, and sociocultural factors interact. Typically, the first major life problem from excessive alcohol use appears in early adulthood, followed by periods of exacerbation and remission; the lifespan of the alcoholic is shortened by an average of 15 years due to increased risk of death from heart disease, cancer, accidents, or suicide.

Clinical Features

As 20% of the average physician's pts will suffer from alcoholism, routine medical care requires attention to potential alcohol-related illness:

1. Neurologic—blackouts, seizures, delirium tremens, cerebellar degeneration, neuropathy, myopathy
2. Gastrointestinal—esophagitis, gastritis, pancreatitis, hepatitis, cirrhosis, GI hemorrhage
3. Cardiovascular—hypertension, cardiomyopathy
4. Hematologic—macrocytosis, folate deficiency, thrombocytopenia, leukopenia
5. Endocrine—gynecomastia, testicular atrophy, amenorrhea, infertility
6. Skeletal—fractures, osteonecrosis
7. Infectious

However, most alcoholic pts will not have dramatic physical symptoms and instead will present with psychosocial difficulties. Marital difficulties, job problems (tardiness, absenteeism), and legal problems resulting from driving while intoxicated are common. A positive answer to any of the CAGE questions, indicates a high probability of alcoholism: Are you . . . *C*utting down, or feel the need to? *A*nnoyed when people criticize your drinking? *G*uilty about your drinking? *E*ye-opening with a drink in the morning? Typically, pts will describe a host of difficulties but will then deny that they have a problem with alcohol abuse. Denial is a characteristic, if not the core, symptom of alcoholism.

Alcohol is a CNS depressant that acts on receptors for

gamma-aminobutyric acid (GABA), the major inhibitory neurotransmitter in the nervous system. Behavioral, cognitive, and psychomotor changes can occur at blood alcohol levels as low as 4–7 mmol/L (20–30 mg/dL). Mild to moderate intoxication occurs at 17–43 mmol/L (80–200 mg/dL). Incoordination, tremor, ataxia, confusion, stupor, coma, and even death occur at progressively higher blood alcohol levels.

Chronic alcohol use produces CNS dependence. In such individuals, the earliest sign of alcohol withdrawal is *tremulousness* ("shakes" or "jitters"), which usually occurs in the first 8–24 h after the last drink. This may be followed by generalized seizures ("rum fits") in the first 24–48 h; these do not require the initiation of anti-seizure medications. With severe withdrawal, autonomic hyperactivity ensues (sweating, hypertension, tachycardia, tachypnea, fever), accompanied by insomnia, nightmares, anxiety, and GI symptoms.

Delirium tremens (DTs), which may begin 3–5 days after the last drink, is a very severe withdrawal syndrome characterized by profound autonomic hyperactivity, extreme confusion, agitation, vivid delusions, and hallucinations (often visual and tactile); mortality is 5–15%. *Wernicke's encephalopathy* is an alcohol-related syndrome characterized by ataxia, ophthalmoplegia, and confusion, often with associated nystagmus, peripheral neuropathy, cerebellar signs, and hypotension; there is impaired short-term memory, inattention, and emotional lability. *Korsakoff's syndrome* follows as the encephalopathy and ocular findings resolve; it is characterized by anterograde and retrograde amnesia and confabulation. *Wernicke-Korsakoff's syndrome* is caused by chronic thiamine deficiency, resulting in damage to thalamic nuclei, mamillary bodies, and brainstem and cerebellar structures.

Laboratory Findings

Clues to alcoholism include mild anemia with macrocytosis, folate deficiency, thrombocytopenia, granulocytopenia, abnormal LFTs, hyperuricemia, and elevated triglycerides. Decreases in serum K, Mg, Zn, and PO_4 levels are common. Diagnostic studies such as GI radiology or endoscopy, abdominal ultrasound or CT, liver-spleen scan, liver biopsy, ECG, echocardiogram, brain CT or MRI, EEG, and nerve conduction studies may show evidence of alcohol-related organ dysfunction.

℞ TREATMENT

Acute Withdrawal Acute alcohol withdrawal is treated with thiamine (50–100 mg IV or 100 mg PO daily for 5 d) to replenish depleted stores; if Wernicke-Korsakoff's syndrome is suspected, the IV route must be used, since intestinal absorption is unreliable in alcoholics. CNS depressant drugs that enhance GABA-mediated inhibition are used when seizures or autonomic hyperactivity are present. These drugs halt the rapid state of withdrawal in the CNS and allow for a slower, more controlled reduction of the substance. Low-potency benzodiazepines with long half-lives are the medication of choice (e.g., diazepam, chlordiazepoxide), because they produce fairly steady blood levels of drug and there is a wide dose range within which to work. These benefits must be weighed against the risk of overmedication and oversedation, which occur less commonly with shorter-acting agents (e.g. oxazepam, lorazepam). Typical doses are diazepam 5–10 mg or chlordiazepoxide 25–50 mg PO every 1–4 h prn objective signs of alcohol withdrawal (such as pulse > 90). Extremely high doses are sometimes required for the chronic alcoholic.

In severe withdrawal or DTs, the physician must also look for evidence of trauma or infection that may be masked by prominent withdrawal symptoms or that contribute to the patient's debilitated state. Fluid and electrolyte status and blood glucose levels should be closely followed as well. Cardiovascular and hemodynamic monitoring are crucial, as hemodynamic collapse and cardiac arrhythmia are not uncommon.

Recovery and Sobriety   Treatment of alcoholism requires confrontation of the pt's denial, followed by a motivation to change. A stage of recovery (early abstinence) is followed by ongoing sobriety. The physician must counsel the pt about the need for abstinence and recommended regular participation in self-help resources such as AA as a primary treatment goal.

Disulfiram (Antabuse), a drug that inhibits aldehyde dehydrogenase and results in toxic symptoms (nausea, vomiting, diarrhea, tremor) if the pt consumes alcohol, is used in some centers but is not an effective therapy in the absence of psychosocial intervention. Preliminary studies show that naltrexone and acamprosate may reduce recidivism in abstinent alcoholics.

For a more detailed discussion, see Schuckit MA: Alcohol and Alcoholism, Chap. 386, p. 2503, in HPIM-14.

195

NARCOTIC ABUSE

Narcotics, or opiates, bind to specific opioid receptors in the CNS and elsewhere in the body. These receptors mediate the opiate effects of analgesia, euphoria, respiratory depression, and constipation. Endogenous opiate peptides (enkephalins and endorphins) are natural ligands for the opioid receptors and appear to play a role in analgesia, memory, learning, reward, mood regulation, and stress tolerance.

The prototypic opiates, morphine and codeine, are derived from the juice of the opium poppy, *Papaver somniferum*. The semisynthetic drugs produced from morphine include hydromorphone (Dilaudid), diacetylmorphine (heroin), and oxycodone. Purely synthetic agents are meperidine (Demerol), propoxyphene (Darvon), and methadone. All of these substances produce analgesia and euphoria as well as physical dependence when taken in high enough doses for prolonged periods of time.

1% of the U.S. population meets criteria for narcotic abuse or dependence at some time in their lives. 70% of narcotic-addicted individuals have another psychiatric disorder (usually depression, alcoholism, or a personality disorder). Three groups of abusers can be identified: (1) "medical" abusers—pts with chronic pain syndromes who misuse their prescribed analgesics; (2) physicians, nurses, dentists, and pharmacists with easy access to narcotics; and (3) "street" abusers. The street abuser is typically a higher functioning individual who began by using tobacco, alcohol, and marijuana and then moved on to opiates.

Clinical Features

Acutely, all opiates have the following CNS effects: sedation, euphoria, decreased pain perception, decreased respiratory drive, and vomiting. In larger doses, markedly decreased respirations, bradycardia, pupillary miosis, stupor, and coma ensue. Additionally, the adulterants used to "cut" street drugs (quinine, phenacetin, strychnine, antipyrine, caffeine, powdered milk) can produce permanent neurologic damage, including peripheral neuropathy, amblyopia, and myelopathy. The shared use of contaminated needles is a major cause of brain abscesses, acute endocarditis, hepatitis B, AIDS, septic arthritis, and soft tissue infections. At least 25% of street abusers die within 10–20 years of starting active opiate abuse.

Chronic use of opiates will result in tolerance (requiring higher doses to achieve psychotropic effects) and physical dependence. With shorter-acting opiates such as heroin, morphine, or oxycodone, withdrawal signs begin 8–12 h after the last dose, peak at 2–3 days, and subside over 7–10 days. With longer-acting opiates such as methadone, withdrawal begins 2–4 days after the last dose, peaks at 3–4 days, and lasts several weeks.

Withdrawal produces diarrhea, coughing, lacrimation, rhinorrhea, diaphoresis, twitching muscles, piloerection, fever, tachypnea, hypertension, diffuse body pain, insomnia, and yawning. Relief of these exceedingly unpleasant symptoms by narcotic administration leads to more frequent narcotic use. Eventually, all of the person's efforts are consumed by drug-seeking behavior.

℞ TREATMENT

Overdose High doses of opiates, whether taken in a suicide attempt or accidentally when the potency is misjudged, are frequently lethal. Toxicity occurs immediately after IV administration and with a variable delay after oral ingestion. Symptoms include miosis, shallow respirations, bradycardia, hypothermia, stupor or coma, and pulmonary edema. Treatment requires cardiorespiratory support and administration of the opiate antagonist naloxone (0.4 mg IV repeated in 3–10 min if no or only partial response). Because the effects of naloxone diminish in 2–3 h compared with longer-lasting effects of heroin (up to 24 h) or methadone (up to 72 h), pts must be observed for at least 1–3 days for reappearance of the toxic state.

Withdrawal or Abstinence Syndromes Clonidine is effective in decreasing the sympathetic nervous system hyperactivity observed in opiate withdrawal. Doses of 0.3–0.5 mg/d are used for the 2–3 weeks of the withdrawal period. Although it is highly unpleasant, opiate withdrawal is not physically dangerous per se in adults (unlike alcohol withdrawal). However, withdrawal syndromes in newborns of street abusers are fatal in 3–30% of cases.

Methadone maintenance (to avoid withdrawal or abstinence syndromes) is a widely used treatment strategy in the management of opiate addiction. Long-acting oral methadone is most convenient: 1 mg methadone is equivalent to 3 mg morphine, 1 mg heroin, or 20 mg meperidine. Most pts receive 10–25 mg methadone bid, with higher doses given if withdrawal symptoms break through. Although methadone has mood-elevating effects in some individuals, maintenance nevertheless leads to reduced opiate and nonopiate drug use, reduced criminal behavior, and decreased depressed symptoms.

L-Alpha-acetylmethadol (LAAM) is a long-acting synthetic narcotic that may be given only 3 times a week; however, some pts experience nervousness and stimulation on LAAM. Buprenorphine is a partial receptor agonist that blocks some of the subjective effects of narcotics and that may be as effective as low-dose methadone in maintenance treatment.

To help prevent relapses in the abstinent pt, the oral antagonist naltrexone is used in doses of 50–150 mg/d. It blocks the euphoric and analgesic effects of the opiate when a pt relapses and uses narcotics.

Chronic Pain Syndromes Physicians should avoid establishing narcotic addiction in pts with chronic pain syndromes. Once tolerance and physical dependence are established, withdrawal and abstinence syndromes will intensify the pt's pain and confuse the management of an already difficult problem. Pts must be educated that medications will be used to minimize the effects of pain on physical function but not to abolish pain entirely. Nonpharmacologic approaches to pain management must be part of the pt's treatment.

Identification of the Chronic Narcotic User Blood and urine screens for opiates, or the naloxone challenge test, can be used to identify chronic narcotic users. In the naloxone challenge test, 0.4 mg is given slowly IV over 5 min, and the pt is observed for 1–2 h for signs of withdrawal.

For any pt, realistic expectations for rehabilitation are possible only when the pt is motivated to make a long-term commitment to a drug-free lifestyle. Specialized counseling and peer programs, including Narcotics Anonymous, are a mainstay of treatment. In many cases, adjunctive pharmacologic management is helpful, either to block the euphoric effects of opiates or to impede withdrawal/abstinence syndromes (discussed above).

Special issues exist for medical staff. Physicians should never prescribe opiates for themselves or members of their families. Medical organizations need to be prepared to identify and rehabilitate substance-impaired physicians as quickly as possible.

For a more detailed discussion, see Shucket MA, Segal DS: Opioid Drug Abuse and Dependence, Chap. 387, p. 2508, in HPIM-14.

196

ADVERSE DRUG REACTIONS

Adverse drug reactions are among the most frequent problems encountered clinically and represent a common cause for hospitalization. They occur most frequently in pts receiving multiple drugs and are caused by

1. Errors in self-administration of prescribed drugs (quite common in the elderly).
2. Exaggeration of intended pharmacologic effect (e.g., hypotension in a pt given antihypertensive drugs).
3. Concomitant administration of drugs with synergistic effects (e.g., aspirin and warfarin).
4. Cytotoxic reactions (e.g., hepatic necrosis due to acetaminophen).
5. Immunologic mechanisms (e.g., quinidine-induced thrombocytopenia, hydralazine-induced SLE).
6. Genetically determined enzymatic defects (e.g., primaquine-induced hemolytic anemia in G6PD deficiency).
7. Idiosyncratic reactions (e.g., chloramphenicol-induced aplastic anemia).

RECOGNITION History is of prime importance. Consider (1) nonprescription drugs and topical agents as potential offenders; (2) previous reaction to identical drugs; (3) temporal association between drug administration and development of clinical manifestations; (4) subsidence of manifestations when the agent is discontinued or reduced in dose; (5) recurrence of manifestations with cautious readministration (for less hazardous reactions); (6) *rare:* (a) biochemical abnormalities, e.g., red cell G6PD deficiency as cause of drug-induced hemolytic anemia, (b) abnormal serum antibody in pts with agranulocytosis, thrombocytopenia, hemolytic anemia.

Table 196-1 lists a number of clinical manifestations of adverse effects of drugs. It is not designed to be complete or exhaustive.

Table 196-1

Clinical Manifestations of Adverse Reactions to Drugs

MULTISYSTEM MANIFESTATIONS

Anaphylaxis
  Cephalosporins
  Dextran
  Insulin
  Iodinated drugs or
    contrast media
  Lidocaine
  Penicillins
  Procaine
Angioedema
  ACE inhibitors
**Drug-induced lupus
  erythematosus**
  Cephalosporins
  Hydralazine
  Iodides
  Isoniazid
  Methyldopa

  Phenytoin
  Procainamide
  Quinidine
  Sulfonamides
  Thiouracil
Fever
  Aminosalicylic acid
  Amphotericin B
  Antihistamines
  Penicillins
Hyperpyrexia
  Antipsychotics
Serum sickness
  Aspirin
  Penicillins
  Propylthiouracil
  Sulfonamides

ENDOCRINE MANIFESTATIONS

Addisonian-like syndrome
  Busulfan
  Ketoconazole
Galactorrhea (may also
  cause amenorrhea)
  Methyldopa
  Phenothiazines
  Tricyclic antidepressants
Gynecomastia
  Calcium channel
    antagonists
  Digitalis
  Estrogens
  Griseofulvin
  Isoniazid
  Methyldopa
  Phenytoin
  Spironolactone
  Testosterone
Sexual dysfunction
  Beta blockers
  Clonidine
  Diuretics

  Guanethidine
  Lithium
  Major tranquilizers
  Methyldopa
  Oral contraceptives
  Sedatives
**Thyroid function tests,
  disorders of**
  Acetazolamide
  Amiodarone
  Chlorpropamide
  Clofibrate
  Colestipol and nicotinic
    acid
  Gold salts
  Iodides
  Lithium
  Oral contraceptives
  Phenothiazines
  Phenylbutazone
  Phenytoin
  Sulfonamides
  Tolbutamide

(*continued*)

Table 196-1 (*Continued*)

Clinical Manifestations of Adverse Reactions to Drugs

METABOLIC MANIFESTATIONS

Hyperbilirubinemia
  Rifampin
Hypercalcemia
  Antacids with absorbable
    alkali
  Thiazides
  Vitamin D
Hyperglycemia
  Chlorthalidone
  Diazoxide
  Encainide
  Ethacrynic acid
  Furosemide
  Glucocorticoids
  Growth hormone
  Oral contraceptives
  Thiazides
Hypoglycemia
  Insulin
  Oral hypoglycemics
  Quinine
Hyperkalemia
  ACE inhibitors
  Amiloride
  Cytotoxics
  Digitalis overdose
  Heparin
  Lithium
  Potassium preparations
    including salt substitute
  Potassium salts of drugs
  Spironolactone
  Succinylcholine
  Triamterene
Hypokalemia
  Alkali-induced alkalosis

Amphotericin B
Diuretics
Gentamicin
Insulin
Laxative abuse
Mineralocorticoids, some
  glucocorticoids
Osmotic diuretics
Sympathomimetics
Tetracycline
Theophylline
Vitamin B_{12}
Hyperuricemia
  Aspirin
  Cytotoxics
  Ethacrynic acid
  Furosemide
  Hyperalimentation
  Thiazides
Hyponatremia
  1. Dilutional
      Carbamazepine
      Chlorpropamide
      Cyclophosphamide
      Diuretics
      Vincristine
  2. Salt wasting
      Diuretics
      Enemas
      Mannitol
Metabolic acidosis
  Acetazolamide
  Paraldehyde
  Salicylates
  Spironolactone

DERMATOLOGIC MANIFESTATIONS

Acne
  Anabolic and androgenic
    steroids
  Bromides

Glucocorticoids
Iodides
Isoniazid
Oral contraceptives

(*continued*)

Table 196-1 (*Continued*)

Clinical Manifestations of Adverse Reactions to Drugs

DERMATOLOGIC MANIFESTATIONS (*Cont.*)

Alopecia
  Cytotoxics
  Ethionamide
  Heparin
  Oral contraceptives
    (withdrawal)
Eczema
  Captopril
  Cream and lotion
    perservatives
  Lanolin
  Topical antihistamines
  Topical antimicrobials
  Topical local anesthetics
Erythema multiforme or
Steven-Johnson syndrome
  Barbiturates
  Chlorpropamide
  Codeine
  Penicillins
  Phenylbutazone
  Phenytoin
  Salicylates
  Sulfonamides
  Sulfones
  Tetracyclines
  Thiazides
Erythema nodosum
  Oral contraceptives
  Penicillins
  Sulfonamides
Exfoliative dermatitis
  Barbiturates
  Gold salts
  Penicillins
  Phenylbutazone
  Phenytoin
  Quinidine
  Sulfonamides
Fixed drug eruptions
  Barbiturates

Captopril
  Phenylbutazone
  Quinine
  Salicylates
  Sulfonamides
Hyperpigmentation
  Bleomycin
  Busulfan
  Chloroquine and other
    antimalarials
  Corticotropin
  Cyclophosphamide
  Gold salts
  Hypervitaminosis A
  Oral contraceptives
  Phenothiazines
Lichenoid eruptions
  Aminosalicylic acid
  Antimalarials
  Chlorpropamide
  Gold salts
  Methyldopa
  Phenothiazines
Photodermatitis
  Captopril
  Chlordiazepoxide
  Furosemide
  Griseofulvin
  Nalidixic acid
  Oral contraceptives
  Phenothiazines
  Sulfonamides
  Sulfonylureas
  Tetracyclines, particularly
    demeclocycline
  Thiazides
Purpura (see also
  thrombocytopenia)
  Allopurinol
  Ampicillin

(*continued*)

Table 196-1 (*Continued*)

Clinical Manifestations of Adverse Reactions to Drugs

DERMATOLOGIC MANIFESTATIONS (*Cont.*)

Purpura (*Cont.*)
  Aspirin
  Glucocorticoids
Rashes (nonspecific)
  Allopurinol
  Ampicillin
  Barbiturates
  Indapamide
  Methyldopa
  Phenytoin
Skin necrosis
  Warfarin
Toxic epidermal necrolysis (bullous)
  Allopurinol

  Barbiturates
  Bromides
  Iodides
  Nalidixic acid
  Penicillins
  Phenylbutazone
  Phenytoin
  Sulfonamides
Urticaria
  Aspirin
  Barbiturates
  Captopril
  Enalapril
  Penicillins
  Sulfonamides

HEMATOLOGIC MANIFESTATIONS

Agranulocytosis (see also pancytopenia)
  Captopril
  Carbimazole
  Chloramphenicol
  Cytotoxics
  Gold salts
  Indomethacin
  Methimazole
  Oxyphenbutazone
  Phenothiazines
  Phenylbutazone
  Propylthiouracil
  Sulfonamides
  Tolbutamide
  Tricyclic antidepressants
Clotting abnormalities/ hypothrombinemia
  Cefamandole
  Cefoperazone
  Moxalactam
Eosinophilia
  Aminosalicylic acid
  Chlorpropamide

  Erythromycin estolate
  Imipramine
  L-Tryptophan
  Methotrexate
  Nitrofurantoin
  Procarbazine
  Sulfonamides
Hemolytic anemia
  Aminosalicylic acid
  Cephalosporins
  Chlorpromazine
  Dapsone
  Insulin
  Isoniazid
  Levodopa
  Mefenamic acid
  Melphalan
  Methyldopa
  Penicillins
  Phenacetin
  Procainamide
  Quinidine
  Rifampin
  Sulfonamides

(*continued*)

Table 196-1 (*Continued*)

Clinical Manifestations of Adverse Reactions to Drugs

HEMATOLOGIC MANIFESTATIONS (*Cont.*)

**Hemolytic anemias in
  G6PD deficiency**
  See Table 49-41
Leukocytosis
  Glucocorticoids
  Lithium
Lymphadenopathy
  Phenytoin
  Primidone
Megaloblastic anemia
  Folate antagonists
  Nitrous oxide
  Oral contraceptives
  Phenobarbital
  Phenytoin
  Primidone
  Triamterene
  Trimethoprim
**Pancytopenia (aplastic
  anemia)**
  Carbamazepine
  Chloramphenicol
  Cytotoxics
  Gold salts
  Mephenytoin
  Phenylbutazone
  Phenytoin
  Quinacrine
  Sulfonamides

Trimethadione
Zidovudine (AZT)
Pure red cell aplasia
  Azathioprine
  Chlorpropamide
  Isoniazid
  Phenytoin
Thrombocytopenia (see
  also pancytopenia)
  Acetazolamine
  Aspirin
  Carbamazepine
  Carbenicillin
  Chlorpropamide
  Chlorthalidone
  Furosemide
  Gold salts
  Heparin
  Indomethacin
  Isoniazid
  Methyldopa
  Moxalactam
  Phenylbutazone
  Phenytoin and other
    hydantoins
  Quinidine
  Quinine
  Thiazides
  Ticarcillin

CARDIOVASCULAR MANIFESTATIONS

Angina exacerbation
  Alpha blockers
  Beta blocker withdrawal
  Ergotamine
  Excessive thyroxine
  Hydralazine
  Methysergide
  Minoxidil
  Nifedipine

Oxytocin
Vasopressin
Arrhythmias
  Adriamycin
  Antiarrhythmic drugs
  Atropine
  Anticholinesterases
  Beta blockers
  Digitalis

(*continued*)

Table 196-1 (*Continued*)

Clinical Manifestations of Adverse Reactions to Drugs

CARDIOVASCULAR MANIFESTATIONS (*Cont.*)

Arrhythmias (*Cont.*)
Emetine
Lithium
Phenothiazines
Sympathomimetics
Thyroid hormone
Tricyclic antidepressants
Verapamil
AV block
Clonidine
Methyldopa
Verapamil
Cardiomyopathy
Adriamycin
Daunorubicin
Emetine
Lithium
Penothiazines
Sulfonamides
Sympathomimetics
**Fluid retention or
congestive heart failure**
Beta blockers
Calcium antagonists
Estrogens
Indomethacin
Mannitol
Minoxidil
Phenylbutazone
Steroids

Hypotension
Calcium antagonists
Citrated blood
Diuretics
Levodopa
Morphine
Nitroglycerin
Phenothiazines
Protamine
Quinidine
Hypertension
Clonidine withdrawal
Corticotropin
Cyclosporine
Glucocorticoids
Monoamine oxidase
inhibitors with
sympathomimetics
NSAIDs
Oral contraceptives
Sympathomimetics
Tricyclic antidepressants
with sympathomimetics
Pericarditis
Emetine
Hydralazine
Methysergide
Procainamide
Thromboembolism
Oral contraceptives

RESPIRATORY MANIFESTATIONS

Airway obstruction
Beta blockers
Cephalosporins
Cholinergic
drugs
NSAIDs
Penicillins
Pentazocine
Streptomycin

Tartrazine (drugs with
yellow dye)
Cough
ACE inhibitors
Pulmonary edema
Contrast media
Heroin
Methadone
Propoxyphene

(*continued*)

Table 196-1 (*Continued*)

Clinical Manifestations of Adverse Reactions to Drugs

RESPIRATORY MANIFESTATIONS (*Cont.*)

Pulmonary infiltrates
Acyclovir
Amiodarone
Azathioprine
Bleomycin
Busulfan
Carmustine (BCNU)
Chlorambucil
Cyclophosphamide
Melphalan
Methotrexate
Methysergide
Mitomycin C
Nitrofurantoin
Procarbazine
Sulfonamides

GASTROINTESTINAL MANIFESTATIONS

Cholestatic jaundice
Anabolic steroids
Androgens
Chlorpropamide
Erythromycin estolate
Gold salts
Methimazole
Nitrofurantoin
Oral contraceptives
Phenothiazines
Constipation or ileus
Aluminum hydroxide
Barium sulfate
Calcium carbonate
Ferrous sulfate
Ion exchange resins
Opiates
Phenothiazines
Tricyclic antidepressants
Verapamil
Diarrhea or colitis
Antibiotics (broad-spectrum)
Colchicine
Digitalis
Magnesium in antacids
Methyldopa
Diffuse hepatocellular damage
Acetaminophen (paracetamol)
Allopurinol
Aminosalicylic acid
Dapsone
Erythromycin estolate
Ethionamide
Glyburide
Halothane
Isoniazid
Ketoconazole
Methimazole
Methotrexate
Methoxyflurane
Methyldopa
Monoamine oxidase inhibitors
Niacin
Nifedipine
Nitrofurantoin
Phenytoin
Propoxyphene
Propylthiouracil
Pyridium
Rifampin
Salicylates
Sodium valproate
Sulfonamides
Tetracyclines
Verapamil
Zidovudine (AZT)
Intestinal ulceration
Solid KCl preparations

(*continued*)

Table 196-1 (*Continued*)

Clinical Manifestations of Adverse Reactions to Drugs

GASTROINTESTINAL MANIFESTATIONS (*Cont.*)

Malabsorption
Aminosalicylic acid
Antibiotics (broad-
spectrum)
Cholestyramine
Colchicine
Colestipol
Cytotoxics
Neomycin
Phenobarbital
Phenytoin
Nausea or vomiting
Digitalis
Estrogens
Ferrous sulfate
Levodopa
Opiates
Potassium chloride
Tetracyclines
Theophylline
Oral conditions
1. Gingival hyperplasia
   Calcium antagonists
   Cyclosporine
   Phenytoin
2. Salivary gland swelling
   Bretylium
   Clonidine
   Guanethidine
   Iodides
   Phenylbutazone

3. Taste disturbances
   Biguanides
   Captopril
   Griseofulvin
   Lithium
   Metronidazole
   Penicillamine
   Rifampin
4. Ulceration
   Aspirin
   Cytotoxics
   Gentian violet
   Isoproterenol
   (sublingual)
   Pancreatin
Pancreatitis
Azathioprine
Ethacrynic acid
Furosemide
Glucocorticoids
Opiates
Oral contraceptives
Sulfonamides
Thiazides
**Peptic ulceration or
hemorrhage**
Aspirin
Ethacrynic acid
Glucocoricoids
NSAIDs

RENAL/URINARY MANIFESTATIONS

Bladder dysfunction
Anticholinergics
Disopyramide
Monoamine oxidase
inhibitors
Tricyclic antidepressants

Calculi
Acetazolamide
Vitamin D

(*continued*)

Table 196-1 (*Continued*)

Clinical Manifestations of Adverse Reactions to Drugs

RENAL/URINARY MANIFESTATIONS (*Cont.*)

Concentrating defect with polyuria (or nephrogenic diabetes insipidus)
Demeclocycline
Lithium
Methoxyflurane
Vitamin D
Hemorrhagic cystitis
Cyclophosphamide
Interstitial nephritis
Allopurinol
Furosemide
Penicillins, esp.
  methicillin
Phenindione
Sulfonamides
Thiazides
Nephropathies
Due to analgesics (e.g.,
  phenacetin)
Nephrotic syndrome
Captopril
Gold salts
Penicillamine

Phenindione
Probenecid
Obstructive uropathy
Extrarenal: methysergide
Intrarenal: cytotoxics
Renal dysfunction
Cyclosporine
NSAIDS
Triamterene
Renal tubular acidosis
Acetazolamide
Amphotericin B
Degraded tetracycline
Tubular necrosis
Aminoglycosides
Amphotericin B
Colistin
Cyclosporin
Methoxyflurane
Polymyxins
Radioiodinated contrast
  medium
Sulfonamides
Tetracyclines

NEUROLOGIC MANIFESTATIONS

Exacerbation of myasthenia
Aminoglycosides
Polymyxins
Extrapyramidal effects
Butyrophenones, e.g.,
  haloperidol
Levodopa
Methyldopa
Metoclopramide
Oral contraceptives
Phenothiazines
Tricyclic antidepressants
Headache
Ergotamine (withdrawal)

Glyceryl trinitrate
Hydralazine
Indomethacin
Peripheral neuropathy
Amiodarone
Chloramphenicol
Chloroquine
Chlorpropamide
Clofibrate
Demeclocycline
Disopyramide
Ethambutol
Ethionamide
Glutethimide
Hydralazine

(*continued*)

Table 196-1 (*Continued*)

Clinical Manifestations of Adverse Reactions to Drugs

NEUROLOGIC MANIFESTATIONS (*Cont.*)

Isoniazid
Methysergide
Metronidazole
Nalidixic acid
Nitrofurantoin
Phenytoin
Polymyxin, colistin
Procarbazine
Streptomycin
Tolbutamide
Tricyclic antidepressants
Vincristine
Pseudotumor cerebri (or intracranial hypertension)
Amiodarone
Glucocorticoids, mineralocorticoids
Hypervitaminosis A

Oral contraceptives
Tetracyclines
Seizures
Amphetamines
Analeptics
Isoniazid
Lidocaine
Lithium
Nalidixic acid
Penicillins
Phenothiazines
Physostigmine
Theophylline
Tricyclic antidepressants
Vincristine
Stroke
Oral contraceptives

OCULAR MANIFESTATIONS

Cataracts
Busulfan
Chlorambucil
Glucocorticoids
Phenothiazines
Color vision alteration
Barbiturates
Digitalis
Methaqualone
Streptomycin
Thiazides
Corneal edema
Oral contraceptives
Corneal opacities
Chloroquine
Indomethacin
Vitamin D

Glaucoma
Mydriatics
Sympathomimetics
Optic neuritis
Aminosalicylic acid
Chloramphenicol
Ethambutol
Isoniazid
Penicillamine
Phenothiazines
Phenylbutazone
Quinine
Streptomycin
Retinopathy
Chloroquine
Phenothiazines

(*continued*)

Table 196-1 (*Continued*)

Clinical Manifestations of Adverse Reactions to Drugs

EAR MANIFESTATIONS

Deafness
  Aminoglycosides
  Aspirin
  Bleomycin
  Chloroquine
  Erythromycin
  Ethacrynic acid

  Furosemide
  Nortriptyline
  Quinine
Vestibular disorders
  Aminoglycosides
  Quinine

MUSCULOSKELETAL MANIFESTATIONS

Bone disorders
  1. Osteoporosis
     Glucocorticoids
     Heparin
  2. Osteomalacia
     Aluminum hydroxide
     Anticonvulsants
     Glutethimide

Myopathy or myalgia
  Amphotericin B
  Chloroquine
  Clofibrate
  Glucocorticoids
  Oral contraceptives
Myositis
  Gemfibrozil
  Lovastatin

PSYCHIATRIC MANIFESTATIONS

**Delirious or confusional
states**
  Amantadine
  Aminophylline
  Anticholinergics
  Antidepressants
  Cimetidine
  Digitalis
  Glucocorticoids
  Isoniazid
  Levodopa
  Methyldopa
  Penicillins
  Phenothiazines
  Sedatives and hypnotics
Depression
  Amphetamine withdrawal
  Beta blockers
  Centrally acting
    antihypertensives

  (reserpine, methyldopa,
    clonidine)
  Glucocorticoids
  Levodopa
Drowsiness
  Antihistamines
  Anxiolytic drugs
  Clonidine
  Major tranquilizers
  Methyldopa
  Tricyclic antidepressants
Hallucinatory states
  Amantadine
  Beta blockers
  Levodopa
  Meperidine
  Narcotics
  Pentazocine
  Tricyclic antidepressants

(*continued*)

Table 196-1 (*Continued*)

Clinical Manifestations of Adverse Reactions to Drugs

PSYCHIATRIC MANIFESTATIONS (*Cont.*)

Hypomania, mania, or excited reactions	Glucocorticoids
Glucocorticoids	Levodopa
Levodopa	Lysergic acid
Monoamine oxidase inhibitors	Monoamine oxidase inhibitors
Sympathomimetics	Tricyclic antidepressants
Tricyclic antidepressants	**Sleep disturbances**
Schizophrenic-like or paranoid reactions	Anorexiants
Amphetamines	Levodopa
Bromides	Monoamine oxidase inhibitors
	Sympathomimetics

SOURCE: Adapted from Wood AJJ: HPIM-14, pp. 424–429.

For a more detailed discussion, see Wood AJJ: Adverse Reactions to Drugs, Chap. 69, p. 422, in HPIM-14.

197

LABORATORY VALUES OF CLINICAL IMPORTANCE

The system of international units (SI, Système International d'Unités) is now used in most countries and in virtually all medical and scientific journals. However, clinical laboratories in some countries report values in traditional units. Therefore, both systems are utilized for the Appendix. Values in SI units appear first, and *traditional units appear in parentheses* after the SI units. This dual system is also followed in large part in the text. In those instances in which the numbers remain the same but only the terminology is changed (mmol/L for meq/L or IU/L for mIU/mL), only the SI units are given. In all other instances in the text the SI unit is followed by the traditional unit in parentheses. For a more complete listing, consult the Appendix of HPIM-14.

$$mmol/L = \frac{mg/dL \times 10}{atomic\ weight}$$

$$mg/dL = \frac{mmol/L \times atomic\ weight}{10}$$

BODY FLUIDS AND OTHER MASS DATA

Body fluid, total volume: 50% (in obese) to 70% (in lean) of body weight
  Intracellular: 30–40% of body weight
  Extracellular: 20–30% of body weight
Blood:
  Total volume:
    Males: 69 mL/kg body weight
    Females: 65 mL/kg body weight
  Plasma volume:
    Males: 39 mL/kg body weight
    Females: 40 mL/kg body weight
  RBC volume:
    Males: 30 mL/kg body weight (1.15–1.21 L/m² body surface area)

Females: 25 mL/kg body weight (0.95–1.00 L/m² body surface area)

$$\text{Body surface area (m}^2) = \frac{(\text{wt in kg})^{0.425} \times (\text{ht in cm})^{0.725}}{139.315}$$

CSF

Glucose 2.2–3.9 mmol/L (40–70 mg/dL)
Total protein 0.2–0.5 g/L (20–50 mg/dL)
    Albumin 0.066–0.442 g/L, (6.6–44.2 mg/dL)
    IgG 0.009–0.057 g/L (0.9–5.7 mg/dL)
    IgG index* 0.29–0.59
    Oligoclonal bands (OCB) <2 bands not present in matched serum sample
CSF pressure 50–180 mmH₂O
Leukocytes:
    Total <5 per μL
    Differential:
    Lymphocytes 60–70%
    Monocytes 30–50%
    Neutrophils None

CHEMICAL CONSTITUENTS OF BLOOD

Albumin, serum: 35–55 g/L (3.5–5.5 g/dL)
Aldolase: 0–100 nkat/L (0–6 U/L)
Aminotransferases, serum:
    Aspartate (AST, SGOT): 0–0.58 μkat/L (0–35 U/L)
    Alanine (ALT, SGPT): 0–0.58 μkat/L (0–35 U/L)
Ammonia, as NH_3, plasma: 6–47 μmol/L (10–80 μg/dL)
Amylase, serum: 0.8–3.2 μkat/L (60–180 U/L)
Arterial blood gases:
    [HCO_3^-]: 21–28 mmol/L
    P_{CO_2}: 4.7–6.0 kPa (35–45 mmHg)
    pH: 7.38–7.44
    P_{O_2}: 11–13 kPa (80–100 mmHg)
Bilirubin, total, serum (Malloy-Evelyn): 5.1–17 μmol/L (0.3–1.0 mg/dL)
    Direct, serum: 1.7–5.1 μmol/L (0.1–0.3 mg/dL)
    Indirect, serum: 3.4–12 μmol/L (0.2–0.7 mg/dL)
Calcium, ionized: 1.1–1.4 mmol/L (4.5–5.6 mg/dL)
Calcium, plasma: 2.2–2.6 mmol/L (9–10.5 mg/dL)

$$*\text{IgG index} = \frac{\text{CSF IgG(mg/dL)} \times \text{serum albumin(g/dL)}}{\text{Serum IgG(g/dL)} \times \text{CSF albumin(mg/dL)}}$$

Carbon dioxide content, plasma (sea level): 21–30 mmol/L
Carbon dioxide tension (P_{CO_2}), arterial blood (sea level): 4.7–5.9 kPa (35–45 mmHg)
Chloride, serum: 98–106 mmol/L
Cholesterol, plasma:
   Desirable: <5.20 mmol/L (<200 mg/dL)
   Borderline: 5.20–6.18 mmol/L (200–239 mg/dL)
   Undesirable: ≥6.21 mmol/L (≥240 mg/dL)
Complement, serum:
   C3: 0.55–1.20 g/L (55–120 mg/dL)
   C4: 0.20–0.50 g/L (20–50 mg/dL)
Creatine kinase, serum (total):
   Females: 0.17–1.17 μkat/L (10–70 U/L)
   Males: 0.42–1.50 μkat/L (25–90 U/L)
Creatinine, serum: <133 μmol/L (<1.5 mg/dL)
Digoxin, serum:
   Therapeutic level: 0.6–2.8 nmol/L (0.5–2.2 ng/mL)
   Toxic level: >3.1 nmol/L (>2.4 ng/mL)
Ethanol, plasma:
   Behavioral changes: >4.3 mmol/L (>20 mg/dL)
   Legal intoxication: >17 mmol/L (>80 mg/dL)
   Coma and death: >65 mmol/L (>300 mg/dL)
Ferritin, serum:
   Women: 10–200 μg/L (10–200 ng/mL)
   Men: 15–400 μg/L (15–400 ng/mL)
Glucose (fasting), plasma:
   Normal: 4.2–6.4 mmol/L (75–115 mg/dL)
   Diabetes mellitus: >7.8 mmol/L (>140 mg/dL) (on more than one occasion)
   [>7.0 mmol/L (>126 mg/dL) on more than one occasion according to the American Diabetes Association]
Glucose, 2-h postprandial, plasma:
   Normal: <7.8 mmol/L (<140 mg/dL)
   Impaired glucose tolerance: 7.8–11.1 mmol/L (140–200 mg/dL)
   Diabetes mellitus: >11.1 mmol/L (>200 mg/dL) (on more than one occasion)
Hemoglobin A_{1c}: Up to 6% of total hemoglobin
Immunoglobulins, serum:
   IgA: 0.9–3.2 g/L (90–325 mg/dL)
   IgD: 0–0.08 g/L (0–8 mg/dL)
   IgE: <0.00025 g/L (<0.025 mg/dL)
   IgG: 8.0–15.0 g/L (800–1500 mg/dL)
   IgM: 0.45–1.5 g/L (45–150 mg/dL)
Iron, serum: 9.0–27 μmol/L (50–150 μg/dL)
Iron-binding capacity, serum: 45–66 μmol/L (250–370 μg/dL)
   Saturation: 20–45%

Lactate dehydrogenase, serum: 1.7–3.2 μkat/L (100–190 μ/L)
Lipoproteins, plasma (desirable):
    LDL cholesterol: <3.36 (<130 mg/dL)
    HDL cholesterol: >1.8 mmol/L (>70 mg/dL)
Magnesium, serum: 0.8–1.2 mmol/L (1.8–3 mg/dL)
Osmolality, plasma: 285–295 mmol/kg serum water
Phenytoin, plasma:
    Therapeutic range: 40–80 μmol/L (10–20 mg/L)
    Toxic level: >120 μmol/L (>30 mg/L)
Phosphatase, acid, serum: <0.90 nkat/L (<5.5 U/L)
Phosphatase, alkaline, serum: 0.5–2.0 μkat/L (30–120 U/L)
Phosphorus, inorg., serum: 1.0–1.4 mmol/L (3–4.5 mg/dL)
Potassium, serum: 3.5–5.0 mmol/L
Protein, total, serum: 55–80 g/L (5.5–8.0 g/dL)
Protein fractions, serum:
    Albumin: 35–55 g/L (3.5–5.0 g/dL) (50–60%)
    Globulin: 20–35 g/L (2.0–3.5 g/dL) (40–50%)
    Alpha$_1$: 2–4 g/L (0.2–0.4 g/dL) (4.2–7.2%)
    Alpha$_2$: 5–9 g/L (0.5–0.9 g/dL) (6.8–12%)
    Beta: 6–11 g/L (0.6–1.1 g/dL) (9.3–15%)
    Gamma: 7–17 g/L (0.7–1.7 g/dL) (13–23%)
Sodium, serum: 136–145 mmol/L
Triglycerides, plasma: <1.8 mmol/L (<160 mg/dL)
Urea nitrogen, serum: 3.6–7.1 mmol/L (10–20 mg/dL)
Uric acid, serum:
    Men: 0.15–0.48 mmol/L (2.5–8.0 mg/dL)
    Women: 0.09–0.36 mmol/L (1.5–6.0 mg/dL)

FUNCTION TESTS

Circulation

Cardiac output (Fick): 2.5–3.6 L/m^2 body surface area per min
Ejection fraction, stroke volume/end-diastolic volume (SV/EDV): Normal range: 0.55–0.78, average 0.67
Pulmonary vascular resistance: 2–12 kPa·s/L [(20–120 (dyn·s)/cm^5]
Systemic vascular resistance: 77–150 (dyn·s)/cm^5 [(770–1500 (kPa·s)/L]

Gastrointestinal

D-Xylose absorption test: After an overnight fast, 25 g xylose is given PO in aqueous solution; urine collected for the following 5 h should contain 33–53 mmol (5–8 g) xylose (or >20% of ingested dose); serum xylose should be 1.7–2.7 mmol/L (25–40 mg per 100 mL) 1 h after the oral dose.

Gastric juice:
  Volume:
    24 h: 2–3 L
    Nocturnal: 600–700 mL
    Basal, fasting: 30–70 mL/h
  pH: 1.6–1.8
  Acid output:
    Basal:
      Women (mean ± 1 SD): 0.6 ± 0.5 μmol/s (2.0 ± 1.8 meq/h)
      Men (mean ± 1 SD): 0.8 ± 0.6 μmol/s (3.0 ± 2.0 meq/h)
    Maximal (after subcutaneous histamine acid phosphate 0.004 mg/kg and preceded by 50 mg promethazine; or after beta-zole 1.7 mg/kg or pentagastrin 6 μg/kg):
      Women (mean ± 1 SD): 4.4 ± 1.4 μmol/s (16 ± 5 meq/h)
      Men (mean ± 1 SD): 6.4 ± 1.4 μmol/s (23 ± 5 meq/h)
Secretin test (pancreatic exocrine function): 1U/kg body weight, IV:
  Volume (pancreatic juice): >2.0 mL/kg in 80 min
  Bicarbonate concentration: >80 mmol/L
  Bicarbonate output: >10 mmol in 30 min

Metabolic and Endocrine

Adrenal steroids, plasma:
  Cortisol:
    8 A.M. 140–690 nmol/L (5–25 μg/dL)
    4 P.M. 80–330 nmol/L (3–12 μg/dL)
Adrenal steroids, urinary excretion:
  Aldosterone: 14–53 nmol/d (5–19 μg/d)
  Cortisol, free: 55–275 nmol/d (20–100 μg/d)
  17-Hydroxycorticosteroids: 5.5–28 μmol/d (2–10 mg/d)
  17-Ketosteroids:
    Men: 24–88 μmol/d (7–25 mg/d)
    Women: 14–52 μmol/d (4–15 mg/d)
Estradiol:
  Women: 70–220 pmol/L (20–60 pg/mL), higher at ovulation
  Men: <180 pmol/L (<50 pg/mL)
Progesterone:
  Men, prepubertal girls, preovulatory women, and postmeno-pausal women: <6 nmol/L (2 ng/mL)
  Women, luteal, peak: 6–60 nmol/L (2–20 ng/mL)
Testosterone:
  Women: <3.5 nmol/L (<1 ng/mL)

Men: 10–35 nmol/L (3–10 ng/mL)
Prepubertal boys and girls: 0.17–0.7 nmol/L (0.05–0.2 ng/mL)
Thyroid function tests:
Radioactive iodine uptake, 24 h: 5–30% (range varies in different areas due to variations in iodine intake)
Resin T_3 uptake: 25–35% (varies among laboratories)
Thyroid-stimulating hormone (TSH): 0.4–5 mU/L (0.4–0.5 μU/mL)
Thyroxine (T_4), serum radioimmunoassay: 64–154 nmol/L (5–12 μg/dL)
Triiodothyronine (T_3), plasma: 1.1–2.9 nmol/L (70–190 ng/dL)

Renal

Clearances (corrected to 1.72 m^2 body surface area):
Insulin clearance (mean ± 1 SD):
Men: 2.1 ± 0.4 mL/s (124 ± 25.8 mL/min)
Women: 2.0 ± 0.2 mL/s (119 ± 12.8 mL/min)
Endogenous creatinine clearance: 1.5–2.2 mL/s (91–130 mL/min)
Concentration and dilution test:
Specific gravity of urine:
After 12-h fluid restriction: 1.025 or more
After 12-h deliberate water intake: 1.003 or less

HEMATOLOGIC EXAMINATIONS

(See also "Chemical Constituents of Blood")
Carboxyhemoglobin:
Nonsmoker: 0–2.3%
Smoker: 2.1–4.2%
CD4+ T lymphocytes: 600–1200/μL
Haptoglobin, serum: 0.5–2.2 g/L (50–220 mg/dL)
Hemoglobin, adults
Women: 7.4–9.9 mmol/L (12–16 g/dL)
Men: 8.1–11.2 mmol/L (13–18 g/dL)
Leukocytes, total, adults: 4.3–10.8 × 10^9/L (4300–10,800/μL)

Differential count	Approx % of total
Segmented neutrophils	45–74
Bands	0–4
Lymphocytes	16–45
Monocytes	4–10
Eosinophils	0–7
Basophils	0–2

Platelets and coagulation parameters
  Fibrinogen: 2–4 g/L (200–400 mg/dL)
  Platelets 130–400 $\times$ 10^9/L (130,000–400,000/μL)
  Bleeding time (Ivy): 2.5–10 min
Sedimentaton rate:
  Westergren, <50 years of age:
    Men: 0–15 mm/h
    Women: 0–20 mm/h
  Westergren, >50 years of age:
    Men: 0–20 mm/h
    Women: 0–30 mm/h

URINE

Creatinine: 8.8–14 mmol/d (1.0–1.6 g/d)
Protein: <0.15 g/d (<150 mg/d)
Potassium: 25–100 mmol/d (varies with intake)
Sodium: 100–260 mmol/d (varies with intake)

INDEX

Numbers in bold refer to whole sections; t and f refer to table and figure, respectively.